OCULAR PATHOLOGY
Clinical Applications and
Self-Assessment

OCULAR PATHOLOGY

Clinical Applications and
Self-Assessment
FIFTH EDITION

David J. Apple, MD
Professor and Chairman Emeritus, Department of Ophthalmology
Pawek-Vallotton Chair of Biomedical Engineering and Director of Research
Albert Florens Storm Eye Institute, Medical University of South Carolina, Charleston,
  South Carolina;
Director, Ocular Pathology Laboratory and Center for Research in Ocular Therapeutics
  and Biodevices;
Director, World Health Organization (WHO) Collaborating Centre for Prevention
  of Blindness;
Distinguished Senior U.S. Scientist Awardee, Alexander von Humboldt Foundation.
Formerly: Professor of Ophthalmology and Pathology, University of Utah Health Sciences Center, Salt
  Lake City, Utah

Maurice F. Rabb, MD, Dsc (Hon)
Professor of Ophthalmology
Department of Ophthalmology, Eye and Ear Infirmary
University of Illinois at Chicago, College of Medicine, Chicago, Illinois;
Chairman, Department of Ophthalmology
Mercy Hospital and Medical Center, Chicago, Illinois;
Medical Director, Prevent Blindness America

with 930 illustrations and 243 color plates

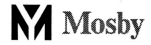 Mosby

St. Louis Baltimore Boston Carlsbad Chicago Minneapolis New York Philadelphia Portland
London Milan Sydney Tokyo Toronto

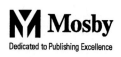

Senior Editor: Laurel Craven
Developmental Editor: Kimberley J. Cox
Project Manager: Chris Baumle
Production Editor: Marian S. Hall
Design Manager: Carolyn O'Brien
Manufacturing Manager: William A. Winneberger, Jr.

Cover illustrations, demonstrating the concept of clinicopathologic correlation.

Front Cover: Primary intraocular tumor, retinoblastoma. *Top,* clinical leukokoria. *Middle,* gross photograph showing exophytic tumor growth. *Bottom,* photomicrograph showing tumor calcification, DNA deposition within a tumor stromal vessel, and Flexner-Wintersteiner rosettes.

Back Cover: Secondary intraocular tumor, adenocarcinoma metastatic from the thyroid to the choroid. *Top,* fundus photograph showing a minimally elevated amelanotic mass temporal to the optic nerve head, with overlying pigment changes. *Middle,* gross photograph showing solid choroidal mass. *Bottom,* photomicrograph showing tumor with differentiation toward thyroid follicles.

FIFTH EDITION
Copyright © 1998 by Mosby-Year Book, Inc.

Previous editions copyrighted 1974, 1978, 1985, 1991

Printed in the United States of America
Composition by Maryland Composition
Printing/binding by Maple-Vail Book Manufacturing Group

Mosby-Year Book, Inc.
11830 Westline Industrial Drive
St. Louis, Missouri 63146

Library of Congress Cataloging in Publication Data

Apple, David J., 1941–
    Ocular pathology : clinical applications and self-assessment /
  David J. Apple, Maurice F. Rabb.—5th ed.
      p.   cm.
    Includes bibliographical references and index.
    ISBN 0-8151-0592-4
    1. Eye—Diseases. 2. Eye—Diseases—Atlases.   I. Rabb, Maurice
  F.   II. Title.
    [DNLM: 1. Eye Diseases—pathology.   WW 140 A648o   1998]
  RE48.A66   1998
  617.7′1—dc21
  DNLM/DLC
  for Library of Congress   97-41914
                                                          CIP

98 99 00 01 02/9 8 7 6 5 4 3 2 1

To our parents.

Foreword to the Fifth Edition

The Fifth Edition of any academic publication these days is a testament to readability and quality combined with desire on the part of the authors to be willing to repeat the arduous process of revision yet one more time. Each edition is somewhat like the delivery of a new child, with anxious parents wondering if the child will be whole and accepted in society. Such is clearly the case for this fifth edition, which builds on the strengths of the past and (as one would expect) has vital new information.

The most notable additions are an update on small-incision cataract surgery and intraocular lens (IOL) implantation and a brand new chapter on the pathology of refractive surgery. Refractive surgery is exploding in ophthalmology and is not without its complications. Just as Dr. Apple did in the field of IOLs and Dr. Rabb did in the field of medical retina in the previous editions, the clinicopathologic correlations and histopathologic illustrations in this text provide a solid basis for understanding clinical problems.

As a friend and mentor from years ago and a colleague with tremendous respect for the work of David Apple, I have followed the achievements of both authors for many years and am, indeed, honored to be asked to write this foreword. I am particularly pleased that this edition again strives to bridge the barrier between the private/corporate sector and academic medicine. For example, it was amazing how few people were willing to consider a career understanding IOLs as one worthy of any consideration in academia despite the fact that IOLs are a vital part of cataract surgery, the single most important surgery in ophthalmology. David Apple took this challenge and the rest is history. The IOL section of this edition, updated to include the latest small-incision foldable lens technology, is a testament indeed to this body of work.

I remember a professor many years ago in medical school who pointed out to us that the time when we are unwilling to learn new things in medicine is the time to call it quits. There is much interesting and new here, and I challenge my colleagues to read through the material to find the pearls and clinicopathologic gems that literally pepper this edition. To Drs. Apple and Rabb, as anxious parents, the birthing process was well worth the wait.

Respectfully submitted,

Randall J. Olson, M.D.
John A. Moran Professor of Ophthalmology
Department Chairman and Director
John A. Moran Eye Center
Chairman, Faculty Practice Organization
University of Utah School of Medicine
Salt Lake City, Utah

Foreword to the First Edition

He from thick films shall purge the visual ray, and on the sightless eyeball pour the day.

Alexander Pope

By reading this book, we become the beneficiaries of the professional skills and avocations of two dedicated eye physicians. For years, Maurice Rabb has perseveringly recorded by stereophotography the incredible variety of human ocular disease. Similarly, David Apple has documented, utilizing similar stereoscopic techniques, the appearance of gross pathologic specimens and has carefully studied the diseased eye with the techniques and perspective of the general pathologist. Utilizing the resources of the University of Illinois Eye and Ear Infirmary, these authors have successfully blended their interests and skills with their ophthalmic knowledge. The result is a book with widespread appeal. Practicing ophthalmologists will enjoy the stereoscopic presentation of clinical and gross pathologic specimens. Pathologists will enhance their knowledge of eye disease. Medical students will marvel at the diversity of ways in which the human eye manifests abnormal processes. Most important, ophthalmology resident physicians will have available a readable introductory text with highly informative illustrations.

Morton F. Goldberg, MD
1974

Preface to the Fifth Edition

Since its inception in 1974, the major goal of this text has been to provide a didactic, illustrated overview of ophthalmic pathology. In this Fifth Edition, we continue to offer this teaching and reference source based on the principle of clinicopathologic correlation. As the book has evolved over the past quarter century, we have gradually added sections on the pathology of various ophthalmic surgical procedures. These additions supplement the core discussions on diseases of the eye and we continue this trend in this edition.

In the preface to the Fourth Edition (1989), we noted that "the various keratorefractive operations that are being applied and popularized today remain experimental. Definite data about the operations that are most useful and a well catalogued collection of pathologic material are not yet available." Since that time the field of refractive surgery has advanced remarkably! Therefore one of the high points of this Fifth Edition is the addition of a new chapter covering Pathology of Refractive Surgery (Chapter 5). This chapter represents the first comprehensive publication on clinicopathologic correlation of refractive surgery, and the material and illustrations have not been published elsewhere. This was made possible because of the invaluable input of David G. Kent, F.R.A.C.O., a research fellow working in our laboratory.

Cataract surgery with intraocular lens implantation continues to be a highly successful procedure, and the chapter on the pathology of the lens, cataract surgery, and intraocular lenses (Chapter 4) has been updated to include modern small-incision surgery and foldable lens technology. These are the procedures that have become the gold standard for the treatment of cataract. Knowledge of the pathology of complications is required as we continue to fine-tune these procedures.

We have updated the text and added references covering almost all topics in the book. For the busy clinician who seeks rapid access to information and "pearls," we recommend focusing on the text and selectively bypassing the detailed references. The book then functions as a handbook that provides concise, clinically relevant and practical information regarding eye conditions. Alternatively, some readers and researchers may wish to obtain in-depth background information and thorough detail covering various topics. This can be accomplished by utilizing the comprehensive references distributed throughout the book. We have increased the total number of references from 5026 in the previous edition to 9181 in this edition, covering the period through the first quarter of 1997.

The number of self-assessment questions and answers has been increased from a total of 350 in the Fourth Edition to 550 in this edition (50 per chapter). There are 930 black-and-white illustrations, an increase of 107 from the previous edition. The number of color illustrations has been increased from 158 to 239 images.

Special thanks to Qun Peng, M.D., senior postdoctoral fellow in the ocular pathology laboratory, who holds the position of Cornelia Ayer Endowed Fellow in Ophthalmology at the Storm Eye Institute, for her tireless effort and important input in preparing this new edition.

In addition to Drs. Kent and Peng, and the individuals cited in the first four editions of this text, we thank Teddy Redmon and Sherrie Nesbitt, Administrative Specialists, who spent many hours organizing, typing and proofing the manuscript.

We are pleased that this text has evolved over the years to a point where we are now producing this Fifth Edition. It has been gratifying to speak to innumerable successful ophthalmology and pathology Board Candidates and others who have benefited from this publication. It also has been especially satisfying to know and work with eye specialists worldwide whose patients have benefited from our clinicopathologic studies related to ocular diagnosis and surgery. We hope that this edition will be useful to all individuals interested in ophthalmology and the visual sciences as our specialty continues to grow and provide enhanced vision care to the populations of the world as we enter the new millenium.

David J. Apple, M.D.
Maurice F. Rabb, M.D.

Contents

CHAPTER 1

INTRODUCTION

Basic ocular structure*

The eye is composed of three primary layers† (Fig. 1-1). We follow conventional terminology, designating the outer aspect of the globe as the outside layer that borders the orbit and the inner layer as the center layer that faces toward the vitreous. In all subsequent photomicrographs involving structures of the ocular fundus, the outer scleral aspect is at the bottom of the photograph; the inner aspect is toward the top.

The outer coat, the **tunica fibrosa,** is composed primarily of collagen-elastic tissue and provides a protective outer wall. The cornea forms the anterior one sixth of this layer and the scleral forms the posterior five sixths. The sclera is white and opaque as a result of the random, irregular layering of its collagen fibers. In contrast, the corneal collagen lamellae are arranged in a parallel fashion and therefore have a geometrically regular appearance. This renders the cornea transparent to incoming light.

The uvea, or **tunica vasculosa,** is the middle layer of the eye and lies immediately inside the sclera. This richly vascular and pigmented tissue consists of three parts: the iris, the ciliary body, and the choroid. When the uveal tissues are separated from the other layers of the eye and examined grossly, they reveal a purple color and rounded contour that resembles a grape (hence the name *uvea,* which is derived from the Latin word for grape). The most important function of the uvea is to provide the vascular supply to the eye, particularly to the outer portion of the sensory retina via the choriocapillaris.

The inner layer of the eye, the **tunica nervosa,** composed of sensory retina, pigment epithelium, and the optic nerve, develops embryologically as an anteriorly protruding portion of the brain. This tunic is derived from the two-layered neuroectodermal optic cup (p. 8, see Figs. 1-9 and 1-10). In the posterior aspect of the eye, the original inner layer of the optic cup forms the sensory retina and the outer layer develops the retinal pigment epithelium. The space between these layers, the original cavity of the optic vesicle, forms the subretinal space in the adult eye. In the adult, it is normally merely a potential space and reappears only in cases of pathologic retinal detachment (p. 9). The anterior aspect of the **tunica nervosa** develops into the two-layered epithelia of the iris and ciliary body.

Techniques of examination

GROSS EXAMINATION OF THE EYE

The eye is a sphere that measures roughly 24 to 25 mm in each diameter (Figs. 1-1 to 1-3). The cornea, which

---

* General references in ocular embryology and anatomy,[1-31] pathology,[32-106] and selected general ophthalmology textbooks that pertain to these subjects[107-152] are listed at the end of this chapter.
† References 8-11, 15, 21-23, 26, 27, 50.

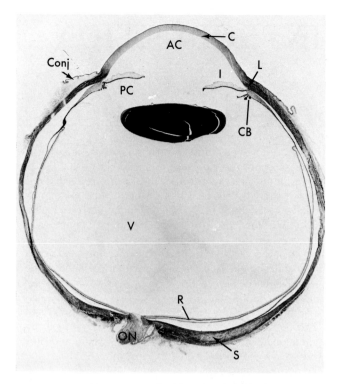

Fig. 1-1. Histologic section through a child's globe demonstrating the three major tunics. The outer fibrous tunic consists of the cornea *(C)*, which is continuous with the sclera *(S)* at the limbus *(L)*. The bulbar conjunctival epithelium *(Conj)* is continuous with the corneal epithelium. The middle (uveal) tunic consists of the iris *(I)*, ciliary body *(CB)*, and choroid. The sensory retinal *(R)* fibers enter the optic nerve *(ON)* posteriorly. *AC,* anterior chamber; *PC,* posterior chamber; *V,* vitreous. (H & E stain; ×6.)

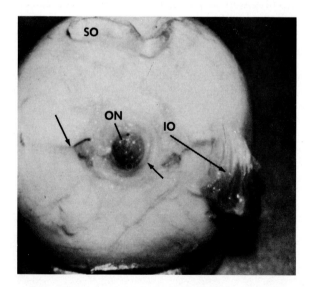

Fig. 1-2. Posterior aspect of an enucleated right eye. The superior oblique *(SO)* muscle insertion is tendinous; the fleshy inferior oblique *(IO)* muscle inserts directly onto the temporal sclera. *Long arrow,* Prominent nasal long posterior ciliary vessel; *ON,* optic nerve; *short arrow,* dural sheath of the nerve.

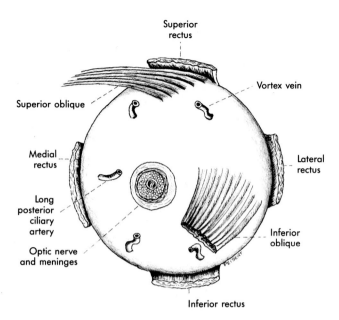

Fig. 1-3. Normal right globe, posterior external aspect.

occupies approximately the anterior sixth of the globe, has a lesser radius of curvature than the sclera. The anterior aspect of the globe contains the refractive media and accessory structures of the visual apparatus. The perceptive tissues and nervous elements are largely confined to the posterior aspect.

Identification of major landmarks on the exterior of the unopened enucleated globe allows the pathologist to differentiate the right from the left eye, determine the horizontal-vertical orientation of the globe, and define the site of clinically observed intraocular lesions. These determinations are necessary to ensure proper sectioning of the globe (Fig. 1-4).

The adult cornea normally measures approximately 12 by 11 mm. It is actually round but appears oval because the superior and inferior conjunctiva at the limbus partly overlie the cornea at these sites. Because the apparently long axis lies in the horizontal plane, the shape of the cornea readily identifies the horizontal axis.

Examination of the posterior aspect of the eye (Fig. 1-2) confirms the direction of the horizontal plane. At least one of the two long posterior ciliary vessels is visible as they course horizontally, emanating from the region of the optic nerve. The nasal one is almost always more prominent than the temporal; this observation aids in determining the globe's nasal aspect.

The inferior oblique muscle has a muscular rather than a tendinous insertion into the sclera. It is identifiable at a point just temporal to the optic disc, overlying the macula. Observation of this muscle with its thick fleshy appearance and the superior oblique muscle, which is in the superotemporal quadrant and has a tendinous insertion, allows differentiation of the right and left globes.

When intraocular tumors such as choroidal malignant melanoma° (see Chapter 7) are suspected, the location of

---

° References 40-42, 52, 90-92, 116, 119, 125, 140, 142.

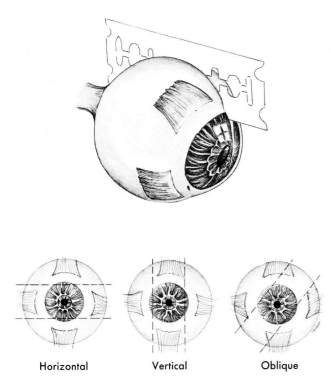

Fig. 1-4. Technique of gross sectioning of the globe. (From Naumann GOH and Apple DJ: In Doerr W, Seifert G, and Uehlinger E, editors: Handbuch der speziellen pathologischen Anatomie, Band Auge, Berlin, 1980, Springer-Verlag; modified and redrawn by Dr Steven Vermillion, University of Iowa.)

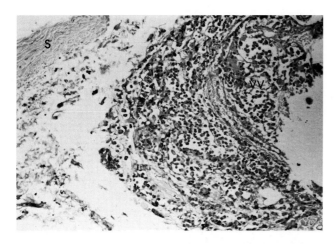

Fig. 1-5. Photomicrograph showing extension of malignant melanoma cells through a vortex vein. This nodule was shaved off the epibulbar surface before sectioning of the globe. *S,* Adjacent scleral tissue; *VV,* vortex vein containing myriad epithelioid cells. (H & E stain; ×220.)

the mass can often be determined by transillumination before the globe is sectioned. In addition, in cases of intraocular melanoma, it is important to examine the vortex veins or scleral emissaria (Fig. 1-3). A suspected tumor that may have extended onto the epibulbar surface (Fig. 1-5, Color Plate 1-1) can be excised from the external surface of the globe and submitted separately for a microscopic examination.

HISTOLOGIC STAINS

Specific staining techniques[49,82,98] make possible the recognition of characteristic structures within the eye and are invaluable for complete evaluation of certain disease entities (Table 1-1). The theory of special staining is simple: the various components of the eye have an affinity for certain stains so that each structure under study can be identified by the color imparted by the stain (which is essentially a tissue dye). Because reference is commonly made to these various techniques in the literature, it is useful to be aware of the major categories of stains available to the ophthalmic pathologist.

For routine histopathologic examination of ocular tissue, specimens are cut from a paraffin block and stained by the hematoxylin and eosin technique. Hematoxylin imparts a basophilic (blue) stain to nuclear elements and structures containing nucleic acid, whereas eosin renders most cytoplasmic organelles a light pink.

Tissue prepared for electron microscopy is not normally embedded in paraffin; it must be embedded in special plastics to achieve satisfactory preservation for ultrastructural analysis. This type of embedding is advantageous both for light microscopy and thin-section electron microscopy. Cellular organelles are much better preserved by this method (compare, for example, Figs. 8-3 and 8-5); however, the adaptability of special staining techniques after plastic embedding is limited. For plastic-embedded tissue, most laboratories use dyes that give a blue color to the tissue (hence the names *toluidine blue, methylene blue,* and *Mallory blue,* which appear frequently in the literature). Plastic-embedding techniques are mainly used when electron microscopy is to be performed or when special details in the tissue must be critically studied without artifact. The technique is too tedious for routine use.

If plastic-embedded tissue is further processed for thin-section electron microscopy, it is usually fixed and stained by three agents: osmium tetroxide, uranyl acetate, and lead citrate. These compounds contain heavy metals that have an affinity for cell membranes and cell organelles. Contrast of cell structures is thus attained because most cell organelles are derived from such unit membranes (see Fig. 10-5).

The most important special stain used by ophthalmic pathologists is the periodic acid-Schiff (PAS) stain. The PAS stain has an affinity for certain mucopolysaccharides and glycoproteins and is particularly useful in demonstrating ocular basement membranes. Such structures stain a brilliant red and have enhanced visibility in contrast to the poorly staining background tissue. The important basement membranes in the eye include Descemet's membrane (see Figs. 3-2 and 3-4), the lens capsule (the thickest basement membrane in the body (see Figs. 4-6 and 4-7), the basement membrane of the ciliary processes, the internal limiting membrane of the retina, Bruch's membrane (see Fig. 8-13), and the basement membrane of all vessels—that of intraocular vascular endothelial cells and pericytes (see Fig. 8-12).

The trichrome stain of Masson or a similar trichrome technique devised by Gomori is invaluable for identifying

Table 1-1. Routine and special stains used in ocular pathology.*

Staining technique	Substances, cellular components, and tissues that are stained	Staining characteristics
Paraffin embedding (fixation with 10% buffered formaldehyde)		
Hematoxylin	Nucleic acids within cellular nuclei	Basophilic (blue)
Eosin	Cytoplasmic organelles (e.g., mitochondria)	Eosinophilic (pink)
Periodic acid-Schiff	Mucopolysaccharides and glycoproteins (e.g., ocular basement membranes, glycogen)	Brilliant red or rose
Trichrome	Collagen (e.g., sclera or cornea)	Blue
	Smooth muscle (e.g., ciliary muscle)	Red
Van Gleson	Collagen	Collagen—red; Muscle—yellow
Verhoeff's elastic stain	Elastic fibers	Elastic—black; Collagen—red; Muscle—yellow
Mallory's phospho-tungstic acid hematoxylin (PTAH)	Cross striation in skeletal muscle, rhabdomyosarcoma, fibrils in smooth muscle fibrin, glial elements	Muscle, glial, filaments—blue; Collagen—purple; Elastin—brown
Alcian blue, colloidal iron	Mucopolysaccharides, hyaluronic acid (e.g., vitreous, mucin)	Blue
Prussian (Berlin) blue, Mallory, Perl, and Lillie stains	Iron (hemosiderin) (e.g., iron foreign bodies, blood products)	Blue
Mayer's Mucicamine	Acid mucopolysaccharide, cryptococcus	Mucin and capsule of crutococus-red
Alizarin red, von Kossa	Calcium	Red
Kluver-Barrera, Luxol fast blue	Myelin (e.g., optic nerve)	Blue
Weigert	Myelin	Black
Bodian, Cajal, Golgi	Neurons	Dark red or black
Holzer's stain	Glial fibers	Deep violet
Oil red O, Sudan	Lipid (e.g., meibomian [sebaceous] gland secretions and carcinoma)	Red
Congo red	Amyloid (e.g., lattice corneal dystrophy)	Pale red
Thioflavine T	Amyloid	Fluorescence
Crystal violet	Amyloid	Metachromasia
Silver stains (reticulum, Grocott's modification of Gomori's methenamine silver [GMS])	Reticular fibrils, fungal walls, melanin derivatives	Black
Fontana	Melanin granules	Black
Gram	Bacteria	Gram positive—blue; gram negative—pink
Gridley fungus	Fungus	Mycelia—purple and rose; Conidia—blue
Giemsa	Rickettsia, chlamydia	Rickettsia—black/purple; Chlamydia, bacteria—blue
Calcafluor white	Acanthamoeba, fungus	White fluorescence
Ziehl-Neelsen	Acid fast	Acid fast bacteria—bright red

* Courtesy of David J. Apple, M.D., and James Reidy, M.D.

intraocular structures of different compositions. For example, collagenous tissues such as sclera and cornea stain blue, whereas smooth muscle such as the ciliary muscle assumes a dull red hue (see Fig. 6-3). Pathologic deposits seen in some diseases (e.g., granular corneal dystrophy; see Fig. 3-46) have an affinity for components of the trichrome stain. This contrast in tissue staining improves visualization and differentiation of diverse tissues.

Numerous stains assist in the differentiation of several groups of mucopolysaccharides. They generally exhibit a blue color when results are positive. Such stains are important in analyzing deposits of mucopolysaccharide in specific disease states, such as macular corneal dystrophy (see Fig. 3-47) or the systemic mucopolysaccharides. Hyaluronic acid, the normal substance present in the vitreous, is stained positively with this type of procedure. The commonly used stains include Alcian blue and colloidal iron.

The Prussian blue stain for iron is invaluable for differen-

tiation of intraocular pigments. The presence of iron, as observed in intraocular siderosis (see Figs. 3-64 and 3-65) and in the various corneal iron lines or as occurs after hemorrhage, contrasts readily with normal intraocular melanin pigment. Melanin granules may resemble iron in routinely stained sections, but the blue color imparted to iron particles in this staining reaction ensures easy identification in most cases.

The various stains for myelin are useful in assessing the degree of optic nerve disease or atrophy (see Figs. 10-26 and 10-27). The more commonly used stains include the Luxol fast blue stains and the Weigert stain. These stains are taken up by normal myelin. A defect in stain uptake is created at a site of demyelination, as in multiple sclerosis (see Fig. 10-27).

Lipid structures normally do not stain in routinely prepared hematoxylin and eosin sections because the lipid is removed during technical processing through paraffin. Lipid

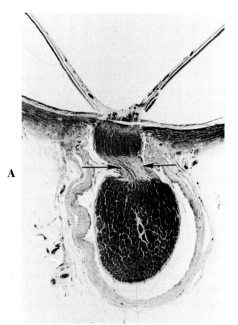

A

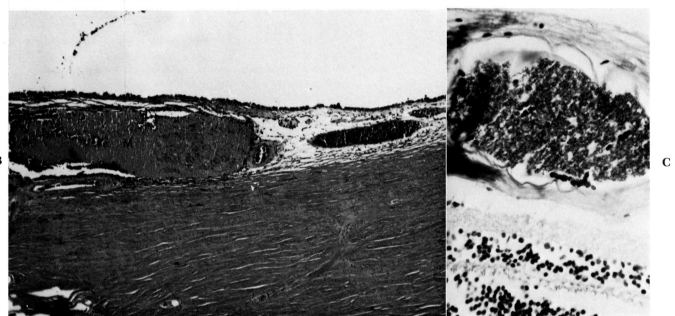

B

C

Fig. 1-6. A, Photomicrograph of an optic nerve of an enucleated eye showing a site of decreased diameter of the nerve where it was constricted *(arrows)* during surgical removal, expressing myelin onto the optic nerve head and into the retina. The myelin is deeply stained in this photograph. The lack of stain uptake between the arrows resulted from the expression of myelin from the constricted area. (Luxol fast blue stain; ×75.) **B,** Photomicrograph of the choroid of the same case as **A,** showing massive deposits of myelin *(M)* within this layer. (H & E stain; ×150.) **C,** High-power photomicrograph through a retinal vessel containing myelin from the same case as **A.** (Luxol fast blue stain; ×275.)

can be demonstrated on freshly frozen tissue by using special stains, the most important of which are the Sudan stains and the oil red O technique. Such techniques are important in evaluating disease states involving lipid-secreting tissues such as the meibomian glands (see Fig. 11-53).

Important stains for amyloid are available; the best known is Congo red. Histopathologic diagnosis of lattice corneal dystrophy (p. 91) is readily accomplished by use of amyloid stains.

Certain structures possess a molecular structure that, when stained and viewed through polarizing lenses, appears to glow (double refraction, or birefringence). Major examples are amyloid (see Figs. 3-50, *B* and 3-51, *B*) and numerous types of foreign material such as wood (see Fig. 3-62) and insect hairs (see Fig. 3-63).

An important artifact occasionally observed after enucle-

ation of a globe is the so-called myelin artifact of the optic disc and retina, first described in 1958 by Cogan and Kuwabara,[53] and elaborated on by Zimmerman and Fine[104] in 1965. The myelin artifact results from compression of the optic nerve by the surgical instruments as the eye is removed (Fig. 1-6, *A*). This compression may express myelin from the optic nerve to the epipapillary or peripapillary area and into the choroid (Fig. 1-6, *B*) or into retinal vessels (Fig. 1-6, *C*). The expression occurs in a manner somewhat analogous to squeezing toothpaste out of its tube. The myelin can be readily identified with the Luxol fast blue stain (Table 1-1). This phenomenon is significant because during gross examination, the white myelin may occasionally be misinterpreted by the pathologist as an epipapillary mass or tumor. It may also erroneously suggest occluded retinal blood vessels.

Although transmission electron microscopy traditionally has been an important research technique, in experienced hands, it also is an effective tool for resolving diagnostic dilemmas, such as tumor identification.[68,74,78] Transmission electron microscopy may be regarded as an extension of routine light microscopy. Tissues for light and electron microscopy are prepared in different manners (i.e., formalin versus glutaraldehyde fixation). It is therefore important to make arrangements with the histology laboratory before submitting tissue.

IMMUNOHISTOCHEMICAL STAINS[*]

Immunohistology, such as immunohistochemical stains, is used for the identification and localization of specific cells, tissues, or causative agents in disease (Table 1-2). Immunoperoxidase and immunofluorescent techniques use antibodies that bind to and define specific antigens. Components that may be demonstrated are endogenous cellular substances such as lineage-specific cytoplasmic filaments, DNA, immunoglobulin, hormones, cell surface receptors, tumor-specific antigens, or exogenous agents such as bacteria and viruses. Monoclonal or polyclonal antibodies are labeled with substances that allow the colorimetric or fluorescent visualization of the antigen of interest.

Immunoperoxidase methods, which detect the presence of monotypic immunoglobulin or specific cytofilaments, are often used for tumor analysis. Cytofilaments are the structural components of the cell cytoskeleton and have been classified by ultrastructural parameters. These protein filaments are specific for certain tissues and include the cytokeratins found in epithelial tissue and the neurofilaments present in all neurons of the central and peripheral nervous system.

Other proteins that can be detected by immunoperoxidase staining, which may be useful in ophthalmic diagnosis, include leukocyte common antigen (LCA) present on lymphoreticular cell surfaces, S-100 protein (Color Plate 1-2) in neural crest-derived cells and non-neural cells (e.g., Langerhans cells), and glial fibrillary acidic protein (GFAP) present in glial and Schwann cells. Antibodies specific for these filaments and proteins can be used to categorize tumors. For example, antibody to the leukocyte common antigen (LCA or CD45) may be invaluable in the diagnosis of a malignant lymphoma. Neurofilaments and GFAP are present in many primitive tumors of neuroblastic origin and can be found in retinoblastomas and neuroblastomas. Glial fibrillary acidic protein often is present in optic nerve gliomas. S-100 protein is commonly found in nevi, melanomas, and histiocytosis X disease.

Immunohistochemical studies that detect monoclonal expression of immunoglobulin light or heavy chains may be performed on cryostat sections of orbital or conjunctival tissue. Monoclonal antibodies to B- and T-cell surface markers are also commercially available. The presence of monotypic immunoglobulin expression may help to differentiate benign from malignant B-cell lymphoid infiltrates when histologic features of malignancy such as cytologic atypia or Dutcher bodies are not found. If immunohisto-

Table 1-2. Immunohistochemical stains[*]

Staining technique	Substances, cellular components, and tissues that are stained
Kermix	Keratin, epithelial cells
Vimentin	Intermediate filaments, mesenchymal cells
S-100 protein	Neural crest-derived cells
Desmin	Intermediate filaments, muscle cells
HMB-45	Melanocytic cells, nevus, melanoma
Factor VIII	Endothelial cells
Leukocyte common antigen (LCA)	White blood cells, lymphoma, leukemia, myeloma, inflammation
Lysozyme	Polymorphonuclear neutrophils (PMN), histiocytes, monocytes, leukemia
L26	B-cells
UCHL-1	T-cells
Kappa and lambda	Cytoplasmic light chain immunoglobulin
LEU M1	Reed-Sternberg cells, macrophages, granulocytes
Neurofilament protein (NFP)	Neuronal cell axons
Glial fibrillary acidic protein (GFAP)	Glial cells - glioma
Leu 7	T-cell marker, nonspecific reactivity for Schwann cells, oligodendroglia, Mueller cell foot processes
Neuron specific enolase (NSE)	Retinoblastoma, neuroblastoma
BrEP4	Epithelial tumors
Immunoglobulin	IgG, IgM, IgA

STAINS FOR SPECIFIC TUMORS THAT MAY BE METASTATIC TO OCULAR TISSUE

alpha-fetoprotein (AFP)	Germ cells, gonadal tumors
alpha 1-antitrypsin	Hepatic carcinoma
Carcinoembryonic antigen (CEA)	Gastrointestinal carcinoma
Chromogranin	Neuroendocrine tumors, carcinoids
Gonadotropin	Choriocarcinoma
Thyroglobulin	Thyroid carcinoma

[*] Best on frozen tissue, but most also will work on formalin-fixed, paraffin-embedded tissue.

chemical studies are nondiagnostic, gene rearrangement analysis may provide clarification.

Many hospital laboratories can now analyze cell surface antigens and cellular DNA content by flow cytometry. Single-cell suspensions made from fresh tissue are stained with fluorescent or phycobiliprotein-tagged monoclonal antibodies, which are specific for cell surface antigens. Immunophenotypic features of lymphoid tissue can be determined, and the results can often be used to differentiate between benign reactive polyclonal lymphoid hyperplasia and monoclonal malignant lymphoma.

Origin and development of the eye[†]

The three layers of the globe exist and function in close connection with the adnexal structures of the eye and the

[*] References 51, 56, 58, 59, 72, 77, 79, 86, 88, 99, 106.

[†] References 2-4, 7, 8, 14, 16, 17, 25, 28, 110.

central visual tracts and cortical receptive areas in the brain. These structures are characterized by a complicated embryonic developmental process caused by intricate interactions of the various germ layers. Knowledge of the embryology of the eye is necessary to understand the structure of the normal adult eye and to explain the pathogenesis of the numerous congenital defects and anomalies that may occur (see Chapter 2).

This section describes the origin and early development of the eye as a whole. Detailed embryology and histology of the individual ocular tissues are described in subsequent chapters: sclera and cornea, Chapter 3; lens, Chapter 4; anterior segment and angle, Chapter 6; uvea, Chapter 7; retina and vitreous, Chapter 8; optic nerve, Chapter 10; and conjunctiva and eyelid, Chapter 11.

OPTIC VESICLE AND OPTIC CUP

The eye forms directly from the anlage of the brain by means of an outgrowth of the anterolateral part of the embryonic neutral tube at the diencephalic level (Fig. 1-7). The neuroectodermal parts of the eye—the future retina and pigment epithelium—develop from the primitive neural tube ependyma at an early point (within the first 2 to 3 weeks). At this time, the apical (anterior) neural tube has not yet closed.

The first evidence of eye development occurs as two anterolateral depressions of the neural plate: the optic grooves. They enlarge rapidly to form the optic vesicles (Fig. 1-7, A). The cavity of the evaginated optic vesicle is originally in broad communication with the lumen of the diencephalon. However, the connection between the brain and vesicle eventually contracts to form the optic stalk, the anlage of the future optic nerve (Fig. 1-7, B). The distal (anterior) wall of the optic nerve vesicle is destined to form the sensory retina. The proximal (posterior) wall represents the primordia of the future retinal, ciliary, and iris pigment epithelia.

At approximately the end of the first month, the distal (anterior) wall of the optic vesicle makes contact with the outer epithelial lining of the embryo, the surface ectoderm. The primordium of the future lens develops from cells of this surface layer at the point of contact (see Fig. 4-1). Not only the lens but also the future epithelia of the cornea, the conjunctiva, and the entire integument are derived from this single layer of surface epithelium.

The neuroectodermal anlage of the eye is, in all stages of its development, completely surrounded by several layers of mesoderm, or mesectoderm (neural crest mesenchyme) (Fig. 1-7, A). This is the "middle tissue," situated between the core of neuroectoderm and the outer lining of surface ectoderm. The anterior portion of the mesectoderm forms a portion of the future cornea (with the exception of the corneal epithelium), the stroma of the iris and ciliary body, and the structures of the anterior chamber filtration apparatus. Important structures that develop from the mesectoderm posteriorly are the stroma and vessels of the choroid, the sclera, and the bulk of the orbital tissues.

The primary optic vesicle is transformed into the optic cup between the fourth and sixth weeks of gestation (Figs. 1-7, B to 1-11). The optic cup forms by an invagination of the anterior (distal) and inferior wall of the optic vesicle.

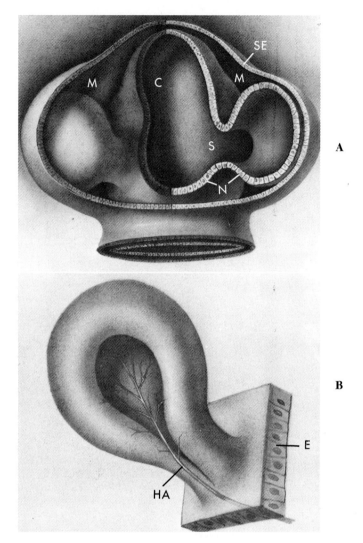

A

B

Fig. 1-7. A, Schematic illustration of the forebrain with formation of the optic vessel in the first month of gestation. Two lateral outpouchings of neuroectoderm form the vesicles. *SE,* Surface ectoderm lining the embryo; *N,* neuroectoderm derived from the neural tube, forming an ependymal lining of the forebrain and primitive eye; *M,* mesectoderm filling the space between *SE* and *N; C,* cavity of the forebrain, which is continuous with the cavity of the optic vesicle through the optic stalk *(S).* **B,** Schematic illustration of the optic cup. The hyaloid artery *(HA)* enters the cup through the inferior embryonic ocular fissure. *E,* Ependymal lining of the diencephalon.

This epithelium folds posteriorly in the direction of the cavity of the optic vesicle and immediately begins to increase in thickness to form the sensory retina (see Fig. 8-1). The invagination extends from the anterior aspect of the cup all the way posteriorly to the optic stalk. In so doing, a cleft forms along the inferior margin of the eye, the embryonic ocular fissure (Figs. 1-7, B and 1-10). The fissure develops because the invagination that transforms the vesicle into the cup occurs not only in an anteroposterior direction but also from underneath or ventral to the optic vesicle.

The older terms *fetal* fissure and *choroidal* fissure are incorrect because the developing organism is technically

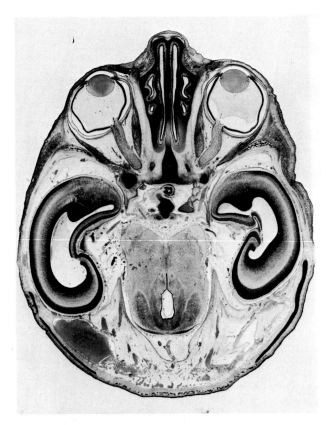

Fig. 1-8. Horizontal section through fetal head showing advanced development of optic cups. (H & E stain; ×5.) (From the collection of Professor Wolfgang Stock, Tübingen, West Germany, and from Naumann GOH and Apple DJ: In Doerr W, Seifert G, and Uehlinger E, editors: Handbuch der speziellen pathologischen Anatomie, Band Auge, Berlin, 1980, Springer-Verlag.)

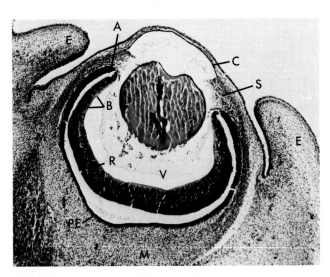

Fig. 1-9. Human embryonic eye at the 23 mm stage (approximately 7 weeks' gestation). **A,** Anterior margin of the two-layered cup, the future iris; **B,** site of the future epithelium of the ciliary body. Posteriorly, the inner layer forms the sensory retina (*R*) and the outer layer forms the retinal pigment epithelium (*PE*). *C,* Cornea; *E,* eyelid buds; *S,* stroma of the future iris and ciliary body; *V,* primary vitreous; *M,* mesectoderm surrounding the cup and differentiating toward the choroid and sclera. (H & E stain; ×40.)

an embryo at this stage rather than a fetus. Furthermore, the cleft is formed from the neuroectodermal layers, not the choroid, which at this stage barely exists.

The formation of the embryonic ocular fissure is necessary for two reasons. The fissure creates a ventral defect or groove through which the trunk of the transient embryonic intraocular vessels (hyaloid vessel) is able to grow into the eye from the inferior orbit (Fig. 1-7, *B*). The hyaloid vascular contributes to the primary vitreous (p. 7, also see Chapter 2, p. 28). This ingrowth would not be possible without the fissure. The fissure also provides a pathway for the ganglion cells in the sensory retina to send their processes from the retina into the brain through the optic stalk. If the fissure were not present, the walls of the optic cup would form a barrier to growth of these axons into the brain.

Once the embryonic vessels and nerve fibers complete their passage through the cleft, the lips of the fissure fuse together. The closure normally occurs at approximately 6 weeks of gestation, corresponding approximately to the 15-mm crown-rump length of the fetus (see Fig. 2-1). This is a critical time in embryogenesis, not only in the eye but also in the entire body. At 6 weeks of gestation, the anlagen of most body tissues are formed. Development after 6 weeks is actually a process of cell differentiation and tissue

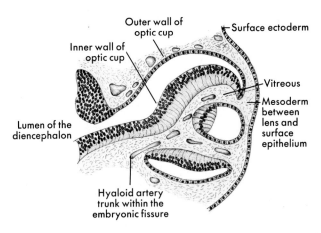

Fig. 1-10. Drawing of sagitally sectioned optic cup. (Modified from Salzmann M: The anatomy and histology of the human eyeball in the normal state, Chicago, 1912, University of Chicago Press. [Translated by EVL Brown.])

maturation. As a general rule, endogenous or exogenous insults[35,47,65] before this time are expected to cause more severe defects. Noxious influences occurring at later stages, well after formation and early differentiation of the tissues, are expected to be less dangerous, not only as a threat to the life of the fetus but also in the severity of the anomalies they may induce.

Closure of the fissure normally initially occurs in the middle regions of the optic cup near the region of the midperiphery of the retina. Later closure of the fissure subsequently occurs in the anterior and posterior segments of the optic cup: the iris and optic nerve head region,

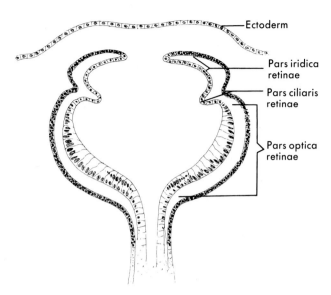

Ectoderm

Pars iridica
retinae

Pars ciliaris
retinae

Pars optica
retinae

Fig. 1-11. The three major subdivisions of the neuroectodermal optic cup. The inner and outer neuroblastic layers of the retina are beginning to form at the posterior (peripapillary) aspect of the inner layer of the optic cup. The transient noncellular layer is termed *Chievitz layer* (see Chapter 7).

respectively. This sequence of closure explains the frequency of formation of the various types of typical coloboma[39,47] that occur when the fissure fails to close (p.00).

The optic cup is crescent shaped, with the anterior lips, or margins, delineating the margins of the future pupillary aperture. Because of the selective growth and specialization, the original cuboidal epithelium of the cup is transformed into three distinct segments (Figs. 1-9 and 1-11):

1. Both layers of the cup become heavily pigmented at the anterior (pupillary) margin, forming the iris epithelium (pars iridica retinae) (Figs. 1-9, *A* and 1-11). These two layers are so heavily pigmented that they appear as a single layer clinically and histopathologically. The dilator and sphincter muscles of the iris arise from the iris epithelium and migrate into the iris stroma just anterior to the epithelium. These muscles, like the erector muscles of the hairs, have the distinction of being of ectodermal rather than mesodermal derivation.

2. A small segment of the optic cup epithelium just posterior to the future iris undergoes a convolution, or folding movement, and becomes the epithelium of the ciliary body (pars ciliaris retinae) (Figs. 1-9, *B* and 1-11). The outer layer is pigmented; the inner layer remains nonpigmented. Both cell layers retain the simple cuboidal pattern.

3. The large segment of the two-layered cup posterior to the ciliary body zone (pars optica retinae; Fig. 1-11) develops into the outer, single-layered retinal pigment epithelium and inner sensory retina, which, after complex cell migrations, eventually differentiates into nine layers.[13,18-20,24,31] The most posterior segment of the optic cup and the stalk, which connect the cup with the forebrain, represent the primordia of the optic disc and optic nerve, respectively.

The lens plate, the thickening of the surface ectoderm induced by earlier contact with the optic vesicle, begins to invaginate from the epithelial surface, forming the lens groove at approximately the same time that the optic cup is developing from the optic vesicle (see Fig. 4-1). As the lens groove develops into the lens vesicle and separates from the surface ectoderm, the anterior margins of the optic cup move forward and form the rudiments of the future papillary margins (Figs. 1-9 and 1-10). The lens vesicle is therefore almost totally surrounded by the neural ectoderm of the optic cup and separated from the overlying surface ectoderm and adjacent anterior mesectoderm. The lens capsule (a PAS-positive basement membrane) forms at the lens vesicle stage. Of surgical importance,[48] the anterior lens capsule becomes relatively thick; the posterior capsule remains very thin (see also Chapter 4, p. 120). The primary vitreous (p. 28) begins to develop behind the lens, between the lens and the inner layer of the optic cup (Figs. 1-9, 1-10, 2-23, and 2-24).

The embryonic germ layer components of the visual system are summarized in the following outline:

I. Neuroectoderm
  A. Optic cup
    1. Sensory retina
    2. Pigment epithelium
    3. Inner layers of Bruch's membrane
    4. Ciliary epithelium
      a. Inner layer; nonpigmented
      b. Outer layer; pigmented
    5. Iris epithelium
    6. Iris dilator muscle
    7. Iris sphincter muscle
      a. Vitreous
        (1) Primary
        (2) Secondary
        (3) Tertiary
  B. Optic stalk and forebrain
    1. Optic nerve, chiasm, tract
    2. Lateral geniculate body
    3. Visual radiations
    4. Cortical visual centers
  C. Neural crest (pp. 288 and 307) (Because the neural crest represents the cell of origin of many diverse types of tissue [see Fig. 7-4], many types of tumors[92,105] may be derived from this embryonic cell line. Some of the most important examples are the melanocytic tumors of the uvea [see Chapter 7[40-42,76,90]], the phacomatoses [see Chapter 9], and the conjunctiva and eyelids [see Chapter 11]).
    1. Uveal melanocytes (chromatophores)
    2. Peripheral nerves and Schwann cells of the eye and its adnexa
    3. Sympathetic ganglion cells
    4. Pial and arachnoid sheaths of the optic nerve meninges
II. Mesectoderm (neural crest mesenchyme) and Mesoderm (vessels)
  A. Cornea (except for epithelium)
    1. Bowman's layer
    2. Stroma
    3. Descemet's membrane
    4. Endothelium
  B. Sclera
  C. Episclera

D. Tenon's capsule
E. Anterior chamber angle filtration structures
   1. Scleral spur
   2. Trabecular meshwork
   3. Schlemm's canal
   4. Schwalbe's line
F. Iris stroma (except for chromatophores, clump cells, and iris muscles)
G. Ciliary body stroma and ciliary muscles (except for chromatophores)
H. Choroid (except for chromatophores)
I. Outer layers of Bruch's membrane
J. Hyaloid artery and its branches (transient embryonic intraocular vessels), a major component of the primary vitreous (probably a true mesoderm)
K. All vessels of the eye and its adnexa (probably a true mesoderm)
L. All muscles of the eye and its adnexa (except for the iris muscles)
M. Fat and connective tissue of the orbit
III. Surface ectoderm
A. Corneal epithelium
B. Conjunctival epithelium
C. Eyelid epidermis
D. Appendages of the eyelid skin
   1. Eccrine glands
   2. Hair
   3. Sebaceous glands (meibomian and Zeis glands)
   4. Glands of Moll
   5. Primary and accessory lacrimal glands (glands of Wolfring and Krause)
E. Caruncle epithelium and appendages
F. Lens (an evagination of the surface epithelium)
G. Vitreous
   1. Primary
   2. Tertiary (not yet proved)

EYE OF THE NEWBORN, GROWTH, AND AGING CHANGES

The size of a newborn's eye[7] varies considerably, with the sagittal diameter ranging between 16 and 19 mm. The eye grows most rapidly during the first year of life, particularly the anterior segment.[12] Growth thereafter is much slower. The cornea at birth is relatively large; its size ratio to the long axis of the eye in newborns is approximately 1:1.8. In adults, this ratio is 1:2. The infantile cornea is more dome shaped than that of an adult.

The stroma of the uveal tract is poorly pigmented in the newborn. Chromatophores are initially confined primarily to the peripapillary region, which explains why the iris of the newborn is almost always gray-blue. Time is required for development of these pigmented cells, which migrate in from the neural crest (see Fig. 7-4). Although the pigmentation of the middle and anterior aspects of the uvea proceeds rapidly during the first days of life, the development of the definitive iris color may require several weeks.

The stroma of the uveal tract is extremely cellular in the newborn. The ciliary muscle is well developed at birth and shows prominent and numerous cellular nuclei within the muscle parenchyma. This cellularity decreases gradually as an aging process until the ciliary muscle appears relatively "hyalinized" in eyes of elderly persons. For this reason, the

pathologist is often able to histologically examine the ciliary muscle and estimate the approximate age of the patient, at least in an attempt to differentiate the eye of a child from that of a teenager, middle-aged, or older aged person.

The lens of a newborn is more spheric (greater anteroposterior diameter) than that of an adult. For this reason, the anterior chamber is relatively shallow, and the angle is correspondingly narrow. The uveal meshwork retains in large part its fetal character; delicate processes may persist shortly after birth (see Fig. 6-1).

The retina is well developed at birth[1] but shows evidence of fetal character in two locations: the foveal region and the far periphery. In the newborn, the foveal depression is underdeveloped and often poorly visualized histologically. Development of the fovea to its mature configuration (see Fig. 8-8) usually requires 4 or more weeks.[37] In sections of the peripheral retina[57,60] in infants, the retina at the ora serrata often detaches from the pigment epithelium (Fig. 1-12). It forms a circular (Lange's) fold[64] that protrudes in the direction of the vitreous. This fold, or elevation, is a consistent artifact of preparation caused by unequal shrinkage of the retina and adjacent tissues during tissue preparation.

Full myelination of the optic nerve up to the level of the lamina cribrosa may require 1 to several months after birth. Remnants of the trunk of the hyaloid artery and its sheath, Bergmeister's papilla, are often present on the optic nerve head for weeks or months after birth (see Figs. 2-27 and 10-1).

Many physiologic aging changes within the eye actually begin in childhood and gradually develop throughout life. Examples are nuclear sclerosis of the lens and cystoid degeneration of the retina.

Certain other changes usually occur in elderly persons and are not commonly seen before age 50. These include corneal arcus senilis, certain lens opacities, and drusen of Bruch's membrane. When such changes are seen in young individuals, they are sometimes considered pathologic. In elderly persons, they are usually considered physiologic or, when more severe, may likewise induce pathologic changes with visual loss.

Arcus senilis is an opacity confined to the peripheral

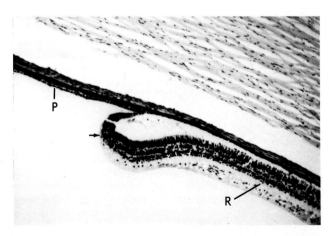

Fig. 1-12. Fetal ora serrata with Lange's fold *(arrow). P,* Pars plana epithelium; *R,* peripheral retina. (H & E stain; ×285.)

reaches of the cornea. A border of clear cornea remains around the lesion adjacent to the limbus.

Pinguecula and pterygia occur in persons exposed to extremes in environmental influences (p. 574). The conjunctival stroma and the superficial corneal and scleral stromal collagen undergo a hyalinization and collagenelastic degeneration. A thickening and yellowing of the subepithelial stroma occurs. Infiltration of lipid, calcium, or both occurs as a secondary phenomenon.

So-called keratinoid degeneration (p. 574; see Fig. 11-19) consists of a deposition of "droplets" within the superficial stromal layers of the conjunctiva or cornea. These droplets are nonspecific degenerative changes caused by environmental influences such as sun, wind, and dust and are generally not responsible for visual difficulties except in rare instances when the visual axis is involved.

Hyperplasia and proliferation of the ciliary epithelium, including Fuchs' adenoma (see Fig. 7-70) and cysts of the pars plana and pars plicata (see Fig. 8-65), occur as benign aging processes.

Lens opacities, including small or peripheral opacities that do not affect vision, and frank cataracts that do lead to decrease in vision are discussed in Chapter 4.

The various basement membranes of the eye show a tendency to thicken with age. This thickening may be diffuse or may occur as local wartlike thickenings or excrescences. The lens capsule typically shows a diffuse thickening. Descemet's membrane normally becomes diffusely thicker in its central portions and characteristically reveals focal excrescences in its peripheral reaches. The latter are termed Hassall-Henle warts (see Fig. 3-4); they represent a physiologic aging process and do not affect vision. Hassall-Henle warts are analogous in structure to the pathologic guttata seen in Fuchs' combined dystrophy (see Fig. 3-49).

Drusen of Bruch's membrane (see Figs. 8-89 and 8-90) occasionally occur as a dominant hereditary process; they more commonly appear as nonspecific degenerative changes. They are small, white-yellow, round lesions that represent secretory and degenerative products of the pigment epithelium and its basement membrane. Angiographically, drusen reveal hyperfluorescence caused by the window defect created by the atrophy of pigment epithelium. As long as the drusen are confined to the periphery of the fundus, there is very little visual loss. Even when involvement of the macula occurs, vision may remain good for long periods. However, age-related disciform macular degeneration (p. 442) and visual loss may ensue.

The retina of almost all people older than 40 years of age reveals a constant gradual decrease in the amount of nervous elements with corresponding replacement by glial tissue.[128] This decrease probably depends on a very slow atrophy and insufficiency of the choriocapillaris and of the retinal capillaries. Chorioretinal adhesions and pigmentary lesions are common aging processes in the retinal periphery and at the ora serrata. The vascular insufficiency is probably largely responsible for the formation of peripheral microcystic degenerative lesions, which occur in all retinas after the teenage years (see Figs. 8-10, 8-67, and 8-68). In flat preparations, these spaces are seen as numerous communicating channels that vary in width and cover a several-millimeter-wide surface posterior to the ora serrata. Histologic sections reveal that the cystic spaces (Blessig-Iwanoff cysts) are localized primarily within the outer plexiform layer, are lined by Müller cells, and contain mucopolysaccharides. In advanced stages, they can affect almost all layers of the retina. Confluent spaces progress toward "senile" retinoschisis.

REFERENCES°

Embryology and anatomy

1. Abramov I and others: The retina of the newborn infant, Science 217:265, 1982.
2. Bach L and Seefelder R: Atlas zur Entwicklungsgeschichte des menschlichen Auges, Leipzig, 1914, Wilhelm Engelmann.
3. Badtke G: Die normale Entwicklung des menschlichen Auges. In Velhagen K, editor: Der Augenarzt, Leipzig, 1958, VEB Thieme.
4. Barber AN: Embryology of the human eye, St Louis, 1955, The CV Mosby Co.
5. Cunha-Vaz J: The blood-ocular barriers, Surv Ophthalmol 23:279, 1979.
6. Cunha-Vaz JG, editor: The blood-retinal barriers, NATO Advanced Study Institutes Series, Series A, Life Sciences, vol 32, New York, 1980, Plenum Press.
7. Drualt A and Drualt S: Eye of the newborn, Ann Oculist 179:375, 1946.
8. Duke-Elder S and Cook C: System of ophthalmology, vol III, Normal and abnormal development, part 1, Embryology, St Louis, 1963, The CV Mosby Co.
9. Duke-Elder S and Wybar KC: System of ophthalmology, vol II, The anatomy of the visual system, St Louis, 1961, The CV Mosby Co.
10. Fine B and Yanoff M: Ocular histology: a text and atlas, New York, 1979, Harper & Row, Publishers.
11. Hogan M, Alvarado J, and Weddell J: Histology of the human eye, Philadelphia, 1971, WB Saunders Co.
12. Isenberg SJ, ed. The Eye in Infancy, ed 2, St Louis, 1994, Mosby-Year Book.
13. Jakus M: Ocular fine structure, Boston, 1964, Little, Brown & Co.
14. Kollmann J: Handatlas der Entwicklungsgeschichte des Menschen, Jena, 1907, Gustay Fischer.
15. Kolmer W and Lauber H: Haut und Sinnesorgane, Band Auge. In Mollendorf W, editor: Handbuch der Mikroskopischen Anatomie des Menschen, Berlin, 1936, Julius Springer.
16. Mann I: The development of the human eye, London, 1969, William Clowes & Sons, Ltd.
17. Ozanics V and Jakobiec FA: Prenatal development of the eye and its adnexa. In Duane TD and Jaeger EA, editors: Biomedical foundations of ophthalmology, vol 1, Philadelphia, 1982, Harper & Row, Publishers.
18. Polyak S: The retina, Chicago, 1941, University of Chicago Press.
19. Polyak S: The vertebrate visual system, Chicago, 1957, University of Chicago Press.
20. Pouliquen Y: Atlas d'histologie et d'ultrastructure du globe oculaire, Paris, 1969, Masson & Cie., Editeurs.
21. Renard G, Masson C, and Saraux II: Anatomie de l'oiel et de ses annexes, Paris, 1965, Masson & Cie., Editeurs.
22. Rohen J: Das Auge und seine Hilfsorgane. In Mollendorf W and Bargmann W, editors: Handbuch der microskopischen Anatomie des Menschen, vol III/4, Berlin, 1964, Springer-Verlag.
23. Rohen J: Anatomie des Auges. In Velhagen K, editor: Der Augenarzt 2 Aufl, vol 1, Leipzig, 1969, VEB Thieme.
24. Rohen J: Funktionelle Anatomie des Nervensystems, Stuttgart, 1971, FK Schattauer Verlag, GmbII.
25. Rohen J: Morphologie und Embryologie des Sehorgens. In Francois J and Hollwich F, editors: Augenheilkunde in Klinik und Praxis, Stuttgart, 1977, Georg Thieme Verlag.

° These references are confined to several major works of ocular embryology, histology, anatomy, pathology, and general ophthalmology. The reader is referred to these large reference works for further direction to individual journal publications. Many of the older listings are classics that are not only of historic interest but remain valid and of interest to today's reader because of their abundant illustrations and thorough discussions of ocular disease.

26. Salzmann M: Anatomie und Histologie des menschlichen Auges, Leipzig, 1912, Franz Deuticke.

27. Salzmann M: The anatomy and histology of the human eyeball in the normal state, Chicago, 1912, University of Chicago Press. (Translated by EVL Brown.)

28. Seefelder R: Entwicklung des menschlichen Auges. In Schieck F and Bruckner A, editors: Kurzes Handbuch der Ophthalmologie, vol 1, Berlin, 1930, Julius Springer.

29. Waitzman MB: Possible new concept relating prostaglandins to various ocular functions, Surv Ophthalmol 14:301, 1970.

30. Wolff E: Anatomy of the eye and orbit, ed 7, Philadelphia, 1976, WB Saunders Co.

31. Zinn K, editor: Ocular fine structure for the clinician, Int Ophthalmol Clin 13(3):1, 1973.

Pathology

32. Albert D and Puliafito C, editors: Foundations of ophthalmic pathology, New York, 1979, Appleton-Century-Crofts.

33. Alt A: Compendium der normalen und pathologischen Histologie des Auges, Wiesbaden, 1880, JF Bergmann.

34. American Academy of Ophthalmology: Ophthalmic Pathology and Intraocular Tumors, Basic and Clinical Science Course, Section 4, 1996/97.

35. Apple DJ: Chromosome-induced ocular disease. In Goldberg MF, editor: Genetic and metabolic eye disease, Boston, 1974, Little, Brown & Co.

36. Apple DJ: Histopathology of xenon-arc and argon laser photocoagulation. In L'Esperance FA Jr, editor: Current diagnosis and management of chorioretinal diseases, St Louis, 1977, The CV Mosby Co.

37. Apple DJ: Anatomy and histology of the macular region, Int Ophthalmol Clin 21(3):1, 1981.

38. Apple DJ: Pathology. In L'Esperance FA Jr and James WA Jr, editors: Diabetic retinopathy: clinical evaluation and management, St Louis, 1981, The CV Mosby Co.

39. Apple DJ: New aspects of coloboma and optic nerve anomalies, Int Ophthalmol Clin 24(1):109, 1984.

40. Apple DJ and Blodi FC: Pathological observations and clinical approach to uveal melanoma. In Nicholson DH, editor: Ocular pathology update, New York, 1980, Masson Publishing USA, Inc.

41. Apple DJ and Blodi FC: Uveal melanocytic tumors: a grouping according to phases of growth and prognosis with comments on current theories of nonenucleation treatment, Int Ophthalmol Clin 20(2): 33, 1980.

42. Apple DJ and Boutros G: Tumors of the eye and adnexa. In Reed J and Wilensky J, editors: Ophthalmology for the general practitioner, Philadelphia, 1984, WB Saunders Co.

43. Apple DJ and Rabb MF: Clinicopathologic correlation of ocular disease: a text and stereoscopic atlas, St Louis, 1974, The CV Mosby Co.

44. Apple DJ and Rabb MF: Clinicopathologic correlation of ocular disease: a text and stereoscopic atlas, ed 2, St Louis, 1978, The CV Mosby Co.

45. Apple DJ and Rabb MF: Ocular pathology. Clinical applications and self-assessment, ed 3, St Louis, 1985, The CV Mosby Co.

46. Apple DJ and Rabb MF: Ocular pathology. Clinical applications and self-assessment, ed 4, St Louis, 1991, Mosby Year Book.

47. Apple DJ, Rabb MF, and Walsh PM: Congenital anomalies of the optic disc, Surv Ophthalmol 27:3, 1982.

48. Apple DJ and others: Intraocular lenses. Evolution, designs, complications, and pathology, Baltimore, 1989, Williams & Wilkins.

49. Armed Forces Institute of Pathology: Laboratory Methods in Histotechnology, Washington DC, 1992, American Registry of Pathology.

50. Barsky D: Color atlas of pathology of the eye, New York, 1966, McGraw-Hill Book Co.

51. Battifora H and Kopinski M: The influence of protease digestion and duration of fixation on the immunostaining of keratins: a comparison of formalin and ethanol fixation, J Histochem Cytochem 34: 1095, 1986.

52. Bornfeld N and others: Tumors of the eye, New York, 1991, Kugler Publications.

53. Cogan D and Kuwabara T: Some common artifacts in the retina, J Histochem Cytochem 6:290, 1958.

54. Cohen IK and others: Wound healing: biochemical & clinical aspects, New York, 1994, Marcel Dekker, Inc.

55. Collins ET and Mayou MS: Pathology and bacteriology of the eye, ed 2, Philadelphia, 1925, P Blakiston's Son & Co.

56. Corwin DJ and Gown M: Review of selected lineage-directed antibodies useful in routinely processed tissues, Arch Pathol Lab Med 113:645, 1989.

57. Daicker B: Anatomie und Pathologie der menschlichen retinoziliaren Fundusperipherie, Basel, 1972, S Karger, AG.

58. Deegan MJ: Membrane antigen analysis in the diagnosis of lymphoid leukemias and lymphomas: differential diagnosis, prognosis as related to immunophenotype, and recommendations for testing, Arch Pathol Lab Med 113:606, 1989.

59. DeLellis RA: Advances in immunohistochemistry, New York, 1988, Raven Press.

60. Eisner G: Biomicroscopy of the peripheral fundus, New York, 1973, Springer Publishing Co, Inc.

61. Friedenwald JS and others: Ophthalmic pathology: an atlas and textbook, Philadelphia, 1952, WB Saunders Co.

62. Garner A and Klintworth GK: Pathobiology of ocular disease: a dynamic process, New York, 1982, Marcel Dekker, Inc.

63. Garner A and Klintworth GK, editors: Pathobiology of ocular disease: a dynamic approach, ed 2, New York, 1994, Marcel Dekker, Inc.

64. Gartner S and Henkind P: Lange's folds: a meaningful ocular artifact, Ophthalmology 88:1307, 1981.

65. Gieser SC, Apple DJ, and Carey JC: Pathology of chromosome-induced ocular disease. In Goldberg MF and Renie W, editors: Genetic and metabolic eye disease, ed 2, Boston, 1985, Little, Brown & Co.

66. Greer C: Ocular pathology, Oxford, 1963, Blackwell Scientific Publications, Ltd.

67. Greer C: Ocular pathology, ed 3, Oxford, 1979, Blackwell Scientific Publications, Ltd.

68. Henderson DW, Papadimitriou JM, and Coleman M: Ultrastructural appearances of tumours, ed 2, Edinburgh, 1986, Churchill Livingstone, Inc.

69. Henke F and Lubarsch O, editors: Handbuch der Speziellen Pathologischen Anatomie und Histologie, vols I to III, Berlin, 1928, Julius Springer.

70. Hogan M and Zimmerman LE: Ophthalmic pathology, ed 2, Philadelphia, 1962, WB Saunders Co.

71. Iris L: Histopathologie oculaire, Paris, 1972, Masson & Cie., Editeurs.

72. Kincaid MC, Grossniklaus HE: Immunohistochemical staining in ophthalmic pathology, Ophthalmol Clin N Am 8:17, 1995.

73. Klintworth G and Launders M III: The eye: structure and function in disease, Baltimore, 1976, The Williams & Wilkins Co.

74. Mackay B and Osborne BM: The contribution of electron microscopy to the diagnosis of tumors, Pathobiol Ann 8:359, 1978.

75. Margo CE, Grossniklaus HE: Ocular histopathology: a guide to differential diagnosis, Philadelphia, 1991, WB Saunders Co.

76. McLean IW and others: Tumors of the eye and ocular adnexa, Washington, DC: Armed Forces Institute of Pathology, 1994.

77. Medeiros LJ and Harris NL: Lymphoid infiltrates of the orbit and conjunctiva: a morphologic and immunophenotypic study of 99 cases, Am J Surg Pathol 13:459, 1989.

78. Mierau GW and Favara BE: Rhabdomyosarcoma in children: ultrastructural study of 31 cases, Cancer 46:2035, 1980.

79. Nadji M and Morales MR: Immunoperoxidase techniques: a practical approach to tumor diagnosis, Chicago, 1986, American Society of Clinical Pathologists Press.

80. Naumann GOH and Apple DJ: Pathologie des Auges. In Doerr W, Seifert G, and Uehlinger L, editors: Handbuch der speziellen pathologischen Anatomie, Band Auge, Berlin, 1980, Springer-Verlag.

81. Naumann GOH and Apple DJ: Pathology of the eye, New York, 1985, Springer-Verlag, Inc. (Translation, modification, and update of *Pathologie des Auges* by DJ Apple.)

82. Ni C and others: Rapid paraffin fixation for use in histologic examinations, Ophthalmology 88:1372, 1981.

83. Nicholson DH, editor: Ocular pathology update, New York, 1980, Masson Publishing USA, Inc.

84. Offret G and others: Anatomie pathologique de l'oeil et de ses annexes, Paris, 1974, Masson & Cie., Editeurs.

85. Parsons J: The pathology of the eye, vols 1 to 4, New York, 1904, GP Putnam's Sons.

86. Perentes E and Rubinstein LJ: Recent applications of immunoperoxidase histochemistry in neuro-oncology: an update, Arch Pathol Lab Med 111:115, 1987.
87. Radnot M: Pathologie des Auges, Budapest, 1951, Hungarian Academy of Sciences.
88. Rahi A and Garner A: Immunopathology of the eye, Philadelphia, 1976, JB Lippincott Co.
89. Samuels B and Fuchs A: Clinical pathology of the eye, New York, 1952, Paul B Hoeber, Inc, Medical Book Department of Harper & Brothers.
90. Sandborn GE and others: Atlas of intraocular tumors, Philadelphia, 1994, WB Saunders Co.
91. Shields JA: Diagnosis and management of intraocular tumors, St Louis, 1983, The CV Mosby Co.
92. Shields JA and Shields CL: Intraocular tumors: a text and atlas, Philadelphia, 1992, WB Saunders Co.
93. Smith M, editor: Ocular pathology, Int Ophthalmol Clin 2(3):1, 1971.
94. Sobel HJ and others: Tumors and tumor-like conditions of soft tissues, bones, and joints, New York, 1981, McGraw-Hill.
95. Sommers I: Histology and histopathology of the eye, New York, 1949, Grune & Stratton.
96. Spencer WH, editor: Ophthalmic pathology: an atlas and textbook, ed 3, vol 2, Philadelphia, 1985, WB Saunders Co.
97. Stock W: Pathologische Anatomie des Auges, Stuttgart, 1939, Ferdinand Enke Verlag.
98. Torezynski E: Preparation of ocular specimens for histopathologic examination, Ophthalmology 88:1367, 1981.
99. Trojanowski JQ, Lee VM-Y, and Schlaepfer WW: An immunohistochemical study of human central and peripheral nervous system tumors, using monoclonal antibodies against neurofilaments and glial filaments, Hum Pathol 15:248, 1984.
100. Wolff E: A pathology of the eye, ed 2, London, 1944, HK Lewis.
101. Yanoff M and Fine BS: Ocular pathology: a text and atlas, Philadelphia, 1975, Harper & Row, Publishers.
102. Yanoff M and Fine BS: Ocular pathology: a text and atlas, ed 2, Philadelphia, 1982, Harper & Row, Publishers.
103. Yanoff M and Fine M: Ocular pathology, ed 4, Barcelona, 1996, Mosby-Wolfe.
104. Zimmerman LE and Fine BS: Myelin artifacts in the optic disc and retina, Arch Ophthalmol 74:394, 1965.
105. Zimmerman LE and Sobin LH: International histological classification of tumours, No 24, Histological typing of tumours of the eye and its adnexa, Geneva, 1980, World Health Organization.
106. Zollinger H and Mihatsch MJ, editors: Light, electron immunofluorescent microscopy, pathology and biopsy, Berlin, 1978, Springer-Verlag.

General references

107. Albert DM and Jakobiec FA, editors: Principles and practice of ophthalmology, Philadelphia, 1994, WB Saunders Co.
108. Allansmith MR: The eye and immunology, St Louis, 1982, The CV Mosby Co.
109. Apple DJ: Chromosome-induced ocular disease. In Goldberg MF, editor: Genetic and metabolic eye disease, Boston, 1974, Little, Brown & Co.
110. Apple DJ and Hamming NA: Embryology and anatomy of the eye. In Peyman GA, Sanders DR, and Goldberg MF, editors: Principles and practice of ophthalmology, Philadelphia, 1980, WB Saunders Co.
111. Axenfeld T: Lehrbuch und Atlas der Augenheilkunde, Jena, 1912, Gustav Fischer.
112. Blodi FC, editor: Current concepts in ophthalmology, vol 4, St Louis, 1974, The CV Mosby Co.
113. Duane T, editor: Clinical ophthalmology, ed 5, New York, 1981, Harper & Row, Publishers.
114. Duane T and Jaeger E, editors: Biomedical foundations of ophthalmology, New York, 1982, Harper & Row, Publishers.
115. Duke-Elder S, editor: System of ophthalmology, vols I to XV, St Louis, 1958 to 1971, The CV Mosby Co.
116. Ferry AP, editor: Ocular and adnexal tumors, Int Ophthalmol Clin 12(1):1, 1972.
117. François J and Hollwich F, editors: Augenheilkunde in Klinik und Praxis, Stuttgart, 1977, Georg Thieme Verlag.
118. Fuchs E: Lehrbuch der Augenheilkunde, Vienna, 1889, Franz Deuticke.
119. Gass JDM: Differential diagnosis of intraocular tumors: a stereoscopic presentation, St Louis, 1974, The CV Mosby Co.
120. Geeraets W: Ocular syndromes, ed 3, Philadelphia, 1976, Lea & Febiger.
121. Gieser SC, Apple DJ, and Carey JC: Pathology of chromosome-induced ocular disease. In Goldberg MF and Renie W, editors: Genetic and metabolic eye disease, ed 2, Boston, 1985, Little, Brown & Co.
122. Harley R, editor: Pediatric ophthalmology, Philadelphia, 1975, WB Saunders Co.
123. Hollwich F: Ophthalmology: a short textbook, Chicago, 1979, Year Book Medical Publishers, Inc.
124. Hollwich F: Pocket atlas of ophthalmology, Chicago, 1981, Year Book Medical Publishers, Inc. (Translated by FC Blodi.)
125. Jakobiec F: Ocular and adnexal tumors, New York, 1978, Aesculapius Publishers, Inc.
126. Larsen H: The ocular fundus: a color atlas, Philadelphia, 1976, WB Saunders Co.
127. Leydhecker W: Grundriss der Augenheilkunde, ed 19, Berlin, 1976, Springer-Verlag.
128. Marshall J and others: Convolution in human rods: an aging process, Br J Ophthalmol 63:181, 1979.
129. Mausolf F, editor: The eye and systemic disease, St Louis, 1975, The CV Mosby Co.
130. Meyner E: Atlas der Spaltlampenphotographie, Stuttgart, 1976, Ferdinand Enke Verlag.
131. Nema II: Ophthalmic syndromes, Ontario, 1973, Butterworth & Co (Canada), Ltd.
132. Newell FW: Ophthalmology: principles and concepts, ed 4, St Louis, 1979, The CV Mosby Co.
133. Newell FW: Ophthalmology: principles and concepts, ed 5, St Louis, 1982, The CV Mosby Co.
134. Newell FW and Ernest JT: Ophthalmology: principles and concepts, ed 3, St Louis, 1974, The CV Mosby Co.
135. Oeller J: Atlas seltener ophthalmoskopischer Befunde, Wiesbaden, 1903, JF Bergmann.
136. Offret G and Haye C: Tumeurs de l'oeil et des annexes oculaires, Paris, 1971, Masson & Cie., Editeurs.
137. Pau H, editor: Axenfeld's Lehrbuch und Atlas der Augenheilkunde, Stuttgart, 1973, Gustav Fischer Verlag.
138. Pau H: Differential diagnose der Augenkrankheiten, Stuttgart, 1974, Georg Thieme Verlag.
139. Pau H: Differential diagnosis of eye diseases, Philadelphia, 1978, WB Saunders Co. (Translated by G Cibis.)
140. Peyman GA, Apple DJ, and Sanders DR, editors: Intraocular tumors, New York, 1977, Appleton-Century-Crofts.
141. Peyman GA, Sanders DR, and Goldberg MF, editors: Principles and practice of ophthalmology, Philadelphia, 1980, WB Saunders Co.
142. Reese AB: Tumors of the eye, ed 3, New York, 1976, Harper & Row, Publishers.
143. Roy F: Ocular differential diagnosis, Philadelphia, 1975, Lea & Febiger.
144. Ryan S and Smith R, editors: The eye in systemic disease, New York, 1974, Grune & Stratton, Inc.
145. Ryan SJ: Retina, ed 2, vols 1 to 3, St Louis, 1994, Mosby-Year Book, Inc.
146. Schatz H and others: Interpretation of fundus fluorescein angiography, St Louis, 1978, The CV Mosby Co.
147. Scheie HG and Albert DM: Adler's textbook of ophthalmology, ed 8, Philadelphia, 1969, WB Saunders Co.
148. Scheie HG and Albert DM: Textbook of ophthalmology, ed 9, Philadelphia, 1977, WB Saunders Co.
149. Schwartz B and Ericson E, editors: Ophthalmic reviews, vol IV, 1982, Boston, Survey of Ophthalmology, Inc.
150. Spalton DJ and others: Atlas of clinical ophthalmology, ed 2, London, 1994, Mosby-Year Book Europe Limited.
151. Thiel R: Atlas of diseases of the eye, vols 1 and 2, Amsterdam, 1963, Elsevier Publishing Co. (Translated by D Guerry, W Geeraets, and H. Wiesinger.)
152. Vaughn D and Asbury T: General ophthalmology, ed 8, Los Altos, 1977, Lange Medical Publications.

DEVELOPMENTAL ANOMALIES

Introduction

In this chapter we describe a group of congenital and developmental eye lesions that are characterized by distinct structural changes.[1-44] Although oversimplified, it is useful to classify these lesions as shown in Fig. 2-1, which correlates the normal development of the eye in the various stages of gestation with the age of the embryo of fetus and with the anomaly that originates at the various stages. For example, specific noxious influences, such as x-rays, chromosome defects,[17-20,24,31,40] alcohol,[8,10,15,37,38] or teratogenic drugs,* may be introduced and cause anomalies at specific times in development. We will discuss the anomalies according to the scheme outlined in Fig. 2-1. This chapter considers general maldevelopments of the globe as a whole; anomalies of the various individual tissue components of the eye are described in other chapters.

The anterolateral outpouching, or evagination, of the primitive brainstem to form the optic vesicle is one of the earliest events in the differentiation of the embryonic neural tube, occurring during the first weeks of gestation (Tables 2-1 and 2-2). Any significant abnormality in this evagination process produces a severe ocular malformation. Four anomalies associated with defective embryogenesis at this stage are anophthalmia, cyclopia (synophthalmia), congenital cystic eye, and congenital nonattachment of the retina.

Anophthalmia

Anophthalmia (Figs. 2-2 and 2-3)[36,45,48-52,56,58] is either primary, in which no evagination from the forebrain occurs and no ocular anlage forms, or degenerative (consecutive), in which an optic vesicle forms but does not develop or regresses because of various kinds of disruption. Rudiments of an eye (e.g., retina, ciliary epithelium, or pigment

Table 2-1. Correlation of gestational age with fetal length

Gestational age (mo.)	Crown-rump length (mm)
1	0–8
2	10–30
3	31–70
4	71–110
5	111–150
6	151–190
7	191–240
8	241–280
9	280–320

* References 1, 2, 5, 9, 29, 30, 68, 69.

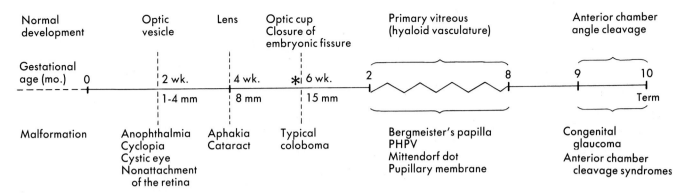

Fig. 2-1. Correlation of selected congenital diseases with gestational age.

Table 2-2. Correlation of congenital disease with gestational age

Crown-rump length (mm)	Gestational age	Normal development	Malformation or disease
2–4	0–2 weeks	Optic vesicle forms	Anopthalmia; cyclopia
4–8	2–4 weeks	Optic cup forms; lens vesicle forms	Congenital cystic eye; congenital nonattachment of the retina; congenital aphakia
8–15	4–6 weeks	Fissure closes	Typical coloboma
10–320	5 weeks to term	Primary vitreous develops	PHPV
320	9–10 months	Cleavage of anterior chamber angle structures	Congenital glaucoma; anterior chamber cleavage syndromes

PHPV, persistent hyperplastic primary vitreous.

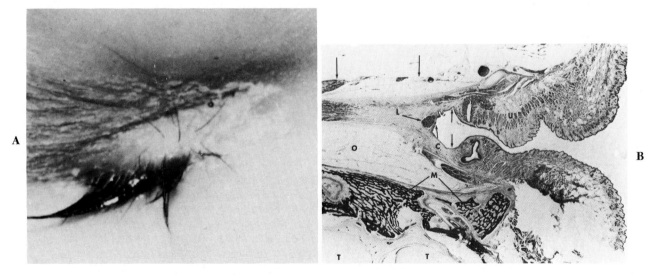

Fig. 2-2. A, Clinical anophthalmia showing a shrunken socket and fused, hypoplastic eyelids. **B,** Primary anophthalmia. Serial sections, such as this one through the orbit of a stillborn infant, revealed no traces of embryonic optic vesicle derivatives. This sagittal section reveals a cluster of ectopic lacrimal gland acini (*L*) at the place where the globe should be situated. *C,* Undeveloped corneal epithelium; *U,* upper lid; *small arrows,* conjunctival fornices; *large arrows,* roof of the orbit; *O,* orbital fat; *M,* maxillary bones forming floor of orbit; *T,* maxillary teeth. (H & E stain; ×15.)

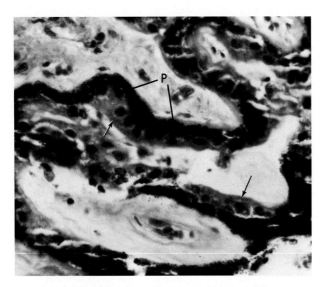

Fig. 2-3. Secondary anophthalmia. The eye socket from a 60-year-old man with "congenital anophthalmia" contains convoluted rudiments of primitive ocular neuroepithelium that resembles ciliary epithelium. *P,* Pigment epithelium; *arrows,* nonpigmented layer. (H & E stain; ×400.)

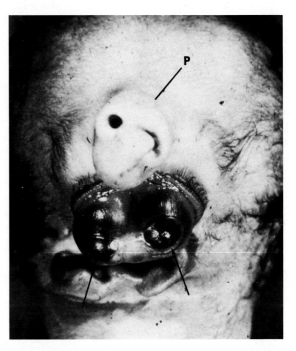

Fig. 2-4. Photograph taken at necropsy, demonstrating a case of "cyclopia"—in actuality, a synophthalmia in which the eyes (*arrows*) are fused medially. The sclera is extremely rudimentary, and the anteriorly protruding globes appear deeply pigmented because of exposed uveal and pigment epithelial layers. *P,* Midline proboscis above the orbit.

epithelium) may be present in the latter type, indicating the presence of a previously formed optic vesicle (Fig. 2-3).[56] Diagnosis of primary anophthalmia requires serial histologic sectioning of orbital tissue obtained by biopsy or during autopsy. In the absence of histopathologic verification, one always should consider the condition to be a clinical anophthalmia or an extreme microphthalmia (Fig. 2-2, *A*).

Bilateral cases comprise 75% of cases of primary anophthalmia and generally are unassociated with a positive family history or other systemic defects. Typically, the lids are partially fused, but lid structures are otherwise present. The lacrimal gland is present but often is larger than normal because of an uninhibited overgrowth (Fig. 2-2, *B*).

The nonectodermal contents of the globe—choroid, sclera, and orbital tissues such as the extraocular muscles—are present but are disorganized and hypoplastic. Often cartilaginous metaplasia of the orbital mesoderm occurs. The central pathways generally are absent or hypoplastic.

Obviously, no appropriate treatment is available for the condition other than introduction of serial orbital implants to enhance normal orbital growth for cosmetic purposes.

In cryptophthalmos,[36,50] although an eye may show all ranges of size, from normal to apparent anophthalmia, most affected globes are maldeveloped and microphthalmic. This condition should be considered in the differential diagnosis of anophthalmia or extreme microphthalmia. The characteristic clinical findings consist of a complete absence of the lids (ablepharon), the cilia, and the palpebral fissure. A smooth skin without normal appendages covers the orbit and merges with the surrounding skin of the cheeks and forehead. Most cases are bilateral.

Cyclopia (synophthalmia)

The region of the apical or rostral forebrain contains the olfactory and ocular primordia. The malformations caused by maldevelopment of this region form a spectrum of conditions including cyclopia (synophthalmia),[46,47,53-55,57,59-61] ethmocephaly, cebocephaly, and arrhinencephaly. These severe forebrain lesions often are accompanied by severe systemic malformations, and affected infants rarely survive.

Cyclopia is characterized by anomalous development of the ocular primordia during the first month. Most instances involve a fusion of the two optic vesicles, or synophthalmia (Figs. 2-4 and 2-5). True cyclopia with a solitary optic anlage is extremely rare.

Neither true cyclopia nor synophthalmia is compatible with life because an anomalous development of the brain is involved. Typically the division of the telencephalon in the two hemispheres fails, often leaving a median dorsal cyst lined by ependyma. In cases of synophthalmia, the eyes may exhibit varying degrees of fusion (Fig. 2-5); this may involve merely the optic nerves or a portion of the medial sclera, or more extensive portions of the globes. In addition to the ectodermal aberrations affecting the brain and eyes, there is abnormal development of the mesodermal structures of the face, leading to creation of the proboscis above the medial eye or eyes (Fig. 2-4).

Ethmocephaly is a similar condition in which the eyes are separated more widely than in synophthalmia. The proboscis often is present, and the eyes may show equally severe malformations. Cebocephaly, in contrast, is an exaggerated separation of the eyes with a maldeveloped nose in between. The eyes themselves also are severely malformed, and a true or incomplete anophthalmia may occur.

The common denominator of the various types of arrhinencephaly is a defect in the olfactory apparatus of the

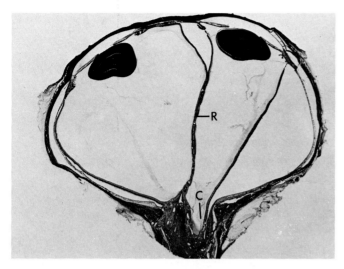

Fig. 2-5. Synophthalmia. The medial sclera-choroid is absent. The eyes share a common medial retina *(R)*. *C*, Colobomatous defect of the optic nerve. (H & E stain; ×12.)

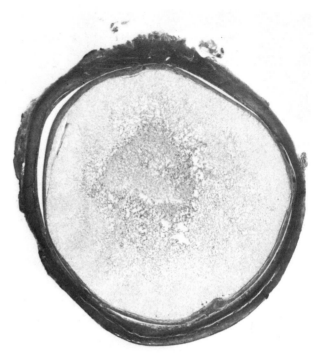

Fig. 2-6. Congenital orbital cyst filled with serous fluid, lined by undifferentiated neuroepithelium and sclera. (H & E stain; ×20.)

telencephalon, often with absence of the olfactory nerve. Infants with arrhinencephaly characteristically have cleft lip and palate, heart defects, polydactyly, spina bifida, and maldevelopment of the lung and adrenal glands. Arrhinencephaly commonly is seen in the trisomy 13 syndrome (p. 45). Furthermore, recent studies have shown that most patients with cyclopia have abnormal chromosome patterns, usually a trisomy 13 (55% of cases).[371]

Congenital cystic eye and congenital nonattachment of the retina

During the period of transformation of the optic vesicle into the optic cup, the growth of the eye can be misdirected, leading to congenital cystic eye or congenital nonattachment of the retina (Fig. 2-1).[56] The cause is not clear, and such anomalies are extremely rare.

A partial or complete failure of invagination of the primary optic vesicle leads to a congenital cystic eye or congenital orbital cyst (Fig. 2-6). The primary optic vesicle develops, but the anterior part of the vesicle (the future sensory retina) remains separated from the pigment epithelium. The cavity of the optic vesicle persists between these layers, and a cyst remains. These primary congenital cystic eyes must be differentiated pathogenically from colobomatous cysts that form secondarily to colobomatous defects (p.00; see Fig. 2-15).

When the secondary invagination of the optic vesicle occurs in an incomplete form in which the two anterior and posterior layers approach each other but do not come into contact, the subretinal space persists and produces a congenital nonattachment of the retina. Most such eyes are extremely microphthalmic or may produce a clinical anophthalmia. Because these also occur early in gestation, other intraocular anomalies, such as persistent hyperplastic primary vitreous (PHPV) or colobomas, often occur concurrently.

Typical colobomas

After development of the embryonic optic vesicle, development of the eye proceeds by a secondary invagination

of the anterior wall of the vesicle, forming the optic cup and the embryonic ocular fissure (see Figs. 1-7 to 1-10 and 2-7).[62] The fissure is a transient cleft along the ventral aspect of the cup and in effect functions to create a defect, or notch, in the inferior wall. This defect provides an entrance and exit for the transient embryonic blood vessels and creates a temporary slit in the optic stalk through which the retinal nerve fibers pass from the ganglion cell layer of the retina into the brain.

Fusion of the lips of the embryonic ocular fissure, critically important in the normal development of the eye, leads to closure of the cleft and formation of an intact, complete globe. This event normally occurs at the 15-mm stage, corresponding to approximately 6 weeks' gestation (Fig. 2-1). This is a critical point in the development of the eye and body as a whole because the primordia of most body tissues are formed by this time and the basic structure of all organs is essentially defined.

Defective closure of the embryonic ocular fissure produces the typical coloboma[62-94] (Gr. *koloboma*, mutilation). The choice of this term underscores the fact that investigators for years had observed significantly deformed eyes in which the pathogenesis of the deformities remained undefined. Only after the definitive studies of von Szily[90,91] was it clear that defective closure of the fissure was the underlying basis for the numerous abnormalities.

Most typical colobomas arise sporadically. Occasionally, they may be transmitted as an irregular dominant trait with incomplete penetrance; other genetic transmissions also are known. They usually are isolated and commonly are not involved in systemic disease. Exceptions are notable; trisomy 13 syndrome, thalidomide embryopathy syn-

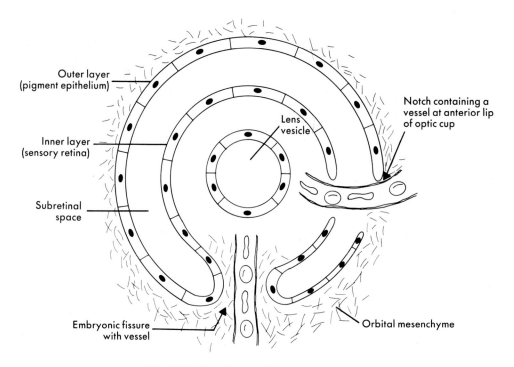

Fig. 2-7. Frontal view of the embryonic cup.

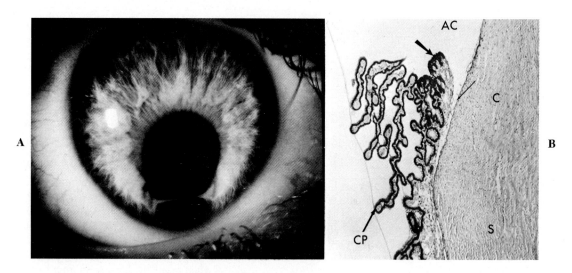

Fig. 2-8. A, Typical iris coloboma with a small bridge of tissue. **B,** Coloboma of the iris with almost complete absence of the iris leaf *(large arrow)*. The only iris tissue present is a short portion of the root. The histopathologic pattern of this type of localized iris coloboma is similar to that seen in microsections of aniridia (Fig. 2-21, *B*). *C,* Cornea; *S,* sclera; *AC,* anterior chamber; *CP,* ciliary processes; *small arrow,* incompletely developed anterior chamber angle. (H & E stain; ×100.) (**A** from Meyner E: Atlas der Spaltlampenphotographie, Stuttgart, 1976, Ferdinand Enke Verlag.)

drome,[29,30,68] and lysergic acid diethylamide (LSD) embryopathy.[2,5,9,64,65,69]

Because the embryonic fissure normally courses along the inferonasal aspect of the eye, the typical colobomatous defect occupies the same position.

IRIS AND CILIARY BODY COLOBOMAS

The coloboma defect may involve the iris, creating the so-called keyhole pupil (Fig. 2-8 and Color Plate 2-1). Colobomas of the ciliary body are much less common than those of the iris and are more difficult to see clinically. They are best visualized by scleral depression, indirect ophthalmoscopy, gonioscopy, or transillumination. Coloboma of the ciliary body is one of the most important malformations in the trisomy 13 syndrome (pp. 45-48). Typical colobomas of the lens (Color Plate 2-2) usually are caused by defective zonule development at the site of a ciliary body coloboma, leading to notching of the lens.

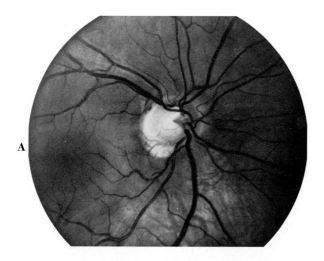

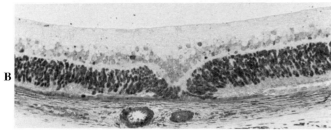

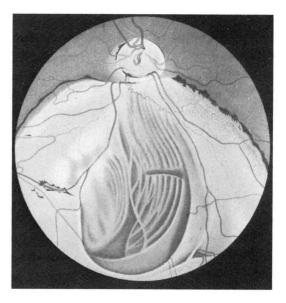

Fig. 2-10. Drawing of a typical coloboma of the fundus showing marked involvement of the inferior retina. (From Oeller J: Atlas seltener ophthalmoskopischer Befunde, Wiesbaden, 1903, JF Bergmann.)

Fig. 2-9. A, Very small inferior nasal coloboma just below the optic disc (coloboma spurium, or Fuchs' coloboma).[97] **B,** Photomicrograph through the retina at the site of the embryonic fissure showing a microscopic focus of irregularity of the retinal layers at the site of malclosure of the embryonic fissure. (Mallory blue stain; ×150.)

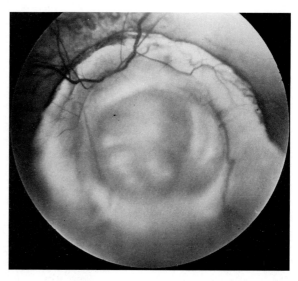

Fig. 2-11. Massive coloboma involving the optic disc (*upper left*) and a major portion of the inferior fundus. The white color of the involved area is caused primarily by maldevelopment of the pigment epithelium and choroid. This facilitates visualization of the white sclera. Abnormal retinal tissue and retinal vessels are present. There is no visual function in the field of the defect.

FUNDUS COLOBOMAS

Fundus colobomas (Color Plate 2-3) range in size from a minimal focus or conus just below the disc (coloboma spurium, or Fuchs' coloboma[122]; Fig. 2-9) to an extension over the entire length of the embryonic ocular fissure, including ciliary body and iris (Figs. 2-10 and 2-11). The observation that colobomas involving the most posterior aspect of the optic cup (the disc and peripapillary retina) (Color Plate 2-4) or the most anterior reach of the cup (the iris) are more common than those of the intermediate areas of the ciliary body and midfundus can be explained by the fact that fissure closure during normal embryogenesis begins in the midzone and later extends posteriorly and anteriorly. The peripheral segments of the fissure normally remain open for a longer time and therefore are more susceptible to teratogenic insults.

A bridge coloboma (Color Plate 2-5) spares intervening areas of retina. The margins of a fundus coloboma in most cases are sharply demarcated, and the region of the coloboma itself typically is white because of baring of the sclera.

Thus, hypoplastic retinal tissue overlies the area of absent pigment epithelium and choroid. Retinal holes and retinal detachments, which may be difficult to repair and often require extensive vitreous surgery, have been estimated to be associated with fundus colobomas in as many as 40% of cases.[78,84]

OPTIC NERVE COLOBOMAS, ECTATIC COLOBOMAS, AND COLOBOMATOUS CYSTS

Congenital anomalies of the optic disc have been considered in detail with an extensive review of the literature by Apple, Rabb, and Walsh.[3]

Optic disc colobomas (Figs. 2-11 to 2-14, Color Plate 2-6) are not rare.[3,7] The Fuchs' coloboma[122] often has been described as a forme fruste or partial coloboma involving the inferior aspect of the optic nerve head (Fig. 2-9, *A*).

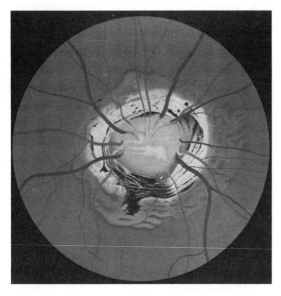

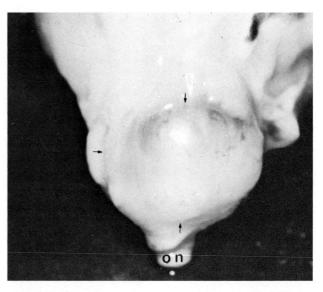

Fig. 2-12. Historical photograph of a colobomatous defect of the optic nerve, which we now term the *morning glory syndrome.* There is deep excavation of the optic nerve head with abnormal peripapillary tissue showing gliosis and foci of pigmentation. (From Oeller J: Atlas seltener ophthalmoskopischer Befunde, Wiesbaden, 1903, JF Bergmann.)

Fig. 2-13. Posterior external view of the inferior aspect of a globe with an ectatic optic nerve coloboma (morning glory syndrome). The cyst *(arrows)* is confined to the inferior aspects of the optic nerve *(ON)* along the line of the embryonic fissure. It is lined by a hypoplastic, poorly differentiated neuroglial membrane derived from the optic cup. (Courtesy Dr. Samuel Vainisi.)

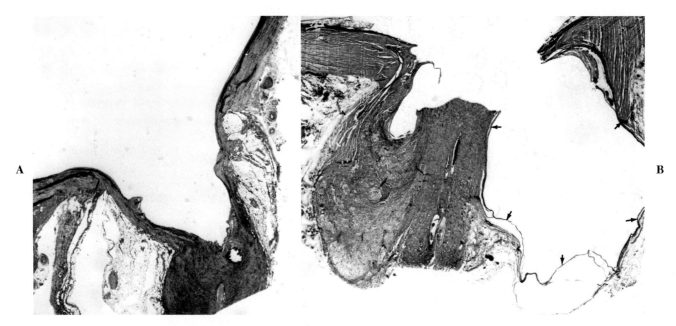

Fig. 2-14. A, Optic nerve coloboma with mild ectasia (H & E stain; ×100.) **B,** Optic nerve coloboma with severe ectasia and cyst formation *(arrows).* (H & E stain; ×125.)

In most cases, the coloboma is associated with an inferior conus or crescent. Most of these eyes are otherwise normal, and resultant visual problems are rare.

The inferior crescent or conus may vary in size depending on the absence of the pigment epithelium and choroid at the inferior edge of the disc. A larger inferior conus may be accompanied by a staphylomatous posterior bowing of the fundus inferior to the defect. Such cases actually represent a part of the spectrum of the congenital tilted disc syndrome (p. 00).

Areas of pigment clumping often appear at the border of the junction of normal fundus and the colobomatous defect (Fig. 2-12; Color Plate 2-6). When significant areas of retinal tissue are involved in the colobomatous defect, holes and tears can form at the border of the defect, which may lead to retinal detachment.

The retinal vessels may course around the coloboma, but in many cases pass directly over the defect and appear in sharp contrast to the white background. The "superior rim syndrome" is the configuration of an intact superior optic disc rim with extensive colobomatous involvement of the temporal, inferior, and nasal rims. The vessels emerge from the center of the disc and extend up and over the superior rim, while vessels coursing inferiorly pass directly downward, resulting in a north-south axis of the retinal vessels. The "situs inversus" of the congenital tilted disc syndrome (p. 22) is considered to be an intermediate retinal vessel configuration between that of the "superior rim syndrome" (vertical or north-south axis) and that of the normal optic disc (horizontal or nasal-temporal axis). Anomalous vessels also are especially prominent in the so-called morning glory syndrome (Fig. 2-12; Color Plates 2-6 and 2-7).

In fundus or optic nerve colobomas in which scleral thinning and staphyloma formation have occurred in the region of the defect (Figs. 2-12 to 2-14), the posterior bulging can be severe, up to 10 diopters (D) or greater. Such an "ectatic" fundus coloboma can be considered a mild or early form of colobomatous cyst (Color Plate 2-6). The cyst is caused by a protrusion, or herniation, or retinoglial tissue through the colobomatous defect into the orbit. Such colobomatous cysts may enlarge tremendously, occasionally replacing the eye within the orbit (Fig. 2-15).

In general, there are three types of congenital orbital cysts: (1) colobomatous cysts, (2) cysts caused by a primary failure of growth of the optic vesicle, and (3) cysts that are enrelated to the eye. Most of the third type are inclusion cysts derived from the epithelium of respiratory or sinus mucosa, including mucoceles.

Because the development of the neuroectodermal tissue along the lines of the fissure is faulty, aberrant induction of adjacent structures often results in multiple secondary intraocular changes within many colobomatous eyes. Such changes include dysplasia and rosette formation in the involved peripapillary retina or aberrant differentiation of the adjacent choroid, often leading to formation of ectopic tissue, for example, cartilage, bone, muscle, or fat.[3,62,63,66,72,74,94] Intraocular adipose tissue is seen not only in association with colobomatous defects of the fundus and optic nerve but also sometimes in phthisis bulbi, where it is localized within spaces like bone marrow. It also is occasionally

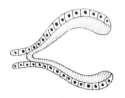

1. Normal

Failure to invaginate to form optic cup

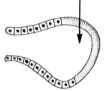

2. Congenital cystic eye

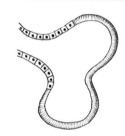

3. Colobomatous cyst

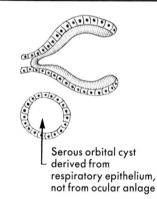

Serous orbital cyst derived from respiratory epithelium, not from ocular anlage

4. Serous orbital cyst

Fig. 2-15. Pathogenesis of retinal-orbital cysts.

seen in PHPV, where the term *pseudophakia lipomatosa* has been applied (p. 32; see Fig. 2-33).

Clinical symptoms in cases of fundus and optic nerve colobomas depend primarily on the extent of the lesion and whether other intraocular findings are present. When the macula is not involved, one may simply find a scotoma confined to the site of the defect. Sometimes the visual field defect resulting from a coloboma mimics that of intracranial disease (p. 23). When other abnormalities such as microphthalmia and persistence of the embryonic vessels are present, or when the colobomatous defect is broad in its extent, vision may decrease sharply.

Aicardi syndrome, characterized by infantile spasms, agenesis of the corpus callosum, severe mental retardation, and X-linked inheritance pattern, often reveals a clinical microphthalmia and colobomatous defect. Hypoplasia of the optic nerves, coloboma of the juxtapapillary choroid and optic disc, neural retinal detachment, retinal dysplasia, chorioretinal lacunae with focal thinning, and atrophy of the retinal pigment epithelium and choroid have been found.[73,75,81,93]

MORNING GLORY SYNDROME[95-115]

Although the characteristic fundus picture (Figs. 2-12 to 2-14; Color Plate 2-7) has long been recognized,[3,105,112,113] the term *morning glory syndrome*, which designates a specific type of optic nerve anomaly, was first used by Kindler[108] in 1970. This condition is characterized by an excavation of the optic nerve associated with characteristic retinal vascular anomalies, glial proliferation, and metaplasia, and peripapillary pigmentary changes. Apple and co-workers[3,62,63] have observed that it seems reasonable to speculate that this condition might be created when the most superior aspect of the embryonic fissure fails to close (analogous to a focal defect in closure of a zipper), allowing posterior prolapse of the tissues at the disc and peripapillary region into the colobomatous defect.

In the morning glory syndrome, the disc is displaced posteriorly within the depths of a funnel-shaped staphylomatous excavation involving the nerve proper and the peripapillary retina. The surrounding area usually is elevated, and there often is a surrounding elevated annulus of chorioretinal pigmentary clumping. The vessels usually show anomalous patterns and may branch, loop, or form arcade patterns. The demarcation of the elevated peripapillary tissue and normal retina is indistinct. The peripheral retina usually is normal.

A few patients with morning glory syndrome have surprisingly good vision, but the majority suffer from marked visual loss, often with an associated amblyopia. There is a tendency toward a myopic, astigmatic refractive error. Fortunately, the morning glory syndrome is only rarely bilateral; however, the contralateral eye sometimes demonstrates other anomalies, such as microphthalmia, anterior chamber cleavage syndrome, hyaloid remnants, or other types of coloboma. To date, there is no compelling evidence for a hereditary factor in this condition. Eustis and associates[101] have described this syndrome in association with endocrine and central nervous system anomalies.

The most common severe complication of the morning glory syndrome is retinal detachment.[98,103,104,115] The detachment characteristically occurs around the deeply excavated disc and usually is confined to the posterior or pole of the retina. In contrast to the rhegmatogenous retinal detachment associated with colobomas, no tears, holes, or vitreoretinal adhesions were noted in eight cases investigated by Hamada and Ellsworth.[104] They believed that the detachments were tractional as a result of tugging caused by the abnormal glial tissue within the lesion.

CONGENITAL TILTED DISC SYNDROME*

The congenital tilted disc syndrome (Color Plate 2-8) is an abnormality consisting, in full-blown cases, of inferonasal "tilting" of the optic disc, usually with an associated inferonasal crescent (conus),[122] thinning of the retinal pigment epithelium and choroid in the inferonasal fundus, posterior staphyloma of the affected inferonasal region of the fundus, and situs inversus of the retinal vessels. The most important clinical correlates of these lesions are a myopic astigmatism (most pronounced in the region of the staphyloma where the axial length of the eye is increased) and superotemporal, bitemporal, or superior altitudinal visual field defects caused by the anomalous development of the inferonasal aspect of the optic nerve and retina.

The seemingly endless nomenclature used to designate this syndrome (reviewed by Apple, Rabb, and Walsh)[3]—for example, oblique disc, inverted disc, dysverted disc, inferior conus, coloboma of the disc, nasal conus, and wet-stone papilla—demonstrates the lack of understanding of the pathogenesis of this condition. The descriptive term *congenital tilted disc* seems the most appropriate. Controversy regarding the nature, cause, and pathogenesis of tilted discs still exists. However, strong evidence indicates that this anomaly is a form of congenital typical coloboma that arises because of varying degrees of malclosure of the embryonic ocular fissure.[3,62,63,122] This congenital, inferior lesion should be distinguished from the acquired, usually temporal, lesions seen in most myopic eyes.

Following is a summary of the clinical characteristics of the congenital tilted disc syndrome[3]:

1. These eyes usually are mildly to moderately myopic. Astigmatism with an oblique axis often is present. In contrast to acquired pathologic high myopia (characterized by marked elongation and streaking of the eye), the myopia is not progressive.

2. The disc usually appears tilted downward and nasal.

3. An inferior or inferonasal crescent or conus almost always is present (Fuchs' coloboma).

4. Situs inversus often is present. The vessels emerge from the temporal rather than the nasal side of the disc and course nasally before sweeping out in the usual temporal distribution.

5. There is pallor of the inferonasal fundus, representing a probable "formefruste" manifestation of a typical coloboma. These changes generally are described as an "atrophy" of the tissues, particularly the pigment epithelium, but because the lesion is congenital, we believe the term *hypoplasia* would be more appropriate.

6. A posterior, inferonasal staphyloma is present. These may range from 6 to 9 D by retinoscopy and correspond to the region of fundus pallor. The degree of posterior bulging can be confirmed by computed tomography (CT) scan and B mode echograms.

7. A superior temporal or bitemporal visual field defect (the latter resembling a bitemporal hemianopsia of pituitary disease, but without respect of the midvertical line of

---

* Summarized in part from Apple DJ, Rabb MF, and Walh PM: Surv Ophthalmol 27:3, 1982.[3,116-141]

the field) can occur; these subtend the area of the inferonasal defect.°

8. A diminished response on electroretinogram sometimes can be elicited.

The syndrome appears with equal frequency in both sexes, and no significant association with systemic or neurologic disease has been documented consistently.

The ophthalmoscopic appearance of a tilt results from the fact that, instead of the vertically oval appearance of the normal disc where the superior pole of the disc appears near the 12 o'clock position, the orientation of the disc is shifted so that the superior aspect of the nerve appears to be dislocated nasally to the superonasal quadrant. The tilt can be moderate in degree or may extend up to almost 90 degrees so that the long axis of the disc approaches the horizontal meridian (Fig. 2-16, *A*). In such cases, the inferior pole of the disc appears to be pointing toward the macula. No rotation actually occurs, but because the nerve tissue inferonasally has been hollowed out as the staphylomatous coloboma forms, the inferior pole of the disc seems to have rotated because the long axis of the disc is no longer vertical. Only the heaped-up superotemporal portion of the disc actually is perceived ophthalmoscopically as the disc proper (Fig. 2-16). The entire inferonasal aspect of the disc is scooped out and emerges with the inferonasal conus. A clinical awareness of this condition is important for three reasons:

1. This anomaly and its many variations rank with acquired myopic disc changes (p. 37) as the most common disc lesions that can mimic the nerve head changes of glaucoma. Also, when central glaucomatous changes are superimposed on a disc with the congenital tilted disc syndrome, it becomes difficult to separate the two and to clinically follow the status and progress of the glaucoma. The staphylomatous "scooping out" of the inferior aspect of the disc frequently is confused with the pathologic excavation of glaucoma.

2. The myopic astigmatism of this disease is an annoying clinical problem, but fortunately it often is clinically insignificant because central vision usually is not affected or is corrected easily. Also, unlike an acquired high myopia, which can be progressive and lead to ominous tissue changes, the congenital tilted disc syndrome is not progressive and tissue changes, apart from the initial congenital defect itself, do not appear.

3. The previously described inferior, inferonasal, or predominantly nasal disc-fundus defects can create visual field abnormalities in the superior, superotemporal, and temporal fields, respectively.† More than one instance of intracranial operative intervention for a suspected pituitary tumor or other prechiasmal mass lesions has occurred based on the bitemporal hemianopsia caused by this otherwise totally benign fundus lesion. Recognition of the colobomatous defect usually is simple and should obviate the need for a major neurologic workup, much less surgery.

Unlike the visual field defect in pituitary tumors, the visual field in the congenital tilted disc syndrome usually does not respect the vertical meridian but usually will cross

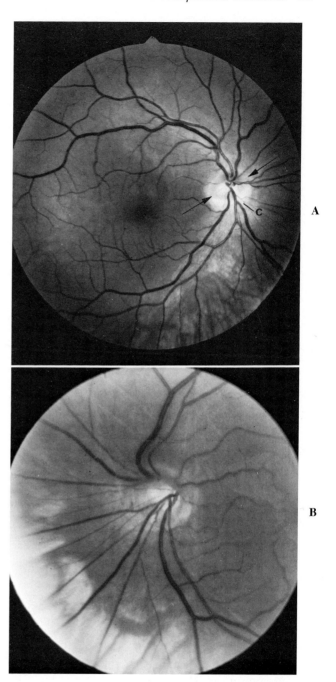

Fig. 2-16. A, Congenital tilted disc syndrome, OD. The long axis of the disc is oblique approaching the horizontal meridian (*arrows*). The inferior pole of the disc "points toward the macula." *C*, Inferior crescent (Fuchs' coloboma). Note the "albinoid" appearance of the inferior nasal fundus with increased visibility of the underlying choroidal vessels due to retinal pigment epithelial deficiency. **B,** Clinical appearance of a left fundus from different patient with a congenital tilted disc syndrome. The "tilted" superior and inferior poles of the disc are at approximately 11 and 5 o'clock, respectively. Note fundus depigmentation in the inferior nasal quadrant. (From Apple DJ, Rabb MF, and Walsh PM: Surv Ophthalmol 27:3, 1982.)

° References 3, 116, 123, 127, 128, 131-133, 136, 138, 140.
† References 3, 116, 123, 127, 128, 131, 133, 136, 138, 140.

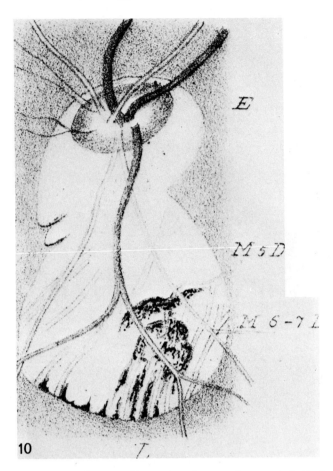

Fig. 2-17. Schematic illustration of a typical congenital tilted disc syndrome, OS. There is an associated fully developed inferior coloboma of the fundus. The changes in refraction induced by the inferior staphylomatous defect were appreciated by Fuchs.[97] At the level of the disc, the eye was emmetropic (*E*). Inferiorly, the myopia (*M*) gradually increased from 5 to 7 D. (From Fuchs E: Graefes Arch Ophthalmol 28:139, 1882.)

it at one site or another. In some cases but not all, the field defect improves with refractive correction of the myopia. As indicated in Fig. 2-17, refractive changes within the inferior staphylomatous defect may vary over a wide range: in this case, from emmetropia (*E*) to −7 D inferiorly. In more severe cases, the vision and field over the site of the defect cannot be improved so readily with minus lenses. This especially is true when the affected disc and fundus are damaged too severely by an extensive associated coloboma.

In 1882, Fuchs[122] was the first to explain this syndrome as being nothing more than a form of typical coloboma with defective closure of the fissure in the involved regions. His ideas were not widely accepted[137]; indeed, they often are ridiculed by many, including such experts as Elschnig, Schnabel, and other famous contemporaries.[120] To this day, the controversy exists. We now believe, however, that Fuchs, as usual, was correct.[122] The reasons are as follows[3,62,63]:

1. The few histopathologic specimens of this condition available show the characteristic features of a typical coloboma.

2. An extensive review of the literature back to the nineteenth century has revealed that more than 99% of reported cases of true congenital tilted disc syndrome show the disc-fundus lesion to be within the domain of the former embryonic fissure—most commonly inferonasal. The coincidence is too great for one to ascribe the pathogenesis of these cases to any cause unrelated to the fissure.

3. Finally, a review of the literature and, in particular, detailed ophthalmic atlases over the past 120 years, have documented in numerous instances the association of congenitally tilted discs with definite colobomas.

One may conclude that the spectrum of changes seen in this syndrome depends on the degree of vigor of closure of the embryonic ocular fissure at the 6-week stage of gestation. The spectrum ranges from a minimal (forme fruste) defect to a frank unmistakable coloboma.

Atypical colobomas

An atypical coloboma is a developmental defect occurring at any site other than inferiorly along the line of the embryonic fissure.[142-218] Such lesions resemble or are identical morphologically to typical colobomas but, because of their location in other quadrants of the globe, cannot be explained on the basis of malclosure of the fissure. Three specific forms of atypical colobomas are noteworthy: optic pits, iris colobomas, and macular colobomas.

OPTIC PITS

In 1882, Wiethe[217] described abnormalities in both optic discs of a 62-year-old woman. His description of dark-gray depressions in the optic nerve heads probably was the first report of optic disc pits. Since Wiethe's initial description, excavations of the optic nerve head have been described variously as craters, holes, cavities, and, most recently, congenital pits of the optic nerve head.

Optic pits[165-218] (Color Plates 2-9 and 2-10) are congenital defects within the substance of the optic nerve head. They are slitlike, triangular, polygonal, or oblong. Pits usually have steep walls and reach depths ranging from 1 to 25 D. They also vary in diameter, but on average are approximately 0.3 disc-diameters in width. They usually are gray, gray-olive, gray-yellow, or blue. The hue in each instance probably results from the variable amounts of pigmentation and shadows within the pit. Often, tissue lies within or over the pit; pulsation of such veils has been observed, probably because of the motion of the surrounding vessels. Centrally located pits often are associated with a temporal disc pallor. The incidence of pits is reported to be from approximately 1:7000 to 1:65,000, with a figure of 1:11,000 accepted by most authors.

Several reports have detailed the location of pits within the disc.[175] The majority (approximately 70%) occur temporally. Most fundi of eyes with optic pits show abnormal peripapillary pigment epithelial changes, particularly when the pit is located temporally. The pit can be bilateral or unilateral and usually occurs singly. However, pits can be multiple and may also occur in conjunction with a classic inferonasal typical coloboma of the optic nerve and retina (Fig. 2-18, *A* and *B* and Color Plate 2-11). There is neither a tendency toward a specific refractive error associated with optic pits nor a sexual, racial, or hereditary predilection. Pit-like localized cupping of the optic nerve (so-called

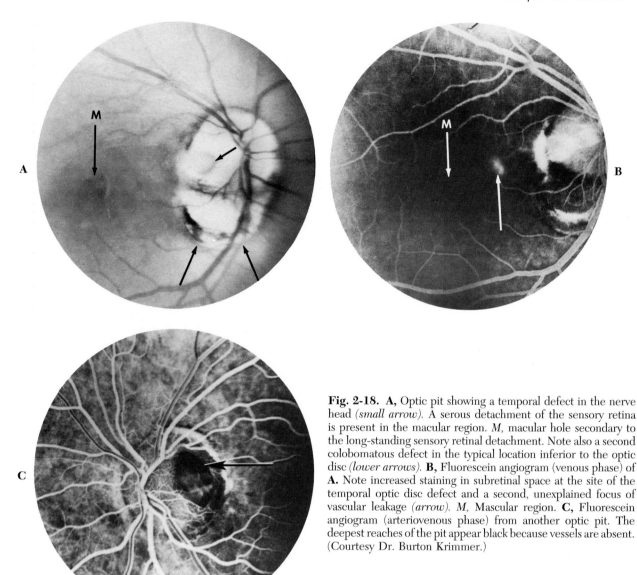

Fig. 2-18. A, Optic pit showing a temporal defect in the nerve head *(small arrow).* A serous detachment of the sensory retina is present in the macular region. *M,* macular hole secondary to the long-standing sensory retinal detachment. Note also a second colobomatous defect in the typical location inferior to the optic disc *(lower arrows).* **B,** Fluorescein angiogram (venous phase) of **A.** Note increased staining in subretinal space at the site of the temporal optic disc defect and a second, unexplained focus of vascular leakage *(arrow). M,* Macular region. **C,** Fluorescein angiogram (arteriovenous phase) from another optic pit. The deepest reaches of the pit appear black because vessels are absent. (Courtesy Dr. Burton Krimmer.)

acquired pit[189]) has been reported in glaucoma, especially the low-tension form.[202]

Various defects in the visual fields have been described[210] but are not necessarily explicable by serous maculopathy, which is the most important complication associated with optic pits (detailed next). At least half of patients with optic pits exhibit some abnormality in visual fields, including an enlarged blind spot, nasal steps, arcuate scotomas, paracentral scotomas, centrocecal scotomas, and generalized field constriction.

Chang[178] summarized the different fluorescein angiographic patterns in cases of true central serous maculopathy and in cases of serous macular detachment associated with optic pits. Optic pits show hyperfluorescence that fades late (Fig. 2-18).

In 1908, Reis[204] described a case of an optic nerve pit with associated maculopathy. However, this association was not taken seriously until Petersen[200] in 1958 described sev-

eral patients with what he called craterlike holes in the optic disc who also had a central serous chorioretinopathy. This relationship was firmly emphasized by Kranenburg[194] in 1960, who described 24 cases of optic disc pits. One third of these patients had serous retinal detachments, and another third had macular changes that he interpreted as reflecting a previous episode of nonrhegmatogenous serous retinal detachment.

In temporally located optic pits that are associated with a serous detachment of the macula,[145,195] secondary macular edema, retinoschisis, and macular hole occasionally also may develop (Fig. 2-18, *A* and *B*). Larger but not necessarily deeper pits are associated with a higher incidence of serous maculopathy. Macular edema or detachment eventually will develop in 40% to 60% of patients with an optic pit. Posterior vitreous detachment often is observed in cases of detached retina accompanying optic pits.

The pathogenesis of the macular involvement has been

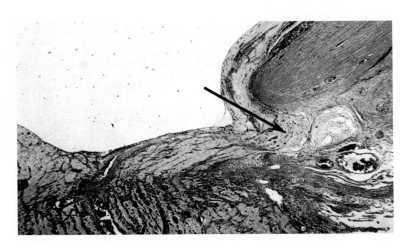

Fig. 2-19. Histologic section through an optic pit. On the right side of the photomicrograph the nerve fibers dig deep into the sclera at the margin of the papilla. (From Blodi FC and Allen L: Stereoscopic manual of the ocular fundus in local and systemic disease, vol I, St. Louis, 1964, The CV Mosby Co.)

debated extensively. A few investigators[181,187] have suggested that cerebrospinal fluid may leak from the optic nerve subarachnoid space into the optic pit, and from there into the subretinal space. However, intrathecal fluorescein injections in human subjects, in animals, and in histologic studies have failed to demonstrate any such connections. A gray fibroglial membrane appears to overlie the pit in many cases. This membrane may be intact or may incompletely cover the pit. The fact that patients with serous macular detachments also invariably have defects in their diaphanous membrane has prompted theories on how the optic nerve pit leads to the development of serous macular detachment. Recent studies on collie dogs and clinical observations of a series of 75 eyes with optic pits have led Brown and co-workers[176] to conclude in substantial agreement with Sugar's (1962)[211-213] and Brockhurst's (1975)[172] theory that the subretinal fluid arises from liquefied vitreous and gains entrance to the subretinal space through the pit. Vogel and Wessing[216,217] also believe that the fluid arises in the vitreous. Chang has reviewed the evidence for these various theories.[178] Differences of opinion continue to exist on the natural course of serous maculopathy associated with optic pits and the value of photocoagulation in preventing loss of visual acuity.[188,193,214]

Histopathologically, an optic pit consists of a pocket-like depression or herniation of rudimentary or degenerative neuroectodermal tissue (Fig. 2-19). In many cases, it contains elements of sensory retina, pigment epithelium, and glial tissue, which project into the defect within the optic nerve substance. The defect usually is surrounded by a connective tissue capsule that lies in conjunction with the meninges.

The differential diagnoses of optic pits include tumors of the optic nerve head, such as melanocytomas and astrocytic hamartomas, glaucoma (when the pit is extensive), optic neuritis, central serous choroidopathy, presumed ocular histoplasmosis syndrome, and other types of disc colobomas.

The pathogenesis of optic pits is not entirely clear.[172] Sugar[211,212] believes that optic pits located temporally or in other "atypical" locations are related to colobomas and may be caused by incomplete closure of an abnormally located, twisted, or shifted embryonic fissure, resulting in the usual temporal disc defect. Such an atypical location of the embryonic fissure has been seen in animals but not confirmed in humans. Apple and colleagues[3,167,168] have emphasized that because the normal fissure completely surrounds and encompasses the developing optic disc, it would seem reasonable to thus consider an optic pit lesion as another form of typical coloboma. Thus, any defect in the "zippering effect" of closure of the fissure might be expected to create potential defects, not only inferonasally, but also at any site on the disc, including the temporal aspect, where most optic pits are situated.

IRIS COLOBOMAS

Atypical iris colobomas are much less common than their typical counterparts. They are atypical because they may occur in any quadrant and therefore cannot be explained by nonclosure of the embryonic fissure.[142,155,156]

They may be manifest as a solitary defect (Fig. 2-20) or may consist of multiple lesions. They range in severity from a small notch in the pupillary margin to an iris defect involving a large sector. Sometimes half or more of the iris is involved, and the severity of the lesion approaches an aniridia.

Remnants of the anterior hyaloid system and pupillary membrane often are seen in association with atypical iris defects. This persistent fibrovascular tissue may impede the anterior growth of the optic cup, thereby being partly responsible for the pathogenesis of these defects (see Figs. 2-20, A, and 2-23 for diagrams of these embryonic vessels).

Aniridia, either occurring in a sporadic form or transmitted as an autosomal dominant trait, also might be considered a form of atypical iris coloboma* (Fig. 2-21; Color Plate 2-12). In reality, aniridia is an iris hypoplasia rather than an aplasia. A small rudimentary bud of iris root is present, and the embryonic iris primordium fails to grow anteriorly and centrally toward the pupillary region.

Congenital glaucoma occurs in approximately one third of patients with aniridia. Other intraocular defects include congenital cataracts and macular aphasia, which often induce nystagmus as a result of congenitally poor vision.

An inexplicable coexistence of sporadically occurring aniridia and Wilms' tumor (nephroblastoma) has been reported in a statistically significant number of cases (Miller's syndrome),[161] indicating that this association is more than

---

* References 143, 144, 146-152, 154, 157, 159, 161-163.

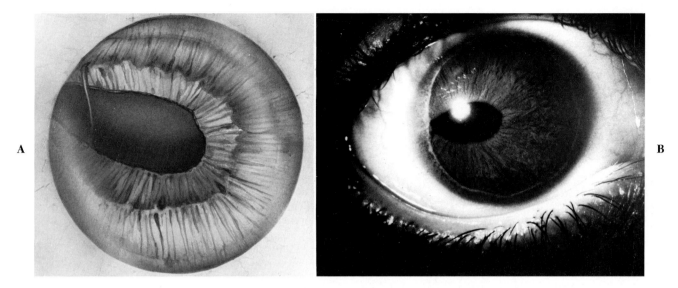

Fig. 2-20. A, Schematic illustration of atypical iris coloboma with hyaloid vascular remnant coursing through the defect. **B,** Atypical iris coloboma. A prominent posterior embryotoxon (anteriorly displaced, enlarged Schwalbe's line, p. 61) encircles the peripheral cornea. (From Meyner E: Atlas der Spaltlampenphotographie, Stuttgart, 1976, Ferdinand Enke Verlag.)

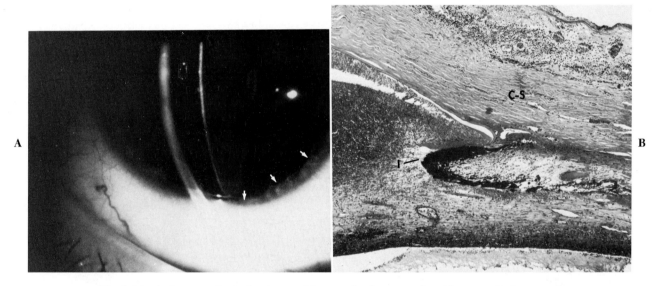

Fig. 2-21. A, Congenital aniridia. *Arrows,* Margins of rudimentary, hypoplastic iris. **B,** Congenital aniridia, photomicrograph of iris stump *(I).* The anterior chamber membrane *(left* and *below)* is a result of nonrelated trauma. *C-S,* Corneoscleral junction. (H & E stain; ×50.) (From Naumann GOH and Apple DJ: In Doerr W, Seifert G, and Uehlinger E, editors: Handbuch der speziellen pathologischen Anatomie, Band Auge, Berlin, 1980, Springer-Verlag.)

a coincidence. This association usually does not occur in the familial form of aniridia. In individuals without Wilms' tumor, the incidence of aniridia is 1 in 50,000; in those with Wilms' tumor, the incidence is 1 in 73. Aniridia with Wilms' tumor has been found in various chromosome anomalies.

Microscopically, aniridia is similar to that of the typical iris coloboma. The iris defect in aniridia may be visible microscopically for 360 degrees regardless of the plane of section. The iris defect in a typical coloboma is visible only inferiorly (Fig. 2-8, *B*).

The multiple iris defects seen in advanced cases of essential iris atrophy (so-called ICE syndrome) may resemble those of congenital atypical iris colobomas, but they are distinguished easily from the latter by the clinical history. Essential iris atrophy is a relatively infrequent cause of secondary angle-closure glaucoma, for which the etiology is obscure. This unilateral condition is an example of an abiotrophy, in which the mesectodermally derived tissues of the iris, the trabecular meshwork, and the corneal endothelium undergo a spontaneous, slowly progressive atrophy. Thinning and hole formation in the midperiphery of the iris are followed by displacement of the pupil. Thereafter, peripheral anterior synechiae form adjacent to the holes on the side opposite pupil displacement. As the atrophic process spreads around the iris, the synechiae extend until the angle is closed sufficiently to induce glaucoma.

These "ICE syndromes" are discussed and illustrated on pages 266-268.

MACULAR COLOBOMAS

Colobomas of the macula (Fig. 2-22, Color Plate 2-13) probably are not always developmental anomalies in the true sense of the word; they often may represent instances of scarring, pigmentation, and atrophy following intrauterine inflammation.

Most macular colobomas occur bilaterally, and the visual acuity almost always is decreased severely. Passage in families has been described. Some of the familial cases probably represent various types of heritable macular dystrophies.

The macula shows a round or oval, white, craterlike depression with pigmented borders. It may be associated with inflammatory scars in other parts of the fundus, thus suggesting that many cases are postinflammatory, for example, after congenital toxoplasmosis or syphilis.

Macular colobomas seldom have been studied histopathologically, but it can be assumed that at least some cases show changes similar to those seen in acquired postinflammatory chorioretinal scars—for example, in toxoplasmosis (see Chapter 8).

Anomalies based on persistence of the transient embryonic vasculature[219-259]

The embryonic fissure of the optic cup creates a notch or temporary defect that allows ingrowth of vascular elements into the eye (see Figs. 1-7, *B,* 1-10, and 2-7). These transient vessels, which are necessary for growth and development of the eye during the fetal period (Fig. 2-1), include a hyaloid artery trunk and its tributaries (Figs. 2-23 and

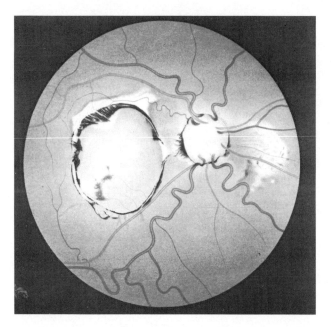

Fig. 2-22. Historical photograph of a so-called coloboma of the macula. (See also Color Plate 2-13.) (From Oeller J: Atlas seltener ophthalmoskopischer Befunde, Wiesbaden, 1903, JF Bergmann.)

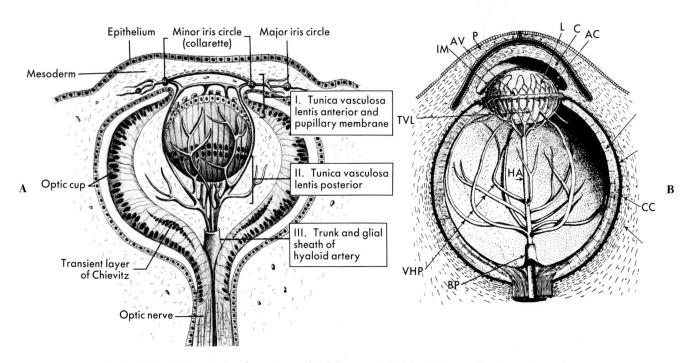

Fig. 2-23. A, Transient embryonic vessels of the eye. **B,** Original schema of embryonal vessels. (From Kollmann J: Handatlas der Entwicklungsgeschichte des Menschen, Jena, 1907, Gustav Fischer.)

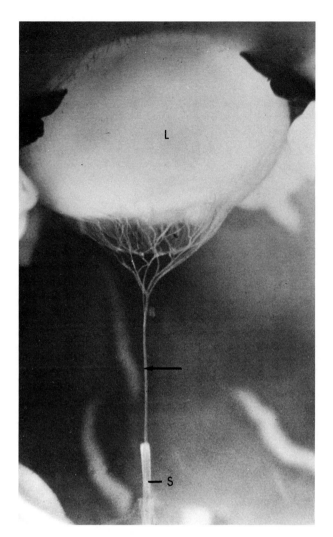

Fig. 2-24. Gross photograph of main hyaloid trunk *(arrow)* and retrolental tunica vasculosa lentis. *L,* Lens; *S,* perivascular sheath.

2-24), the precursors of the central retinal arterial system (reviewed by Apple and co-workers).[220,235]

The hyaloid vascular system, together with a scaffolding of delicate fibrillar strands, forms the primary vitreous (see Fig. 8-14). This fills the entire vitreous space during early gestation. Thereafter, the avascular secondary, or adult, vitreous forms and proceeds to occupy an increasingly greater proportion of the vitreous space. The tertiary vitreous, or zonules of Zinn, also begins to form around the fourth month of gestation. Eventually the primary vitreous is confined to a small area (Cloquet's canal), extending from the disc to the back of the lens.

The embryonic intraocular vascular system may be divided into two main components: an anterior system in front of the lens and a posterior component within the vitreous (Fig. 2-23). This division is useful for descriptive purposes but is somewhat artificial because all components are interrelated structurally in rich anastomoses and functionally in development and regression.

The pupillary membrane is formed by small, blind buds from the annular vessel (minor iris circle) that grow centrally to vascularize the mesoderm anterior to the lens. These vessels form the anterior vascular tunic of the lens (see Fig. 7-1). This central portion is destined to disappear during fetal life. The peripheral pupillary membrane and remnants of the annular vessel persist throughout life as the collarette. Persistence of the pupillary membrane is one of the most common, albeit usually clinically innocuous, congenital malformations of the eye[233,243] (Figs. 2-25 and 2-26). Congenital pupillary membranes always arise at the collarette. Acquired (postinflammatory or post-traumatic) membranes arise on any portion of the iris. When the persistence and hyperplasia are severe, as seen in Fig. 2-25, the condition is designated a congenital hyperplasia of the iris stroma.

The posterior tunica vasculosa lentis (Figs. 2-23 and 2-24) is formed by the terminal branches of the main trunk of hyaloid artery. The artery grows anteriorly from the optic nerve head toward the lens, where its terminal branches envelop the posterior surface of the lens and extend around

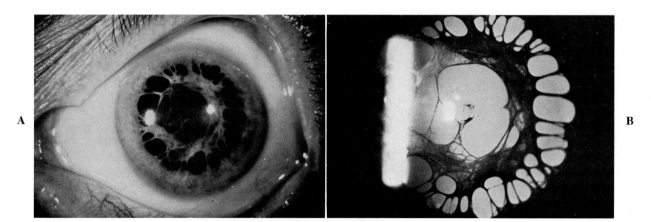

Fig. 2-25. Extreme degree of persistence of the pupillary membrane. **A,** Direct illumination. **B,** Retroillumination. Note superficial resemblance to essential iris atrophy (Fig. 6-10, *A*). (From Gutmann E and Goldberg M: Arch Ophthalmol 94:156, 1976. Copyright 1976, American Medical Association.)

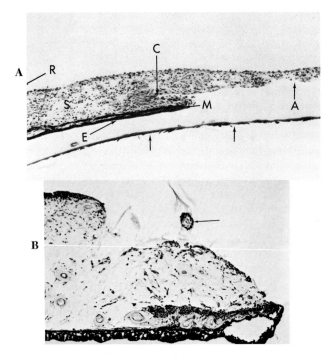

Fig. 2-26. Persistence of the pupillary membrane, one of the most common congenital abnormalities. **A,** It originates from the iris stroma at the collarette *(C)*. This contrasts to most acquired pupillary membranes, which arise from the pupillary margin *(M)* or elsewhere. *A,* Pupillary aperture, partially covered by the delicate strand of a pupillary membrane; *R,* direction of angle recess; *S,* iris stroma; *E,* iris pigment epithelium; *arrows,* anterior lens capsule. (H & E stain; ×100.) **B,** Note cross-section of strand of pupillary membrane *(arrow).* (H & E stain; ×150.)

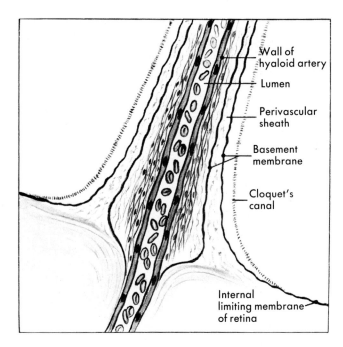

Fig. 2-27. Schematic illustration of embryonic optic nerve head with origin of hyaloid vessel and its sheaths (Bergmeister's papilla).

the equator of the lens as the lateral tunica vasculosa lentis or capsulopupillary vessels. This route provides an anastomosis with the anterior tunica vasculosa lentis and a drainage system through the annular vessel and, later in gestation, the ciliary vessels. The intravitreal branches located outside the narrow confines of the posterior tunica vasculosa lentis are termed the *vasa hyaloidea propria.*

By the end of gestation, the retrolental vascular tunic of the lens usually is almost entirely atrophied, except for its anterior termination, which may form a clinically insignificant opacity on the posterior lens surface, the Mittendorf dot.[244,245]

The glial sheath of Bergmeister (Figs. 2-23, 2-24, 2-27, and 2-28) envelops the posterior third of the hyaloid artery. It begins to atrophy at approximately the seventh month of gestation, even before the main vessel itself atrophies (Fig. 2-28, *B*). The extent of this atrophy below the surface of the disc may be partially responsible for the depth of the physiologic cup. If the atrophy of the sheath is less complete, a tuft of glial tissue may be seen throughout life as persistent Bergmeister's papilla (p. 34; see Fig. 2-35).

PERSISTENT HYPERPLASTIC PRIMARY VITREOUS (PHPV)

Persistent hyperplastic primary vitreous is one of the most frequent causes of a white pupillary reflex that may mimic a retinoblastoma (Figs. 2-29 to 2-33).[220] It therefore

is an important factor in the differential diagnosis of leukokoria and pseudoretinoblastoma (see Chapter 9).

For many years, PHPV was described by several different terms, such as persistence and thickening of the posterior fibrovascular sheath of the lens, persistent tunica vasculosa lentis, persistent hyaloid canal and artery, congenital membrane behind the lens, pseudophakia fibrosa, and retrolental fibroplasia. The last term is now reserved for the blinding condition caused by extended, high-concentration oxygen therapy in premature infants (p. 496).

In 1955, Reese[251] suggested *persistent hyperplastic primary vitreous* as a more appropriate term, thus emphasizing that the entity involved not only the posterior tunica vasculosa lentis but all components of the primary vitreous, including the main hyaloid trunk. Persistent hyperplastic primary vitreous is defined as an idiopathic persistence and proliferation of normally transient vasculature of the primary vitreous, in particular the posterior tunica vasculosa lentis, often leading to formation of a retrolental mass with subsequent visual loss.

The clinical appearance of PHPV may vary, depending on the amount and character of the hyperplasia of the embryonic vitreous components and the extent and nature of the secondary complications. The Mittendorf dot[244,245] is common, but because it is so innocuous, it does not warrant classification as PHPV.

In most cases of PHPV, the abnormality is unilateral in a fully developed, full-term otherwise normal infant with no apparent predisposition to sex or race. Most cases are isolated and sporadic with no apparent hereditary influence. Leukokoria is the most common initial sign (Fig. 2-29). In rare instances, the presenting sign may be nystagmus or squint caused by maldevelopment of visual function. The affected eye usually is microphthalmic, which is

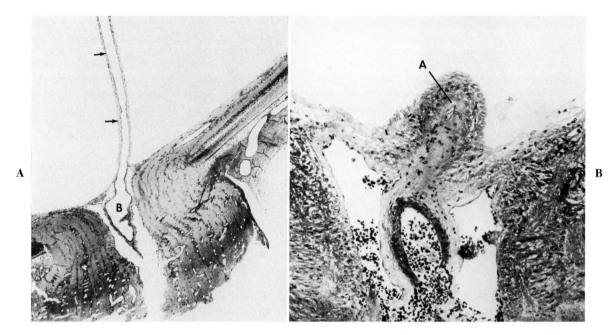

Fig. 2-28. Fetal monkey optic nerve head. **A,** Patent hyaloid artery *(arrows). B,* Bulbous dilatation at origin of the artery. (Mallory blue stain; ×70.) **B,** Hyaloid artery *(A)* after obliteration and regression. (Mallory blue stain; ×220.) (From Hamming NA and others: Invest Ophthalmol 16: 408, 1977.)

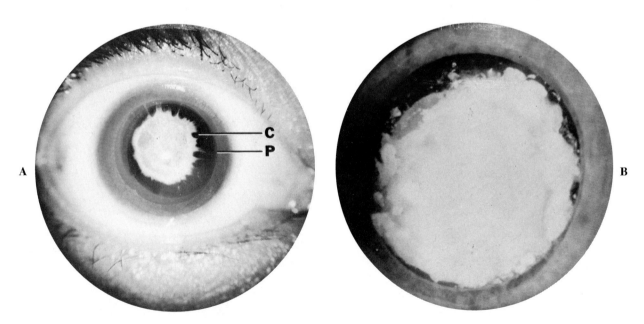

Fig. 2-29. Persistent hyperplastic primary vitreous. **A,** Retrolental membrane. *P,* Pupillary margin; *C,* elongated ciliary processes. **B,** Secondary cataract in PHPV. (**A** courtesy Dr. Michael Goldbaum, San Diego.)

one of the important features differentiating PHPV from retinoblastoma.

The leukokoria initially results from the opacity induced by a funnel-shaped mass of fibrovascular tissue occupying the retrolental space and the site of Cloquet's canal (Figs. 2-31 to 2-33). The retrolental mass may vary in size from a small localized plaque just nasal of center to a complete covering of the posterior surface of the lens. The stem of the funnel often contains remnants of the hyaloid artery. Identification of the hyaloid artery, which may be patent or occluded, is extremely useful in confirming the diagnosis and in differentiating this lesion from other causes of a funnel-shaped retrolental mass (see Chapter 9).

The tissue usually is richly vascular (Figs. 2-30 and 2-31), and repeated hemorrhages within the retrolental mass, the vitreous, and the perilenticular area are common. The vessels characteristically are delicate and friable. Furthermore, the tension between the contracting fibrovascular membrane and the ciliary body may induce rupture of the vessels in these structures.

With mydriasis, elongated, stretched ciliary processes may be seen to extend centrally within the pupillary aperture (Figs. 2-29, *A,* and 2-30). This finding, in conjunction with microphthalmia, constitutes one of the better clinical methods of differentiating PHPV from retinoblastoma and the other causes of leukokoria.

Several iris abnormalities may be clinically apparent. The pupil usually dilates poorly, and with advanced, long-term cases, ectropion uveae occurs. Although not a common feature, remains of the fetal pupillary membrane may simultaneously persist. Rarely, a large vessel derived from the tunica vasculosa lentis may extend anteriorly around the equator of the lens through the pupil, anastomosing with iris stromal vasculature. As might be expected with

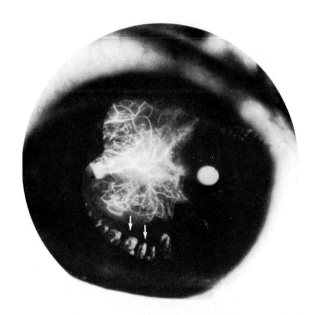

Fig. 2-30. Fluorescein angiogram of PHPV. Because the lens has resorbed, the remnants of the posterior tunica vasculosa lentis are clearly visible. Note elongated ciliary processes. (Courtesy Drs. David Gieser and Morton Goldberg.)

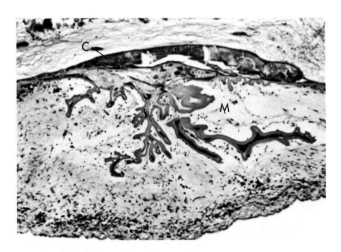

Fig. 2-32. PHPV. *C,* Cataractous lens; *M,* retrolental mass. Coiled fragments of ruptured lens capsule are enmeshed within the mass. (PAS stain; ×200.)

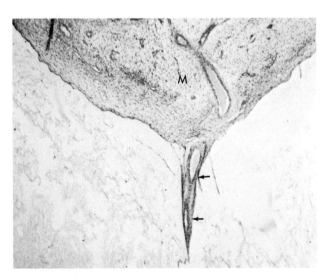

Fig. 2-31. PHPV. Photomicrograph of junction of hyaloid artery *(arrows)* with fibrovascular retrolental mass *(M).* (H & E stain; ×200.)

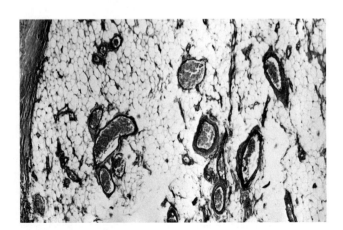

Fig. 2-33. PHPV with adipose metaplasia of the retrolental mass. (H & E stain; ×175.)

persistence of such remnants, atypical colobomas of the iris and lens may ensue (p. 18).

The lens usually is initially clear but with time becomes cataractous, usually because of rupture of the posterior capsule (Figs. 2-29, *B*, and 2-32). The fibrovascular tissue eventually invades the lens cortex, creating cortical fiber degeneration, liquefaction, and cataract formation. This often is accompanied by swelling of the lens, which in turn may lead to secondary closed-angle pupillary block glaucoma. In long-standing, severe cases, the lens cortex may slowly resorb, leaving only remnants of calcified cortex or a wrinkled capsule adjacent to the fibrovascular mass (so-called pseudophakia fibrosa or membranous cataract) (Fig. 2-32).

Because the retrolental mass is composed primarily of tissue of mesenchymal origin, it is not surprising that other mesodermally derived heteroplastic tissues may form as the aberrant proliferative process continues. An interesting form of metaplasia occasionally occurs in which adipose tissue is derived from the mass[227] (Fig. 2-33). Fat may be observed in the plaque, the vitreous body, and even the lens after capsular rupture (so-called pseudophakia lipomatosa). In trisomy 13, a cartilaginous metaplasia of the PHPV tissue commonly occurs (p. 47; see Fig. 2-57).

When the fundus can be seen through the retrolental mass, the retina appears normal in early stages. In more advanced cases, signs of old and recent intravitreal hemorrhage in various stages of organization may be seen. As the fibrovascular mass contracts, the retina may be drawn peripherally by traction onto the pars plana or ciliary processes. This typically induces numerous folds in the retinal periphery. However, severe retinal detachment is relatively unusual.

Clinical course and treatment

After diagnosis of PHPV, the immediacy and type of treatment chosen by the physician is critical because of the constantly changing and complication-ridden course of this syndrome. Untreated cases of full-blown PHPV almost always progress to phthisis bulbi. In the past, most affected eyes did not survive to adult life, either because of phthisis bulbi or because they were enucleated for fear of a retinoblastoma. A case of PHPV in a 71-year-old man[254] represents the most spectacular exception to the rule that affected eyes usually undergo early enucleation. The unrelenting, often rapid progression of secondary complications may create sequelae that force enucleation. These sequelae include unrelenting absolute glaucoma, recurrent massive hemorrhages, retinal detachment and atrophy, and phthisis bulbi.

Because the natural course of PHPV is ill-fated, early intervention is extremely important. Current concepts of surgery are based on the fact that hemorrhage may occur relatively early in life; it appears that "conservative, watchful waiting" only results in eventual progression, necessitating a more radical surgical procedure or even future enucleation. Although details regarding surgical techniques are beyond the scope of this chapter, the reader should be aware of the most important discussions of surgical treatment of PHPV, including the reports of Acers and

Coston[219]; Gass[229]; Nankin and Scott[246]; Peyman, Sanders, and Nagpal[248]; Reese[251]; van Selm[252]; Smith and Maumenee[253]; and Stark and coworkers.[256]

The basic surgical approach is twofold: the aspiration of all lens material and the creation of a clear pupillary space by excision of part of the retrolental membrane. Recent advances in the technique of vitrectomy have greatly improved the prognosis in this disease.[256]

Even if the final visual acuity is poor, sometimes globes are salvaged and enucleation is not necessary. Cosmetically acceptable results can be achieved, thus justifying use of these techniques.

POSTERIOR PHPV AND EPIPAPILLARY AND PERIPAPILLARY LESIONS

Any of the vascular or ectodermal components of the primary vitreous in the posterior segment of the eye may persist.[237] The appearance of each posterior polar anomaly is determined by the degree of retention of one or more of these components.

Persistence of the hyaloid trunk at the posterior pole may occur, ranging from a very short stump of persistent trunk arising from the disc to a longer trunk that may be relatively straight or tortuous, extending up to the posterior aspect of the lens. The persistent vascular strand may be patent or occluded.

The pathogenesis of so-called vascular loops or corkscrew vessels arising from the optic disc is unclear (Fig. 2-34). Some investigators believe that such loops are totally unrelated to persistence of any component of the hyaloid system (reviewed by Bisland[221] and Bruckner, Michaels, and Fine[224]). However, when one considers that the retinal and hyaloid vessels arise from a common embryologic vascular bulb in the optic nerve (Fig. 2-28, *A*), such neglect of the hyaloid artery in the pathogenesis of vascular loops appears arbitrary and actually is a matter of semantics. It

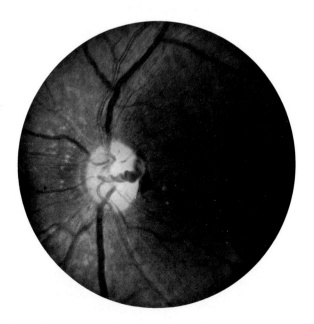

Fig. 2-34. Anomalous "corkscrew" vessel arising from the optic disc and protruding into the vitreous.

is likely that the vascular loop is derived at least partially from the proximal trunk of the hyaloid artery.

The term *persistent Bergmeister's papilla* is used loosely to describe a variety of conditions. Recalling that Bergmeister's papilla is a structure with two components, the central vascular core surrounded by the fibroglial sheath (Figs. 2-23, 2-27, and 2-28), one theoretically could expect persistence of either component. Therefore, a persistent Berg-

meister's papilla might represent a simple vascular remnant usually associated with fibroglial tissue or the fibroglial component alone.

Persistence of at least a minimal component of Bergmeister's papilla is such a common phenomenon that it actually is an anatomic variant (Fig. 2-35). Retention of elements of the glial sheath of Bergmeister usually is clinically manifest by the formation of epipapillary or peripapillary, delicate, white-to-gray membranes or glial cysts[225,230, 247,257] (Fig. 2-36). Such membranes rarely present visual difficulties but are important in relation to the differential diagnosis of lesions on and around the optic nerve, particularly small retinoblastomas. Inflammatory membranes, drusen and hamartomas of the nerve, and medullated retinal nerve fibers must be differentiated from persistent Bergmeister's papilla.

The fibrils of the primary vitreous insert into the sensory retina not only in the region of the optic disc but also in the midperiphery and periphery of the fundus. Therefore, retention and proliferation of these elements occasionally may lead to thickening of the nerve fiber layer and formation of small inner retinal or preretinal fibroglial tufts.[242,259] Pruett and Schepens[249,250] classify this as posterior hyperplastic primary vitreous. Traction exerted by shrinkage of these fibroglial remnants at the vitreoretinal interface may produce retinal folds anywhere in the fundus. Thus, one can explain the attachment of abnormal vitreous fibrils to any portion of the retina as far anteriorly as the ora serrata.

Traction produced by such abnormal vitreoretinal development may create giant retinal tears. Pruett and Schepens[249,250] and Hamada and Ellsworth[234] also postulate that some congenital remnants of the primary vitreous may be operative in the causation of retinal detachment. Furthermore, preretinal proliferation of these membranes may explain the presence of preretinal, intravitreal, or epipapillary cysts that form a distinct clinical entity.[225,228]

CONGENITAL FALCIFORM FOLD

Pruett and Schepens[250] believe that congenital falciform fold is a form of posterior hyperplastic primary vitreous. This condition is a rare cause of leukokoria or pseudoglioma[220] (see Chapter 8). It is clinically recognizable as an elongated folding or tenting of retinal tissue, usually coursing from the optic nerve head toward the retinal periphery or ciliary region[241,258] (Color Plate 2-14). It sometimes is inherited as an autosomal recessive characteristic, often is bilateral, and usually affects the lower temporal quadrant.

Falciform folds are sometimes associated with abnormal persistence of the hyaloid artery, and the artery may be located along the apex of the ridge of retina. Most authors postulate that traction exerted by the persistent components of the primary vitreous on the inner aspect of the retina creates a tenting of the retina. The disease usually is progressive; eventual massive retinal detachment and phthisis bulbi can occur.

Congenital retinal fold and cicatricial retinopathy of prematurity (ROP, retrolental fibroplasia) are strikingly similar; some observers have considered them the same entity. However, retinopathy of prematurity more typically occurs in infants of low birth weight who have been maintained in an incubator for a time. Such a history is not obtained in patients with congenital retinal folds. Microscopic exam-

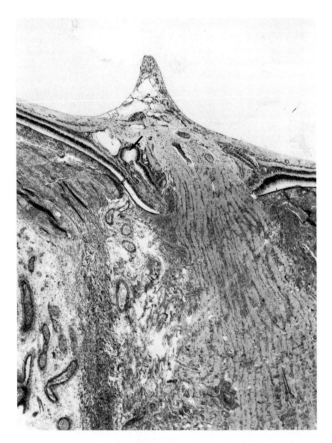

Fig. 2-35. Mound of glial tissue (persistent Bergmeister's papilla) on the optic nerve head. *Arrow,* Focus of retinal dysplasia. (H & E stain; ×100.)

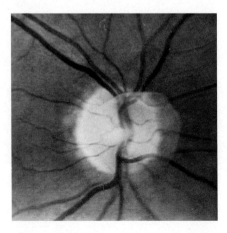

Fig. 2-36. Epipapillary glial membrane (persistent Bergmeister's papilla).

ination of histologic sections provides another reason for segregating these two entities. The retina in congenital falciform fold contains abundant dysplastic rosettes, indicating an early disturbance in embryogenesis, whereas in retrolental fibroplasia, the retina shows secondary gliotic and degenerative changes caused by mechanical traction exerted by the neovascular preretinal membranes. Nematode endophthalmitis caused by *Toxocara canis* also may produce a picture of a "dragged disc" with a retinal fold (p. 99).

Anterior chamber cleavage syndromes

The ophthalmic literature during the past 75 years has produced a myriad of confusing terminology and eponyms relating to conditions in which the anterior chamber angle structures that form the normal filtration apparatus have a faulty cleavage.[260-292] Reese and Ellsworth[281] in 1966 and Waring, Rodrigues, and Laibson[292] in 1975 simplified the concept considerably by lumping many of these conditions under various subdivisions termed the *anterior chamber cleavage syndromes*.[281] These conditions have in common a faulty separation or cleavage of the tissues that form the future cornea and iris. The angle recess and anterior chamber angle filtration structures do not develop normally.

Used with the broadest meaning, this category would include all forms of congenital glaucoma (see Chapter 6), but the term *anterior chamber angle cleavage syndromes* usually is reserved for specific entities such as the three important prototypes that may but do not invariably cause glaucoma: Axenfeld's anomaly,[262] Rieger's syndrome,[282-284] and Peter's anomaly.[280]

Axenfeld's anomaly and Rieger's syndrome are conditions that are inherited in an autosomal-dominant manner and reveal similar anterior segment changes. Because of the defect in cleavage and differentiation of the anterior segment tissues that previously were believed to be mesodermal in origin, they sometimes have been termed *indocorneal mesodermal dysgenesis*. Most authors now believe that the involved tissue is derived from the neural crest (neural crest mesenchyme or mesectoderm), so these conditions now simply are termed iridocorneal dysgenesis.

Axenfeld's anomaly or peripheral dysgenesis of cornea and iris[262] (Figs. 2-37 and 2-38) consists of two distinct

features: posterior embryotoxon (to be distinguished from anterior embryotoxon, which is synonymous with arcus juvenilis (p. 62), and abnormal iris processes that course across the face of the angle between the iris and the posterior cornea. Posterior embryotoxon is defined as a central or anterior displacement and enlargement of Schwalbe's line. The enlarged Schwalbe's line is similar in appearance to that illustrated in Fig. 6-2 in a normal globe. This figure therefore demonstrates that an enlarged Schwalbe line also can appear as a normal anatomic variant (see also Fig. 2-20, *B*).

Clinically, the prominent, anterocentral displacement of Schwalbe's line appears as an arcuate white line or bow (Gr. *toxon,* bow), as illustrated in Figs. 2-20, *B*, and 2-37. In addition to displacement, the enlargement of Schwalbe's line, which is the termination of Descemet's membrane, is histopathologically manifest as a bulbous swelling of this membrane (Fig. 2-38).

Rieger's syndrome,[282-284] also a form of peripheral dysgenesis of cornea and iris, shows posterior corneal and angle changes similar to those of Axenfeld's anomaly. In

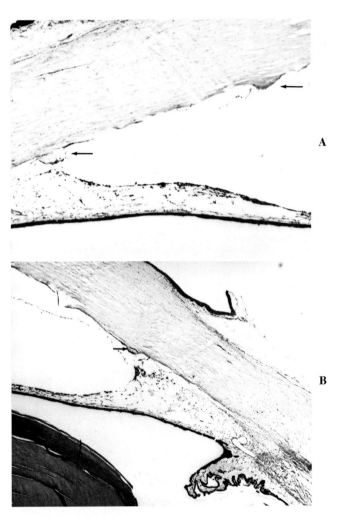

Fig. 2-38. Posterior embryotoxon and Axenfeld's anomaly. **A,** Double posterior embryotoxon *(arrows).* (H & E stain, ×95.) **B,** The iridocorneal adhesion is emphasized. *Arrow,* Posterior embryotoxon. (H & E stain; ×80.)

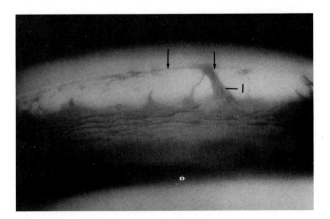

Fig. 2-37. Axenfeld's anomaly. Gonioscopic view of iris processes *(I)* adherent superiorly to an enlarged Schwalbe's line *(arrows).* (From Meyner E: Atlas der Spaltlampenphotographie, Stuttgart, 1976, Ferdinand Enke Verlag.)

addition, patients with Rieger's syndrome usually also exhibit gross malformations of the iris, such as ectropion of the pupil pseudopolycoria, corectopia, and colobomas. Ectodermal abnormalities, particularly dental anomalies, often are present. Glaucoma usually develops during the first to third decades and rarely is present in infancy, whereas infantile glaucoma may occur in Axenfeld's syndrome.

Peter's anomaly,[280] or central corneal dysgenesis (Fig. 2-39), usually transmitted as an autosomal recessive trait, is described classically as a defect induced by delayed separation of the lens vesicle from the surface ectoderm. The embryonic lens is derived from the surface ectoderm after induction from the optic vesicle (see Fig. 4-1). The lens vesicle pinches off from the surface epithelium and migrates posteriorly to its normal posterior chamber location in the eye.

In his original descriptions, Peters[280] reasoned that the combination of a defect or opacity in the posterior aspect of the cornea (sometimes known as a posterior or internal ulcer of von Hippel) associated with cataractous changes at the anterior pole of the lens (such as anterior polar or pyramidal cataract) could be explained by the embryologic mechanism of delayed separation. This theory has not been fully confirmed experimentally or by analysis of sufficient pathologic material to be considered final.

Histologically, the posterior defect reveals absence of

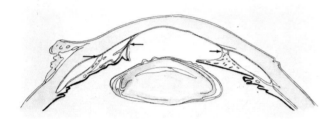

Fig. 2-39. Peters' anomaly. *Arrows,* Corneoiridal processes. (From Peters A: Klin Monatsbl Augenheilkd 44:27, 1906. Redrawn by Dr. Steven Vermillion, University of Iowa.)

endothelium and Descemet's membrane and varying amount of posterior stroma. As with the other examples of mesodermal dysgenesis of the anterior segment, iris anomalies such as corectopia or iridocorneal adhesions occur. Glaucoma may result from the iridocorneal processes and associated hypoplasia of the anterior chamber angle filtration structures.

Anomalies in the size of the eye[293-317]

DECREASED SIZE
Microphthalmia

Microphthalmia, one of the most common ocular developmental anomalies (Fig. 2-40), is classified as follows:

A. Isolated, idiopathic microphthalmia (including nanophthalmia)[293] occurring in the absence of other ocular or systemic changes.[315]
B. Colobomatous microphthalmia, in which growth of the eye is retarded by malclosure of the embryonic fissure[314] (p. 17). These cases often show generalized intraocular changes.
C. Microphthalmia associated with other intraocular anomalies in the absence of proved colobomas, for example:
   1. Sclerocornea
   2. PHPV (p. 30)
   3. Pupillary anomalies
      a. Corectopia
      b. Ectopia pupillae
D. Microphthalmia associated with ocular and systemic diseases[299,300,306] and syndromes such as the following:
   1. Infectious diseases, for example:
      a. Maternal rubella syndrome (p. 132)
      b. Toxoplasmosis
      c. Cytomegalic inclusion disease
   2. Chromosomal anomalies, for example, trisomy 13 (p. 45)
   3. Pupillary anomalies
      a. Corectopia
      b. Ectopia pupillae
   4. Toxic syndromes
      a. Thalidomide syndrome
      b. LSD syndrome
   5. Hallermann-Streiff syndrome

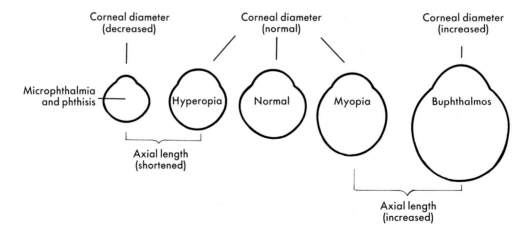

Fig. 2-40. Variations in size of the eye. (From Naumann GOH and Apple DJ: In Doerr W, Seifert G, and Uehlinger E, editors: Handbuch der speziellen pathologischen Anatomie, Band Auge, Berlin, 1980, Springer-Verlag.)

6. Pierre Robin syndrome
7. Waardenburg syndrome
8. Oculodentodigital (Meyer-Schwickerath and Weyers) syndrome
9. Anterior chamber cleavage syndromes
10. Treacher Collins' syndrome

E. Dominantly inherited microphthalmia with congenital cataract.

F. Isolated inherited microphthalmia (dominant or recessive).

All degrees of microphthalmia can be seen,[294,302] ranging from minimal microphthalmia that is very difficult to diagnose clinically to a severe form that falls into the differential diagnosis of a clinical anophthalmia. Congenital microphthalmia should be distinguished from phthisis bulbi, which usually represents an *acquired* shrinkage of the eye after trauma, inflammation, and other conditions rather than a primary developmental defect.

The degree of microphthalmia often depends on the time at which noxious influences affect the developing embryo or fetus. Defects occurring early in gestation at the time of the development of the optic vesicle or optic cup characteristically lead to severe microphthalmia and widespread intraocular changes, whereas changes occurring later in gestation lead to a mild microphthalmia with few or sometimes no intraocular changes (Fig. 2-1).

Nanophthalmia

Nanophthalmia is a congenital retardation in growth of the eye in which the eye is smaller than normal but otherwise well developed without severe intraocular changes.[421] All parts of the globe are reduced in size equally but usually reveal an otherwise normal appearance. Special surgical techniques must be used for such conditions, as cataract[293] and glaucoma.[303] Abnormal scleral growth has been noted.[312,316]

Hyperopia

Hyperopia (hypermetropia or farsightedness) usually is due to a relative decrease in axial length of the eye (Fig. 2-40); less commonly, it is due to a decrease in power of the refractive media. In contrast to high myopia, the anatomic-pathologic changes within the eye are relatively few. Whereas myopia may be a progressive disease in which secondary intraocular degenerative changes may occur later in life, hyperopia is a congenital condition, almost always present at least transiently at birth, which rarely creates significant structural changes in the eye.

Occasionally, the optic nerve head appears elevated in hyperopia; this can be confused with papilledema or papillitis (p. 537).

ENLARGEMENT OF THE GLOBE

Macrophthalmia

A true macrophthalmia represents a harmonically enlarged globe without associated changes. However, a primary enlargement of the globe in the absence of other ocular defects or increased intraocular pressure (p. 273) is extremely rare. The globe may appear clinically enlarged in cases of megalocornea, but the posterior segment is normal in size.

Myopia

STATIONARY MYOPIA

Stationary, or simple, myopia, often transmitted as an autosomal dominant characteristic, is a refractive error of low degree, usually less than 6 to 8 D, which usually develops during the first two decades and fails to progress significantly after completion of body growth.* The refractive error is caused by variations in structure of the optic system, such as increased axial length of the globe, increased curvature of corneal or lens surfaces, or a high refractive capability of the lens. As a rule, with the exception of a myopic conus, there is little significant change in the globe.

PATHOLOGIC MYOPIA

Pathologic (degenerative) myopia is characterized by degenerative changes occurring particularly in the posterior segment of a highly myopic eye, often associated with lengthening of the anteroposterior axis of the globe[54] (Figs. 2-40 to 2-48; Color Plates 2-15 and 2-16). In contrast to simple myopia, which involves a limited degree of ametropia in a relatively healthy globe, pathologic myopia connotes an extreme axial elongation in which degenerative changes are superimposed.

High myopia is slightly more likely to develop in women than men. Whereas the lower degrees of myopia generally are transmitted as a dominant trait, in higher degrees of myopia, which often begin at a relatively early age, a reces-

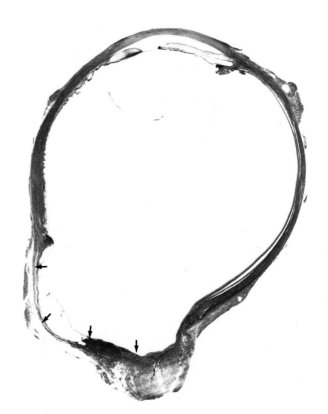

Fig. 2-41. Degenerative myopia with enlargement of the globe and posterior staphyloma *(arrows).* (H & E stain; ×1.)

---

* References 295, 296, 308, 311, 313, 317.

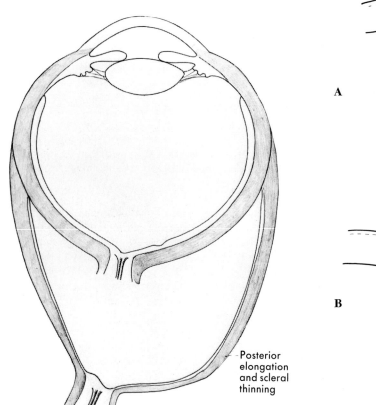

Fig. 2-42. Emmetropic eye superimposed on a myopic eye.

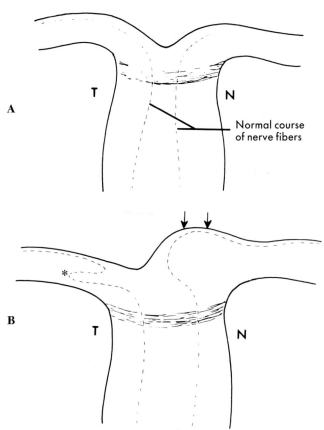

Fig. 2-44. Comparison of the course of optic nerve fibers in a normal (**A**) and myopic (**B**) optic nerve. *Arrows,* nasal supertraction; *asterisk,* temporal loop of Weiss.

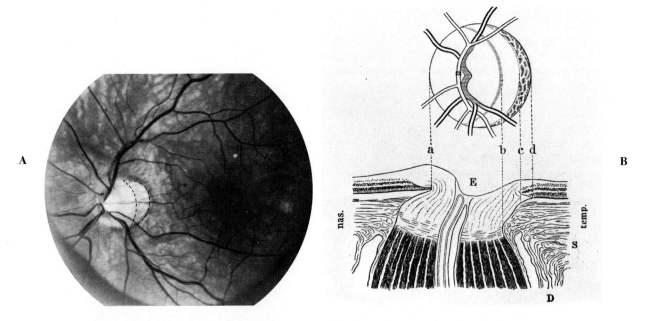

Fig. 2-43. A, Myopic temporal conus *(interrupted line).* **B,** Schematic diagram of myopic conus, showing early termination of pigment epithelium *(d)* and choroid *(c). a* and *b,* Disc margins; *E,* physiologic excavation; *S,* sclera. (From von Graefe A and Saemisch T: Handbuch der gesammten Augenheilkunde, Leipzig, 1974, Wilhelm Engelmann.)

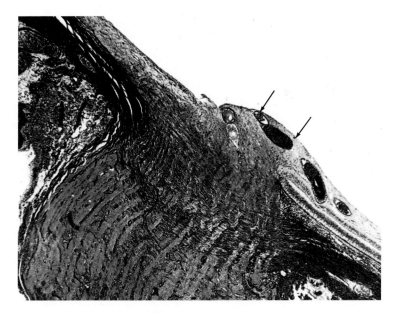

Fig. 2-45. Cross-section of an optic nerve head in severe myopia. The temporal margin (on the left side of the photomicrograph) is flat, and the physiologic excavation is shallow. On that side, choroid, pigment epithelium and retina do not reach the disc margin (temporal crescent). On the nasal side there is supertraction. The retina is pulled over onto the disc *(arrows).* (H & E stain; ×80.) (From Blodi FC and Allen L: Stereoscopic manual of the ocular fundus in local and systemic disease, vol I, St. Louis, 1964, The CV Mosby Co.)

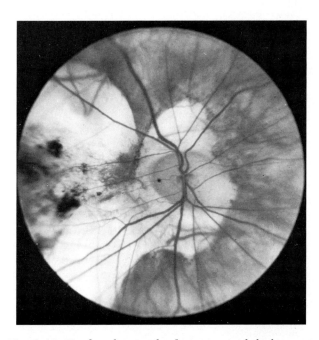

Fig. 2-46. Fundus photograph of a patient with high myopia showing an almost complete ring crescent around the optic disc and deformity of the nerve head. Chorioretinal atrophy is severe with pigmentary changes, particularly in the temporal quadrants.

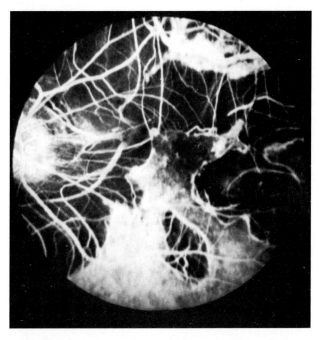

Fig. 2-47. Fluorescein angiogram from another patient with myopia showing marked chorioretinal atrophy with baring of large choroidal vessels.

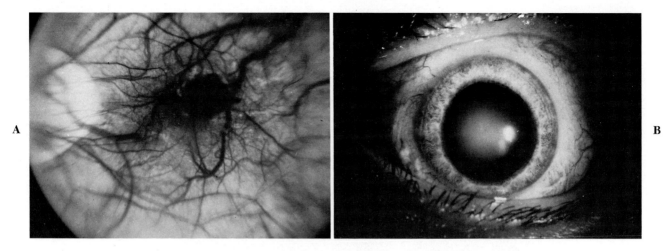

Fig. 2-48. Complications of severe myopia. **A,** Severe choroidal atrophy with baring of large choroidal vessels and sclera and with a Förster-Fuchs black spot at the macula. **B,** Cataracta complicata in myopia. (**A** from Naumann GOH and Apple DJ: In Doerr W, Seifert G, and Uehlinger E, editors: Handbuch der speziellen pathologischen Anatomie, Band Auge, Berlin, 1980, Springer-Verlag. **B** from Meyner E: Atlas der Spaltlampenphotographie, Stuttgart, 1976, Ferdinand Enke Verlag.)

sive transmission is more common. Anisometropia, an unequal degree of myopia in each eye, is the rule in most cases of high pathologic myopia, but gross inequalities greater than 3 D are relatively unusual.

In pathologic myopia, the degenerative and atrophic intraocular changes clearly diminish the prognosis for good visual acuity. Not only does the occurrence of sudden calamities, such as macular lesions, intraocular hemorrhage, or retinal detachment, pose a serious problem with regard to vision, patients with high myopia often experience visual discomfort, strain, and fatigue. The increased tendency toward formation of degenerated and liquefied vitreous and vitreous floaters in myopic eyes adds to the discomfort.

The most common form of pathologic myopia is the isolated development form. Whereas in simple myopia the myopic tendency is restrained after puberty, in developmental pathologic myopia, the nearsightedness may increase even more rapidly during adolescence and the axial enlargement may even slowly increase during adulthood into the 40s and 50s, with eventual genesis of atrophic and degenerative intraocular changes leading to visual loss and possibly blindness.

Congenital axial pathologic myopia also may occur. This frequently is associated with other congenital defects such as colobomas and anomalies of pigmentation of the retina or choroid (see congenital tilted disc syndrome, p. 22). The most common associated fundus conditions resemble partial albinism. Varying degrees of myopia commonly are associated with ROP (retrolental fibroplasia), microphthalmia, microcornea, microphakia, buphthalmos, the tapetoretinal dystrophies, and Down syndrome.

Clinically, a severe myopic eye generally appears large and prominent. The gross appearance of the highly myopic eye is characteristic in size and shape. Instead of being spheric, it is egg- or pear-shaped and significantly enlarged (Figs. 2-40 to 2-42). The cornea may be abnormally flat, the anterior chamber is somewhat deeper than normal, and

the ciliary muscles are atrophic. The ciliary muscle in a person with high myopic often is smaller than normal, probably because the myopic individual requires less use of the muscles of accommodation.

The major changes are confined almost entirely to the posterior pole. The relatively normal appearance of the anterior segment in high myopia is markedly different from that of the buphthalmic globe, in which the globe is enlarged in all dimensions equally and the anterior chamber is correspondingly distorted with a stretched cornea and a deep anterior chamber (Fig. 2-40).

The first to correlate the histologic changes in myopia with the ophthalmoscopic changes was von Graefe.[21] These changes are summarized as follows:

1. Scleral changes: posterior enlargement of the globe and thinning of the sclera at the posterior pole with scleral ectasia and posterior staphyloma.[297]

2. Changes in the epipapillary and peripapillary region: oblique entrance of the optic nerve, tilted disc, myopic crescent, nasal supertraction.

3. Changes in the choroid and retina[301]: atrophy and thinning, particularly affecting the posterior pole and periphery. These changes include atrophy and/or proliferation of the pigment epithelium, formation of the Förster-Fuchs spot at the macula, retinal microcystoid degeneration, and occasional peripheral retinal break formation with subsequent detachment.

4. Degenerative changes in the vitreous and vitreous detachment.

Scleral changes

Scleral thinning with occasional formation of a posterior bulging or staphyloma of the sclera is common.[297] The staphyloma may surround the optic nerve head and extend temporally to involve the posterior pole and sometimes even the equator. The normal sclera progressively thickens from the equator backward, becoming thickest at the posterior pole. In a globe with severe myopia the opposite situation occurs; the sclera becomes progressively thinner posteriorly in the peripapillary region. When present, a staphyloma (Fig. 2-41) is lined by a thin, atrophic choroid, and the margins of the staphyloma usually reveal a relatively abrupt edge. Scleral staphylomas encroaching on the optic nerve head must be histologically differentiated from a congenital coloboma (see congenital tilted disc syndrome, p. 22) or pit of the optic disc, as well as a glaucomatous pathologic excavation.

Changes in the epipapillary and peripapillary regions

Ophthalmoscopically, the optic nerve head in acquired myopia is ovoid with the long axis in the vertical direction. It may appear oblique (tilted disc) and typically is flattened on the temporal side but reveals an exaggeration or supertraction of the normally raised nasal edge (Figs. 2-43 to 2-45 and Color Plate 2-15). The course of the nerve through the optic canal affects the ophthalmoscopic appearance of the disc; usually this course forms a right angle to the surface of the eye. In the typical myopic eye, the nerve axis is oblique toward the temporal side, and the disc appears tilted with the temporal side flattened and the temporal optic nerve canal wall becoming visible. In addition to being flattened temporally, the temporal aspect of the disc often is surrounded by a concentric or crescent-shaped area or areas of relative fundus depigmentation.

The myopic crescent (Figs. 2-43 and 2-45) may be present at birth but usually becomes evident about puberty. It almost invariably occurs in later years in patients with myopia greater than 6 D. It is, however, not exclusively confined to myopic eyes. It usually appears initially as a white, sharply defined area lying on the temporal side of the optic disc where the inner surface of the sclera (and even the wall of the scleral canal when the disc is tilted) is directly seen. The sclera is visible because of an absence of pigment epithelium and choroid, both of which fail to extend to the temporal margin of the disc. This failure presumably results from mechanical factors caused by enlargement of the posterior globe. Sometimes a transitional region of brownish red pigment appears immediately temporal to the white crescent (Fig. 2-43, *B*). This pigmented and vascular choroidal crescent corresponds to an area where the choroid still is partially present and its vessels are rendered visible; the choroid extends closer toward the temporal margin of the disc than does the pigment epithelium.

The crescents of acquired myopia are located temporally in approximately 80% of cases. In 10% of cases, the crescent may extend to become annular (Fig. 2-46), surrounding the entire disc, sometimes even spreading to include a large area of the fundus with envelopment of the macular area. In rare instances, the myopic crescent is situated on the nasal side of the disc (inverse crescent). The inferior crescent seen in the nonprogressive congenital tilted disc syndrome has a different pathogenesis. It represents a colobomatous defect.

In some myopic eyes, the retinal nerve fibers course in a peculiar manner on the temporal side. They transverse the optic nerve head in an obliquely nasal direction. The temporal nerve fibers often then form a loop (loop of Weiss) running away from the nerve and then turning back at a sharp angle to reach the optic nerve (Fig. 2-44, *asterisk*).

Changes in the choroid and retina

Atrophy of the choroid occurring predominantly near the posterior pole is an almost consistent feature of severe pathologic myopia (Figs. 2-46 to 2-48, A; Color Plate 2-16). Initially the retinal pigment epithelium becomes attenuated and the choroidal vessels become visible. In advanced stages, many choroidal vessels as well as the choroidal stroma and melanocytes disappear so that circumscribed white areas of sclera become ophthalmoscopically visible. Simultaneous proliferation of pigment occurs in scattered areas, leading to alternating patches of hyperpigmentation and hypopigmentation. Splits may develop in Bruch's membrane. These form clefts (lacquer cracks[304] or lightning figures [German *Lacksprunge* and *Blitzfiguren*]), which seem to branch and have a reticular appearance. Chorioretinal scars may develop after actual breaks in Bruch's membrane.[304,307]

Atrophic changes in the retina progress simultaneously with those in the choroid. Atrophy, hyperpigmentation, and hypopigmentation of the pigment epithelium are among the earlier changes. Retinal thinning and photoreceptor and pigment epithelial degeneration are especially prominent in the posterior staphylomatous areas.

Macular degeneration[307] in pathologic myopia is common and highly incapacitating. Macular degeneration may occur independently of the scleral conus or may be caused by enlargement of a temporal conus involving the macular region. A central circular dark spot, the Förster-Fuchs spot (Fig. 2-48, A; Color Plate 2-16), occasionally is a characteristic feature at the macula. First described by Förster in 1862 (reviewed by Rabb, Garoon, and LaFranco[307]) and later extensively studied by Fuchs, it probably is caused by a combination of proliferation of pigment epithelium and deposition of blood pigment after subpigment epithelial neovascularization and choroidal hemorrhage. The Förster-Fuchs spot usually appears rapidly in the fourth to fifth decade and develops in association with splits (lacquer cracks) in Bruch's membrane.

In addition to retinal changes at the posterior pole and macula, extensive peripheral retinal changes often develop in patients with high pathologic myopia: microcystoid degeneration of the retina, thinning of the retina, and a tendency toward retinal tear formation. These patients are more prone to formation of peripheral retinal breaks, which predispose to subsequent retinal detachment.[308]

Degenerative changes in the vitreous

Vitreous changes resemble those typically seen in aging eyes, including liquefaction, microfibrillar degeneration, and formation of opacities and floaters (muscae volitantes). Posterior detachment of the vitreous commonly occurs, probably because of stretching of the enlarged globe, leaving a gap between the posterior vitreous and the posterior pole of the eye. The reflex streak of Weiss is a concentric, finely striated reflex on the nasal side of the optic nerve head that occurs in advanced myopia and probably corresponds to a focus of posterior detachment of the vitreous.

Complications

Complications of pathologic myopia typically appear in adult life after myopia has been long established.

Rhegmatogenous retinal detachment is one of the most common complications, showing a progressively greater tendency with increasing myopia. This is particularly facilitated by the occurrence of peripheral retinal degeneration and by the degenerative vitreous changes described previously. The vitreous opacities, always present in some degree in high myopia, may therefore progress from being a nuisance to being a contributor to the pathogenesis of the retinal detachment.

Choroidal thromboses and hemorrhages occur frequently because of obliteration of the choroidal vessels in progressive stages of the disease.

Cataract is a complication of high myopia, occurring particularly in later life and typically affecting the posterior pole of the lens (Fig. 2-48, *B*).

Chronic simple glaucoma occurs in a significant percentage of cases of high myopia. Because the anterior chamber angle in persons with myopia typically is widely open, closed-angle glaucoma is relatively rare. Glaucoma typically is insidious and difficult to diagnose.[4] The appearance of the optic disc also frequently is misleading as a result of the thinness of the precribriform glial tissue, and it sometimes is difficult to differentiate the previously described myopic changes on the optic nerve head from the pathologic changes of an associated glaucoma.

Pigment anomalies[318-368]

ALBINISM

Albinism is a hereditary derangement in melanin pigment metabolism that may occur in humans and many animal species.° The most common metabolic disturbance consists of a deficiency of tyrosinase, which transforms the amino acid tyrosine into dihydroxyphenylalanine (dopa) within chromatophores and epithelial cells. The pigment cells themselves are present; the defect lies in the lack of pigmentation within these cells.[324]

Genetic classification[366]
  I. Oculocutaneous
    A. Tyrosinase-negative
      1. Complete (perfect)
    B. Tyrosinase-positive
      1. Incomplete (imperfect)
      2. With neuropathy and leukopenia (Chédiak-Steinbrinck-Higashi syndrome)
      3. With thrombocyte-serotonin defect
    C. Yellow mutant (tyrosinase test variable)
 II. Ocular albinism
III. Cutaneous (partial albinism)
    A. Without deafness (e.g., Menkes' syndrome)
    B. With deafness (e.g., Waardenburg syndrome)[319,337]

In both the oculocutaneous and ocular forms of albinism, the changes in the eye are especially prominent. Oculocutaneous albinism usually is a simple autosomal-recessive trait. Ocular albinism (Nettleship-Falls) is transmitted more typically as an X-linked recessive characteristic.[327,333,334,353,367] The clinical and pathologic eye findings are similar in both forms; they differ only in that the albinotic changes are confined to the eye in ocular albinism, without cutaneous changes.

Oculocutaneous albinism is divided into the tyrosinase-negative and tyrosinase-positive forms. They can be differentiated by the tyrosinase hair-root test and the dopa test. Tyrosinase-negative (complete or perfect) albinism represents an absolute absence of pigmentation and is rare. Tyrosinase-positive albinism (incomplete or imperfect albinism) involves partial pigmentation rather than complete absence of melanin.

The forms of albinism that affect the skin are characterized by extreme lightness of the skin, blondness (including the eyebrows and cilia), and absence of browning of the skin in sunlight.

In all forms of albinism that affect the eyes (oculocutaneous or ocular albinism), the major change is a lack of pigment in the retina and uvea (Fig. 2-49). The defect is clinically most readily observed by transillumination of the affected iris (Color Plate 2-17). One can see the ciliary processes and lens through the eye, and the pupil appears red. The fundus typically is light red, and the retinal and choroidal vessels appear prominent against the white scleral background. Common symptoms are photophobia, refractive errors of the eye, strabismus, and nystagmus. Poor vision and nystagmus often result from a hypoplasia or aplasia of the fovea centralis.

Histopathologically, one does not observe a decrease in pigment cells within the eye, but rather a partial (or rarely an absolute) lack of melanin granules within the uveal and pigment epithelial cells (Fig. 2-49, *B*). Microscopic sections of the foveal region have shown that development of the foveal depression (foveola) can fail, and the foveal region consists entirely of a six- to eight-layered ganglion cell layer typical of the macular region. The foveal aplasia in albinism is similar in appearance to that which sometimes occurs in aniridia (p. 26).[340]

A special form of oculocutaneous tyrosinase-positive albinism is Chédiak-Steinbrinck-Higashi syndrome.° It is a rare metabolic disturbance that is transmitted as an autosomal-recessive trait in which an enzymatic block in tryptophan metabolism leads to pigment disturbances and abnormalities in leukocytes, including granulation disturbances and inclusion bodies in myelocytic leukocytes. A predisposition to recurrent pyogenic infections is involved. The prognosis is poor because of neurologic defects and septicemia, particularly in childhood. The eye symptoms and pathologic findings are similar to those of other forms of albinism.

MELANOSIS OCULI

Congenital melanosis oculi is a condition in which the pigmentation of the uveal tract is greatly increased (Figs. 2-50 and 2-51).† Congenital melanosis oculi should be differentiated from acquired or precancerous melanosis, which is described in Chapter 11.[427,435,442]

° References 325, 326, 328, 332, 334, 336, 342, 346, 347, 349, 355, 366.

° References 320, 323, 330, 344, 358, 363.
† References 318, 322, 329, 335, 338, 339, 341, 356, 357, 361, 362, 364, 368.

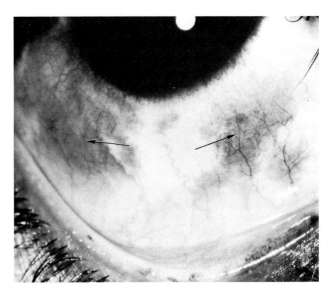

Fig. 2-50. Oculodermal melanocytosis (nevus of Ota). Separate foci of diffuse pigmentation are seen on the bulbar conjuctiva *(arrows)*. Hyperpigmentation of the skin and uveal thickening are also commonly observed in this form of congenital melanosis. Malignant transformation of the skin, mucous membrane, and uveal lesions occurs but is very rare.

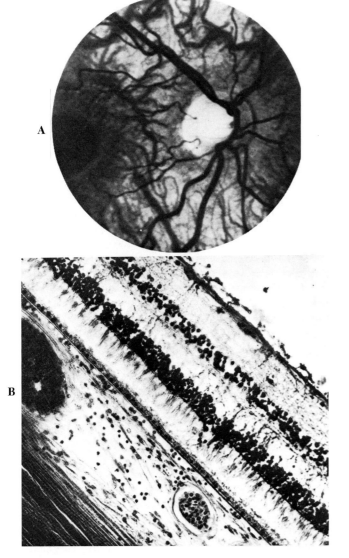

Fig. 2-49. Albinism. **A,** Fundus photograph. The choroidal vessels can be seen clearly against the white background of the sclera. **B,** Cross-section through an albinotic fundus. The retina is normal. There is decreased pigmentation in the retinal pigment epithelium and choroid. (H & E stain; ×200.) (From Blodi FC and Allen L: Stereoscopic manual of the ocular fundus in local and systemic disease, vol I, St. Louis, 1964, The CV Mosby Co.)

The absolute number of normal dendritic melanocytes is increased within the tissue. Affected are the chromatophores of the iris, ciliary body, choroid, conjunctival stroma, sclera, and episclera. Following are the three principal signs of congenital melanosis:

1. Pigmentation of the sclera and episclera;
2. Pigmentation of the iris;
3. A dark appearance of the fundus.

Clinically, the involved portions appear as diffuse broad patches of brown to light blue discoloration. Neither the epithelial pigment cells of the eye nor the conjunctival and skin epithelium are involved primarily; rather, the disease is characterized by involvement of the stomal chromato-

phores that are derived embryologically from the neural crest.

The two basic types of congenital melanosis oculi are (1) that in which the pigmentation is confined to the globe and epibulbar structures and (2) oculodermal melanocytosis, or nevus of Ota. Nevus of Ota (Figs. 2-50 and 2-51) involves the globe, epibulbar structures, and, particularly in Asian persons, the skin.[*] The skin pigmentation occurs in the distribution of the ophthalmic, maxillary, and occasionally mandibular branches of the trigeminal nerve. It almost always is unilateral.[357] Associated findings[361-363] in the involved eye include glaucoma,[361-363] uveitis, and heterochromia iridis. It is common in black and Asian people, but unusual in white people. The condition generally is benign, but rare malignant melanomas of the uvea, skin, or conjunctiva have been reported, mostly in white patients.[339,356]

HETEROCHROMIA IRIDUM AND IRIDIS

In uniocular heterochromia (heterochromia iridis),[331] different parts of the iris of one eye may have areas of different coloration because of either hyperpigmentation of a sector of the iris (e.g., focal melanosis) or a relative hypopigmentation of a portion of iris, as is seen in partial albinism. A clinically insignificant sector of hyperpigmentation in one or both irises is extremely common, occurring in as much as 75% of the population. Although usually occurring spontaneously and sporadically, uniocular heterochromia iridis may be transmitted as a dominant trait. No significant clinical sequelae or associated ocular defects occur with uniocular heterochromia.

Heterochromia iridium is defined as a condition in which the two irises are of different colors. Binocular hetero-

[*] References 318, 335, 339, 341, 356, 357, 361, 362, 364, 368.

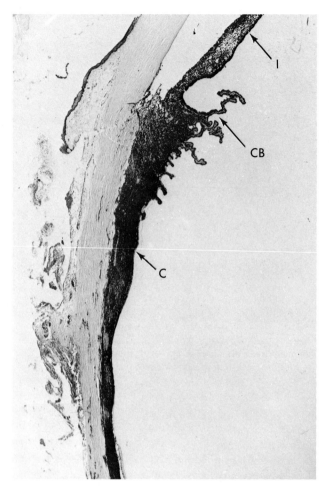

Fig. 2-51. Microscopic section of a globe with congenital oculodermal melanocytosis (nevus of Ota). Note the slight thickening and hyperpigmentation of the iris *(I)*, ciliary body stroma *(CB)*, and choroid *(C)*. This uveal pigmentation is associated with pigmentation in the episclera and conjunctiva and with pigmentation of the eyelid skin. (H & E stain; ×15.)

chromia iridis may occur in a simple form, either sporadically or in an inherited pattern. It is much more common among animals than humans. A relative hyperpigmentation (darker iris) of an iris may occur as a result of many conditions, including congenital ocular or oculodermal melanocytosis, diffuse iris nevus or melanoma (p. 308), ICE syndrome, paradoxical Fuchs' heterochromic iridocyclitis, post-traumatic hemorrhage with deposition of blood breakdown products; in association with melanocytic neoplasms (nevi and malignant melanoma) (p. 308); or after iron deposition or siderosis (p. 82). A relative hypopigmentation (lighter iris) is seen with Fuchs' heterochromic iridocyclitis, amelanotic tumor (nevus, melanoma, metastatic tumor) covering the iris, congenital or acquired Horner's syndrome, chronic iritis, juvenile xanthogranuloma (p. 294), and Waardenburg's syndrome.[337]

Heterochromic iridocyclitis of Fuchs* is one of the more common causes of heterochromia and usually occurs con-

---

* References 321, 331, 343, 351, 352, 354, 359.

genitally or in early life, although cases may develop later in life. Usually the iridocyclitis is mild and unilateral. The heterochromia is such that the involved iris is relatively depigmented and becomes the lighter iris. (The same is true in the heterochromia iridis caused by sympathoparesis associated with Horner's syndrome that is congenital or acquired in infancy.) The hypochromia of the involved eye results from iris stromal atrophy and stromal pigment loss. Secondary glaucoma and cataract are important accompanying features.

Histopathologically, rubeosis iridis, a chronic inflammation within the iris and ciliary body, and stromal atrophy of the iris develop. The atrophy may be so severe that the posterior iris pigment epithelium may become visible, resulting in a paradoxical heterochromia in which the involved eye becomes the darker eye. The anterior segment cellular infiltrate usually is very rich in plasma cells. In addition, inflammatory cell infiltrates occur within the trabeculum and keratitic precipitates form on the posterior corneal surface. Unlike other diseases associated with iris neovascularizations, peripheral anterior synechiae are conspicuously absent. Therefore, the glaucoma probably is a result of the infiltration of cells within the trabecular meshwork. Fortunately, cataract surgery using modern extracapsular techniques, phacoemulsification, and posterior chamber intraocular lens implantation can be performed safely in most patients with this condition.

Chromosomal anomalies[369-447]

The normal diploid human cell possesses 46 chromosomes* 23 are derived from each parent. Of the 46 chromosomes, 44 are autosomes, and 2, the X and Y chromosomes, are the sex chromosomes.

Chromosomes may be isolated from a cell nucleus and stained in metaphase. Such a preparation is called a metaphase plate (Fig. 2-52). The chromosomes may be arranged in a systemic manner in relation to size and shape variations. This arrangement is termed a karyotype: 46 XX signifies 46 chromosomes with a female pattern; 46 XY signifies a male karyotype.

Abnormalities of many of the chromosomes produce ocular defects.† However, three trisomies are particularly relevant for the ophthalmologist because of their high incidence in the population and their characteristic eye findings: trisomies 13, 18, and 21. The most pronounced changes are found in persons with trisomy 13, and the least are found in trisomy 21. Most authors agree that the process of nondisjunction during gametogenesis (Fig. 2-53) is responsible for the creation of the trisomies. Apple and associates[372] have reported a full-blown case of this syndrome in conjunction with an unbalanced D3/D (13/13) translocation.

TRISOMY 13

Trisomy 13 (Patau's syndrome)‡ is the chromosomal aberration most closely associated with severe intraocular ab-

---

* References 371, 374, 393, 407, 413, 430, 442, 445, 446.
† References 369, 379, 386-388, 390, 395, 400, 405, 406, 411, 412, 414, 418, 419, 427, 431, 438.
‡ References 372, 396, 399, 402-404, 415, 420, 423, 424, 427, 428, 435, 436, 441, 443, 444.

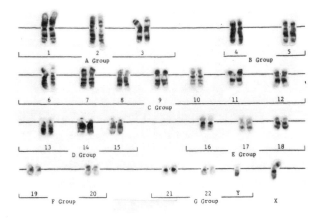

Fig. 2-52. Chromosome analysis by karyotyping showing G-banding pattern. Chromosomes are arrested during cell division in metaphase. They are then separated from the cell nucleus, isolated on a slide, and stained, forming a karyotype. This normal male karyotype shows 22 pairs of autosomes, one X chromosome, and one Y chromosome. The G-banding (Giemsa) technique provides easy identification of each chromosome and the means for recognition of chromosome abnormalities ranging from minute defects to complex rearrangements. (Courtesy Drs. John Carey and Stephen Gieser, University of Utah School of Medicine.)

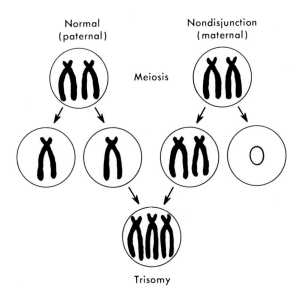

Fig. 2-53. Mechanism of trisomy formation. During reduction division (gamete formation), each sperm or egg normally acquires one member of each chromosome group. If nondisjunction occurs, the daughter cell acquires both members of the pair and, after fertilization, forms an anomalous pattern with three members. (From Gieser SC, Apple DJ, and Carey JC: Pathology of chromosome-induced ocular disease. In Goldberg MF and Renie W, editors: Genetic and metabolic eye disease, ed 2, Boston, 1985, Little, Brown & Co.)

normalities (Figs. 2-54 to 2-58). Most affected infants die in the first few months of life. Therefore, this condition rarely is seen in the ophthalmologic clinic or office. It is observed more frequently by the pediatrician or the pathologist at necropsy. However, the presence of the wide vari-

ety of embryonic defects observed in this syndrome renders it highly instructive as a model demonstrating the pathogenesis of several various forms of congenital ocular disease.

Modern techniques of chromosome analysis enabled Patau and coworkers[424] in 1960 to formulate one unifying pathogenetic basis to what had been a chaotic, heterogeneous, uncategorized complex of abnormalities (reviewed by Gieser et al[393]). Patau and colleagues correlated this complex of abnormalities with a specific chromosomal abnormality based on a nondisjunction-induced trisomy of the acrocentric chromosomes of the 13-15 (D) group. It has since been demonstrated by autoradiography that chromosome 13 (also termed D_1) is specifically involved (Fig. 2-54, *B*). A review of the numerous case reports published during the past century shows beyond doubt that even in the absence of karyotype confirmation, many of the cases described under varying nomenclatures actually represented unquestionable cases of trisomy 13.

Systemic findings of this syndrome include cleft lip and palate (Fig. 2-54), arrhinencephaly (holoprosencephaly; Fig. 2-55), syndactyly or polydactyly, cardiovascular anomalies, facial angiomas, cryptorchidism, transverse palmar creases, renal dysgenesis, and death in the first months of life.[371,420,436]

Bilateral ocular involvement (Figs. 2-56 to 2-58) is present in almost all cases of the full-blown trisomy 13 syndrome* (see the ocular findings list). Microphthalmia, which always is present, may be relatively mild or may be severe with an ocular diameter of less than 8 mm. When the eye is extremely small, this condition often is mistaken for anophthalmia.

Ocular findings[393]

1. Microphthalmia; sometimes apparent (clinical) anophthalmia.
2. Colobomas (usually of ciliary body and iris, less commonly of fundus and optic nerve) are seen in almost all affected eyes.
3. Persistent hyperplastic primary vitreous (communication of extraocular connective tissue of mesodermal origin with intraocular hyaloid system and tunica vasculosa lentis via ciliary body coloboma; sometimes pigmented).
4. Intraocular cartilage formed in mesoderm within the ciliary body coloboma; ingrowth of uveal melanocytes into globe through the coloboma.
5. Retinal dysplasia, including abnormal, anteriorly dislocated sensory retinal tissue formed over pars plana.
6. Cataracts; primary aphakia (rare).
7. Rudimentary differentiation of angle structures.
8. Corneal opacities; posterior corneal ulcers (rare).
9. Optic nerve hypoplasia, atrophy; occasional coloboma of the optic nerve.
10. Cyclopia (rare).

The myriad lesions seen in eyes affected by trisomy 13 are best explained by regarding the basic pathogenetic defect as a deviation from the pathway of normal tissue migration and closure of the ocular fissure during the first 6 weeks of gestation. Very small, retarded eyes that exhibit severe widespread abnormalities result from grossly abnor-

---

* References 371, 372, 396, 404, 413, 428, 444.

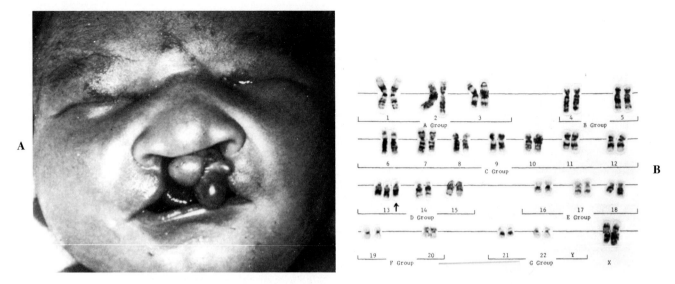

Fig. 2-54. A, The facies of an infant with trisomy D₁ is characterized by a microphthalmia or apparent anophthalmia and defective fusion of facial midline structures, leading to formation of cleft palate and lip. **B,** Karyotype of trisomy 13 showing an extra chromosome 13 *(arrow).* The extra chromosome produces a state of aneuploidy (2n + 1), or a total of 47 chromosomes. **(A** from Gieser SC, Apple DJ, and Carey JC: Pathology of chromosome-induced ocular disease. In Goldberg MF and Renie W, editors: Genetic and metabolic eye disease, ed 2, Boston, 1985, Little, Brown & Co; **B** courtesy Dr. John Carey, University of Utah School of Medicine.)

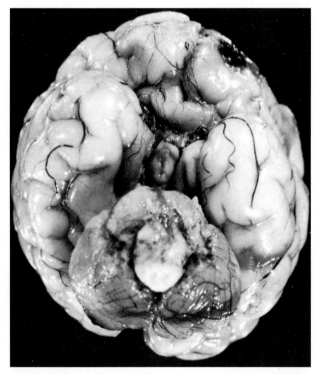

Fig. 2-55. Base of the brain from a patient who died of trisomy 13. The frontal lobes are fused (holoprosencephaly), and the olfactory nerve is absent (arrhinencephaly). The optic nerve and chiasm have been removed. (From Gieser SC, Apple DJ, and Carey JC: Pathology of chromosome-induced ocular disease. In Goldberg MF and Renie W, editors: Genetic and metabolic eye disease, ed 2, Boston, 1985, Little, Brown & Co.)

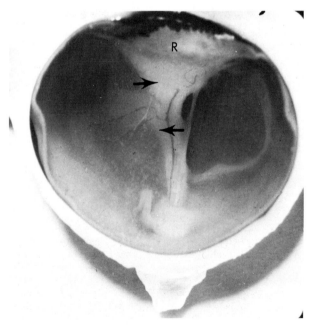

Fig. 2-56. Globe from a patient with trisomy 13. The funnel-shaped retinal detachment extends from the optic nerve to the retrolental region. The retrolental mass *(R)* is composed of a persistent tunica vasculosa lentis (primary vitreous) as well as dysplastic retina. *Arrows,* Persistent embryonic hyaloid artery. (From Gieser SC, Apple DJ, and Carey JC: Pathology of chromosome-induced ocular disease. In Goldberg MF and Renie W, editors: Genetic and metabolic eye disease, ed 2, Boston, 1985, Little, Brown & Co.)

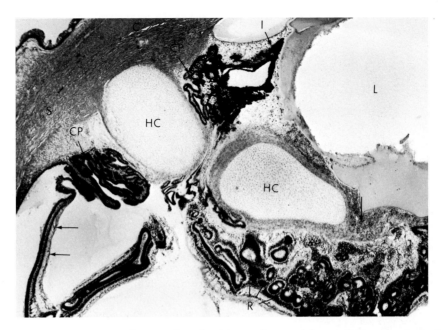

Fig. 2-57. Trisomy 13. Hyaline cartilage *(HC)* lies within a coloboma of the ciliary body. The colobomatous defect is demarcated by a large gap in the epithelium of the ciliary processes *(CP)*. The cornea *(C)* and sclera *(S)* communicate with the retrolental persistent hyperplastic primary vitreous *(right arrow)* through the colobomatous gap. *I*. Malformed iris rudiment. The bulk of the retrolental mass is composed of dysplastic retina characterized by rosette formation *(R)*. The sensory retina *(left arrows)* has developed in lieu of normal simple cuboidal epithelium at the parts plana, a feature often seen in this syndrome. The lens *(L)* artifactitiously shattered during preparation. (H & E stain; ×10.) (From Gieser SC, Apple DJ, and Carey JC: Pathology of chromosome-induced ocular disease. In Goldberg MF and Renie W, editors: Genetic and metabolic eye disease, ed 2, Boston, 1985, Little, Brown & Co.)

mal, misdirected invagination of the optic vesicle. In almost all instances the embryonic ocular fissure fails to close. This usually is manifest as a typical coloboma of the iris and ciliary body (Fig. 2-57). This primary neuroectodermal aberration is largely responsible for the initiation of the secondary changes creating the total clinicopathologic picture.

Two major intraocular findings of trisomy 13 relate to aberrations in tissue induction along the locus of the colobomatous defect: cartilage formation and retinal dysplasia.

Although the presence of intraocular cartilage has been noted in microphthalmic eyes in otherwise healthy individuals[443] (most cases of severe microphthalmia with severe ocular disorganization must have represented bona fide cases of trisomy 13) by many investigators for many years, the association of intraocular cartilage with the trisomy 13 syndrome only recently has been emphasized. The cartilage typically is situated within the ciliary body coloboma (Figs. 2-57 and 7-25).

Although ocular cartilage has been reported in embryonal medulloepithelioma (p. 330), in chromosome 18 deletion defect, in angiomatosis retinae, and in an otherwise healthy individual,[443] it is not present in these conditions within a coloboma of the ciliary body. Therefore, intraocular cartilage within a coloboma of the ciliary body seems to be diagnostic of trisomy 13.

The mass of dysplastic retina, which produces a clinical leukokoria (see Chapter 9), is easily visible grossly as a funnel-shaped white retrolental mass (Fig. 2-56). Because it presents several interesting patterns microscopically that

have intrigued investigators for years, it probably is the most frequently described and best known component of the trisomy 13 syndrome. In the prekaryotype era, the disease often was termed the *retinal dysplasia syndrome*. Retinal dysplasia (p. 401), defined simply as abnormal growth and differentiation of embryonic retina, is best considered to be a lesion, not a specific disease. If a noxious insult affects the retina before a certain point in gestation, dysplastic growth of the embryonic neuroepithelial cells occurs.

Regardless of the disease, histopathologic analysis of globes affected with retinal dysplasia may reveal several morphologic patterns (Figs. 2-57 and 2-58; also see Figs. 8-53, 8-54, and 9-37). These include (1) rosette formation (an abortive attempt to form retinal rods and cones); (2) aimless proliferations of ciliary epithelium, both pigmented and nonpigmented; (3) proliferation of cords of tissue that closely resemble primitive optic cup neuroepithelium; and (4) aberrant formation of glial tissue.

Abnormalities of the 13 chromosome, particularly 13 group deletion, also have been described in association with retinoblastoma. The "malignant" Flexner-Wintersteiner rosette of retinoblastoma is compared with the "benign" dysplastic rosette on page 486 and in Figs. 9-10 and 9-11.

Anomalous differentiation of the anterior chamber angle is a constant finding in trisomy 13. In severe cases of the trisomy 13 syndrome, there is almost complete absence of anterior chamber angle filtration structures. Figure 6-19

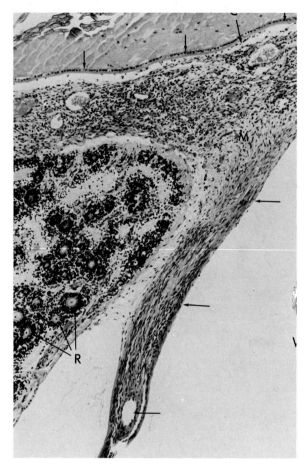

Fig. 2-58. Trisomy 13. This photomicrograph of the retrolental region demonstrates a persistent hyperplastic primary vitreous. The hyaloid artery *(arrows*—note cross-section of the lumen by the bottom arrow) is continuous anteriorly with the retrolental fibrous membrane *(M),* a remnant of the tunica vasculosa lentis. The lens is cataractous, as indicated by migration of lens epithelium to the posterior pole *(small arrows).* The retinal dysplasia is focused with rosettes *(R)* at the left. *C,* Lens capsule; *V,* vitreous. (H & E stain; ×63.) (From Gieser SC, Apple DJ, and Carey JC: Pathology of chromosome-induced ocular disease. In Goldberg MF and Renie W, editors: Genetic and metabolic eye disease, ed 2, Boston, 1985, Little, Brown & Co.)

shows faulty cleavage of the mesoderm, which normally is destined to form the iris and the collagenous structures of the corneoscleral junction, including the trabecular meshwork. There is total absence of Schlemm's canal in this illustration. Most cases of trisomy 13, however, do not develop the full-blown picture of congenital or infantile glaucoma because the syndrome almost invariably is associated with maldevelopment of the ciliary processes, which thus may secrete an inadequate amount of aqueous. Also, patients affected with this syndrome rarely live more than a few months and therefore there is not time for sequelae of increased intraocular pressure to develop.

TRISOMY 18[*]

In 1960, Edwards and coworkers[384] described a new syndrome associated with trisomy of an E group chromosome.

---

[*] References 376, 384, 389, 391, 397, 401, 402, 408, 421, 429, 436.

Cytologic studies have demonstrated that the extra chromosome is number 18. The trisomy probably results from a nondisjunction in gametogenesis.

Trisomy 18 is second only to trisomy 21 as the most frequently occurring autosomal trisomy in newborns. Estimates of its frequency range from 1 in 3500 births to 1 in 14,000 births. Female infants are three times more likely to have this trisomy. Affected infants often are born to women of advanced maternal age and have a limited capacity for survival. More than 50% of these patients die within 2 months of birth, and only 1 in 10 survive the first year of life. The oldest patient reported with trisomy 18 was 15 years of age.

The systemic findings are characteristic, particularly the facies, the shape of the cranium, the low-set, malformed ears, and the finger and foot deformities.

Initial reports emphasized the clinical ocular findings. Ginsberg and coworkers[397] presented the first comprehensive study of the ocular histopathology of trisomy 18. Subsequently, many additional ocular pathologic findings have been described. The most commonly reported affected ocular structures appear to be the cornea (see Fig. 3-53), the anterior uveal tract, the lens, and the retina. Anomalies of all corneal layers have been described. Immaturity of the angle structures and anomalies of the ciliary process and iris frequently are described. Cataractous changes also have been noted. Retinal folds are the single most common histopathologic finding. Other common retinal observations are hypopigmentation of the posterior pigment epithelium, dysplasia, and areas of hemorrhage and gliosis.

Because one third of trisomy 18 babies are born prematurely, differentiation of the pathologic changes of this syndrome from those of prematurity alone is important. For example, at birth, the corneal stroma and choroid show increased cellularity. During the ninth month in the healthy fetus, anterior chamber mesoderm has disappeared only up to the trabecular meshwork, and certain ciliary muscle fibers still are developing. The hyaloid system does not fully disappear until the middle of the eighth month of gestation. Exact determination of fetal age and a variability in ocular development may lead to difficulties in interpretation of several of the reported findings. However, the presence of colobomas or retinal dysplasia, for example, clearly is pathologic, whereas incomplete angle cleavage or corneal stromal hypercellularity may represent developmental findings alone.

Systemic findings[371]

General

Death within first year of life
Mental deficiency, delay of psychomotor development
Decreased growth rate
Cardiac abnormalities
Cryptorchidism
Inguinal or umbilical hernia
Musculoskeletal system
Hypoplasia of skeletal muscle and subcutaneous and adipose tissue
Prominent occiput, narrow bifrontal diameter
Low-set, malformed ears
Micrognathia, receding chin
Small oral opening (microstomia) with narrow palatal arch

Hypertonicity with limbs in flexion; flexion contractures of the
  fingers (camptodactyly)
Clenched hand with tendency for overlapping of index finger over
  third, fifth finger over fourth
Rocker-bottom feet
Small pelvis with limited hip abduction
Hypoplasia of nails, especially on fifth finger and toes

Ocular findings[397,408,421]

Prominent epicanthal folds
Blepharophimosis with unusually small or oblique palpebral fis-
  sures
Unusually thick lower lid
Ptosis; exophthalmos
Hypertelorism; occasional hypotelorism
Hypoplastic supraorbital ridges
Corneal and lens opacities with thickening of Bowman's layer
  (Fig. 3-53)
Microphthalmia
Congenital glaucoma
Uveal colobomas
Myopia
PHPV
Retinal folds and dysplasia

TRISOMY 21 (DOWN SYNDROME)*

  The chromosomal basis of Down syndrome[383,425,447] was
predicted in 1932 by Waardenburg.[438] This astute prediction, made long before human chromosome analysis was
clinically available, was confirmed by Lejeune and coworker-
ers in 1959 (reviewed by Gieser et al[393]). They confirmed
the basic chromosome abnormality of Down syndrome as
an aneuploidy (abnormal number of chromosomes) consisting of 47 chromosomes rather than the normal 46.
Down syndrome is by far the most common autosomal
trisomy condition. In children of younger mothers, the condition is seen in as high as 1 in 600 births. The incidence
sharply increases to 1 in 40 births when the maternal age
is 45 years or older.[377]

  Following are the systemic findings of Down syndrome
(Fig. 2-59) and the general ocular and adnexal abnormalities.[370,371,380,381,385,432,434]

Systemic findings

General

With respect to prognosis, two populations: one with significant
  mortality the first year, the other living into adulthood
Mental deficiency; often euphoria
Small stature
Defective, awkward gait
Cardiac abnormalities
Dry, rough skin
Susceptibility to stress and infection

Head

Brachycephaly
Thin cranium; delayed fontanelle closure
Frontal and perinasal sinus hypoplasia
Small nose with low nasal bridge
Small, round external ear with defective lobules

---

* References 370, 373, 375, 377, 378, 380-383, 385, 392, 394, 398, 403,
409, 410, 416, 417, 422, 425, 426, 432-434, 437, 439, 440, 447.

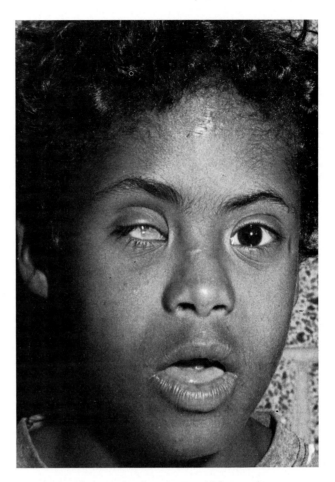

Fig. 2-59. Photograph of a 12-year-old boy with Down syndrome showing several of the classic facial features, including
epicanthus, small nose with low nasal bridge, tendency to open
mouth, and a short neck. This child also had a congenital cataract
in the right eye and at age 5 underwent lens extraction with
insertion of an intraocular lens. Although temporary success was
achieved, visual loss rapidly ensued less than a year after surgery.
The eye has had no light perception for almost 7 years. It now
shows a disfiguring phthisis bulbi with corneal opacification and
associated ptosis.

Tendency toward open mouth, with a thick, roughened protrud-
  ing tongue
Dental hypoplasia
Short, thick neck

Trunk and extremities

Hypotonia; hyperextensible joints
Pelvic hypoplasia
Diastasis recti abdominis
Small, broad, stubby hands, incurved little finger
Characteristic dermatoglyphic findings (simian crease)
Short, broad feet with poorly developed arch, wide gap beneath
  first and second toes

Genitourinary system

Renal hemangiomas
Infertility
Undescended testes
Absent or defective spermatogenesis
Abnormal development of labia

Irregular menses
Ovarian hypoplasia

Gastrointestinal system
Duodenal atresia
Cleft lip and palate

Ocular findings

General ocular and adnexal abnormalities
Mongoloid slant (palpebral fissures slant upward and outward)
Almond-shaped palpebral fissure
Epicanthus
External hypertelorism
Narrowed interpupillary distance
Convergent strabismus (35%)
Blepharitis
Ectropion
Myopia

Specific intraocular pathologic lesions
Cataracts (60%); develop after 8 to 10 years of age
Brushfield's spot (85%) (24% of healthy persons also)
Iris hypoplasia (usually peripheral iris)
Keratoconus, sometimes acute; occurs in adults

The most commonly observed clinically significant intraocular lesions are cataracts, iris lesions, and keratoconus.[380]

Cataracts

The cataracts of persons with Down syndrome are of many diverse types and are best observed by slit-lamp biomicroscopy rather than by examination of pathologic specimens.[378] They usually become manifest after puberty. Attempts have been made to remove these cataracts early in life and insert an intraocular lens, but results have been disappointing to date (Fig. 2-59). Following are the three main groups of lens opacity[416,417]:

1. Arcuate opacities, the most distinctive type. The opaque lens fibers arch around the equator of the early layers of the fetal nucleus. Such cataracts may form in relation to abnormal capsulopupillary vessels of the tunica vasculosa lentis (p. 29); the embryonic vessels normally are transient and should begin a regression in the fourth fetal month. This type of cataract is the earliest to be seen in Down syndrome.

2. Sutural cataracts (Fig. 4-31, *B*). Although such opacities are typically observed along the line of the original Y sutures formed before birth, they are seldom seen early. They become manifest much later, often in the teens.

3. Flake opacities. The nature of this type of cataract remains obscure. Many are deep to the capsule, but in a certain percentage the lens capsule has true thickenings of excrescences. Flake opacities are also observed in Lowe's syndrome (p. 125).

Iris lesions

Brushfield's spots occur in 85% to 90% of persons with Down syndrome, whereas healthy individuals show an incidence of only 24% or less.[375,382] Such spots in healthy persons are often termed *Wolfflin-Kruckmann spots*. The irises in Down syndrome generally contain a greater number of spots than in healthy individuals. Brushfield's spots commonly are found in the midzone, whereas the spots

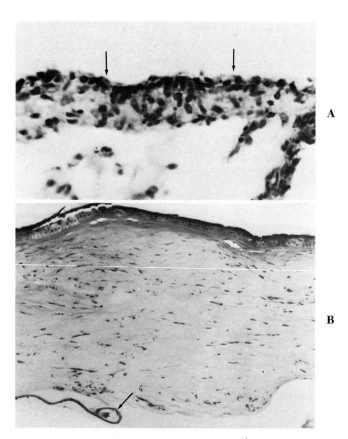

Fig. 2-60. Down syndrome. **A,** Brushfield's spot. Anterior iris surface with proliferation of sheets of stromal cells *(arrows)*. (H & E stain; ×250.) **B,** Acute keratoconus with corneal edema and scarring and rupture of Descemet's membrane *(arrow)* (see also p. 85). (H & E stain; ×175.) (From Gieser SC, Apple DJ, and Carey JC: Pathology of chromosome-induced ocular disease. In Goldberg MF and Renie W, editors: Genetic and metabolic eye disease, ed 2, Boston, 1985, Little, Brown & Co.)

found in healthy individuals are situated more peripherally. Spotting occurs almost as frequently in brown-eyed as in blue-eyed patients with Down syndrome.

Histopathologically, a Brushfield spot consists of an increased density of connective tissue cells on the anterior surface of the stroma (Fig. 2-60, *A*). This tissue is not only white of itself but also covers and shields the pigmented layers of the iris.

Keratoconus

Keratoconus (see also Chapter 3) occurs in approximately 5% of persons with Down syndrome. Nonaffected patients have a much lower incidence of keratoconus. Acute keratoconus (corneal hydrops) is a rare condition in any circumstance, but it is now well established that the acute form is seen with far greater frequency in individuals with Down syndrome than in the general population.

In its initial stages, simple keratoconus is characterized pathologically by fragmentation of the corneal epithelial basement membrane and fibrillation of Bowman's layer and the anterior stroma. Eventual thinning of the entire corneal stroma can occur, especially at the apex of the cone. Ruptures and folds in Descement's membrane often lead to a disturbance in corneal hydration, resulting in either chronic edema of the cone or, as is seen with greater frequency in patients with Down syndrome, the full-blown syndrome of acute keratoconus (Fig. 2-60, *B*).

REFERENCES

Introduction

1. Apple DJ and Boutros GJ: Visual impairments. In Abroms KI and Bennett JW, editors: New directions for exceptional children: genetics and exceptional children, San Francisco, 1981, Jossey-Bass, Inc, Publishers.
2. Apple DJ and Bennett TO: Multiple systemic and ocular malformations associated with maternal LSD usage, Arch Ophthalmol 92:302, 1974.
3. Apple DJ, Rabb MF, and Walsh PM: Congenital anomalies of the optic disc, Surv Ophthalmol 27:3, 1982.
4. Blodi FC and Allen L: Stereoscopic manual of the ocular fundus in local and systemic disease, vol I, St Louis, 1964, The CV Mosby Co.
5. Bogdanoff B and others: Brain and eye abnormalities: possible sequelae to prenatal use of multiple drugs including LSD, Am J Dis Child 123:145, 1972.
6. Brodsky MC: Congenital optic disk anomalies: major review, Surv Ophthalmol 39:89, 1994.
7. Brown G and Tasman W: Congenital anomalies of the optic disk, New York, 1983, Grune & Stratton, Inc.
8. Carones FC, and others: Corneal endothelial anomalies in the fetal alcohol syndrome, Arch Ophthalmol 110:1128, 1992.
9. Chan CC, Fishman M, Egbert PR: Multiple ocular anomalies associated with maternal LSD ingestion, Arch Ophthalmol 96:282, 1978.
10. Cook CS, Nowotny AZ, and Sulik KK: Fetal alcohol syndrome: eye malformations in a mouse model, Arch Ophthalmol 105:1576, 1987.
11. Daicker B: Anatomie und Pathologie der Menschlichen retinoziliaren Fundusperipherie, Basel, 1972, S Karger, AG.
12. Deutman A: The hereditary dystrophies of the posterior pole of the eye, Assen, The Netherlands, 1971, Van Gorcum, BV.
13. Donaldson D: Atlas of external diseases of the eye, vol I, Congenital anomalies and systemic diseases, St. Louis, 1966, The CV Mosby Co.
14. Duke-Elder S: System of ophthalmology, vol III, Normal and abnormal development, part 2, Congenital deformities, St. Louis, 1963, The CV Mosby Co.
15. Edward DP and others: Diffuse corneal clouding in siblings with fetal alcohol syndrome, Am J Ophthalmol 115:484, 1993.
16. Francois J: Heredity in ophthalmology, St. Louis, 1961, The CV Mosby Co.
17. Goldberg M: An introduction to basic genetic principles applied to ophthalmology, Trans Am Acad Ophthalmol Otolaryngol 76:1137, 1972.
18. Goldberg MF, editor: Genetic and metabolic eye disease, Boston, 1974, Little, Brown & Co.
19. Goldberg MF and Renie W, editors: Genetic and metabolic eye disease, ed 2, Boston, 1984, Little, Brown & Co.
20. Goodman R: Genetic disorders of man, Boston, 1970, Little, Brown & Co.
21. von Graefe A and Saemisch T: Handbuch der gesammten Augenheilkunde, Leipzig, 1874, Wilhelm Engelmann.
22. Harley RD, editor: Pediatric ophthalmology, Philadelphia, 1975, WB Saunders Co.
23. Harley RD: Pediatric ophthalmology, vols I and II, ed 2, Philadelphia, 1983, WB Saunders Co.
24. Kertesz ED and Falls HF: Genetic applications to pediatric ophthalmology. In Liebman SD and Gellis SS, editors: The pediatrician's ophthalmology, St. Louis, 1966, The CV Mosby Co.
25. Kollmann J: Handatlas der Entwicklungsgeschichte des Menschen, Jena, 1907, Gustav Fischer.
26. Mann I: Developmental abnormalities of the eye, ed 2, Philadelphia, 1957, JB Lippincott Co.
27. Meyer E and others: Eye pathology in anencephalic babies, Ophthalmic Paediatr Genet 1:219, 1982.
28. Meyner E: Atlas der Spaltlampenphotographie, Stuttgart, 1976, Ferdinand Enke Verlag.

29. Miller MT: Thalidomide embryopathy: a model for the study of congenital incomitant horizontal strabismus, Trans Am Ophthalmol Soc 89:623, 1991.
30. Miller MT, Stromland K: Ocular motility in thalidomide embryopathy, J Pediatr Ophthalmol Strabis 28:47, 1991.
31. Milunsky A: The prenatal diagnosis of hereditary disorders, Springfield, III, 1973, Charles C Thomas, Publisher.
32. Naumann GOH and Apple DJ: Pathology of the eye, New York, 1985, Springer-Verlag, Inc. (Translation, modification, and update of Pathologie des Auges by DJ Apple.)
33. New Orleans Academy of Ophthalmology: Symposium on surgical and medical management of congenital anomalies of the eye: transactions of the New Orleans Academy of Ophthalmology, St. Louis, 1968, The CV Mosby Co.
34. Oeller J: Atlas seltener ophthalmoskopischer Befunde, Wiesbaden, 1903, JF Bergmann.
35. Ophthalmologic Staff of the Hospital for Sick Children, Toronto: The eye in childhood, Chicago, 1967, Year Book Medical Publishers, Inc.
36. Pe'er J and BenEzra D: Heterotopic smooth muscle in the choroid of two patients with cryptophthalmos, Arch Ophthalmol 104:1665, 1986.
37. Streissguth AP and others: Fetal alcohol syndrome in adolescents and adults, JAMA 265:1961, 1991.
38. Strömland K: Contribution of ocular examination to the diagnosis of foetal alcohol syndrome in mentally retarded children, J Ment Def Res 34:429, 1990.
39. Tasmen W: Retinal diseases in children, New York, 1971, Harper & Row, Publishers.
40. Waardenburg P, Franceschetti A, and Klein D: Genetics and ophthalmology, vol 2, Springfield, III, 1963, Charles C Thomas, Publisher.
41. Warburg M: Diagnosis of metabolic eye diseases, Copenhagen, 1972, Munksgaard, International Booksellers & Publishers, Ltd.
42. Warkany J: Congenital malformations, Chicago, 1971, Year Book Medical Publishers, Inc.
43. Yanoff M, Fine BS, Gass JD: Ocular Pathology, ed 4, London, England, 1996, Mosby-Wolfe.
44. Zimmerman LE and Font R: Congenital malformations of the eye: some recent advances in knowledge of the pathogenesis and histopathological characteristics, JAMA 196:684, 1966.

Anophthalmia, cyclopia (synophthalmia), congenital cystic eye, and congenital nonattachment of the retina

45. Apple DJ, Rabb MF, and Walsh PM: Congenital anomalies of the optic disc, Surv Ophthalmol 27:3, 1982.
46. Arstikaitis MJ: Synophthalmia: a case report, J Pediatr Ophthalmol Strabismus 17:412, 1980.
47. Boniuk V, Ho PK: Ocular findings in anencephaly, Am J Ophthalmol 88:613, 1979.
48. Brunquell PJ and others: Sex-linked hereditary bilateral anophthalmos: pathologic and radiologic correlation, Arch Ophthalmol 102:108, 1984.
49. Collins E: On anophthalmus, Ophthalmol Hosp Rep 11:429, 1886.
50. Gupta SP and Saxena RC: Cryptophthalmos, Br J Ophthalmol 46:629, 1962.
51. Haberland C and Perou M: Primary bilateral anophthalmia, J Neuropathol Exp Neurol 28:337, 1969.
52. von Hippel E: Über Anophthalmus congenitus, Graefes Arch Ophthalmol 47:227, 1899.
53. Karseras AG, Laurence KM: Eyes in arrhinencephalic syndromes, Br J Ophthalmol 80:939, 1975.
54. Kinsey JA and Streeten BW: Ocular abnormalities in the median cleft face syndrome, Am J Ophthalmol 83:261, 1977.
55. Kuchle M, Kraus J, Rummelt C and others: Synophthalmia and holoprosencephaly in chromosome. 18p deletion defect. Arch Ophthalmol 109:136, 1991.
56. Pasquale LR, Nongart R, Kubacki J, Johnson MH, Chan GH: Congenital cystic eye with multiple ocular and intracranial anomalies, Arch Ophthalmol 109:985, 1991.
57. O'Ranilly R, Miller F: Interpretation of some median anomalies as illustrated by cyclopia and symmelia, Teratology 40:409, 1989.

58. Sassani JW and Yanoff M: Anophthalmos in an infant with multiple congenital anomalies, Am J Ophthalmol 83:43, 1977.
59. Torezynski E, Jakociec FA, Johnston MC and others: Synophthalmia and cyclopia: a histopathologic, radiographic, and organogenetic analysis, Doc Ophthalmol 44,2:311, 1977.
60. Vare AM: Cyclopia, Am J Ophthalmol 75:880, 1973.
61. Yanko L and Zaifrani S: Synophthalmos in a fullterm newborn child: an anatomic and pathologic study, J Pediatr Ophthalmol 10:65, 1973.

Typical colobomas

62. Apple DJ: New aspects of colobomas and optic nerve anomalies, Int Ophthalmol Clin 24(1):109, 1984.
63. Apple DJ: Pathologie des Nervus opticus unter besonderer Berücksichtigung kolobomatöser Anomalien, Fortschr Ophthalmol 80:19, 1983.
64. Apple DJ and Bennett TO: Multiple systemic and ocular malformations associated with maternal LSD usage, Arch Ophthalmol 92: 301, 1974.
65. Apple DJ and Bennett TO: Multiple systemic and ocular malformations associated with maternal LDS usage (letter), Arch Ophthalmol 93:1061, 1975.
66. Apple DJ and others: Anomalous intraocular and periocular formation of adipose tissue, Am J Ophthalmol 94:344, 1982.
67. Bock E: Die angeborenen Kolobome des Augapfels, Vienna, 1893, Joseph Safar.
68. Casanovas J and Carbonell M: Malformaciones oculares en la embriopatia thalidomidica, Arch Soc Oftalmol Hisp Am 24:947, 1964.
69. Chan CC, Fishman M, and Egbert PR: Multiple ocular anomalies associated with maternal LSD ingestion, Arch Ophthalmol 96:282, 1978.
70. Chestler RJ and France TD: Ocular findings in CHARGE syndrome, Ophthalmology 95:1613, 1988.
71. Coats G: The pathology of coloboma at the nerve entrance, R Lond Ophthalmol Hosp Rep 17:178, 1908.
72. Crawford B: Heterotopic adipose tissue and smooth muscle in the optic disc, Arch Ophthalmol 88:139, 1972.
73. Del Pero RA and others: Anomalies of retinal architecture in Aicardi syndrome, Arch Ophthalmol 104:1659, 1986.
74. Font R and Zimmerman LE: Intrascleral smooth muscle in coloboma of the optic disc: electron microscopic verification, Am J Ophthalmol 72:452, 1971.
75. Font RI and others: Aicardi syndrome: a clinicopathologic case report including electron microscopic observations, Ophthalmology 98:1727, 1991.
76. Foxman S and Cameron JD: The clinical implications of bilateral microphthalmos with cyst, Am J Ophthalmol 97:632, 1984.
77. Goldberg M and McKusick V: X-linked colobomatous microphthalmos and other congenital anomalies, Am J Ophthalmol 71: 1128, 1971.
78. Gopal L and others: Pattern of retinal breaks and retinal detachments in eyes with choroidal coloboma, Ophthalmology 98:1727, 1991.
79. von Hippel E: Embryologischen Untersuchungen über die Entstehungsweise der typischen angeborenen Spaltbildung (Kolobome) des Augapfels, Graefes Arch Ophthalmol 55:507, 1903.
80. Hird B: An exhaustive treatise on the various colobomas, Ophthalmol Rev 31:162, 1912.
81. Hoyt CS and others: Ocular features of Aicardi's syndrome, Arch Ophthalmol 96:291, 1978.
82. Mann I: Coloboma iridis and its embryology, Trans Ophthalmol Soc UK 44:161, 1924.
83. Margolis S, Scher BM, and Carr RE: Macular colobomas in Leber's congenital amaurosis, Am J Ophthalmol 83:27, 1977.
84. McDonald HR and others: Vitreous surgery for retinal detachment associated with choroidal coloboma, Arch Ophthalmol 109:1399, 1991.
85. Mullaney J: Complex sporadic colobomata, Br J Ophthalmol 62:384, 1978.
86. Pagon RA: Ocular coloboma, Surv Ophthalmol 25:223, 1981.
87. Pasman FMH and Pinckers A: Hereditary macular coloboma, Ophthalmic Paediatr Genet 2:67, 1983.
88. Smith B and Guberina C: Coloboma in progressive hemifacial atrophy, Am J Ophthalmol 84:85, 1977.

89. Soong HK and Raizman MB: Corneal changes in familial iris coloboma, Ophthalmology 93:335, 1986.
90. von Szily A: Die Ontogenese der Iriskolobom, Klin Monatsbl Augenheilkd 45:422, 1907.
91. von Szily A: Die Ontogenese der idiotypischen (erbbildlichen) Spaltbildungen des Auges, des Mikrophthalmus und der Orbitalcysten, Z Ges Anat 74:1, 1924.
92. Warburg M: Diagnostic precision in microphthalmos and coloboma of heterogeneous origin, Ophthalmic Paediatr Genet 1:37, 1981.
93. Weber RG, Lovrien EW, and Isom JB: Aicardi's syndrome, Arch Ophthalmol 96:285, 1978.
94. Willis R and others: Heterotopic adipose tissue and smooth muscle in the optic disc: association with isolated colobomas, Arch Ophthalmol 88:139, 1972.

Morning glory syndrome

95. Akiyama K, Azuma N, Hida T, and others: Retinal detachment in morning glory syndrome, Ophthal Surg 15:841, 1984.
96. Apple DJ and others: Intra- and periocular infiltration of heteroplastic adipose tissue, Am J Ophthalmol 94:344, 1982.
97. Beyer WB, Quencer RM, and Osher RH: Morning glory syndrome: a functional analysis including fluorescein angiography, ultrasonography, and computerized tomography, Ophthalmology 89:1362, 1982.
98. Chang S and others: Treatment of total retinal detachment in morning glory syndrome, Am J Ophthalmol 97:596, 1984.
99. Cogan DG: Coloboma of optic nerve with overlay of peripapillary retina, Br J Ophthalmol 62:347, 1978.
100. Corbett JJ and others: Cavitary developmental defects of the optic disc: visual loss associated with optic pits and colobomas, Neurology 37:210, 1980.
101. Eustis HS, Sanders MR, and Zimmerman T: Morning glory syndrome in children. Arch Ophthalmol 112:204, 1994.
102. Goldhammer Y and Smith JL: Optic nerve anomalies in basal encephalocele, Arch Ophthalmol 93:115, 1975.
103. Haik BG and others: Retinal detachment in the morning glory anomaly, Ophthalmology 91:1638, 1984.
104. Hamada S and Ellsworth RM: Congenital retinal detachment and the optic disc anomaly, Am J Ophthalmol 71:460, 1971.
105. Handmann M: Erbliche, vermutlich angeborene zentrale gliose Entartung des Sehnerven mit besonderer Beteilingung der Zentralgefasse, Klin Monatsbl Augenheilkd 83:145, 1929.
106. Jensen PE and Kalina RE: Congenital anomalies of the optic disk, Am J Ophthalmol 82:27, 1976.
107. Kawano K and Fujita S: Duane's retraction syndrome associated with morning glory syndrome, J Pediatr Ophthalmol Strabismus 18: 51, 1981.
108. Kindler P: Morning glory syndrome: unusual congenital optic disk anomaly, Am J Ophthalmol 69:376, 1970.
109. Koenig SG, Naidich TP, and Lissner G: The morning glory syndrome associated with sphenoidal encephalocele, Ophthalmology 89:1368, 1982.
110. Krause U: Three cases of the morning glory syndrome, Acta Ophthalmol 50:188, 1972.
111. Pedler C: Unusual coloboma of the optic nerve entrance, Br J Ophthalmol 45:803, 1961.
112. Reis W: Eine wenig bekannte typische Missbildung am Sehnerveneintritte, Unschriebene Augenheilkd 19:505, 1908.
113. Rieger G: Zum Krankheitsbild der Handmannschen Sehnervenanomalie: "Windenbl⟨um⟩uten" ("morning glory") syndrome? Klin Monatsbl Augenheilkd 170:697, 1977.
114. Steinkuller PG: The morning glory disk anomaly: case report and literature review, J Pediatr Ophthalmol Strabismus 17:81, 1980.
115. von Fricken MA and Dhungel R: Retinal detachment in the morning glory syndrome: pathogenesis and management, Retina 4:97, 1984.

Congenital tilted disc syndrome

116. Berry H: Bitemporal depression of the visual fields due to an ocular cause, Br J Ophthalmol 47:441, 1963.
117. Caccamise WC: Situs inversus of the optic disc with inferior conus and variable myopia: a case report, Am J Ophthalmol 38:845, 1954.
118. Dorrell D: The tilted disc, Br J Ophthalmol 62:16, 1978.

119. Duke-Elder S and Wybar KC: System of ophthalmology, vol II, The anatomy of the visual system, St Louis, 1961, The CV Mosby Co.
120. Elschnig A: Colobom am Sehnerveneintritte und der Conus nach unten, Graefes Arch Ophthalmol 51:391, 1900.
121. Fuchs A: Atlas of the histopathology of the eye, vol 1, Leipzig, 1924, Franz Deuticke.
122. Fuchs E: Beitrag zu den Angeborenen Anomalien des Sehnerven, Graefes Arch Ophthalmol 28:139, 1882.
123. Graham MV and Wakefield GJ: Bitemporal visual field defects associated with anomalies of the optic disc, Br J Ophthalmol 57:307, 1973.
124. Hittner HM, Borda RP, and Justice J Jr: X-linked recessive congenital stationary night blindness, myopia, and tilted discs, J Pediatr Ophthalmol Strabismus 18:15, 1981.
125. Jaeger E: Ophthalmoskopischer Hand-Atlas, Leipzig, 1890, Franz Deuticke.
126. Malinowski SM and others: The protective effect of the tilted disc syndrome in diabetic retinopathy, Arch Ophthalmol 114:230, 1996.
127. Manor RS: Temporal field defects due to nasal tilting of discs, Ophthalmologica 168:269, 1974.
128. Odland M: Bitemporal defects of the visual fields due to anomalies of the optic discs, Acta Neurol Scand 43:630, 1967.
129. Pinckers A, Lion F, and Notting JGA: X-chromosomal recessive night blindness and tilted disk anomaly: a case report, Ophthalmologica 176:160, 1978.
130. Quevillon A, Brouillette G, and Aube M: Syndrome du tilted disc tomographie axiale: presentation d'un cas, Can J Ophthalmol 12:261, 1977.
131. Riise D: Visual field defects in optic disc malformation with ectasia of the fundus, Acta Ophthalmol 44:906, 1966.
132. Riise D: Neuro-ophthalmological patients with bitemporal hemianopsia: follow-up on etiology, Acta Ophthalmol 48:685, 1970.
133. Schmidt T: Perimetric relativer Skotome, Ophthalmologica 129:303, 1955.
134. von Szily A: Ueber den "Conus" in heterotypischer Richtung, Graefes Arch Ophthalmol 110:183, 1922.
135. von Szily A: Die Ontogenese der idiotypischen (erbbildlichen) Spaltbildungen des Auges, des Mikrophthalmus und der Orbitalcysten, Z Ges Anat 74:1, 1924.
136. Veirs ER: Inversio papillae with altitudinal fields: report of a case, Am J Ophthalmol 34:1596, 1951.
137. Vossius A: Beitrag zur Lehre von den angeborenen Conus, Klin Monatsbl Augenheilkd 23:137, 1885.
138. Walsh FB and Hoyt WF: Clinical neuro-ophthalmology, vols 1 and 2, ed 3, Baltimore, 1969, The Williams & Wilkins Co.
139. de Wecker L: Trait(ac)e des maladies du fond de l'oeil et atlas d'ophthalmoscopie, Paris, 1870, A Delahaye.
140. Young SE, Walsh FB, and Know DL: The tilted disk syndrome, Am J Ophthalmol 82:16, 1976.
141. Zimmerman LE and Font R: Congenital malformations of the eye: some recent advances in knowledge of the pathogenesis and histopathological characteristics, JAMA 196:684, 1966.

Atypical colobomas

142. Badtke G: Uber das Wesen und die Genesis der sogenannten atypischen Kolobome der inneren Augenhaute und des Sehnerven, Klin Monatsbl Augenheilkd 131:1, 1957.
143. Bateman JB and others: Aniridia: enzyme studies in an 11p-chromosomal deletion, Invest Ophthalmol Vis Sci 25:612, 1984.
144. Bonetta L and others: Wilms tumor locus on 11p13 defined by multiple CpG island-associated transcripts, Science 250:994, 1990.
145. Brodsky MC: Congenital optic disk anomalies: major review, Surv Ophthalmol 39:89, 1994.
146. Burch U and others: Aniridia-Wilms' tumor syndrome with deletion of the short arm of chromosome 11, Ophthalmic Paediatr Genet 1:183, 1982.
147. Delleman JW and Winkelman JE: The significance of atypical colobomata and defects of the iris for the diagnosis of the hereditary aniridia syndrome, Klin Monatsbl Augenheilkd 63:528, 1973.
148. Dowdy SF and others: Suppression of tumorigenicity in Wilms tumor by the p15.5-p14 region of chromosome 11, Science 254:293, 1991.
149. Elsas FJ and others: Familial aniridia with preserved ocular function, Am J Ophthalmol ••:718, 1977.
150. François J, Verschraegen-Spae MR, and DeSutter E: The aniridia-Wilms' tumor syndrome and other associations of aniridia, Ophthalmic Paediatr Genet 1:125, 1982.
151. Grant W and Walton D: Progressive changes in the angle in congenital aniridia, with development of glaucoma, Trans Am Ophthalmol Soc 72:207, 1974.
152. Halcken B and Miller D: Simultaneous occurrence of congenital aniridia, hamartoma and Wilms' tumor, J Pediatr 78:497, 1971.
153. Hamada S and Ellsworth R: Congenital retinal detachment and the optic disk anomaly, Am J Ophthalmol 71:460, 1971.
154. Haung A and others: Tissue, developmental, and tumor-specific expression of divergent transcripts in Wilms tumor, Science 250:991, 1990.
155. Hayreh S and Cullen J: Atypical minimal peripapillary choroidal colobomata, Br J Ophthalmol 56:86, 1972.
156. Hess C: Ein Beitrag zur Kenntnis der nicht nach unten gerichteten angeborenen Iriscolobome, Klin Monatsbl Augenheilkd 30:109, 1892.
157. Hittner HM and others: Variable expressivity in autosomal dominant aniridia by clinical, electrophysiologic and angiographic criteria, Am J Ophthalmol 89:531, 1980.
158. Klien B: The pathogenesis of some typical colobomas of the choroid, Am J Ophthalmol 48:597, 1959.
159. Kolata GB: Genes and cancer: the story of Wilms' tumor. Science 207:970, 1980.
160. Magli A and others: Coloboma of the lens associated with coloboma of the alar nasal cartilages in a pair of female monozygotic twins: a new syndrome? Ophthalmic Paediatr Genet 2:83, 1983.
161. Miller D, Froumeni J, and Manning M: Association of Wilms' tumor with aniridia, hemihypertrophy, and other congenital malformations, N Engl J Med 270:922, 1964.
162. Nelson LB and others: Aniridia: a review, Surv Ophthalmol 28:621, 1984.
163. Pilling F: Wilms' tumor in seven children with congenital aniridia, J Pediatr Surg 10:87, 1975.
164. Rones B: The genesis of atypical colobomas, Am J Ophthalmol 17:883, 1934.

Optic Pits

165. Akiba J and others: Vitreous findings in cases of optic nerve pits and serous macular detachment, Am J Ophthalmol 116:38, 1993.
166. Apple DJ, Rabb MF, and Walsh PM: Congenital anomalies of the optic disc, Surv Ophthalmol 27:3, 1982.
167. Apple DJ: Pathologie des Nervus opticus unter besonderer Berücksichtigung kolobomatöser Anomalien, Fortschr Ophthalmol 80:19, 1983.
168. Apple DJ: New aspects of colobomas and optic nerve anomalies, Int Ophthalmol Clin 24(1):109, 1984.
169. Blodi FC and Allen L: Stereoscopic manual of the ocular fundus in local and systemic disease, vol I, St Louis, 1964, The CV Mosby Co.
170. Bonnet M: Serous macular detachment associated with optic nerve pits, Graefes Arch Clin Exp Ophthalmol 229:526, 1991.
171. Borodic GE and others: Peripapillary subretinal neovascularization and serous macular detachment: association with congenital optic nerve pits, Arch Ophthalmol 102:229, 1984.
172. Brockhurst RJ: Optic pits and posterior retinal detachment, Trans Am Ophthalmol Soc 73:264, 1975.
173. Brown GC and Augsburger JJ: Congenital pits of the optic nerve head and retinochoroidal colobomas, Can J Ophthalmol 15:144, 1980.
174. Brown GC, Shields JA, and Goldberg RE: Congenital pits of the optic nerve head. II. Clinical studies in humans, Ophthalmology 87:51, 1980.
175. Brown GC and others: Congenital pits of the optic nerve head. I. Experimental studies in collie dogs, Arch Ophthalmol 97:1341, 1979.
176. Brown GC, Tasman WS: Congenital anomalies of the optic disk, New York, 1983, Grune & Stratton.
177. Chang M: Pits and crater-like holes of the optic disc, Ophthalmic Semin 1:21, 1976.
178. Eisum EF: Crater-like holes in the optic disc, Acta Ophthalmologica 35:200, 1957.

179. Ferry A: Macular detachment associated with congenital pit of the optic nerve head: pathologic findings in two cases simulating malignant melanoma of the choroid, Arch Ophthalmol 70:346, 1963.

180. Gass JDM: Serous detachment of the macula secondary to congenital pit of the optic nerve head, Am J Ophthalmol 67:821, 1969.

181. Gass JDM: In discussion of Brockhurst R: Optic pits and posterior retinal detachment, Trans Am Ophthalmol Soc 73:264, 1975.

182. Gorden R and Chatfield K: Pits in the optic disc associated with macular degeneration, Br J Ophthalmol 53:481, 1969.

183. Grear J: Pits, or crater-like holes, in the optic disc, Arch Ophthalmol 28:467, 1942.

184. Grimson BS, Mann JD, and Pantell JP: Optic nerve pit during papilledema, Arch Ophthalmol 100:99, 1982.

185. Henkind P: Crater-like holes in the optic nerve, Am J Ophthalmol 55:613, 1963.

186. Irvine AR and others: The pathogenesis of retinal detachment with morning glory disc and optic pit, Retina 6:146, 1986.

187. Jack M: Central serous retinopathy with optic pit treated with photocoagulation, Am J Ophthalmol 67:519, 1969.

188. Javitt JC and others: Acquired pits of the optic nerve, Ophthalmology 97:1038, 1990.

189. Johnson W, Smith J, and Hart L: Macular changes with pit of optic disc; fluorescein photography, Am J Ophthalmol 55:1070, 1963.

190. Kalina RE, Conrad WC: Intrathecal fluorescein for serous macular detachment, Arch Ophthalmol 94:1421, 1976.

191. Kayazawa F: A case of an optic pit, Ann Ophthalmol 13:865, 1981.

192. Kottow M: Photocoagulation of optic disc pits, Ophthalmologica 184:26, 1982.

193. Krankenburg E: Crater-like holes in the optic disc and central serous retinopathy, Arch Ophthalmol 64:912, 1960.

194. Lin CCL, Tso MOM, and Vygantas CM: Coloboma of optic nerve associated with serous maculopathy: a clinicopathologic correlative study, Arch Ophthalmol 102:1651, 1984.

195. Lincoff H and others: Retinoschisis associated with optic nerve pits, Arch Ophthalmol 106:61, 1988.

196. Miller SA and Bresnik G: Familial bilateral macular colobomata, Br J Ophthalmol 62:261, 1978.

197. Mustonen E and Varonen T: Congenital pit of the optic nerve head associated with serous detachment of the macula Acta Ophthalmol 50:689, 1972.

198. Pahwa V: Optic pit and central serous detachment, Indian J Ophthalmol 33:175, 1985.

199. Petersen HP: Pits or crater-like holes in the optic disc, Acta Ophthalmologica 36:435, 1958.

200. Pfaffenbach D and Walsh F: Central pit of the optic disc, Am J Ophthalmol 73:102, 1972.

201. Radius RL, Maumenee AE, and Green WR: Pitlike changes of the optic nerve head in open-angle glaucoma, Br J Ophthalmol 62:389, 1978.

202. Regenbogen L, Stein R, and Lazar M: Macular and juxtapapillary serous retinal detachment associated with pit of optic disc, Ophthalmologica 148:247, 1964.

203. Reis W: Eine wenig bejkannte typische Missbildung am Sehnerveneintritt: Umschriebene Grubenbildung auf der Papilla n. optici, Z Augenheilkd 19:505, 1908.

204. Rubinstein K and Ali M: Complications of optic disc pits, Trans Ophthalmol Soc UK 98:195, 1978.

205. Savir H and Rosen E: Congenital pit of the optic disc with acquired retinal cyst, Ann Ophthalmol 4:756, 1972.

206. Schatz H, McDonald HR: Treatment of sensory retinal detachment associated with optic nerve pit or coloboma, Ophthalmology 95:178, 1972.

207. Seefelder R: Ein pathologische-anatomischer Beitrag zur Frage der Kolobome und umschriebenen Grubenbildungen am Sehnerveneintritte, Arch Ophthalmol 90:129, 1915.

208. Simpson DE: Optic nerve pit, J Am Optom Assoc 58:118, 1987.

209. Slusher MM and others: The spectrum of cavitary optic disc anomalies in a family, Ophthalmol 96:342, 1989.

210. Sobol WM and others: Long-term visual outcome in patients with optic nerve pit and serous retinal detachment of the macula, Ophthalmology 97:1539, 1990.

211. Sugar H: Congenital pits on the optic disc with acquired macular pathology, Am J Ophthalmol 53:307, 1962.

212. Sugar H: Congenital pits in the optic disc, Am J Ophthalmol 63:298, 1967.

213. Sugar HS: An explanation for the acquired macular pathology associated with congenital pits of the optic disc, Am J Ophthalmol 57:833, 1964.

214. Theodossiadis G: Evolution of congenital pit of the optic disk with macular detachment in photocoagulated and nonphotocoagulated eyes, Am J Ophthalmol 84:620, 1977.

215. Theodossiadis GP: Visual acuity in patients with optic nerve pit(letter), Ophthalmology 98:563, 1991.

216. Vogel H: Macular changes associated with pits in the optic disc, Klin Monatsbl Augenheilkd 164:90, 1974.

217. Wiethe T: Eil Fall von angeborener Deformität der Sehnervenpapille, Arch Augenheilkd 11:4, 1982.

218. Vogel H and Wessing A: Maculaveranderungen bei Grubenpapille. In Deutsche Ophthalmologische Gesellschaft (1973 Congress): Erkrankungen der Macula, Munich, 1975, JF Bergmann.

Anomalies based on persistence of the transient embryonic vasculature

219. Acers T and Coston T: Persistent hyperplastic primary vitreous, Am J Ophthalmol 63:734, 1967.

220. Apple DJ, Hamming NA, and Gieser DK: Differential diagnosis of leukocoria. In Peyman GA, Apple DJ, and Sanders DR, editors: Intraocular tumors, New York, 1977, Appleton-Century-Crofts.

221. Bisland T: Vascular loops in the vitreous, Arch Ophthalmol 49:514, 1953.

222. Blodl FC: Preretinal glial nodules in persistence and hyperplasia of primary vitreous, Arch Ophthalmol 87:531, 1972.

223. Braekevelt CR and Hollenberg MJ: Comparative electron microscopic study of development of hyaloid and retinal capillaries in albino rats, Am J Ophthalmol 69:1032, 1970.

224. Bruckner A, Michaels R, and Fine S: Congenital retinal arterial loops and vitreous hemorrhage, Am J Ophthalmol 84:220, 1977.

225. Bullock I: Development vitreous cysts, Arch Ophthalmol 91:83, 1974.

226. Degenhart W and others: Prepapillary vascular loops, Ophthalmology 88:1126, 1981.

227. Font R, Yanoff M, and Zimmerman L: Intraocular adipose tissue and persistent hyperplastic primary vitreous, Arch Ophthalmol 82:43, 1969.

228. François J: Prepapillary cyst developed from remnants of the hyaloid artery, Br J Ophthalmol 34:365, 1951.

229. Gass JDM: Surgical excision of persistent hyperplastic primary vitreous, Arch Ophthalmol 82:163, 1970.

230. Gieser DK and others: Persistent hyperplastic primary vitreous in an adult: case report with fluorescein angiography finds, J Pediatr Ophthalmol Strabismus 15:213, 1978.

231. Gloor B: Zur Entwicklung des Glaskorpers und der Zonula, Graefes Arch Clin Exp Ophthalmol 186:299, 1973.

232. Goldberg MF and Mafee M: Computed tomography for diagnosis of persistent hyperplastic primary vitreous (PHPV), Ophthalmology 90:442, 1983.

233. Gutmann F and Goldberg M: Persistent pupillary membrane and other ocular anomalies, Arch Ophthalmol 94:156, 1976.

234. Hamada S and Ellsworth R: Congenital retinal detachment and the optic disc anomaly, Am J Ophthalmol 71:460, 1971.

235. Hamming NA and others: Ultrastructure of the hyaloid vasculature in primates, Invest Ophthalmol Vis Sci 16:408, 1977.

236. Jack R: Regression of the hyaloid vascular system: an ultrastructural analysis, Am J Ophthalmol 74:261, 1972.

237. Joseph N, Ivry M, and Oliver M: Persistent hyperplastic primary vitreous at the optic nerve head, Am J Ophthalmol 73:580, 1972.

238. Kollmann J: Handatlas der Entwicklungsgeschichte des Menschen, Jena, 1907, Gustav Fischer.

239. Mann I: The relations of the hyaloid canal in the fetus and in the adult, J Anat 62:290, 1928.

240. Mann I: A case of congenital abnormality of the retina, Trans Ophthalmol Soc UK 48:383, 1928.

241. Mann I: Congenital retinal fold, Br J Ophthalmol 19:641, 1935.

242. Manschot W: Persistent hyperplastic primary vitreous, Arch Ophthalmol 59:188, 1958.

243. Merin S, Crawford J, and Cardarelli J: Hyperplastic persistent pupillary membrane, Am J Ophthalmol 72:717, 1971.

244. Mittendorf W: On the frequency of posterior capsular opacities at the place of attachment of the hyaloid artery, Trans Am Ophthalmol Soc 6:413, 1892.

245. Mittendorf W: Punctate or hyaline opacities of the posterior lens capsule, Ophthalmol Rec 15:489, 1906.

246. Nankin S and Scott W: Persistent hyperplastic primary vitreous, Arch Ophthalmol 95:240, 1977.

247. Petersen H: Persistence of the Bergmeister papilla with glial overgrowth, Acta Ophthalmol 46:430, 1968.

248. Peyman GA, Sanders DR, and Nagpal K: Management of persistent hyperplastic primary vitreous by pars plana vitrectomy, Br J Ophthalmol 11:756, 1976.

249. Pruett R: The pleomorphism and complications of posterior hyperplastic primary vitreous, Am J Ophthalmol 80:625, 1975.

250. Pruett R and Schepens C: Posterior hyperplastic primary vitreous, Am J Ophthalmol 69:534, 1970.

251. Reese AB: Persistent hyperplastic primary vitreous, Am J Ophthalmol 40:317,1955.

252. van Selm J: Surgery for retinal dysplasia and hyperplasia of the persistent primary vitreous, Trans Ophthalmol Soc UK 89:545, 1970.

253. Smith R and Maumenee A: Persistent hyperplastic primary vitreous, results of surgery, Trans Am Acad Ophthalmol Otolaryngol 78:911, 1974.

254. Spaulding A: Persistent hyperplastic primary vitreous humor: a finding in a 71-year-old man, Surv Ophthalmol 12:448, 1967.

255. Spaulding A and Naumann G: Persistent hyperplastic primary vitreous in an adult, Arch Ophthalmol 77:666, 1967.

256. Stark WJ and others: Persistent hyperplastic primary vitreous: surgical treatment, Ophthalmology 90:452, 1983.

257. Tower P: Congenital prepapillary cyst, Arch Ophthalmol 48:433, 1952.

258. Warburg M: Norrie's disease and falciform detachment of the retina. In Goldberg MF, editor: Genetic and metabolic eye disease, Boston, 1974, Little, Brown & Co.

259. Wolter J and Flaherty N: Persistent hyperplastic vitreous, Am J Ophthalmol 47:491, 1959.

Anterior chamber cleavage syndromes

260. Alkemade P: Dysgenesis mesodermalis of the iris and the cornea, Springfield, III, 1969, Charles C Thomas, Publisher.

261. Allen L, Burian H, and Braley A: A new concept of the anterior chamber angle, Arch Ophthalmol 53:783, 1955.

262. Axenfeld T: Embryotoxon corneae posterius, Ber Dtsch Ophthalmol Ges 42:301, 1920.

263. Bann CF and others: Classification of corneal endothelial disorders based on neural crest origin, Ophthalmology 91:558, 1984.

264. Bateman JB, Maumenee IH, and Sparkes RS: Peters' anomaly associated with partial deletion of the long arm of chromosome 11, Am J Ophthalmol 97:11, 1984.

265. Beauchamp GR: Anterior segment dysgenesis keratolenticular adhesion and aniridia, J Pediatr Ophthalmol Strabismus 17:55, 1980.

266. Burian H, Braley A, and Allen L: External and gonioscopic visibility of the ring of Schwalbe and the trabecular zone: interpretation of the posterior corneal embryotoxon and the so-called congenital hyaline membranes on the posterior corneal surface, Trans Am Ophthalmol Soc 52:389, 1955.

267. Cibis GW and others: Peters' anomaly in association with ring 21 chromosomal abnormality, Am J Ophthalmol 100:733, 1985.

268. deRespinis PA, Wagner RS: Peters' anomaly in father and son, Am J Ophthalmol 104:545, 1987.

269. vanDorp DB and others: Oculocutaneous albinism and anterior chamber cleavage malformations, Clin Genet 26:440, 1984.

270. Fagle JA and others: Peripheral Peters' anomaly: a histopathologic case report, J Pediatr Ophthalmol Strabismus 15:71, 1978.

271. Ferguson JG and Hicks EL: Rieger's anomaly and glaucoma associated with partial trisomy 16q, Arch Ophthalmol 105:323, 1987.

272. Gregor Z and Hitchings RA: Reiger's anomaly: a 42-up, Br J Ophthalmol 64:56, 1980.

273. Henkind P, Seige I, and Carr R: Mesodermal dysgenesis of the anterior segment: Rieger's anomaly, Arch Ophthalmol 73:810, 1965.

274. Hiltner HM and others: Variable expressivity of autosomal dominant anterior segment mesenchymal dysgenesis in six generations, Am J Ophthalmol 93:57, 1982.

275. Judisch GF and others: Rieger's syndrome: a case report with a 15-year follow-up, Arch Ophthalmol 97:2120, 1979.

276. Kenyon KR: Mesodermal defects in Peters' anomaly, sclerocornea and congenital endothelial dystrophy, Exp Eye Res 21:125, 1975.

277. Kivlin JD and others: Peters' anomaly as a consequence of genetic and nongenetic syndromes, Arch Ophthalmol 104:61, 1986.

278. Kleinmann RE and others: Primary empty sella and Reiger's anomaly of the anterior chamber of the eye: a familial syndrome, N Engl J Med 304:90, 1981.

279. Lee CF and others: Immunohistochemical studies of Peters' anomaly, Ophthalmology 96:958, 1989.

280. Peters A: Ueber angeborene Defektbildungen der Descemetschen Membran, Klin Monatsbl Augenheilkd 44:27, 1906.

281. Reese A and Ellsworth R: The anterior chamber cleavage syndrome, Arch Ophthalmol 75:307, 1966.

282. Rieger H: Beiträge zur Kenntnis seltener Missbildungen der Iris. I. Membrana iridopupillaris persistens, Graefes Arch Ophthalmol 131:523, 1934.

283. Rieger H: Beiträge zur Kenntnis seltener Missbildungen der Iris. II. Ueber Hypoplasie des Irisvorderblattes mit Verlagerung und Entrundung per Pupille, Graefes Arch Ophthalmol 133:602, 1935.

284. Rieger H: Erbfragen in der Augenheilkunde, Graefes Arch Ophthalmol 143:227, 1941.

285. Scheie HG, Yanoff M: Peters' anomaly and total posterior coloboma of retinal pigment epithelium and choroid, Arch Ophthalmol 87:525, 1972.

286. Shields MB and others: Axenfeld-Rieger syndrome: a spectrum of developmental disorders, Surv Ophthalmol 29:387, 1985.

287. Steinsapir DK and others: Systemic neurocristopathy associated with Rieger's syndrome, Am J Ophthalmol 110:437, 1990.

288. Stone D and others: Congenital central corneal leukoma (Peters' anomaly), Am J Ophthalmol 81:173, 1976.

289. Townsend W, Font R, and Zimmerman L: Congenital corneal leukomas. II. Histopathologic findings in 19 eyes with central defect in Descemet's membrane, Am J Ophthalmol 77:192, 1974.

290. Townsend W, Font R, and Zimmerman L: Congenital corneal leukomas. III. Histopathologic findings in 13 eyes with noncentral defect in Descemet's membrane, Am J Ophthalmol 77:400, 1974.

291. Traboulsi EI and Maumenee IH: Peter's anomaly and associated congenital malformations, Arch Ophthalmol 110:1739, 1992.

292. Waring GO, Rodrigues MM, and Laibson PR: Anterior chamber cleavage syndrome: a stepladder classification, Surv Ophthalmol 20:3, 1976.

Anomalies in the size of the eye

293. Brockhurst RJ: Cataract surgery in nanophthalmic eyes, Arch Ophthalmol 108:965, 1990.

294. Codere F, Brownstein S, and Chen MF: Cryptophthalmos syndrome with bilateral renal agenesis, Am J Ophthalmol 91:737, 1981.

295. Curtin B: Myopia: a review of its etiology, pathogenesis, and treatment, Surv Ophthalmol 15:1, 1970.

296. Curtin B and Karlin D: Axial length measurements and fundus changes of the myopic eye, Am J Ophthalmol 71:42, 1971.

297. Curtin BS, Inamoto T, and Renaldo DP: Normal and staphylomatous sclera of high myopia: an electron microscopic study, Arch Ophthalmol 97:912, 1979.

298. Diaz AG, Alonso MJ, and Borda M: Oculodentodigital dysplasia, Ophthalmic Paediatr Genet 1:227, 1982.

299. François J, Pallotta R, and Gallenga PE: Microphthalmos and malformative syndromes, Ophthalmic Paediatr Genet 2:201, 1983.

300. Fujiki K and others: Genetic analysis of microphthalmos, Ophthalmic Paediatr Genet 1:139, 1982.

301. Hotchkiss ML and Fine SL: Pathologic myopia and choroidal neovascularization, Am J Ophthalmol 91:117, 1981.

302. Howard RO and others: Unilateral cryptophthalmia, Am J Ophthalmol 87:556, 1979.

303. Jin JC, Anderson DR: Laser and unsutured sclerotomy in nanophthalmos, Am J Ophthalmol 109:575, 1990.

304. Klein R and Curtin B: Lacquer crack lesions in pathologic myopia, Am J Ophthalmol 79:386, 1975.

305. Moro F and others: X-linked recessive myopia associated with nyctalopia in a Sicilian family, Ophthalmic Paediatr Genet 1:173, 1982.

306. Nissenkorn I and others: Myopia in premature babies with and without retinopathy of prematurity, Br J Ophthalmol 67:170, 1983.

307. Rabb MF, Garoon I, and LaFranco FP: Myopic macular degeneration, Int Ophthalmol Clin 21(3):51, 1981.

308. Scott JD: Congenital myopia and retinal detachment, Trans Ophthalmol Soc UK 100:69, 1980.

309. Sperduto RD and others: Prevalence of myopia in the United States, Arch Ophthalmol 101:405, 1983.

310. Spitznas M, Gerke E, and Bateman JB: Hereditary posterior microphthalmos with papillomacular fold and high hyperopia, Arch Ophthalmol 101:413, 1983.

311. Stansbury F: Pathogenesis of myopia, Arch Ophthalmol 39:273, 1948.

312. Stewart DH and others: Abnormal scleral collagen in nan-ophthalmos. An ultrastructural study, Arch Ophthalmol 109:1017, 1991.

313. Stocker F: Pathologic anatomy of the myopic eye with regard to newer theories of etiology and pathogenesis of myopia, Arch Ophthalmol 30:476, 1943.

314. Waring G III, Roth A, and Rodrigues M: Clinicopathologic correlation of microphthalmos with cyst, Am J Ophthalmol 82:714, 1976.

315. Weiss AH and others: Simple micro-ophthalmos, Arch Ophthalmol 107:1625, 1989.

316. Yue BYJT and others: Nanophthalmic sclera. Fibronectin studies, Ophthalmology 95:56, 1988.

317. Zadnik K and others: The effect of parental history of myopia on children's eye size, JAMA 271:1323, 1994.

Pigment anomalies

318. Balmaceda CM and others: Nevus of Ota and leptomeningeal melanocytic lesions, Neurology 43:381, 1983.

319. Bard LA: Heterogeneity in Waardenburg's syndrome: report of a family with ocular albinism, Arch Ophthalmol 96:1193, 1978.

320. BenEzra D and others: Chédiak-Higashi syndrome ocular findings, J Pediatr Ophthalmol Strabismus 17:68, 1980.

321. Bloch-Michel E: Physiopathology of Fuchs' heterochromic cyclitis, Trans Ophthalmol Soc UK 101:384, 1981.

322. Blodi FC: Ocular melanocytosis and melanoma, Am J Ophthalmol 80:389, 1975.

323. Blume R and Wolff S: The Chódiak-Higashi syndrome; studies in four patients and a review of the literature, Medicine 51:247, 1972.

324. Broodbakker JTW, Westerhof W, and Van Dorp DB: Ultrastructure of the skin of human albinos, Ophthalmic Paediatr Genet 2:95, 1983.

325. Carr RE and others: Albinism, Ophthalmology 88:377, 1981.

326. Castronuovo S and others: Variable expression of albinism within a single kindred, Am J Ophthalmol 111:419, 1991.

327. Cortin P and others: X-linked ocular albinism: relative value of skin biopsy, iris transillumination and funduscopy in identifying affected males and carriers, Can J Ophthalmol 16:121, 1981.

328. Creel DJ and others: Visual anomalies associated with albinism, Ophthalmic Paediatr Genet 11:193, 1990.

329. Donerty W: Cases of melanosis oculi with microscopic findings, Am J Ophthalmol 10:1, 1927.

330. Donohue W and Bain H: Chédiak-Higashi syndrome, a lethal familial disease with anomalous inclusions in the leukocytes and constitutional stigmata: report of a case with necropsy, Pediatrics 20:416, 1957.

331. Duke-Elder S: Heterochromia. System of ophthalmology, vol. III, part 2, St. Louis, 1964, The CV Mosby Co.

332. van Dorp DB, Haeringen NJ, and Glasius E: Evaluation of hairbulb incubation test and tyrosinase assay in the classification of albinism, Ophthalmic Paediatr Genet 1:189, 1982.

333. Falls H: Sex-linked ocular albinism displaying typical fundus changes in the female heterozygote, Am J Ophthalmol 34:41, 1951.

334. Falls H: Albinism, Trans Am Acad Ophthalmol Otolaryngol 57:324, 1953.

335. Fitzpatrick T and others: Ocular and dermal melanocytosis, Arch Ophthalmol 56:830, 1956.

336. Fulton AB, Albert DM, and Craft JL: Human albinism: light and electron microscopy study, Arch Ophthalmol 96:305, 1978.

337. Goldberg M: Waardenburg's syndrome with fundus and other abnormalities, Arch Ophthalmol 76:797, 1966.

338. Gonder JR and others: Ocular melanocytosis: a study to determine the prevalence rate of ocular melanocytosis, Ophthalmology 89:950, 1982.

339. Gonder and others: Uveal malignant melanoma associated with ocular oculodermal melanocytosis, Ophthalmology 89:950, 1982.

340. Gregor Z: The perifoveal vasculature in albinism, Br J Ophthalmol 62:554, 1978.

341. Helmick E and Pringle R: Oculocutaneous melanosis or nevus of Ota, Arch Ophthalmol 56:833, 1956.

342. Hittner HM and others: Oculocutaneous albinoidism as a manifestation of reduced neural crest derivatives in the Prader-Willi syndrome, Am J Ophthalmol 94:328, 1982.

343. Jain IS and others: Fuchs' heterochromic cyclitis: some observations on clinical picture and cataract surgery, Ann Ophthalmol 15:640, 1983.

344. Johnson D and others: Histopathology of eyes in Chédiak-Higashi syndrome, Arch Ophthalmol 75:84, 1966.

345. King RA and others: Brown oculocutaneous albinism. Clinical, ophthalmological, and biochemical characterization, Ophthalmology 92:1496, 1985.

346. Kinnear PE, Jay B, and Witkop CJ Jr: Albinism, Surv Ophthalmol 30:75, 1985.

347. Kugelman T and Van Scott EJ: Tyrosinase activity in melanocytes of human albinos, J Invest Dermatol 37:73, 1961.

348. LeeS-T and others: Mutations of the P gene in oculocutaneous albinism, and Prader-Willi syndrome plus albinism, N Eng J Med 330:529, 1994.

349. Lewen RM: Ocular albinism, Arch Ophthalmol 106:120, 1988.

350. Mietz H and others: Foveal hypoplasia in complete oculocutaneous albinism, Retina 12:254, 1992.

351. Liesgang TJ: Clinical features and prognosis in Fuchs' uveitis syndrome, Arch Ophthalmol 100:1622, 1982.

352. O'Connor GR: Heterochromic iridocyclitis, Trans Ophthalmic Soc UK 104:218, 1985.

353. O'Donnell F and others: X-linked ocular albinism, Arch Ophthalmol 94:1883, 1976.

354. Perry H, and others: Fuchs' heterochromic iridocyclitis, Arch Ophthalmol 93:337, 1975.

355. Rawles M: Origin of the mammalian pigment cell and its role in the pigmentation of hair. In Gordon M, editor: Conference on the biology of normal and atypical pigment cell growth, ed 3, New York, 1953, Academic Press, Inc.

356. Sang DN and others: Nevus of Ota with contralateral cerebral melanoma, Arch Ophthalmol 95:1820, 1977.

357. Skalka HW: Bilateral oculodermal melanocytosis, Ann Ophthalmol 8:565, 1976.

358. Spencer W and Hogan M: Ocular manifestations of Chédiak-Higashi syndrome, report of a case with histopathologic examination of ocular tissue, Am J Ophthalmol 50:1197, 1960.

359. Tabbot BR and others: Fuchs' heterochromic iridocyclitis in blacks, Arch Ophthalmol 106:1688, 1988.

360. Taylor WOG: Visual disabilities of oculocutaneous albinism and their alleviation: Edridge-Green lecture, Trans Ophthalmol Soc UK 98:423, 1978.

361. Teekhasaenee C and others: Glaucoma in oculodermal melanocytosis, Ophthalmology 97:562, 1990.

362. Teekhasaenee C and others: Ocular findings in oculodermal melanocytosis, Arch Ophthalmol 108:1114, 1990.

363. Valenzuela R and Morningstar WA: The ocular pigmentary disturbance of human Chédiak-Higashi syndrome, Am J Clin Pathol 75:591, 1981.

364. Velazquez N and Jones IS: Ocular and oculodermal melanocytosis associated with uveal melanoma. Ophthalmology 90:1472, 1983.

365. Wack MA and others: Electroretinographic findings in human oculocutaneous albinism, Ophthalmology 96:1778, 1989.

366. Witkop CJ Jr: Albinism. In Harris H and Hirschhorn K, editors: Advances in human genetics, vol 2, New York, 1971, Plenum Press.

367. Wong L, O'Donnell FE Jr, and Green WR: Giant pigment granules in the retinal pigment epithelium of a fetus with X-linked ocular albinism, Ophthalmic Paediatr Genet 2:47, 1983.

368. Yanoff M, Zimmerman LE: Histogenesis of malignant melanomas of the uvea. III. The relationship of congenital ocular melanocytosis and neurofibromatosis to uveal melanomas, Arch Ophthalmol 77:331, 1967.

Chromosomal anomalies

369. Adhikary HP: Ocular manifestations of Turner's syndrome, Trans Ophthalmol Soc UK 101:395, 1981.

370. Ahmad A and Pruett R: The fundus in mongolism, Arch Ophthalmol 94:772, 1976.

371. Apple DJ: Chromosome-induced ocular disease. In Goldberg MF, editor: Genetic and metabolic eye disease, Boston, 1974, Little, Brown & Co.

372. Apple DJ, Holden J, and Stallworth B: Ocular pathology of Patau's syndrome with an unbalanced D/D translocation, Am J Ophthalmol 70:383, 1960.

373. Awan K: Uncommon ocular changes in Down's syndrome (mongolism), J Pediatr Ophthalmol 14:215, 1977.

374. Boue J and others: The eyes of embryos with chromosomal abnormalities, Am J Ophthalmol 78:167, 1974.

375. Brushfield T: Mongolism, Br J Child Dis 21:241, 1924.

376. Calderone JP and others: Intraocular pathology of trisomy 18 (Edwards' syndrome): report of a case and review of the literature, Br J Ophthalmol 67:162, 1983.

377. Christianson R: Down syndrome and maternal age, Lancet 2:1198, 1976.

378. Cogan D and Kuwabara T: Pathology of cataracts in mongolism idiocy, Doc Ophthalmol 16:73, 1962.

379. Cotlier E, Reinglass H, and Rosenthal I: The eye in the partial trisomy 2g syndrome, Am J Ophthalmol 84:251, 1977.

380. Cullen J: Blindness in mongolism (Down's syndrome), Br J Ophthalmol 47:331, 1963.

381. Cullen J and Butler H: Mongolism (Down's syndrome) and keratoconus, Br J Ophthalmol 47:321, 1963.

382. Donaldson D: The significance of spotting of the iris in mongoloids: Brushfield's spots, Arch Ophthalmol 65:26, 1961.

383. Down J: Observation of ethnic classification of idiots, Clin Lect Rep Lond Hosp 3:259, 1866.

384. Edwards J and others: A new trisomic syndrome, Lancet 1:787, 1960.

385. Eissler R and Longenecker C: The common eye findings in mongolism, Am J Ophthalmol 54:398, 1962.

386. Falls H: The role of the sex chromosome in hereditary ocular pathology, Trans Am Ophthalmol Soc 50:421, 1952.

387. Ferry AP, Marchevsky A, and Strauss L: Ocular abnormalities in deletion of the long arm of chromosome 11, Ann Ophthalmol 13:1373, 1981.

388. François J, Berger R, and Saraux H: Chromosomal aberrations in ophthalmology, Assen, The Netherlands, 1975, Van Gorcum, BV.

389. Fulton AB and others: Retinal anomalies in trisomy 18, Graefes Arch Clin Exp Ophthalmol 213:195, 1980.

390. Gallie BL and Phillips RA: Multiple manifestations of the retinoblastoma gene, Birth Defects 18:689, 1982.

391. Garcia-Castro JM and Reyes de Torres LC: Nictitating membrane in trisomy 18 syndrome, Am J Ophthalmol 80:550, 1975.

392. Gaynon MW and Schimek RA: Downs syndrome: a ten-year group study, Ann Ophthalmol 9:1493, 1977.

393. Gieser SC, Apple DJ, and Carey JC: Pathology of chromosome-induced ocular disease. In Goldberg MF and Renie W, editors: Genetic and metabolic eye disease, ed 2, Boston, 1985, Little, Brown & Co.

394. Ginsberg J and others: Further observations of ocular pathology in Down's syndrome, J Pediatr Ophthalmol Strabismus 17:166, 1980.

395. Ginsberg J, Ballard ET, and Soukup S: Pathologic features of the eye in triploidy, J Pediatr Ophthalmol Strabismus 18:48, 1981.

396. Ginsberg J and Bove K: Ocular pathology of trisomy 13, Ann Ophthalmol 6:113, 1974.

397. Ginsberg J and others: Ocular pathology of trisomy 18, Ann Ophthalmol 3:273, 1971.

398. Ginsberg J and others: Pathologic features of the eye in Down's syndrome with relationship to other chromosomal anomalies, Am J Ophthalmol 83:874, 1977.

399. Ginsberg J and others: Ocular abnormality associated with partial duplication of chromosome 13, Ann Ophthalmol 13:189, 1981.

400. Ginsberg J, Soukup S, and Ballard ET: Pathologic features of the eye in trisomy 9, J Pediatr Ophthalmol Strabismus 19:37, 1982.

401. Guterman C and others: Micro-ophthalmos with cyst and Edward's syndrome, Am J Ophthalmol 109:228, 1990.

402. Hinzpeter EN and others: Buphthalmus bei Trisomie-13 Syndrom, Ophthalmologica 170:381, 1975.

403. Hoepner J and Yanoff M: Craniosynostosis and syndactylism (Apert's

404. Hoepner J and Yanoff M: Ocular anomalies in trisomy 13-15: an analysis of 13 eyes with two new findings, Am J Ophthalmol 74:729, 1972.

405. Howard RO: Ocular abnormalities in the cri du chat syndrome, Am J Ophthalmol 73:949, 1972.

406. Howard RO: Chromosome errors in retinoblastoma, Birth Defects 18:703, 1982.

407. Howard RO and others: The eyes of embryos with chromosomal abnormalities, Am J Ophthalmol 78:167, 1974.

408. Huggert A: The trisomy 18 syndrome: a report of three cases in the same family, Acta Ophthalmol 44:186, 1966.

409. Jacoby B and others: Malignant glaucoma in a patient with Down's syndrome and corneal hydrops, Am J Ophthalmol 74:729, 1972.

410. Jaeger EA: Ocular findings in Down's syndrome. Trans Am Ophthalmol Soc 78:808, 1980.

411. Johnson MP and others: Retinoblastoma and its association with a deletion in chromosome #13; a survey using high-resolution chromosome techniques, Cancer Genet Cytogenet 6:29, 1982.

412. Kapoor S and DasGupta J: Chromosomal anomaly in female patient with anterior lenticonus, Ophthalmologica 179:271, 1979.

413. Keith C: The ocular findings in the trisomy syndromes, Proc R Soc Med 61:251, 1968.

414. Kusnetsova EE and others: Similar chromosomal abnormalities in several retinoblastomas, Hum Genet 61:201, 1982.

415. Lichter PR and Schmickel RD: Posterior vortex vein and congenital glaucoma in a patient with trisomy-13 syndrome, Am J Ophthalmol 80:939, 1975.

416. Lowe R: The eye in mongolism, Br J Ophthalmol 33:131, 1949.

417. Lowe R: The arcuate lens opacities of mongolism and cataracts of similar appearance, Br J Ophthalmol 34:484, 1950.

418. Mets MB and Maumenee IH: The eye and the chromosome (review), Surv Ophthalmol 28:20, 1983.

419. Motegi T and others: Retinoblastoma in a boy with a de novo mutation of a 13/18 translocation: the assumption that the retinoblastoma locus is at the 13q141, particularly at the distal portion of it, Hum Genet 60:193, 1982.

420. Mottet N and Jensen H: The anomalous embryonic development associated with trisomy 13-15, Am J Clin Pathol 43:334, 1965.

421. Mullaney J: Ocular pathology in trisomy 18 (Edwards' syndrome), Am J Ophthalmol 76:246, 1973.

422. Orellana J, Palumbo J, and Ritch R: Mesenchymal dysgenesis in a patient with Down's syndrome, J Pediatr Ophthalmol Strabismus 19:144, 1982.

423. Pap Z and others: Hochgradiger Mikrophthalmus beim Patau-Syndrome, Klin Monatsbl Augenheilkd 173:342, 1978.

424. Patau K and others: Multiple congenital anomaly caused by an extra autosome, Lancet 1:790, 1960.

425. Penrose L and Smith G: Down's anomaly, Edinburgh, 1966, Churchill Livingstone, Inc.

426. Robb RM and Marchevsky A: Pathology of the lens in Down's syndrome, Arch Ophthalmol 96:1, 1978.

427. Rochels VR: Ophthalmologische Symptomatik der autosomalen Trisomien; ein Beitrag sur Differentialdiagnose, Fortschr Med 101:55, 1983.

428. Rodrigues M, Valdes-Dapena M, and Kistenmacher M: Ocular pathology in a case of 13 trisomy, J Pediatr Ophthalmol 10:54, 1973.

429. Rodrigues MM and others: Retinal pigment epithelium in a case of trisomy 18, Am J Ophthalmol 76:265, 1973.

430. Schmickel RD: The genetic basis for ophthalmological disease, Surv Ophthalmol 25:37, 1980.

431. Schwartz D: Noonan's syndrome associated with ocular abnormalities, Am J Ophthalmol 73:955, 1972.

432. Skeller E and Oster J: Eye symptoms in mongolism, Acta Ophthalmol 29:149, 1951.

433. Slusher M, Laibson P, and Mulberger R: Acute keratoconus in Down's syndrome, Am J Ophthalmol 66:1137, 1968.

434. Solomon G and others: Four common eye signs in mongolism, Am J Dis Child 110:46, 1965.

435. Stoll C and others: An unusual partial trisomy 13, Clin Genet 9:1, 1976.

436. Taylor A: Autosomal trisomy syndromes; a detailed study of 27 cases

of Edwards' syndrome and 27 cases of Patau's syndrome, J Med Genet 5:227, 1968.

437. Traboulsi EI and others: Infantile glaucoma in Down's syndrome (trisomy 21). Am J Ophthalmol 117:411, 1994.

438. Waardenburg P: Das menschliche Auge und seine Erbanlagen, The Hague, 1932, Martinus Nijhoff.

439. Walsh SZ: Keratoconus and blindness in 469 institutionalized subjects with Down syndrome and other causes of mental retardation, J Ment Defic Res 25:243, 1981.

440. Williams RDB: Brushfield spots and Wolfflin nodules in the iris, an appraisal in handicapped children, Dev Med Child Neurol 23:646, 1981.

441. Wilson L and others: Cytogenetic analysis of a case of "13q syndrome" (46, XX, del 13) using banding techniques, J Pediatr Ophthalmol Strabismus 17:63, 1980.

442. Wilson WA, Alfi OS, and Donnell GN: Ocular findings in cytogenetic syndromes, Ophthalmology 86:1184, 1978.

443. Yanoff M, Font R, and Zimmerman L: Intraocular cartilage in a microphthalmic eye of an otherwise healthy girl, Arch Ophthalmol 81:238, 1969.

444. Yanoff M, Frayer W, and Scheie H: Ocular findings in a patient with 13-15 trisomy, Arch Ophthalmol 70:372, 1963.

445. Yunis JJ and Chandler ME: The chromosomes of man—clinical and biologic significance, Am J Pathol 88:466, 1977.

446. Zellweger H: Cytogenetic aspects of ophthalmology, Surv Ophthalmol 15:77, 1970.

447. Zellweger H and Simpson J: Mongolism (Down's syndrome). In Conn HF and Conn RB Jr, editors: Current diagnosis, Philadelphia, 1974, WB Saunders Co.

CHAPTER 3
CORNEA

Anatomy and histology[1-55]

The cornea and sclera form the outer layer of the globe, providing a protective fibrous capsule.

The sclera consists of intertwining, closely packed lamellae of collagen; a calcified scleral plaque occasionally occurs as an aging process.[8] Scattered dendritic melanocytes are present on the inner side of the sclera adjacent to the choroid, forming the lamina fusca. The sclera is continuous externally with the episclera and, in the region of the insertion of the extraocular muscles, with the connective tissue of Tenon's capsule.

The thickness of the sclera varies considerably in individuals and with age. In newborns, the sclera typically is white-blue because the color of the underlying pigmented uvea is visible through the relatively transparent, thin infantile scleral tissues. The adult sclera is thinnest immediately posterior to the insertion of the extraocular muscles (0.45 mm). At the limbus the sclera measures roughly 0.6 to 0.7 mm, and at the posterior pole it measures approximately 1.1 to 1.3 mm.

The sclera is continuous with the dura mater at the site of penetration of the optic nerve into the eye (see Fig. 10-6). It also continues across the optic nerve head, forming the sieve-like lamina cribrosa (see Figs. 10-2, 10-4, and 10-6). It also is penetrated by fine channels, the emissaria (see Figs. 1-3 and 7-5), which contain penetrating vessels from the uvea (the ciliary vessels and the vortex veins), and branches of the ciliary nerves. The emissaria are important because they provide a passage for extraocular extension of intraocular tumors (p. 325; see Figs. 7-60 and 7-61; Color Plate 1-1).

The nerve loop of Axenfeld,[10] a normal anatomic variation, is an outward bowing of the anterior ciliary nerves in the region behind the limbus (Fig. 3-1). The nerve courses superficially to the episcleral surface and penetrates again into the scleral substance. It sometimes is of clinical significance because the nerves occasionally are accompanied by pigmented chromatophores, which may produce a pigmented spot on the sclera. Because this might be interpreted as a melanotic neoplasm,[10] it must be included in the differential diagnosis of primary or metastatic malignant melanoma occurring in this region.

The cornea is the most important refractive medium of the eye. Its transparency depends on the fact that it is relatively acellular and free of vessels and reveals a smooth, regular contour. It differs from the sclera in that it is covered by two layers, one anterior epithelial and one posterior mesothelial. These cellular layers from semipermeable interfaces, which make possible an active metabolic interchange with the tear film externally as well as with the aqueous humor posteriorly.

Proper hydration of the corneal stroma partially depends on the normally functioning tear-forming apparatus. The tear film forms three layers on the corneal surface:

1. The outer layer consists of an oily secretory product, formed primarily by the sebaceous glands of the lid (the meibomian and Zeis glands; see Fig. 11-3).

2. The middle layer consists of a watery fluid secreted primarily by the lacrimal glands, including the accessory lacrimal glands in the eyelids (see Fig. 11-3).

3. The inner layer consists of mucopolysaccharides secreted primarily by the goblet cells in the conjunctiva (see Fig. 11-2, *A*) and partially from the lacrimal glands.

Deficiencies in the tear film can be demonstrated clinically by use of the rose bengal stain.

The cornea consists of five layers (Fig. 3-2). It is covered by a multilayered nonkeratinized squamous epithelium that develops from the embryonic surface ectoderm. The epithelium is continuous at the limbus with that of bulbar conjunctiva. The more superficial layers of the five- to six-layered epithelium are flattened, whereas the basal layer consists of cuboidal-cylindric cells, whose long axes are oriented perpendicularly to the base of the cell. Between the overlying squamous epithelial cells and the basal layer are cells that show elongated cytoplasmic processes, which in sagittal sections resemble wings; hence the term "wing-cell layer." The epithelial cells are connected to one another by intercellular bridges. Disruption of the epithelial layer and the intercellular junctions is best demonstrated clinically by the use of fluorescein staining.

The basal cell layer elaborates a very thin basement membrane that is best demonstrated by the PAS stain. This true basement membrane of the epithelium should not be confused with Bowman's layer, which is situated directly underneath the basement membrane. Bowman's layer is not a basement membrane but is a hyalinized, modified anterior layer of the stroma. With connective tissue stains such as Masson trichrome, Bowman's layer stains in a manner almost identical to that of the stroma. The corneal epithelium is attached firmly to the underlying Bowman layer or hemidesmosomes, an anatomic feature that is important in the pathogenesis of epithelial corneal dystrophies (p. 86), recurrent erosions (p. 78), and bullous keratopathy (p. 72). More details regarding corneal wound healing are provided in Chapter 5 in the discussion of excimer laser refractive surgery.

Bowman's layer covers almost the entire cornea except for the far peripheral rim, which is approximately 1 mm

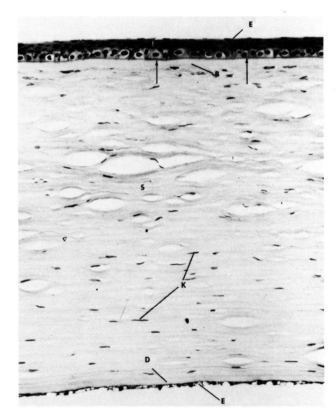

Fig. 3-2. Normal cornea. The epithelium (upper *E*) is five to six layers thick. The basal layer is cuboidal; the remaining cells are flattened and elongated, forming a nonkeratinized, stratified squamous epithelium. A very thin epithelial basement membrane *(arrows)* separates epithelium from Bowman's layer. Bowman's layer *(B)* is a zone with a hyaline appearance and is composed of tissue similar to that of the collagenous stroma. *K,* Keratocyte nuclei. The clefts within the stroma *(S)* are preparation artifacts, not stromal edema. Descemet's membrane *(D)* is faintly visible in routine preparations but is more readily seen by PAS staining because it is true basement membrane. The corneal endothelium (lower *E*) is a flat, single-layered cuboidal epithelium that often appears vacuolated as an artifact of preparation. The degree of autolysis seen in this section should not be confused with endothelial disease. (H & E stain; ×170.)

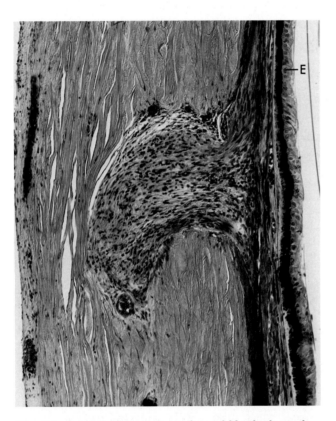

Fig. 3-1. Intrascleral nerve loop of Axenfeld. The long ciliary nerve deviates from the pars plana stroma *(right)* toward the episclera *(left)* and returns to continue anteriorly. The actual breakthrough onto the scleral surface *(left)* is not visible in this plane of section. *E,* Bilayered epithelium of the pars plana. (H & E stain; ×275.)

from the edge of the cornea. The peripheral termination of Bowman's layer is the beginning of the limbus. (The histologic limbus is defined as a zone of approximately 1 to 1 ½ mm in width, the medial aspect of the limbus being the outer border of Bowman's layer. In sagittal histologic sections, the central border of the limbus is represented by a concave line drawn between the terminations of Bowman's layer anteriorly and Descemet's membrane posteriorly.)

Portions of Bowman's layer destroyed by trauma, ulcers, or other causes cannot regenerate. The defects normally are filled in by ingrowth of epithelium or stromal collagen. Defects in Bowman's layer that are filled in by the epithelium are called *epithelial facets* (Fig. 3-3). These are visible focal illumination as a distortion of the corneal light reflex. In contrast, a nebula, defined as a diffuse cloud-like opacity with indistinct borders counts of collagenous scar tissue found predominately in the superficial stroma. A macula is well-circumscribed dense opacity, also found in the stroma. A leukoma is a larger area of white, opaque stromal scarring. When an interconnection between a corneal scar and tissue posterior to the scar (iris or lens) is present, the lesion is termed an adherent leukoma (see Figs. 3-61 and 4-11).

The corneal epithelium and superficial stroma contain abundant nonmyelinated nerve fibers,[28] which usually are not visible in routine histologic stains but require heavy metal impregnation such as the Hortega or Cajal method. These fibers apparently exert a sustaining or trophic effect on the metabolism of the cornea. Damage to these nerves, for example, in neuroparalytic keratitis, causes extensive corneal degeneration. These nerves may enlarge in some disease states, such as Hansen's disease or von Recklinghausen's neurofibromatosis (see Fig. 9-51).

The corneal stroma consists of multiple lamellae of parallel-coursing collagen fibers that are admixed with a mucopolysaccharide ground substance, primarily keratan sulfate and chondroitin sulfate. The stroma makes up 90% of the corneal thickness. The stromal collagen is elaborated by fixed fibrocyte-like cells termed *keratocytes*. In addition to normal collagen and ground substance formation, in pathologic processes these cells participate in phagocytosis and repair. Although blood vessels are present in the limbus, the normal stroma is totally avascular.

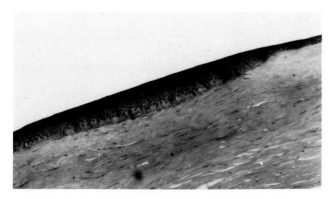

Fig. 3-3. Epithelial facet, a localized corneal epithelial thickening at a site of injury. (H & E stain; ×325.)

Descemet's membrane is a true periodic acid-Schiff (PAS)-positive basement membrane formed by the corneal endothelium. It terminates peripherally at Schwalbe's line, forming at this point the anterior border of the trabecular meshwork (see Figs. 6-2 and 6-3). Descemet's membrane can regenerate partially after breaks. When broken, it shows a tendency to coil or roll into a scroll shape, a morphologic finding that is pathognomonic of a previous disruption.

The corneal endothelium consists of a single row of cuboidal cells that are hexagonal when viewed in a flat preparation. Descemet's membrane lines the anterior surface of the endothelial layer; the anterior chamber forms the posterior aspect. The endothelium typically undergoes rapid autolysis after enucleation; artifactitious vacuolization is a common finding and should not be confused with true endothelial disease (Fig. 3-2).

In contrast to other endothelial cells, the "endothelial cells" of the cornea are roughly rectangular in sagittal or cross-section, rather than elongated or spindle-shaped. They actually are more correctly called a *mesothelium* because they are analogous to the mesothelial cells lining the various fluid-containing body cavities, for example, the pericardium or peritoneum. Technically, the term *endothelium* should be reserved for the cellular linings of blood and lymph vessels. However, the term *corneal endothelium* remains firmly entrenched in clinical usage.

The endothelial layer functions as a regulator of corneal water content. Endothelial cells, which are rich with mitochondria,[17] represent an active metabolic pump that performs this function in conjunction with the tear film. The cornea must remain relatively dehydrated to retain its transparency. If the water content of the ground substance increases significantly, the stroma will become edematous and opaque, and the two most important optical functions of the cornea, transparency and refractive power, may be altered severely.

In addition to endothelial competence that adjusts water content, the transparency of the cornea depends on the regular, parallel arrangement of the stromal collagen lamellae, the maintenance of smooth anterior and posterior border layers of the cornea, and the paucity of cellular elements and blood vessels within the stroma.

Nourishment to the cornea is provided by a limbal vascular arcade in conjunction with direct diffusion of nutrients from the tear film and the aqueous humor. Because the cornea is avascular, generally good transplantation results can be attained; it is relatively unresponsive to blood vessel-mediated immunologic rejection reactions. Only in pathologic states, for example, long-standing inflammation (keratitis), does one observe new vessel formation and vascularization within the cornea, usually caused by ingrowth from the limbal vessels (see Figs. 3-17, *B,* and 3-24).

Two commonly occurring aging processes in the cornea are noteworthy. Hassall-Henle warts—local, well-circumscribed excrescences on Descemet's[164] membrane in the periphery—commonly are seen in older individuals (Fig. 3-4). Because they do not occur within the optical axis, they do not have a significant effect on vision. Hassall-Henle warts are histologically identical in appearance to guttata. The latter are Descemet's membrane thickenings that are observed in the combined endothelial-epithelial

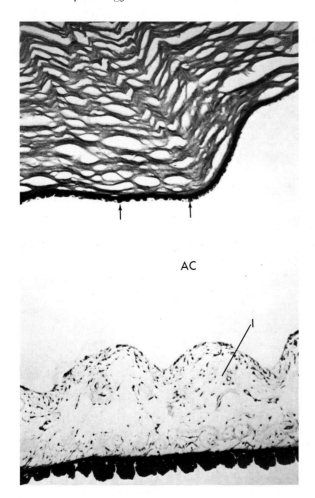

Fig. 3-4. Posterior peripheral cornea showing Hassall-Henle warts *(arrows)*, focal thickenings of Descemet's membrane, which are a normal aging phenomenon without visual significance. These excrescences are histopathologically identical in appearance to the endothelial guttata of Fuchs'' dystrophy. *AC,* Anterior chamber; *I,* iris stroma. (PAS stain; ×280.) (From Naumann GOH and Apple DJ: In Doerr W, Seifert G, and Uehlinger E, editors: Handbuch der speziellen pathologischen Anatomie, Band Auge, 1980, Springer-Verlag.)

dystrophy of Fuchs' (p. 92), or as sequelae to other causes of endothelial decompensation in which the dehydration mechanism of the corneal endothelium is destroyed and corneal edema occurs.

Arcus senilis (gerontoxon) often is seen as an aging process. This white bow or ring, which sometimes occurs only as a partial or half ring, is separated from the limbus by a small outer rim of clear cornea. Because the arcus typically is located peripherally, no visual difficulties result. Arcus senilis is a local aging change and in most instances has little or no connection to generalized metabolic defects, hyperlipidemia, arteriosclerosis, or tendency toward myocardial infarct. Histologically, fat droplets are situated within the stromal lamella and are best demonstrated by frozen sectioning and special fat stains.

Arcus senilis should be differentiated from the limbal girdle of Vogt, a symmetrical, yellow-white opacity forming a half-moonlike arc running concentrically within the lim-

bus superficially in the interpalpebral zone. It is composed of basophilic deposits on Bowman's membrane and superficial stroma.

Arcus juvenilis (anterior embryotoxon) is a similar process in which the lipid infiltrates are present at birth or develop in childhood. It is more likely to be associated with serum lipid abnormalities. It must be differentiated from posterior embryotoxon, which is described on page 35.

Inflammation

GENERAL DISCUSSION

Inflammation is the response of a tissue to either exogenous or endogenous noninfectious agents or infectious agents. A discussion of general inflammation is included here not only because the cornea commonly is involved in inflammatory processes but also in preparation for the description of ocular inflammatory diseases in subsequent chapters.

Histopathologic evaluation of tissue from patients with intraocular inflammation often requires identification of the various types and proportions of inflammatory cells in the lesion. This evaluation frequently is useful in determining a specific cause or pathogenesis. The following outline, which gives a partial listing of a wide variety of ocular diseases, illustrates the important major categories of inflammation. Classification of a particular case in one of these categories establishes a beginning in determining the cause or pathogenesis of the condition.

Selected ocular diseases exemplifying varying categories of inflammation

I. Acute inflammation
  A. Suppurative
    1. Acute bacterial, parasitic, viral, or fungal keratitis and corneal ulcers
    2. Purulent endophthalmitis, vitreous abscess, and panophthalmitis
  B. Nonsuppurative
    1. Acute nonpurulent anterior uveitis (iridocyclitis)
II. Chronic inflammation
  A. Nongranulomatous
    1. Chronic iridocyclitis
    2. Chronic nonspecific choroiditis or chorioretinitis
  B. Granulomatous
    1. Chalazion
    2. Reaction to a foreign body
    3. Sarcoidosis
    4. Sympathetic ophthalmia
    5. Toxoplasmosis
    6. Lens-induced endophthalmitis (phacoanaphylaxis)
    7. Tuberculosis
    8. Fungal keratitis or endophthalmitis
    9. Parasitic infestation
    10. Orbital pseudotumor
    11. Leprosy
    12. Syphilis
    13. Giant cell (temporal arteritis)
    14. Disciform keratitis with granulomatous reaction to Descemet's membrane
    15. Reaction of intraocular lens materials.

Acute inflammation, characterized by an immediate phase of redness (rubor), heat (color), mass (tumor), pair (dolar), and loss of function, is initiated by release of histamine from most cells and various plasma factors, including kinins, plasmins, complement, prostaglandins[127] human leukocyte antigen (HLA), and nonspecific factors such as cytokines. If an acute inflammation is suppurative, a characteristic formation of purulent material occurs with infiltration by polymorphonuclear neutrophils (see Figs. 3-9, 7-10, and 7-11).

Polymorphonuclear neutrophils are drawn to a site of injury by chemotaxisal function to remove noxious material and/or microorganisms by phagocytosis and liposomal digestion.

Most cases of acute nonspecific iridocyclitis are examples of a nonsuppurative acute inflammatory reaction. The majority of these cases are believed to result from an allergic or hypersensitivity reaction. They are characterized by protein and cells (including neutrophils) in the anterior segment rather than by a purulent exudate.

In contrast to the polymorphonuclear neutrophil that characterizes acute inflammation, the hallmark of chronic inflammation is the mononuclear cell. Chronic inflammation is divided into nongranulomatous and granulomatous forms.

Chronic nongranulomatous inflammation generally is characterized by infiltration of lymphocytes and other mononuclear cells such as plasma cells within the affected tissue. Nonspecific chronic iridocyclitis and nonspecific chronic choroiditis are prime examples of this form of chronic inflammation (see Fig. 7-8). Such primary uveal inflammations frequently are seen in clinical practice, but affected eyes rarely require enucleation. In the ocular pathology laboratory, these conditions are seen more commonly in association with trauma or other disease processes elsewhere within the eye.

Chronic granulomatous inflammation is of particular importance to the pathologist because examination of microscopic sections often can pinpoint a specific etiologic or pathogenetic factor in such cases. The preceding outline lists major conditions that may elicit a granulomatous reaction in the eye. The tissue pattern is so specific in many of these conditions that tissue examination alone may provide an unequivocal diagnosis. The hallmark of the granulomatous inflammatory reaction is the epithelioid cell and the closely related giant cell.

All cases of granulomatous inflammation are *not* necessarily chronic. Three noteworthy exceptions are Wegener's granulomatosis, mucormycosis, and the Tolosa-Hunt syndrome.

MORPHOLOGY OF INFLAMMATORY CELLS

Five types of inflammatory cells require individual mention: polymorphonuclear neutrophil, eosinophils, lymphocytes, plasma cells, and epithelioid-giant cells.

The polymorphonuclear neutrophil is the hallmark of acute inflammation. The nucleus of the cell often is composed of three to five lobes. The polymorphonuclear neutrophil can reach quickly the site of tissue irritation by chemotaxis and therefore is prominent in acute inflammatory processes.

The eosinophil is a bilobed cell containing eosinophilic (pink-staining) granules in the cytoplasm.[203] In contrast to the neutrophil, an eosinophil nucleus never contains more than two lobes. Increased numbers of eosinophils typically occur in two major categories of disease: hypersensitivity (allergic) states and parasitic infestations.

The lymphocyte is recognized in tissue sections by its deep-staining, discrete, round nucleus with only scanty cytoplasm. This cell is the hallmark of chronic inflammation, both the nongranulomatous type, in which it is not associated with epithelioid cells, and the granulomatous form, in which it is present in varying proportions with epithelioid cells and giant cells.

The plasma cell is especially important to the ophthalmic pathologist because it frequently is seen in various forms of intraocular inflammation, particularly uveitis. It is a major producer of antibody. This cell is recognizable by five criteria (Fig. 3-5):

1. It is elliptical.
2. It has an eccentric nucleus.
3. The nuclear chromatin characteristically clumps around the peripheral margin of the nucleus. These punctate, deep-staining dots resemble a clock face or the spokes of a wheel.
4. The cytoplasm exhibits an area of decreased staining intensity adjacent to the nucleus. Early pathologists designated this area *the hof* (halo). The hof is the site of the Golgi apparatus.
5. The remainder of the cytoplasm is basophilic in routinely stained sections. This differs from the usual eosinophilic-staining cytoplasm seen in the most cellular elements of the body. This basophilia results from the rich quantity of rough endoplasmic reticulum within the cytoplasm. These organelles contain basophilic-staining RNA. The endoplasmic reticulum synthesizes protein, and, because this cell is the site of formation of antibody protein (primarily gamma globulin), it is not surprising that this cell is rich in protein-forming machinery.

As the plasma cell continues to form immunoproteins, the endoplasmic reticulum in the cytoplasm slowly disintegrates and is replaced by eosinophilic-staining deposits, which represent the proteinaceous products of secretion of the cell—the immunoglobulins. This intermediate form of the plasma cell is the plasmacytoid cell (Fig. 3-5). Eventually, after synthesis of increased amounts of protein and subsequent degeneration of most intracytoplasmic organelles, the nucleus of the plasma cell is extruded, forming a hyaline, amorphous mass known as the Russell body.[112] The presence of numerous plasmacytoid cells and Russell bodies in a tissue section signifies a chronic, long-standing process.

The epithelioid cell (Figs. 3-6, 3-7; see also Figs. 7-13 to 7-19, and 11-14) is the primary indicator of granulomatous inflammation.[211] This mononuclear cell, derived from the reticuloendothelial system, has a large, pale, often indented nucleus that is shaped like a kidney or sausage. The cytoplasm stains a very pale pink. In routine tissue sections, the plasma membrane (the outer cell border of the individual epithelioid cell) is not visible. The cells therefore are arranged in a syncytium, in which all of the cells appear to be fused. The epithelioid cells of chronic granulomatous inflammation should not be confused with the malignant epithelioid cells of uveal malignant melanoma (see Figs. 7-53, 7-57, and 7-58).

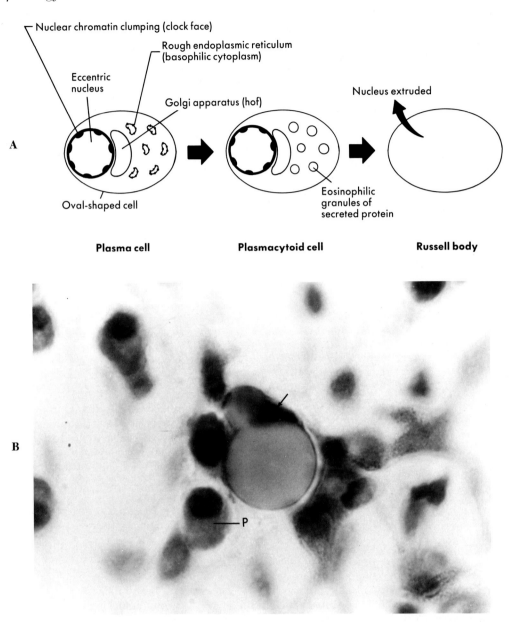

Fig. 3-5. A, Transformation of the plasma cell into a plasmacytoid cell and a Russell body. The latter stages are characterized by the retention of protein within the plasma membrane. **B,** Formation of a Russell body. The plasma cell cytoplasm is transformed into a large eosinophilic hyaline mass, and the nucleus is being extruded *(arrow).* Compare the Russell body in size with the plasma cell *(P).* (H & E stain; ×500.) (Courtesy Dr. Roland Sabates, University of Iowa.)

The giant cell of granulomatous inflammation is a derivative of the epithelioid cell. It either represents a fusion of several epithelioid cells or may have formed by amitotic nuclear division of a single epithelioid cell. The Langhans giant cell shows an arrangement of nuclei around the circumference of the cell. The foreign body giant cell is characterized by a more diffuse dispersion of nuclei throughout the cytoplasm of the cell and a more irregular cell shape. The differentiation between the two is arbitrary, however, because each form occurs interchangeably in a wide variety of types of granulomatous inflammation. Actually, a foreign body giant cell is recognized best by the demonstration of phagocytosed or adjacent foreign material that has induced the granulomatous response.[103,110]

The third specific form of giant cell, the Touton giant cell (see Fig. 7-16), occurs in xanthomatous diseases. Juvenile xanthogranuloma is an important example. It is a granulomatous disease that affects the skin and iris. Hemorrhage from the iris lesion is a significant cause of spontaneous hyphema in young persons. The Touton giant cell is recognized by the presence of lipid within the cellular cytoplasm. The lipid in sections routinely stained with hematoxylin and eosin does not take up the stain but appears as a clear area. It is deposited between the peripheral row of nuclei of the giant cell and the outer plasma membrane of the cell.

There are three basic patterns of granulomatous inflammation. Sympathetic uveitis (p. 298) and juvenile xantho-

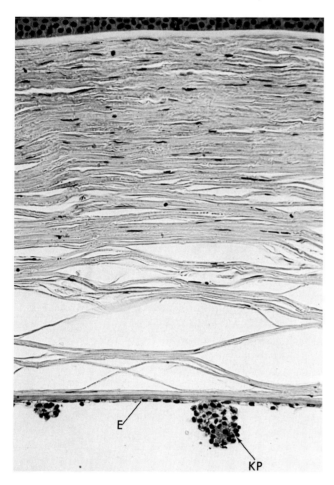

Fig. 3-6. Cornea with keratic precipitates *(KP)* deposited on the endothelium *(E).* These cellular clusters are composed of epithelioid cells that clinically present the familiar mutton-fat appearance (see also Figs. 7-13 and 7-14). (H & E stain; ×120.)

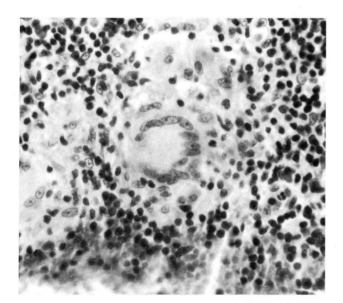

Fig. 3-7. Giant cells in granulomatous inflammation. (H & E stain; ×880.)

granuloma (p. 294), Vogt-Koyanagi-Harada syndrome (p. 299), and toxoplasmosis (p. 395) typically reveal the *diffuse* type, in which the epithelioid/giant cells are randomly distributed against a background of mononuclear cells. Sarcoidosis (p. 293) and tuberculosis typically reveal the *discrete* form, in which the epithelial/giants cells form discreati nodules. The *zonal* form consists of an arrangement of epithelioid/giant cells around a central nidus of foreign material or lens material as occurs in phacoanaphylactic endophthalmitis (see Chapter 4, p. 138).

Aggregates of epithelioid cells in different positions in the eye in various diseases are categorized by specific clinical terms, depending on their location. Keratic precipitates (Fig. 3-6, see also Figs. 7-13 and 7-14) are clusters of epithelioid cells on the posterior surface of the cornea in granulomatous anterior uveitis (mutton-fat precipitates). Koeppe nodules and Busacca nodules are similar accumulations on the iris surface in uveitis. The Dalen-Fuchs' nodule of sympathetic ophthalmia consists of aggregates of epithelioid cells and/or proliferating pigment epithelial cells that are deposited immediately beneath the retinal pigment epithelium (see Fig. 7-19, *B*). The candle-wax lesion of sarcoid consists of focal aggregates of epithelioid cells on the retina. The snowball lesions of pars planitis are clusters of epithelioid cells in the vitreous.

Inflammatory conditions

CORNEAL ULCERS

Corneal ulcers, classified as primary site of involvement as central and peripheral, are caused by a wide variety of insults, including bacterial, fungal, or viral infections, trauma; immunologic alterations[63,75,76,187]; or exposure to physical-chemical agents. An initial destruction of epithelium and Bowman's layer may be followed by varying degrees of destruction of the stroma. Stromal destruction probably is enhanced by collagenase, which is produced by the injured epithelial cells and keratocytes. When stromal destruction is massive and involves the entire thickness down to Descemet's membrane, a descemetocele may be produced (see Fig. 3-13).

In the earliest stages, the prominent histopathologic features are edema, infiltration of polymorphonuclear neutrophils, necrosis, and hypopyon. The late sequelae of corneal inflammatory disease, both ulcerative and nonulcerative, include cicatrization and opacity formation, vascularization, pannus, band keratopathy, ectasia and/or staphyloma, descemetocele, perforation, adherent leukoma, corneal keloid (exposure keratitis xerosis), and lipid degeneration. These conditions are described individually elsewhere.

CENTRAL ULCERS

Bacterial

Bacterial infections* are common and potentially dangerous forms of corneal ulceration (Figs. 3-8 and 3-9; Color Plate 3-1).[59] *Pseudomonas aeruginosa* corneal ulceration[176] is particularly noteworthy because it typically produces a virulent ulceration that may rapidly perforate. Other major agents causing central corneal ulceration include *Staphylo-*

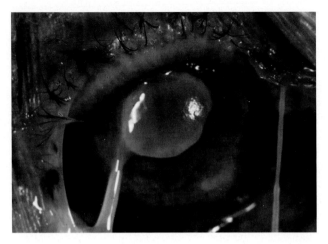

Fig. 3-8. Bacterial corneal ulcer with an acute, purulent inflammatory reaction.

coccus aureus, pneumococcus, streptococcus, and gramnegative rods such as *Escherichia coli, Proteus* species, and *Klebsiella pneumoniae.* Some strains of myocobacteria may rarely cause corneal ulceration, which usually occurs as a complication of corticosteroid therapy.

An intact corneal epithelium usually suffices as a barrier to entry of organisms into the cornea. Therefore, many cases arise after eye injuries that create an epithelial defect. Bacterial ulcers also are common in persons severely debilitated by other diseases, after corticosteroid or immunosuppressive therapy, or as a secondary superinfection to a primary viral keratitis.

The histopathologic hallmarks of acute corneal ulceration caused by bacterial infection, including invasions of polymorphonuclear neutrophils, are illustrated in Fig. 3-9. Occasionally the invasions of organisms may be so intense that bacterial colonies are formed in the tissue and may be observed in routinely stained sections. More commonly, specific diagnosis requires demon-stration of the organisms by culture or by Gram staining of tissue sections.

Fungal

Corneal ulceration caused by fungus° may occur after trauma involving vegetative material and has become increasingly prevalent because of the more widespread use of corticosteroid and immunosuppressive therapy. An unexplained delay in healing of any corneal ulcer should provoke awareness of a fungal keratitis. After trauma, the onset of the ulcer is delayed and usually is first seen 8 to 15 days after the injury. Prominent causative organisms are yeasts such as *Candida albicans* and *Aspergillus,* a mold. Other less frequent causes are *Cephalosporium, Fusarium,* and *Mucorales* species.

The case in Fig. 3-10 illustrates a typical clinical history and clinical appearance of a fungal ulcer, which is best distinguished from a bacterial ulcer by subtle variations in clinical appearance such as formation of characteristic satellite lesions around a central "dry" ulcer and an immune ring of Wessely, which is an infiltration of polyps

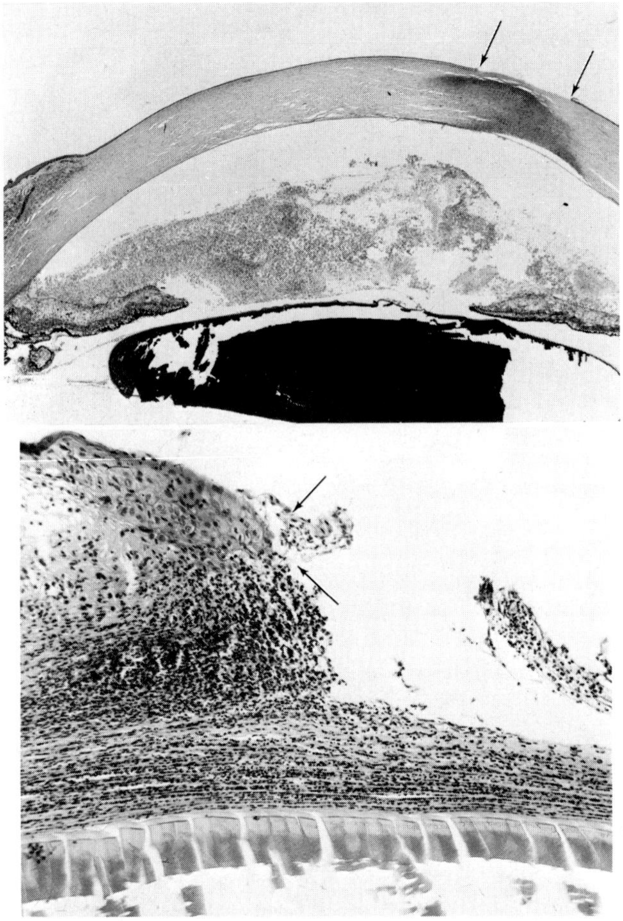

° References 82, 92, 107, 109, 113, 118, 161, 191, 220.

Fig. 3-9. A, Corneal ulcer with hypopyon. Note the defect in the corneal epithelium *(arrows)* and the increased staining intensity of the underlying stroma, which represents stromal collagen necrosis and acute neutrophilic infiltration. The anterior chamber is filled with polymorphonuclear neutrophils. (H & E stain; ×80.) **B,** Margin of a bacterial corneal ulcer. The corneal stroma to the left contains dense aggregates of polymorphonuclear neutrophils, but the overlying epithelium remains intact. The epithelium terminates abruptly at the margin of the ulcer *(arrows),* and the crater of the ulcer *(lower right)* contains a diffuse permeation of acute inflammatory cells. When polymorphonuclear cells invade the corneal stroma, they are compressed by the closely adjacent collagenous lamellae, thus making individual cells slightly more difficult to recognize. An exudate (fragmented because of a preparation artifact) is present immediately posterior to the cornea. (H & E stain; ×115.)

and plasma cells around the central lesion with an intervening area of relatively uninvolved tissue. Occasionally the mycelia within the stroma may be seen by biomicroscopy. Identification of the fungus by scrapings is best accomplished by obtaining tissue at the margin and depths of the lesion as opposed to the necrotic central region.

The histopathologic appearance of such ulcers may be similar to that of acute bacterial lesions. Sometimes abundant eosinophils are present, and the organism occasionally may initiate a granulomatous response. A hypopyon almost always is present. The organisms are best demonstrated in tissue sections using the Grocott modification of the Go-

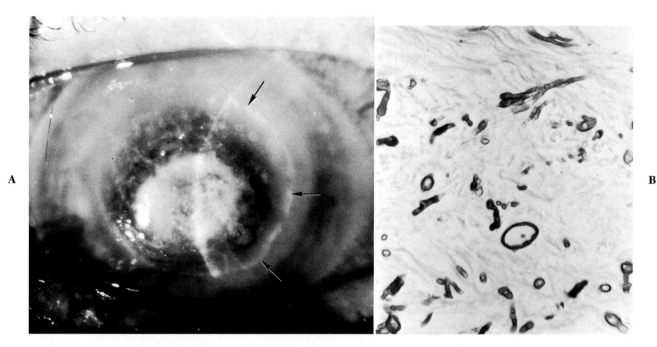

Fig. 3-10. A, Fungal ulcer resulting from trauma: a farmer was struck in the eye by a tree branch. He received subsequent corticosteroid treatment. The ulcer is hyphal, with small linear branches coming from its margin, especially below. Small satellite lesions within the stroma are visible, and an immune ring of Wessely *(arrows)* is beginning between the ulcer and the limbus. **B,** Fungal corneal ulcer and endophthalmitis. *Aspergillus, Fusarium, Candida,* and *Cephalosporium* organisms form hyphae as seen here. These should be contrasted with other fungi with thick walls or capsules, such as *Cryptococcus* and *Rhinosporidium* species. (Gridley fungus stain; ×400.) (Courtesy Dr. Herbert Kaufman.)

mori methenamine silver, Gridley, or PAS techniques (Fig. 3-10, *B;* see Table 1-1).

Acanthamoeba keratitis

Although initially recognized in 1973, case reports of *Acanthamoeba* keratitis* (Color Plates 3-2 to 3-4) were rare over the next decade until the early 1980s, when published reports of this disease increased,[196] implying an increased recognition and increased incidence. It soon became clear that contact lens wear was an important factor in the pathogenesis of this condition.[119,155]

Acanthamoeba is a genus of the order Amoebida. The organism has been isolated from fresh water, well water, sea and brackish water, hot tubs, sewage, soil, wheat, barley, feces of domestic animals, swimming pools and London air. At least 22 species have been distinguished by cyst morphology, immunofluorescent antibody testing, or isoenzyme profiles. The organism is ubiquitous and exists in nature and tissue in two forms: a uninucleated, motile trophozoite, measuring 14 to 45 µg with a wrinkled outer wall (ectocyst) and a stellate, polygonal inner wall (endocyst). The ability of the trophozoite to encyst in adverse conditions renders *Acanthamoeba* highly resistant to freezing, desiccation, standard chlorination of water supplies, and a variety of antimicrobial agents.[119]

Some of the factors proposed as being responsible for

contact lens-associated bacterial and fungal keratitis relate to *Acanthamoeba* infection[155,156]: disruption of the corneal epithelium by lens wear or handling; enhanced adherence of the organism to the lens, lens deposits, or cornea; and contamination of the lens and lens care solutions. Because *Acanthamoeba* may ingest or flourish in a substrate of gram-negative bacilli, bacterial contamination of contact lens materials may enhance the likelihood of *Acanthamoeba* infection. Most cases of contact lens-associated *Acanthamoeba* keratitis occur in patients wearing daily-wear soft contact lenses; many of these patients used saline, distilled water, and salt tablets to cleanse lenses.

Although the presence of a ring-shaped stromal infiltrate of advanced infection[199] is almost pathognomonic, the initial signs of *Acanthamoeba* keratitis may be nonspecific.[119] Patchy epithelial irregularity[93,133] or focal and multifocal pleomorphic epithelial ulceration occur. Mild, but sometimes painful, stromal keratitis and iritis develop. The keratitis has a waxing and waning course but generally is progressive over several months. The stromal inflammation may simulate a herpes simplex disciform stromal keratitis. The ring-shaped infiltrate presumably is caused by interaction of polymorphonuclear leukocytes with intact organisms, antigen, or byproducts of infection. The central stroma within the ring appears coarsely granular. Discrete round or oval zones of relative sparing (lacunae) may appear within areas of the stromal infiltration. Inflammatory cells collect around corneal nerves.[154] Posterior scleritis has been observed.[139] Severe iritis and hypopyon may develop.

---

* References 58, 78, 81, 83, 89, 93, 117, 119, 123, 133, 137, 139, 140, 142, 143, 155–157, 170, 173, 182, 192, 193, 196, 199, 209, 234, 242.

Advanced infection produces necrotizing stromal suppuration and corneal perforation, resembling bacterial or fungal keratitis. Bacterial superinfection and concurrent herpes simplex viral infection have occurred. Hematogenous dissemination from an infected cornea of a patient with *Acanthamoeba* keratitis that produced a chorioretinitis in the opposite eye has been reported.[117]

One must contemplate laboratory investigations in many eyes otherwise diagnosed to be atypical or severe forms of herpes simplex or other immunogenic keratitis.[119] Although *Acanthamoeba* can be identified by Gram and Giemsa staining of corneal scrapings and grows readily on standard blood agar, special methods should be used in suspected *Acanthamoeba* keratitis. Corneal biopsy with a 1.5- or 2-mm trephine may be required to obtain deep material for culture, histopathology, and electron microscopy.[142] Nomarski interference microscopy with phase-contrast illumination is ideal for direct examination for cysts and trophozoites but requires special equipment and must be performed immediately. The calcofluor white stain is useful in detecting cysts in direct smear or biopsy material.[193,209] The organism may be visualized using fluorescein-conjugated lectins[182] and indirect fluorescent antibody staining.[89] A polyclonal antibody for indirect immunofluorescent staining of intact organisms and antigen in corneal smears is available.

Among 74 cases of *Acanthamoeba* keratitis reported or known to Jones,[119] only 39 (52%) were identified by corneal scraping or biopsy before surgery. The organism can also be identified by confocal microscopy. The remainder were diagnosed after therapeutic keratoplasty (31 cases) or enucleation (4 cases). The mean interval from onset of symptoms to diagnosis in all cases was 22 weeks and ranged from 2 to 68 weeks. At the Cullen Eye Institute, *Acanthamoeba* was identified in each of 10 confirmed cases by smear or culture of corneal scrapings or biopsy material. In four, cysts were detected only by the calcofluor white stain. Of the nine culture-positive infections, amebic tracts appeared on horse blood agar in four within 24 hours after inoculation.

The preferred treatment of *Acanthamoeba* keratitis has not been determined. Some investigators have reported improvement after administration of topical neomycin sulfate and propamidine isethionate, oral ketoconazole, natamycin, and paromomycin.[63] Driebe and associates[83] recently reported a potential role for topical clotrimazole, an antifungal agent, in combination chemotherapy of this disease.

Viral

The most frequent type of virus-induced corneal ulceration results from herpes simplex type I virus (Fig. 3-11; Color Plate 3-5); herpes zoster dendritic ulcer is less common (Fig. 3-12).* Following are the ocular manifestations of herpes simplex:

1. Superficial ulcerative keratitis
   a. Dendritic keratitis with or without stromal involvement
   b. Geographic epithelial keratitis

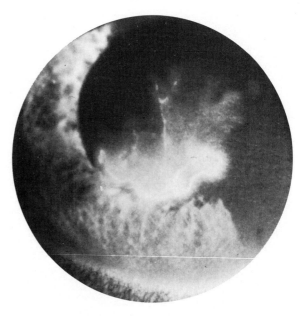

Fig. 3-11. Herpes simplex keratitis with dendritic ulcer.

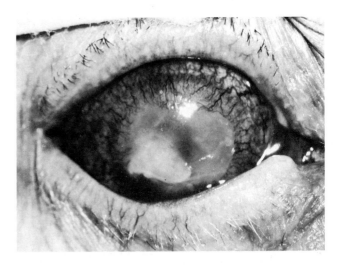

Fig. 3-12. Herpes zoster keratouveitis.

2. Deep keratitis
   a. Endothelitis
   b. Stromal disciform keratitis, perforating or nonperforating, with or without ulceration
   c. Stromal leukoma
3. Uveitis[105,179]
   a. Uveitis without keratitis
   b. Uveitis with keratitis, with or without ulceration

The dendritic ulcer affects the corneal epithelium with or without involvement of the underlying stroma. Geographic keratitis signifies a patchy destruction of epithelium. Individuals who have atopic dermatitis are particularly susceptible to herpes simplex infections. Verification of the diagnosis may be confirmed by corneal scrapings and Giemsa staining or by histopathologic examination of excised tissue. When present, two structures in the involved epithelium and superficial keratocytes are diagnos-

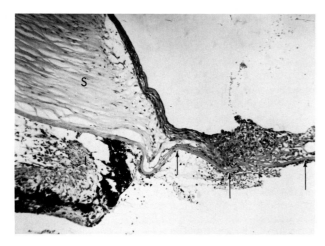

Fig. 3-13. Descemetocele caused by acute viral keratitis and corneal ulcer. The stroma *(S)* abruptly terminates centrally where the corneal thickness is reduced to a thin membrane composed of Descemet's membrane *(arrows)* and necrotic inflammatory debris. Note the fibrin (delicate fibrils in a spider-web arrangement and cells in the anterior chamber. *I,* Iris with an anterior synechia. (H & E stain; ×820.)

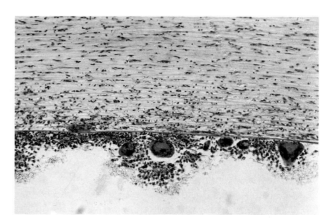

Fig. 3-14. Disciform herpes simplex keratitis, a granulomatous reaction to Descemet's membrane. (H & E stain; ×320.) (From Naumann GOH and Apple DJ. In Doerr W, Seifert G, and Uehlinger E, editors: Handbuch der speziellen pathologischen Anatomie, Band Auge, Berlin, 1980, Springer-Verlag.)

tic: multinucleated giant cells and distinctive intranuclear inclusions, the so-called inclusion of Lipschütz or type A Cowdry inclusions. This inclusion is similar to the intranuclear inclusion of cytomegalic inclusion disease (p. 396) in that it consists of a densely staining, round mass within the nucleus surrounded by an area of decreased stain intensity (peri-inclusion halo). Particles are found in both nucleus and cytoplasm by electron microscopy.

The cellular infiltration may vary with the aggressiveness of the disease, showing a varying proportion of acute inflammatory cells and mononuclear chronic inflammatory cells. A postherpetic chronic ulcer may progress and involve the deeper corneal lamellae down to Descemet's membrane. A descemetocele (Fig. 3-13) may form, and corneal perforation is a distinct hazard.

The virus resides in sensory ganglia, especially the trigeminal, and transmission along axons appears to be a source of recurrent infections.

In addition to postherpetic ulceration of the superficial tissues, a disciform keratitis may occur, either as a complication of an original ulcer or in the absence of an ulcer. This actually is an example of a deep or stromal keratitis in which the stromal lamellae are affected by a chronic, slowly healing inflammatory process and corneal vascularization that may persist for years. Viruses have been demonstrated in the corneal stroma by electron microscopy. Disciform keratitis is thought to be related to the increased use of corticosteroids; it actually may signify only a prolongation of the natural course of herpes by suppression of the normal immune response by steroid therapy. Bullous keratopathy (metaherpetic phase) may occur with epithelial edema that may accompany the stromal involvement.

A characteristic histopathologic feature of long-standing disciform keratitis and some other forms of recurrent keratitis is a granulomatous reaction to Descemet's membrane[103,110] (Fig. 3-14). A mixed inflammatory reaction in which epithelioid cells and giant cells predominate occurs

along Descemet's membrane. The microscopic appearance resembles that which occurs at the lens capsule in phacoanaphylactic endophthalmitis (p. 138; see Fig. 4-43, *B*). Both probably represent an autosensitivity reaction.

Peripheral ulcerations

Four ulceroinflammatory conditions primarily involve the corneal periphery: marginal (catarrhal) ulcer, ring ulcer, ring abscess, and Mooren's ulcer.*

Fuchs' marginal degeneration[69,134,195,198] (chronic peripheral furrow keratitis) should not be confused with the peripheral ulcers because it represents more of a degenerative autoimmune process rather than an inflammatory process, and the epithelium remains intact. It consists of a bilateral corneal opacity that begins superiorly with thinning of the peripheral stroma similar in location to that of arcus senilis. It usually occurs in males younger than 40 years of age and develops slowly over decades. The thinning may be severe, but perforation is rare.

Marginal ulcer. The marginal ulcer consists of numerous small foci of involvement, which may appear in multiple peripheral sectors of the cornea. It occurs in association with eyelid inflammations or conjunctivitis and usually is a hypersensitivity reaction to the toxins produced by staphylococcal blepharitis. The Morax Axenfeld bacillus, staphylococci, or the Koch-Weeks bacillus also may produce peripheral corneal ulcerations by direct invasion.

Retention of normal areas of intervening cornea between each individual ulceration often is a distinguishing feature. This lesion is confined to the very superficial stroma or epithelium in the periphery, and there is little tendency toward significant tissue destruction and loss of vision.

Ring ulcer. In ring ulcer, a complete or almost complete ring of involvement forms around the corneal periphery, often resulting from coalescence of several marginal

---

* References 60, 61, 65, 69, 91, 95, 102, 134, 151–153, 185, 195, 198, 214, 215, 218.

ulcers.[215] It usually is associated with *Staphylococcus aureus* or in rare instances, is a complication of trachoma.

A separate category of ring ulcers has been described in autoimmune endogenous diseases such as rheumatoid arthritis, Wegener's granulomatosis,[91] and other collagen diseases. The exact course of these ulcerations is not known,[61] but they probably result from a hypersensitivity state.

A complete ring may develop from coalescence of individual lesions. Because ulceration may rarely spread centrally and induce a greater degree of necrosis, the ring ulcer is more destructive than the marginal ulcer. However, ring ulcers are confined to the superficial areas of the cornea and do not tend to invade the deeper stroma; therefore, perforation occurs rarely. To date, no histopathologic findings are available that indicate a specific etiologic diagnosis. The destruction of epithelium and formation of a crater is sometimes similar to that seen with a mild infectious ulcer or Mooren's ulcer (Fig. 3-16).

Ring abscess. The ring ulcer should be distinguished clearly from the ring abscess (Fig. 3-15), which is characterized by extensive florid necrosis of the cornea and has a very poor prognosis. Most cases of ring abscess result from accidental or surgical corneal wounds. Metastatic bacterial or fungal invasion after septicemia also may cause a ring abscess. Initially, the peripheral cornea shows small acute inflammatory infiltrate with associated florid necrosis of layers. The far periphery of the cornea remains clear, and the central portion is clear initially but later becomes hazy because of necrosis. Panophthalmitis usually follows.

Mooren's ulcer. Mooren's ulcer (ulcus rodens, chronic serpiginous ulcer),[95,102,134,152,214,218] an uncommon condition, occurs primarily in middle-aged persons and is unilateral in approximately two thirds of cases (Color Plate 3-6). There are two forms, one that is relatively benign, usually occurring in older persons, which often responds to constructive therapy. The classic type, however, often is painful, dramatically progressive, and refractory to therapy. The ulcer begins as an excavating ulceration in the limbal area and extends centrally (Fig. 3-16). Sometimes it also involves the scleral portion of the limbus. It typically has a raised border and an overhanging ridge at the advancing edge. The ulcer may extend for 360 degrees around the periphery. There is a filtration of the lymphocytes and plasma cells. The uninvolved portions of the cornea usually remain clear and transparent. In early stages, the inflammatory reaction affects the epithelium, Bowman's layer, and the anterior stroma; in more severe cases, the infiltration extends deeply into the stroma. As many as a third of the ulcers that involve the limbal sclera in addition to the cornea may progress to perforation.

Microscopically, the cornea is thickened at the margin of the ulcer because of invasion of acute and chronic inflammatory cells into the anterior layers of the stroma and within the epithelium at the edge of the ulcer (Fig. 3-16). The overhanging edge adjacent to the advancing ulcer is characteristic but not always demonstrated well in microscopic sections. Extensive necrosis occurs in the involved epithelium and stroma. Although immunoglobulins in affected corneas have been demonstrated and suggest an autoimmune process, histopathologic studies to date have not successfully implicated a specific etiologic agent or process.

NONULCERATIVE CORNEAL INFLAMMATIONS

Examples of nonulcerative keratitis include infectious crystalline keratopathy, superficial punctate keratitis, epidemic keratoconjunctivitis, and interstitial keratitis.

Infectious crystalline keratopathy

In 1983, Gorovay and coworkers[101] reported the presence of progressive branching, needle-like stromal opacities within the corneal transplant of a patient who had undergone penetrating keratoplasty for aphakic bullous keratopathy. The patient had received topical corticosteroids for a prolonged period of time. Analysis of the corneal

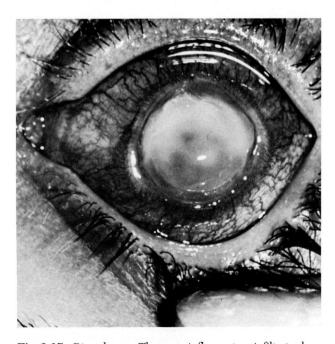

Fig. 3-15. Ring abscess. The acute inflammatory infiltrates have caused a diffuse haze of the entire cornea.

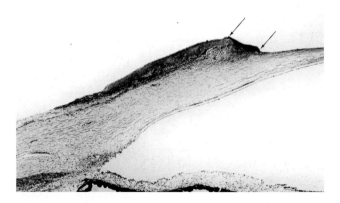

Fig. 3-16. Mooren's ulcer. Note the junction (*arrows*) of the intact corneal epithelium and the broad base or crater of the ulcer on the right. The inflammatory response is nonspecific and reveals no consistent or reliable clues to the origin of the disease. (H & E stain; ×25.)

button by light microscopy disclosed a localized epithelial ingrowth into the stroma at a suture tract accompanied by intrastromal pockets of gram-positive cocci. No inflammatory reaction was found in the areas of bacterial colonization. Cultures were not obtained because the infectious etiology of the lesion was not recognized.

Meisler and coworkers in 1984[148,149] coined the term *infectious crystalline keratopathy* for this entity (Color Plate 3-7). These authors described three patients with this condition, which was characterized by an insidious appearance of white, branching crystalline stromal opacities that increased in size slowly and with little associated corneal inflammation. In two of the three cases, histopathologic studies disclosed accumulation of colonies of gram-positive cocci insinuated between corneal stroma lamellae, *Streptococcus viridans* was isolated in culture. A nonbacterial form of postkeratopathy crystalline keratopathy has also been reported.[207]

Streptococcus viridans has been identified as the cause of the infiltrate in most of the previously reported cases.* Clinically, the disease is characterized by discrete anterior stromal opacities that appear white, branching, and proceed insidiously to create the distinct lesion, usually associated with little or no corneal inflammation.[148,149] It is difficult to account for the crystalline appearance in this entity. The most logical source for the crystalline shape would seem to be bacteria proliferating between corneal lamellae. Local immunosuppression may play a role in the pathogenesis of crystalline keratopathy.[190] The majority of patients had been receiving long-term topical corticosteroid therapy after corneal transplantation or as treatment for recurrent herpes simplex keratitis.

Laboratory confirmation is essential in establishing the diagnosis. Superficial scrapings of corneal surface may fail to show the infectious process. A lamellar keratectomy may be necessary to recover the organisms for culture and microscopy. The usual causative organism, hemolytic streptococcus, is easily recognizable by Gram stain, and transmission electron microscope has disclosed the characteristic trimalleolar structure of the bacterial cell wall. Other bacteria include hemophilus prophilus and aphrophilus.[104]

Therapy for infectious crystalline keratopathy resulting from bacterial infection requires discontinuation of topical corticosteroids and frequent application of broad spectrum antibiotics. However, the infection often is progressive despite intensive antibiotic therapy.

There are several noninfectious causes of crystalline corneal dystrophy,[67] including Schnyder's crystalline corneal dystrophy, Bietti's crystalline dystrophy, cystinosis,† chronic renal failure, dysproteinemia and monoclonal gammopathy hyperkalemia,[15,62,74,86,166] and lipid keratopathy[42] after surgery[204] and after long-term drug therapy.

Superficial punctate keratitis

Superficial punctate keratitis of Thygeson[56,129,197,201] is a bilateral condition showing multiple discrete epithelial opacities, which may number 20 or more and are most common centrally in the pupillary area. The opacities usually are not visible grossly but are seen easily with biomicroscopy. Clinical symptoms include indolent tearing, pain, and photophobia.

Fluorescein staining easily identifies these strictly intraepithelial, nonulcerative lesions. Corneal sensation sometimes is reduced but not to the degree, for example, as that seen in herpes simplex. The actual cause is unknown, although a virus is suspected.[129] Superficial punctate keratitis responds to frequent topical instillation of steroids. Bandage lenses and cyclosporine drops can also be helpful. The histopathologic picture is nonspecific but generally shows mild epithelial edema, early transient acute infiltration of polymorphonuclear neutrophils, and later mild infiltration of lymphocytes and other chronic inflammatory cells.

Epidemic keratoconjunctivitis

Epidemic or subepithelial keratoconjunctivitis, often called *shipyard conjunctivitis* because of epidemics among shipyard personnel, usually is attributed to infection by adenovirus type 8.* The virus is transferred by hand from eye to eye by the physician or nurse during examination. Usually the preauricular lymph nodes are enlarged.

The corneal lesions usually are unilateral, multiple, and more concentrated at the pupillary area. The infiltrates occur in the subepithelial stroma and appear 15 or more days after the onset of an accompanying conjunctivitis. The range of corneal involvement begins with diffuse punctate keratitis, which progresses to focal epithelial keratitis in 6 to 10 days and is followed by the development of subepithelial opacities and eventual formation of the gray epithelial infiltrates. Corneal sensitivity is not affected in most cases. Histopathologically, the early lesions are characterized by edema followed by nonspecific infiltration of lymphocytes, which may create tiny opacities in the affected region. Viral particles have been demonstrated in the involved areas by electron microscopy. It is not clear whether the inflammatory infiltrates represent a direct response to the virus or a focal hypersensitivity reaction.

Interstitial keratitis

Interstitial keratitis† may arise occasionally as an allergic sequela of bacterial infection. Syphilis and, to a lesser extent, tuberculosis and leprosy are the bacterial diseases most commonly associated with interstitial keratitis.[167] In addition, herpes simplex disciform keratitis, herpes zoster, varicella, lymphogranuloma venereum, mumps, and other viruses[144] have been implicated. Onchocerciasis (river blindness), caused by the nematode *Onchocerca volvulus*,[113] is one of the leading causes of blindness in the world and may produce an interstitial keratitis. Diffuse inflammatory involvement of the stroma also occurs in sarcoidosis, mycosis fungoides, and Hodgkin's disease. A foreign body-induced interstitial keratitis (ophthalmia nodosa and nummular keratitis) may be caused by introduction of hairs or vegetable foreign bodies into the cornea (Figs. 3-62 and 3-63). Interstitial keratitis also has been found to follow

* References 104, 114, 124, 125, 135, 145, 147-149, 159, 165, 183, 190, 207, 210.
† References 12, 80, 97, 99, 121, 184.

* References 57, 79, 100, 128, 136, 171.
† References 85, 98, 130, 167, 186, 194, 206, 208.

long-term heavy metal therapy, for example, arsenic or gold.

The overwhelming majority of cases of interstitial keratitis result from congenital syphilis[98] (Fig. 3-17, *A*). The corneal involvement almost always is bilateral. (The occurrence of the unusual unilateral form indicates a high probability of an acquired syphilis rather than the congenital form.) The corneal lesions rarely are present at birth; they typically occur in late childhood or during the teenage years and are most prominent in the third and fourth decades of life.

The major systemic findings of congenital syphilis[98,115,186,194] are partial deafness, Hutchinson's teeth,[115] prominent frontal eminences, saddle-shaped nose, rhagades at the edge of the mouth, and saber shins or tibial periosteitis. Cogan's syndrome shows features similar to those of acquired syphilis, including deafness and interstitial keratitis, and occasionally is associated with periarteritis nodosa.

Histopathologically,[208] interstitial keratitis is characterized by an infiltration of inflammatory cells into the corneal stroma in the absence of overlying ulceration (Fig. 3-17, *B* and *C*). These cells separate the corneal lamellae, and corneal vascularization is extensive. The vascularization in late lesions is responsible for ghost vessels, an important clinical sign.

In the late stage of syphilitic interstitial keratitis, the cornea has red areas. These "salmon patches" represent areas of vascularization in the superficial and deep corneal stromal layers. By the fifth and sixth decades, the endothelium often becomes involved, and large areas may become atrophic.[206] As a result, corneal guttata that are morphologically similar to those seen in Fuchs' dystrophy (see Fig. 3-49) may develop. Progressive edema and opacification of the deeper layers of the stroma result from endothelial decompensation. Secondary band keratopathy, lipid deposition in the stroma, and secondary glaucoma[130] are complications of long-standing cases.

Degenerations[221-342]

AGING AND ENVIRONMENTAL CHANGES

The two most common aging changes occurring in the cornea are Hassall-Henle warts[256] (Fig. 3-4) and arcus senilis[223,224,238,331] (p. 62).

Keratitis sicca is caused by a defect in the watery part of the tear film, causing punctate epithelial erosion. Schirmer's test results are invariably positive. Most patients

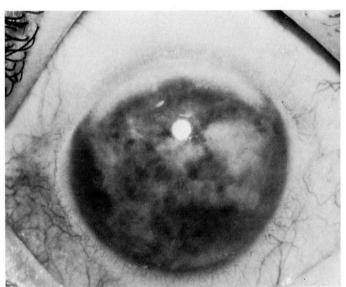

Fig. 3-17. Interstitial keratitis. **A,** Following congenital syphilis in a 20-year-old man. This lesion is the prototype of a keratitis in which the cellular infiltrate is primarily located in the corneal stroma. **B,** Acute form. (H & E stain; ×200.) **C,** Chronic stage with extensive stromal vascularization. (H & E stain; ×220.)

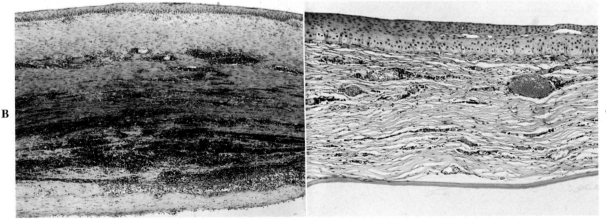

have excess tear film mucous; positive rose bengal staining may demonstrate pre-existing diseases such as staphylococcal conjunctivitis or blepharitis. It may occur as Sjogren's syndrome (keratoconjunctivitis sicca) xerostomia, and connective tissue disease such as rheumatoid arthritis. The filaments of filamentary keratitis consist primarily of degenerated epithelial cells and mucous.

Pinguecula and pterygium and so-called keratinoid degeneration[252,258,282,300] of the superficial corneal-conjunctival stroma share a common pathogenesis because they are induced by constant exposure to sun, wind, dust, and other environmental influences (see Chapter 11).

CORNEAL DELLEN, EDEMA, AND BULLOUS KERATOPATHY

The corneal endothelium is of prime importance in maintaining proper corneal dehydration.[152,170,194] The endothelial cells, rich with mitochondria, serve as an active metabolic pump. In conjunction with the tear film and epithelium anteriorly, they maintain a relative state of detumescence of the cornea. A delle (pl. dellen)[291] is the opposite of corneal edema. It is a localized area of corneal dehydration and thinning caused by a defect transient in continuity of the tear film that is caused by an elevation of surrounding tissues. The break can result from a localized lesion or mass, for example, a pterygium or tumor.

Although corneal edema[222,231,257,263] may result from primary or secondary damage to the epithelium, it usually is caused by diseases affecting the integrity of the endothelium and Descemet's membrane. Such an endothelial decompensation causes an unregulated imbibition of fluid into the cornea, with resultant decrease in transparency (Fig. 3-18). The endothelial dystrophy of Fuchs' (see Fig. 3-49) is a classic example of a disease in which stromal and epithelial edema occur as a direct result of failure of endothelial cell function.

The incidence of intraocular lens (IOL) implantation is increasing dramatically. The advent of this technique has not been without complications; it has led to an increasing

incidence of iatrogenic or postinsertion endothelial damage that causes corneal decompensation and pseudophakic bullous keratopathy[298] (p. 167; see Fig. 4-92). This was especially true with early iris-supported IOLs and poorly designed anterior chamber IOLs. According to Jakobiec,[255] in the 1980s corneal transplantation was performed more often for pseudophakic bullous keratopathy than for any other disease. Waring[298] termed this an epidemic of pseudophakic corneal decompensation. Although newer intraocular designs have lessened the incidence of this complication, it still occurs. Following are many causes of endothelial decompensation (corneal edema):

Primary endothelial disease
    Fuchs' combined dystrophy
    Congenital hereditary endothelial dystrophy
    Schlichting's deep posterior polymorphous dystrophy
Secondary endothelial disease
    After surgical and nonsurgical trauma (birth injury, hyphema, chemical burns, corneal transplant rejection, vitreous touch syndrome after lens extraction, implantation of intraocular lenses
    After glaucoma
    After keratitis, particularly interstitial keratitis
    After uveitis
    Complication of corneal stromal dystrophies, particularly lattice dystrophy
    Complication of retrocorneal fibrous membrane
After rupture of Descemet's membrane
    Congenital glaucoma (Haab's striae)
    Birth trauma (forceps injury)
    Acute keratoconus
    High myopia

Stromal edema is readily appreciated clinically (Fig. 3-18); however, in the majority of cases, it may be more difficult to confirm histopathologically. The fluid permeates the mucopolysaccharide ground substance of the stroma and creates a separation of the collagen lamellae. However, this microscopic diagnosis usually is tenuous because during routine processing, the normally hydrated cornea often shows artifactitious formation of interlamellar clefts (Fig. 3-2). Corneal scarring and vascularization are sequelae of long-standing stromal edema.

Epithelial edema, however, is easily recognized microscopically (Fig. 3-19). The fluid sometimes is found between corneal epithelial cells (intercellular edema) or is imbibed into the epithelial cells, usually involving the basal layer initially and leading to intracellular edema. This hydropic swelling may lead to necrosis of the affected cells and the formation of intraepithelial microcysts.

Bullous keratopathy[178,222,257] (Figs. 3-20 and 3-21) leads to severe visual loss[178] and irregular astigmatism because of irregularity of the corneal surface. As noted previously, the incidence of pseudophakic bullous keratopathy[178,298,299] has increased greatly in recent years and is becoming a major cause of corneal decompensation. The bulla, or cavity, is created when a cleavage plane forms between the corneal epithelium and the underlying Bowman's layer.[222] Degeneration of the epithelial basement membrane occurs with loss of hemidesmosomes. The latter structures are specialized cell junctions, visible only at the

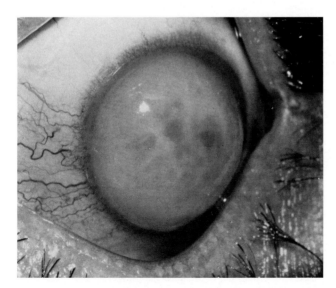

Fig. 3-18. Keratoconus with hydrops. Total opacity has resulted from edema of the epithelium and stroma.

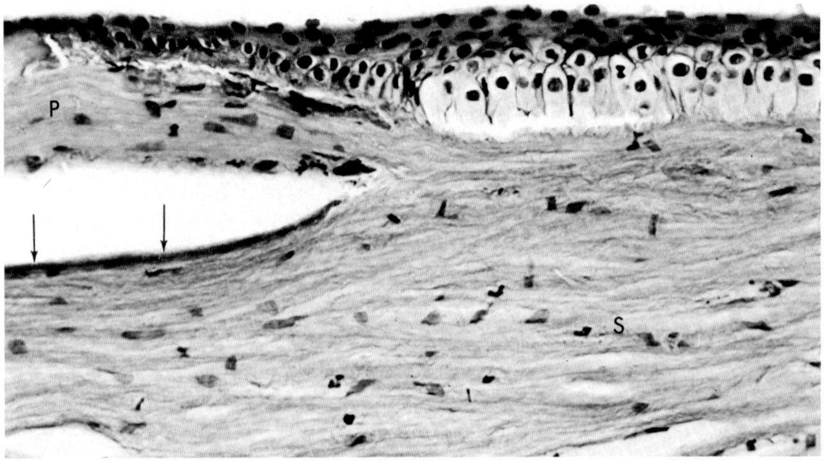

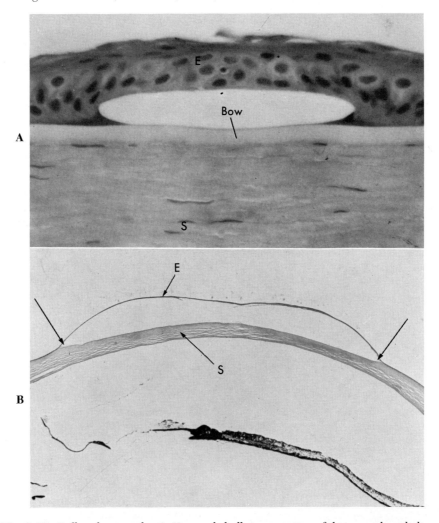

Fig. 3-19. Corneal epithelial edema in long-standing glaucoma. The bloated, poorly staining cells of the basal layer of corneal epithelium have undergone hydropic swelling. A plaque resembling a fibrovascular pannus *(P)* separates the epithelium from Bowman's layer. This is the site of an old bullous keratopathy. *Arrows,* Calcification (increased staining) of Bowman's layer; *S,* extensive scarring of the stroma. (H & E stain; ×190.)

Fig. 3-20. Bullous keratopathy. **A,** Very early bullous separation of the corneal epithelium. The corneal epithelium *(E)* is separated from the underlying Bowman's layer *(Bow)*, forming a small vesicle. *S,* Stroma. (H & E stain; ×280.) **B,** Advanced case with separation of the corneal epithelium *(E)* from the underlying stroma *(S)*. *Arrows,* Margins of the plane of separation of the epithelium. (H & E stain; ×65.)

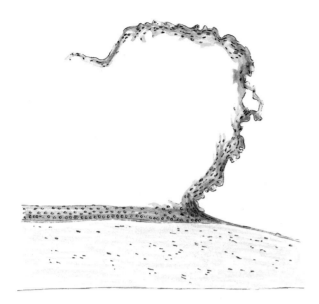

Fig. 3-21. Schematic illustration of splitting and separation of the corneal epithelium (filamentary keratopathy). (Redrawn by Dr. Steven Vermillion, University of Iowa, from von Hippel E: In Henke F and Lubarsch O, editors: Handbuch der speziellen Pathologischen Anatomie und Histologie, Berlin, 1928, Julius Springer.)

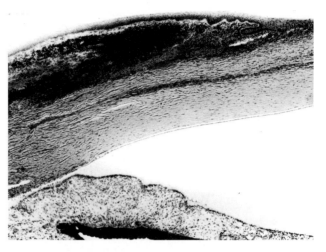

Fig. 3-22. Inflammatory pannus, characterized by ingrowth of inflammatory cells from the limbus, leading to a separation of the corneal epithelium from the underlying Bowman's layer. (H & E stain; ×88.)

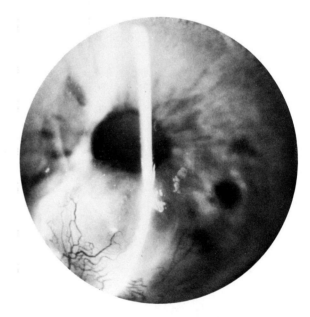

Fig. 3-23. Degenerative (fibrovascular) pannus in keratoconus. Note the vascular ingrowth from the inferior limbus.

ultrastructural level, that attach the epithelium to Bowman's layer.

In late stages, the bullous cavity is replaced by organized fibrous tissue interposed between the epithelium and Bowman's layer. Histopathologic sections of such a fibrous plaque resemble that of a long-standing degenerative pannus. However, as usually defined, a pannus is a limbal ingrowth of connective tissue, whereas the degenerative plaque resulting from old bullous epithelial separation is caused by in situ fibrosis and degeneration of the involved area.

PANNUS

A pannus[232,239] is an ingrowth of tissue from the limbus onto the peripheral cornea. The infiltration occurs between the corneal epithelium and Bowman's layer, thereby creating a separation of these two layers. Bowman's layer often is destroyed. An inflammatory pannus (Fig. 3-22) occurs in many forms of ulcerative or nonulcerative keratoconjunctivitis. As this term suggests, the pannus is composed of inflammatory cells in the peripheral, subepithelial stratum of the cornea. Its chronic phases involve secondary scarring and further opacification of the cornea. Sometimes in late stages, the inflammatory cells are replaced by fibrous tissue, and the true nature of the lesion is therefore obscured.

An inflammatory pannus is distinguished from a degenerative, or fibrovascular, pannus (Figs. 3-23 and 3-24). This ingrowth of collagen and vessels occurs as a nonspecific response to a wide variety of insults, such as long-standing glaucoma, bullous keratopathy, exposure keratitis, and trauma.

Fatty plaques often are deposited within the substance of a degenerative pannus (Fig. 3-25). When the infiltrates

are prominent, it is termed a *lipid keratopathy* (secondary lipid degeneration, lipidosis corneae).[237,280,303] These processes are distinguished from a primary lipid degeneration, or so-called lipid dystrophy (p. 86).

BAND-SHAPED KERATOPATHY

Band keratopathy° (Figs. 3-19 and 3-26) may occur as a secondary response (dystrophia calcification) to any degenerative or inflammatory process affecting the anterior layers of the cornea—for example, trauma, chronic kerati-

° References 227, 236, 241, 251, 261, 265, 270, 272, 274, 275, 296.

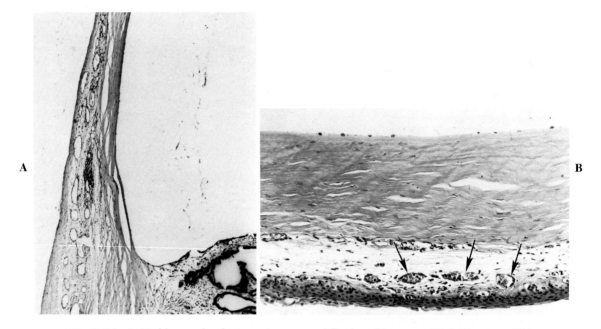

Fig. 3-24. A, Highly vascular degenerative pannus following old trauma. (H & E stain; ×15.)
B, Degenerative (fibrovascular) pannus. The corneal epithelium and Bowman's layer are separated
by an ingrowth of fibrovascular tissue (*arrows,* vessels), which occurs as a nonspecific finding in
many degenerative conditions, such as trauma or glaucoma. Bowman's layer has been destroyed.
(H & E stain; ×230.)

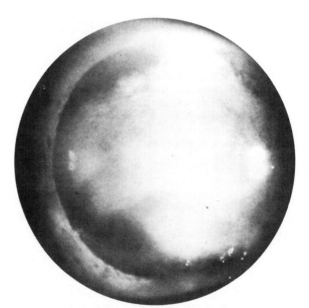

Fig. 3-25. Lipid keratopathy. **A,** Diffuse lipid infiltrates throughout the entire cornea. **B,** Nonstaining lipid deposits within the superficial stroma. (H & E stain; ×220.)

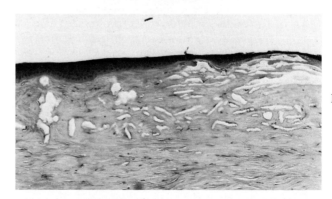

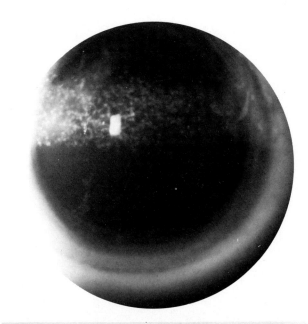

A

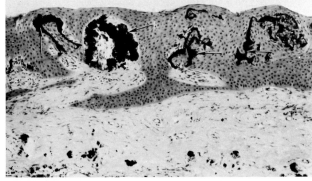

B

Fig. 3-26. A, Clinical photograph of band keratopathy caused by a horizontally coursing deposition of calcium in Bowman's layer in the region corresponding to the margins of the palpebral fissures. **B,** Band keratopathy (calcific deposits at the level of Bowman's layer and the epithelium, *arrows*) resulting from long-standing glaucoma. The epithelium is significantly irregular. Calcification of a diseased focus is termed *dystrophic calcification.* Metastatic calcification occurs in normal tissue when serum calcium levels are increased because of any factor. (H & E stain; ×280.)

Table 3-1. Corneal iron lines

Name of line	Associated tissue changes
Hudson-Stahli	Iron line seen centrally in the aging cornea or seen as a nonspecific degenerative response to trauma or inflammation; courses horizontally just inferior to the center of the palpebral fissure
Stocker	Iron line in front of the head of pterygium
Fleischer	Iron line seen at the cone base in kerataconus
Ferry	Iron line in front of filtering bleb
Coat's white ring (unproved)	White ring usually in the inferior half of the cornea; pathogenesis unknown

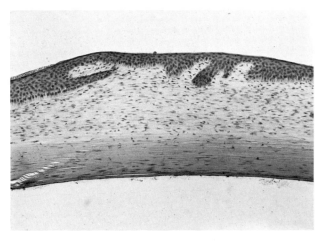

Fig. 3-27. Dense fibrosis of the anterior two thirds of the corneal stroma and significant epithelial irregularities. (H & E stain; ×180.)

tis or uveitis, long-standing glaucoma, sarcoidosis, or rheumatoid arthritis.

Calcification of a normal Bowman's layer (metastatic calcification) sometimes occurs when the patient has high serum calcium levels.[236,296] This phenomenon occurs in such conditions as hypervitaminosis D, renal insufficiency,[274] Fanconi's syndrome, the milk-alkali syndrome, and hyperparathyroidism.[275] In rare instances, band keratopathy results from gout or ichthyosis or is transmitted in families (see Table 3-2). The line of calcification forms a horizontal band because the exposed, unprotected interpalpebral portion of the cornea is more susceptible. Small circular clear areas within the semiopaque band sometimes can be seen by biomicroscopy; these probably correspond to the sites of passage of the corneal nerves as they pass through Bowman's layer.

The calcium is deposited primarily in Bowman's layer

and may extend into the epithelium or occasionally into the superficial stroma. It is basophilic by hematoxylin and eosin stain but stains brilliantly by the alizarin red technique (Table 3-1).

SCARRING AND VASCULARIZATION

The most common acquired causes of cicatrization (Fig. 3-27) and vascularization of the cornea are trauma, keratitis, corneal edema, and chronic glaucoma. A nebula is a very small corneal scar that can be seen only by biomicroscopy. A corneal opacity of intermediate size and density is a macula. More dense and usually larger corneal opacities are termed leukomas. These scars are most frequently seen after penetrating or perforating corneal trauma.

A corneal keloid[235,273] (Fig. 3-28) exemplifies a greatly exaggerated fibrous overgrowth of the cornea, which usually follows trauma. This type of scar occasionally is present at birth and may be confused with a large corneal dermoid. Histopathologically, large dense bundles of collagen in disarray replace the corneal stroma.

Formation of new corneal vessels probably is mediated through a chemical angiogenic factor that is released by damaged corneal tissue, but to date this has not been

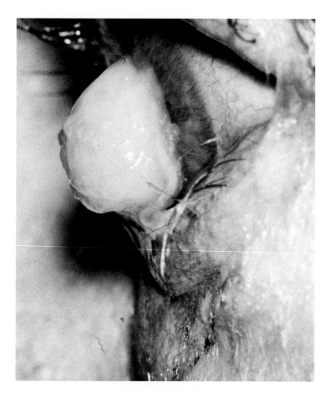

Fig. 3-28. Corneal keloid. This lesion probably represents a massive production of collagen in response to a corneal injury. This response is not unlike that which occurs after injury to the skin. (Courtesy Drs. Harold Kirk and Richard O'Grady.)

identified. Ingrowth of vessels occurs most readily in edematous corneas in which the stromal lamellae become separated, allowing an unimpeded route for spread of vessels.

Vascularization of the cornea is of two types: superficial and deep. Superficial vascularization occurs by ingrowth of a pannus from the limbus (Figs. 3-23 and 3-24). Deep vascularization is a common sequela of interstitial keratitis (Fig. 3-17, *C*).

SALZMANN'S NODULAR DEGENERATION

Formerly known as Salzmann's nodular "dystrophy," Salzmann's nodular degeneration usually occurs as a reactive process after corneal injury or keratitis and is better classified as a degeneration.[279,295] It consists of gray-blue superficial nodular masses, most commonly seen in elderly women. Histopathologic features include alternating thickening and thinning of the epithelium, increase in thickness of the subepithelial basement membrane, pannus formation, and hyaline thickening of the superficial stroma by deposition of nodular collagen masses.

RETROCORNEAL FIBROUS MEMBRANE

Formation of a retrocorneal fibrous membrane (Figs. 3-29 and 3-30) can result from many causes. These include fibrous organization of a hyphema (Figs. 3-29, *A*, and 3-30, *A*), organization of inflammatory debris within the anterior chamber (Figs. 3-29, *B*, and 3-30, *B*), alkali burns (p. 104), ingrowth of fibrous tissue through a perforating corneal wound, or corneal transplantation (Fig. 3-30, *C*; see also Figs. 4-84 to 4-86).

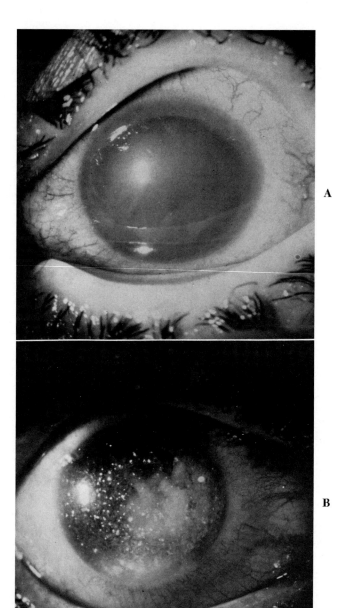

Fig. 3-29. Causes of retrocorneal fibrous membrane. **A,** Hyphema. **B,** Inflammatory debris in anterior chamber. (From Meyner E: Atlas der Spaltlampenphotographie, Stuttgart, 1976, Ferdinand Enke Verlag.)

Apparently, irritation of the corneal endothelium by such factors has chemical burns or surgical trauma sometimes stimulates a fibrous metaplasia of corneal endothelium, that is, a transformation of the flat cuboidal endothelial cell into a fibrocyte. In some cases, the membrane may result from ingrowth of fibrous tissue that gains access to the retrocorneal space through a defect in Descement's membrane.

SUPERFICIAL EPITHELIAL EROSIONS

Superficial epithelial erosions (recurrent erosions) usually are precipitated by corneal injury with breakdown of

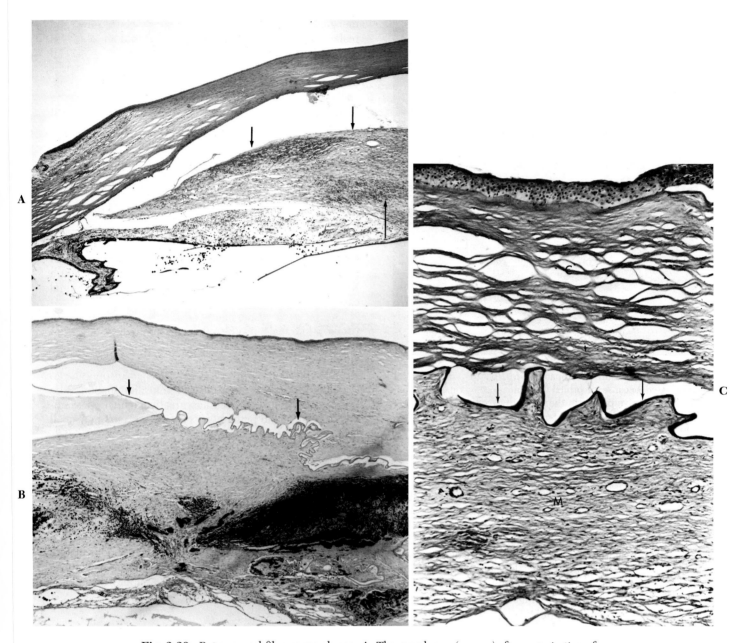

Fig. 3-30. Retrocorneal fibrous membrane. **A,** The membrane *(arrows)* after organization of a hyphema. (H & E stain; ×7.) **B,** The membrane caused by organization of inflammatory debris in the anterior chamber. The deeply staining foci are residual inflammatory cell infiltrates. *Arrows,* Detached, wrinkled Descemet's membrane. (H & E stain; ×8.) **C,** The membrane *(M)* caused by ingrowth of fibrovascular tissue through the wound following a corneal graft. *Arrows,* Wrinkled Descemet's membrane; *C,* corneal stroma. (PAS stain; ×180.)

hemidesmosomes, but this condition also can be inherited as an autosomal-dominant trait (see Table 3-2, p. 87). In the latter situation, the changes usually are bilateral. Similar painful recurrent erosions also follow inflammatory keratitis, such as herpes simplex, and are common complications of other corneal dystrophies (see Table 3-2), particularly the epithelial microcystic dystrophies[388,542] and lattice dystrophy (p. 91).

Recurrent erosion may be a prominent complication of neuroparalytic keratitis. The corneal disturbances result from a loss of the sustaining or trophic effect that occurs after a lesion of the ophthalmic division of the trigeminal nerve. Untreated cases may slowly progress to desquamation of the epithelium, secondary infection, and perforation.

CORNEAL EPIDERMALIZATION

The two most common causes of corneal epidermalization are exposure keratopathy and keratomalacia.

Exposure keratopathy may follow any lesion that pre-

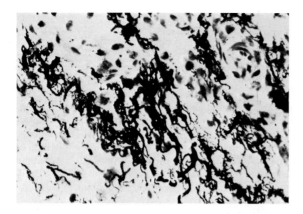

Fig. 3-35. Argyrosis of the conjunctival stroma following long-term silver protein (Argyrol) therapy. The densely staining silver has impregnated the elastic tissue. (Silver stain; ×250.)

smooth because the stain is resorbed at an equal rate around the entire circumference of the lesion. The stain may resorb within months in favorable cases or may remain for several years.

Intact erythrocytes are not seen in the cornea. The erythrocytes disintegrate in the anterior chamber, and blood breakdown products diffuse into the cornea, particularly when the intraocular pressure is elevated or the endothelium is damaged. This process itself may irritate and partially destroy the endothelium. Small, light brown to orange irregular granules are microscopically visible within the corneal stroma (Fig. 3-37). These granules sometimes penetrate as far anteriorly as the epithelial surface. The granules within the corneal stroma represent freed hemoglobin and its breakdown products. In later stages, if resorption is incomplete, the Prussian blue stain for iron eventually may become positive because of further degradation of the blood products to hemosiderin (see Table 1-1).

Siderosis resulting from an iron foreign body is discussed on page 99.

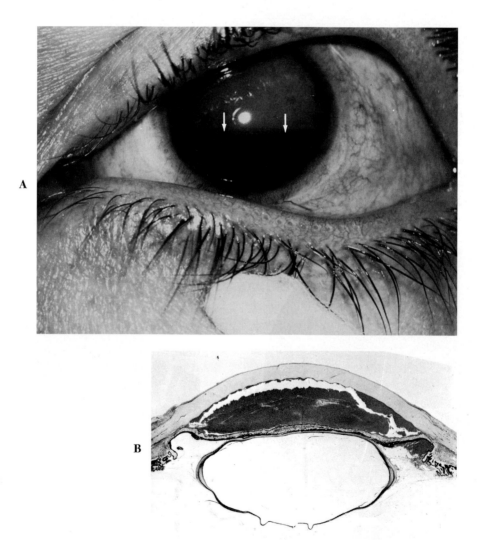

Fig. 3-36. Hyphema. **A,** The blood has gravitated inferiorly. *Arrows,* Aqueous-blood fluid level.
B, Photomicrograph of a total hyphema. (H & E stain; ×15.)

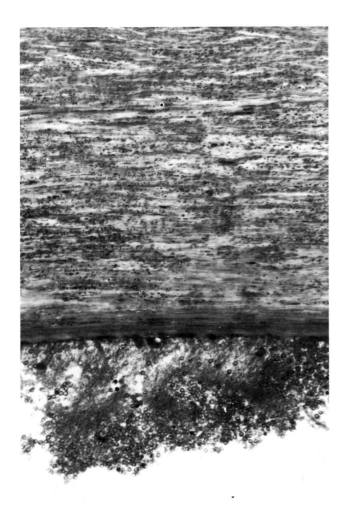

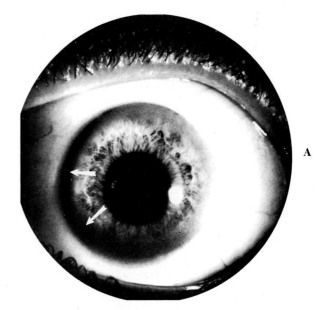

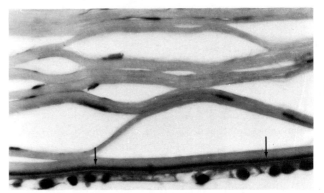

Fig. 3-37. Bloodstaining of the cornea. A residual hyphema with degenerating erythrocytes is present in the anterior chamber. The pigmented granules within the corneal stroma represent breakdown products (hemoglobin) from the blood within the anterior chamber. The endothelium is almost absent. (H & E stain; ×150.)

Fig. 3-38. Kayser-Fleischer ring. **A,** Arrows demarcate a partial brown ring in the corneal periphery. **B,** The pigment is deposited on Descemet's membrane *(arrows).* (H & E stain; ×300.) (**A** from Meyner E: Atlas der Spaltlampenphotographie, Stuttgart, 1976, Ferdinand Enke Verlag.)

IRON LINES

In the corneal iron lines, the iron typically is deposited within the epithelium.[225,312,314,318,333] Routinely stained histopathologic sections reveal faint light brown to yellow granules, and the iron sometimes is difficult to differentiate from melanin pigment. Prussian blue staining demonstrates the iron by imparting a blue color to the granules. Table 3-1 lists five named iron lines and the degenerative or pathologic conditions with which they are associated.

KAYSER-FLEISCHER RING

The Kayser-Fleischer ring,* not to be confused with the Fleischer iron line of the cornea (Table 3-1), is a deposit of copper in Descemet's membrane (Fig. 3-38). To a lesser extent, copper also may be deposited in the lens capsule. The brown copper deposits form a ring at the corneal periphery (Fig. 3-38, *A*). Usually a clear area intervenes between the ring and the limbus.

The ring is associated with Wilson's disease (hepatolenticular degeneration),* which usually is an autosomal recessively inherited increase in serum copper levels caused by a deficiency in copper-binding serum ceruloplasmin. In Wilson's disease, the rings are bilateral, usually present by the second decade of life, and sometimes associated with a sunflower cataract.[309]

A copper intraocular foreign body (chalcosis)[243,339] may cause a Kayser-Fleischer ring, which is histopathologically identical to that of Wilson's disease. However, the ring in chalcosis typically is unilateral in the injured eye only.

Abnormalities in size and shape[343-376]

MICROCORNEA

Microcornea,[348] defined as a corneal diameter of less than 11 mm, often is seen in conjunction with microphthalmia, sclerocornea,[352,366,375] or both, but it also occurs in

---

* References 317, 319, 320, 327, 335, 339.

* References 310, 315, 322, 324, 340, 341.

otherwise normal eyes. It occasionally is seen in chromosome anomalies and in the anterior chamber cleavage syndromes. When an associated malformation of the anterior chamber angle is severe, congenital glaucoma may ensue.

MEGALOCORNEA

An enlarged, stretched cornea may be seen in association with congenital glaucoma (buphthalmos), but when enlargement of the cornea (greater than 13 mm) occurs as an isolated phenomenon, it is known as megalocornea.[374] Most cases are isolated and generally do not produce symptoms apart from axial myopia. Cataract and lens dislocation can develop in adulthood.

CORNEA PLANA

The cornea is flattened abnormally, with or without opacities. It is most common in sclerocornea and microphthalmia of various causes.[359]

ANTERIOR CHAMBER CLEAVAGE SYNDROMES (IRIDOCORNEAL DYSGENESIS)

Anomalies in transparency,[360,364,371] size, and shape (iridocorneal dysgenesis) of the cornea may be seen in association with the anterior chamber cleavage syndrome (p. 35).

STAPHYLOMA AND ECTASIA

Any condition that creates a focal weakness of the cornea or sclera (e.g., a penetration, perforation, or ulceration) predisposes to ectasia or staphyloma formation.[344] The major causes of corneoscleral ectasia and staphyloma are trauma (Fig. 3-39; see Color Plate 3-10), corneal and scleral

inflammatory diseases (Fig. 3-40), such as rheumatoid arthritis, corneoscleral melting diseases[267] (Fig. 3-41; Color Plate 3-11), and advanced glaucoma.

An ectasia refers to a protrusion of the cornea or sclera, which by definition does not contain prolapsed uvea.

Strictly defined, a staphyloma consists of an outward bulging, or protruding, of the outer fibrous tissue of the globe with simultaneous bulging of the underlying uvea (Fig. 3-39; Color Plates 3-10 and 3-11). The adjacent uveal tissue usually adheres to the posterior aspect of the weak-

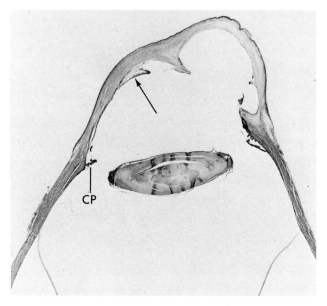

Fig. 3-40. Congenital anterior staphyloma, probably caused by an intrauterine inflammatory process. Remnants of atrophic iris pigment and stroma *(arrow)* adhere to the protruding cornea. An intrauterine keratitis or corneal ulcer is thought to weaken the cornea and render it susceptible to anterior stretching and protrusion. *CP,* Atrophic ciliary processes. (H & E stain; ×7.)

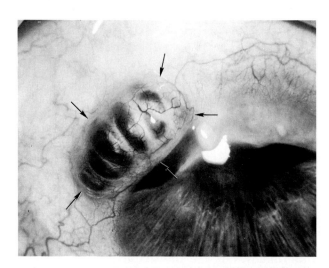

Fig. 3-39. Posttraumatic staphyloma of the limbus. The sclera has become extremely thin. *Arrows,* Protrusions of dark blue-appearing uvea. A simple ectasia consists of a protrusion of bulging of the corneal or scleral coat but not of the uvea. Disruption of the uvea and/or prolapse of uveal tissue into a perforating wound are generally considered prerequisite to subsequent development of sympathetic ophthalmia. Fortunately, this complication occurs in only a very small percentage of cases.

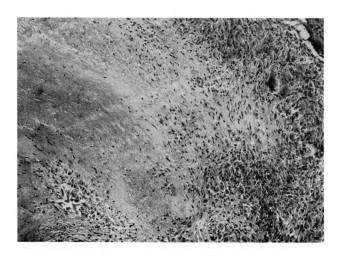

Fig. 3-41. Zonular granulomatous inflammation in a case of rheumatoid keratoscleritis showing focal necrosis of collagen centrally with a border consisting of round cells, epithelioid cells, and giant cells. This type of lesion occurs in several "melting" diseases. (See Color Plate 3-11.)

ened and typically thinned cornea or sclera (Fig. 3-40). The dark blue to purple color of a staphylomatous protrusion imparted by the pigmentation of the underlying iris or ciliary body resembles that of a grape, hence the term *staphyloma* (Gr. *staphyle*, grape). Staphylomas are designated according to their location, for example, corneal, limbal (intercalary), equatorial, or posterior. Posterior staphyloma is a frequent complication of pathologic myopia (see Chapter 2).

Some cases of congenital anterior staphyloma[278] (Fig. 3-40) seem to be caused by a maldevelopment of the cornea or anterior segment structures. Familial transmission and association with other congenital malformations suggest a primary developmental anomaly. However, many such cases probably result from intrauterine corneal inflammatory processes in which the pathogenesis of the staphyloma is similar to that in adults with ocular inflammation.

In some anterior segment, fundus, and optic nerve colobomas, scleral thinning and staphyloma formation occur in the region of the inferonasal defect. The sclera becomes stretched and bulges posteriorly and inferiorly (see Figs. 2-12 to 2-14; Color Plate 2-6). These ectatic, or staphylomatous, defects represent an early stage of a colobomatous cyst. They may enlarge tremendously, occasionally replacing the eye within the orbit (p. 21; Fig. 2-15).

KERATOCONUS

Keratoconus[*] (Color Plate 3-12) often is classified as an ectatic corneal dystrophy; both a recessive and a dominant mode of inheritance has been reported. However, in most cases, no inheritance pattern is present, and we prefer to separate this condition from the heredofamilial dystrophies. The disease is characterized by bilateral thinning, scarring, and conical ectasia of the central cornea. A painless progressive decrease in vision caused by scarring and irregular myopic astigmatism may result (Fig. 3-42). The majority of affected patients are female. The ectasia becomes manifest in the first or second decades, progresses for 4 to 6 years, and then tends to subside.

The apex of the cone usually is slightly inferior and nasal to the center of the cornea. Munson's sign occurs when the lower lid bulges on downward gaze. Vogt's vertical lines are in within the stroma.

Clinically, some cases progress from a stage of mild visual loss caused by myopic astigmatism, which often can be corrected by hard contact lenses, to a stage of more severe corneal ectasia and thinning. Penetrating keratoplasty is required in more advanced cases in which the cornea is scarred or becomes too steep for a contact lens.

Fleischer's ring, an intraepithelial iron line that is best seen with a cobalt-blue filter on the slit lamp (Table 3-1), forms at the base of the cone.[351] Bowman's layer may rupture early, and scarring and rupture of Descemet's membrane may occur in later stages. In exceptional cases, particularly in keratoconus associated with Down syndrome (p.00), corneal edema (acute keratoconus, hydrops) may occur (see Figs. 2-60, *B*, 3-18, and 3-43, *B*). This usually signifies an influx of aqueous through the rupture in Descemet's membrane into the stromal lamellae.

---

[*] References 343, 346, 347, 349, 351, 353-358, 361-363, 367-369, 372, 373, 376.

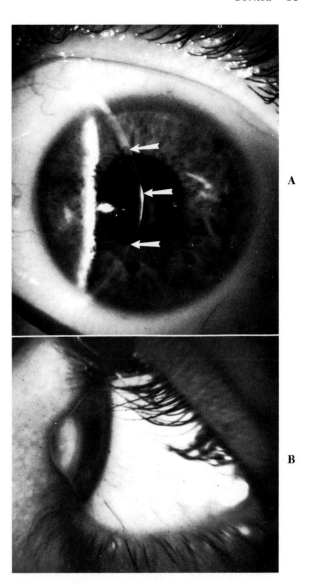

Fig. 3-42. Keratoconus. **A,** Slitlamp view of the conical cornea *(arrows).* **B,** Side view showing typical conical shape and extensive scarring. (See Color Plate 3-12.)

Keratoconus is sometimes associated with other ocular abnormalities such as tapetoretinal degeneration, aniridia, and Marfan's syndrome. Pellucid degeneration of the cornea usually represents an inferior conical protrusion of the cornea, which some physicians classify as a form of inferior keratoconus.[347,357]

Microscopic analysis[346] of a corneal button from a patient with keratoconus typically reveals thinning of the central stroma (Fig. 3-43, *A*). The peripheral cornea is of normal thickness or even slightly thicker because of secondary scarring except in advanced cases. Some histopathologic studies have suggested that the primary weakness of the cornea resides at the levels of the epithelial basement membrane and Bowman's layer.[346] Discontinuities in these layers are seen consistently in tissue sections from patients with keratoconus. If this hypothesis is correct, the well-known changes such as corneal stretching and conical ectasia, corneal opacification, subsequent rupture of Descem-

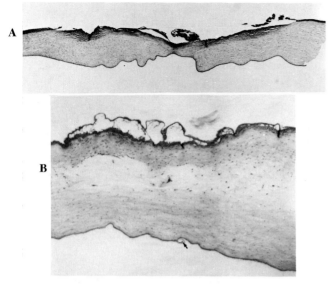

Fig. 3-43. Keratoconus. **A,** Simple type. The epithelium and Bowman's layer have degenerated, and the central portion of the cornea has thinned significantly. (H & E stain; ×6.) **B,** Acute form with hydrops. Epithelial edema with microcyst formation and marked rarefaction of stroma caused by fluid influx through a ruptured Descemet's membrane *(arrow)* have occurred. (H & E stain; ×50.)

Fig. 3-44. Schematic drawing of microscopic configuration of corneal epithelial microcysts. (Redrawn by Dr. Steven Vermillion, University of Iowa, from von Hippel E: In Henke F and Lubarsch O, editors: Handbuch der speziellen pathologischen Anatomie und Histologie, Berlin, 1928, Julius Springer.)

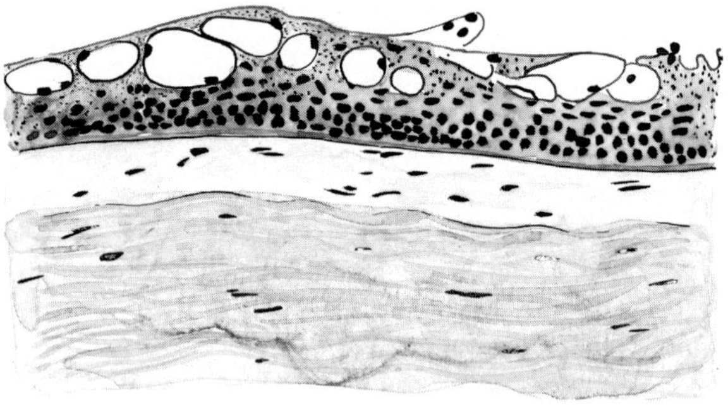

et's membrane, and abnormalities in hydration are results of this primary defect. Other studies have suggested that the disease is caused by faulty development of the corneal stroma, including its ground substance.

Keratoglobus[345] is a rare condition that differs from keratoconus because the stromal thinning extends from limbus to limbus and is more marked in the periphery. It may be stationary and may be associated with other conditions such as keratoconjunctivitis, blepharitis with eye rubbing, and postpenetrating keratopathy. Pellucid margin degeneration[347,353,357,365] is a bilateral condition with inferior peripheral thinning as opposed to the central thinning of keratoconus.

Dystrophies[377-555]

Unlike the numerous corneal degenerative diseases that usually are acquired, the corneal dystrophies usually are primary, bilateral, heredofamilial affections of the cornea unaccompanied by systemic disease.* Affected corneas show no new vessels or primary inflammation, although secondary inflammation may occur. Several conditions that are known as corneal dystrophies do not fulfill these requirements and are better categorized as degenerations. These include so-called lipid dystrophies of the cornea (usually a secondary lipid degeneration) (p. 75) and Salzmann's nodular corneal dystrophy (p. 78).

The most convenient classification (Table 3-2) of the corneal dystrophies is according to the primary layer of involvement:

1. Primary involvement of epithelium, epithelial basement membrane, and/or Bowman's layer (so-called anterior membrane dystropies);
2. Primary involvement of the stroma;
3. Primary involvement of the endothelium and Descemet's membrane.

Bron and Tripathi[389] and Waring, Rodrigues, and Laibson[546,547] provide excellent, comprehensive classifications and reviews of the clinical and pathologic features of most of the corneal dystrophies.

This section is limited to a discussion of (1) the epithelial microcystic dystrophies (Meesmann's, Cogan's, and inherited recurrent erosion syndrome) and a dystrophy primarily affecting Bowman's layer (Reis-Bümcklers); (2) the three classic stromal dystrophies (granular, macular, and lattice); and (3) an example of endothelial dystrophy (Fuchs' combined dystrophy). The recurrent erosion syndrome,[230,301,305,391,541] which results from corneal injury or various corneal diseases more frequently than does its dystrophic form, is described on page 78.

Keratoconus, classified as a nonfamilial dystrophy by some physicians, is described on page 85.

EPITHELIAL DYSTROPHY

*Microcystic dystrophies**

The clinical and histopathologic features of corneal-conjunctival disorders characterized by the formation of intraepithelial cysts (Fig. 3-44) have been reviewed by Bron and Tripathi.[388] Meesmann's dystrophy (Stocker-Holt dystrophy[429]), Cogan's dystrophy, and the inherited form of recurrent erosion syndrome are examples. The microcysts clinically show a globular profile and a smooth outline. They generally are located in the middle and superficial regions of the epithelium. The cysts usually contain degenerate epithelial cells, and a typical cyst is lined by the plasma membranes of adjacent epithelial cells (Fig. 3-44).

Tripathi and Bron postulate two pathogenetic mechanisms for the formation of intraepithelial cysts. First, in

* References 393, 406, 425, 426, 428, 434, 449, 481.

* References 360, 382, 387, 388, 395, 407, 412, 414, 419, 421, 422, 436-438, 446, 457, 462, 468, 474, 488, 495, 500, 508, 511, 534, 541-544, 553.

Table 3-2. Classification of selected corneal dystrophies

Nomenclature	Hereditary transmission	Symptoms	Clinical appearance	Primary histopathologic alteration
Epithelium-Bowman's layer				
Meesmann's (Stocker-Holt) juvenile epithelial dystrophy	Autosomal dominant	Irritation; late impairment of vision, late erosions	Epithelial microcysts and vesicles	Intraepithelial microcysts containing periodic acid-Schiff (PAS)-positive granules (glycogen)
Cogan's microcystic (dot, fingerprint, geographic) dystrophy	None (rarely dominant)	None, or late erosions	Epithelial microcysts and vesicles, fingerprintlike lines	Epithelial microcysts and vesicles; loose epithelium eventually peels of apparently abnormal basement membrane; loss of hemidesmosomes
Recurrent erosion syndrome (Franceschetti)	Autosomal dominant	Recurrent attacks of pain; lacrimation; photophobia, usually upon awakening	Epithelial microcysts and vesicles	Same as Cogan's dystrophy
Hereditary anterior membranous dystrophy of Grayson-Wilbrandt	Autosomal dominant	Slow decrease in visual acuity	Flat, membranelike opacity level of epithelium	Defects in epithelial basement membrane
Subepithelial mucinous corneal dystrophy (SMCD)	Autosomal dominant	Decrease in visual acuity, recurrent erosions	Subepithelial haze involving entire cornea	PAS and Alcian-blue positive mucin material anterior to Bowman's layer
Ring dystrophy of Reis-Bücklers	Autosomal dominant	Decrease in visual acuity; recurrent erosions	Fine, white, thread-like opacities arranged in maplike or granular configurations	Defects in epithelial basement membrane and Bowman's layer; loss of hemidesmosomes; abnormal proliferation of stromal keratocytes anterior to Bowman's layer
Anterior crocodile shagreen of Vogt	Autosomal dominant	Very slow decrease in visual acuity	Polygonal gray opacities forming a mosaic	Fine, granular deposits (breaks) in Bowman's layer
Primary dystrophic band keratopathy	Autosomal dominant or X-linked recessive	Early onset but slowly progressive decrease in visual acuity	White band-shaped deposits in Bowman's layer within region of palpebral fissure	Calcification of Bowman's layer; later pannus
Keratoconus	Usually none	Decreased acuity, irregular myopic astigmatism, later acute corneal edema (hydrops)	Cone-shaped, thinned cornea; later opacification	Pathogenesis unclear, probably defective basement membrane and Bowman's layer; stromal endothelial changes secondary
Stroma Granular (Bücklers I, Groenouw I) dystrophy	Autosomal dominant	Vision may or may not be seriously affected; in later stages pain may result from recurrent erosions	Milk-white, crumblike spots; intervening and peripheral cornea clear	Hyaline protein deposition, first in superficial stroma, later in deep stroma; readily diagnosed with Masson trichome stain
Macular (Bücklers II, Groenouw II) dystrophy	Autosomal dominant	Progressive, severe decrease in visual acuity caused by diffuse stromal opacification; recurrent erosions may occur	Large, diffuse confluent gray opacities extending to limbus and deep stroma	Mucopolysaccharide deposition; readily diagnosed with colloidal iron or Alcian blue stain
Lattice (Bücklers III, Bibaer-Haab-Dimmer) dystrophy	Autosomal dominant	Eventual marked decrease in visual acuity; high incidence of recurrent epithelial erosion	Spider weblike opacities; network of transparent tubes	Amyloid deposition; readily diagnosed with Congo red, thioflavine T, polarized light

Continued

Table 3-2. Classification of selected corneal dystrophies—cont'd

Nomenclature	Hereditary transmission	Symptoms	Clinical appearance	Primary histopathologic alteration
Epithelium-Bowman's layer—cont'd				
Central stromal crystalline dystrophy of Schnyder (lipid dystrophy)	Autosomal dominant	Minimal decrease in visual acuity	Disc-shaped to ring-like crystalline or needle-shaped opacities of superficial stroma	Cholesterol and neutral fat deposition in superficial stroma
Fleck (speckled) dystrophy of Francois and Neetens	Autosomal dominant	Asymptomatic	Snowflake-like flecks in all stromal layers, clear between the opacities	Vacuolated keratocytes possibly contain mucopolysaccharides
Posterior crocodile shagreen (central cloudy dystrophy of Francois)	Autosomal dominant	Usually asymptomatic	Large gray polygord gray lesions separated by clear areas	Irregular collagen configuration
Endothelium, Descemet's membrane				
Congenital hereditary endothelial dystrophy (CHED) (Maumenee)	May be transmitted in dominant and recessive modes	Early severe loss of visual acuity	Blue-gray, ground glass appearance of entire stroma	Thickening and reduplication of Descemet's membrane; paucity or absence of endothelium; stromal edema
Fuchs' combined dystrophy	Sometimes transmitted as autosomal-dominant trait	Eventual progression to stromal and epithelial edema, progressive visual loss	Hammered appearance of Descemet's membrane (guttata)	PAS-positive excrescences of Descemet's membrane; later progression to epithelial edema
Posterior polymorphous dystrophy (Schlichting)	Autosomal dominant or recessive	Minimal impairment of vision in most cases	Vesicles and polymorphous opacities in Descemet's membrane and posterior stroma	Endothelium may contain microvilli; excrescences in Descemet's membrane

Modified and expanded from an unpublished classification of Dr. William F. Hughes, former Chairman, Department of Ophthalmology, Presbyterian-St. Luke's Medical Center, Professor of Ophthalmology, University of Illinois, Abraham Lincoln School of Medicine, Chicago, Ill.

some instances, an abnormally weak adherence of adjacent epithelial cells results from faulty desmosomes or intercellular bridges. Also, the attachment between the epithelial cells and underlying Bowman's layer may be tenuous because of defective hemidesmosomes between these structures. The cells are separated from each other (spongiosis or acantholysis), and the cysts are derived from openings within the widened extracellular spaces. Second, any condition that gives rise to increased corneal hydration may produce intraepithelial cysts. Excessive entry of fluid into the corneal epithelium may occur from either of two sources: the tear film or the aqueous. The latter follows decompensation of affected endothelial cells, forming a nidus for cyst formation.

Later stages of the microscopic dystrophies involve abnormal laying down of new epithelial basement membrane material and superficial stromal scarring that occasionally may affect vision.

Reis-Bücklers ring dystrophy[360,393,394,398]

The ring dystrophy of Reis-Bücklers is a dominantly inherited condition in which fine, white threadlike opacities are arranged in maplike configurations on the corneal surface.[380] The dystrophy involves defects in the epithelial basement membrane and deposition of a finely fibrillar substance in Bowman's layer. The major decrease in visual acuity results from passage of stromal keratocytes through Bowman's layer forming superficial collagen plaques. Loss of hemidesmosomes between the epithelium and Bowman's layer leads to painful recurrent erosions that begin in early childhood.

STROMAL DYSTROPHIES

The three important inherited stromal dystrophies[459,486,546] (Table 3-2) resemble one another in their early onset, progressive nature, and involvement of the anterior stroma in the early stages. Granular dystrophy and lattice dystrophy are dominantly inherited; macular dystrophy is transmitted in an autosomal-recessive manner.

Granular dystrophy°

Granular (Bücklers I, Groenouw I) dystrophy is an autosomal-dominant inherited condition in which the corneal changes usually become visible at puberty. Vision slowly deteriorates but usually is not affected seriously until after the fifth decade of life. The discrete crumblike white to gray opacities (Fig. 3-45 and Color Plate 3-13) appear in the anterior stromal layers of the axial cornea. The central opacities penetrate deep but usually do not affect the deep-

---

° References 379, 392, 424, 440, 456, 496, 514, 515, 519.

est layers of the stroma. Although the lesions spread peripherally, the outer 2 to 3 mm of the stroma are not affected. The areas of corneal tissue between the granules remain clear and optically transparent. Therefore, although the opacities involve the central cornea, the prognosis for useful vision is much better than in the other two major corneal dystrophies.

The histopathologic and ultrastructural features of granular dystrophy are listed in Table 3-3.[459] The granular hyaline material seen in microscopic sections (Fig. 3-46) is believed to represent a proteinaceous secretory product of stromal keratocytes. The nature of this protein substance, which stains a brilliant red with Masson trichrome stain (Fig. 3-46, *A*, and Color Plate 3-14) remains obscure.

Macular dystrophy*

Because macular (Bücklers II, Groenouw II) dystrophy is responsible for the most visual impairment, it is fortunate that it is inherited only as an autosomal-recessive trait. The recessive pattern dictates that both parents must be carriers of the disease, rather than only one.

Diffuse clouding of the cornea (Fig. 3-47, *A* and Color Plate 3-15) is first seen in affected patients during the latter portion of the first decade of life. Initially, the opacification affects the superficial stromal layers, but by the second or third decade, it usually involves the entire thickness of the cornea. In contrast to granular and lattice dystrophies, the peripheral cornea is not spared. About the third decade, ill-defined nodular opacities of varying size sometimes appear within the cloudy stroma. Visual deterioration usually is rapid, and most patients are essentially blind by 40 years of age.

Microscopically, the accumulation of opaque material is most severe in the superficial axial cornea (Fig. 3-47, *B* and Color Plate 3-16). The deposits are situated in keratocytes, in endothelial cell, and in small pools between stromal lamellae. The lesions sometimes extend through defects in Bowman's layer into the subepithelial space so that the corneal surface becomes irregular. The lesion may extend deeply through the entire thickness of the stroma, even reaching the endothelium, producing secondary corneal guttata. Special staining techniques (Table 3-3) show that the stromal opacities are composed of mucopolysaccharides.

Ultrastructural studies have revealed a primary defect in the metabolism of the keratocytes that leads to increased

---

* References 408, 415, 416, 430, 453, 458, 472, 492, 519, 536, 538, 539, 554.

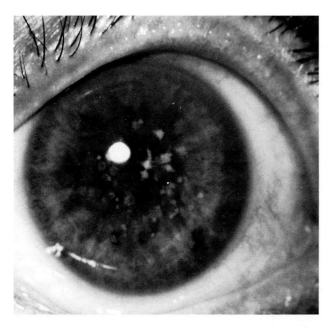

Fig. 3-45. Granular corneal dystrophy. The periphery is unaffected. The unaffected zones between the crumblike opacities are clear, and visual acuity may be relatively intact for many years.

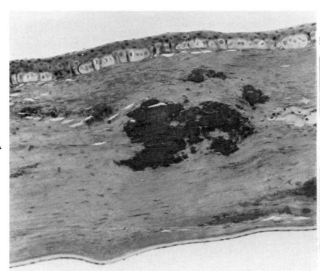
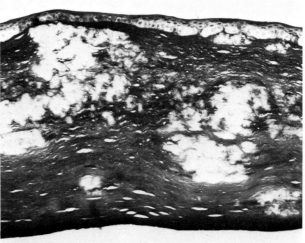

A **B**

Fig. 3-46. Granular dystrophy. **A,** Stromal hyaline deposits are intensely positive when stained with Masson trichrome. (Masson trichrome; ×150.) **B,** The stromal deposits do not stain (white patches) with the PAS technique. (PAS stain; ×150.)

Table 3-3. Histopathologic and ultrastructural features of the three major corneal dystrophies

Method	Granular dystrophy	Macular dystrophy	Lattice dystrophy
Microscopic appearance, formalin-fixed tissue	Granular hyaline	Granular nonhyaline	Fibrillar hyaline
Hematoxylin-eosin	Pink to red	Pale gray	Pink
Crystal violet	± ±	+ + +	+ + +
Congo red	– – –	– – –	+ + +
Birefringence	– – –	– – –	+ + +
Dichroism	– – –	– – –	+ + +
Coupled tetrazonium	+ + +	– – –	+ + +
Thioflavin - T	– – –	– – –	+ + +
Masson trichrome	+ + +	– – –	+ – –
PAS	– – –	+ + +	+ +
Alcian blue	– – –	+ + +	– – –
Weigert's resorcin	– – –	+ + +	– – –
Electron microscopy (ultrastructure)	Electron-dense, rod-shaped, and trapezoidal amorphous "crystals"	Mucopolysaccharide; fine filamentous and granuloamorphous deposits	Fine fibrils characteristic of amyloid

From Bron AJ and Tripathi RC: In Goldberg MF, editor: Genetic and metabolic eye disease, Boston, 1974, Little, Brown & Co.

Fig. 3-47. Macular dystrophy. **A,** Although patchy densely opaque foci are present in this 21-year-old man, the corneal opacification is much more diffuse than in granular dystrophy, in which the intervening areas are clear. Note the diffuse clouding of the entire cornea. **B,** Faint subepithelial accumulation of mucopolysaccharide *(arrows).* (Alcian blue; ×160.)

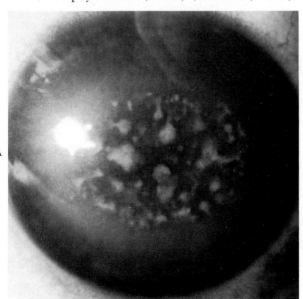

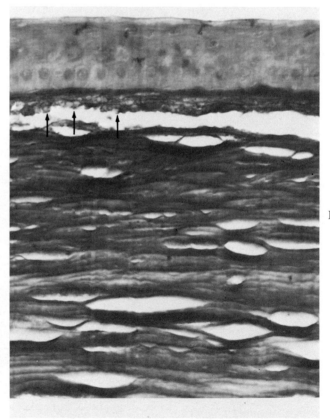

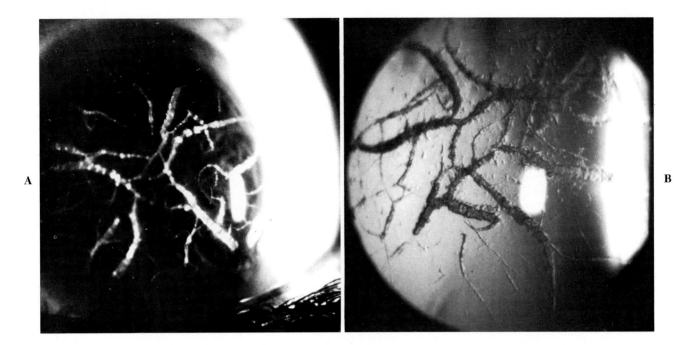

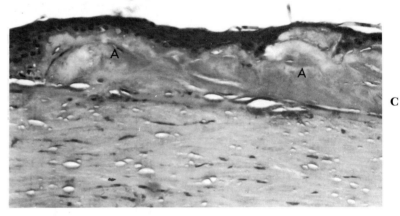

Fig. 3-48. Lattice dystrophy. **A,** The lattice lines in this case are thick and beaded (punctate nodules). In other cases the lines may be thinner and more delicate. **B,** Retroillumination study. **C,** Amyloid (*A*) is deposited between the thinned epithelium and anterior stroma. (H & E stain; ×300.)

mucopolysaccharide storage within the cells. The storage material is found in the cisternae of the rough-surfaced endoplasmic reticulum of the cells. Cotlier and Hughes[408] have demonstrated a deficiency of the enzyme α-glactosidase in cultured keratocytes and limbal fibroblasts. Therefore, this dystrophy is now regarded as a genetically determined local enzyme deficiency similar to the systemic mucopolysaccharide disorders (p. 94). However, in the latter disorders, the mucopolysaccharide accumulates within lysosomal vacuoles rather than within the endoplasmic reticulum. The mucopolysaccharides are considered to be inherited disorders of the lysosomal enzymes affecting multiple tissues in the body. Deposition of mucopolysaccharides in tissues other than the cornea rarely is observed in macular corneal dystrophy.

Lattice dystrophy

Lattice (Bücklers III, Biber-Haab-Dimmer) dystrophy*usually appears at the end of the first decade of life with symptoms of recurrent erosion or visual disturbances. The changes in this dominantly inherited condition begin in the anterior and middle portions of the axial stroma. The lattice lines resemble tubes arranged in a spiderweblike pattern (Fig. 3-48, *A* and *B* and Color Plate 3-17). The double-contoured, relucent branching filaments often are arranged in a radial disposition, interlacing and overlapping at different levels. The limbal region is spared. The lines, which branch dichotomously, resemble corneal nerves. They may be relatively thick and show focal nodularity but sometimes are much more delicate than is illustrated (Fig. 3-48, *A* and *B*). Deterioration of vision is not as rapid as is characteristic of macular dystrophy, but it is more severe than is seen in granular dystrophy.

Histochemical analysis, polarizing microscopy, immunofluorescent techniques, and electron microscopy have revealed that the stromal deposits are composed of amyloid (Fig. 3-48, *C* and Color Plate 3-18, Table 3-3). Amyloid is a fine fibrillar proteinaceous material that has a distinctive appearance by electron microscopy.

Lattice dystrophy of the cornea usually occurs as an iso-

---

*References 442, 447, 470, 471, 475, 487, 489, 490, 497, 504, 505, 519, 529, 532, 533, 555.

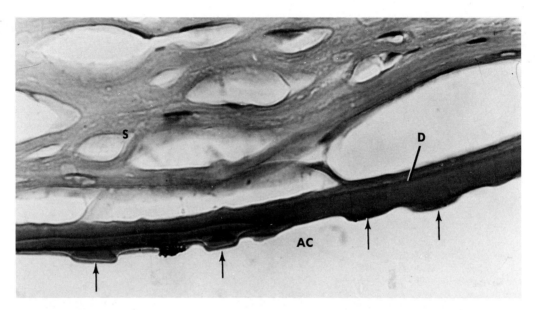

Fig. 3-49. Fuchs' endothelial guttata. This section of the posterior aspect of a cornea stained by the PAS technique delineates the wartlike excrescences or thickenings of Descemet's membrane *(arrows)*. The total degeneration and absence of the endothelium is largely responsible for the stromal and epithelial edema. *S,* Corneal stroma with numerous clefts between lamellae, probably caused by corneal edema; *D,* Descemet's membrane; *AC,* anterior chamber. (PAS stain; ×400.)

lated disorder. However, it may on rare occasions be associated with primary or secondary systemic amyloidosis.

Two variations of lattice dystrophy are primary gelatinous drop-like dystrophy[352,397] and polymorphic amyloid degeneration. Lattice dystrophy should be differentiated from primary familial corneal amyloidosis (pp. 93 and 94; Figs. 3-50 and 3-51). A combined granule-lattice dystrophy has been observed from patients who have traced their origins to Avellino, Italy.[423,443,448,479,522] Corneas from individuals with Avellino granule-lattice dystrophy show both trichome positive granule deposits and Congo-red positive amyloid deposits.

ENDOTHELIAL DYSTROPHY°

Fuchs' endothelial dystrophy

Most cases of Fuchs' endothelial dystrophy (Fuchs' combined dystrophy)[429] are regarded as an age-related degeneration of relatively late onset, but an autosomal-dominant mode of inheritance has been reported in a number of pedigrees.[269] Women usually are affected more than men. The clinical hallmark of this condition consists of corneal guttata (Fig. 3-49), fine wartlike excrescences on Descemet's membrane that begin centrally and spread peripherally with age. They are readily seen on specular reflection during biomicroscopy. The edema results from a decreased pumping and barrier function of the disordered endothelium (p. 61). In its earliest asymptomatic stage, corneal guttata are seen, but otherwise the cornea appears normal. As the disease slowly progresses, there is a painless de-

crease in visual acuity and glare, associated with mild stromal and mild intraepithelial edema (corneal bedewing). Cells eventually grow superficially through Bowman's layer, sometimes forming a degenerative pannus. Pain and more severe stromal and epithelial edema marked the stage of bullous keratopathy—severe pain often resulting from bullous rupture. In end stages, the bullae disappears and pain thus subsides, but opacification and increased pannus formation and scarring further reduce vision.

Microscopic studies reveal corneal endothelial degeneration, with variation in cell size and an absolute decrease in numbers of endothelial cells. The endothelial cells show nuclear pyknosis and vacuolation of the cytoplasm, with eventual disappearance of the cells, particularly over the warts. The wartlike excrescences on Descemet's membrane (the basement membrane of the endothelium) form concurrently with the endothelial cell damage (Fig. 3-49). The excrescences probably are secretory or degenerative products of the damaged endothelial cell. They morphologically resemble and show similar staining characteristics of Descemet's membrane. In essence, the individual warts represent the addition of newly formed basement membranelike material to the pre-existing basement membrane.

Guttata are microscopically identical in appearance to the Hassall-Henle wart that occurs in the peripheral cornea as a normal aging process (Fig. 3-4). In contrast to the centrally located guttata associated with endothelial disease that is responsible for marked overhydration of the cornea (corneal edema), the Hassall-Henle wart is of little significance. Other causes of focal thickening of Descemet's membrane include congenital hereditary endothelial dystrophy,[466,467,469] Schlichting's posterior polymorphous dystrophy,[385,446] focal excrescences after trauma (e.g., forceps

---

° References 377, 378, 381, 384-386, 391, 397, 402-404, 409, 429, 433, 441, 445, 447, 451, 452, 454, 455, 461, 463, 464, 467, 473, 476, 477, 480, 482, 498, 502, 509, 512, 513, 516, 521, 522, 524, 526, 528, 547, 552.

injury at birth), postsurgical corneal decompensation (e.g., pseudophakic bullous keratoplasty, see Fig. 4-92; Color Plate 4-44), and Haab's striae seen in congenital glaucoma.

The corneal edema (p. 72) after endothelial degeneration is first manifest in the posterior stromal layers. Although the stroma clinically exhibits a random separation of collagen fibrils by fluid deposition, this change is difficult to evaluate microscopically because such clefts frequently occur as artifacts in sections of normal corneas. Epithelial edema (Fuchs' combined dystrophy) first appears in the basal layers; later it affects the more superficial layers. With chronic edema, a bullous keratopathy may ensue (Fig. 3-20). The rupture of epithelial bullae accounts for the repeated attacks of pain.

Amyloidosis[556-595]

In addition to amyloid deposits in lattice corneal dystrophy (p. 91), the cornea and conjunctiva also may be involved in other forms of amyloidosis. These include systemic and localized forms as well as involvement in plasma cell myeloma (Table 3-4).[556-595] Amyloid has two major biochemical forms.[560] One probably is derived from immunoglobulins. This is referred to as amyloid of immunoglobulin origin (AIO) or amyloid-B. The immunoglobulin-like amyloid-B generally is found in primary amyloidosis and plasma cell dyscrasias like multiple myeloma. A second form of amyloid is designated amyloid of unknown origin (AUO) or amyloid-A. Amyloid-A usually is found in the remaining types of amyloidoses.

Amyloid is an eosinophilic, glassy, hyaline, amorphous extracellular substance that stains pale pink with the hematoxylin and eosin stain (Fig. 3-50, *A*; see Tables 1-1 and 3-3).[583] It is orthochromatic when stained with toluidine blue, although it shows metachromasia when treated with crystal violet or methyl violet. The periodic acid-Schiff (PAS) stain gives a violet hue. Congo red is used most extensively for staining amyloid; sections stained with formalin-fixed Congo red show a unique green birefringence (double refraction) when viewed through a polarizing microscope (Fig. 3-50, *B* and 3-51, *B*). This procedure is the most useful for establishing the presence of amyloid. Thioflavine T dye also is a sensitive indicator of amyloid, causing a fluorescence of the substance. It generally is used for screening only because it has a relative lack of specificity.

Ophthalmologic lesions in amyloidosis (Table 3-4) range from isolated localized subconjunctival deposits to infiltrations or papules on the eyelids, which may represent only one lesion among many in a multisystemic disease that may be fatal. The latter condition is an example of primary systemic amyloidosis. The most commonly involved site in the body is the eyelid. In fact, the finding of amyloid in skin lesions of the eyelid is an indication for a general examination of a patient to search for primary systemic amyloidosis.

Secondary systemic amyloidosis is associated with a wide variety of infectious, inflammatory, and other diseases (Table 3-4). In contrast to primary systemic amyloidosis, involvement of the eye and its adnexa is extremely rare. Although systemic amyloidosis develops in about 10% of patients with plasma cell myeloma,[389] it closely mimics primary amyloidosis with regard to the biochemical nature of the amyloid, as well as the systemic and ocular findings.

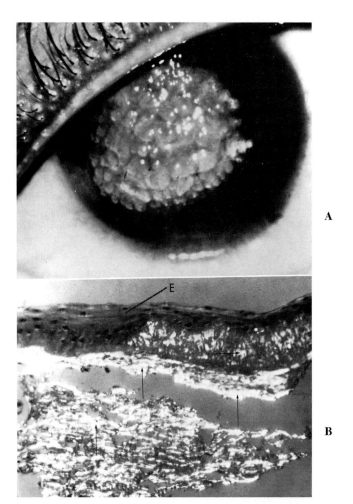

Fig. 3-50. Familial primary amyloidosis of the cornea. **A,** This gelatinous, mulberrylike lesion involves the central portion of the cornea. Vision is greatly reduced because of the opacity of the mass and scarring of the underlying anterior cornea. **B,** Photomicrograph of the amyloid deposits from the case in **A.** The amyloid material was subjected to the Congo red stain and photographed through polarizing lenses. *Arrows,* Birefringence: the molecular structure of the material is such that it "glows" when viewed with the polarizing lenses. *E.* Corneal epithelium. (See Color Plate 3-10.) (Congo red stain; ×300.) (From Kirk HQ and Rabb M; Hattenhauer J and Smith R: Trans Am Acad Ophthalmol Otolaryngol 77:411, 1973.)

Localized amyloidosis[556,557,558,568,564,570] may also be divided into primary and secondary types (Table 3-4). Figure 3-50, *B* shows two cases of familial primary localized amyloidosis of the cornea. Both types are without life-threatening systemic amyloid infiltrates. Whereas primary localized amyloidosis involving the eye may mimic a neoplasm or may require surgical extirpation or penetrating keratoplasty, deposits resulting from preexisting diseases such as infections, environmental exposure (e.g., within pterygia or in so-called ligneous conjunctivitis) or trauma are generally without clinical significance.

Systemic disorders causing corneal clouding in childhood[596-649]

Following are major causes of corneal clouding in childhood, many of which are described individually in their

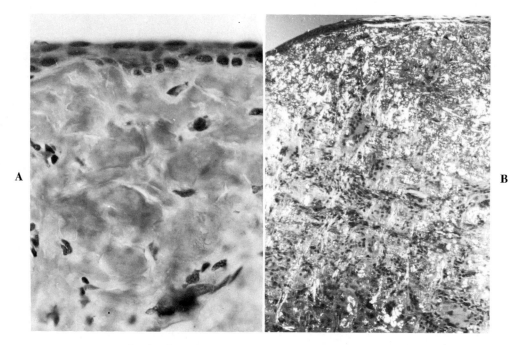

Fig. 3-51. Primary localized amyloidosis of the conjunctiva that appeared as a case of clinical ligneous conjunctivitis. **A,** The amyloid deposits, admixed with scattered inflammatory cells, exhibit an amorphous pattern. (H & E stain; ×150.) **B,** Birefringence of the amyloid deposits as viewed with crossed polarizing filters. Scattered giant cells are also present. (Congo red stain; ×100.)

respective chapters (the mucopolysaccharidoses and Bowman's layer dysplasia, a newly recognized disease, are discussed in this section):

1. Trauma (intrauterine and after birth injury)
2. Intrauterine inflammation
3. Congenital glaucoma
4. Microphthalmia and sclerocornea
5. Anterior chamber cleavage syndromes
6. Congenital anterior staphyloma
7. Corneal dermoid
8. Rubella embryopathy
9. Congenital hereditary endothelial corneal dystrophy
10. Anterior embryotoxon (arcus juvenilis)
11. Mucopolysaccharidoses and mucolipidoses
12. Sphingolipidoses (e.g., Fabry's disease, metachromatic leukodystrophy)
13. Lipidoses (e.g., Refsum's syndrome, Tangier disease)
14. Errors of amino acid metabolism (e.g., cystinosis)
15. Bowman's layer dysplasia

MUCOPOLYSACCHARIDOSES[596-638]

The mucopolysaccharidoses are a group of genetically determined systemic disorders of mucopolysaccharide metabolism in which these substances accumulate in multiple body tissues and are excreted in excess in the urine. Affected patients show a coarse, gargoylelike facies (Fig. 3-52, *A*), variable mental impairment, skin and visceral changes, and skeletal dysplasia. Several types of this disorder may show corneal clouding, congenital glaucoma,[628] optic atrophy, papilledema,[596] pigmentary degeneration of the retina, anterior polar cataract, and megalocornea.

The seven forms of mucopolysaccharidoses are classified according to the pattern of inheritance, phenotypic expression, and biochemical disturbance. Hunter's syndrome is inherited as an X-linked recessive trait. The others are transmitted as an autosomal-recessive trait. The old classification has been revised (Table 3-5) so that Scheie's syndrome (formerly type V) now is classified as type I-S.

Mucopolysaccharides have been demonstrated in the liver, brain, skin, cornea (Fig. 3-52, *B*), conjunctiva, and other tissues. The tinctorial features of the corneal deposits seen microscopically are similar to those of macular corneal dystrophy (Table 3-5). The histopathologic features of the mucopolysaccharidoses are discussed in detail by Kenyon.[609] Ultrastructural studies have shown that the mucopolysaccharide accumulates in lysosomal vacuoles within affected cells. This finding suggests that the inherited enzymatic defect may represent a deficiency of lysosomal acid hydrolases, which normally function to degrade mucopolysaccharides in cells. Deficiency of tissue galactosidases has been demonstrated in several types of mucopolysaccharide storage disease.

Hurler's syndrome (gargoylism, type I-H) is the classic form of mucopolysaccharidosis, with coarse facial features, mental deficiency, and early death. It is inherited as an autosomal-recessive trait. The cornea has a severe, progressive ground-glass appearance. Abnormally high levels of chondroitin sulfate and heparin sulfate are present. The deposition of mucopolysaccharides is seen most commonly in the posterior corneal stroma. Only in Hunter's and Sanfilippo's syndromes is the cornea usually spared.

Hunter's syndrome (type II) shows the clinical features of a classic Hurler's syndrome but usually in a less severe form. Most patients live until at least early middle age. The cornea usually is clear in young patients, but cloudiness may be observed by biomicroscopy in older patients. Because Hunter's syndrome is transmitted as an X-linked recessive trait, it rarely is observed in females.

Table 3-4. Classification of amyloidosis

Type	Systemic findings (organs involved)	Associated or predisposing systemic disease	Ocular findings
Primary systemic Nonfamilial Familial	Primarily affects muscles (especially heart, tongue, and gastrointestinal tract), skin, nerves (chronic sensorimotor polyneuropathy), and blood vessels	Usually no underlying disease	Eyelid nodules, blepharoptosis, purpura, and ecchymoses of eyelid skin and conjunctiva Vitreoretinal deposits, plaque-like infiltrates in retinal and uveal vessels, secondary glaucoma Extraocular muscle and orbital infiltrates, external ophthalmoplegia Tigeminal nerve involvement, neuroparalytic keratitis Pupillary abnormalities resulting from neuropathy
Secondary systemic (most common form with systemic involvement)	Primarily affects kidneys, spleen, liver, adrenal glands	Usually associated with underlying effusive pyogenic or granulomatous inflammatory disease: tuberculosis, rheumatoid arthritis, leprosy, osteomyelitis, syphilis, collagen disease associated with malignancies	Eye involvement rare
Plasma cell myeloma°	Amyloid deposits same as in primary systemic anyloidosis	Amyloid deposits develop in 10% of patients with myeloma	Amyloid deposits in eye and milky white, nonamyloid cysts of the pars plana (see Fig. 8-66)
Primary localized (so-called tumor-forming amyloidosis)	Predilection for localized deposits in certain sites: skin	None	Localized nodular deposits in cornea, eyelid, conjunctiva, and orbit; sometimes produces blepharoptosis, exophthalmos, decreased tearing, trigeminal nerve involvement
Secondary localized (most common form with eye involvement)	None	None	Associated with previous localized eyelid, conjunctival disease; basal cell carcinoma and other tumors, previous infections, trachoma, blepharitis, degenerative diseases, trauma, formation in a corneal scar
Latice corneal	None	None	Localized form of hereditary amyloidosis; characteristic lattice lines in corneal stroma, recurrent erosions

° Although strictly speaking this is a form of "secondary" amyloidosis, it is classified separately because the distribution of the amyloid deposit more closely resembles that of primary amyloidosis.
Modified by Dr. Loren Barrus, University of Utah, from Brownstein MH, Elliott R, and Hellwig EG: Am J Ophthalmol 69:423, 1970, and Blodi FC and Apple DJ: Am J Ophthalmol 88:346, 1979.

HEREDITARY BOWMAN'S LAYER DYSPLASIA[639-649]

Few reports of corneal clouding caused by thickening of Bowman's layer are available. Scattered publications report an association with such conditions as trisomy 18[639] (Fig. 3-53), Smith-Lemli-Opitz syndrome,[644] anterior segment mesodermal dysgenesis,[648,649] and a case of mucopolysaccharide accumulation in Bowman's membrane[647] differing from systemic mucopolysaccharidosis.

We have described hereditary Bowman's layer dysplasia, a condition characterized by bilateral diffuse, ground-glass corneal clouding at birth that rapidly progresses to total opacification.[640-645] The disease is always rapidly recurrent within several months after keratoplasty.

The primary histopathologic feature of this condition, which may be transmitted as an autosomal-recessive trait, is a generalized nodular thickening of Bowman's layer three to four times that observed in normal corneas (Fig. 3-

54). Bowman's layer not only is thickened, it also undergoes qualitative changes that appear to make this disease unique and that are responsible for the relentless corneal clouding that is the hallmark of Bowman's layer dysplasia. Bowman's layer normally is almost completely acellular. Figure 3-54 clearly demonstrates that this layer in a patient affected with this disease contains myriad cells with spindle-shaped nuclei. Electron microscopy shows these cells to be modified keratocytes or fibroblasts that are actively elaborating abnormal irregularly arrayed collagen (Fig. 3-54, *C*). In essence, Bowman's layer over the entire surface of the cornea is peppered with these microscopic foci of collagen formation. As an aggregate, they render the cornea opaque.[640]

This profile is reminiscent of that seen on a fetal cornea during the process of differentiation of Bowman's layer.[641] The subepithelial region in the fetal cornea also contains

Table 3-5. Differential features of the systemic mucopolysaccharidoses*

MPS type	Genetics	Systemic features		Ocular features			Urinary AMP excess			Deficient enzyme
		Skeletal dysplasia	Mental retardation	Corneal clouding	Retinal pigmentary degeneration	Optic atrophy	Heparan sulfate	Dermatan sulfate	Keratan sulfate	
I-H: Hurler	AR (allelic)	+++	+++	+++	R	R	++	+++	--	α-L-Iduronidase
I-S: Scheie (formerly MPS V)	AR (allelic)	+	±	+++	R	R	++	+++	--	α-L-Iduronidase (partial)
I-H/S: Phenotype intermediate between Huler and Scheie				+++						
II: Hunter	XR (allelic)									
A: Severe phenotype		+++	+++	--	R	R	++	++	--	Iduronate sulfate sulfatase
Mild phenotype		++	±	+†	R	R	++	++	--	Iduronate sulfate sulfatase
III: Sanfilippo	AR (nonallelic)									
A.		±	+++	--	R	R	+++	--	--	Heparan sulfate sulfatase
B.		±	+++	--	R	R	+++	--	--	N-Acetyl-α-D-glucosaminidase
C.										α-Glucosaminidase-N-acetyltransferase
D.										N-Acetylglucosamine-6-sulfatase
IV: A: Morquio	AR	+++	±	++	NR	R	--	--	+++	Hexosamine-6-sulfatase
B: Morquio-like syndrome, less severe changes										
V: Vacant; now MPS I-S										
VI: Maroteaux-Lamy	AR (allelic)									
A: Severe phenotype		+++	--	++	NR	R	--	+++	--	N-Acetylgalactosamine-4-sulfatase (arylsulfatase B)
B: Mild phenotype		+	--	++	NR	NR	--	+++	--	N-Acetylgalactosamine-4-sulfatase (arylsulfatase B)
VII: β-Glucuronidase deficiency	Homozygous for mutant gene at β-glucuronidase locus	+++	+++	--	NR	NR	--	+++	--	N-Acetylgalactosamine-4-sulfatase (arylsulfatase B)

* AR, autosomal recessive; XR, X-linked recessive; R, reported; NR, not reported; –, absent/not elevated; ±, variable; +, mild; ++, moderate; +++, marked.
† Positive by biomicroscopy in some older patients.
Modified by Dr. Stephen Gieser from Kenyon KR: In Goldberg MF, editor: Genetic and metabolic eye disease, Boston, 1974, Little, Brown & Co.

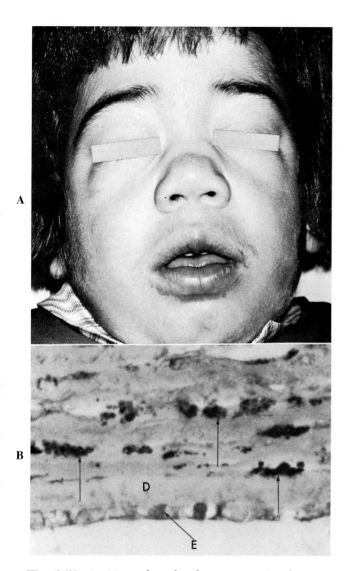

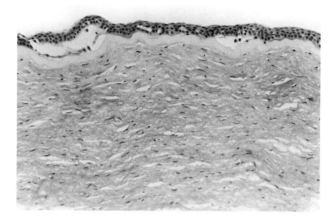

Fig. 3-53. Cornea from a child with trisomy 18 showing significant thickening and irregularity of Bowman's layer. (H & E stain; ×120.) (From Apple DJ: In Goldberg MF and Renie W, editors: Genetic and metabolic eye disease, ed 2, Boston, 1985, Little, Brown & Co.)

Fig. 3-52. A, Mucopolysaccharidosis type I (Hurler's syndrome). **B,** Corneal clouding in mucopolysaccharidosis. The posterior stroma contains deeply staining deposits *(arrows),* which are dispersed through the corneal stroma. They stain positively for mucopolysaccharides. The mucopolysaccharides are within the cytoplasm of keratocytes. The accumulation of this material in the corneal stroma is analogous to that seen in corneal macular dystrophy (p. 89). *D,* Descemet's membrane; *E,* corneal endothelium. (Colloidal iron stain; ×300.) (Courtesy Dr. Morton F Goldberg.)

abundant proliferating fibroblasts similar to that seen in this condition. Although the exact origin of Bowman's layer still is disputed (epithelial origin versus stromal fibroblasts), this dysplastic condition may represent an atavistic phenomenon in which the anterior corneal layers retain this fetal configuration. In other words, the appearance of Bowman's layer resembles that seen in the developing fetus during formation of Bowman's layer. Therefore, this process of continued proliferation and thickening of Bowman's layer, when it normally has no regenerative capacity except in utero, may be the persistent manifestation of a fetal event.

The histopathologic appearance of Bowman's layer dysplasia clearly differs from that of Reis-Bückler's dystrophy,[646] which also has been shown to affect Bowman's layer. In Reis-Bückler's dystrophy short, curled filaments of abnormal material are interspersed among normal collagen fibrils in Bowman's zone associated with areas of focal loss of Bowman's layer. These foci contain subepithelial plaques of fibrous tissue.

Trauma[650-731]

PERFORATING TRAUMA

Before and up to the first edition of this textbook (1974), trauma[684,704,705,730] accounted for more than 75% of all globes processed in most ocular pathology laboratories (Fig. 3-55).[681] However, with the advent of improved surgical techniques, such as improved anterior segment reconstruction techniques and modern vitreoretinal surgery, the request to remove eyes after each severe trauma has been reduced. Good surgical repair also decreases the risk of sympathetic ophthalmia. Erie and associates[681] noted that nonsurgical and surgical trauma now accounts for 35% of enucleation. The tissue of reference is important in differentiating a penetrating from a perforating injury.[667-669,711,714,728] A penetrating injury by definition extends only partially through the tissue of reference; a perforation is complete passage of a foreign device through the tissue of reference. For example, a perforation of the cornea represents a mere penetration of the globe (Fig. 3-56). A perforation of a tissue thus signifies the presence of not only an entrance wound but also an exit wound at a second site.

Corneoscleral laceration, with perforation of these structures and associated complications, is the most common form of trauma that leads to enucleation. A common sequela of corneoscleral perforation is prolapse or extrusion of intraocular contents into the wound tract.[702] Prolapse of uveal tissue into such a wound is common (Fig. 3-57, *A*) and leads to the possibility of sympathetic ophthalmia (p. 298). Prolapse of retinal tissue into a corneal or scleral wound (Fig. 3-57, *B*) is a much more ominous prognostic sign than prolapse of uveal tissue. Extrusion of the sensory

Fig. 3-54. Bilateral diffusely cloudy cornea in a child. **A,** Photomicrograph through the cornea showing extensive thickening of Bowman's layer and presence of numerous keratocytes within this layer. (H & E stain; ×175.) **B,** Higher-power photomicrograph showing marked thickening and irregularity of Bowman's layer. (H & E stain; ×250.) **C,** Electron micrograph through Bowman's layer showing an area where a fibroblast and surrounding dense collagenous tissue *(arrows)* interrupts the normal delicate fibrillar structure of Bowman's layer. Multiple lesions such as these have created the diffuse opacity. (Uranyl acetate lead citrate; ×2000.) (From Apple DJ and others: Corneal opacification secondary to Bowman's layer dygenesis, Am J Ophthalmol 93:320, 1984.)

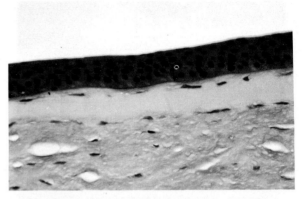

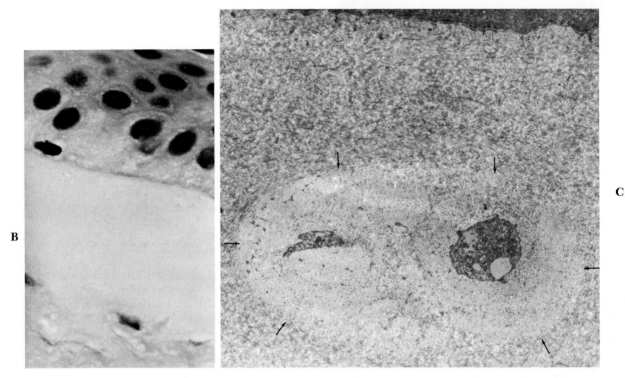

retina implies massive retinal detachment. Such eyes are very difficult to treat.

Histopathologic recognition of a corneal or scleral perforation is easy in the acute phase after nonsurgical or surgical trauma.[651,652,655,657] However, identification of a previous corneal penetration or perforation in an eye enucleated many years after the original trauma is much more difficult. Such identification occasionally is necessary for medicolegal purposes. Serial sectioning of the cornea may be required to locate the site of the injury, which, after healing, often is difficult to identify, even microscopically.

A study of changes at various levels of the cornea may provide clues to the nature of the injury (Fig. 3-58).

When Bowman's layer is disrupted, it cannot regenerate, and a permanent defect or gap in this layer results. Furthermore, as the epithelium regrows, the superficial surface of the epithelium remains smooth. The newly formed epithelium assumes the contour of the corneal surface to prevent optic aberration. However, epithelial growth over the defect in Bowman's layer is irregular, and deeply grow-

ing epithelial cells typically fill the gap. The focus of epithelial thickening at the site of the wound is known as an epithelial facet (Figs. 3-3 and 3-58).

Complete corneal perforation always interrupts Descemet's membrane. However, this membrane also may rupture as a secondary effect of blunt trauma. Evidence of previous damage to Descemet's membrane is attained easily in microscopic sections: the membrane appears broken, coiled, and wrinkled, and may protrude anteriorly into the corneal stroma (Fig. 3-58). Descemet's membrane, a true basement membrane, is best studied by the PAS stain. Other corneal changes indicative of a previous wound include localized calcification of Bowman's layer (band keratopathy) and scarring and/or vascularization of the corneal stroma along the edges of the wound tract.

Epithelial ingrowth,[662,693,731] which may follow accidental or surgical trauma, is an ominous complication of perforating corneal or scleral trauma. A relentless ingrowth of epithelium through the wound tract onto the posterior surface of the cornea (Fig. 3-59) forms an opaque sheath that

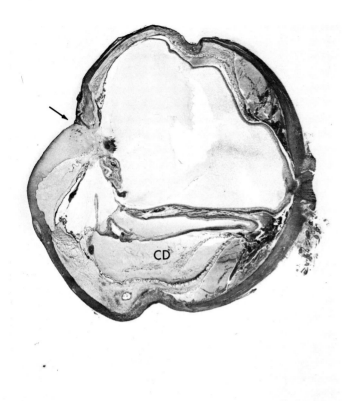

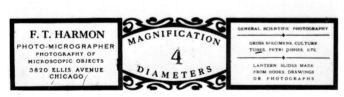

Fig. 3-55. Photomicrograph of a globe with a limbal perforation, one of the earliest specimens obtained and prepared by Dr. GD Theobald, a pioneering American ophthalmic pathologist in Chicago. This slide shows a healed scar at the limbus *(arrow)*, total retinal detachment, and a marked choroidal detachment *(CD)* inferiorly. (H & E stain; ×4.) (From the original collection of the late Dr. Georgiana Dvorak, University of Illinois Eye and Ear Infirmary, Chicago.)

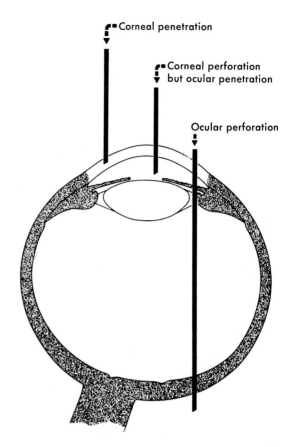

Fig. 3-56. When penetration is differentiated from perforation, the tissue of reference is of critical importance. Because the cornea is the tissue of reference, a corneal perforation is considered an ocular penetration (because the whole eye is the tissue of reference).

may extend across the anterior chamber angle, inducing a secondary glaucoma. The sheets of ingrowing epithelium are composed of a nonkeratinized, stratified squamous epithelium similar to that usually found on the cornea or conjunctival epithelium. The membrane also may grow onto the iris as far as the pupillary margin, and in rare instances, the epithelium grows through the pupillary aperture into the posterior chamber as far posteriorly as the ciliary body. The prognosis of severe epithelial ingrowth is grave. Although treatment with cryotherapy has shown encouraging results, this disease remains extremely difficult to manage.

Anterior chamber cysts (Fig. 3-60) form by a pathogenesis similar to that of epithelial ingrowth. After formation of a perforating wound tract through the cornea or sclera, clusters of epithelial cells from the corneal or conjunctival epithelium may be deposited through the wound tract into the anterior chamber. The aqueous fluid serves as an excellent tissue culture medium, permitting proliferation of the epithelial cells within the anterior chamber. As the cells

proliferate, a central cavitation of the mass of cells often occurs, leading to the formation of a cyst.[655,657,670]

This pathogenesis of an anterior chamber inclusion cyst should be distinguished from the rare development cysts that form as a result of separation of the two epithelial layers of the iris (the cavity of the embryonic optic cup). Drug-induced cysts are caused by hyperplasia of iris epithelial cells. They are much smaller than epithelial or congenital cysts and generally occur on the pupillary margin in patients undergoing therapy with echothiophate (Phospholine) iodide (see Fig. 7-3).[655]

Perforating corneal wounds[655] commonly produce corneal opacities. A tiny opacity that can be seen only with the slit lamp is termed a nebula, an opacity of intermediate size is a macula, and larger opacities are categorized as leukomas. An adherent leukoma (leukoma adhaerens; Figs. 3-61 and 4-11, *A*) is an adherence, usually by a fibrous band, between the cornea and structures posterior to the cornea. These posterior structures usually include the iris and an intact or cataractous lens. In addition, in aphakic eyes, the fibrous band may insert onto a cyclitic membrane or even onto the anterior face of the vitreous.

Intraocular foreign bodies[689]

After perforating injury to the cornea or sclera, foreign bodies often become lodged within the globe. Some for-

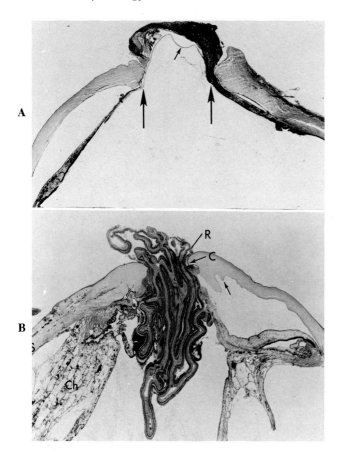

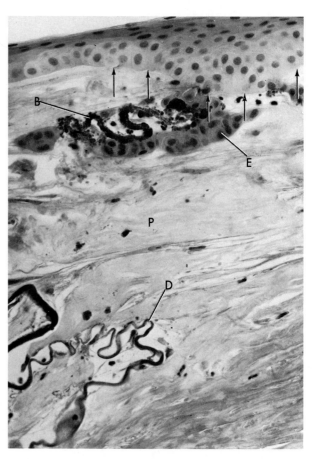

Fig. 3-57. A, Corneal perforation with uveal prolapse. The basement membrane-like structure *(small arrow)* represents residual lens capsule. The smooth edges of the wound *(large arrows)* resulted from a perforation caused by a sharp knife. The identification of uveal tissue will influence the decision whether to enucleate in cases in which sympathetic ophthalmia might subsequently develop. (H & E stain; ×15.) **B,** Perforating corneal wound with prolapse of a major portion of sensory retina *(R)* into the wound. Impending, or frank, phthisis bulbi is apparent histopathologically by marked swelling of the choroid *(Ch)*, which signifies hypotony. Retinal prolapse usually signifies widespread destruction of intraocular structures and usually terminates in phthisis bulbi. *S,* Sclera; *C,* cornea at the margin of the perforating wound; *arrow,* wrinkled Descemet's membrane. (H & E stain; ×15.)

Fig. 3-58. Anterior aspect of the cornea several months after a perforating injury. Five major changes prove the existence of previous injury: (1) the epithelial defect at the site of the wound entrance is filled in by an epithelial facet *(arrows)*; (2) epithelial inclusions *(E)* are embedded within the corneal stroma; (3) band keratopathy or calcification of Bowman's layer *(B)* is seen; (4) there is marked scarring of the corneal stroma along the line of the perforation *(P)*; and (5) Descemet's membrane *(D)*, which is prolapsed into the stroma, characteristically becomes wrinkled and coiled after rupture. Such wrinkling is a result of the rich elastic tissue content of this membrane. Rupture of Descemet's membrane does not necessarily imply corneal perforation. Blunt trauma can sufficiently distort the cornea to cause stretching and rupture of the membrane. (H & E stain; ×250.)

eign bodies are relatively inert. Glass, for example, incites only minimal inflammatory reaction. Even these inert substances may lead to loss of the eye as a result of a tissue disruption caused by the initial injury or introduction of infectious agents into the eye by the foreign material. Probably the two most common types of foreign bodies that enter the eye are vegetable matter and metal.

Intraocular vegetable foreign bodies are often readily visualized by histopathologic examination (Fig. 3-62, *A*).[679,703] In cases in which the foreign material is extremely minute or in which a massive inflammatory reaction tends to obscure the presence of the foreign body, the technique of polarizing microscopy is extremely useful to the pathologist. Figs. 3-62, *B*, and 3-63 illustrate the concept of tissue birefringence when this technique is used. The foreign material in these cases is large and clearly visualized in regular

hematoxylin and eosin sections but becomes even more apparent when viewed through polarizing lenses.

As noted on page 5, polarizing lenses are useful when studying material made of molecules that possess a regular or crystalline-like arrangement. When the cross-polarizing filters are placed on a microscope, noncrystallinelike structures are filtered out and appear as a dark background. Most normal tissues in the eye fall into this category. In contrast, tissues with a regular geometric molecular arrangement, such as some vegetable materials, appear to glow (show birefringence) when viewed through these filters. Therefore, a small structure that might otherwise be missed becomes readily apparent to the microscopist. Other structures that show birefringence through polarizing lenses include amyloid (Fig. 3-50, *B*), calcium oxalate

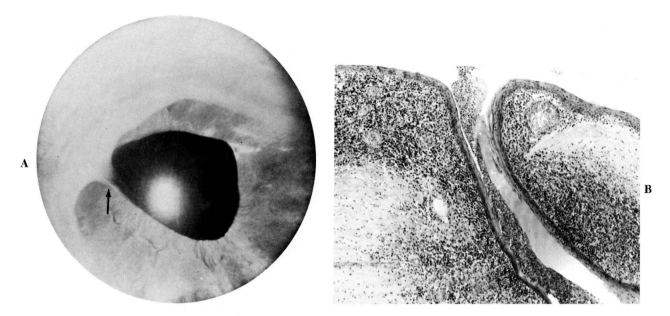

Fig. 3-59. A, Epithelial ingrowth. A diffuse white semiopaque membrane is growing downward on the posterior aspect on the cornea from the superonasal limbus through the distorted pupil onto the posterior iris surface *(arrow).* **B,** Anterior half of a cornea after corneal perforation. Epithelial ingrowth has occurred along the line of the wound track, which courses obliquely through the center of the section. The epithelium is derived directly from the corneal epithelium (above). Intensive secondary acute and chronic inflammation and vascularization have occurred within the corneal stroma along the borders of the wound tract. (H & E stain; ×125.)

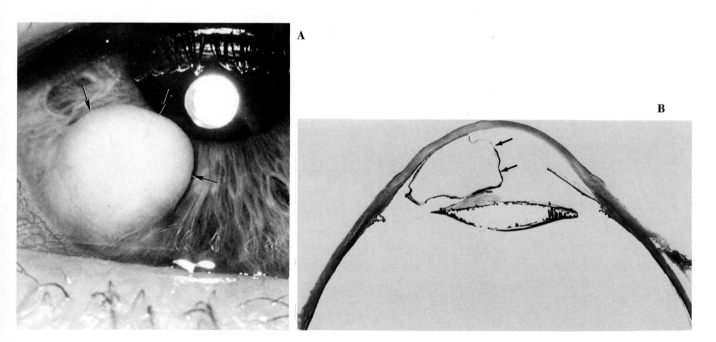

Fig. 3-60. A, Anterior chamber cyst *(arrows)* on the surface of the iris. The epithelial lining of such a cyst is usually of the nonkeratinized, stratified squamous type, similar to that of the normal corneal or conjunctival epithelium. **B,** Photomicrograph of an anterior chamber cyst *(arrows).* (H & E stain; ×5.)

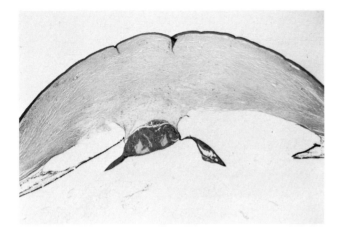

Fig. 3-61. Corneal scarring caused by central corneal perforation, with adherent leukoma. The significantly cataractous lens is fused with the posterior cornea. (H & E stain; ×10.)

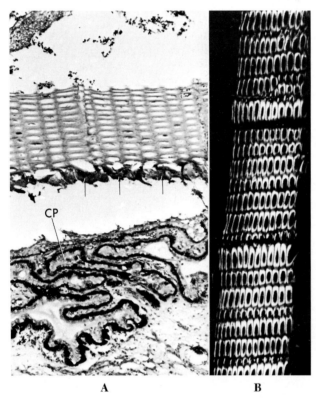

A   B

Fig. 3-62. A, Photomicrograph of an eye enucleated after corneal perforation and entrance of a vegetable (wood) foreign body into the vitreous. Note the distorted ciliary processes (*CP*), blood, and fibrin adjacent to the foreign body. The wood fibers have a parallel, lattice, or trellislike arrangement. Small arrows identify a row of foreign body giant cells that attempt to surround the foreign material. (H & E stain; ×100.) **B,** Intraocular wood foreign body seen by microscopy with polarizing lenses (same structure as in **A**). Polarizing lenses filter out all light except that passing through the crystalline-like, regularly arranged molecules of the foreign body. Therefore the foreign material appears to glow (show birefringence) against the dark background. This technique is useful in the differentiation of various forms of foreign bodies. (H & E stain; ×90.)

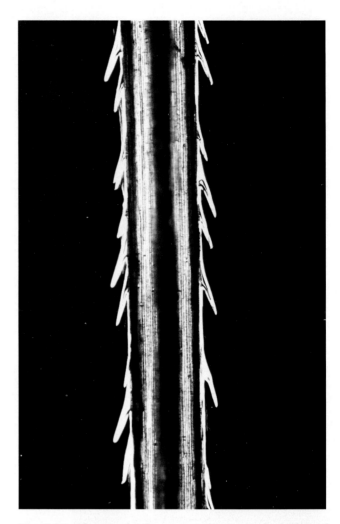

Fig. 3-63. Photograph of an intraocular foreign body derived from an insect. Distinct details of the substructure are visible through polarizing lenses. (×350.)

crystals within a hypermature lens (see Fig. 4-24), silicone implants, and many types of suture material.

Iron-containing foreign bodies (Fig. 3-64) may lead to siderosis bulbi.* Iron uptake within ocular structures generally is more prominent in, but not confined to, the epithelially derived elements of the eye. Thus, the structures most commonly affected in siderosis bulbi include the epithelium of the lens (siderosis lentis) (Fig. 3-65, *A*), the sensory retina (Fig. 3-65, *B*) and pigment epithelium, the epithelium of the iris and ciliary body, and the epithelially derived smooth muscles of the iris.

In histopathologic sections, iron pigment appears light brown and granular and usually is easy to differentiate from the more deep brown to black pigmentation of melanin. (Figs. 8-62 and 8-63, *B*, show the typical appearance of melanin pigment deposited within the perivascular spaces of the retina.) In equivocal cases, intraocular iron can be demonstrated in tissues by the Prussian blue stain (Fig. 3-65), which imparts a blue color to the iron deposits. The marked destruction of intraocular tissues in siderosis seems

---

* References 336, 660, 665, 666, 675, 698, 723, 725.

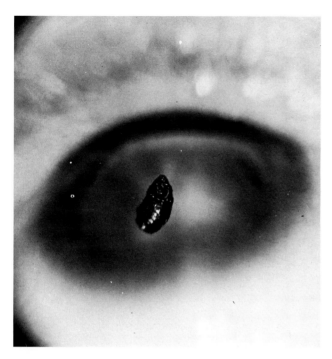

Fig. 3-64. Metallic foreign body in the anterior chamber with a secondary cataract caused by siderosis.

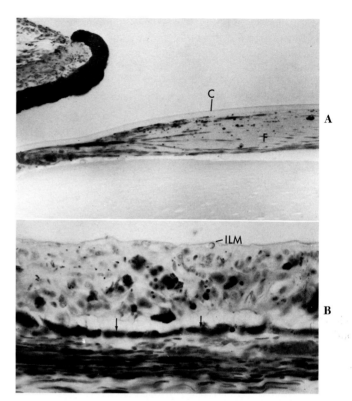

Fig. 3-65. Siderosis bulbi. **A,** Siderosis lentis, with granules of iron deposited in an anterior subcapsular fibrous plaque *(F)*. *C,* Lens capsule. The iris margin is at the upper left. (Prussian blue stain; ×275.) **B,** Retinal degeneration resulting from iron deposition (dark granules). Almost all neuronal elements are absent, and the pigment epithelium *(arrows)* is atrophic. *ILM,* Internal limiting membrane. (Prussian blue stain; ×320.) (From Naumann GOH and Apple DJ: In Doerr W, Seifert G, Uehlinger E, editors: Handbuch der speziellen pathologischen Anatomie, Band Auge, Berlin, 1980, Springer-Verlag.)

to result from a direct toxic effect of the iron deposits on the tissue. Intraretinal deposits of iron in siderosis bulbi may be so extensive as to mimic retinitis pigmentosa. In such cases, however, because the iron is deposited in a diffuse manner throughout the sensory retina rather than in a perivascular distribution (p. 403), the bone spicule pattern of pigmentary retinopathy is not as prominent.

Choleosis[713] due to copper foreign body is described under Kaiser-Fleischer's ring (p. 83).

NONPERFORATING TRAUMA[655,676,716]

A contusion injury[663] of the cornea or sclera is a nonperforating blunt injury that may cause mechanical distortion of the various tunics of the globe. The most severe intraocular changes are caused by sudden stretching and compression of the various layers of the globe that result from sudden increases in pressure within the globe. Secondary open-angle glaucoma results from excessive cleavage of the angle recess, the so-called contusion deformity of the angle.[690,710,717,720,729] Contusion injuries in children[653,654,680,696,712] and adults may cause a wide variety, including corneal damage,[416] secondary cataracts (cataracta complicata), dislocation of the lens, hyphema, eightball hemorrhage, blood staining of the cornea (Figs. 3-36 and 3-37), hemophthalmos, and iridocyclitis. Phacoanaphylactic endophthalmitis (p. 138) may follow lens capsular rupture. Retinal changes such as commotio retinae (Berlin's edema), macular hole formation, choroidal rupture (see Fig. 8-118),[650] and chorioretinal hemorrhage also result from blunt trauma.° Most of these lesions are described separately in other chapters.

RETROCORNEAL FIBROUS MEMBRANE

Formation of a retrocorneal fibrous membrane° (Figs. 3-29 and 3-30) can result from many causes. These include fibrous organization of a hyphema (Figs. 3-29, *A,* and 3-30, *A*), organization of inflammatory debris within the anterior chamber (Figs. 3-29, *B,* and 3-30, *B*), alkali burns (p. 104), ingrowth of fibrous tissue through a perforating corneal wound, or corneal transplantation (Fig. 3-30, *C,* see also Figs. 4-84 to 4-86).

Apparently, irritation of the corneal endothelium by such factors as chemical burns or surgical trauma sometimes stimulates a fibrous metaplasia of corneal endothelium,[297] that is, a transformation of the flat cuboidal endothelial cell into a fibrocyte. In some cases, the membrane may result from ingrowth of fibrous tissue that gains access to the retrocorneal space through a defect in Descemet's membrane.

FAILED PENETRATING KERATOPLASTY[697,722,724]

Failed corneal graft due to homograft reaction is now relatively infrequent, but the incidence is increased with

---

° References 658, 661, 671, 672, 676, 686, 687.

° References 228, 259, 260, 271, 281, 283, 284, 293, 294, 656.

grafting and vascularized cornea. An immune reaction usually starts within a month of surgery and is characterized
by iridocyclitis with fine keratic precipitates and vascularization that extends centrally from the periphery, with the
eventual stromal edema. There is infiltration of polymorphonuclear neutrophils and central necrosis and eventual
necrosis of the central zone of the donor cornea. This is
surrounded by deposition of leukocytes and plasma cells.

Retrocorneal membrane is found in as many as 50% of
graphs that require retreatment. It not only occurs after
homograft rejection, but also after poor wound deposition.
The cells of the membrane originate either from a fibrous
metaplasia of endothelial cells or from proliferation of fibrous cells in the wound or keratocytes.

CHEMICAL BURNS*

Alkali burns of the cornea are much more destructive
than acid burns and are significant cause of retrocorneal
fibrous membrane. Acid solutions do not readily penetrate
the corneal epithelium because the acid groups are re-
pelled by the lipoprotein cell walls of the corneal epithelial
cells and keratocytes. Therefore, acid burns of the cornea
usually are sharply demarcated and superficial because of
the limited spread of the solution and the buffering action
of the tissues.

Solutions with an alkaline pH rapidly penetrate and
spread deep into the corneal stroma and into the anterior
chamber. Most alkali burns are caused by lye (NaOH or
KOH) and ammonia (NH_4OH) or lime (CaO).

It appears that there are two basic mechanisms for retrocorneal fibrous membrane: 1) irritation of the corneal endothelium by such factors as chemical burns or surgical
trauma stimulate a fibrous metaplasia of corneal endothelium,[192] that is, transformation of the endothelial cells into
a fibrocyte; and 2) in some cases, the membrane may result
from ingrowth of fibrous tissue that gains access to the
retrocorneal space through a defect in Descemet's membrane.

Hughes[691,692] has described in detail the clinical and histopathologic features of corneal alkali burns. During the
early stages of the burn, the cornea appears nearly normal.
However, the solution quickly penetrates the entire thickness of the cornea and cannot be removed easily by irrigation. The alkali produces rapid loosening and sloughing of
the corneal epithelium and thus facilitates rapid penetration. Penetration of the alkaline fluid leads to extensive
florid necrosis of all corneal layers (Fig. 3-66). The cornea
softens and exhibits a gelatinous consistency. Edema of the
cornea and conjunctiva results from endothelial damage. In
the acute stage, diffuse coagulation necrosis of all corneal
lamellae occurs, with pyknosis and eventual disappearance
of epithelial and keratocytic nuclei. Polymorphonuclear
neutrophils enter the burned stroma from the limbal vessels within hours. Mucopolysaccharides within the stroma
are lost. The intraocular pressure may increase within minutes but may decrease after several hours or days. Iritis is
common.

In a later stage (the stage of reparation), the conjunctival
and corneal edema subsides. The peripheral epithelium

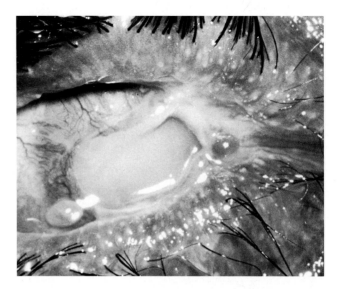

Fig. 3-66. Alkali burns of the cornea cause a florid necrosis of
most anterior segment structures. Pseudopterygium, symblepharon, and ankyloblepharon are common sequelae in the cicatricial
stage, which follows the initial necrosis.

regenerates abnormally, and the newly formed epithelial
basement membrane is abnormal or absent. Craters or irregular defects composed of broken-down collagen develop. Further infiltration of polymorphonuclear neutrophils occurs. Proteolytic enzymes such as collagenase are
produced in excessive amounts by the abnormal epithelium
and leukocytes. Enzyme levels are increased by local administration of steroids. Although collagenase usually is
present in the cornea and is important in healing of corneal
wounds, alkali-burned corneas seem to be particularly susceptible to damage by this enzyme.

In partial burns, a retrocorneal fibrous membrane forms
within 2 to 3 weeks. The retrocorneal membrane arises
after fibrous metaplasia of residual corneal endothelial
cells.* At 6 weeks, a new endothelium covers the retrocorneal membrane and a new Descemet's membrane is
formed, with later resorption of the retrocorneal membrane. In severe total burns, in which no endothelial cells
remain, the fibrous retrocorneal membrane probably arises
from the connective tissue of the angle, and a new endothelium does not appear.

Within 1 to 2 weeks, vascularization of the cornea develops in association with reduction in the edema and cellular
infiltration. In late stages, the cornea remains opacified and
vascularized. The final cicatricial stage is characterized by
formation of a vascularized membrane (pseudopterygium),
symblepharon, and ankyloblepharon. Recurrent corneal ulcerations, which sometimes progress to corneal perforation, are common.[437] Secondary descemetocele or perforation, anterior uveitis, secondary cataract, secondary
glaucoma, and loss of the tear film also are frequent complications.

* References 659, 673, 688, 691, 692, 709.

* References 603, 694, 695, 699-701, 706, 707, 715, 718, 726.

REFERENCES

General references

1. Barr CC, Grelender H, and Font RL: Corneal crystalline deposits associated with dysproteinemia: report of two cases and review of the literature, Arch Ophthalmol 98:884, 1980.
2. Berliner ML: Biomicroscopy of the eye, New York, 1966, Hafner Publishing Co.
3. Bond WI, Monroe LD, and Morgan KS: Idiopathic breaks in Descemet's membrane, J Pediatr Ophthalmol Strabismus 19:386, 1979.
4. Braley AE and others: Stereoscopic atlas of slit-lamp biomicroscopy, vol 1, St. Louis, 1970, The CV Mosby Co.
5. Braude LS and Chandler JW: Corneal allograft rejection: the role of the major histocompatibility complex, Surv Ophthalmol 27:290, 1983.
6. Bron AJ and Tripathi RC: Corneal disorders. In Goldberg MF, editor: Genetic and metabolic eye disease, Boston, 1974, Little, Brown & Co.
7. Busacca A: Biomicroscopie et histopathologie de Foeil, Zurich, 1952, Schweizer Druck & Verlagshaus.
8. Cogan DG, Hurlbut CS, and Kuwabara T: Crystalline calcium sulfate (gypsum) in scleral plaques of a human eye, J Histochem Cytochem 6:142, 1958.
9. Colosi NJ and Yanoff M: Reactive corneal endothelialization, Am J Ophthalmol 83:219, 1977.
10. Crandall A, Yanoff M, and Schaffer D: Intrascleral nerve loop mistakenly identified as a foreign body, Arch Ophthalmol 95:497, 1977.
11. Diaz-Araya CM and others: Immunohistochemical and topographic studies of dendritic cells and macrophages in human fetal cornea, Invest Ophthalmol Vis Sci 36:644, 1995.
12. Dodd MJ, Pusin SM, and Green WR: Adult cystinosis: a case report, Arch Ophthalmol 96:1054, 1977.
13. Donaldson DD: Atlas of external diseases of the eye, vol III, Cornea and sclera, ed 2, St. Louis, 1980, The CV Mosby Co.
14. Duke-Elder S, editor: System of ophthalmology, vol VIII, Diseases of the outer eye, part 1, Conjunctiva; part 2, Cornea and sclera, St. Louis, 1965, The CV Mosby Co.
15. Eiferman RA and Rodrigues MM: Unusual superficial stromal corneal deposits in IgG kappa monoclonal gammmopathy, Arch Ophthalmol 98:78, 1980.
16. Elliott JH and others: Hereditary sclerocornea, Arch Ophthalmol 103:676, 1985.
17. Feenstra RPG, Tseng SCG: Comparison of fluorescein and rose bengal staining, Ophthalmol 99:605, 1992.
18. Feldon SE and others: Clinical manifestations of brawny scleritis, Am J Ophthalmol 85:781, 1978.
19. Fishman and others: Cornea plana: a case report, Ann Ophthalmol 14:47, 1982.
20. Gandhi SS, Lamberts DW, and Perry HD: Donor to host transmission of disease via corneal transplantation, Surv Ophthalmol 25:306, 1981.
21. Geroski DH and others: Pump function of the human corneal endothelium: effects of age and cornea guttata, Ophthalmology 92:759, 1985.
22. Goldberg MF and Renie W, editors: Genetic and metabolic eye disease, ed 2, Boston, 1985, Little, Brown & Co.
23. Grayson M: Diseases of the cornea, ed 2, St. Louis, 1983, The CV Mosby Co.
24. Grayson M and Keates R: Manual of diseases of the cornea, Boston, 1969, Little, Brown & Co.
25. Harbin RL and others: Sclerocornea associated with the Smith-Lemli-Opitz syndrome, Am J Ophthalmol 84:72, 1977.
26. Henke F and Lubarsch O: Handbuch der speziellen pathologischen Anatomie und Histologie, Berlin, 1928, Julius Springer.
27. King JH Jr and McTigue JW, editors: The Cornea World Congress, London, 1965, Butterworth & Co (Publishers), Ltd.
28. Klauss V and Riedel K: Bilateral and unilateral mesodermal corneal metaplasia, Br J Ophthalmol 67:320, 1983.
29. Laing RA and others: Evidence for mitosis in the adult corneal endothelium, Ophthalmology 91:1129, 1984.
30. Mackool RJ and Holtz SJ: Descemet's membrane detachment, Arch Ophthalmol 95:459, 1977.
31. Marshall J and Grindle CFJ: Fine structure of the cornea and its development, Trans Ophthalmol Soc UK 98:320, 1978.
32. Meesmann A: Die Mikroskopie des lebenden Auges: vorderen Abschnittes, Munich, 1927, Urban & Schwarzenberg.
33. Mensher JH: Corneal nerves, Surv Ophthalmol 19:1, 1974.
34. Meyner E: Atlas der Spaltlampenphotographie, Stuttgart, 1976, Ferdinand Enke Verlag.
35. Naumann GOH and Apple DJ: Pathology of the eye, Berlin, 1985, Springer-Verlag. (Translation, modification, and update of Pathologie des Auges by DJ Apple.)
36. New Orleans Academy of Ophthalmology: Symposium on the cornea: transactions of the New Orleans Academy of Ophthalmology, St. Louis, 1972, The CV Mosby Co.
37. Orellana J and Friedman AH: Ocular manifestations of multiple myeloma, Waldenström's macroglobulinemia and benign monoclonal gammopathy, Surv Ophthalmol 26:157, 1981.
38. Pirie A: Effect of vitamin A deficiency on the cornea, Trans Ophthalmol Soc UK 98:357, 1978.
39. Polack F, editor: Corneal and external disease, Springfield, Ill, 1970, Charles C Thomas, Publisher.
40. Polack F: Contributions of electron microscopy to the study of corneal pathology, Surv Ophthalmol 20:376, 1976.
41. Rich LF and others: Keratocyte survival in keratophakia lenticules, Arch Ophthalmol 99:677, 1981.
42. Rodrigues MM and others: Posterior corneal crystalline deposits in benign monoclonal gammopathy: a clinicopathologic case report, Arch Ophthalmol 97:124, 1979.
43. Shamsuddin AKM and others: Is the corneal posterior cell layer truly endothelial? Ophthalmology 93:1298, 1986.
44. Schaumburg-Lever G, Leven WF: Color atlas of histopathology of the skin, Philadelphia, 1988, JB Lippincott.
45. Slansky HH and Dohlman CH: Collagenase and the cornea, Surv Ophthalmol 14:402, 1970.
46. Sprague JB and Forstot SL: Bilateral corneal leukomas, J Pediatr Ophthalmol Strabismus 17:251, 1980.
47. Straub W and Rossman H: Atlas der Erkrankungen des vorderen Abschnittes, Munich, 1982, Verlag Urban & Schwarzenberg.
48. Sturrock GD, Sherrard ES, and Rice NSC: Specular microscopy of the corneal endothelium, Br J Ophthalmol 62:809, 1978.
49. Vogt A: Lehrbuch und Atlas der spaltlampenmikroskopie des lebenden Auges, vols I and II, ed, Berlin, 1930-1931, Julius Springer.
50. Waring GO III and Rodrigues MM: Patterns of pathologic response in the cornea, Surv Ophthalmol 31:262, 1987.
51. Waring GO III and others: The corneal endothelium, Ophthalmology 89:531, 1982.
52. Watson PG and Hazleman MB: The sclera and systemic disorders: major problems in ophthalmology, vol 2, Philadelphia, 1976, WB Saunders Co.
53. Wong S and others: Color specular microscopy of disorders involving the corneal epithelium, Ophthalmology 91:1176, 1984.
54. Yamamoto GK and others: Long term ocular changes in cystinosis: observations in renal transplant recipients, J Pediatr Ophthalmol Strabismus 19:21, 1979.
55. Yanoff M, Fine BS: Ocular pathology: a color atlas, ed. 2, New York, 1992, Gower Medical Publishing.

Inflammatory conditions

Inflammation, corneal ulcers and nonulcerative inflammation

56. Abbott RL, Forster RK: Superficial punctate keratitis of Thygeson associated with scarring and Salzmann's nodular degeneration, Am J Ophthalmol 87:296, 1979.
57. Adenovirus keratoconjunctivitis (editorial), Br J Ophthalmol 61:73, 1977.
58. Aitken D and others: Amebic keratitis in a wearer of disposable contact lenses due to a mixed vahlkampfia and hartmannella infection, Ophthalmol 103:485, 1996.
59. Allen HC: Current status of prevention, diagnosis and management of bacterial corneal ulcers, Ann Ophthalmol 3:235, 1971.
60. Aronson SB and others: Pathogenic approach to therapy of peripheral corneal inflammatory disease, Am J Ophthalmol 70:65, 1970.
61. Austin P and others: Peripheral corneal degeneration and occlusive vasculitis in Wegener's granulomatosis, Am J Ophthalmol 85:311, 1978.
62. Barr CC and others: Corneal crystalline deposits associated with dysproteinemia. Report of two cases and review of the literature, Arch Ophthalmol 98:884, 1980.
63. Bernauer W and others: The management of corneal perforations

associated with rheumatoid arthritis: an analysis of 32 eyes, Ophthalmol 102:1325, 1995.

64. Binder P: Herpes simplex keratitis, Surv Ophthalmol 21:313, 1977.

65. Binder P, Zavala EY, and Stainer GA: Noninfectious peripheral corneal ulceration: Mooren's ulcer or Terrien's marginal degeneration? Ann Ophthalmol 14:425, 1982.

66. Boerner CF and others: Electron microscopy for the diagnosis of ocular viral infections, Ophthalmology 88:1377, 1981.

67. Brooks AMV and others: Determination of the nature of corneal crystals by specular microscopy, Ophthalmol 95:448, 1988.

68. Brown DC: Ocular herpes simplex, Invest Ophthalmol 10:210, 1971.

69. Brown SI, Grayson M: Marginal furrows: characteristic corneal lesion of rheumatoid arthritis, Arch Ophthalmol 79:563, 1968.

70. Bullington RH and others: Nontuberculous mycobacterial keratitis. Report of two cases and review of literature. [review] Arch Ophthalmol 110:519, 1992.

71. Buus DR and others: Lymphogranuloma venereum conjunctivitis with a marginal corneal perforation, Ophthalmology 95:799, 1988.

72. Chandler JW and Milam DF: Diphtheria corneal ulcers, Arch Ophthalmol 96:53, 1978.

73. Charles NC, Bennett TW, and Margolis S: Ocular pathology of the congenital varicella syndrome, Arch Ophthalmol 95:2034, 1977.

74. Cherry PMH and others: Corneal and conjunctival deposits in monoclonal gammopathy, Can J Ophthalmol 18:142, 1983.

75. Claman HN: The biology of the immune response, JAMA 268:2790, 1992.

76. Collin HB and others: The fine structure of nuclear changes in superior limbic keratoconjunctivitis, Invest Ophthalmol Vis Sci 17: 791, 1978.

77. Coster DJ: Herpetic keratitis and corneal destruction, Trans Ophthalmol Soc UK 98:372, 1978.

78. Davis and others: Acanthamoeba keratitis and infectious crystalline keratopathy, Arch Ophthalmol 105:1524, 1987.

79. Dawson CR, Hanna L, and Togni B: Adenovirus type 8 infections in the United States. IV. Observations on the pathogenesis of lesions in severe eye disease, Arch Ophthalmol 87:258, 1972.

80. Dodd MJ and others: Adult cystinosis: a case report, Arch Ophthalmol 96:1054, 1978.

81. Dougherty PJ and others: Acanthamoeba sclerokeratitis, Am J Ophthalmol 117:475, 1994.

82. Doughman DJ and others: Fungal keratitis at the University of Minnesota: 1971-1981, Trans Am Ophthalmol Soc 80:235, 1982.

83. Driebe WT Jr and others: *Acanthamoeba* keratitis: potential role for topical clotrimazole in combination chemotherapy, Arch Ophthalmol 106:1196, 1988.

84. Dugel PU and others: *Microbacterium fortuitum* keratitis, Am J Ophthalmol 105:661, 1988.

85. Edmonds C and Iwamoto T: Electron microscopy of late interstitial keratitis, Ann Ophthalmol 4:693, 1972.

86. Eiferman RA, Rodrigues MM: Unusual superficial stromal corneal deposits in IgG γ monoclonal gammopathy, Arch Ophthalmol 98: 78, 1980.

87. Eiferman RA, Ogden LL, and Snyder J: Anaerobic peptostreptococcal keratitis, Am J Ophthalmol 180:335, 1985.

88. Eltner VM and others: Intercellular adhesion molecule-1 (icam-1) and hla-dr antigens in herpes keratitis, Ophthalmol 97:1194, 1990.

89. Epstein RJ: Rapid diagnosis of *Acanthamoeba* keratitis from corneal scrapings using indirect fluorescent antibody staining, Arch Ophthalmol 104:1318, 1986.

90. Falcon MG and Williams HP: Herpes simplex kerato-uveitis and glaucoma, Trans Ophthalmol Soc UK 98:101, 1978.

91. Ferry AP, Leopold IH: Marginal (ring) corneal ulcer as presenting manifestation of Wegener's granuloma: clinicopathologic study, Trans Am Acad Ophthalmol Otolaryngol 74:1276, 1970.

92. Fine BS: Mycotic keratitis. In King JH Jr and McTigue JW, editors: The Cornea World Congress, London, 1965, Butterworth & Co (Publishers), Ltd.

93. Florakis GJ and others: Elevated corneal epithelial lines in *Acanthamoeba* keratitis, Arch Ophthalmol 106:1202, 1988.

94. Font RL: Chronic ulcerative keratitis caused by herpes simplex virus, Arch Ophthalmol 90:382, 1973.

95. Foster CS and others: The immunopathology of Mooren's ulcer, Am J Ophthalmol 88:149, 1979.

96. Foster CS and others: Immunopathology of atopic keratoconjunctivitis, Ophthalmol 98:1190, 1991.

97. Frazier PD, Wong VG: Cystinosis. Histologic and crystallographic examination of crystals in eye tissues, Arch Ophthalmol 80:87, 1968.

98. Friedenwald JS: Ocular lesions in fetal syphilis, Bull Johns Hopkins Hosp 46:185, 1930.

99. Gahl WA and others: Cystine transport is defective in isolated leukocyte lysosomes from patients with cystinosis, Science 217:1263, 1982.

100. Ginsberg HS: Adenoviruses, Am J Clin Pathol 57:771, 1972.

101. Gorovoy MS: Intrastromal noninflammatory bacterial colonization of a corneal graft, Arch Ophthalmol 101(11), 1983.

102. Gottsch JD and others: Mooren's ulcer and evidence of stromal graft rejection after penetrating keratoplasty, Am J Ophthalmol 113:412, 1992.

103. Green WR and Zimmerman LE: Granulomatous reaction to Descemet's membrane, Am J Ophthalmol 64:555, 1967.

104. Groden LR, Pascucci SE, and Brinser JH: *Haemophilus aphrophilus* as a cause of crystalline keratopathy, Am J Ophthalmol 104:89, 1987.

105. Gupta K and others: Pseudomelanoma of the iris in herpes simplex keratoiritis, Ophthalmol 93:1524, 1986.

106. Guyer DR and others: Climatic droplet keratopathy, Surv Ophthalmol 36:241, 1992.

107. Haggerty TE and Zimmerman LE: Mycotic keratitis, South Med J 51:453, 1958.

108. Hedges TR III and Albert DM: The progression of the ocular abnormalities of herpes zoster: histopathologic observations of nine cases, Ophthalmology 89:165, 1982.

109. Hirst LW and others: *Nocardia asteroides* keratitis, Br J Ophthalmol 63:449, 1979.

110. Holbach LM and others: Herpes simplex stromal and endothelial keratitis. Granulomatous cell reactions at the level of Descemet's membrane, the stroma, and Bowman's layer, Ophthalmol 97:722, 1990.

111. Holbach LM and others: Recurrent herpes simplex keratitis with concurrent epithelial and stromal involvement, Arch Ophthalmol 109:692, 1991.

112. Hsu S-M and others: Russell bodies: a light and electron microscopic immunoperoxidase study, Am J Clin Pathol 77:26, 1982.

113. Hunter GW III, Frye WW, and Swartzwalder JC, editors: A manual of tropical medicine, ed 4, Philadelphia, 1966, WB Saunders Co.

114. Hunts JH and others: Infectious crystalline keratopathy: the role of bacterial exopolysaccharide, Arch Ophthalmol 111:1057, 1993.

115. Hutchinson J: A clinical memoir on certain diseases of the eye and ear, consequent on inherited syphilis, London, 1863, J Churchill.

116. Hykin PG and others: The natural history of recurrent corneal erosion: a prospective randomized trial, Eye 8:35, 1994.

117. Johns KJ, O'Day DM, and Feman SS: Chorioretinitis in the contralateral eye of a patient with *Acanthamoeba* keratitis, Ophthalmology 95:635, 1988.

118. Jones DB: Pathogenesis of bacterial and fungal keratitis, Trans Ophthalmol Soc UK 98:367, 1978.

119. Jones DB: *Acanthamoeba*-the ultimate opportunist? (editorial), Am J Ophthalmol 102:527, 1986.

120. Jones BR and others: Symposium on herpes simplex eye disease: objectives in therapy of herpetic eye disease, Trans Ophthalmol Soc UK 97:305, 1977.

121. Katz B and others: Recurrent crystal deposition after keratoplasty in nephropathic cystinosis, Am J Ophthalmol 104:190, 1987.

122. Kaufman HF, Centifanto-Fitzgerald YM, and Varnell ED: Herpes simplex keratitis, Ophthalmology 90:700, 1983.

123. Key SN III and others: Keratitis due to *Acanthamoeba castellani*: a clinicopathologic case report, Arch Ophthalmol 98:475, 1980.

124. Kincaid MC and Snip RC: Antibiotic resistance of crystalline bacterial ingrowth in a corneal graft, Ophthalmic Surg 18:268, 1987.

125. Kincaid MC and others: Infectious crystalline keratopathy after relaxing incisions, Am J Ophthalmol 111:374, 1991.

126. Krachmer JH and others: *Helminthosporium* corneal ulcers, Am J Ophthalmol 85:666, 1978.

127. Kuehl FA and Egan RW: Prostaglandins, arachidonic acid and inflammation, Science 210:978, 1980.

128. Laibson PR and others: Corneal infiltrates in epidemic keratoconjunctivitis, Arch Ophthalmol 84:36, 1970.

129. Lemp MA, Chambers RW, and Lundy J: Viral isolate in superficial punctate keratitis, Arch Ophthalmol 91:8, 1974.

130. Lichter PR and Schaffer RM: Interstitial keratitis and glaucoma, Am J Ophthalmol 68:241, 1969.

131. Liesegang TJ: Corneal complications from herpes zoster ophthalmicus, Ophthalmology 92:316, 1985.

132. Liesegang TJ: Biology and molecular aspects of herpes simplex and varicella-zoster virus.

133. Lindquist TD, Sher NA, and Doughman DJ: Clinical signs and medical therapy of early *Acanthamoeba* keratitis, Arch Ophthalmol 106: 73, 1988.

134. Lopez JS and others: Immunohistochemistry of Terrien's and Mooren's corneal degeneration, Arch Ophthalmol 109:988, 1991.

135. Lubniewski and others: Posterior infectious crystalline keratopathy with Staphylococcus epidermidis, Ophthalmology 97:1454, 1990.

136. Lund OE and Stefani FH: Corneal histology after epidemic keratoconjunctivitis, Arch Ophthalmol 96:2085, 1978.

137. Lund OE, Stefani FH, and Dechant W: Amoebic keratitis: a clinicopathological case report, Br J Ophthalmol 62:373, 1978.

138. Maguire LJ and others: Corneal topography of pellucid marginal degeneration, Ophthalmology 94:519, 1987.

139. Mannis MJ and others: *Acanthamoeba* sclerokeratitis: determining diagnostic criteria, Arch Ophthalmol 104:1313, 1986.

140. Marines HM and others: The value of calcofluor white in the diagnosis of mycotic and Acanthamoeba infections of the eye and ocular adnexa, Ophthalmology 94:23, 1987.

141. Martin RG and others: Herpes virus in sensory and autonomic ganglia after eye infection, Arch Ophthalmol 95:2053, 1977.

142. Mathers W and others: Immunopathology and electron microscopy of *Acanthamoeba* keratitis, Am J Ophthalmol 103:626, 1987.

143. Mathers WD and others: Outbreak of keratitis presumed to be caused by Acanthamoeba, Am J Ophthalmol 121:129, 1996.

144. Matoba AY, Wilhelmus KR, and Jones DB: Epstein-Barr viral stromal keratitis, Ophthalmology 93:746, 1986.

145. Matoba AY and others: Infectious crystalline keratopathy due to Streptococcus pneumoniae: possible association with serotype, Ophthalmology 101:1000, 1994.

146. Maudgal PC and Missotten L: Histopathology of human superficial herpes simplex keratitis, Br J Ophthalmol 62:46, 1978.

147. McDonnell PJ and others: Characterization of infectious crystalline keratitis caused by a human isolate of Streptococcus mitis, Arch Ophthalmol 109:1147, 1991.

148. Meisler DM and others: Infectious corneal crystalline formation, ARVO Abstracts, Suppl Invest Ophthalmol Vis Sci, Philadelphia, 1984, JB Lippincott.

149. Meisler DM and others: Infectious crystalline keratopathy, Am J Ophthalmol 97:337, 1984.

150. Meyers-Elliott RH, Pettit TH, and Maxwell WA: Viral antigens in the immune ring of herpes simplex stromal keratitis, Arch Ophthalmol 98:897, 1980.

151. Mondino BJ: Inflammatory diseases of the peripheral cornea, Ophthalmology 95:463, 1988.

152. Mondino BJ and others: Cellular immunity in Mooren's ulcer, Am J Ophthalmol 85:788, 1978.

153. Mondino BJ and others: Peripheral corneal ulcers with herpes zoster ophthalmicus, Am J Ophthalmol 86:611, 1978.

154. Moore MB, Newton C, and Kaufman HE: Chronic keratitis caused by *Mycobacterium gordonae*, Am J Ophthalmol 102:516, 1986.

155. Moore MB and others: *Acanthamoeba* keratitis associated with soft contact lenses, Am J Ophthalmol 100:396, 1985.

156. Moore MB and others: Radial keratoneuritis as a presenting sign in *Acanthamoeba* keratitis, Ophthalmology 93:1310, 1986.

157. Moore MB and others: *Acanthamoeba* keratitis: a growing problem in soft and hard contact lens wearers, Ophthalmology 94:1654, 1987.

158. Nagy RM and others: Scanning electron microscope study of herpes simplex virus experimental disciform keratitis, Br J Ophthalmol 62: 838, 1978.

159. Nanda M and others: Intracorneal bacterial colonization in a crystalline pattern, Graefes Arch Clin Exp Ophthalmol 224:251, 1986.

160. Naumann G, Gass JDM, and Font RL: Histopathology of herpes zoster ophthalmicus, Am J Ophthalmol 65:533, 1968.

161. Naumann G, Green WR, and Zimmerman LE: Mycotic keratitis, Am J Ophthalmol 64:668, 1967.

162. O'Brien TP and others: Efficacy of ofloxacin vs cefazolin and tobramycin in the therapy for bacterial keratitis—report from the bacterial keratitis study research group, Arch Ophthalmol 113:1257, 1995.

163. Ohl J, editor: Herpes virus infections, Surv Ophthalmol 1:81, 1976. (Special symposium issue.)

164. Ormerod LD and others: Microbial keratitis in children, Ophthalmology 93:449, 1986.

165. Ormerod LD and others: Infectious crystalline keratopathy, Ophthalmology 98:159, 1991.

166. Ormerod LD and others: Paraprotein crystalline keratopathy, Ophthalmology 95:202, 1988.

167. Patterson A: Interstitial keratitis, Br J Ophthalmol 50:612, 1966.

168. Pavan-Langston D and Hettinger ME: Ocular herpes: an update, Ann Ophthalmol 13:1213, 1981.

169. Pavan-Langston D and McCulley JP: Herpes zoster dendritic keratitis, Arch Ophthalmol 89:25, 1973.

170. Perry HD and others: Decreased corneal sensation as an initial feature of Acanthamoeba keratitis, Ophthalmology 102:1565, 1995.

171. Pettit TH and Holland GN: Chronic keratoconjunctivitis associated with ocular adenovirus infection, Am J Ophthalmol 88:748, 1979.

172. Peyman GA and others: Intraocular injections of gentamicin: toxic effects and clearance, Arch Ophthalmol 92:42, 1974.

173. Pfister DR and others: Confocal microscopy findings of Acanthamoeba keratitis, Am J Ophthalmol 121:119, 1996.

174. Pineros O and others: Long-term results after penetrating keratoplasty for Fuchs' endothelial dystrophy, Arch Ophthalmol 114:15, 1996.

175. Prebenga LW and Laibson PR: Dendritic lesions in herpes zoster ophthalmicus, Arch Ophthalmol 90:268, 1973.

176. Raber IM: *Pseudomonas* corneoscleral ulcers, Am J Ophthalmol 92: 353, 1981.

177. Raman SBK, van Slyck EJ: Nature of intracytoplasmic crystalline inclusions in myeloma cells (morphologic, cytochemical, ultrastructural, and immunofluorescent studies), Am J Clin Pathol 80:224, 1983.

178. Rao GN and others: Pseudophakic bullous keratopathy: relationship to preoperative corneal endothelial status, Ophthalmology 91:1135, 1984.

179. Rao NA and others: Basic principles. In Rao N, Forster DJ, and Augsburger JJ, editors: The Uvea, vol 2. In Podos SM and Yanoff M, editors: Textbook of Ophthalmology, New York, 1992, Gower Medical Publishing.

180. Rao NA and others: Chalcosis in the human eye: a clinicopathologic study, Arch Ophthalmol 94:1379, 1976.

181. Rennie AGR and others: Ocular vaccinia, Lancet 2:273, 1974.

182. Robin JB, Chan R, and Anderson BR: Rapid visualization of *Acanthamoeba* using fluorescein-conjugated lectins, Arch Ophthalmol 106:1273, 1988.

183. Reiss GR, Campbell RJ, and Bourne WM: Infectious crystalline keratopathy, Surv Ophthalmol 31:69, 1986.

184. Richler M and others: Ocular manifestation of nephropathic cystinosis, cystinosis, Arch Ophthalmol 109:359, 1991.

185. Robin JB and others: Peripheral corneal disorders, Surv Ophthalmol 31:1, 1986.

186. Robinson RCV: Congenital syphilis, Arch Dermatol 99:399, 1969.

187. Roitt IM and others: Immunology, ed 2, London, 1989, Gower Medical Publishing.

188. Rosenthal AR and others: Chalcosis: a study of natural history, Ophthalmology 86:1956, 1979.

189. Russell RG and others: Role of T-lymphocytes in the pathogenesis of herpetic stromal keratitis, Invest Ophthalmol Vis Sci 25:938, 1984.

190. Samples JR, Baumgartner SD, and Binder PS: Infectious crystalline keratopathy: an electron microscope analysis, Cornea 4:118, 1985-1986.

191. Schwartz JN, Donnelly EH, and Klintworth GK: Ocular and orbital phycomycosis, Surv Ophthalmol 22:2, 1977.

192. Sharma S and others: Acanthamoeba keratitis in noncontact lens wearers, Arch Ophthalmol 108:676, 1990.

193. Silvany RE, Luckenbach MW, and Moore MB: The rapid detection of *Acanthamoeba* in paraffin-embedded sections of corneal tissue with calcofluor white, Arch Ophthalmol 105:1366, 1987.

194. Smith JI: The current status of ocular syphilis, Surv Ophthalmol 14: 176, 1969.

195. Soong HK and others: Corneal hydrops in Terrien's marginal degeneration, Ophthalmology 93:340, 1986.

196. Stehr-Green JK, Bailey TM, and Visvesvara GS: The epidemiology of *Acanthamoeba* keratitis in the United States, Am J Ophthalmol 107:331, 1989.

197. Tabbara KF and others: Thygeson's superficial punctate keratitis, Ophthalmology 88:74, 1981.

198. Terrien F: Dystrophie marginale symjetrique des deux cornjes avec astigmatisme rjgulier consjcutif et fujrique par la cautjrisation ignje, Arch Ophthalmol (Paris) 20:12, 1900.

199. Theodore KH and others: The diagnostic value of a ring infiltrate in Acanthamoebic keratitis, Ophthalmology 92:1471, 1985.

200. Thomas MA and others: Rebleeding after traumatic hyphema, Arch Ophthalmol 104:206, 1986.

201. Thygeson P: Superficial punctate keratitis, JAMA 144:1544, 1950.

202. Tripathi RC, Bron AJ: Ultrastructural study of nontraumatic recurrent corneal erosion, JAMA 144:1544, 1950.

203. Trocme SD, Aldave AJ: The eye and the eosinophil, Surv Ophthalmol 39:241, 1994.

204. Uchida Y, Kaneko M, and Hayashi K: Varicella dendritic keratitis, Am J Ophthalmol 89:259, 1980.

205. Uusitalo R and others: Management of traumatic hyphema in children, Arch Ophthalmol 106:1207-1209, 1988.

206. Waring GO and others: Alterations of Descemet's membrane in interstitial keratitis, Am J Ophthalmol 81:773, 1976.

207. Welsenthal RW and others: Postkeratoplasty crystalline deposits mimicking bacterial infectious crystalline keratopathy, Am J Ophthalmol 105:70, 1988.

208. Weskamp C: Histopathology of interstitial keratitis due to congenital syphilis, Am J Ophthalmol 32:793, 1949.

209. Wilhelmus KR and others: Rapid diagnosis of *Acanthamoeba* keratitis using calcofluor white, Arch Ophthalmol 104:1309, 1986.

210. Wilhelmus KR, Robinson NM: Infectious crystalline keratopathy caused by Candida albicans, Am J Ophthalmol 112:322, 1991.

211. Williams GT, Willaims WJ: Granulomatous inflammation—a review, J Clin Pathol 85:160, 1983.

212. Wolken SH: Acute hemorrhagic conjunctivitis, Surv Ophthalmol 19:71, 1974.

213. Wolter JR and others: Acquired autosensitivity to degenerating Descemet's membrane in a case with anterior uveitis in the other eye, Am J Ophthalmol 72:782, 1971.

214. Wood TO and Kaufman HE: Mooren's ulcer, Am J Ophthalmol 71:417, 1971.

215. Wood WJ and Nicholson DH: Corneal ring ulcer as the presenting manifestation of acute monocytic leukemia, Am J Ophthalmol 76:69, 1973.

216. Yanoff M and Perry HD: Juvenile xanthogranuloma of the corneoscleral limbus, Arch Ophthalmol 113:915, 1995.

217. Yassa NH and others: Corneal immunoglobulin deposition in the posterior stroma: a case report including immunohistochemical and ultrastructural observations, Arch Ophthalmol 105:99, 1987.

218. Young RD and Watson PG: Light and electron microscopy of corneal melting syndrome (Mooren's ulcer), Br J Ophthalmol 66:341, 1982.

219. Zaidman GW and others: The histopathology of filamentary keratitis, Arch Ophthalmol 103:1178, 1985.

220. Zimmerman LE: Keratomycosis, Surv Ophthalmol 8:1, 1963.

Degenerations

221. Adamis AP and others: Anterior corneal disease of epidermolysis bullosa simplex, Arch Ophthalmol 111:499, 1993.

222. Allen TD: On the pathology of bullous keratitis, Trans Am Ophthalmol Soc 30:391, 1932.

223. Barchiesi BJ and others: The cornea and disorders of lipid metabolism, Surv Ophthalmol 36:1, 1991.

224. Barchlesi BJ and others: The cornea and disorders of lipid metabolism [published erratum appears in Surv Ophthalmol 1992 Jan-Feb; 36(4): 324]. [review] Surv Ophthalmol 36:1, 1991.

225. Barraquer-Somers E, Chan CC, and Green WR: Corneal epithelial iron deposition, Ophthalmology 90:729, 1983.

226. Baum JL and Rao G: Keratomalacia in the cachectic hospitalized patient, Am J Ophthalmol 82:435, 1976.

227. Binder PS, Deg JK, and Kohl FS: Calcific band keratopathy after intraocular chondroitin sulfate, Arch Ophthalmol 105:1243, 1987.

228. Bloomfield SE, Jakobiec FA, and Iwamoto T: Fibrous ingrowth with retrocorneal membrane, Ophthalmology 88:459, 1981.

229. Brooks HL Jr and others: Xerophthalmia and cystic fibrosis, Arch Ophthalmol 108:354, 1990.

230. Brown N and Bron A: Recurrent erosion of the cornea, Br J Ophthalmol 60:84, 1976.

231. Brown SI: Peripheral corneal edema after cataract extraction, Am J Ophthalmol 70:326, 1970.

232. Chan WK and Weissman BA: Corneal pannus associated with contact lens wear, Am J Ophthalmol 121:540, 1996.

233. Chuck RS and others: Recurrent corneal ulcerations associated with smokeable methamphetamine abuse, Am J Ophthalmol 121:571, 1996.

234. Chynn EW and others: Acanthamoeba keratitis—contact lens and noncontact lens characteristics, Ophthalmology 102:1369, 1995.

235. Cibis GW and others: Corneal keloid in Lowe's syndrome, Arch Ophthalmol 100:1795, 1982.

236. Cogan DG, Albright F, and Bartler FC: Hypercalcemia and band keratopathy: report of nineteen cases, Arch Ophthalmol 40:624, 1948.

237. Cogan DG and Kuwabara T: Lipid keratopathy and atheroma, Circulation 18:519, 1958.

238. Cogan DG and Kuwabara T: Arcus senilis: its pathology and histochemistry, Arch Ophthalmol 61:353, 1959.

239. Crowell D and Jakobiec FA: Hemorrhagic corneal pannus simulating a spontaneous expulsive hemorrhage, Ophthalmology 88:693, 1981.

240. Croxatto JO, Dodds CM, and Dodds R: Bilateral and massive lipoidal infiltration of the cornea (secondary lipoidal degeneration), Ophthalmology 92:1686, 1985.

241. Curslno JW and Fine BS: A histologic study of calcific and noncalcific band keratopathies, Am J Ophthalmol 82:395, 1976.

242. Daversa G and others: Diagnosis and successful medical treatment of acanthamoeba keratitis, Arch Ophthalmol 113:1120, 1995.

243. Delaney WV Jr: Presumed ocular chalcosis: a reversible maculopathy, Ann Ophthalmol 7:378, 1975.

244. Dutt S and others: Secondary localized amyloidosis in interstitial keratitis, Ophthalmol 99:817, 1992.

245. Eagle RC and Yanoff M: Cholesterolosis of the anterior chamber, Graefes Arch Ophthalmol 193:121, 1975.

246. Eagle RC and Yanoff M: Anterior chambr cholesterolosis, Arch Ophthalmol 108, 1990.

247. Fine BS, Berkow JW, and Fine S: Corneal calcification, Science 162:129, 1968.

248. Fine BS and others: Primary lipoidal degeneration of the cornea, Am J Ophthalmol 78:12, 1974.

249. Font RL, Yanoff M, and Zimmerman LE: Benign lymphoepithelial lesion of the lacrimal gland and its relationship to Sjogren's syndrome, Am J Clin Pathol 48:365, 1967.

250. Fraunfelder FT and others: Corneal mucus plaques, Am J Ophthalmol 83:191, 1977.

251. Freddo TF and Leibowitz HM: Bilateral acute corneal calcification, Ophthalmology 92:537, 1985.

252. Hida T and others: Familial band-shaped spheroid degeneration of the cornea, Am J Ophthalmol 97:651, 1984.

253. Hidayat AA and Risco J: Amyloidosis of cornea stroma in patients with trachoma, Ophthalmology 96:1203, 1989.

254. Hyndiuk RA and others: Neurotropic corneal ulcers in diabetes mellitus, Arch Ophthalmol 95:2193, 1977.

255. Jakobiec FA: I want to say one word to you . . . plastics (editorial), Ophthalmology 90(4):29A, 1983.

256. Johnson DH, Bourne WM, and Campbell RJ: The ultrastructure of Descemet's membrane. I. Changes with age in normal corneas, Arch Ophthalmol 100:1942, 1982.

257. Johnson DH, Bourne WM, and Campbell RJ: The ultrastructure of Descemet's membrane. II. Aphakic bullous keratopathy, Arch Ophthalmol 100:1948, 1982.

258. Johnson GJ and Overall M: Histology of spheroidal degeneration of the cornea in Labrador, Br J Ophthalmol 62:53, 1978.

259. Kampik A, Patrinely JR, and Green WR: Morphologic and clinical feature of retrocorneal melanin pigmentation and pigmented pupillary membranes: a review of 225 cases, Surv Ophthalmol 27:161, 1982.

260. Karal A, Mustakallio AH, and Kaufman H: Electron microscopic studies of corneal endothelium: the abnormal endothelium associated with retrocorneal membrane, Ann Ophthalmol 4:564, 1972.

261. Kennedy RE and others: Further observations on atypical band keratopathy in glaucoma patients, Trans Am Ophthalmol Soc 72:107, 1974.

262. Klintworth GK, Bredchoeft SJ, and Reed JW: Analysis of corneal crystalline deposits in multiple myeloma, Am J Ophthalmol 86:303, 1978.

263. Krachmer JH, Schnitzer JI, and Fratkin J: Cornea pseudoguttata: a

clinical and histopathologic description of endothelial cell edema, Arch Ophthalmol 99:1377, 1981.

264. Krachmer JH and others: Corneal posterior crocodile shagreen and polymorphic amyloid degeneration: a histopathologic study, Arch Ophthalmol 101:54, 1983.

265. Kremer I, Ingber A, and Ben-Sira I: Corneal metastatic calcification in Werner's syndrome, Am J Ophthalmol 106:221, 1988.

266. Levine RA and Rabb MF: Bitot's spot overlying a pinguecula, Arch Ophthalmol 86:525, 1971.

267. Lloyd-Jones D and Hembry RM: Destructive corneal disease in the connective tissue disorders: comparison with an experimental model, Trans Ophthalmol Soc UK 98:383, 1978.

268. Mannis MJ and others: Polymorphic amyloid degeneration of the cornea: a clinical and histopathologic study, Arch Ophthalmol 99:1217, 1981.

269. McDonnell PJ and others: Blood staining of the cornea: light microscopic and ultrastructural features, Ophthalmology 92:1668, 1985.

270. Meisler DM and others: Familial band-shaped nodular keratopathy, Ophthalmology 92:217, 1985.

271. Michels RG, Kenyon KR, and Maumenee AE: Retrocorneal fibrous membrane, Invest Ophthalmol 11:822, 1972.

272. O'Connor GR: Calcific band keratopathy, Trans Am Ophthalmol Soc 70:58, 1972.

273. O'Grady RB and Kirk HQ: Corneal keloids, Am J Ophthalmol 73:206, 1972.

274. Porter R and Crombie AL: Corneal and conjunctival calcification in chronic renal failure, Br J Ophthalmol 57:339, 1973.

275. Porter R and Crombie AL: Corneal calcification as a presenting and diagnostic sign in hyperparathyroidism, Br J Ophthalmol 57:665, 1973.

276. Ramsey MS and others: Localized corneal amyloidosis: case report with electron microscopic observations, Am J Ophthalmol 73:560, 1972.

277. Savino DF and others: Primary lipidic degeneration of the cornea, Cornea 5:191, 1986.

278. Schanzlin DJ and others: Histopathologic and ultrastructural analysis of congenital corneal staphyloma, Am J Ophthalmol 95:506, 1983.

279. Severine M, Kirchhof B: Recurrent Salzmann's corneal degeneration, Graefes Arch Clin Exp Ophthalmol 228:101, 1990.

280. Shapiro LA and Farkas TC: Lipid keratopathy following corneal hydrops, Arch Ophthalmol 95:456, 1977.

281. Silbert AM and Baum JL: Origin of retrocorneal membrane in the rabbit, Arch Ophthalmol 97:1141, 1979.

282. Singh D and Singh M: Climatic keratopathy, Trans Ophthalmol Soc UK 98:10, 1978.

283. Snif RC and others: Posterior corneal pigmentation and fibrous proliferation by iris melanocytes, Arch Ophthalmol 99:1232, 1981.

284. Snif RC, Kenyon KR, and Green WR: Retrocorneal fibrous membrane in the vitreous touch syndrome, Am J Ophthalmol 79:233, 1975.

285. Sommer A: Effects of vitamin A deficiency on the ocular surface, Ophthalmology 90:592, 1983.

286. Sommer A: Xerophthalmia, keratomalacia and nutritional blindness, Int Ophthalmol 14:195, 1990.

287. Sommer A and others: Clinical characteristics of vitamin A responsive and nonresponsive Bitot's spots, Am J Ophthalmol 90:160, 1980.

288. Sommer A, Green WR, and Kenyon KR: Bitot's spots responsive and nonresponsive to vitamin A: clinicopathologic correlations, Arch Ophthalmol 99:2014, 1981.

289. Sommer A, Green WR, and Kenyon KR: Clinicohistopathologic correlations in xerophthalmic ulceration and necrosis, Arch Ophthalmol 100:953, 1982.

290. Sommer A and Sugana T: Corneal xerophthalmia and keratomalacia, Arch Ophthalmol 100:404, 1982.

291. Soong HK and Quigley HA: Dellen associated with filtering blebs, Arch Ophthalmol 102:139, 1995.

292. Suan EP and others: Corneal perforation in patients with vitamin A deficiency in the United States, Arch Ophthalmol 108:350, 1990.

293. Sutton DF and others: Retrocorneal smooth-muscle proliferation on rejected corneal graft, Arch Ophthalmol 101:429, 1983.

294. Swan KC, Meyer SL, and Lyman J: Retrocorneal pigment proliferation after cataract extraction, Ophthalmology 86:732, 1979.

295. Vannas A, Hogan MJ, and Wood I: Salzmann's nodular degeneration of the cornea, Am J Ophthalmol 79:211, 1975.

296. Walsh FB and Howard JE: Conjunctival and corneal lesions in hypercalcemia, J Clin Endocrinol Metab 7:644, 1947.

297. Waring G, Laibson P, and Rodrigues M: Clinical and pathologic alterations of Descemet's membrane, with emphasis on endothelial metaplasia, Surv Ophthalmol 18:325, 1974.

298. Waring GO III: The 50-year epidemic of pseudophakic corneal edema, Arch Ophthalmol 107:657, 1989.

299. Waring GO III and others: Results of penetrating keratoplasty in 123 eyes with pseudophakic or aphakic corneal edema, Ophthalmology 90:25, 1983.

300. Waring GO and others: Climatic proteoglycan stromal keratopathy, a new corneal degeneration, Am J Ophthalmol 120:330, 1995.

301. Weene LE: Recurrent corneal erosion after trauma: a statistical study, Ann Ophthalmol 17:521, 1985.

302. Weiss JS and others: Panstromal Schnyder's corneal dystrophy. Ultrastructural and histochemical studies, Ophthalmol 99:1972, 1992.

303. Wilhelmus KR and others: Corneal lipidosis in patients with the acquired immunodeficiency syndrome [see comments], Am J Ophthalmol 119:14, 1995.

304. Wilson SE and others: Edema of the corneal stroma induced by cold in trigeminal neuropathy, Am J Ophthalmol 107:52, 1989.

305. Wood TO and others: Recurrent erosion, Trans Am Ophthalmol Soc 82:850, 1984.

306. Zaidman GW and others: The histopathology of filamentary keratitis, Arch Ophthalmol 103:1178, 1985.

Pigmentations

307. Blodi F: Über einen Fall von querliegender Krukenbergscher Spindel, Acta Ophthalmol 26:374, 1948.

308. Broderick JD: Corneal blood staining after hyphaema, Br J Ophthalmol 56:589, 1972.

309. Cairns JE, Williams HP, and Walshe JM: Sunflower cataract in Wilson's disease, Br Med J 3:95, 1969.

310. Cartwright GE: Diagnosis of treatable Wilson's disease, N Engl J Med 298:1347, 1978.

311. Coles WH: Traumatic hyphema, South Med J 61:813, 1968.

312. Ferry AP: A "new" iron line of the superficial cornea: occurrence in patients with filtering blebs, Arch Ophthalmol 79:142, 1968.

313. Ferry AP and Zimmerman LE: Black cornea: a complication of topical use of epinephrine, Am J Ophthalmol 58:205, 1964.

314. Gass JDM: The iron lines of the superficial cornea, Arch Ophthalmol 71:348, 1964.

315. Goldberg MF and von Noorden GK: Ophthalmologic findings in Wilson's hepatolenticular degeneration, Arch Ophthalmol 75:162, 1966.

316. Hanna C, Fraunfelder FT, and Sanchez J: Ultrastructural study of argyrosis of the cornea and conjunctiva, Arch Ophthalmol 92:18, 1974.

317. Harry J and Tripathi R: Kayser-Fleischer ring: a pathological study, Br J Ophthalmol 54:794, 1970.

318. Iwamoto T: Electron microscopical study of the Fleischer ring, Arch Ophthalmol 94:1579, 1976.

319. Johnson BL: Ultrastructure of the Kayser-Fleischer ring, Am J Ophthalmol 76:455, 1973.

320. Johnson RE and Campbell RJ: Wilson's disease: electron microscopic, x-ray energy spectroscopic, and atomic absorption spectroscopic studies of corneal copper deposition and distribution, Lab Invest 46:564, 1982.

321. Kampik A, Sani JN, and Green WR: Ocular ochronosis: clinicopathological, histochemical, and ultrastructural studies, Arch Ophthalmol 98:1441, 1980.

322. Kashani AA: Ocular manifestations of Wilson's disease in Iran, Trans Ophthalmol Soc UK 97:18, 1977.

323. Madge GE, Geeraets WJ, and Guerry DP: Black cornea secondary to topical epinephrine, Am J Ophthalmol 71:402, 1971.

324. Martin NF and others: Ocular copper deposition associated with pulmonary carcinoma, IgG monoclonal gammopathy and hyperenpremia: a clinicopathological correlation, Ophthalmology 90:110, 1983.

325. McCormick SA and others: Ocular chrysiasis, Ophthalmology 92:1432, 1985.

326. McDonnell PJ and others: Blood staining of the cornea: light microscopic and ultrastructural features, Ophthalmology 92:1668, 1985.

327. Mitchell AM and Heller GL: Changes in Kayser-Fleischer ring dur-

ing treatment of hepatolenticular degeneration, Arch Ophthalmol 80:622, 1968.

328. Rakusin W: Traumatic hyphema, Am J Ophthalmol 74:285, 1972.

329. Read J and Goldberg MF: Comparison of medical treatment for traumatic hyphema, Trans Am Acad Ophthalmol Otolaryngol 78: OP 799, 1974.

330. Reinecke RD and Kuwabara T: Corneal deposits secondary to topical epinephrine, Arch Ophthalmol 70:170, 1963.

331. Rifkind BM: Corneal arcus and hyperlipoproteinaemia, Surv Ophthalmol 16:295, 1972.

332. Searl SS and others: Corneal hematoma, Arch Ophthalmol 102: 1647, 1984.

333. Steinberg EB and others: Stellate iron lines in the corneal epithelium after radial keratotomy, Am J Ophthalmol 98:416, 1984.

334. Sternlieb I: The Kayser-Fleischer ring, Med Radiogr Photogr 42: 14, 1966.

335. Sussman W and Scheinberg IH: Disappearance of Kayser-Fleischer rings: effects of penicillamine, Arch Ophthalmol 82:738, 1963.

336. Tawara A: Transformation and cytotoxicity of iron in siderosis bulbi, Invest Ophthalmol Vis Sci 27:226, 1985.

337. Tesluk GC and Spaeth GL: The occurrence of primary open-angle glaucoma in the fellow eye of patients with unilateral angle-cleavage glaucoma, Ophthalmol 92:904, 1986.

338. Tonjum AM and Thylefors B: Aspects of corneal changes in onchocerciasis, Br J Ophthalmol 62:458, 1978.

339. Tso MOM, Fine BS, and Thorpe HE: Kayser-Fleischer ring and associated cataract in Wilson's disease, Am J Ophthalmol 79:479, 1975.

340. Walshe JM: Wilson's disease: its diagnosis and management, Br J Hosp Med 4:91, 1970.

341. Wilson SAK: Progressive lenticular degeneration: a familial nervous disease associated with cirrhosis of the liver, Brain 34:295, 1912.

342. Yanoff M and Scheie HG: Argyrosis of the conjunctiva and lacrimal sac, Arch Ophthalmol 72:57, 1964.

Abnormalities in size and shape

343. Beardsley TL and Foulks GN: An association of keratoconus and mitral valve prolapse, Ophthalmology 89:35, 1982.

344. Berney A and others: Bilateral, congenital, dermis-like choristomas overlying corneal staphylomas, Arch Ophthalmol 99:1995, 1981.

345. Biglan AW, Brown SI, and Johnson BL: Keratoglobus and blue sclera, Am J Ophthalmol 83:225, 1977.

346. Chi HH, Katzin HM, and Teng CC: Histopathology of keratoconus, Am J Ophthalmol 42:847, 1956.

347. François J, Hanssens M, and Stockmans L: Dégénérescence marginale pellucide de la cornée, Ophthalmologica 155:337, 1968.

348. Hyams SW and Neuman E: Congenital microcornea and combined mechanism glaucoma, Am J Ophthalmol 68:326, 1969.

349. Ihalainen A: Clinical and epidemiological features of keratoconus. Genetic and external factors in the pathogenesis of the disease, Acta Ophthalmol 64:5, 1986.

350. Ingraham HJ and others: Keratoconus with spontaneous perforation of the cornea, Arch Ophthalmol 109:1651, 1991.

351. Iwamoto T, DeVoe AG: Electron microscopical study of the Fleischer ring, Arch Ophthalmol 94:1579, 1976.

352. Kanai A and others: The fine structure of sclerocornea, Invest Ophthalmol 10:687, 1971.

353. Kayazawa F and others: Keratoconus with pellucid marginal corneal degeneration, Arch Ophthalmol 102:895, 1984.

354. Kennedy RH and others: A 48-year study clinical and epidemiologic study of keratoconus, Am J Ophthalmol 101:267, 1986.

355. Krachmer JH, Feder RS, and Belin MW: Keratoconus and related noninflammatory corneal thinning disorders, Surv Ophthalmol 28: 293, 1984.

356. Krachmer JH, Feder RS, and Belin MW: Keratoconus and related noninflammatory corneal thinning disorders (review), Surv Ophthalmol 28:293, 1984.

357. Krachmer JH: Pellucid marginal corneal degeneration, Arch Ophthalmol 96:1217, 1978.

358. Krachmer JH and Rodrigues MM: Posterior keratoconus, Arch Ophthalmol 96:1867, 1978.

359. Larson V and Eriksen A: Cornea plana, Acta Ophthalmol 27:295, 1949.

360. Lee C-F and others: Immunohistochemical studies of Peters' anomaly, Ophthalmology 96:958, 1989.

361. Lipman RM and others: Keratoconus and Fuchs'' corneal endothelial dystrophy in a patient and her family, Arch Ophthalmol 108: 993, 1990.

362. Nauheim JS and Perry HD: A clinicopathologic study of contact lens-related keratoconus, Am J Ophthalmol 100:543, 1985.

363. Perry HD and others: Round and oval cones in keratoconus, Ophthalmology 87:905, 1980.

364. Polack FM and Grave EL: Scanning electron microscopy of congenital corneal leukomas (Peters' anomaly), Am J Ophthalmol 88:169, 1979.

365. Pouliquen Y and others: Degenerscence pellucide marginale de la corne ou keratocone marginal, J Fr Ophthalmol 3:109, 1980.

366. Rodrigues MM, Calhoun J, and Weinreb S: Sclerocornea with an unbalanced translocation, Am J Ophthalmol 78:49, 1974.

367. Sawaguchi S and others: Lysosomal enzyme abnormalities in keratoconus, Arch Ophthalmol 107:1507, 1989.

368. Shapiro MB and others: Anterior clear spaces in keratoconus, Ophthalmology 93:1316, 1986.

369. Stone DL and others: Ultrastructure of keratoconus with healed hydrops, Am J Ophthalmol 82:450, 1976.

370. Topilow HW and others: Bilateral corneal dermis-like choristomas: an X chromosome-linked disorder, Arch Ophthalmol 99:1387, 1981.

371. Townsend WM: Congenital cornea leukomas. I. Central defect in Descemet's membrane, Am J Ophthalmol 77:80, 1974.

372. Tuft SJ and others: Acute corneal hydrops in keratoconus, Ophthalmology 101:1738, 1994.

373. Tuft SJ and others: Prognosis factors for the progression of keratoconus, Ophthalmology 101:439, 1994.

374. Vail DT: Adult hereditary anterior megalophthalmus sine glaucoma: a definite disease entity, Arch Ophthalmol 6:39, 1931.

375. Waring GO and Rodrigues MM: Ultrastructure and successful keratoplasty of sclerocornea in Mieten's syndrome, Am J Ophthalmol 90:469, 1980.

376. Yanoff M: Discussion of Perry HD et al: Round and oval cones in keratoconus, Ophthalmology 87:909, 1980.

Dystrophies

377. Abbott RL and others: Specular microscopic and histologic observations in nonguttate corneal endothelial degeneration, Ophthalmology 88:788, 1981.

378. Adamis AP and others: Fuchs' endothelial dystrophy of the cornea. (review), Surv Ophthalmol 38:149, 1993.

379. Akiya S and Brown SI: Granular dystrophy of the cornea, Arch Ophthalmol 84:179, 1970.

380. Akiya S and Brown SI: The ultrastructure of Reis-Bücklers' dystrophy, Am J Ophthalmol 72:549, 1971.

381. Alexander RA, Grierson I, and Garner A: Oxytalan fibers in Fuchs'' endothelial dystrophy, Arch Ophthalmol 99:1622, 1981.

382. Alkemade PPH and Van Balen ATM: Hereditary epithelial dystrophy of the cornea, Mecsmann type, Br J Ophthalmol 50:603, 1966.

383. Apple DJ and others: Congenital corneal opacification secondary to Bowman's layer dysgenesis, Am J Ophthalmol 98:320, 1984.

384. Bahn CF and others: Classification of corneal endothelial disorders based on neural crest origin, Ophthalmology 91:558, 1984.

385. Boruchoff SA and Kuwabara T: Electron microscopy of posterior polymorphous degeneration, Am J Ophthalmol 72:879, 1971.

386. Bourne WM, Johnson DH, and Campbell RJ: The ultrastructure of Descemet's membrane. III. Fuchs'' dystrophy, Arch Ophthalmol 100:1952, 1982.

387. Broderick JD: Anterior membrane dystrophy following cataract extraction, Br J Ophthalmol 63:331, 1979.

388. Bron AJ and Tripathi RC: Cystic disorders of the corneal epithelium. I. Clinical aspects, Br J Ophthalmol 57:361, 1973.

389. Bron AJ and Tripathi RC: Corneal disorders. In Goldberg MJ, editor: Genetic and metabolic eye disease, Boston, 1974, Little, Brown & Co.

390. Brooks AMV and others: Differentiation of posterior polymorphous dystrophy from other posterior corneal opacities by specular microscopy, Ophthalmology 96:1639, 1989.

391. Brown N and Bron AJ: Recurrent erosion of the cornea, Br J Ophthalmol 60:84, 1976.

392. Brownstein S and others: Granular dystrophy of the cornea—light and electron microscopic confirmation of recurrence in a graft, Am J Ophthalmol 77:701, 1974.

393. Bücklers M: Die erblichen Hornhautdystrophien: Dystrophiae corneae hereditariae, Stuttgart, 1938, Ferdinand Enke.

394. Bücklers M: Ueber eine weitere familiare Hornhautdystrophie, Klin Monatsbl Augenheilkd 114:386, 1949.

395. Burns R: Meesmann's corneal dystrophy, Trans Am Ophthalmol Soc 66:530, 1968.

396. Burns RP and others: Cholesterol turnover in hereditary crystalline corneal dystrophy of Schnyder, Trans Am Ophthalmol Soc 76:184, 1978.

397. Burns RR and others: Endothelial function in patients with cornea guttata, Invest Ophthalmol 20:77, 1981.

398. Caldwell DR: Postoperative recurrence of Reis-Bücklers corneal dystrophy, Am J Ophthalmol 85:567, 1978.

399. Cameron JA: Keratoglobus, Cornea 12:124, 1993.

400. Campbell RJ and Bourne WM: Unilateral central corneal epithelial dysplasia, Ophthalmology 88:1231, 1981.

401. Carpel EF, Sigelman RJ, and Doughman DJ: Posterior amorphous corneal dystrophy, Am J Ophthalmol 83:629, 1977.

402. Chi HH, Teng CC, and Katzin HM: Histopathology of primary endothelial-epithelial dystrophy of the cornea, Am J Ophthalmol 45:518, 1958.

403. Cibis GW and others: The clinical spectrum of posterior polymorphous dystrophy, Arch Ophthalmol 95:1529, 1977.

404. Cibis GW, Tripathi RC: The differential diagnosis of Descemet's tears (Haab's striae) and posterior polymorphous dystrophy bands: a clinicopathologic study, Ophthalmology 89:614, 1982.

405. Cibis GW, Waeltermann J, and Harris DJ: Peters' anomaly in association with ring 21 chromosomal abnormality, Am J Ophthalmol 100:733, 1985.

406. Clark WB: Hereditary and constitutional dystrophies of the cornea, Am J Ophthalmol 33:692, 1950.

407. Cogan DG and others: Microcystic dystrophy of the corneal epithelium, Trans Am Ophthalmol Soc 62:213, 1964.

408. Cotlier E and Hughes WF: Enzymatic deficiency in macular corneal dystrophy (Groenouw II), Paper presented at the meeting of the Association for Research on Vision and Ophthalmology, Sarasota, Fla, April 1972.

409. Cross HE, Manmenee AE, and Cantolino SE: Inheritance of Fuchs'' endothelial dystrophy, Arch Ophthalmol 85:268, 1971.

410. Dangel ME, Bremer DL, and Rogers GL: Treatment of corneal opacification in mucolipidosis IV with conjunctival transplantation, Am J Ophthalmol 99:137, 1985.

411. Dark AJ: Bleb dystrophy of the cornea: histochemistry and ultrastructure, Br J Ophthalmol 61:65, 1977.

412. Dark AJ: Cogan's microcystic dystrophy of the cornea: ultrastructure and photomicroscopy, Br J Ophthalmol 62:821, 1978.

413. Doughman DJ: Ocular amyloidosis, Surv Ophthalmol 13:133, 1968.

414. Eagle RC and others: Epithelial abnormalities in chronic corneal edema: a histopathology study. Trans Am Ophthalmol 87:107, 1989.

415. Edward DP and others: Macular dystrophy of the cornea: a systemic disorder of keratan sulfate metabolism, Ophthalmology 97:1194, 1990.

416. Edward DP and others: Heterogeneity in macular corneal dystrophy, Arch Ophthalmol 106:1579, 1988.

417. Falls HL and others: Ocular manifestations of hereditary primary systemic amyloidosis, Arch Ophthalmol 54:660, 1955.

418. Feder RS and others: Subepithelial mucinous corneal dystrophy. Clinical and pathological correlations, Arch Ophthalmol 111:1106, 1993.

419. Fine BS and others: Meesmann's epithelial dystrophy of the cornea, Am J Ophthalmol 83:633, 977.

420. Fine BS and others: Primary lipoidal degeneration of the cornea, Am J Ophthalmol 78:12, 1974.

421. Fogle JA, Green WR, and Kenyon KR: Anterior corneal dystrophy, Am J Ophthalmol 77:529, 1974.

422. Fogle JA and others: Defective epithelial adhesion in anterior corneal dystrophies, Am J Ophthalmol 79:925, 1975.

423. Foldberg R and others: The relationship between granular, lattice type 1, and Avellino corneal dystrophies: a histopathologic study, Arch Ophthalmol 112:1080, 1994.

424. Foldberg R and others: Clinically atypical granular corneal dystrophy with pathologic features of lattice-like amyloid deposits: a study of three families, Ophthalmology 95:46, 1988.

425. Franceschetti A: Classification and treatment of hereditary corneal dystrophies, Arch Ophthalmol 52:1, 1954.

426. Franceschetti A and Babel J: The heredofamilial degenerations of the cornea, XVI Concil Ophthalmol 1:245, 1951.

427. Franceschetti A and Forni S: The heredofamilial degenerations of the cornea, XVI Concil Ophthalmol 1:193, 1950.

428. François J: Heredo-familial corneal dystrophies, Trans Ophthalmol Soc UK 86:367, 1966.

429. Fuchs' E: Dystrophia epithelialis cornea, Graefes Arch Ophthalmol 76:478, 1910.

430. Garner A: Histochemistry of corneal macular dystrophy, Invest Ophthalmol 8:475, 1969.

431. Garner A and Tripathi RC: Hereditary crystalline stromal dystrophy of Schnyder. II. Histopathology and ultrastructure, Br J Ophthalmol 56:400, 1972.

432. Gandhi SS, Lamberts DW, and Perry HD: Donor to host transmission of disease via corneal transplantation, Surv Ophthalmol 25:306, 1981.

433. Gasset AR and Zimmerman TJ: Posterior polymorphous dystrophy associated with keratoconus, Am J Ophthalmol 78:535, 1974.

434. Goar EL: Dystrophies of the cornea, Am J Ophthalmol 33:674, 1950.

435. Goldberg MF and others: Variable expression in flecked (speckled) dystrophy of the cornea, Ann Ophthalmol 9:889, 1977.

436. Grayson M and Wilbrandt H: Dystrophy of the anterior limiting membrane of the cornea (Reis-Bücklers' type), Am J Ophthalmol 61:345, 1966.

437. Griffith DG and Fine BS: Light and electron microscopic observations in a superficial corneal dystrophy, probably early Reis-Bücklers' type, Am J Ophthalmol 63:1659, 1967.

438. Guerry D III: Observations on Cogan's microcystic dystrophy of the corneal epithelium, Trans Am Ophthalmol Soc 63:320, 1965.

439. Guerry D III: Observations of Cogan's microcystic dystrophy of the corneal epithelium, Am J Ophthalmol 62:65, 1966.

440. Haddad R, Font RL, and Fine BS: Unusual superficial variant of granular dystrophy of the cornea, Am J Ophthalmol 83:213, 1977.

441. Henriquez AS and others: Morphologic characteristics of posterior polymorphous dystrophy: a study of nine corneas and review of the literature, Surv Ophthalmol 29:139, 1984.

442. Hida T, Proia AD, Kigasawa K, et al: Histopathologic and immunochemical features of lattice corneal dystrophy type III, Am J Ophthalmol 104:249, 1987.

443. Hida T, Tsubota K, Kigasawa K, et al: Avellino corneal dystrophy, Ophthalmology 99:1564, 1992.

444. Hida T and others: Clinical features of a newly recognized type of lattice corneal dystrophy, Am J Ophthalmol 104:241, 1987.

445. Hogan MJ and Bietti G: Hereditary deep dystrophy of the cornea (polymorphous), Am J Ophthalmol 68:777, 1969.

446. Hogan MJ and Wood I: Reis-Bücklers' corneal dystrophy, Trans Ophthalmol Soc UK 91:41, 1971.

447. Hogan MJ, Wood I, and Fine M: Fuchs'' endothelial dystrophy of the cornea, Am J Ophthalmol 78:363, 1974.

448. Holland EJ and others: Avellino corneal dystrophy, Ophthalmology 99:1564, 1992.

449. Hughes WF: The treatment of corneal dystrophies by keratoplasty, Am J Ophthalmol 50:1100, 1960.

450. Ingraham HJ and others: Progressive Schnyder's dystrophy, Ophthalmology 100:1824, 1993.

451. Iwamoto T and DeVoe AG: Electron microscopic studies of Fuchs'' combined dystrophy. I. Posterior portion of cornea, Invest Ophthalmol 10:9, 1971.

452. Iwamoto T and DeVoe AG: Electron microscopic studies of Fuchs'' combined dystrophy. II. Anterior portion of cornea, Invest Ophthalmol 10:29, 1971.

453. Johannsson JH and Jonasson F: Methenamine-silver staining in macular corneal dystrophy, Am J Ophthalmol 106:630, 1988.

454. Johnson AT and others: The pathology of posterior amorphous corneal dystrophy [see comments], Ophthalmol 97:104, 1990.

455. Johnson BL and Brown SI: Posterior polymorphous dystrophy: a light and electron microscopic study, Br J Ophthalmol 62:89, 1978.

456. Johnson BL, Brown SI, and Zaidman GW: A light and electron microscopy study of recurrent granular dystrophy of the cornea, Am J Ophthalmol 92:49, 1981.

457. Jones ST and Stauffer LK: Reis-Bücklers' corneal dystrophy: a clinicopathologic study, Trans Am Acad Ophthalmol Otolaryngol 74:417, 1970.

458. Jones ST and Zimmerman LE: Macular dystrophy of the cornea (Groenouw type II), Am J Ophthalmol 47:1, 1959.

459. Jones ST and Zimmerman LE: Histopathologic differentiation of granular, macular and lattice dystrophies of the cornea, Am J Ophthalmol 51:394, 1961.

460. Judisch GF and Maumenee IH: Clinical differentiation of recessive congenital hereditary endothelial dystrophy and dominant hereditary endothelial dystrophy, Am J Ophthalmol 85:606, 1978.

461. Kanai A and Kaufman HE: Further electron microscopic study of hereditary corneal edema, Invest Ophthalmol 10:545, 1971.

462. Kanai A, Kaufman HE, and Polack FM: Electron microscopic study of Reis-Bücklers' dystrophy, Ann Ophthalmol 5:953, 1973.

463. Kayes J and Holmberg A: The fine structure of the cornea in Fuchs'' endothelial dystrophy, Invest Ophthalmol 3:47, 1964.

464. Kenyon KR: Mesenchymal dysgenesis in Peter's anomaly, sclerocornea and congenital endothelial dystrophy, Exp Eye Res 21:125, 1975.

465. Kenyon KR and Antine B: The pathogenesis of congenital hereditary endothelial dystrophy of the cornea, Am J Ophthalmol 72:787, 1971.

466. Kenyon KR and Maumenee AE: The histological and ultrastructural pathology of congenital hereditary corneal dystrophy: case report, Invest Ophthalmol 7:475, 1968.

467. Kenyon KR and Maumenee AE: Further studies of congenital hereditary endothelial dystrophy of the cornea, Am J Ophthalmol 76:419, 1973.

468. King RG Jr and Geeraets R: Cogan-Guerry microcystic corneal epithelial dystrophy: a clinical and electron microscopic study, Med Col Va Q 8:241, 1972.

469. Kirk HQ and others: Primary familial amyloidosis of the cornea, Trans Am Acad Ophthalmol Otolaryngol 77:411, 1973.

470. Klintworth GK: Lattice corneal dystrophy: an inherited variety of amyloidosis restricted to the cornea, Am J Pathol 50:371, 1967.

471. Klintworth GK and others: Recurrence of lattice corneal dystrophy type 2 in the corneal grafts of two siblings, Am J Ophthalmol 94:540, 1982.

472. Klintworth GK and others: Recurrence of macular corneal dystrophy within grafts, Am J Ophthalmol 95:60, 1983.

473. Krachmer JH and others: Corneal posterior crocodile shagreen and polymorphic amyloid degeneration: a histopathologic study, Arch Ophthalmol 101:54, 1983.

474. Kuwabara T and Cicarelli EG: Meesmann's corneal dystrophy: a pathologic study, Arch Ophthalmol 71:676, 1964.

475. Lanier JD, Fine M, and Togni B: Lattice corneal dystrophy, Arch Ophthalmol 94:921, 1976.

476. Liakos GM and Casey TA: Posterior polymorphous keratopathy, Br J Ophthalmol 62:39, 1978.

477. Lipman RM and others: Keratoconus and Fuchs'' corneal endothelial dystrophy in a patient and her family, Arch Ophthalmol 108:993, 1990.

478. Lisch W: Primary hereditary band-shaped corneal dystrophy and its association with other hereditary corneal lesions, Klin Monatsbl Augenheilkd 169:717, 1976.

479. Lucarelli MH and Adamis AP: Avallino corneal dystrophy, Arch Ophthalmol 112:418, 1994.

480. MaGovern M and others: Inheritance of Fuchs'' combined dystrophy, Ophthalmology 86:1897, 1979.

481. Malbran ES: Corneal dystrophies: a clinical, pathological, and surgical approach, Trans Am Acad Ophthalmol Otolaryngol 76:573, 1972.

482. Mandell RB and others: Corneal hydration control in Fuchs'' combined dystrophy, Invest Ophthalmol Vis Sci 30:845, 1989.

483. Maumenee AE: Congenital hereditary corneal dystrophy, Am J Ophthalmol 50:114, 1960.

484. McCarthy M and others: Panstromal Schnyder corneal dystrophy. A clinical pathologic report with quantitative analysis of corneal lipid composition, Ophthalmology 101:895, 1994.

485. McPherson SD Jr, Kiffney GT Jr, and Freed CC: Corneal amyloidosis, Trans Am Ophthalmol Soc 64:148, 1966.

486. McTigue JW: The human cornea: a light and electron microscopic study of the normal cornea and its alterations in various dystrophies, Trans Am Ophthalmol Soc 65:591, 1967.

487. McTigue JW and Fine BS: The stromal lesion in lattice dystrophy of the cornea, Invest Ophthalmol 3:355, 1964.

488. Meesmann A and Wilke F: Klinische und anatomische Untersuchungen über eine bisher unbekannte, dominant vererbte Epitheldystrophie der Hornhaut, Klin Monatsbl Augenheilkd 103:361, 1939.

489. Mehta RF: Unilateral lattice dystrophy of the cornea, Br J Ophthalmol 64:53, 1980.

490. Meisler DM and Fine M: Recurrence of the clinical signs of lattice corneal dystrophy (type I) in corneal transplants, Am J Ophthalmol 97:210, 1984.

491. Mullaney PB and others: Congenital hereditary endothelial dystrophy associated with glaucoma, Ophthalmology 102:186, 1995.

492. Newsome DA and others: Biochemical and histological analysis of recurrent macular corneal dystrophy, Arch Ophthalmol 100:1125, 1982.

493. Nicholson DH and others: A clinical and histopathological study of François-Neetens speckled corneal dystrophy, Am J Ophthalmol 83:554, 1977.

494. Nirankari VS and others: Recurrence of keratoconus in donor cornea 22 years after successful keratoplasty, Br J Ophthalmol 67:23, 1983.

495. Olson RJ and Kaufman HE: Recurrence of Reis-Bücklers' corneal dystrophy in a graft, Am J Ophthalmol 85:349, 1978.

496. Owens SL and others: Superficial granular corneal dystrophy with amyloid deposits, Arch Ophthalmol 110:175, 1992.

497. Panjawani N and others: Lectin receptors of amyloid in corneas with lattice dystrophy, Arch Ophthalmol 105:688, 1987.

498. Paolo de Felice G and others: Posterior polymorphous dystrophy of the cornea, Graefes Arch Clin Exp Ophthalmol 223:265, 1985.

499. Paton D and Duke JB: Primary familial amyloidosis, Am J Ophthalmol 61:736, 1966.

500. Perry HD, Fine BS, and Caldwell DR: Reis-Bücklers' dystrophy: a study of eight cases, Arch Ophthalmol 97:664, 1979.

501. Perry HD, Leonard ER, and Yourish NB: Superficial reticular degeneration of Koby, Ophthalmology 92:1570, 1985.

502. Polack FM and others: Scanning electron microscopy of posterior polymorphous corneal dystrophy, Am J Ophthalmol 89:575, 1980.

503. Purcell JJ, Krachmer JH, and Weingeist TA: Fleck corneal dystrophy, Arch Ophthalmol 95:440, 1977.

504. Purcell JJ and others: Lattice corneal dystrophy associated with familial systemic amyloidosis (Meretoja's syndrome), Ophthalmology 90:1512, 1983.

505. Rabb MF, Blodi F, and Boniuk M: Unilateral lattice dystrophy of the cornea, Am J Ophthalmol 78:440, 1974.

506. Reed JW, Cashwell LF, and Klintworth GK: Corneal manifestations of hereditary benign intraepithelial dyskeratosis, Arch Ophthalmol 97:297, 1979.

507. Reis W: Familiäre, fleckige Hornhautentartung, Dtsch Med Wochenschr 43:575, 1917.

508. Rice NSC and others: Reis-Bücklers' dystrophy: clinicopathological study, Br J Ophthalmol 52:577, 1968.

509. Richardson WP and Hettinger ME: Endothelial and epithelial-like cell formations in a case of posterior polymorphous dystrophy, Arch Ophthalmol 103:1520, 1985.

510. Riedel KG and others: Ocular abnormalities in mucolipidosis IV, Am J Ophthalmol 99:125, 1985.

511. Rodrigues MM and others: Disorders of the corneal epithelium: a clinicopathologic study of dot, geographic and fingerprint patterns, Arch Ophthalmol 92:475, 1974.

512. Rodrigues MM and others: Epithelialization of the corneal endothelium in posterior polymorphous dystrophy, Invest Ophthalmol Vis Sci 19:832, 1980.

513. Rodrigues MM and others: Glaucoma due to endothelialization of the anterior chamber angle: a comparison of posterior polymorphous dystrophy of the cornea and Chandler's syndrome, Arch Ophthalmol 98:688, 1980.

514. Rodrigues MM and others: Microfibrillar protein and phospholipid in granular corneal dystrophy, Arch Ophthalmol 101:802, 1983.

515. Rodrigues MM and others: Unusual superficial confluent form of granular corneal dystrophy, Ophthalmology 90:1507, 1983.

516. Rodrigues MM and others: Fuchs'' corneal dystrophy: a clinicopathologic study of the variation in corneal edema, Ophthalmology 93:789, 1986.

517. Rodrigues MM and others: Unesterified cholesterol in Schnyder's corneal crystalline dystrophy, Am J Ophthalmol 104:157, 1987.

518. Rodrigues MM and others: Cholesterol localization in ultrathin frozen sections in Schnyder's corneal crystalline dystrophy, Am J Ophthalmol 110:513, 1990.

519. Rodrigues MM and others: Unesterfied cholesterol in granular, lattice and macular dystrophies, Am J Ophthalmol 115:112, 1993.

520. Rodrigues MM and others: Gelsolin immunoreactivity in corneal amyloid, wound healing, and macular and granular dystrophies, Am J Ophthalmol 115:644, 1993.

521. Rosenblum P, Stark WJ, and Maumenee IH: Hereditary Fuchs" dystrophy, Am J Ophthalmol 90:455, 1980.
522. Rosenwasser GO and others: Phenotypic variation in combined granular-lattice (avellino) corneal dystrophy [see comments], Arch Ophthalmol 111:1546, 1993.
523. Ross JR and others: Immunohistochemical analysis of the pathogenesis of posterior polymorphous dystrophy, Arch Ophthalmol 113:340, 1995.
524. Roth SI and others: Endothelial viral inclusions in Fuchs" corneal dystrophy, Hum Pathol 18:338, 1987.
525. Santo RM and others: Clinical and histopathologic features of corneal dystrophies in japan, Ophthalmol 102:557, 1995.
526. Sekundo W and others: An ultrastructural investigation of an early manifestation of the posterior polymorphous dystrophy of the cornea, Ophthalmology 101:1422, 1994.
527. Sher NA, Letson RD, and Desnick RJ: The ocular manifestations in Fabry's disease, Arch Ophthalmol 97:671, 1979.
528. Small KW and others: Mapping of Reis-Bucklers corneal dystrophy to chromosome 5q, Am J Ophthalmol 121:384, 1996.
529. Smith ME and Zimmerman LE: Amyloid in corneal dystrophies: differentiation of lattice from granular and macular dystrophies, Arch Ophthalmol 79:407, 1968.
530. Snyder WB: Hereditary epithelial corneal dystrophy, Am J Ophthalmol 55:56, 1963.
531. Stainer CA and others: Correlative microscopy and tissue culture of congenital hereditary endothelial dystrophy, Am J Ophthalmol 93:456, 1982.
532. Starck T and others: Clinical and histopathologic studies of two families with lattice corneal dystrophy and familial systemic amyloidosis (Meretoja syndrome), Ophthalmology 98:1197, 1991.
533. Stock EL and others: Lattice corneal dystrophy type IIIa. Clinical and histopathologic correlations, Arch Ophthalmol 109:354, 1991.
534. Stocker W and Holt LB: Rare form of hereditary epithelial dystrophy, Arch Ophthalmol 53:536, 1955.
535. Stone EM and others: Three autosomal dominant corneal dystrophies map to chromosome 5q, Nature 6:47, 1994.
536. Sundar Raj N and others: Macular corneal dystrophy: immunochemical characterization using monoclonal antibodies, Invest Ophthalmol Vis Sci 28:1678, 1987.
537. Takahashi M and others: Unusual inclusions in stromal macrophages in a case of gelatinous drop-like corneal dystrophy, Am J Ophthalmol 99:312, 1985.
538. Teng CC: Macular dystrophy of the cornea: a histochemical and electron microscopic study, Am J Ophthalmol 62:436, 1966.
539. Thonar EJ-MA and others: Absence of normal keratan sulfate in the blood of patients with macular corneal dystrophy, Am J Ophthalmol 102:561, 1986.
540. Ticho U, Lahau M, and Ivry M: Familial band-shaped keratopathy, J Pediatr Ophthalmol Strabismus 19:183, 1979.
541. Tripathi RC and Bron AJ: Ultrastructural study of nontraumatic recurrent corneal erosion, Br J Ophthalmol 56:73, 1972.
542. Tripathi RC and Bron AJ: Cystic disorders of the corneal epithelium. II. Pathogenesis, Br J Ophthalmol 57:376, 1973.
543. Tripathi RC and Bron AJ: Secondary anterior crocodile shargreens of Vogt. Vogt 59:59-175.
544. Trobe JD and Laibson PR: Dystrophic changes in the anterior cornea, Arch Ophthalmol 87:378, 1972.
545. Tuppurainen K and others: Fabry's disease and cornea verticillata, Acta Ophthalmol 59:674, 1981.
546. Waring GO III, Rodrigues MM, and Laibson PR: Corneal dystrophies. I. Dystrophies of the epithelium, Bowman's layer and stroma, Surv Ophthalmol 23:71, 1978.
547. Waring GO III, Rodrigues MM, and Laibson PR: Corneal dystrophies. II. Endothelial dystrophies, Surv Ophthalmol 23:147, 1978.
548. Weingeist TA and Blodi FC: Fabry's disease: ocular findings in a female carrier—a light and electron microscopic study, Arch Ophthalmol 85:169, 1971.
549. Weller RO and Rodger FC: Crystalline stromal dystrophy: histochemistry and ultrastructure of the cornea, Br J Ophthalmol 64:46, 1980.
550. Wilson DJ and others: Bietti's crystalline dystrophy: a clinicopathologic correlative study, Arch Ophthalmol 107:213, 1989.
551. Witschel H and others: Congenital hereditary stromal dystrophy of the cornea, Arch Ophthalmol 96:1043, 1978.
552. Wolter JR, Henderson JW, and Gates K: Endothelial and epithelial dystrophy of the cornea, Am J Ophthalmol 44:191, 1957.
553. Yamaguchi T, Polack FM, and Valenti J: Electron microscopic study of recurrent Reis-Bümcklers' corneal dystrophy, Am J Ophthalmol 90:95, 1980.
554. Yang CJ and others: Immunohistochemical evidence of heterogeneity in macular corneal dystrophy, Am J Ophthalmol 106:65, 1988.
555. Yanoff M and others: Lattice corneal dystrophy: report of an unusual case, Arch Ophthalmol 95:651, 1977.

Amyloidosis

556. Blodi FG and Apple DJ: Amylose conjonctivale localisée, Bull Mem Soc Fr Ophthalmol 91:107, 1979.
557. Blodi FG and Apple DJ: Localized conjunctival amyloidosis, Am J Ophthalmol 88:346, 1979. (Maumenee/Festschrift issue.)
558. Borodic GE and others: Immunoglobulin deposition in localized conjunctival amyloidosis, Am J Ophthalmol 98:617, 1984.
559. Brownstein MH, Elliott R, and Helwig EB: Ophthalmologic aspects of amyloidosis, Am J Ophthalmol 69:423, 1970.
560. Cohen AS: An update of clinical, pathologic, and biochemical aspects of amyloidosis, Int J Dermatol 20:515, 1981.
561. Doughman DJ: Ocular amyloidosis, Surv Ophthalmol 13:133, 1968.
562. Dutt S and others: Secondary localized amyloidosis in interstitial keratitis. Clinicopathologic findings, Ophthalmology 99:817, 1992.
563. Falls HL and others: Ocular manifestations of hereditary primary systemic amyloidosis, Arch Ophthalmol 54:550, 1955.
564. Fett DR and Putterman AM: Primary localized amyloidosis presenting as an eyelid margin tumor, Arch Ophthalmol 104:584, 1986.
565. Finlay K, Rootman J, and Dimmick J: Optic neuropathy in primary orbital amyloidosis, Can J Ophthalmol 15:189, 1980.
566. Gorevic PD and others: Lack of evidence for protein AA reactivity in amyloid deposits of lattice corneal dystrophy and amyloid corneal degeneration, Am J Ophthalmol 98:216, 1984.
567. Gorevic PD and others: Prealbumin: a major constituent of vitreous amyloid, Ophthalmology 94:792, 1987.
568. Hidayat AA and Risco JM: Amyloidosis of corneal stroma in patients with trachoma: a clinicopathologic study of 62 cases, Ophthalmology 96:1203, 1989.
569. Hinzpeter EN and Nauman GOH: Zur sekundaren Amyloidose der Hornhaut ein Klinisch-pathologisches Bericht, Graefes Arch Klin Exp Ophthalmol 192:19, 1974.
570. Jensen JE: Localized amyloidosis in relation to conjunctival haemorrhagic lymphangiectasia and occlusion of the orbital veins: a case report, Acta Ophthalmol 61:254, 1983.
571. Kirk HQ and others: Primary familial amyloidosis of the cornea, Trans Am Acad Ophthalmol Otolaryngol 77:411, 1973.
572. Kivelä T and others: Ocular amyloid deposition in familial amyloidosis, Finnish: an analysis of native and variant gelsolin in Meretoja's syndrome, Invest Ophthalmol Vis Sci 35:3759, 1994.
573. Loeffler KU and others: An immunohistochemical study of gelsolin immunoreactivity in corneal amyloidosis, Am J Ophthalmol 113:546, 1992.
574. Mannis MJ and others: Polymorphic amyloid degeneration of the cornea, Arch Ophthalmol 99:1217, 1981.
575. Marsh WM and others: Localized conjunctival amyloidosis associated with extranodal lymphoma, Ophthalmology 94:61, 1987.
576. McCarthy M and others: Panstromal schnyder corneal dystrophy: a clinical pathologic report with quantitative analysis of corneal lipid composition, Ophthalmology 101:895, 1994.
577. McPherson SD Jr, Kiffney GT Jr, and Freed CC: Corneal amyloidosis, Trans Am Ophthalmol Soc 64:148, 1966.
578. Meisler DM and others: Conjunctival inflammation and amyloidosis in allergic granulomatosis and angiitis (Churg-Strauss syndrome), Am J Ophthalmol 91:216, 1981.
579. Mondino BJ, Rabb MF, and Suger J: Primary amyloidosis of the cornea, Am J Ophthalmol 92:732, 1981.
580. Paton D and Duke JB: Primary familial amyloidosis, Am J Ophthalmol 61:736, 1966.
581. Raflo G, Farrell T, and Sioussat R: Complete ophthalmoplegia secondary to amyloidosis associated with multiple myeloma, Am J Ophthalmol 92:221, 1981.
582. Richlin JJ and Kuwabara T: Amyloid disease of the eyelid and conjunctiva, Arch Ophthalmol 67:138, 1962.
583. Robbins SL and Cotran SC: Pathologic basis of disease, ed 3, Philadelphia, 1984, WB Saunders Co.

584. Schwartz MF and others: An unusual case of ocular involvement in primary systemic nonfamilial amyloidosis, Ophthalmoloy 89:394, 1982.
585. Shimazaki J and others: Long-term follow-up of patients with familial subepithelial amyloidosis of the cornea, Ophthalmology 59:59, 1975.
586. Smith ME and Zimmerman LF: Amyloidosis of the eyelid and conjunctiva, Arch Ophthalmol 75:1966.
587. Stern GA, Knapp A, and Hood CI: Corneal amyloidosis associated with keratoconus, Ophthalmology 95:52, 1988.
588. Takahashi T and others: A case of corneal amyloidosis, Acta Ophthalmol 61:150, 1983.
589. Teekhasaenee C and others: Posterior polymorphous dystrophy and Alport syndrome, Ophthalmology 98:1207, 1991.
590. Threlkeld AB and others: A clinicopathologic study of posterior polymorphous dystrophy: implications for pathogenetic mechanism of the associated glaucoma, Trans Am Ophthalmol Soc 92:133, 1994.
591. Vallat M and others: Primary systemic amyloidosis: an electron microscopic study of the vitreous, Arch Ophthalmol 98:540, 1980.
592. Waring GO III and others: Corneal dystrophies. II. Endothelial dystrophies, Surv Ophthalmol 23:147, 1978.
593. Weber FL and Babel J: Gelatinous drop-like dystrophy: a form of primary corneal amyloidosis, Arch Ophthalmol 98:144, 1980.
594. Wilson DJ and others: Bietti's crystalline dystrophy. A clinicopathologic correlative study, Arch Ophthalmol 107:213, 1989.
595. Wilson SE and others: Aqueous humor composition in Fuchs" dystrophy, Invest Ophthalmol Vis Sci 30:449, 1989.

Systemic disorders causing corneal clouding in childhood

596. Beck M: Papilledema in association with Hunter's syndrome, Br J Ophthalmol 67:174, 1983.
597. Cantor LB and others: Glaucoma in the Maroteaux-Lamy syndrome, Am J Ophthalmol 108:426, 1989.
598. Chan CC and others: Ocular ultrastructural studies of two cases of the Hurler syndrome (systemic mucopolysaccharidosis 1-H), Ophthalmic Paediatr Genet 2:3, 1983.
599. Collins DG and others: Optic nerve head swelling and optic atrophy in the systemic mucopolysaccharidoses, Ophthalmology 97:1445, 1990.
600. Di Ferrante N and others: Deficiencies of glucosamine-6 sulfate or galactosamine-6 sulfate sulfatases are responsible for different mucopolysaccharidoses, Science 199:79, 1980.
601. Emery JM and others: G$_{M1}$-Gangliosidosis: ocular and pathological manifestations, Arch Ophthalmol 85:177, 1971.
602. Gibis GW and others: Mucolipidosis I, Arch Ophthalmol 101:933, 1983.
603. Goldberg MF: A review of selected inherited corneal dystrophies associated with systemic disease, Birth Defects 7:13, 1971.
604. Goldberg MF, Maumenee AE, and McKusick VA: Corneal dystrophies associated with abnormalities of mucopolysaccharide metabolism, Arch Ophthalmol 74:516, 1965.
605. Hambrick GW Jr and Scheie HG: Studies of the skin in Hurler's syndrome, Arch Dermatol 85:455, 1962.
606. Hayasaka S: Lysosomal enzymes in ocular tissues and diseases, Surv Ophthalmol 27:245, 1983.
607. Hogan MJ and Cordes FC: Lipochondrodystrophy (dysostosis multiplex; Hurler's disease): pathologic changes in cornea in three cases, Arch Ophthalmol 32:287, 1944.
608. Jensen OA: Mucopolysaccharidoses type III (Sanfilippo's syndrome): histochemical examination of the eyes and brain with a survey of the literature, Acta Pathol Microbiol Scand [A] 79:257, 1971.
609. Kenyon KR: Ocular ultrastructure of inherited metabolic diseases. In Goldberg MF, editor: Genetic and metabolic eye disease, Boston, 1974, Little, Brown & Co.
610. Kenyon KR and others: The systemic mucopolysaccharides: ultrastructural and histochemical studies of conjunctiva and skin, Am J Ophthalmol 73:811, 1972.
611. Kenyon KR and others: Ocular pathology of the Maroteaux-Lamy syndrome (systemic mucopolysaccharidosis type VI): histologic and ultrastructural report of two cases, Am J Ophthalmol 73:718, 1972.
612. Kenyon KR and others: Mucolipidosis IV: histopathology of conjunctiva, cornea, and skin, Arch Ophthalmol 97:1106, 1979.
613. Keyon KR and Sensenbrenner JA: Mucolipidosis II (I-cell disease): ultrastructural observations of conjunctiva and skin, Invest Ophthalmol 10:555, 1971.
614. Lavery MA and others: Ocular histopathology and ultrastructure of Sanfilippo's syndrome, type III-B, Arch Ophthalmol 101:1263, 1983.
615. Levy LA and others: Ultrastructures of Reilly bodies (metachromatic granules) in the Maroteaux-Lamy syndrome (mucopolysaccharidosis VI). A histochemical study, Am J Clin Pathol 73:416, 1980.
616. Libert J and others: Ocular findings in I-cell disease (mucolipidosis type II), Am J Ophthalmol 83:617, 1977.
617. McDonnell JM and others: Ocular histopathology of systemic mucopolysaccharidosis, type II-A (Hunter syndrome, severe), Ophthalmology 92:1772, 1985.
618. McKusick VA: The mucopolysaccharidoses. In McKusick VA: Heritable disorders of connective tissue, ed 4, St Louis, 1972, The CV Mosby Co.
619. Naumann G: Clearing of cornea after perforating keratoplasty in mucopolysaccharidosis type VI (Maroteaux-Lamy syndrome), N Engl J Med 312:995, 1985.
620. Naumann GOH and Rummelt V: Aufklaren der transplantatnahen Wirtshornhaut nach perforierender keratoplastik beim Maroteaux-Lamy-Syndrome (Mukopolysaccharidose Type VI-A), Klin Monastbl Augenheilkd 203:351, 1993.
621. Newman NJ and others: Corneal surface irregularities and episodic pain in a patient with mucolipidosis IV, Arch Ophthalmol 108:251, 1990.
622. Newman NJ and others: Corneal surface irregularities and episodic pain in a patient with mucolipidosis IV [clinical conference], Arch Ophthalmol 108:251, 1993.
623. O'Brien JF: The lysosomal storage diseases, Mayo Clin Proc 57:192, 1982.
624. Pinnolis M and others: Nosematosis of the cornea: case report, including electron microscopic studies, Arch Ophthalmol 99:1044, 1981.
625. Polack F: Contributions of electron microscopy to the study of corneal pathology, Surv Ophthalmol 20:375, 1976.
626. Quigley HA and Goldberg MF: Conjunctival ultrastructure in mucolipidosis III (pseudo-Hurler polydystrophy), Invest Ophthalmol 10:568, 1971.
627. Quigley HA and Goldberg MF: Scheie syndrome and macular corneal dystrophy: an ultrastructural comparison of conjunctiva and skin, Arch Ophthalmol 85:553, 1971.
628. Quigley HA and Kenyon KR: Ultrastructural and histochemical studies of a newly recognized form of systemic mucopolysaccharidosis (Maroteaux-Lamy syndrome, mild phenotype), Am J Ophthalmol 77:809, 1974.
629. Rummelt V and others: Light and electron microscopy of the cornea in systemic mucopolysaccharidosis type I-S (Scheie's syndrome), Cornea 2:86, 1992.
630. Scheie HG and others: A newly recognized forme fruste of Hurler's disease (gargoylism), Am J Ophthalmol 53:753, 1962.
631. Spellacy E and others: Glaucoma in a case of Hurler disease, Br J Ophthalmol 64:773, 1980.
632. Spranger JW and Wiedemann HR: The genetic mucolipidoses. Diagnosis and differential diagnosis, Humangenetik 9:113, 1970.
633. Summers CG and others: Ocular changes in the mucopolysaccharidoses after bone marrow transplantation, Ophthalmology 96:977, 1989.
634. Süveges I: Histological and ultrastructural studies of the cornea in Maroteaux-Lamy syndrome, Graefes Arch Ophthalmol Clin Ophthalmol 212:29, 1979.
635. Topping TM and others: Ultrastructural ocular pathology of Hunter's syndrome: systemic mucopolysaccharidosis type II, Arch Ophthalmol 86:164, 1971.
636. Vogel MH, Müller KM, and Witting C: Ocular histopathology in mucopoly-saccharidosis III (Sanfilippo), Ophthalmologica 169:311, 1974.
637. Winterbotham CT and others: Unusual mucopolysaccharide disorder with corneal and scleral involvement, Am J Ophthalmol 109: 544, 1990.
638. Zabel RW and others: Scheie's syndrome. An ultrastructural analysis of the cornea, Ophthalmol 96:1631, 1989.

Hereditary Bowman's layer dysplasia

639. Apple DJ: Chromosome-induced ocular disease. In Goldberg MF, editor: Genetic and metabolic eye disease, Boston, 1974, Little, Brown & Co.

640. Apple DJ and others: Corneal opacification secondary to Bowman's layer dysgenesis, Am J Ophthalmol 93:320, 1984.

641. Bach LB and Seefelder R: Atlas zur entwicklungsgeschichte des menschlichen Auges, Leipzig, 1912, Wilhelm Engelmann.

642. Hittner H and others: Variable expressivity of autosomal dominant anterior segment mesodermal dysgenesis in second generation, Am J Ophthalmol 93:57, 1982.

643. Klintworth GK and McCracken JS: Electron microscopy in human medicine: corneal diseases, New York, 1979, McGraw-Hill Book Co.

644. Kretzer FL, Hittner H, and Mehta R: Ocular manifestations of Smith-Lemli-Opitz syndrome, Arch Ophthalmol 99:2000, 1981.

645. Orloff C and others: Angeborene Hornhauttrucbung durch Verdickung der Bowman's chen Membran, Fortsehr Ophthalmol 1984.

646. Perry HD, Fine BS, and Caldwell DR: Reis-Bücklers dystrophy: a study of eight cases, Arch Ophthalmol 97:66-1, 1979.

647. Rodrigues M, Calhoun J, and Harley R: Corneal clouding with increased acid mucopolysaccharide accumulation in Bowman's membrane, Am J Ophthalmol 79:916, 1975.

648. Townsend WAL, Font RL, and Zimmerman LE: Congenital corneal leukomas: histopathologic findings in 19 eyes with central defect in Descemet's membrane, Am J Ophthalmol 77:192, 1974.

649. Waring CO, III, Rodrigues MM, and Laibson PR: Anterior chamber cleavage syndrome: a stepladder classification, Surv Ophthalmol 20:3, 1975.

Trauma

650. Aguilar JP, Green WR: Choroidal rupture: a histopathologic study of 47 cases, Retina 4:269, 1984.

651. Apple DJ and others: Ocular perforation secondary to strabismus surgery, J Pediatr Ophthalmol Strabismus 22(5):184, 1985.

652. Beltman JW Jr: Pathology of complications of intraocular surgery, Am J Ophthalmol 68:1037, 1969.

653. Bergen R and Margolis S: Retinal hemorrhages in the newborn, Ann Ophthalmol 8:53, 1976.

654. Blodi B and others: Purtscher's-like retinopathy after childbirth, Ophthalmology 97:1654, 1990.

655. Bloomfield SE, Jakobiec FA, and Iwamoto T: Traumatic intrastromal corneal cyst, Ophthalmology 87:951, 1980.

656. Bloomfield SE, Jakobiec FA, and Iwamoto T: Fibrous ingrowth with retrocorneal membrane, Ophthalmology 88:459, 1981.

657. Boruchoff SA and others: Epithelial cyst of the iris following penetrating keratoplasty, Br J Ophthalmol 64:440, 1980.

658. Bright R and Hart JCO: Structural changes in the outer retinal layers following blunt mechanical non-perforating trauma to the globe: an experimental study, Br J Ophthalmol 61:573, 1977.

659. Brown SI, Weller CA, and Kiyas A: Pathogenesis of ulcers of the alkaliburned cornea, Arch Ophthalmol 83:204, 1970.

660. Burch PG and Albert DM: Transscleral ocular siderosis, Am J Ophthalmol 81:90, 1977.

661. Burton TC: Unilateral Purtscher's retinopathy, Ophthalmology 87:1096, 1977.

662. Cameron JD and others: In vitro studies of corneal wound healing: epithelial—endothelial interactions, Invest Ophthalmol 95:1189, 1988.

663. Cherry PM: Indirect traumatic rupture of the globe, Arch Ophthalmol 96:252, 1978.

664. Cibis GW, Weingeist TA, and Krachmer JH: Traumatic corneal endothelial rings, Arch Ophthalmol 96:485, 1978.

665. Cibis PA, Brown EG, and Hong S: Ocular effects of systemic siderosis, Am J Ophthalmol 44:158, 1957.

666. Cibis PA, Brown EB, and Hong S: Clinical aspects of ocular siderosis and hemosiderosis, Arch Ophthalmol 62:180, 1959.

667. Cleary PE and Ryan SJ: Posterior perforating eye injury: experimental animal model, Trans Ophthalmol Soc UK 98:34, 1978.

668. Cleary PE and Ryan SJ: Experimental posterior penetrating eye injury in the rabbit. II. Histology of wound, vitreous, and retina, Br J Ophthalmol 63:312, 1979.

669. Cleary PE and Ryan SJ: Histology of wound, vitreous, and retina in experimental posterior penetrating eye injury in the rhesus monkey, Am J Ophthalmol 88:221, 1979.

670. Coburn A and others: Spontaneous intrastromal iris cyst: a case report with immunohistochemical and ultrastructural observations, Ophthalmology 92:1691, 1985.

671. Cogan DG: Pseudoretinitis pigmentosa, Arch Ophthalmol 81:45, 1969.

672. Cox MS and Freeman HM: Retinal detachment due to ocular penetration. I. Clinical characteristics and surgical results, Arch Ophthalmol 96:1354, 1978.

673. Crabb CV: A light microscopic study of ground substance changes in alkali burned corneas, Am J Ophthalmol 86:92, 1978.

674. Crandall A, Yanoff M, and Schaffer D: Intrascleral nerve loop mistakenly identified as a foreign body, Arch Ophthalmol 95:497, 1977.

675. Declercy SS, Meredith PCA, and Rosenthal AR: Experimental siderosis in the rabbit: correlation between electroretinography and histopathology, Arch Ophthalmol 95:1051, 1977.

676. Dolan S and Oliver M: Shallow anterior chamber and uveal effusion after nonperforating trauma to the eye, Am J Ophthalmol 94:782, 1982.

677. Dua HS and Forrester JV: Clinical patterns of corneal epithelial wound healing, Am J Ophthalmol 104:481, 1987.

678. Duke-Elder S and MacFaul PA: System of ophthalmology, vol XIV, Injuries, part I, Mechanical injuries; part II, Nonmechanical injuries, St. Louis, 1972, The CV Mosby Co.

679. Eagle RC Jr and others: Intraocular wooden foreighn body clinically resembling a pearl cyst, Arch Ophthalmol 95:835, 1977.

680. Elner S and others: Ocular and associated systemic findings in suspected child abuse, Arch Ophthalmol 108:1094, 1990.

681. Erie JC and others: Incidence of enucleation in a defined population, Am J Ophthalmol 113:138, 1992.

682. Fenton RH, and Zimmerman LE: Hemolytic glaucoma: an unusual cause of acute open-angle secondary glaucoma, Arch Ophthalmol 70:236, 1963.

683. Fogle JA, Kenyon KR, and Stark WJ: Damage to epithelial basement membrane by thermokeratoplasty, Am J Ophthalmol 83:392, 1977.

684. Freeman HM, editor: Ocular trauma, New York, 1979, Appleton-Century-Crofts, p. 453.

685. Giovinazzo VJ and others: The ocular complications of boxing, Ophthalmology 94:587, 1987.

686. Goldberg MF: Chorioretinal vascular anastomoses after blunt trauma to the eye, Am J Ophthalmol 82:892, 1976.

687. Goldberg MF: Chorioretinal vascular anastomoses after perforating trauma to the eye, Am J Ophthalmol 892, 1976.

688. Grant WM and Kern HL: Action of alkalis on the corneal stroma, Arch Ophthalmol 54:931, 1955.

689. Havener WH and Gloeckner S: Atlas of diagnostic techniques and treatment of intraocular foreign bodies, St. Louis, 1969, The CV Mosby Co.

690. Herschler J: Trabecular damage due to blunt anterior segment injury and its relationship to traumatic glaucoma, Trans Am Acad Ophthalmol Otolaryngol 83:239, 1977.

691. Hughes WF: Alkali burns of the eye. I. Review of literature and summary of present knowledge, Arch Ophthalmol 35:423, 1946.

692. Hughes WF: Alkali burns of the eye. II. Clinical and pathologic course, Arch Ophthalmol 36:189, 1946.

693. Jensen P, Minckler DS, and Chandler JW: Epithelial ingrowth, Arch Ophthalmol 95:837, 1977.

694. Karai A, Mustakallio AH, and Kaufman H: Electron microscopic studies of corneal endothelium: the abnormal endothelium associated with retrocorneal membrane, Ann Ophthalmol 4:564, 1972.

695. Kremer I, Rapuano C, Cohen E, et al.: Retrocorneal fibrous membrane in failed corneal grafts, Am J Ophthalmol 115:4, 1993.

696. Lambert SR, Johnson TE, and Hoyt CS: Optic nerve sheath and retinal hemorrhages associated with the shaken baby syndrome, Arch Ophthalmol 104:1509, 1986.

697. Lang GK, Green WR, and Maumenee AE: Clinicopathologic studies of keratoplasty eyes obtained postmortem, Am J Ophthalmol 101:28, 1986.

698. Levine J: Siderosis bulbi, Arch Ophthalmol 11:625, 1934.

699. Matsuda H and Smelser GK: Endothelial cells in alkali burned corneas, Arch Ophthalmol 89:402, 1973.

700. Matsuda II and Smelser GK: Epithelium and stroma in alkali burned corneas, Arch Ophthalmol 89:396, 1973.

701. Michels RG, Kenyon KR, and Maumenee AE: Retrocorneal fibrous membrane, Invest Ophthalmol 11:822, 1972.

702. McKnight GT and others: Transcorneal extrusion of anterior chamber intraocular lenses: a report of three cases, Arch Ophthalmol 105:1656, 1987.

703. Meyer RF and Hood CI: Fungus implantation with wooden intraocular foreign bodies, Ann Ophthalmol 9:271, 1977.

704. New Orleans Academy of Ophthalmolognhy: Industrial and trau-

matic ophthalmology: transaction of the New Orleans Academy of Ophthalmology, St. Louis, 1964, The CV Mosby Co.

705. O'Grady RB and Kirk HQ: Corneal keloids, Am J Ophthalmol 73: 206, 1972.

706. Olson LE and others: Effects of ultrasound on the corneal endothelium. I. The acute lesion, Br J Ophthalmol 62:134, 1978.

707. Olson LE and others: Effects of ultrasound on the corneal endothelium. II. The endothelial repair process, Br J Ophthalmol 62:145, 1978.

708. Paton D and Goldberg MF: Management of ocular injuries, Philadelphia, 1976, WB Saunders Co.

709. Pfister RR: The effects of chemical injury on the ocular surface, Ophthalmology 90:601, 1983.

710. Pilger IS and Khwarg WG: Angle recession glaucoma: review and two case reports, Ann Ophthalmol 17:197, 1985.

711. Potts AM and Distler JA: Shape factor in the penetration of intraocular foreign bodies, Am J Ophthalmol 100:183, 1985.

712. Riffenburgh R and Sathyavagiswaran L: Ocular findings at autopsy of child abuse victims, Ophthalmology 98:1519, 1991.

713. Rosenthal AR, Appleton B, and Hopkins JL: Intraocular copper foreign bodies, Am J Ophthalmol 78:671, 1974.

714. Runyan TE: Concussive and penetrating injuries of the globe and optic nerve, St. Louis, 1975, The CV Mosby Co.

715. Silbert AM and Baum JL: Origin of retrocorneal membrane in the rabbit, Arch Ophthalmol 97:1141, 1979.

716. Slingsby JC and Forstot SL: Effect of blunt trauma on the corneal endothelium, Arch Ophthalmol 99:1041, 1981.

717. Smith ME and Zimmerman LE: Contusive angle recession in phacolytic glaucoma, Arch Ophthalmol 74:799, 1965.

718. Snif RC, Kenyon KR, and Green WR: Retrocorneal fibrous membrane in the vitreous touch syndrome, Am J Ophthalmol 79:233, 1975.

719. Snip RC, Green WR, and Kreutzer EW: Posterior corneal pigmentation and fibrous proliferation by iris melanocytes, Arch Ophthalmol 99:1232, 1981.

720. Spaeth GL: Traumatic hyphema, angle recession, dexamethasone hypertension and glaucoma, Arch Ophthalmol 78:714, 1967.

721. Sternberg P and others: Ocular BB injuries, Ophthalmology 91:1269, 1984.

722. Hood CA: Epithelial downgrowth following penetrating keratoplasty in the aphake, Arch Ophthalmol 95:464, 1977.

723. Sugar HS, Kobernick SD, and Weingarten JE: Hematogenous ocular siderosis of local cause, Am J Ophthalmol 64:749, 1967.

724. Sutton DF and others: Retrocorneal smooth-muscle proliferation on rejected corneal graft, Arch Ophthalmol 101:429, 1983.

725. Talamo JH and others: Ultrastructural studies of cornea, iris and lens in a case of siderosis bulbi, Ophthalmology 92:1675, 1985.

726. Waring G, Laibson P, and Rodrigues M: Clinical and pathologic alterations of Descemet's membrane, with emphasis on endothelial metaplasia, Surv Ophthalmol 18:325, 1974.

727. Winslow RL, Stevenson W III, and Yanoff MF: Spontaneous expulsive choroidal hemorrhage, Arch Ophthalmol 92:126, 1974.

728. Winthrop SR and others: Penetrating eye injuries: a histopathological review, Br J Ophthalmol 64:809, 1980.

729. Wolff SM and Zimmerman LE: Chronic secondary glaucoma associated with retrodisplacement of iris root and deepening of the anterior chamber angle secondary to contusion, Am J Ophthalmol 54: 547, 1962.

730. Zagora E: Eye injuries, Springfield, III, 1970, Charles C Thomas, Publisher.

731. Zavala EY and Binder PS: The pathologic findings of epithelial ingrowth, Arch Ophthalmol 98:2007, 1980.

CHAPTER 4

LENS AND PATHOLOGY OF INTRAOCULAR LENSES

Embryology and anatomy

The structure of the adult lens can be appreciated only with a knowledge of its embryology (Fig. 4-1).[1–39] It is derived from the embryonic surface ectoderm after contact and interaction of the anterior wall of the neuroectodermal optic vesicle with the epithelial lining of the embryo. Without this critical interaction, induction and, therefore, formation and development of the lens do not occur.[10,23,28,31,36] Such a failure causes a primary congenital aphakia (p. 15). Because the lens is derived from surface ectoderm, many skin diseases may also affect the lens. For example, atopic dermatitis is associated with various forms of cataract.

The first trace of the lens, the lens plate, appears about the third week of gestation in the form of a thickening of the surface ectoderm at the site of previous contact of the optic vesicle. At the next stage, approximately 22 to 23 days, the cells of the lens plate arch posteriorly, forming a concave depression, the lens pit. This area eventually separates from the epithelium, transforming the lens pit into the primary lens vesicle, which is surrounded by a periodic acid-Schiff (PAS)-positive lens capsule. The remaining overlying surface ectoderm reforms to create an uninterrupted layer anteriorly; this layer becomes the corneal epithelium. Soon after the lens vesicle forms, the front (anterior) and rear (posterior) walls of the lens vesicle differentiate into dissimilar structures. The anterior wall remains a single layer of cuboidal epithelium, but the cells of the posterior wall are modified, and development of the primary lens fibers begins. The cells on the posterior wall increase in length and form elongated fibers that project into the lumen of the vesicle (Fig. 4-1). Their nuclei migrate forward from the posterior pole toward the middle of the vesicle. The vesicle remains spheric, but the lumen of the vesicle becomes much smaller and is eventually obliterated by these fibers. This process results in the solid embryonic lens nucleus, which is completely developed by the end of the fourth week.

The formation of all subsequent fibers around the embryonic nucleus occurs in the equatorial region at the lens bow (Figs. 4-2 and 4-3). The anterior lens epithelial cells migrate equatorially, undergo mitotic division, and form elongated new lens fibers concentrically at the equator around the older central fibers. This growth of new fibers is continuous throughout life so that the lens increases in weight and size, although at a much slower rate in later years. As the new fibers are formed, the nuclei of the cells

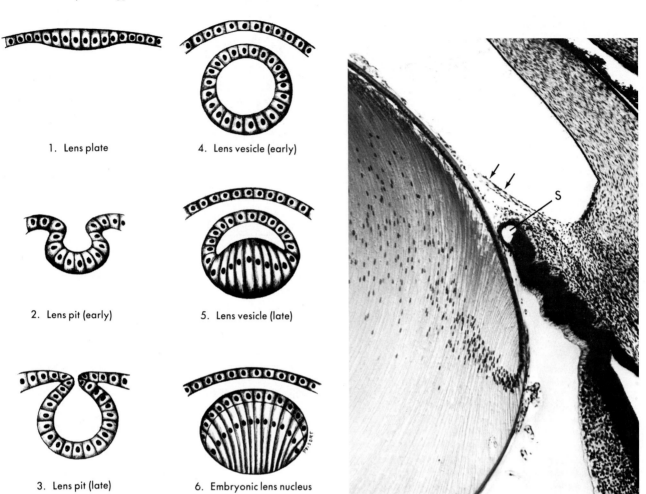

1. Lens plate

4. Lens vesicle (early)

2. Lens pit (early)

5. Lens vesicle (late)

3. Lens pit (late)

6. Embryonic lens nucleus

Fig. 4-1. Stages of growth of the embryonic lens. (From Naumann GOH and Apple DJ. In Doerr W, Seifert G, and Uehlinger E, editors: Handbuch der speziellen pathologischen Anatomie, Band Auge, Berlin, 1980, Springer-Verlag.)

Fig. 4-2. Photomicrograph of a fetal lens at the equator, showing the lens bow where new fibers are laid down. The fiber nuclei disappear toward the center of the lens. *Arrows,* Pupillary membrane; S, marginal sinus of von Szily. (H & E stain; ×120.) (From Naumann GOH and Apple DJ: In Doerr W, Seifert G, and Uehlinger E, editors: Handbuch der speziellen pathologischen Anatomie, Band Auge, Berlin, 1980, Springer-Verlag.)

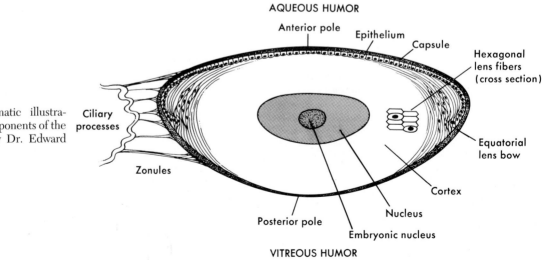

Fig. 4-3. Diagrammatic illustration of the major components of the adult lens. (Courtesy Dr. Edward Cotlier.)

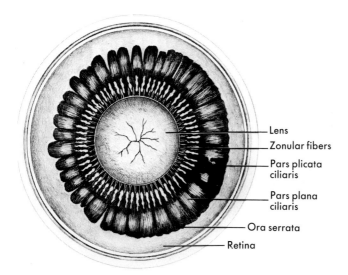

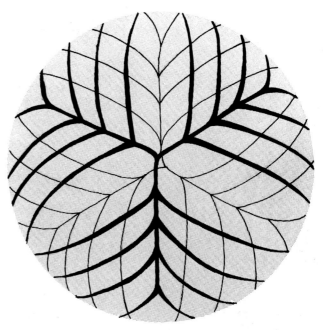

Fig. 4-4. Schematic illustration of the anterior third of the globe as viewed from behind. Note the prominent dendritic pattern of the lens sutures. (Modified from Salzmann M: The anatomy and histology of the human eyeball in the normal state, Chicago, 1912, University of Chicago Press. [Translated by EVL Brown.])

Fig. 4-5. Schematic illustration showing the arrangement of embryonic lens sutures.

gradually disappear, resulting in a lens center normally devoid of cellular nuclei.[10,23,28,31,36]

The lens sutures appear in the second month, immediately after the formation of the primary lens nucleus from the lens vesicle. Initially, at the stage of the primary embryonic nucleus, the lens fibers extend from the anterior to the posterior pole, and the lens is spheric. As growth proceeds, an unequal elongation of the newly formed lens fibers occurs so that pole-to-pole growth is not achieved. This unequal growth phenomenon explains the formation of the sutures. The purpose of the sutures is to ensure that the lens becomes a flattened biconvex sphere rather than retaining its initial spheric shape. The unequal growth rates of individual fibers are indicated by the fact that a newly formed equatorial fiber, which reaches the posterior pole, shows a retardation of growth anteriorly. Thus it never reaches the anterior pole and vice versa. The linear juncture, where the fibers terminate and abut each other, forms the basis of the lens sutures. The sutures are molded together by deposition of ground substance.

Initially two Y-shaped sutures are present: the upright anterior Y suture and the inverted posterior suture (see Fig. 4-31). During later gestation and after birth, the growth of the lens sutures is much more irregular. Instead of a simple Y suture, more complicated dendritic patterns caused by asymmetric fiber growth are observed (Figs. 4-4, 4-5 and 4-37).

The adult lens measures approximately 9 mm in diameter and has the form of a biconvex disc with round peripheral edges. The anterior and posterior poles form the geometric and optical axis of the lens. Although the normal lens is transparent and clear in vivo, it is seldom completely colorless, showing even in youth a slight yellowish tint that often intensifies with age. Opacification of lens specimens always occurs after fixation in formalin and most other preservatives. In globes of infants and children a posterior

polar depression or pitting regularly occurs as a fixation artifact; this should not be confused with a congenital "umbilication" of the lens, which is rare.

The lens consists of three components (Figs. 4-2, 4-3, and 4-6): from the outer surface inward they are the lens capsule, the lens epithelium, and the lens substance. The lens substance is a product of the continuous growth of the epithelium and consists of the cortex and nucleus. The transition between cortex and nucleus is gradual and does not reveal a concise line of demarcation when observed in histologic sections.

The lens does not possess nerves, vessels, or connective tissue. Its nourishment is derived from the circulating anterior chamber aqueous fluid and the vitreous; therefore, disturbances in circulation of these fluids, or inflammatory processes in these chambers, play a large role in the pathogenesis of lens abnormalities. Disturbances in permeability of the lens capsule and epithelium can occur, leading to formation of cataracts.*

CAPSULE

By light microscopy the lens capsule appears as a structureless, elastic membrane, which completely ensheathes the lens. It is a true PAS-positive basement membrane, a secretory product of the lens epithelium. It functions as a metabolic barrier and may be largely responsible for the elasticity and shaping of the lens during accommodation (Fig. 4-6).

The capsule is of variable thickness in various zones (Fig. 4-7). At its thickest regions the lens capsule represents the thickest basement membrane in the body. The relative thickness of the anterior capsule compared with the cap-

---

* References 2, 3, 8–10, 16, 18, 24, 36, 38.

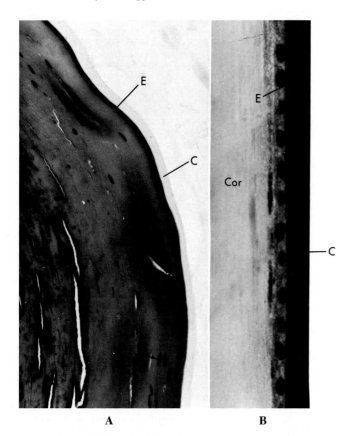

A **B**

Fig. 4-6. A, Equatorial region of the crystalline lens showing the capsule *(C)* situated adjacent to the epithelium *(E)* on the anterior aspect. Epithelial nuclei separate from the capsule at the equator as new fibers are laid down. *Arrows,* Ingrowth of lens nuclei at the equator; each nucleus represents a newly formed fiber. The nuclei disappear as the center of the lens is approached (toward the left). The lens capsule *(C)* is barely visible by routine staining techniques. (H & E stain; ×230.) **B,** Anterior lens surface stained by the PAS technique, which imparts a brilliant red hue to basement membranes. The anterior lens epithelium *(E)* lays down a basement membrane (lens capsule, *C*), which is thick anteriorly; it is the thickest basement membrane in the body. *Cor,* Subepithelial lens cortex. (PAS stain; ×625.)

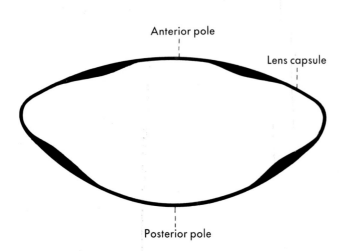

Fig. 4-7. Variations in thickness of the lens capsule.

sule at the posterior pole may be a result of the fact that it is directly adjacent to the epithelium and is actively secreted by it, whereas no lens epithelium is present on the posterior surface of the lens where the capsule is thinner. Because of the danger of rupture of the capsule during intracapsular lens extraction, it is of surgical importance to appreciate exactly where it becomes relatively thin and delicate.

Remnants of the tunica vasculosa lentis are common and appear as light gray opacities (Mittendorf dots) at or near the posterior pole. These opacities are rarely responsible for significant visual loss.

The zonular fibers, the zonules of Zinn, insert on the outermost surface of the equatorial lens capsule (Fig. 4-3). The fibers radiate from the ciliary processes and the valleys between them. The posterior border of insertion of the zonular fibers onto the lens coincides approximately with the insertion of the anterior face of the vitreous (the ligamentum hyaloideo-capsulario, or Wieger's ligament) onto the back of the lens. This 360-degree circular lens-vitreous adhesion corresponds to the outer borders of Cloquet's canal. Contraction of the ciliary muscle during accommodation results in relaxation of the zonular fibers. When this occurs, the lens capsule becomes relaxed and the lens becomes more spheric, increasing its refractive power.

EPITHELIUM

The lens epithelium is confined to the anterior surface and the equatorial lens bow. It consists of a single row of cuboidal-cylindric cells, which can biologically be divided into two different zones. The central zone is not directly concerned with the formation of new lens fibers but under pathologic circumstances has the capability to proliferate (Figs. 4-15 and 4-28). Some forms of anterior polar (Fig. 4-28) or anterior subcapsular cataract result from a reactive fibrous metaplasia of the epithelium (termed *pseudofibrous* by some authors). Although *pseudometaplasia* is technically correct because basement membrane is elaborated within the "fibrous" plaque (the cells are, therefore, not true fibrocytes in the strict sense of the word), the terms *fibrous* and *pseudofibrous metaplasia* are used interchangeably by most clinical ophthalmologists.

The second zone, the cells at the equatorial pole, normally shows mitotic capability, and new lens fibers are continuously produced here. Because cell production in this region is relatively active, the cells are rich in enzymes and have extensive protein metabolism. These cells are responsible for continuous formation of all cortical fibers and account for a constant growth in size and weight of the lens throughout life. During lens enlargement the location of older fibers becomes relatively more central as new fibers are formed at the periphery. The older central fibers become increasingly less curved in contrast to the marked bowing present in newly formed fibers.

The normal absence of posterior epithelium is a reflection of the embryonic development in which the posterior epithelial cells of the lens vesicle migrate forward toward the center of the cavity (Fig. 4-1); therefore, lens epithelium on the posterior surface is seen only in pathologic conditions. The presence of lens epithelial cells, either normal in appearance or bloated and edematous (Wedl, or bladder, cells), reflects a posterior migration of lens epithelium from the equator (Figs. 4-17 and 4-19) and is diagnostic of cataract.

All lens epithelial cells possess the capacity to proliferate and undergo a fibrous metaplasia. With the advent of widespread intraocular lens implantation, this phenomenon has assumed an increasing importance (p. 174). Following extracapsular lens extraction, residual lens epithelial cells around the implanted pseudophakos may undergo such proliferation, thus forming unwanted opaque membranes (often called "cocoon" membranes, p. 145). The most commonly involved site is at the posterior capsule. Recent studies have shown that these membranes may be treated and destroyed by such modern treatment modalities as the Nd:YAG (neodymium-yttrium-aluminum-garnet) laser.

SUBSTANCE (CORTEX AND NUCLEUS)

The lens substance consists of the lens fibers themselves, which are derived from the equatorial lens epithelium. On cross-section these cells are hexagonal (Figs. 4-3 and 4-8) and are bound together by ground substance. After formation, the cellular nuclei of the lens fibers are present only

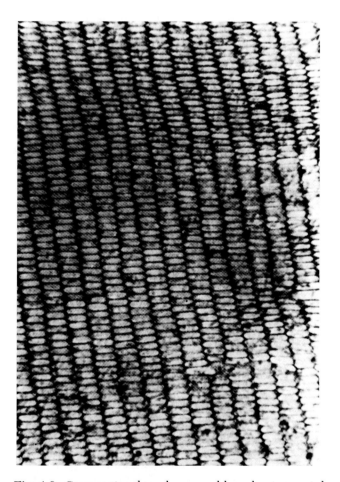

Fig. 4-8. Cross-section through a normal lens showing myriad lens fibers that are roughly hexagonal. Each fiber begins by mitotic division of the lens epithelium at the equator. After elongation of the original cuboidal epithelial cell, the cytoplasm forms elongated fibers and the epithelial cell nucleus eventually disappears. (Mallory blue stain; ×450.) (Courtesy Dr. Edward Cotlier.)

temporarily. Subsequently they disappear so the lens center is devoid of cell nuclei except in certain pathologic situations, for example, the maternal rubella syndrome (p. 134; Fig. 4-35, *B*).

The original lens vesicle represents the primary embryonic nucleus. This is a pinpoint-sized central focus by slit-lamp examination.[24,37] In later stages of gestation the fetal nucleus encircles the embryonic nucleus. The various layers surrounding the fetal nucleus are designated according to stages of growth, for example, infantile, adolescent, and adult nuclei. The most peripherally located fibers, which underlie the lens capsule, form the lens cortex. The designation *cortex* is actually an arbitrary term signifying a peripheral location within the lens rather than specific fibers. For example, the lens cortex in a 3- or 6-month-old child would be incorporated into the nucleus of an adult lens following continuous growth at the periphery.

Growth of the lens by deposition of new fibers occurs throughout the life span. Growth is slower after the second decade, and the lens does not increase much in size thereafter because a relative loss of hydration and shrinkage of the lens nucleus. Resulting nuclear opacities (nuclear sclerosis) may be only a physiologic change or may be sufficiently severe to cause visual difficulties. The lens capsule often thickens with age and loses some inherent elasticity, which is responsible for decreased capacity for accommodation and presbyopia.

Acquired cataracts

The slitlamp appearance of most types of cataract is well recognized.* In this chapter we emphasize the less well-known histopathologic alterations that correlate with the clinically evident opacities. Although clinical examination reveals myriad types of congenital and acquired cataracts, the pathologic reactions to the many possible forms of insults are limited, and the basic tissue alterations occurring in most forms are confined to a relatively few changes involving the major components of the lens: capsule, epithelium, cortex, and nucleus.

So-called senile (better termed *age-related cataracts*) (Fig. 4-9) and lens opacities resulting from trauma are the most common conditions that affect the lens and lead to visual loss. Following are the major types of acquired cataracts classified according to pathogenesis or association with generalized syndromes:

A. So-called senile cataracts
B. Traumatic cataracts
   1. Blunt trauma (contusion cataract, contusion rosette)
   2. Perforating trauma
      a. Perforation rosette
      b. Vossius' ring (deposition of iris pigment on the lens surface)
   3. Foreign bodies in lens
      a. Iron (siderosis lentis)
      b. Copper (chalcosis, sunflower cataract)
   4. Traumatic lens dislocation
   5. Chemical burns
   6. Radiant energy

---

* References 2, 3, 8-10, 16, 18, 19, 21, 24, 31, 35, 38.

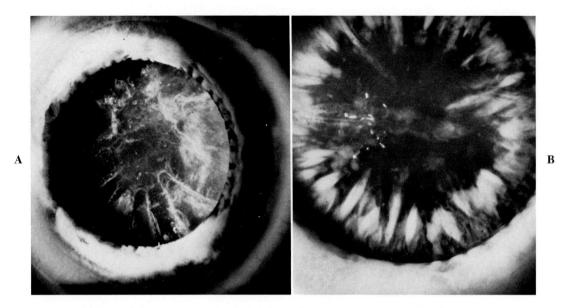

Fig. 4-9. "Senile" cataracts. **A,** Posterior subcapsular opacities. **B,** Cortical spoking. (Courtesy Dr. Ernst Martin Meyner, formerly of University of Tübingen, Tübingen, West Germany.)

    a. Glassblowers' cataract (true exfoliation of the lens capsule) caused by thermal effect of infrared light
    b. Radiograph cataract[20]
    c. Laser cataract
    d. Electric cataract
    e. Solar (ultraviolet) cataract[39]
C. Metabolic disorders (The list on page 129 includes additional cataract types associated with systemic syndrome.)
    1. Diabetes mellitus
        a. Early onset of senile cataract
        b. Snowflake cataract in juvenile diabetics
    2. Hypocalcemic or tetany cataract; seen in hypoparathyroidism, rickets, pregnancy
    3. Myotonic dystrophy
    4. Wilson's disease (sunflower cataract)
    5. Corticosteroid induced
D. Skin disorders
    1. Atopic dermatitis
    2. Neurodermatitis
E. Complicated cataracts[12,29] (opacities caused by associated intraocular disease) such as
    1. Uveitis
    2. Fuchs' heterochromic iridocyclitis
    3. Glaucoma (glaukomflecken)
    4. Retinitis pigmentosa
    5. Retinal detachment
    6. Fuchs' endothelial corneal dystrophy
    7. Intraocular tumors
    8. Myopia
F. Drug-induced cataracts
    1. Corticosteroids (posterior subcapsular or diffuse in type)
    2. Busulfan (Myleran)[19]
    3. Triparanol (MER-29)
    4. Phospholine iodide
    5. Phenothiazines[7]
    6. Antibiotics

The origin of most senile cataracts is still largely unknown. Following are the four main clinical types:

1. Nuclear sclerosis: caused by decrease in nuclear water content, sometimes progressing to a brunescent cataract (brown or yellow discoloration)
2. Cupuliform: most commonly manifest as a posterior cortical subcapsular plaque (Fig. 4-9, *A*)
3. Cuneiform: peripheral cortical "spokes" (Fig. 4-9, *B*) with radially coursing water-filled clefts caused by separation of cortical fiber lamellae
4. Perinuclear punctate cataract: punctate or dust-like opacities in the perinuclear cortex

The clinical staging of senile cataracts is as follows:

1. Incipient: peripheral opacities only
2. Premature: more diffuse opacities but at an early stage
3. Provecta: intumescent, moderately advanced
4. Mature: "ripe," total opacification and liquefaction
5. Hypermature: "overripened," a total cataract, sometimes progressing from the stage of a morgagnian cataract to a shrunken membranous cataract after spontaneous loss of liquid protein and resorption of liquefied cortex (Figs. 4-21–4-23).

The histopathologic changes corresponding to the preceding stages are described in Box 4-1.

Breaks or ruptures

The lens capsule most commonly ruptures after accidental or surgical trauma, inflammatory processes, or other insults (Figs. 4-10, 4-11, 4-12, 4-13; Color Plate 4-1). In histopathologic sections a ruptured capsule typically appears as a wrinkled or coiled membrane (Fig. 4-12, *B*), which is visually enhanced with the PAS stain.

A Soemmering ring cataract (Figs. 4-10 and 4-11; Color Plate 4-1) usually follows rupture of the lens capsule, in most cases as a result of perforating corneal trauma.

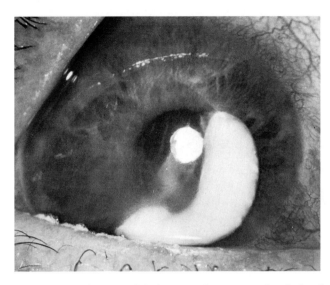

Fig. 4-10. Dislocation of the lens into the anterior chamber and formation of a partial Soemmering ring cataract following corneal perforation and rupture of the anterior lens capsule. In this case the ring is only one-third complete.

Box 4-1. General histopathologic features of cataracts.

Capsule

The lens capsule may undergo the following pathologic alterations:
1. Breaks or ruptures
2. Diffuse or focal thickening
3. Lamellar splitting
4. Pseudoexfoliation
5. Surface deposits
   a. Remnants of the hyaloid vessels
   b. Melanin: in pigmentary dispersion syndrome with a Krukenberg spindle, Vossius' ring after trauma, and melanin deposits after uveitis
   c. Hirschberg-Elschnig pearls

A form of Soemmering's ring is created when a surgeon performs a modern, planned extracapsular extraction (Color Plate 4-1). This is usually done in conjunction with implantation of an intraocular lens. In most cases the surgeon leaves intact the posterior and equatorial portions of the capsule. Even under the best of circumstances, small remnants of epithelial cells and cortical material remain at the equator. These epithelial remnants (analogous to Hirschberg-Elschnig pearls) may later haunt the surgeon by undergoing a proliferation or fibrous metaplasia. This change can lead to unwanted perilenticular, or "cocoon," membranes around the implanted lens (pp. 145 and 146, Figs. 4-54 and 4-55) or, in extremely rare instances, a "toxic lens syndrome" caused by a phacotoxic or phacoanaphylactic endophthalmitis (p. 136).

Figure 4-10 shows a partial Soemmering ring in which about a third of the equatorial cortex remains intact. Clinically, a complete Soemmering ring cataract resembles a doughnut. The center of the doughnut is usually composed

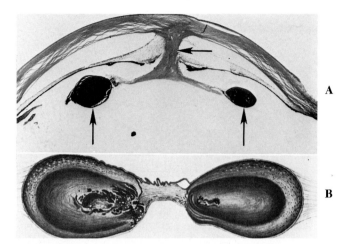

Fig. 4-11. A, Globe enucleated after perforating trauma of the central cornea. *Upper arrow,* Wound track with formation of an adherent leukoma between the cornea and a Soemmering ring cataract. Pupillary block by the fibrous membrane creates an anterior displacement or anterior bowing of the iris. The central contents of the lens have extruded through a rupture in the anterior lens capsule. The only residual lens cortical material is in the equatorial region *(lower arrows).* This barbell shape of the lens in sections correlates with the doughnut shape seen during clinical and gross examination (Color Plate 4-1). (H & E stain; ×15.) **B,** Schematic drawing of a Soemmering ring. (**A:** In Henke F and Lubarsch O, editors: Handbuch der speziellen pathologischen Anatomie und Histologie, Berlin, 1928, Julius Springer; **B** from von Szily.)

of a membrane formed by the residual lens capsule (Color Plate 4-1). Because they share a common pathogenesis, an adherent leukoma and a Soemmering ring cataract often occur in a single eye (Fig. 4-11, *A*).

Microscopic examination of tissue sections reveals that the doughnut-shaped lens clinically or grossly resembles a barbell (Fig. 4-11). The central contents of the lens extrude through the ruptured lens capsule and subsequently are resorbed. The anterior and posterior capsules of the lens are, therefore, in apposition, forming the shaft of the barbell. Because residual lens cortical material usually is retained in the equatorial region, the bulbous prominences remain visible at the equators. Occasionally, the entire contents of the lens are lost and the lens is reduced to a shrunken membranous cataract, a flat membrane composed only of remnants of the capsule and fibrous tissue (Fig. 4-12).

Hirschberg-Elschnig pearls

Hirschberg-Elschnig pearls (Fig. 4-13) occasionally are associated with a rupture of the lens capsule following accidental or surgical trauma and are, therefore, sometimes associated with a Soemmering's ring (Fig. 4-14). As mentioned before, they may occur after planned extracapsular cataract extractions. Disrupted subcapsular lens epithelial cells are displaced through the rent in the capsule into the anterior chamber and settle on the lens or iris surface. Because the anterior chamber fluid is an ideal medium for cell growth, the cells regenerate and proliferate in this abnormal location. Microscopically the pearls resemble clusters of bladder cells (p. 125). The latter also represent

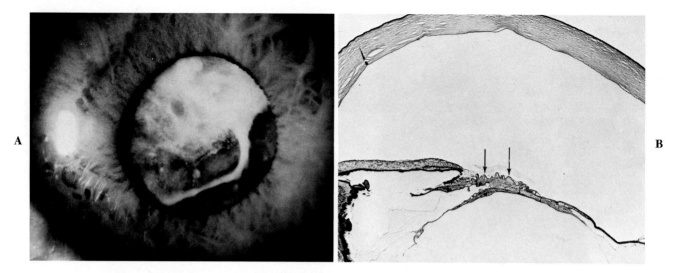

Fig. 4-12. Membranous cataract (after cataract). The lens substance is resorbed after capsular rupture. **A,** Clinical photograph. **B,** The lens substance has almost completely resorbed, leaving only a plaque of fibrous tissue derived from the epithelium sandwiched between the anterior and posterior portions of the capsule. *Arrows,* Folded capsule. (H & E stain; ×10.) (**A** courtesy Dr. Ernst Martin Meyner, formerly of University of Tübingen, Tübingen, West Germany.)

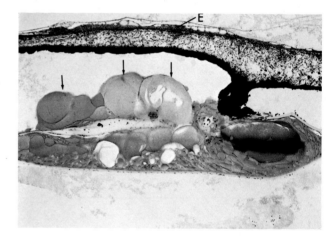

Fig. 4-13. Hirschberg-Elschnig pearls *(arrows).* These clusters of swollen epithelial cells situated on the lens capsule resemble bladder cells. *I,* Iris stroma; *E,* epithelial downgrowth caused by perforating trauma. (From Naumann GOH and Apple DJ: In Doerr W, Seifert G, and Uehlinger E, editors: Handbuch der speziellen pathologischen Anatomie, Band Auge, Berlin, 1980, Springer-Verlag.)

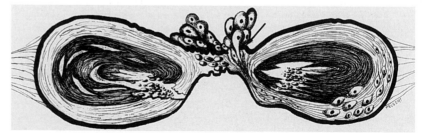

Fig. 4-14. Schematic illustration demonstrating pathogenesis of a Soemmerring's ring cataract. Note the perforation of the anterior lens capsule *(arrow)* with extrusion of lens material, forming Elschnig's pearls. As the central lens substance is extruded, the remaining cortical material peripherally forms the typical pattern of a Soemmerring's ring.

abnormally located lens epithelial cells; they are found within the posterior aspect of a cataractous lens. The pearls become clinically visible when they proliferate sufficiently to produce large clusters of cells (Fig. 4-13).

Diffuse or focal thickening

Diffuse thickening of the capsule occurs as a normal aging process. Focal excrescences have been documented in several types of congenital cataract, particularly in Lowe's syndrome and Down syndrome (p. 49).

Lowe's syndrome is characterized by development of mental retardation, renal rickets, general hypotonia, congenital cataract, and glaucoma.[40,49,65,70,76] Observed only in males, the disease is transmitted as an X-linked recessive trait. These children typically exhibit generalized aminoacidemia and systemic acidosis, with inability to produce ammonia in the kidneys.

The lens of Lowe's syndrome is typically small (microphakia), and wartlike excrescences on the capsule of the lens are an interesting histopathologic finding. Such capsular thickenings are not diagnostic of this syndrome; however, the small snowflake capsular opacities in the female carrier are considered typical of Lowe's syndrome and may be seen in other forms of congenital cataract. Perhaps the generalized amino acid disturbances are responsible for the qualitative changes in the lens protein, which may then create lens fiber opacities. Electrolyte changes in the lens protein may then create lens fiber opacities. Electrolyte changes in serum may result in aqueous humor acidosis and indirectly affect the permeability of the lens, with formation of lens opacities. According to Zimmerman and Font,[83] the glaucoma in Lowe's syndrome may be caused by the small size of the lens, which creates traction on the ciliary processes and apparently retards proper cleavage of the anterior chamber angle structures.

Lamellar splitting

See true exfoliation of the lens capsule, page 139.

Pseudoexfoliation

See page 136.

Surface deposits

Persistence of remnants of the embryonic tunica vasculosa lentis (see Figs. 2-23 and 2-24) can cause minimal to clinically significant polar opacities ranging from minimal to clinically significant (p. 28).

Melanin granules on the lens, usually derived from iris pigment epithelium, are common (1) in the pigmentary dispersion syndrome (p. 268), (2) after trauma (Vossius' ring, a circular ring of melanin on the anterior lens surface just behind the pupil), and (3) after intraocular inflammation. Hirschberg-Elschnig pearls are described earlier in this chapter.

EPITHELIUM

Proliferative changes

Fibrous metaplasia of the anterior or equatorial (lens bow) lens epithelium may lead to opacities.[16] The cuboidal epithelium of the lens has the capacity to transform into typical fibroblasts and fibrocytes, which may create an ante-

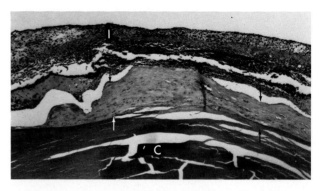

Fig. 4-15. Fibrous metaplasia of the anterior lens epithelium (caused by uveitis) forming an anterior subcapsular plaque *(arrows)*. *I,* Inflammatory membrane in anterior chamber and iris; *C,* lens cortex. (H & E stain; ×50.)

rior subcapsular fibrous plaque (Figs. 3-65, 4-15, and 4-28). This type of cataract is a common response to many types of irritation or disruption of the anterior lens, particularly trauma and uveitis. This is also the mechanism of formation of the so-called reduplication cataract, in which multiple layers of such plaques are laid down with intervening layers of normal cortex.

As noted on page 174, a similar type of proliferation and fibrous metaplasia (pseudometaplasia) of residual lens epithelium following extracapsular lens extraction may occur around an implanted intraocular lens. It may progress to a formation of an opaque fibrous membrane around the lens optic (a form of cocoon membrane). This important complication of intraocular lens implantation can lead to severe visual loss (Figs. 4-64 to 4-69).

One of the most common pathologic reactions of the lens epithelium is an abnormal overgrowth or proliferation of the equatorial cells, creating a posterior migration of the lens epithelium (Figs. 4-16 to 4-19). This reaction occurs in most idiopathic "senile" posterior subcapsular (cupuliform) cataracts.[11,13,17] Epithelial cells are not seen on the posterior surface of a normal lens. Possibly this abnormal proliferation represents an abortive attempt to replace the degenerate, often liquefied lens substance in the cataractous lens (Figs. 4-16 to 4-24).

In addition to simple posterior migration, the epithelial cells typically become bloated or swollen as a result of imbibition of proteinaceous fluid derived from liquefied cortical fibers. These swollen cells are bladder cells or Wedl cells (Fig. 4-17).[38] (See also Hirschberg-Elschnig pearls, p. 123.)

Posterior migration and bladder cell formation signify a histopathologic lesion, not a specific disease. Such diverse conditions as senile cataract, secondary traumatic cataract, and congenital cataract associated with hyaloid vascular remnants therefore, can create an identical tissue reaction (Fig. 4-19).

Degenerative changes

Deposits of iron in the lens epithelium (siderosis lentis; Fig. 3-65, *A*) or copper (chalcosis) may lead to eventual atrophy of these cells.

Glaukomflecken (cataracta disseminata subcapsularis glaucomatosa; p. 275; see Fig. 6-25) are multiple gray-

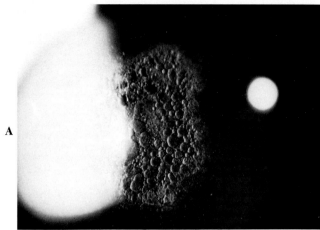

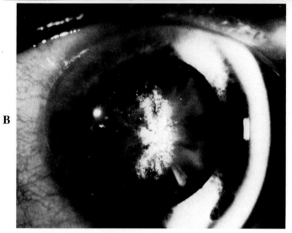

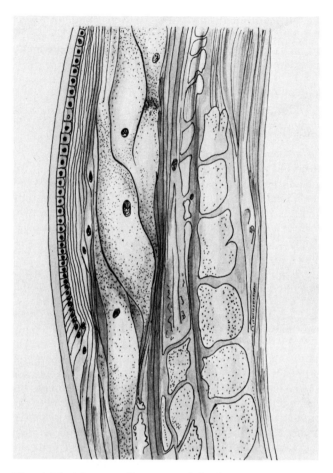

Fig. 4-16. A, Clinical appearance of a steroid cataract with posterior subcapsular cataract. **B,** Posterior subcapsular cortical cataract, "senile" type. (Courtesy Dr Ernst Martin Meyner, formerly of University of Tübingen, Tübingen, West Germany.)

Fig. 4-17. Schematic illustration of the lens equator showing "bladder" or "Wedl" cell formation. (Redrawn by Dr. Steven Vermillion, University of Iowa, from von Szily A: In Henke F and Lubarsch O, editors: Handbuch der speziellen pathologischen Anatomie und Histologie, Berlin, 1928, Julius Springer.)

white opacities. These areas of anterior epithelial and cortical necrosis are caused by interference in normal lens metabolism during acute rises in intraocular pressure.

SUBSTANCE

Nucleus

The bulk of the lens is made up of elongated lens fibers, which form the nucleus and cortex. New lens fibers are continuously laid down at the equatorial lens bow. The nucleus of each individual fiber is lost during maturation of the fiber; therefore, the center of the lens is normally free of cellular nuclei. These nuclei, however, may persist centrally in certain types of congenital cataracts (p. 134; Fig. 4-35, *B*).

Because of a complete encasement of the lens by its capsule, a desquamation or turnover of fibers is impossible. The older fibers are forced into the nucleus of the lens. In elderly persons the protein within the lens fibers denatures, thereby increasing dehydration and deposition of urochrome pigment, which leads to nuclear opacification. This nuclear sclerosis increases the refractive power, causing a lens-induced myopia. The pigment leads to a yellow-brown to black discoloration, cataracta brunescens or cataracta nigra.

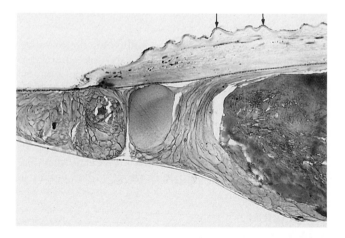

Fig. 4-18. Photomicrograph of a crystalline lens with a dense anterior subcapsular cataract caused by pseudofibrous metaplasia of anterior epithelium membrane at top of photograph. Note also a cortical cataract with marked liquifaction of cortical material. (H & E stain; ×150.)

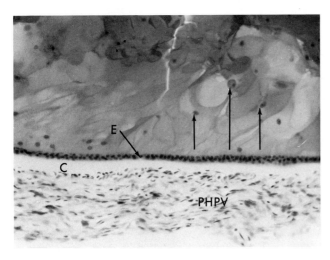

Fig. 4-19. Posterior aspect of a cataractous lens from an infant with persistent hyperplastic primary vitreous (PHPV). The nuclei of several bladder cells are visible in this plane of the section (*arrows*). The cells are swollen lens epithelial cells that have migrated posteriorly from the lens equator. They are pathognomonic of various forms of cataract. Normally no epithelial cell nuclei are present at the posterior pole. *C,* Lens capsule at the posterior pole; *E,* rows of epithelial cells that have undergone an abnormal posterior migration. (H & E stain; ×350.)

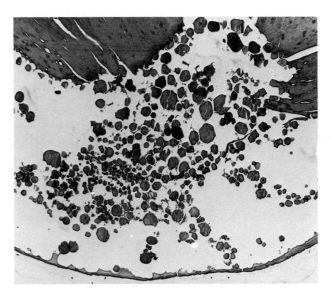

Fig. 4-21. The posterior pole of this lens with a mature cataract shows marked liquefactive degeneration of the cortex, with formation of morgagnian droplets or globules (not to be confused with *morgagnian cataract,* a clinical term, p. 122). (H & E stain; ×80.)

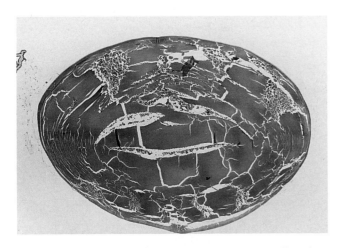

Fig. 4-20. Photomicrograph of a cataractous crystalline lens showing formation of numerous cortical clefts with numerous pockets of cortical liquifaction and degeneration. (H & E stain; ×4.)

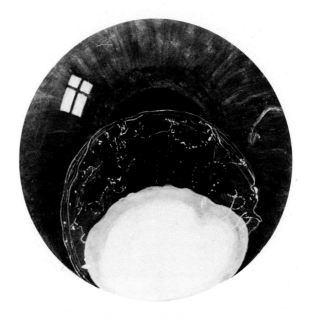

Fig. 4-22. Historical photograph of a morgagnian cataract in which not only is the lens cortex liquefied with suspension of the lens within the lens capsule, but the lens is also anteriorly dislocated. (From the collection of Professor Wolfgang Stock, University of Tübingen, Tübingen, West Germany.)

Histopathologically, nuclear sclerosis is seen as an eosinophilic amorphous mass within the center of the lens. The homogeneous consistency of the mass can be distinguished from the newer fibers of the surrounding cortex because the newer fibers often retain visible outlines of plasma membranes.

Cortex

Cortical liquefactive degeneration is an important histopathologic indication of cataractous change (Figs. 4-19–4-25). Such changes are frequently associated with the epithelial modifications described previously. The liquefac-

tion may be minimal or may advance to a more mature state (p. 128).

In microscopic sections the changes look like clefts between groups of lens fibers. Spheric droplets, termed *morgagnian droplets* or *globules,* often occupy the spaces within the clefts (Figs. 4-20 and 4-21). In vivo, such droplets represent a watery, milky fluid; however, during technical processing the fluid is chemically and physically al-

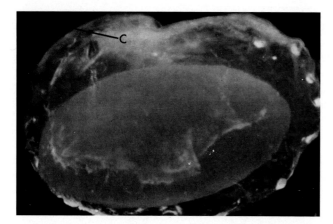

Fig. 4-23. Mature lens with a morgagnian cataract from a patient with phacolytic glaucoma. Following intracapsular extraction (note the intact lens capsule, *C*), the lens was immersed in an aqueous solution for this gross photograph. The nucleus is suspended in a sac of fluid cortex. Leakage of this protein-rich fluid through the intact lens capsule into the anterior chamber may evoke a macrophagic response, with subsequent phacolytic glaucoma. (From Goldberg MF: Br J Ophthalmol 51:847, 1967.)

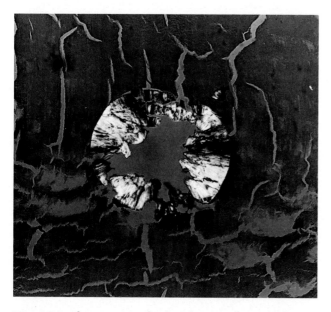

Fig. 4-24. Photomicrograph of a calcium oxalate crystal within a mature lens. The crystals exhibit birefringence—that is, they "glow"—if viewed microscopically through polarizing filters. The background lens cortex remains relatively dark. The crystal was partially shattered during sectioning. (From Goldberg MF: Br J Ophthalmol 51:847, 1967.)

tered in such a way that it assumes the appearance of multiple individual droplets. The morgagnian globule should be distinguished from a morgagnian cataract.[4] The latter is clinically defined as a liquefaction of the cortical lens, leaving a central solid nucleus that may descend by gravity to the base or the lower equatorial region of the lens (Figs. 4-22, 4-23, and 4-25).

Crystals are often present within mature lenses (Fig. 4-24). Many are composed of calcium oxalate and are most

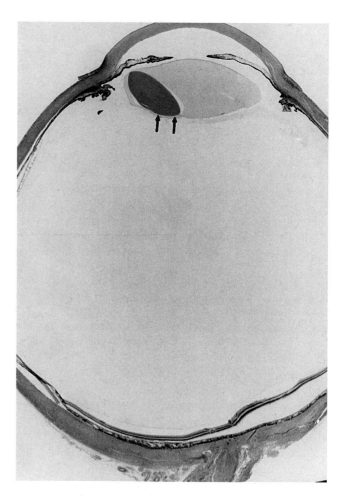

Fig. 4-25. Photomicrograph of a globe with a morgagnian cataract. Note inferior dislocation of the lens nucleus (*arrows*), and total liquifaction of the remaining lens. (H & E; ×1.)

visible by examination of tissue sections on the microslide with polarizing lenses. The precise geometric regularity in the arrangement of the molecules of the crystalline substance causes the crystal to "glow" against the background tissues when viewed by this special technique. Such mature lenses, which occur fairly often in elderly persons, may occasionally produce phacolytic glaucoma (p. 136).[15,28]

Bone formation in the lens (cataracta ossea) occurs as a dystrophic reaction to lens tissue, most commonly after trauma and in phthisis bulbi (see Fig. 7-22).

Deposition of intralenticular or perilenticular adipose tissue (cataracta adiposa or pseudophakia lipomatosa) occurs in a small percentage of cases of persistent hyperplastic primary vitreous (see Fig. 2-33). Embryonic mesenchyme within the retrolental mass enters the lens through a break in the posterior capsule and undergoes metaplastic transformation into adipose tissue (p. 136).

Developmental and congenital anomalies

Developmental and congenital lesions of the lens include absence of the lens, variations in lens size and shape (Fig. 4-26), abnormal locations (subluxation or dislocation) of the lens, and cataracts.[40-84] Approximately a third of all congenital cataracts are genetic. The most common mode of inheritance is autosomal dominant.

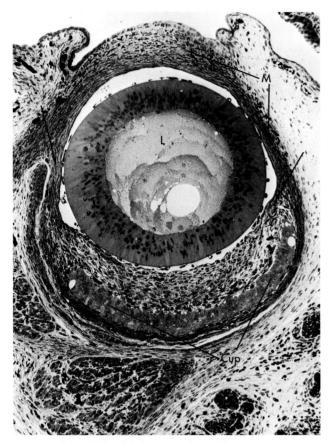

Fig. 4-26. Photomicrograph of an eye showing significant retardation of growth with extreme microphakia in which the lens *(L)* has not grown past the lens vesicle stage (Fig. 4-1). This specimen represents a clinical anophthalmia or an extreme microphthalmia. The development of the optic cup *(Cup)*, primary vitreous, and mesodermal structures *(M)* around the eyes is also greatly stunted. *Arrows,* Area of the surrounding mesoderm that has hindered the forward growth of the embryonic optic cup. (Mallory blue stain; ×300.)

The following outline categorizes congenital cataracts according to pathogenesis or association with systemic syndromes (modified from a classification of Dr. Edward Cotlier, Cornell University, New York; formerly of the Department of Ophthalmology, University of Illinois School of Medicine, Chicago):

1. Genetic disorders
   a. Dominant
   b. Recessive
   c. X-linked[72]
2. Viral disorders
   a. Rubella°
   b. Herpesvirus
   c. Cytomegalic inclusion disease
   d. Mumps
   e. Variola
   f. Vaccinia
3. Inborn errors of metabolism (autosomal recessive)

a. Galactosemia[46]
   b. Galactokinase deficiency
   c. Lowe's syndrome, X-linked°
   d. Phenylketonuria
   e. Mannosidosis
   f. Hypophosphatasia
   g. Tyrosinosis
   h. Aminoaciduria
   i. Hereditary spherocytosis
4. Associated with dislocated lenses (usually autosomal recessive)
   a. Homocystinuria
   b. Hyperlysinemia
   c. Marfan's syndrome
   d. Weill-Marchesani syndrome
5. Trauma
   a. Birth trauma
   b. Blunt trauma
   c. Perforating injuries
   d. Battered-child syndrome
   e. Radiographs (for retinoblastoma)
6. Dermatologic disorders
   a. Rothmund-Thompson syndrome (recessive)
   b. Congenital ectodermal dysplasia (dominant)
   c. Incontinentia pigmenti
   d. Ichthyosis
   e. Ehlers-Danlos syndrome
7. Endocrine disorders
   a. Congenital hypoglycemia
   b. Congenital hypoparathyroidism (recessive, dominant, X-linked)
   c. Laurence-Moon-Bardet-Biedl syndrome (recessive)
   d. Turner's syndrome
   e. Infantile diabetes
8. Neuromuscular disorders
   a. Myotonic dystrophy[50]
   b. Marinesco-Sjögren syndrome
   c. Smith-Lemli-Opitz syndrome[62]
   d. Cerebrohepatorenal syndrome
   e. Norrie's disease (X-linked)
   f. Refsum's disease
   g. Alport's syndrome[74,84]
9. Resulting from any retrolental mass (retinoblastoma, pseudoglioma)
10. Chromosomal anomalies
    a. Trisomy 13
    b. Trisomy 18
    c. Trisomy 21 (Down syndrome)
    d. Cri-du-chat syndrome (5 deletion)
    e. 13 deletion
11. Associated with bone malformations
    a. Chondrodystrophia calcificans (Conradi's disease)
    b. Hallermann-Streiff-François syndrome
    c. Apert's syndrome
    d. Crouzon's disease
    e. Albright's hereditary osteodystrophy
    f. Rubinstein-Taybi syndrome
    g. Ellis–van Creveld syndrome (recessive)
12. Associated with other eye malformations

° References 43–45, 47, 51, 55–57, 59, 63, 64, 71, 73, 74, 77–83.

° References 40, 49, 65, 70, 76, 83.

a. Microphthalmos
b. Rieger's anomaly (dominant)
c. Peters' anomaly (recessive)
d. Henkind's iridogoniodysgenesis (recessive)
e. Meckel syndrome
13. Miscellaneous
a. Cockayne's syndrome
b. Aniridia (sporadic or associated with Wilms' tumor)
c. Treacher Collins' syndrome (dominant)
d. Pierre Robin syndrome (dominant, recessive)
e. de Lange's syndrome
f. Bonnevie-Ullrich syndrome
g. Tuberous sclerosis
h. Resulting from intrauterine irradiation or drug toxicity

Selected lens anomalies are described according to the following classification, which is based on morphologic criteria:

1. Congenital aphakia
2. Variations in size and shape
   a. Lens umbilication
   b. Lens coloboma
   c. Microspherophakia
   d. Anterior and posterior lenticonus (globus)
   e. Disc-shaped cataracts
3. Polar and pyramidal cataracts
4. Nuclear cataracts
5. Sutural cataracts
6. Miscellaneous (clinical designations with unknown or nonspecific histopathology)
   a. Zonular cataracts
   b. Lamellar cataracts
   c. Cataracta pulverulenta (floriformis)
   d. Cataracta coronaria
   e. Cataracta coerulea

CONGENITAL APHAKIA

In primary congenital aphakia the lens vesicle fails to form.[41,68] This is rare and implies a lack of inductive contact between the neuroectodermal optic vesicle and the adjacent surface ectoderm, a contact necessary for lens differentiation (p. 118). Almost always a globe with primary aphakia would be expected to suffer from multiple severe malformations because the defect is induced early in gestation (Fig. 2-1).

Secondary congenital aphakia is more common, particularly in stillborn infants and aborted fetuses. The primary causes of secondary aphakia, in which the lens forms but is completely or partially resorbed, are probably intrauterine trauma and inflammation. Histopathologic examination in such cases reveals lens remnants, such as coiled fragments of lens capsule, which are not clinically evident. In most cases the common pathogenetic factor appears to be a rupture of the lens capsule, with resorption of the lens cortex and nucleus.

VARIATIONS IN SIZE AND SHAPE

Lens umbilication

A congenital umbilication of the lens is rare. Most of these cases represent a fixation artifact that occurs in almost all infantile eyes in which a craterlike depression is present on the posterior lens surface.

Lens coloboma

A congenital notch in the lens (Color Plate 2-2) is usually but not always based on abnormal closure of the embryonic fissure. The primary lesion may be a small coloboma of the adjacent ciliary body with defective development of the zonules and, hence, the lens in that quadrant.

Microspherophakia

Microspherophakia (Fig. 4-27) may be an isolated anomaly but is more commonly associated with conditions such as Lowe's syndrome* or any condition that causes an early arrest in the development of the lens or the eye as a whole.

---

* References 40, 49, 65, 70, 76, 83.

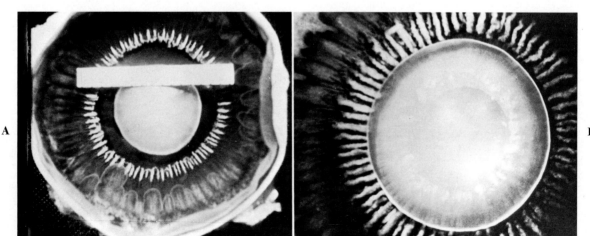

Fig. 4-27. A, Microphakia: view of a gross specimen from behind. The small lens is widely separated from the ciliary processes. (Compare with **B.**) **B,** The equatorial border of this normal-sized lens rests in a normal position in relation to the ciliary processes. (From Daicker B: Anatomie und Pathologie der menschlichen retino-ziliaren Fundusperipherie, Basel, 1972, S Karger, AG.)

An important complication of microspherophakia is the development of congenital or infantile glaucoma (p. 272), possibly as a result of a pupillary block mechanism.[83]

Lenticonus (lentiglobus)

The terms *lenticonus* (cone shape) and the closely related *lentiglobus* (spheric shape) apply to prominent elevation or bulging that may occur on the anterior-to-posterior surfaces of the lens (Fig. 4-28); Color Plate 4-3).[66] In such cases the lens is not necessarily opaque. A pyramid-shaped protrusion from the anterior pole, inducing opacity of the involved fibers, is termed an *anterior pyramidal cataract*.

DISC-SHAPED OR MEMBRANOUS CATARACTS

Probably the most common type of congenital or infantile cataract seen in the ophthalmic pathology laboratory is caused by prenatal or postnatal trauma. In most instances the lens capsule ruptures and the intralenticular contents are extruded. A dumbbell or disc-shaped cataract (Soemmering's ring) may be formed in which residual cortex is present only in the equatorial regions (Figs. 4-10 and 4-11; Color Plate 4-1). In the event that most or all of the

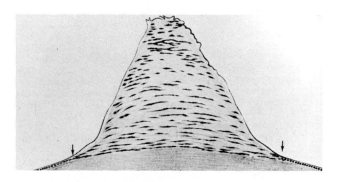

Fig. 4-28. Most anterior polar or anterior pyramidal cataracts are caused by fibrous metaplasia of the anterior lens epithelium (*arrows*) forming a fibrous plaque or mound (Color Plate 4-3). (From von Szily A: In Henke F and Lubarsch O, editors: Handbuch der speziellen pathologischen Anatomie und Histologie, Berlin, 1928, Julius Springer.)

lens substance is resorbed, a so-called membranous cataract results in which only layers of residual lens capsule are apparent. This can also be classified as a secondary congenital or infantile aphakia if the lens is not visible clinically.

POLAR AND PYRAMIDAL CATARACTS

Polar cataracts are opacities located at the anterior or posterior pole of the lens. Anterior polar cataracts (Color Plates 4-3 to 4-5) are often caused by a fibrous metaplasia, or pseudometaplasia, of the anterior lens epithelium (Fig. 4-28; Color Plate 4-2).[58] If the opacity protrudes noticeably, it is termed a *pyramidal cataract*. These types of cataracts may be genetically transmitted, but the disturbed epithelial growth can also result from irritation caused by persistent fibers of the pupillary membrane (see Fig. 7-1), which may insert on the lens surface (Color Plate 4-4). A so-called fleck opacity is a collection of small white or pigmented punctate opacities at the site of the previous insertion of the embryonic pupillary membrane. The epithelial changes may also arise as sequelae to inflammation or trauma.

The Mittendorf dot (p. 30) and congenital posterior polar cataract are often related to irritation or pressure from the insertion of the posterior tunica vasculosa lentis (Figs. 2-23, 2-24, and 4-29) that may persist on the posterior pole of the lens.

The so-called reduplication cataract is characterized by proliferation of the anterior epithelium into several layers. These layers are separated from each other by intervening normal fibers; therefore, several discrete plaques of opacity form near the anterior surface and are separated by optically clear zones. This implies a period of abnormal epithelial growth, a successive period of normal growth, and a further period of renewed abnormal epithelial proliferation leading to the layered pattern of this type of cataract.

CORTICAL AND NUCLEAR CATARACTS

A wide variety of congenital cortical or nuclear cataracts (Figs. 4-30, 4-31, 4-32 and 4-35) occur. The time of formation of a nuclear opacity can be approximated by determin-

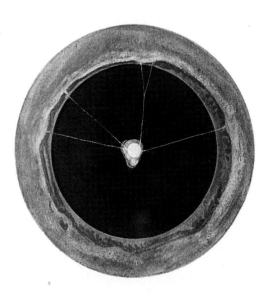

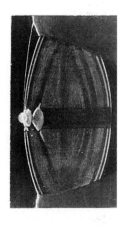

Fig. 4-29. Historical schematic illustration showing congenital anterior polar and subcapsular cataracts (anterior and sagittal view). Note associated delicate remnants of the anterior pupillary membrane.

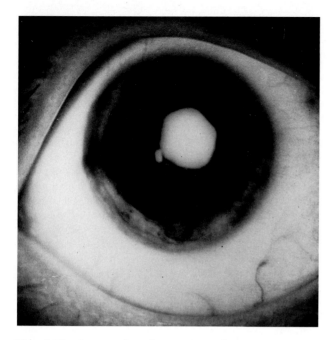

Fig. 4-30. Congenital nuclear cataract. (Courtesy Dr. Ernst Martin Meyner, formerly of University of Tübingen, Tübingen, West Germany.)

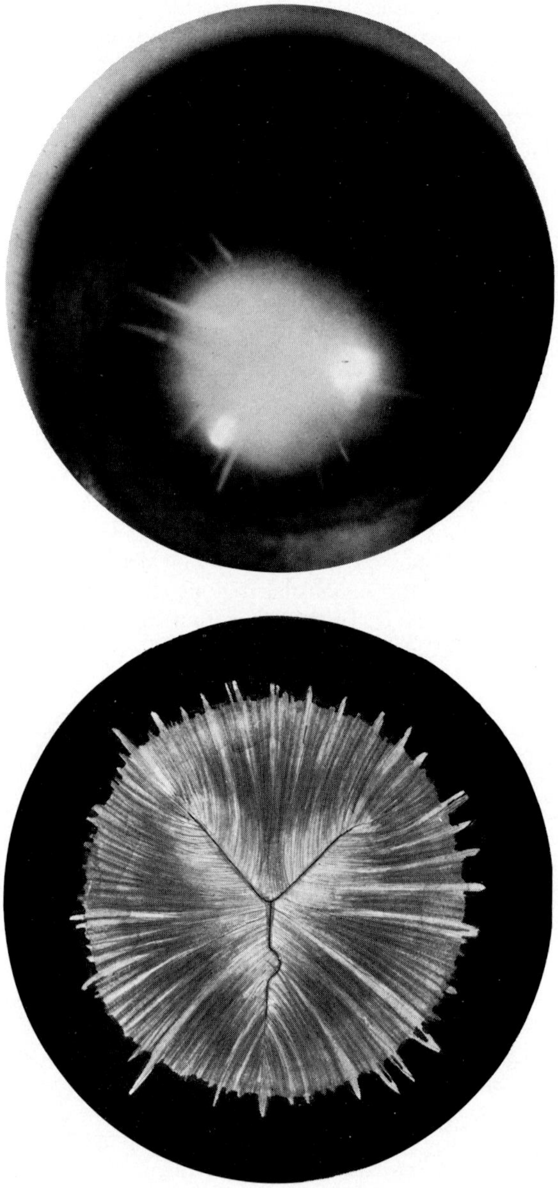

ing the exact location and size of the lesion. A central pinpoint lens opacity might connote involvement of the embryonic nucleus in the original lens vesicle. An opacity involving a broader area of the lens nucleus signifies further opacification during the fetal, infantile, or adolescent period.

The cataract of the maternal rubella syndrome (Figs. 4-33, 4-34, 4-35–4-36) is usually of the nuclear type* (Fig. 4-35). This syndrome, which occurred in epidemic proportions in the United States in the early 1960s, is manifest in its complete form by several systemic findings. These include failure to thrive, deafness, cardiac anomalies, patent ductus arteriosus, and thrombocytopenic rash. A moderate microphthalmia (Fig. 4-33) is common, and congenital cataracts occur in more than 50% of cases.

Three major histopathologic features permit diagnosis of the rubella syndrome by examination of the sectioned eye.

1. A characteristic necrotizing iridocyclitis may be present (Fig. 4-34). Such an inflammatory process is rare in most other conditions of infancy and childhood.

2. The rubella cataract involves a characteristic, although not pathognomonic, pattern of retention of lens fiber nuclei within the lens center (Fig. 4-35, *B*). The lens epithelial cells normally proliferate and generate new lens fibers by growth at the equatorial region of the lens (Figs. 4-2, 4-3, and 4-6). As new fibers are formed, the nucleus of the fiber disintegrates and disappears. In the rubella-infected lens these cells have an abnormal persistence of nuclei (Fig. 4-29, *B*). This retention of nuclear material is a manifestation of virus invasion of the proliferating cells.

---

* References 43–45, 47, 51, 55–57, 59, 63, 64, 71, 73, 74, 77–83.

Fig. 4-31. Congenital nuclear cataracts. **A,** Note "riders." **B,** Note prominent Y sutures. (**A** courtesy Dr. Ernst Martin Meyner, formerly of University of Tübingen, Tübingen, West Germany.)

The organism seems to produce an aberrant maturation of the infected cell nucleus.

3. Rubella embryopathy initiates only moderately severe insults in the globe, and major severe congenital aberrations such as anophthalmia, colobomas, persistent hyperplastic primary vitreous, or retinal dysplasia are noticeably absent.

Some rubella-affected eyes may have anterior chamber angle anomalies and infantile glaucoma. Occasionally a single case may exhibit variable involvement of each eye (Fig. 4-33). Buphthalmos may occur in one eye in which the angle involvement is severe; the other eye may show a moderate degree of microphthalmia, a finding more typical of rubella.

The most common clinical and histopathologic finding

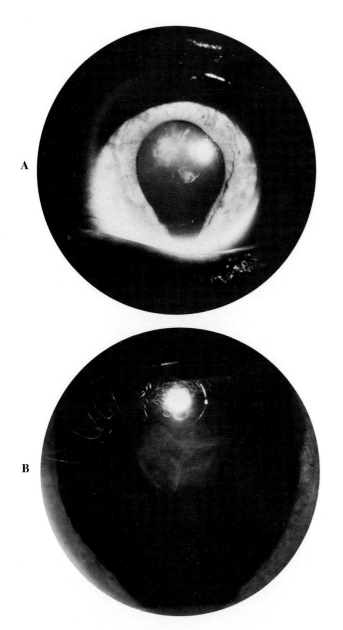

A

B

Fig. 4-32. Bilateral nuclear cataracts associated with typical iris colobomas. **A,** Right eye. **B,** Left eye, with prominent Y̌ suture.

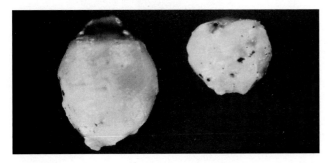

Fig. 4-33. Gross photograph of two globes enucleated at autopsy from an infant with congenital rubella syndrome. The left eye is buphthalmic because of anomalous anterior chamber angle differentiation; the right eye shows a more common finding, a moderate degree of microphthalmia.

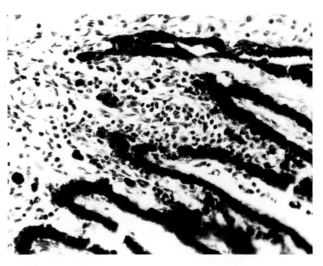

Fig. 4-34. Photomicrograph of the ciliary body in a case of maternal rubella syndrome. The infiltration of lymphocytes, round cells, and plasma cells indicates a necrotizing iridocyclitis. (H & E stain; ×150.)

of rubella is probably the so-called salt-and-pepper fundus (Fig. 4-36).[63,64,81] This pigmentary abnormality does not represent a migration of pigment into perivascular compartments of the sensory retina such as one observes with retinitis pigmentosa (Figs. 8-58 to 8-61). The pigmentary changes result from alternating in situ hyperpigmentation and hypopigmentation of the retinal pigment epithelium. These changes do not cause important clinical sequelae. This salt-and-pepper fundus can also be clearly distinguished from retinitis pigmentosa because the electroretinogram remains normal in patients with rubella retinopathy.

The widespread use of the rubella vaccine has resulted in a significant decrease in the incidence of the congenital rubella syndrome.

SUTURAL CATARACTS

The development and function of the lens sutures (Figs. 4-4, 4-5, and 4-37) were briefly described earlier (p. 119). Sutural opacities may exist as isolated phenomena (Fig. 4-31, *B*) or may occur in association with major systemic syndromes such as Fabry's disease (Fig. 4-37). Abnormal lens growth occurring extremely early in gestation (within the first trimester) produces simple Y̌-shaped sutural cataracts. Sutural opacities that exhibit secondary branching and arborization (Fig. 4-4) reflect a teratologic insult later in gestation, or even after birth, when the sutural pattern is more complicated.

Lens displacement syndromes

Most cases of subluxation (partial dislocation) or luxation (complete dislocation) of the lens occur under three circumstances: (1) most commonly after trauma, (2) in congenital or infantile glaucoma, or (3) on a developmental basis.[85–103]

TRAUMA

Dislocation of the lens is a common sequela to nonperforating or perforating trauma (Fig. 4-38).[90,92] Anterior dis-

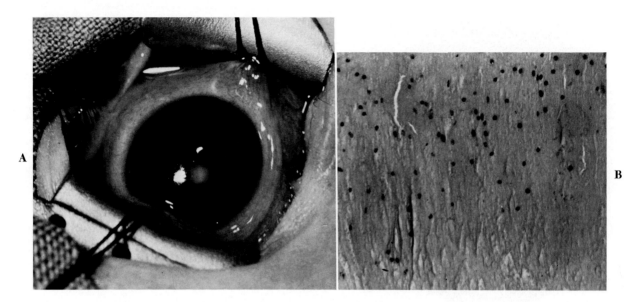

Fig. 4-35. Nuclear cataracts caused by rubella. **A,** Photograph before discission and aspiration. Although the typical rubella cataract is nuclear, more widespread involvement may be seen in certain cases. **B,** Photograph of center of lens. Pyknotic lens fiber nuclei (dark punctate spots) have persisted into the lens nucleus. (H & E stain; ×325.) (**A** courtesy Dr. Edward Cotlier.)

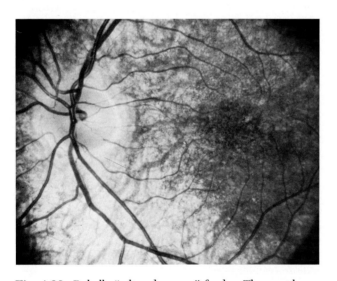

Fig. 4-36. Rubella "salt-and-pepper" fundus. The macular region is surrounded by diffuse pigment epithelial hyperpigmentation.

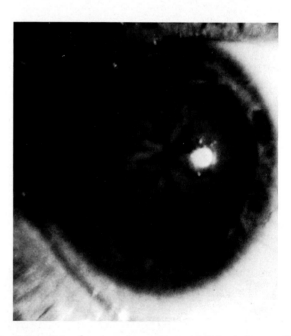

Fig. 4-37. Sutural cataract in a patient with Fabry's disease. The sutures have reached a point of extensive arborization in their formation as compared with the original **Y** sutures. This signifies an insult in development during late gestation or early infancy. (Courtesy Dr. Edward Cotlier.)

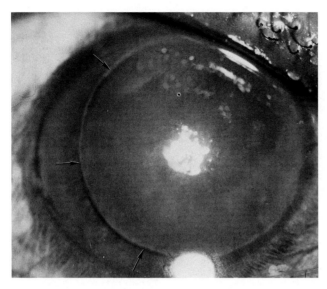

Fig. 4-38. Traumatic dislocation of the lens into the anterior chamber. *Arrows,* Outer margins of the displaced lens.

placement of the lens is extremely ominous because of the high risk of secondary glaucoma in such cases.[86] Secondary glaucoma may also follow posterior dislocation of the lens into the vitreous, but in many cases posterior dislocation is innocuous if the lens is deposited out of the visual axis.[101]

GLAUCOMA

Dislocation in congenital glaucoma is caused by rupture of stretched zonules (see Fig. 6-23).

DEVELOPMENTAL LENS DISPLACEMENT SYNDROMES

The developmental lens displacement syndromes (Color Plate 4-6; Figs. 4-39 and 4-40) in which the abnormality may be congenital or may become manifest long after birth include (1) ectopia lentis simplex, which may occur as an isolated genetically inherited syndrome (usually in an autosomal-dominant pattern); (2) ectopia lentis et pupillae,[87,94,98,102] in which the ectopic lens is accompanied by a displacement of the pupil in the opposite direction from the lens; and (3) ectopia lentis associated with widespread systemic syndromes. Examples of the latter group of diseases are Marfan's syndrome, homocystinuria, and the Weill-Marchesani syndrome. Less common causes are the Ehlers-Danlos syndrome and hyperlysinemia.

Marfan's syndrome, inherited in an autosomal dominant manner, is characterized by widespread skeletal abnormalities including arachnodactyly.[85,88,91,96,99] The most severe cardiovascular abormality is dissecting aortic aneurysm. Ectopia lentis, microspherophakia, iridodonesis, and anterior chamber cleavage anomalies are the significant ocular changes.[85] The lens subluxation of Marfan's syndrome frequently occurs in an upward direction (Fig. 4-39). In contrast, the direction of lens displacement in homocystinuria is more commonly downward and nasal.

Homocystinuria, inherited in an autosomal recessive manner, is an inborn error of metabolism involving a deficiency of cystathionine synthetase, an enzyme that converts

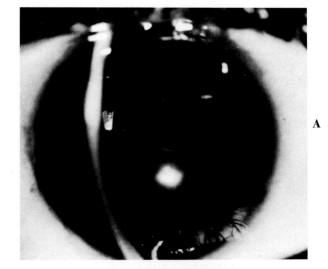

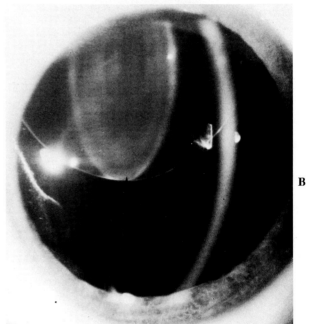

Fig. 4-39. Marfan's syndrome. **A,** Left eye. The upward and outward subluxation of the lens visible here is characteristic of this syndrome, in contrast to the downward, inward subluxation more often associated with homocystinuria. **B,** Right eye, with upward and outward subluxation of lens *(arrows).* (**A** courtesy of Dr. Edward Cotlier.)

methionine to cystine.[88,92,95,100] Patients with homocystinuria typically suffer from vascular thrombotic insults, and most of these patients also have ectopia lentis. In contrast to the partial subluxation seen more commonly in Marfan's syndrome, the propensity of lenses affected with homocystinuria to totally dislocate is probably explained by the fact that the zonular filaments clearly disintegrate. According to morphologic studies to date, the zonular fibrils of Marfan's syndrome appear relatively normal.

The Weill-Marchesani syndrome exhibits a picture of brachycephaly, short stature (in contrast to the tall, thin individual affected by Marfan's syndrome), ectopia lentis, and microspherophakia.[93,95,97,103] As in homocystinuria,

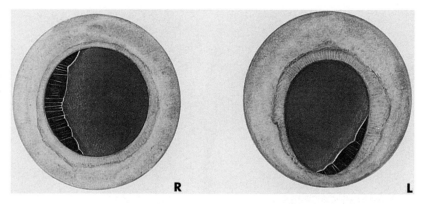

Fig. 4-40. Historic schematic illustration showing a case of bilateral congenital malposition of the crystalline lens. Right eye inward and left eye upward and inward malposition.

the lens more typically undergoes a total dislocation rather than a partial subluxation.

Lens-related ocular diseases

Abnormalities in lens structure or metabolism may play a primary role in the pathogenesis of several potentially severe intraocular diseases.[104–159] Four examples are phacolytic glaucoma, phacoanaphylactic endophthalmitis, pseudoexfoliation of the lens capsule, and true exfoliation of the lens capsule. The first three conditions are occasionally responsible for secondary glaucoma.

PHACOLYTIC GLAUCOMA

Phacolytic glaucoma occurs as a complication of leakage of lens protein from a mature lens (Figs. 4-23 and 4-41) into the anterior chamber and trabecular meshwork.[104–107] The affected patient is usually elderly, has a long-standing senile cataract, and eventually develops an acute congestive glaucoma. Clinical examination typically reveals a deep anterior chamber with flare and cells and a milky-appearing aqueous.

Liquefied proteinaceous material from the hypermature lens diffuses through a usually intact lens capsule into the anterior chamber. A macrophage response to this material occurs within the anterior chamber. These large cells contain small, centrally placed or eccentric nuclei. The cytoplasm of the macrophage that imbibes the lens material is foamy because of the staining characteristics of the ingested lens protein. The cells create a secondary open-angle glaucoma by mechanically blocking the outflow passages of the trabecular meshwork.

When the clinical diagnosis of phacolytic glaucoma is doubtful, an anterior chamber paracentesis is useful.[105,107] Cytologic examination of the aspirated aqueous fluid reveals the characteristic macrophages (Figs. 4-41, *C* and 4-42). Presence of the macrophages substantiates a decision for surgical intervention in such cases. Immediate and correct clinical diagnosis is essential because lens removal is generally curative.

PHACOANAPHYLACTIC ENDOPHTHALMITIS

Phacoanaphylactic endophthalmitis is considered an inflammatory reaction against one's own lens protein.[108–118] It is usually observed after any form of insult that produces rupture of the lens capsule, for example, after accidental trauma or following surgery, such as extracapsular lens extraction. Extracapsular lens extraction, including modern phacoemulsification, is performed much more frequently now than in previous years because of the efficacy of this method in association with intraocular lens implantation. In rare instances, the so-called toxic lens syndrome associated with intraocular lens implantation may actually represent a phacoanaphylactic reaction to the patient's residual lens cortex and not to the pseudophakos (p. 162). This concept is supported by the fact that the severity of some cases of toxic lens syndrome may increase after removal of the pseudophakos.

The reaction is usually unilateral unless the trauma and lens rupture happen to be bilateral. Occasionally, however, the condition may also involve the opposite eye, as a sympathetic response.[109] The reaction is initiated by an autosensitization to lens protein through the ruptured lens capsule. In oversimplified terms, the lens material apparently suddenly functions as a foreign protein or antigen after having been normally sequestered throughout life by the originally intact capsule. The presence of bacteria in the lens, as may occur with accidental trauma associated with contamination or following cataract surgery with localized endophthalmitis (p. 163), may exacerbate the inflammatory response.

A zonal inflammatory reaction is induced about the lens (Fig. 4-43). Varying types of inflammatory cell infiltrates form concentric zones. A central polymorphonuclear reaction around the lens destroys the outer cortex. More peripherally, infiltration of epithelioid cells and giant cells creates a granulomatous response, and the entire mass eventually may be encased in granulation tissue. The anterior uveitis may cause an initial hypotony. As cellular and exudative plugging of the outflow channels evolves, a glaucoma may ensue.

PSEUDOEXFOLIATION OF THE LENS CAPSULE (GLAUCOMA CAPSULARE)

Pseudoexfoliation, first accurately and thoroughly described by Vogt[159] in 1925, involves a deposition of dandruff-like particles (Figs. 4-44 to 4-46) on the tissue surfaces within the anterior segment.[119–159] It was termed *glaucoma capsulare* by Vogt and first designated as pseudoexfoliation by Theobald.[158] It is probably inherited, and it has a high incidence in the Scandinavian countries. In some cases a glaucoma is induced by blockage of the trabecular meshwork by the particulate matter.

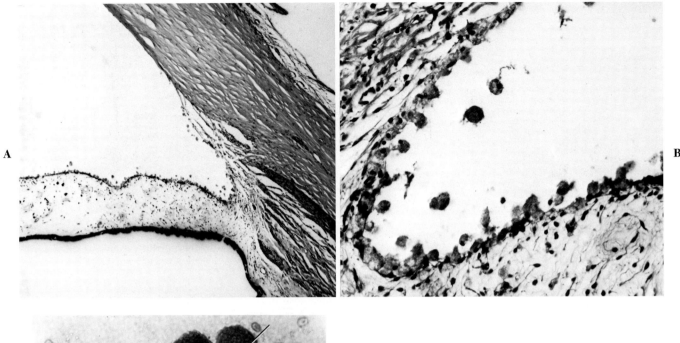

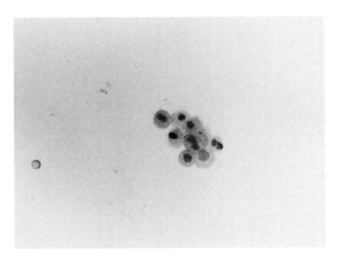

Fig. 4-41. Phacolytic glaucoma. **A,** Low-power photomicrograph of cells on the anterior iris surface and trabecular meshwork. (H & E stain; ×15.) **B,** High-power photomicrograph of the opposite angle of the same eye showing large macrophages in the angle recess. (H & E stain; ×320). **C,** Anterior chamber paracentesis and cytologic analysis of the aspirated aqueous fluid reveals the presence of these round, large macrophages. Such cells are often 40 μm in diameter and are diagnostic of the condition. *Arrow.* Nucleus of macrophage. (From Goldberg MF: Br J Ophthalmol 51:847, 1967.)

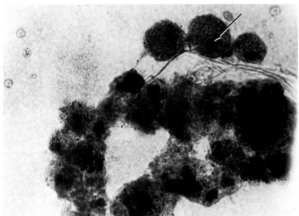

Fig. 4-42. High-power photomicrograph of aspirate from the anterior chamber in a case of phacolytic glaucoma showing large (40μm in diameter) macrophages (Papanicolao stain; ×350.)

Pseudoexfoliation occurs in elderly persons. The deposits on the anterior lens capsule have a characteristic picture in which a central disc of deposits corresponds to the smallest size of the pupil (Fig. 4-44, *A*). This disc is surrounded by a clear zone and a second peripheral band of material that extends to the equator. The clear zone apparently results from movements of the pupil so that the particles cannot accumulate. Material is also deposited on the zonules, iris, and ciliary body epithelium throughout the anterior chamber and trabecular meshwork and around conjunctival blood vessels.

Often a degeneration of iris pigment epithelium occurs with deposits of pigment within the trabecular meshwork similar to that seen in pigmentary glaucoma (Sampaolesi's line). Deposits of pigment also occur in the posterior peripheral cornea.

The mechanism of formation of the dandruff-like material (Fig. 4-44, *B*) has not been clearly elucidated. Major theories of origin include (1) derivation from the lens capsule, (2) formation from the epithelium of the ciliary processes, and (3) precipitation from the aqueous. The chemical nature of the material is unknown, but it probably represents fragmented basement membrane material de-

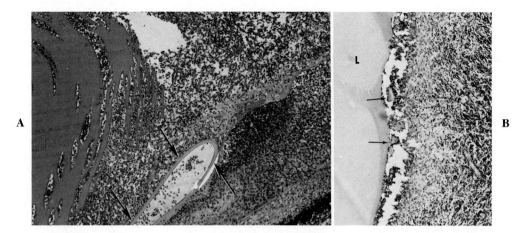

Fig. 4-43. Phacoanaphylactic endophthalmitis (lens-induced uveitis). **A,** Note the characteristic ruptured lens capsule *(arrows)* and infiltration of polymorphonuclear neutrophils into the greatly disrupted cortex of the lens. The pattern of this inflammatory process is characteristically zonal: the central polymorphonuclear infiltrate may be surrounded by concentric zones of granulomatous inflammation, nonspecific subacute and chronic inflammation, or areas of peripheral organization and scarring. Only the central acute focus is illustrated in this micrograph, but other sections more removed from the lens confirmed the presence of an epithelioid cell response. (H & E stain; ×150.) **B,** More chronic phase than in **A.** Numerous giant cells *(arrows)* and epithelioid cells are immediately adjacent to the lens *(L).* (H & E stain; ×250.)

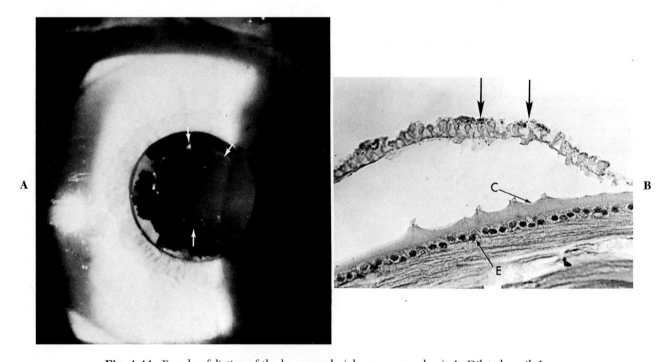

Fig. 4-44. Pseudoexfoliation of the lens capsule (glaucoma capsulare). **A,** Dilated pupil. Large sheets of material are visible at the pupillary margin left and below. The smaller ring of deposits more centrally located *(arrows)* represents a concentration of material laid down adjacent to the margin of the nondilated pupil. **B,** Flakes of so-called dandruff have layered *(large arrows)* above the surface of the lens capsule *(C).* There are three major hypotheses regarding the origin of this material: (1) derivation from the lens capsule, zonules, or both; (2) derivation from the ciliary epithelial basement membrane; and (3) condensation of precipitates from the aqueous. *E.* anterior lens epithelium overlying the lens cortex below. (H & E stain; ×400.)

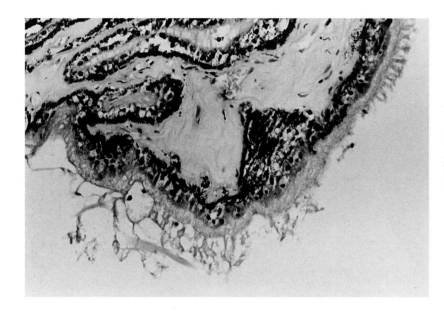

Fig. 4-45. High power photomicrograph of the ciliary body (pars plicata) showing deposition of pseudoexfoliation material derived from the epithelial basement membrane. (H & E stain; ×200.)

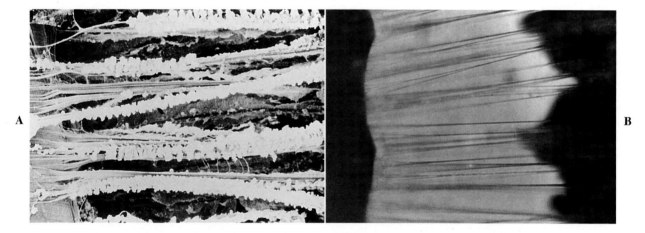

Fig. 4-46. A, Scanning electron micrograph of zonules from a case of pseudoexfoliation glaucoma, showing deposition of material along zonules. (Original magnification ×50; compare with Fig. 4-47, *B*, showing normal zonules.) **B,** High-power gross photograph of normal zonules in a healthy eye (compare with Fig. 4-47, *A*). (Vital staining with PAS; original magnification ×4.)

rived either from the lens capsule or other basement membranes in the anterior segment.

The term *pseudoexfoliation* is slightly misleading because if the material indeed arises from the lens capsule or the ciliary processes, the flaking off of the material would then be a true exfoliation. On the other hand, the so-called true exfoliation, or glassblowers' cataract, is actually not an exfoliative process but rather a lamellar splitting of the lens capsule.

TRUE EXFOLIATION OF THE LENS CAPSULE

True exfoliation is caused by exposure to radiation in the infrared spectral range.[127,129,131] It is an occupational hazard of glassblowers, but it can occur as an aging process in the absence of a definite history of environmental exposure to infrared light. The lens effect is probably caused by thermal shock of radiation on the capsule. The capsule

undergoes a lamellar splitting. The outer aspect of the membrane partially peels away (Fig. 4-47). As the capsule splits, it undergoes coiling because of its inherent elastic properties. The coiling creates the "scroll effect," an important clinical sign. Further opacification of the adjacent cortex may ensue, but in contrast to the three lens-related diseases just discussed, glaucoma is not an important complication.

Intraocular lenses

EVOLUTION OF INTRAOCULAR LENS IMPLANTATION

The magnitude of the cataract problem has been clearly defined in international and federal studies.[330] By the late 1990s, this number had increased to an estimated 20 million and this could double early in the twenty-first cen-

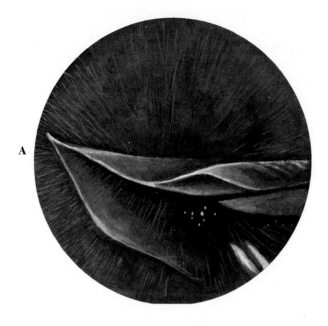

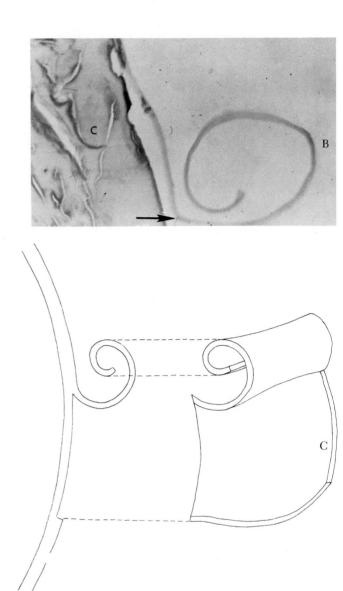

Side view   Frontal view

Fig. 4-47. A, Schematic illustration of so-called true exfoliation of the anterior lens capsule (glassblowers' cataract). **B,** True exfoliation of the lens capsule *(arrow)*. The involved capsule becomes curled on itself because of its inherent elasticity. This creates the scroll appearance seen clinically. *C,* Lens cortex adjacent to the capsule, which is situated on the right of this photomicrograph. (PAS stain; ×430.) **C,** Schematic illustration of pathogenesis of so-called true exfoliation of the lens capsule. Note the lamellar splitting and "scroll" formation of the capsule. (**A** from von Szily A: In Henke F and Lubarsch O, editors: Handbuch der speziellen pathologischen Anatomie und Histologie, Berlin, 1928, Julius Springer.)

tury.[183,295] As of 1984, it was noted that 12 to 15 million people worldwide were blind from cataracts.[330] Cataract is the most prevalent ophthalmic disease in terms of sheer numbers, and, according to the United Nations Population Division, the cataract backlog will continue to rapidly increase during the next five decades as the median age of the population increases.[421] Since the late 1960s, the number of cataract extractions per year has been steadily increasing, especially since the introduction of the intraocular lens (IOL).[160-433]

Although extensive research regarding the pathogenesis of cataracts is ongoing and a pharmacologic preventative treatment for this blinding disease is being sought, the solution still appears to be many years away.* Therefore surgical treatment for cataracts, which increasingly includes IOL implantation, remains the only viable alternative.

---

* References 160, 162, 240, 241, 252, 279, 308, 327, 344, 380, 415, 422, 425.

Intraocular lens (IOL, pseudophakos, phakoprosthesis, lenticulus, intraoculaire kunstlens [Dutch], Kunstlinse [German], or cristallin artificiel [French]) implantation is now a highly successful operation.[121,1121] Although follow-up for longer than 20 to 25 years of a large series of cases implanted with modern anterior and posterior chamber lenses is incomplete, data indicate that the complication rate has been greatly reduced during the last decade.

Treatment of cataracts has been practiced for centuries using various procedures such as medical therapy, couching, intracapsular surgery, and extracapsular techniques.[288,309,426] However, avoidance of complications and attainment of a high-quality postoperative visual rehabilitation in the years before the introduction of modern intraocular lenses was a difficult problem.[221,263,347] Significant dioptric power resides in the crystalline lens, so its removal results in marked visual disability.

Spectacle correction has been prescribed throughout history, but glasses have been less than satisfactory because of the visual distortions inherent in such high-power lenses.* In addition, aphakic spectacles are unsightly with their "Coke-bottle bottom" appearance. The thick lenses induce a Galilean telescopic effect, magnifying the world by an additional one third and thus drastically altering depth perception.

It was not until the late 1940s that the tremendous optical advantages that an IOL could provide in visual rehabilitation were understood and used by Harold Ridley.†

VISUAL REHABILITATION WITH INTRAOCULAR LENSES

In the last few years, several authors, studying large series of patients, have documented that excellent visual rehabilitation results have been achieved with IOLs.[161] Although reports of good short-term visual results with few apparent complications have been published concerning all lens types, analyses of follow-up reports have revealed that certain lens types and styles‡ have distinct advantages over others. As these data have been publicized, some of the less successful lenses have been withdrawn from the market.

Posterior chamber IOLs, following a long period of disfavor after the Ridley lens was discontinued, were reintroduced in the mid-1970s and early 1980s. Jaffe[299,300] and other authors compared posterior chamber lenses to iris-supported lenses and were impressed by the superior results achieved with the former type of lens following an extracapsular cataract extraction (ECCE) technique. Several other surgeons have also documented good visual results with lenses implanted after ECCE.§ The use of posterior chamber IOLs, therefore, is now clearly the treatment of choice, at least in the highly industrialized countries of the world.

In 1978 the Food and Drug Administration (FDA) began regulating IOLs implanted in the United States to collect data concerning IOL safety and effectiveness. Several reports derived from FDA data and other sources have been presented to the American Academy of Ophthalmology, although they are not actually considered official reports. More than 8 million IOLs were implanted in the United States from 1978 up to 1990.‖ As of 1991, at the time of the fourth edition of this text, an estimated 1.1 million IOLs were implanted annually in the United States. By 1998 this number had increased to more than 1.6 million annually. Implantation data from other countries are scanty, but the total number of implantations per year worldwide is increasing rapidly. Studies are still ongoing to determine which lens design will be safest, most practical, and most economical for high-volume use in the less advantaged areas of the world.

---

* References 275, 346, 355, 386, 387, 407, 417, 418.

† Rerenences 171, 184, 232, 294, 343, 355, 376, 377, 379, 381, 405.

‡ The term *lens type* connotes a general classification of IOLs according to the three basic sites of fixation: (1) anterior chamber, (2) iris, and (3) posterior chamber. An *IOL style* refers to the design or configuration of any type of pseudophakos, for example, an anterior chamber lens type may be either rigid of flexible, have open or closed loops, or may be uniplanar or vaulted. A *lens model* refers to the manufacturer's designation for any given lens.

§ References 226, 276, 286, 302, 314, 342, 371.

‖ References 244, 246, 406, 407, 409, 410, 412, 430, 431, 432.

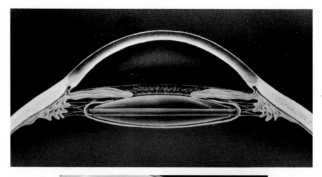

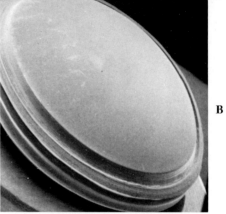

Fig. 4-48. A, Schematic illustration of a sagittal section of the anterior segment of the eye showing the original Ridley biconvex disc posterior chamber IOL implanted in the lens capsular sac following ECCE. **B,** Scanning electron micrograph of a Ridley lens removed from a human eye obtained postmortem. Note the peripheral ridge and the excellent finish quality of the biconvex optical surface. ($\times$10.) (**A,** Krystyna Srodulski, artist.)

Lens design

From the time of Ridley's first lens implantation to the present day, the evolution of IOLs can be arbitrarily divided into five generations.[165,171,178,355]

1. Generation I (1949): Original Ridley posterior chamber lens
2. Generation II (1952–1962): Early anterior chamber lenses
3. Generation III (1953–1973): Iris supported lenses
4. Generation IV (1963–1990): Modern anterior chamber lenses
5. Generation V (1975–present): Early posterior chamber lenses
6. Generation VI (1990–present): Modern capsular lenses, rigid PMMA and soft foldable designs

Generation I. A practical application of the concept of IOLs began with Harold Ridley[171,184] and credit for the introduction of lens implants clearly belongs to him. Ridley's first IOL operation was performed on a 45-year-old woman at St. Thomas Hospital in London on November 29, 1949. His original IOL was a biconvex polymethylmethacrylate (PMMA) disc designed to be implanted after ECCE (Fig. 4-48).

Ridley's first article[376] on IOLs was published in 1951, and his first lecture on the subject in the United States was presented at the fifty-seventh session of the American Academy of Ophthalmology and Otolaryngology, held in

Chicago, Illinois on October 12–17, 1952.[378] There he and his procedure were met with great hostility by several skeptical and critical ophthalmologists.[263] Good results, however, were attained in enough cases to warrant further implantation of the Ridley IOL (Color Plate 4-7). Other surgeons such as Edward Epstein[269,271,611] of South Africa carried on with this design and various modifications.

Generation II. Because of the relatively high frequency of dislocations with the Ridley lens, a new implantation site was considered: the anterior chamber, with fixation of the lens in the angle recess. There was less likelihood of dislocation with implantation in the narrow confines of the anterior chamber. In addition, anterior chamber lenses could be implanted after either an intracapsular cataract extraction (ICCE) or an ECCE. Anterior chamber placement of the pseudophakos was considered a simpler technical procedure than placing the lens behind the iris.[395]

Unlike the original posterior chamber lens, which Ridley inarguably originated, the design of the first generation of anterior chamber IOLs was a synthesis of the ideas of many surgeons who worked on the concept at essentially the same time. Baron,[198] in France, is generally credited as the first designer and implanter of an anterior chamber lens. He first performed this procedure on May 13, 1952 (Fig. 4-56, *A*).

Late endothelial atrophy, corneal decompensation, and pseudophakic bullous keratopathy were initially observed with the original Baron lens and were also seen with many other rigid anterior chamber lens designs. It took many modifications of the haptic/loop configuration and the lens-vaulting characteristics to develop an anterior chamber lens allowing a reasonable prediction of long-term success. This was achieved largely because of advances in lens design by Dr. Peter Choyce[230-239] of England and later by Dr. Charles Kelman[311] of New York. The Choyce lenses produced by his licensed manufacturers were carefully manufactured, finished, and polished. By the mid-to-late 1970s, however, several other manufacturers in the United States produced copies of the Choyce designs with sharp edges and warped foot plates. The entity we now term *uveitis-glaucoma-hyphema (UGH) syndrome* was first described when ocular tissue damage occurred that was clearly caused by these badly manufactured Choyce lens copies.[267,268]

Generation III. Iris-supported or iris-fixated IOLs were introduced in an attempt to overcome the problems with both Ridley's original posterior chamber lens and the anterior chamber lenses available in the early 1950s. Fairly frequent dislocation of the former lens and an unacceptably high rate of corneal decompensation with anterior chamber lenses caused some surgeons to entirely discontinue implantation of IOLS.[260,355]

Dr. Cornelius Binkhorst[200-220] of Holland was an early advocate of iris-supported IOLs. His four-loop iris clip IOL (Color Plate 4-8) design was based on four premises:

1. PMMA was well tolerated within the eye, provided it had been properly cleansed and sterilized.
2. The Ridley posterior chamber IOL had a tendency to dislocate, leading to its disuse.
3. Most anterior chamber lenses caused corneal decompensation.
4. Intraocular lens contact with the posterior surface of the iris did not cause complications.

Premise 4 was not entirely true and problems with iris chafing, pupillary abnormalities, and dislocation continued to be significant difficulties with the iris clip lens.[228,257,265,305] In an effort to circumvent dislocation, Binkhorst made the anterior loops of his four-loop lens longer, but this led to increased corneal decompensation from peripheral touch.[355]

Binkhorst occasionally implanted his four-loop lens following an ECCE rather than an ICCE.[383] His positive experience with this procedure prompted him to modify his iris clip lens for implantation following ECCE. The firm fixation of the lens to both the iris and the remaining lens capsule proved highly efficacious, especially in decreasing the amount of unwanted chafing against uveal tissues and decreasing the incidence of complications such as inflammation.

Binkhorst's change to ECCE and the introduction of his two-loop iridocapsular IOL (Color Plate 4-9) in 1965 were important advances in both IOL design and mode of fixation.[256] In many ways, these innovations culminated in modern capsular (in-the-bag) fixation of posterior chamber IOLs. The experience of Binkhorst and others with the two-loop lens style and its modifications were influential in leading to modern design concepts of IOLs.[197,213,220]

The original iridocapsular lens was produced by Binkhorst by simply removing the two anterior loops of his original four-loop lens design.[201-204] He first implanted this modified version in 1965, and this procedure quickly became his preferred implantation method. By eliminating the two anterior loops in front of the iris, he decreased the incidence of such problems as pupillary distortion, sphincter muscle atrophy, and iris chafing. Capsular fixation of the two loops offered much better stability, and the presence of an intact posterior capsule decreased the marked movement of the vitreous (vitreodonesis) and iris (iridodonesis) that often occurred after ICCE.[254] Sometimes the IOL optic would dislocate behind the pupil, generally a harmless occurrence that effectively rendered this a true in-the-bag posterior chamber lens.

The iridocapsular lens was introduced at a time when the entire future of IOL implantation was in jeopardy. Binkhorst's innovative lens design and his advocacy of ECCE provided the major impetus that set the stage for modern posterior chamber lens implantations.[301]

Generation IV. While iris-supported IOLs were undergoing major modifications in the early 1950s up to the beginning of the 1980s, several new designs of anterior chamber IOLs were being introduced. Well-designed, correctly vaulted, and properly sized anterior chamber lenses can provide excellent long-term results. As with the early generation of anterior chamber IOLs, new lens designs included both haptic (footplate) fixation lenses and small-diameter, round-looped IOLs.

Choyce[230-239] continued improving his anterior chamber lens design and implanted his first Mark VIII lens in 1963 (Fig. 4-61). This lens represented a departure from his seven earlier designs in that it had four foot plates instead of three. With careful surgical technique and proper sizing of the IOL, good results were commonly seen in patients implanted with these carefully finished lenses.

The problems of tenderness and difficulties in correct sizing associated with rigid IOLs were addressed by the development of anterior chamber lenses with more flexible loops or haptics. Unlike the ill-fated, nylon-looped lenses introduced by Dannheim in the early 1950s, the fixation elements of these anterior chamber IOLs were made from more stable polymers, usually PMMA and polypropylene. One of the first modern semiflexible anterior chamber lenses was the rectangular, all-PMMA, closed-loop Surgidev Style 10 Leiske lens introduced in 1978 (see p. 149). Several modifications of this general style were marketed by other IOL manufacturers.[335-374] For reasons to be described (see p. 146), the general class of closed-loop IOLs has been removed from the American market.

Various open-loop, one-piece PMMA designs, such as the three- and four-point fixation Kelman IOLs and their modifications such as proposed by Baikoff in France (phakic IOL) and Clemente in Munich (a three-point fixate design with no position holes in the haptic), have been in use since the late 1970s and 1980s and are the styles most generally implanted today.[771]

Generation V. Shearing[395] identified four major milestones that have marked the evolution of ECCE surgery: (1) microscopic surgical techniques, (2) phacoemulsification, (3) iridocapsular fixation, and (4) flexible posterior chamber lenses.

Without microscopic surgery modern IOL implantations would be far more difficult. Although phacoemulsification was originally promoted because of the small wound, it became clear that if an IOL were to be inserted, the wound would have to be enlarged after removal of the cataract, and thus nonultrasonic methods were refined. By the mid 1970s, implantation of IOLs again began to achieve significant acceptability. A natural marriage between phacoemulsification and implantation of IOLs occurred.[185]

Cornelius Binkhorst's iridocapsular IOL was among the first IOLs to achieve major recognition in this country. He was one of the pioneers in the return to the ECCE procedure.[210,211,218,278] Binkhorst came to believe in the superiority of the ECCE technique, recognizing that an intact posterior capsule enhanced stability, and he recognized the many advantages of implanting the IOL within the capsular sac.

Binkhorst's term *endophthalmodonesis* refers to the lack of stability within the eye from which the lens capsule-zonule barrier has been removed. He believed the absence of this barrier set up turbulence within the aqueous, possibly liquefying the vitreous.[209,210,212,218] Evidence continues to accumulate that cystoid macular edema[414] and retinal detachment[218,403] occur less frequently with ECCE than with ICCE.[218,403,414] It has been suggested that an intact posterior capsule also provides an important barrier against the diffusion of such substances as inflammatory mediators into the posterior segment—mediators that may in part be a cause of cystoid macular edema.

The introduction of flexible posterior chamber lenses designed to be implanted following ECCE largely resolved the debate about ECCE versus ICCE clearly in favor of the extracapsular procedure.

The return to the posterior chamber lens began in 1975.

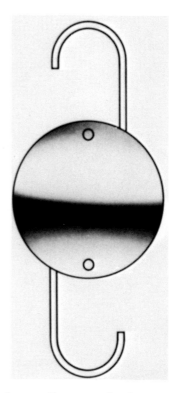

Fig. 4-49. Schematic illustration of a Shearing J-loop posterior chamber IOL, introduced in 1977. The two polypropylene loops were staked into the two injected, molded PMMA optics.

John Pearce[363-369] of England implanted the first uniplanar posterior chamber lens since Ridley. It was a rigid tripod design with the two inferior feet implanted in the capsular bag and the superior foot implanted in front of the anterior capsule and sutured to the iris.

Dr. Steven Shearing[248,291,325,358-360,391-395] of Las Vegas introduced a major lens design breakthrough in early 1977 with his posterior chamber lens (Fig. 4-49). The design consisted of an optic with two flexible J-shaped loops.

William Simcoe of Tulsa publicly introduced his C-looped posterior chamber lens shortly after Shearing's J-loop design appeared[397-399] (Fig. 4-50, *A*). Dr. Robert Sinskey of Santa Monica[400] and Dr. Richard Kratz of Newport Beach, as well as others, introduced various modified J-loop designs (Fig. 4-50, *B*). The original J-loop and modified IOLs had two polypropylene loops staked into an anteriorly convex–posteriorly planar PMMA optic. Dr. John Sheets of Odessa, Texas, and Dr. Aziz Anis of Lincoln, Nebraska, both introduced early closed-loop posterior chamber IOL designs. Dr. Eric Arnott of London was an early advocate of one-piece, all-PMMA posterior chamber IOLs, while Dr. Richard Lindstrom of Minneapolis introduced a modified J-loop lens with a reversed or posterior convex optic and loops made of extruded PMMA (Fig. 4-50, *C*).

The flexible open-loop designs (J loop, modified J loop, C loop or modified C loop) account for the largest number of IOL styles implanted worldwide. Generation VI modern capsular posterior chamber lenses designed specifically for in-the-bag (capsular) fixation now dominate the market. These include rigid PMMA designs and lenses made of

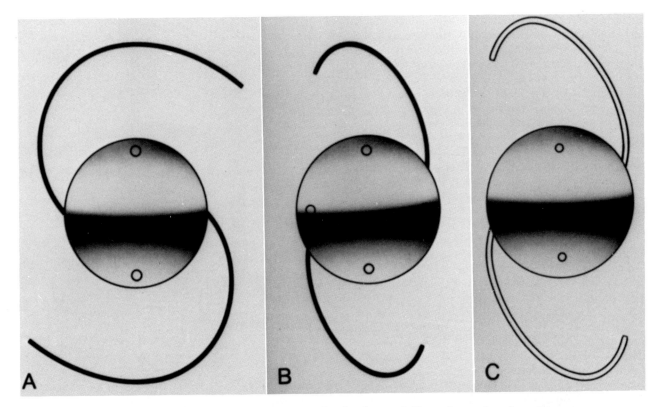

Fig. 4-50. A, The Simcoe **C**-loop posterior chamber lens with blue polypropylene loops introduced in 1977. **B,** The modified **J**-loop lens with blue polypropylene loops. This general design was introduced in 1980, first by Dr. Robert Sinskey and shortly thereafter by Dr. Richard Kratz. **C,** Posterior chamber IOL with extruded PMMA loops was introduced by Dr. Richard Lindstrom. This lens also has a modified **J**-loop design.

soft or malleable material that may be folded and inserted through a small incision. These capsular designs are described on page 156.

LENS FIXATION

In 1967 Binkhorst proposed a detailed classification of the various means of fixation for each IOL type.[207] In a 1985 update of this classification, Binkhorst listed four IOL types according to fixation sites:

1. Iris-supported lenses
2. Anterior chamber angle-supported lenses
3. Posterior chamber angle (ciliary sulcus)-supported lenses
4. Capsule-supported lenses

By common agreement most surgeons, therefore, differentiate lens types as (a) iris-supported lenses, (b) anterior chamber lenses, and (c) posterior chamber lenses.[324]

Iris fixation of iris-supported intraocular lenses

Fixation of the pseudophakos to the iris represented an attempt to avoid lens decentration and dislocation, a complication with Ridley's posterior chamber lens. This led to the development of iris-supported IOLs in 1953. Use of iris-supported IOLs in the United States has declined rapidly and these lenses are now rarely implanted.

Most iris-supported lenses were biplanar, with the optic placed in front of the pupil, such as the Binkhorst four-loop lens, the iris clip lens, the Fyodorov IOL, the

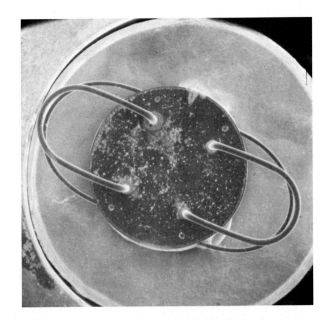

Fig. 4-51. Scanning electron micrograph of a four-loop iris support lens removed because of chronic uveitis. Inflammatory cells and protein deposits are visible on the lens optic surface. (×10).

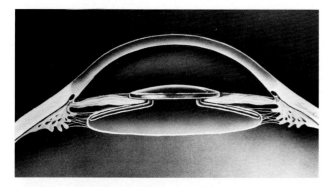

Fig. 4-52. Schematic illustration of a sagittal section of an eye containing a Binkhorst two-loop iridocapsular lens with the loops implanted in the lens capsular sac. (Krystyna Srodulski, artist.)

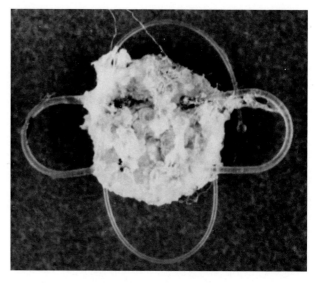

Fig. 4-54. Gross photograph of a removed four-loop iris-supported lens. Visible is a classic cocoon membrane composed of delicate, velvety white tissue that completely surrounds the lens optic. This patient suffered from "endothelial touch syndrome" with corneal decompensation. (From Apple DJ and others: Surv Ophthalmol 29:1, 1984.)

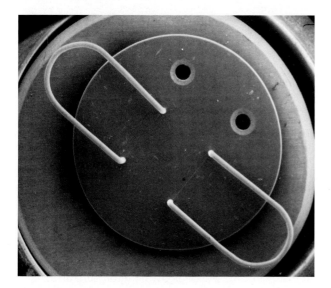

Fig. 4-53. Scanning electron micrograph of a two-loop iris support lens with iris suture holes in the optic. The nylon iris-fixation suture had disintegrated within patient's eye. Removal of the IOL was required when pseudophakodonesis and secondary inflammation developed. (×10.)

Binkhorst two-loop iridocapsular lens, and some lens designs of Jan Worst.[208,250,272,305,370] In general, biplanar IOLs required a larger limbal wound opening for insertion. The Severin lens and some other designs were also biplanar IOLs, but the optic was placed behind the pupil.[382,389,390]

Binkhorst's original four-loop iris clip IOL (Fig. 4-51; Color Plate 4-8) and variations of it were totally dependent on the iris for support.[217,290,300] His two-loop iridocapsular IOL, introduced in 1965, depended largely on the lens capsular sac for fixation (Fig. 4-52; Color Plate 4-9).[208,216,289] The change to capsular fixation after ECCE provided better stability for the pseudophakos. This very important modification was a forerunner to capsular sac (in-the-bag) fixation of modern posterior chamber IOLs (see p. 158).[256] Figure 4-53 shows a modification of the two-loop lens with suturing holes drilled in the optic for iris-fixation sutures.

Binkhorst had originally assumed, based on his previous experience with anterior and posterior chamber lenses, that contact by the IOL with the iris was harmless to the eye (p. 142).[200-204,206] Yet beginning with the first iris-supported lenses, many clinical and subclinical problems emerged, such as dislocation, pupillary deformity and erosion, iris atrophy with transillumination defects, pigment dispersion, uveitis, hemorrhage, and opacification of the media (Fig. 4-54).[420] Many of these complications are now known to be caused by chronic rubbing or chafing of the iris by IOL loops or haptics.[165,171,257] Problems were especially severe with metal loop IOLs (Fig. 4-55) and occurred frequently with multiple-looped lenses because uveal contact and chafing against the mobile iris tissues were unavoidable with these designs.[290]

There was an increased incidence of corneal edema in many cases with iris-supported lens designs.[225,274,303] Throughout the 1970s and 1980s, corneal decompensation and pseudophakic bullous keratopathy were now very common indications for penetrating keratoplasty. A recognized relationship between pseudophakic bullous keratopathy and cystoid macular edema, termed the *corneal-retinal inflammatory syndrome* by Obstabaum and Galin,[356] was described in the late 1970s.

The move to iris fixation was largely based on the fact that subluxation and malpositioning were significant complications, which continue to occur with every type of IOL.* Anterior displacement of an IOL frequently causes contact of the pseudophakos with the corneal endothelium, causing corneal decompensation.[266,298,424] Posterior dislocation toward the vitreous occasionally occurring as a complication with iris-supported IOLs.† In favorable cases a

---

* References 242, 243, 245, 281, 298, 326, 342, 354, 388, 424, 431, 446.
† References 229, 257, 264, 265, 298, 304, 335.

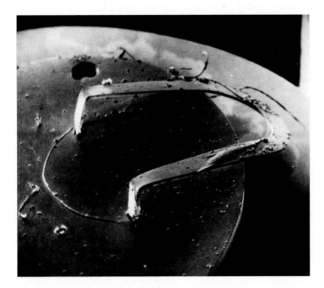

Fig. 4-55. Scanning electron micrograph of a metal-looped Medallion iris-support IOL. Problems caused by metal haptics or loops included tearing of tissue and dislocation of the lens because of the excessive weight of the IOL. Note the sharp edges of both the loop and the optic component at the lower right. (×20.)

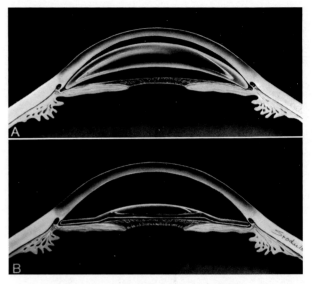

Fig. 4-56. A, Schematic illustration of a sagittal section of the anterior segment of the eye showing the original 1952 Baron anterior chamber lens, with fixation in the angle recess. This one-piece lens was rigid and sizing problems were unavoidable. Note the extremely steep anterior curvature of the lens. Such excessive anterior vaulting invariably caused corneal endothelial problems. **B,** Schematic illustration of a sagittal section of the anterior segment of the eye showing placement of a modern anterior chamber lens fixated in the angle recess. Note the more subtle anterior vaulting of the loops and lens optic. (**B** from Apple DJ and others: Anterior chamber lenses. I. Complications and pathology and a review of designs. II. A laboratory study, J Cataract Refract Surg 13:157, 175, 1987.)

posteriorly dislocated IOL settles on the inferior retina, usually out of the visual axis.

Jan Worst,[427,428,429] in Holland, developed IOLs intended to provide improved stability by suturing the lens to the iris (Fig. 4-53). The fact that nylon was used, however, created a new problem—hydrolytic breakdown of the nylon iris-fixation sutures and subsequent subluxations. In a further attempt to achieve better fixation, various types of clips (e.g., the Worst Platina IOL) were used.[310,320]

Metal-looped lenses (Fig. 4-55) were designed to obviate the biodegradation problem of nylon loops and sutures.[322,323,331] With the use of metal fixation elements, however, complications such as inflammation, hemorrhage, and damage to iris tissue occurred.[318,341]

One must not understate the extreme importance of the advance in the evolution of IOLs that occurred when Binkhorst advocated a return to ECCE with the introduction of his two-loop iridocapsular lens in 1965.* Use of this lens brought an almost immediate reduction in the incidence of complications.

Binkhorst was the first to emphasize the importance of endophthalmodonesis (see p. 142). This phenomenon paradoxically led to difficulties with Binkhorst's original four-loop iris clip lens following ICCE.[306] He found that by not removing the lens capsule, greater stability for the pseudophakos could be achieved. The transition from ICCE to ECCE with iridocapsular fixation undoubtedly decreased the problems associated with endophthalmodonesis and the barrier deprivation syndrome.[208,212,278]

At the time when iris-supported lenses were in widespread use, manufacturing methods and surgical techniques were less sophisticated. A major reason for the de-

cline in the use of these lenses is the unacceptably high incidence of complications caused by mechanical contact and chafing of uveal tissues by the lens components.

There is no doubt that most modern high-quality anterior and posterior chamber IOLs provide better success than IOLs that depend on the iris for support. Surgeons agree that when a patient with an iris-supported IOL develops late complications, such as inflammation or corneal decompensation that does not respond rapidly to conservative therapy, lens explanation or exchange is almost always the best treatment.[414]

Fixation of Anterior Chamber Intraocular Lenses

General considerations. Fixation of lenses into the anterior chamber seemed appealing because of perceived of insertion and low incidence of lens dislocation within its narrow confines.* Only recently has a suitable design been established for this purpose.

Although in the 1950s, implantations with early anterior chamber IOLs were often disappointing, some models of anterior chamber lenses[164,413,433] did provide good success, particularly when the lens was properly sized. Two important factors have led to an improved success rate with some anterior chamber IOL designs by the mid to late 1980s:

1. *Improved lens designs:* More appropriate lens flexi-

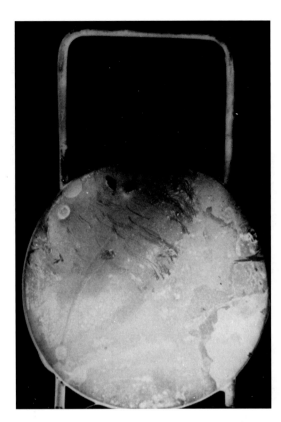

Fig. 4-57. Scanning electron micrograph of a Surgidev Corporation. Leiske closed-loop anterior chamber IOL removed because of severe anterior uveitis and corneal decompensation. The inferior loop had to be amputated at the time of explantation. It is sometimes difficult to surgically remove the residual portion of the loops from dense synechiae in the angle recess. (×15.)

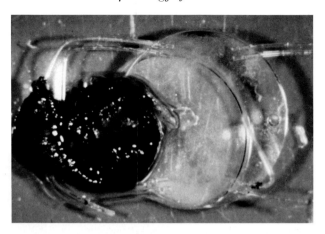

Fig. 4-58. Gross photograph of an explanted Optical Radiation Corporation. Model 11 Stableflex anterior chamber IOL. The patient suffered from secondary glaucoma, and at the time of lens removal there was copious bleeding inferiorly and a sector iridectomy was required. The large amount of tissue removed with the lens is clearly visible. The multiple small-diameter, round loops, characteristic of this IOL, are incarcerated within this hemorrhagic mass.

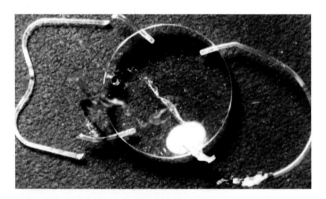

Fig. 4-59. Gross photograph of an IOLAB Corporation Azar 91Z anterior chamber lens removed from a patient with uveitis. Note the pigmented tissue and debris at the margins of the loops: these areas represent the sites of insertion of the loops into the angle recess. (×8.)

bility has now been achieved that decreases the need for perfect sizing. The increased attention given to the anterior-posterior vaulting characteristics of IOLs (compare Fig. 4-56, *A* with 4-56, *B*) has reduced the incidence of intermittent touch and uveal chafing problems. In addition to improving the lens designs, several design flaws in older lens styles have been identified.[259,395] For example, anterior chamber IOLs with round, small-diameter (tubular) loops and a closed-loop design (Figs. 4-57 to 4-60) have been removed from the market in the United States.

2. *Improvements in modern manufacturing and lens finishing techniques:* Tumble polishing of IOLs, particularly one-piece, all-PMMA lenses, produces excellent surface and edge finish (Fig. 4-61). The elimination of sharp optic or haptic edges is absolutely critical in the production of anterior chamber IOLs. This is true even more than with posterior chamber IOLs because anterior chamber IOLs are fixated in a confined space directly adjacent to delicate anterior segment tissues (Fig. 4-62).

Anterior chamber lenses can be implanted after either an ICCE or ECCE, an advantage that was recognized soon after their introduction. These lenses seldom dislocate, although they may become decentered. They can be implanted following such intraoperative complications as vitreous loss or posterior capsule rupture. Thus many surgeons who usually implant posterior chamber lenses still

find anterior chamber IOLs useful as backup when intraoperative complications occur.

Anterior chamber IOLs are also implanted under what may sometimes be difficult circumstances, for example, as a secondary implant or as an IOL exchange procedure. By definition, such procedures are performed on eyes that have been previously opened and manipulated by an initial cataract extraction. It is often difficult to determine if a complication in an eye with an anterior chamber lens occurs because of the IOL itself, a preexisting disease, or variations in surgical technique.

Site of fixation: proximity to adjacent ocular structures. The two major disadvantages of an anterior chamber IOL, compared with posterior chamber lens styles, are (1) the close proximity of the haptics or loops to delicate tissues such as the trabecular meshwork, corneal epithelium anteriorly, and the angle recess and anterior

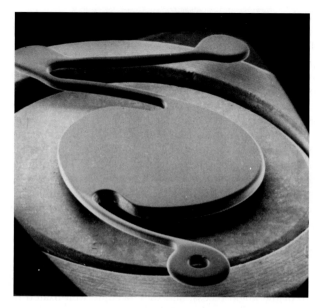

Fig. 4-64. Scanning electron micrograph of the finely polished Iolab Kelman Omnifit, a flexible tripod style anterior chamber lens. Allergan Medical Optics also makes a similar lens, the Kelman Model AC-21. Note the two broad footplates *(above)* and a positioning hole in the inferior haptic. (×10.) (From Apple DJ and others: Anterior chamber lenses. I. Complications and pathology and a review of designs. II. A laboratory study, J Cataract Refract Surg 13:157, 175, 1987.)

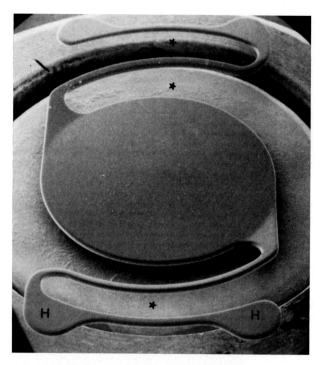

Fig. 4-65. Scanning electron micrograph of an IOLAB Surefit 85J flexible, one-piece, all-PMMA anterior chamber lens. Several other IOL companies produce this basic style of lens with good success. The lens is tumble polished and the surfaces and edges are smooth and rounded. This four-solid haptic *(H)* design is similar to the original Choyce four-point Mark VIII lens (see Fig. 4-61), but this lens is not solid. The interior portions *(asterisks)* are cut out to make the lens more flexible. (×10.)

The closed-loop anterior chamber IOLs* (Figs. 4-57–4-60 and 4-63) did not provide the safety and efficacy achieved by other anterior chamber lens designs, such as finely polished, flexible, one-piece, all-PMMA lenses (Figs. 4-64 and 4-65) (see Boxes 4-2 and 4-3). By 1987 the FDA had placed IOLs of the closed-loop design on core investigational status. This had the effect of removing them from the market in the United States, although this did not prevent the export of such lenses.

Unfortunately, the bad results attained from these poor-quality early designs have unfairly tarnished the reputation of anterior chamber lenses that are capable of providing excellent results. These are the flexible open-loop designs, modifications of the original Kelman anterior chamber IOLs (Color Plates 4-10 and 4-11). These lenses are well-finished by tumble polishing, thereby providing a rounded "tissue-friendly" surface at points of contact with delicate uveal tissues. Although PMMA is classified as a glass-like polymer, the danger of in vivo fracture, a rare problem even in earlier years, has been solved largely by proper design and use of better manufacturing methods. Three-and four-point fixation designs of Kelman style IOLs are available. Dr. Peter Clemente in Munich feels that a more stable and physiologic fit is achieved with the three-piece designs. The relatively long and rectangular four-point fixation designs often cause oval pupil. One-piece IOLs, particularly those with a foot plate design, are usually much easier to explant than IOLs with round, small-diameter loops, either closed-loop or open-loop designs.

Box 4-2. Disadvantages of closed-loop anterior chamber lenses.

1. Lenses may be difficult to size.
2. Lenses may have inappropriate vault-compression ratios. When a lens is compressed, it may vault anteriorly or posteriorly. Either type of response can cause deleterious effects.
3. Small diameter loops may cause a "cheese-cutter effect,: particularly if the lens is too large. Subsequent erosion and chafing can cause uveitis, including cystoid macular edema and pseudophakic bullous keratopathy.
4. Some lenses have a large contact zone over broad areas of the angle with the potential for secondary glaucoma.
5. The poorly finished, sharp edges of some lens models can cause chafing, leading to such sequelae as uveitis or the UGH syndrome.
6. Synechiae formation around the small-diameter loops may make the lens difficult to remove when necessary. Tearing of ocular tissues, hemorrhage, and iridocyclodialysis are possible complications of IOL removal if correct procedures are not used.

From Apple DJ and others: Intraocular lenses: evolution, designs, complications, and pathology, Baltimore, 1989, Williams & Wilkins.

* References 169, 173, 176, 180, 297, 307, 340, 374, 402.

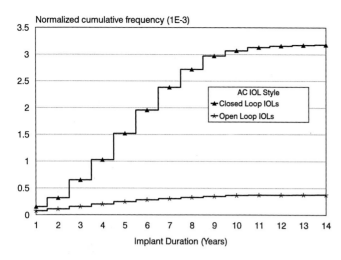

Fig. 4-66. This illustration demonstrates the marked variation in tolerance of the poorly manufactured closed loop AC-IOLs versus the modern well-manufactured open loop AC-IOLs. Note that the frequency of corneal complications and hence explantation is substantially lower over time with the modern open loop styles. (From Auffarth and others.[191])

Box 4-3. Advantages of modern open-loop, one-piece all-PMMA flexible anterior chamber lenses.

1. Most modern lenses have an excellent finish with highly polished smooth surfaces and rounded edges from tumble polishing. Tissue contact by any component of these IOLs is much less prone to cause chafing damage.

2. Sizing is less critical with flexible open-loop designs.

3. In contrast to a closed-loop anterior chamber IOL, the vault engineered into a well-designed, open-loop lens is maintained even under high compression. This minimizes IOL touch against the cornea anteriorly, or against the iris posteriorly.

4. Point fixation is possible since haptic may subtend only small areas of the angle outflow structures.

5. Most open-loop IOL designs are much easier to remove, when necessary, especially those with Choyce-like haptic or foot plate fixation. The well polished surfaces of these lenses usually do not become completely surrounded by goniosynechiae or cocoon membranes, and therefore can usually be removed if necessary without undue difficulty or excessive tissue damage.

From Apple DJ and others: Intraocular lenses: evolution, designs, complications, and pathology, Baltimore, 1989, Williams & Wilkins.

Many anterior chamber lens implantations are associated with complicated cases, for example, cases with intraoperative complications, patients with pre-existing ocular disease, or patients who have had previous surgery. Cases also may be complicated by a wide variation in surgical techniques and expertise and, in many instances, by inferior quality lenses. Now that most poor-quality IOLs have been removed from the market, the overall complication rate for anterior chamber IOLs is measurably reduced (Fig. 4-66).

Iris or scleral fixated sutured posterior chamber IOLs may be used in cases formerly reserved for anterior chamber IOLs. Results have been encouraging (Color Plate 4-12).[*] There is still uncertainty as to whether a retropupillary lens is superior to a modern well-manufactured Kelman-style anterior chamber IOL in such cases as intraoperative capsular rupture or vitreous loss, or as a secondary or exchange procedure. The technique is more difficult than anterior chamber lens insertion and should therefore only be carried out by a surgeon experienced in this technique.

Fixation of posterior chamber intraocular lenses

One obvious major theoretic advantage of an IOL in the posterior chamber versus one in the anterior chamber is its position behind the iris, away from the delicate structures of the anterior segment including the cornea, the aqueous outflow channels, the iris, and the ciliary body.[164] The only type of IOL that has no direct contact with uveal tissues is a posterior chamber IOL implanted entirely within the lens capsular sac.

The return to Harold Ridley's original concept[376] of IOL implantation in the posterior chamber occurred after 1975.[178,258,366,395] The most commonly implanted posterior chamber IOL during the early 1980s was a modified J-loop design (Fig. 4-67). The modified or short C-loop design accounts for the largest number of haptic-style IOLs implanted as we enter the twenty-first century. These IOL styles, which fit well into the capsule bag, are lightweight, and provide better fixation, have greatly increased the safety and efficacy of IOL implantation.

Centration of an IOL depends upon achieving systemic fixation of lens haptics, an objective that was difficult to achieve consistently in the early years of posterior chamber resurgence (1975–1990). As posterior chamber lens implantation evolved, the type of fixation achieved in the early years depended largely on chance or on the surgeon's individual preference. In general, the loops were anchored in one of three ways:

1. Both loops were placed in the ciliary region[†] (Color Plate 4-13; Figs. 4-68 and 4-69). We now know from autopsy studies that true ciliary sulcus fixation of *both* loops was, and still is, achieved much less often than was previously assumed.

2. Both loops were placed within the lens capsular sac. Capsular fixation evolved from the original work of Binkhorst, who advocated and popularized the use of ECCE used in conjunction with his two-loop iridocapsular IOL and its modifications.[178] In the early years of posterior chamber implantation, capsular or "in-the-bag" fixation (Color Plates 4-14 to 4-16; Fig. 4-70) was intentionally performed by only a handful of surgeons; widespread use did not occur until the mid 1980s.

3. One loop (usually the leading or inferior loop) was placed in the capsular sac and the other loop (usually the trailing or superior loop) was placed in a variety of locations *anterior* to the anterior capsular flap (Color Plate 4-17).

---

* References 172, 179, 181, 182, 199, 224, 247, 249, 251, 255, 261, 277, 280, 285, 292, 296, 315, 337, 338, 348, 349, 1208.

† References 163, 165, 168, 172, 176, 227, 282, 283, 345, 362.

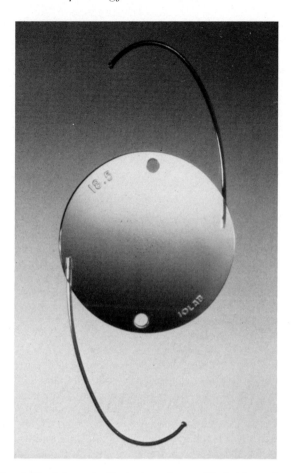

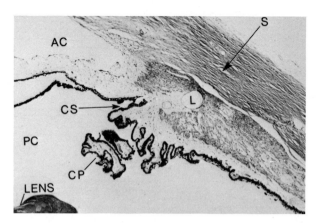

Fig. 4-69. Photomicrograph of the anterior segment of a globe implanted with a ciliary-fixated posterior chamber IOL. The loop (*L*) has eroded almost entirely through the ciliary body stroma, encroaching on the sclera (*S*) where it is situated within the parenchyma of the ciliary muscle. Note the equatorial remnants of the lens capsular sac (lens). Anterior chamber (*AC*), posterior chamber (*PC*), ciliary sulcus (*CS*), ciliary processes (*CP*). (H&E stain; ×20.)

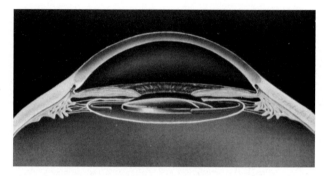

Fig. 4-70. Schematic illustration of a sagittally sectioned anterior segment containing a (in-the-bag) capsular-fixated posterior chamber IOL. The loops are confined behind the anterior capsular flap so that there is no direct contact of the loops with the adjacent uveal tissues.

Fig. 4-67. Schematic illustration of a modified J-loop, three-piece posterior chamber IOL. This lens style, introduced by Dr. Robert Sinskey, in 1980 and manufactured by IOLAB Corporation, had a polymethylmethacrylate (PMMA) optic component and blue polypropylene (Prolene) loops. (Courtesy Mr. Jack V McGrann, IOLAB Corporation, Claremont, Calif.)

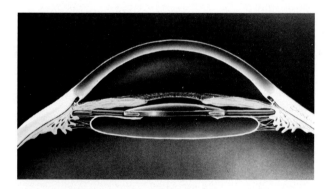

Fig. 4-68. Schematic illustration of a sagittally sectioned anterior segment containing a ciliary-fixated posterior chamber lens. The loops course in front of the peripheral flaps of the anterior capsule and insert into the angle or groove formed by the junction of the iris root and the ciliary body (the anatomic site now referred to as the "ciliary sulcus"). (Krystyna Srodulski, artist.)

This has been the most common type of fixation since the late 1970s when the flexible posterior chamber IOLs were introduced. Retrospective analysis of clinical cases, autopsy studies, and experience with animal implantations have shown that this asymmetric fixation occurs in most implantations when a lens is simply inserted behind the iris, without specific intended placement of the loops. The direction of the lens as it enters the posterior chamber is usually the deciding factor in determining where the loop is fixated. The IOL passes through the pupil in an oblique fashion during the insertion process. Typically the leading or inferior loop passes into the equatorial fornix of the capsular sac at 6 o'clock. Then, as the superior or trailing loop is inserted, often without good visibility, the loop springs into a site behind the iris but anterior to the anterior capsular flap at 12 o'clock.

As Fig. 4-71 illustrates, there are several loop-fixation sites possible with modern flexible-loop posterior chamber IOLs.[172] These fixation sites have been confirmed histolog-

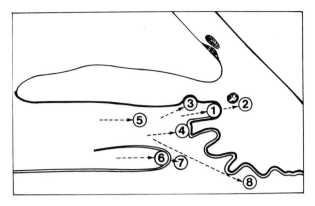

Fig. 4-71. Schematic illustrations showing possible placement sites of posterior chamber lens loops. *Site 1:* Loop in the ciliary sulcus. *Site 2:* Loop after erosion into the ciliary body stroma in the region of the major iris arterial circle. *Site 3:* Loop in contact with the iris root. *Site 4:* Loop attached to a ciliary process. *Site 5:* Loop in aqueous without tissue contact (can cause "windshield wiper" syndrome because of inadequate fixation). *Site 6:* Loop in the lens capsular sac. *Site 7:* Loop ruptured through the lens capsular sac (a rare occurrence). *Site 8:* Loop in the zonular region between the ciliary sulcus and the lens capsular sac. The loop may penetrate the zonules (zonular fixation) or extend as far posteriorly as the pars plana (pars plana fixation). (Krystyna Srodulski, artist.)

ically by analyses of postmortem globes implanted with posterior chamber IOLs. When the loops fixate directly on the surface of the ciliary sulcus, they are secured in the angle formed by the junction of the posterior iris root and the anterior margin of the ciliary processes or pars plicata. This site is theoretically the ideal placement area for uveal fixation because a fibrous encapsulation around the loop often develops, enhancing fixation and preventing deep loop erosion into the ciliary body. Fixation of both IOL loops at this site, however, is achieved in fewer than one in five cases.[172,283]

A major cause of asymmetric fixation and subsequent lens decentration is the "pea-pod" effect in which a loop exits from the capsular sac, either during intraoperative manipulations, such as "dialing," or postoperatively (Figs. 4-72 and 4-73). The major cause of "pea-podding" is the presence of a radial tear in the anterior capsule or too scanty an anterior capsular flap after a large capsulotomy. An abundant anterior flap is necessary to permanently secure the loop in the equatorial fornix. The potential of radial tear formation is lessened by performing a circular smooth-edged continuous tear anterior capsulotomy (continuous curvilinear capsulorhexis [CCC]) (p. 156).

Sulcus fixated haptics (Fig. 4-74) loops may migrate or erode through the ciliary epithelium and into the stromal tissues of the ciliary body.[168,334] This is actually the most common form of uveal fixation. The loops may encroach upon or compress the major iris circle and other vessels in the ciliary vascular plexus. At times a loop may migrate through the ciliary body stroma, become embedded in the ciliary muscle, or may even come to rest on or near the supraciliary space adjacent to the sclera. When such a migration occurs, this may play a role in the pathogenesis of such lens malpositions (Color Plates 4-17 to 4-21) as the

"sunrise" syndrome, particularly after asymmetric implantation of the IOL loops.[177,223,283]

Only when both loops are secured in the lens capsular sac does one achieve a fixation in which IOL contact with uveal tissues (Fig. 4-74) is avoided. Fixation of iris supported, anterior chamber, or uvea-fixated posterior (Fig. 4-72, *A* and *B*, Fig. 4-73, and Fig. 4-71 and Fig. 4-74, respectively) chamber IOLs, by definition, implies direct contact of the loop or haptic with delicate ocular tissues.

If IOL loops are either intentionally or inadvertently placed in front of the capsular sac, which occurs in as many as 8% of cases, the loop may be positioned so that it is neither in the ciliary sulcus nor in the lens capsular sac.[283] The loop may slide between these structures and become entangled in the zonules or may pass through the zonules to settle as far posteriorly as the pars plana (Color Plate 4-21). This may clinically cause a case of zonular rupture and lens decentration.

The excellent success rate now achieved with posterior chamber IOL implantation is associated with improved IOL designs and improved surgical techniques, including meticulous placement of loops,* as shown in Box 4-4.

As noted on Color Plate 4-12, in recent years many surgeons have popularized the implantation of posterior chamber IOLs in lieu of anterior chamber lenses in cases of secondary or exchange implantation when there is a defective or absent capsular bag. Posterior chamber IOLs can be sutured in the ciliary sulcus or with scleral fixation and to the iris sutured as a secondary or exchange procedure.

Explantation of posterior chamber IOLs because of complications is now rarely required—particularly with well-implanted capsule-fixed lenses. Decentration and posterior capsular opacification (PCO), however, are two complications that still occur following posterior chamber IOL surgery (Color Plates 4-17–4-22).† Posterior capsular opacification is discussed in detail on page 174. Because decentration was a major problem with Generation V, the period of transition towards posterior chamber IOLs, it is discussed in detail in this section.

There are several causes of posterior chamber IOL decentration:

1. Asymmetric loop insertion, or one loop in the lens capsular sac, one loop in the ciliary region ("sunrise" syndrome or "east-west" syndrome) (Color Plates 4-17 to 4-21).[283]

2. Escape of a loop initially placed in the lens capsular sac, either intraoperatively, during rotation or "dialing" of the IOL, or postoperatively because of a gaping anterior capsular tear, a too large anterior capsulotomy that does not leave enough anterior capsular flap to hold the lens in place ("pea-pod" effect).

3. Sliding or slippage of a loop that is sandwiched between the iris and anterior capsular flap but not securely fixated in the ciliary sulcus (Color Plate 4-19), for example, a lens that is functionally too short to snuggly fit in the sulcus.

---

* References 165, 166, 168, 170, 172, 173, 179, 209, 520.
† References 165, 168, 171, 172, 223, 282, 362.

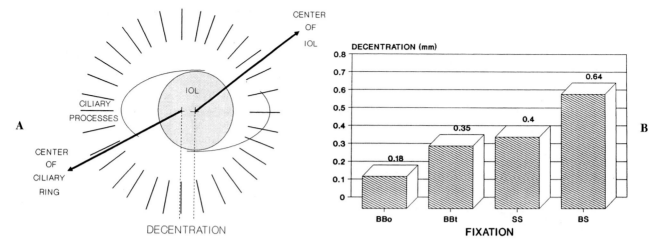

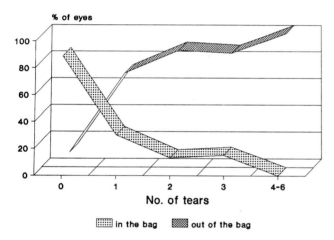

Fig. 4-72. Decentration of an IOL can be determined in an eye obtained postmortem by measuring the distance of the IOL center from the center of the ciliary ring. **A,** Technique analysis of PC-IOL decentration. **B,** Note that the most decentration occurs with asymmetric (bag-sulcus [BS]) fixation. Bag-bag (BB) fixation without tears is slightly better than bag-bag with tears. The latter is similar to that obtained with sulcus (SS) fixation. (From Assia and others.[483])

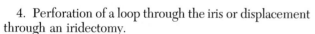

Fig. 4-73. Graph based on an analysis of a large series of eyes obtained postmortem with posterior chamber lenses. It was determined that the success and in-the-bag fixation was best with no or few tears, whereas the number of haptics situated outside of the capsular bag increased with the number of radial tears in each eye. (From Assia and others.[483])

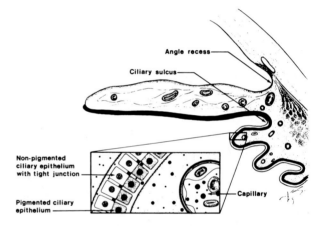

Fig. 4-74. Schematic illustration of the anterior segment of the eye showing the major components that form the surface of the blood-aqueous barrier. These include the epithelia of the ciliary body and the intrastromal vascular channels of the iris and ciliary body. Any disruption of the lining of the blood-aqueous barrier can lead to inflammation and its sequelae. (Krystyna Srodulski, artist.)

4. Perforation of a loop through the iris or displacement through an iridectomy.

5. Optic migration during pupillary capture.

6. Distorting or bending of a loop during insertion, usually during excessive flexion or pronation of the superior loop, causing a difference in loop length and subsequent asymmetric fixation.[187] A haptic or loop may bend in situ within the capsular bag as a result of capsular bag cataractis or fibrosis.

7. Pressure or traction exerted on the loop and/or optical component of the IOL by proliferating residual lens epithelial cells and their derivatives. A fibrous or myoepithelial metaplasia of these cells produces a cicatricial contraction of the capsular sac.[357] This phenomenon may be exacerbated by an asymmetric anterior capsulotomy. The so-called capsulorhexis contraction syndrome is a significant problem with plate style IOLs (Color Plate 4-33).

8. Loop disinsertion at the site where the loop is staked into the loop-optic junction.

9. Loop fracture.

Clinically significant signs and symptoms of decentration include undesirable visual complications such as glare, halo, monocular diplopia, or other visual aberrations. These may occur because of the presence of optic edges or other lens elements such as positioning holes within the pupillary aperture. It is well-documented that these phenomena may be clinically significant.[177] Even in eyes in which postoperative vision is adequate—as determined by a Snellen visual acuity test—the subjective symptoms experienced by the

Box 4-4. Advantages of placing both loops in the lens capsular sac.[194]

1. The IOL is positioned in the proper anatomic site.
2. Both loops can be placed symmetrically in the capsular sac as easily as in the ciliary sulcus.
3. Intraoperative stretching or tearing of zonules by loop manipulations in front of the anterior capsular leaflet is avoided.
4. There is low incidence of lens decentration and dislocation.
5. There is no evidence of spontaneous loop dislocation.
6. The IOL is positioned a maximal distance behind the cornea.
7. The IOL is positioned a maximal distance from the posterior iris pigment epithelium, iris root, and ciliary processes.
8. Iris chafing—caused postoperative pigment dispersion into the anterior chamber is reduced.
9. There is no direct contact by, or erosion of, IOL loops or haptics into ciliary body tissues.
10. Chronic uveal tissue chafing is avoided, and the probability of long-term blood-aqueous barrier breakdown is reduced.
11. Surface alteration of loop material is less likely.
12. IOL implantation is safer for children and young individuals.
13. Posterior capsular opacification may be reduced.
14. The IOL may be easier to explant, if necessary.

patient may be troublesome. The symptoms may be exacerbated in conditions such as dim light when pupillary dilatation occurs.[177] The best means of decreasing such visual aberrations is to decrease the incidence of optic decentration by symmetric loop placement.

With the use of viscoelastic agents and a well-controlled anterior capsulotomy that leaves a large enough anterior capsular flap for good loop support, symmetric placement of both loops in the lens capsular sac is not difficult in most instances. As surgeons gain experience with various implantation techniques, including modern capsulorhexis procedures, a more carefully controlled operation is possible during all stages of IOL implantation. Atraumatic removal of lens substance without damage to the capsular-zonular apparatus is possible. Simple, uncontrolled behind-the-iris, uncontrolled, asymmetric implantation (one loop fixated in the capsule and the opposite loop in the ciliary region) may seem technically easier, but the potential for intraoperative and postoperative complications is increased. Intraoperative tearing of zonules by loops that are manipulated or "dialed" in front of the anterior capsular flaps, as well as rupture through the zonules, can be avoided by placing the loops within the capsule.

In a large series of autopsy eyes with posterior chamber IOLs, Ohmi, Assia, and associates[186,361,852,1043] have shown that the mean crystalline lens diameter was 9.6 mm (standard deviation 0.4 mm), the diameter of the evacuated capsular sac is approximately 10.5 mm, and the diameter of the ciliary sulcus was 11 mm (standard deviation of 0.5 mm). These measurements agree with those of other published studies.[251,375]

The original Shearing posterior chamber IOL measured 12.5 mm in diameter and was not as flexible as today's modified "soft, rounded" J-loop and C-loop designs. If the lens was too small for the eye or if a loop eroded into the ciliary body, the IOL became decentered and "windshield wiper" syndrome and other undesirable IOL movements occurred. These problems prompted most lens designers to increase the total lens diameter. Most three-piece, flexible-looped IOLs in current use measure from 13.75 to 14.5 mm in diameter. These IOLs were originally designed to ensure consistent ciliary region fixation, to provide a snug fit, and thus to prevent the IOL from dislocating. In general, when such IOLs are used with capsular fixation, the flexible loops must bend or crimp sufficiently to conform to the much smaller diameter of the capsular sac. The loop tip may even extend to the edge of or over the optic in such cases.

Many lenses designed specifically for "in-the-bag" placement are one-piece designs with a smaller total diameter (12.0–12.5 mm). As more surgeons now prefer capsular bag implantation, use of these smaller diameter IOLs has increased. This transition to capsular surgery has been very instrumental in reducing incidence of problems associated with severe bending and crimping of lens loops, such as capsular distortion and the spring effect that can occur when the loop is exposed to contractile forces within the capsular bag.

There is now little doubt[287,668,681] that in general, the final configuration of implanted loop IOL loops of all IOL shapes assume a C-shape configuration that conformed to the circular capsule. There is significant compression and bending of a J-loop or modified J-loops. The distal portion of J-loop or modified J-loop IOLs frequently exert a one-directional force that causes stretching and ovaling of the capsular sac.[681] This may result in the formation of folds or striae parallel to the long axis of the lens. These changes occasionally caused such clinically significant problems as glare or a Maddox-rod effect.

Modified or short C-loop lenses, adaptations of the original Simcoe C-loop and variations of the original Sinskey and Kratz designs are now widely used because surgeons find these IOLs easy to insert and the loops conform well to the circular shape of the capsular sac.

Posterior capsular opacification (Elschig pearls, or so-called secondary cataract) is a significant postoperative complication in IOL. Evidence is clear that the concept of a barrier effect to retard PCO is a valid one.[178] Placement of a well-designed posterior chamber lens in the lens capsular sac provides a gentle but taut radial stretch on the posterior capsule.[284,416] Of the present open-loop, flexible IOLs, the one-piece, all-PMMA, posterior chamber designs with posterior convex or biconvex optics appear to be especially effective in providing a symmetric stretch.[167] This aids in minimizing posterior capsular opacification by reducing the folds in the capsular sac and holding the posterior capsule firmly against the posterior surface of the IOL optic. This is sometimes termed the *no space, no cells* concept.[178,188,424] If IOL loops are placed in front of the anterior capsule (i.e., if the loops are not in place to expand or stretch the capsule at the equatorial fornix), there is no mechanical means to prevent shrinkage or corrugation of the capsule. In such cases, as the bag shrinks, traction on the zonules with stretching or rupture may occur. The development of good in-the-bag lenses and modern capsular surgery techniques, including hydrodissection have reduced the incidence of PCO from a level of about 50% in the early 1980s to about 10% to 15% today.

In conclusion, the quality of surgery and the accuracy of loop placement are important factors that affect the outcome of the cataract operation. By the early to mid 1980s new and helpful tools became available to surgeons that not only make precise loop or haptic placement possible but have irreversibly transformed the quality of cataract surgery. Excellent examples are (1) viscoelastics and (2) new methods of controlling the size, shape, and quality of the anterior capsulotomy—especially the CCC technique. These greatly increase the facility to achieve accurate and permanent loop placement. These and other advances have now brought us to a new level of quality—a new generation (generation VI) that was only thought of at the time of preparation of the last edition of this text in the early 1990s.

Modern capsular intraocular lenses: generation VI (1990 to present)

By the end of the 1980s, clinical laboratory studies[°] had clearly demonstrated that cataract surgical techniques and IOL designs and manufacture had shown remarkable advancement. Older techniques such as implantation of IOLs through can-opener incisions after simple extracapsular surgery gave way to more modern techniques. The common denominator was the achievement of safe, permanent, and secure in-the-bag (capsular) fixation of the pseudophakos.[†] The newly developed "capsular lenses" fabricated from both rigid and soft biomaterials were well-suited for implantation with modern techniques.[434-1014]

The many changes in surgical techniques that entered the surgeon's armamentarium by the end of the 1990s included the adjunctive use of viscoelastics,[‡] CCC, which has largely replaced the old can-opener technique (Color Plates 4-22 and 4-23), hydrodissection (Color Plate 4-24), and the increased usage of phacoemulsification. These techniques have not only allowed much safer surgery (compare Color Plates 4-25 and 4-26), but help achieve safe implantation through much smaller incisions than were possible in the early days of extracapsular extraction, for example, as small as 3.0 mm as opposed to 11.0 mm.

The move toward capsular fixation and progress from the can-opener anterior capsulectomy toward CCC (Fig. 4-75) was anticipated by Cornelius Binkhorst, who developed (the envelope or intercapsular technique) what in essence was a two-step capsulorhexis technique. An initial small linear horizontal or smiling incision was prepared, the cataract was removed, and the IOL was inserted through this small incision. The second step was a continuous circular enlargement of the tear that provided a smooth-edged circular anterior capsular opening in front of the IOL optic.

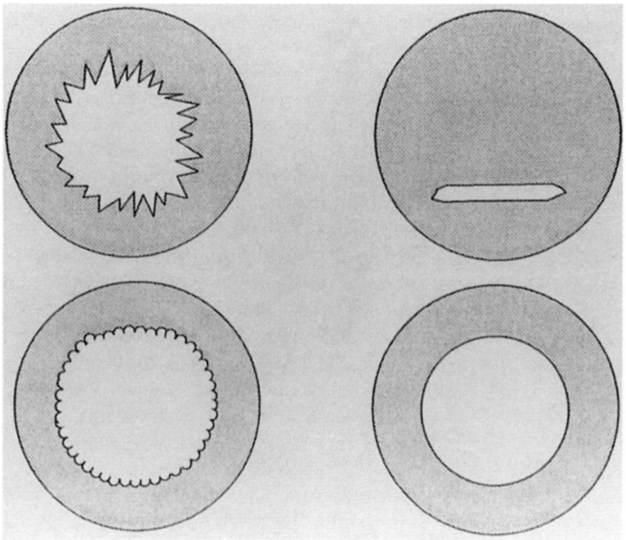

Fig. 4-75. Examples of the various types of anterior capsulectomy available for cataract surgery include: original can opener technique (**A**); the envelope technique in which an initial horizontal incision is made, followed by circular tear made at the end of the operation (**B**); a modified can opener technique with multiple scalloped edges of the incision (**C**); and the modern continuous curvilinear capsulorhexis (CCC), with no jagged edges at the edge of the capsular tear (**D**). (From Assia and others.[471])

This evolved into the single-step CCC described by Gimbel and Neuhann.[°]

There are two clear advantages of the modern CCC over the early can-opener techniques (Figs. 4-76 and 4-77). Firstly, the formation of radial tears at the anterior capsular edge is minimized (Figs. 4-76, *A* and *B*). This in turn helps decrease the incidence of formation of radial tears of the anterior capsule. Such tears tend to reduce the stability of the capsular bag and may even allow exit of haptics out of the capsular bag through the anterior capsular tear (so-called "pea-podding" effect). This increases the risk of IOL decentration. Secondly, and less commonly recognized, capsulorhexis provides a stable capsular bag that allows copious hydrodissection without tearing the capsular edges. Hydrodissection is very helpful in achieving good cortical clean-up. With a frayed anterior capsular edge such as seen with the can-opener technique, hydrodissection is difficult without forming unwanted radial tears.

Hydrodissection was first described by Faust[481,621,625,693] in 1984. Its many variations, for example, cortical cleavage hydrodissection and hydrodilineation, enhance mobilization and removal of lens cells and cortical material. This helps reduce the formation of a Soemmering's ring and this in turn helps minimize the long-term risk of PCO (p. 174).[498,499] The more cells that can be removed at surgery, especially in the region of the equatorial fornix, the less chance of subsequent cellular migration across the visual axis. Autopsy studies have clearly shown that the quality

---

° References 412, 454, 454, 460, 489, 490, 495, 500, 508, 563, 564, 578, 603, 638, 692, 696, 701–703, 710, 711, 744, 762, 763, 764, 888, 892, 919, 933, 946, 962.

† References 214, 215, 445, 447, 459, 460, 473–477, 478, 479, 487, 493, 515, 522, 537, 590, 640, 666, 667, 739, 766, 767, 781, 828, 863.

‡ References 437, 438, 482, 494, 647, 705, 768, 787, 898, 930, 955, 960, 1009.

° References 353, 449, 451, 457, 458, 470–472, 473–477, 480, 483, 484, 491, 496, 497, 642, 671, 690, 691, 843, 844, 868, 872, 894, 945, 970, 985, 998.

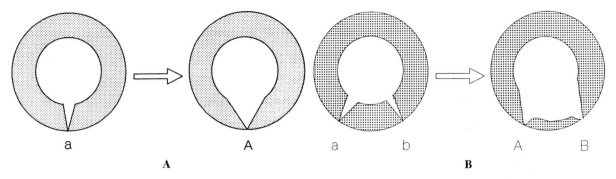

Fig. 4-76. Mechanism of intraocular lens pea podding (exit from the capsular bag) with either one or two radial tears of the anterior capsule). Any extension of an anterior capsular tear forms a large gaping wound through which the IOL haptic, originally situated in the capsular bag, can escape through the defect. **A.** One tear (*a*). **B.** Two tears (*a* and *b*). (Courtesy Dr. Ehud Assia.)

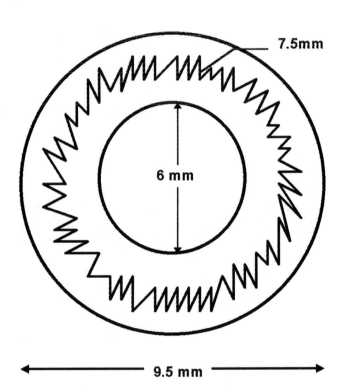

Fig. 4-77. Schematic illustration comparing the appearance of early relatively large can opener capsulectomies (e.g., 7.5 mm), with the preferred modern midsized continuous curvilinear capsulorhexis (CCC). Most surgeons to make the capsulorhexis approximately the same size as the diameter of the IOL optic, in this case illustrated as 6 mm. (Courtesy Dr. Qun Peng.)

of cortical removal from clinical cases had clearly improved by the late 1990s (Color Plate 4-26), as opposed to the years prior to modern capsular surgery, which by definition connotes the period before the widespread use of hydrodissection.

Modern phacoemulsification, pioneered by Charles Kelman, has now made removal of lens material and implantation of IOLs through incisions as small as 3.0 mm in diameter, as opposed to incisions up to 11 to 12 mm in the early days of extracapsular cataract extraction. There are many real advantages of small incision cataract surgery and var-

ious ancillary procedures such as topical anesthesia, temporal incisions, no-stitch (sutureless) surgery, and small clear corneal or corneal-scleral incisions. These include safer healing with less risk of complications such as inflammation or endophthalmitis, more rapid healing, and rapid recovery of visual rehabilitation with less postoperative astigmatism.° These factors are very important now that we have high standards for results following IOL implantation, especially in this era in which IOL implantation is not only considered to be a means of optical rehabilitation after removal of a cataract but is now also considered to be a bona fide refractive procedure.† The development of bi- and multifocal IOL designs is one example of this evolutionary process.‡

Accompanying the developments of the above-mentioned surgical techniques, which allow secure in-the-bag implantation, both rigid PMMA IOLs and soft, foldable IOLs (Color Plates 4-27 and 4-28; Figs. 4-78, *A* and *B*) have evolved simultaneously that work well with these techniques. Figure 4-78, *A* and *B* show examples of modern state-of-the-art, one-piece, all-PMMA IOLs that are designed for in-the-bag implantation.§ These highly biocompatible lenses can be inserted with incisions as small as 5.5 to 6 mm and provide an excellent alternative for the surgeon who remains comfortable with the fact that PMMA has functioned as a reliable lens biomaterial for a half century. Long-term results with these IOLs are excellent, and these IOLs provide the best centration of all designs to date. Although these lenses generally provide slightly better centration than do most of the more modern foldable lenses available at the present time, they, of course, cannot be inserted through ultratiny incisions. The ideal size for a one-piece, all-PMMA IOL design is 12.0 to 12.5 mm, which allows an almost perfect snug fit into the adult capsu-

---

° References 333, 592, 597–599, 610, 613, 614, 626, 636, 641, 653, 719, 720, 722, 723, 731, 760, 761, 773, 779, 793, 794, 797, 810, 835, 836, 841, 858, 865, 880, 904, 916, 926, 927, 947, 953, 958, 959, 963, 967, 978, 989, 1011.
† References 312, 512, 517, 519, 526, 527, 559, 591, 615, 722, 782, 797, 811, 835, 841, 849, 866.
‡ References 436, 455, 643, 684, 685, 695, 718, 727, 778, 951, 990, 993.
§ References 167, 168, 187, 446, 448, 452, 456, 460, 463–465, 476, 501, 506, 507, 510, 604, 655–657, 796, 852.

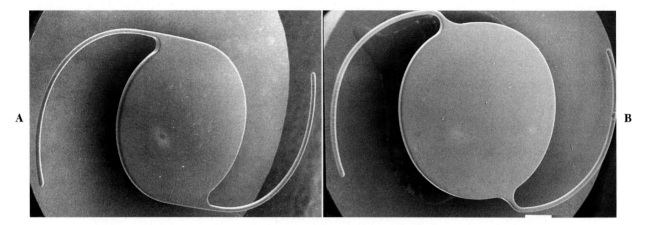

Fig. 4-78. Scanning electron micrographs of two well-finished and well-designed, one-piece, all-PMMA 12-mm diameter capsular lenses. **A,** Flexible design with relatively curved haptics that insures excellent centration in the capsular bag. (SEM ×10.) **B,** Another design that has a slightly more rigid configuration because the haptics course directly off of the optic. (SEM ×10.)

lar bag, which measures about 10.5 mm diameter (Figs. 4-79, *A–C*).[186,273,683] Recall that the diameter of the ciliary sulcus is only slightly larger (approximately 11 mm) and decreases with age.[186,222,852,942]

These rigid PMMA IOL designs have also been found to be very satisfactory in pediatric IOL implantation.* Knowing that 90% of growth of the infantile globe occurs during the first 18 months to 2 years (Fig. 4-80 Color Plate 4-29), it follows that one can safely implant "adult" 12-mm lenses in children this age and older with safe results.[535] This has been verified with experimental studies using the Miyake posterior video technique (Color Plate 4-30).[453,508] A significant problem in the past and still a nuisance with pediatric IOL implantation is that of capsular fibrosis and posterior capsular opacification.[458] This is a not-infrequent cause, which necessitates surgical or Nd:YAG laser secondary posterior capsulotomy (Color Plate 4-31). Most surgeons address this with prophylactic primary posterior capsulotomy, including posterior CCC with lens optic capture.[562] Intense research is ongoing to improve surgical techniques and minimize this problem. Increased use of hydrodissection to improve cortical cleanup may help address this problem.[458]

Similar one-piece, all-PMMA designs are also being developed for use in the underprivileged or developing world where the backlog of cataract blind is huge.[183,295,673,943] Such lenses can now be manufactured in underdeveloped countries at a reasonable price with good quality. There is no doubt that it is imperative to try to increase the incidence of IOL implantation in patients in developing world countries to move forward from the less satisfactory apha-kic-spectacle treatment aphakia, with its inherent problems of visual distortions and lost or broken spectacles (Color Plate 4-32).[183,295]

As small incision surgical techniques have improved and IOL designs have improved, this has led to a natural evolu-

tion toward the other type of modern capsular IOL designed specifically for the in-the-bag fixation—the foldable lens designs, generally manufactured from silicone, hydrogel, or acrylic material (Color Plates 4-33–4-36).*

An early design with widespread clinical usage in the early 1980s was the plate lens design of Mozzacco,[801] known as the Mazzacco taco (named after its appearance after folding in its longitudinal dimension). In early years these were poorly manufactured with sharp edges (Fig. 4-81, *B*) and sometimes with poor optical quality. In the early years before modern capsular surgical techniques the lenses were poorly implanted, especially with asymmetric fixation. Many complications ensued. In recent years manufacture has greatly improved (Figs. 4-82, *A* and *B*), and these lenses are now satisfactory for clinical usage. The best plate lenses are those with large positioning holes that allow in-the-bag synechia formation, which enhances fixation and stability.[461,729] Earlier small-hole designs had often been associated with malpositions such as subluxation and decentration.[560,586,786,833,1010] Plate lenses are, therefore, now providing excellent results.

The other commonly implanted designs at present are three-piece designs with optics fabricated from silicone, acrylic, or hydrogel biomaterials. Foldable lenses implanted through incisions as small as 3.0 mm with various modifications, such as clear corneal incisions and topical anesthesia, provide rapid visual restoration. Such surgery is virtually analogous to arthroscopy of the eye.

Lens design and manufacture has improved to such an extent that the most important factor in achieving a suc-

---

* References 219, 287, 323, 491, 496, 497, 514, 520, 525, 528, 531, 535, 539, 543, 550, 560, 567, 605, 639, 644, 645, 680, 681, 682, 686, 721, 733, 757, 784, 788, 802, 935, 961, 977, 983, 999, 1000, 1012.

---

* References 228, 231, 239, 420–429, 434, 435, 440, 441, 467, 489, 502–505, 509, 523, 533, 534, 542, 545, 546–549, 557, 558, 566, 571, 572, 574, 579–582, 584–587, 589, 593, 595, 596, 606, 608, 618–624, 628, 632, 650, 652, 658, 659, 661, 676–679, 694, 714, 717, 724, 726, 728, 729, 731, 732, 735, 738, 747, 750–752, 765, 770–772, 777, 780, 783, 786, 789, 790, 792, 793, 795, 799, 801, 803–808, 813–816, 820, 833, 834, 837–839, 848, 854–856, 857, 859–861, 864, 871, 876, 877, 882–884, 887, 913, 925, 928, 929, 931, 932, 936–938, 944, 952–969, 976, 981, 986, 987, 991, 994, 996, 1003, 1005, 1007, 1010, 1013, 1014.

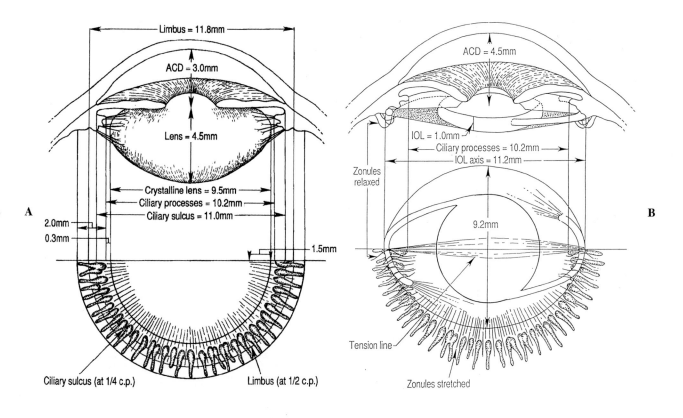

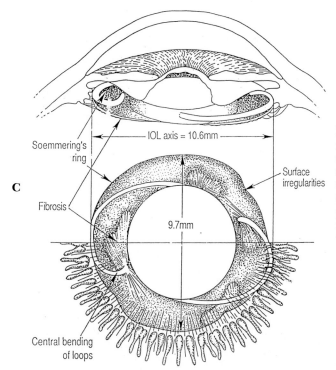

Fig. 4-79. Schematic illustration showing basic measurements of the crystalline lens pre- and postextracapsular cataract extraction and IOL implantation. **A,** Average measurements of adult crystalline lens. **B,** Various tissue measurements immediately after implantation of an IOL immediately postoperatively. **C,** Same measurements, late postoperative stage. Note that over the long-term the originally stretched oval capsular bag becomes more rounded. (From Assia and others.[487])

cessful result is usually not related to the IOL itself but the quality of surgery. It is of utmost importance to achieve good cortical clean-up and symmetrical capsular bag fixation. Color Plates 4-37 and 4-38 show vivid examples of the importance of good surgical technique. Color Plate 4-37 shows an excellent result with a well-centered lens and

a well-cleaned capsular bag. Color Plate 4-38, however, shows a poor result with virtually the same IOL style. Fixation and cortical clean-up were poorly done in the latter case. Placement of one haptic in the capsular bag and one haptic in the ciliary sulcus (asymptomatic fixation) commonly causes lens decentration. Exuberant cortical rem-

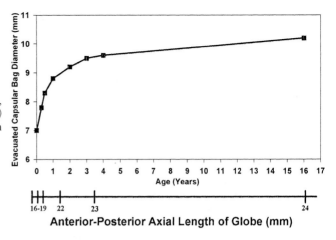

Fig. 4-80. Graph, based on a study of 50 eyes obtained postmortem, demonstrating that the growth of the globe (and lens capsular bag) occurs relatively rapidly during the first 18 months to 2 years. (From Wilson ME and others.[999])

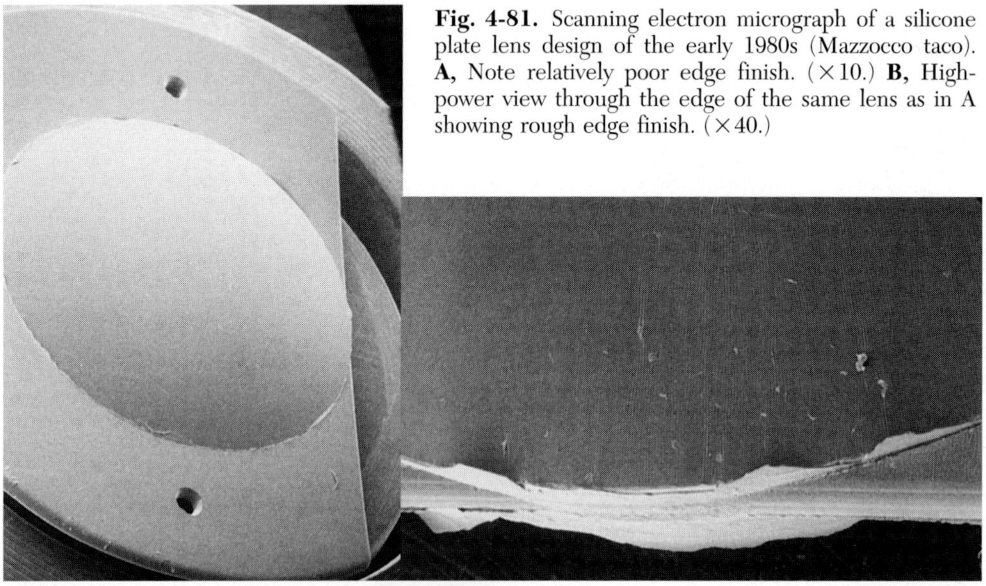

Fig. 4-81. Scanning electron micrograph of a silicone plate lens design of the early 1980s (Mazzocco taco). **A,** Note relatively poor edge finish. (×10.) **B,** High-power view through the edge of the same lens as in A showing rough edge finish. (×40.)

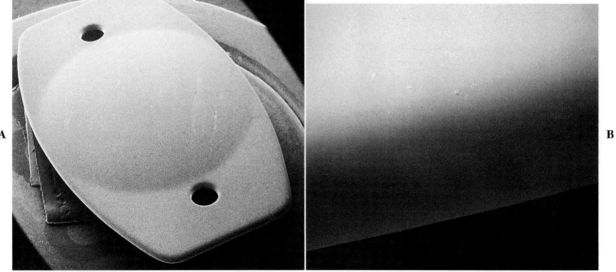

Fig. 4-82. Scanning electron micrograph showing marked improvement of plate lens manufacture by the 1990s. **A,** Note excellent overall design and manufacture finish. (×10.) **B,** High-power view showing excellent edge finish at the optic. (×50.)

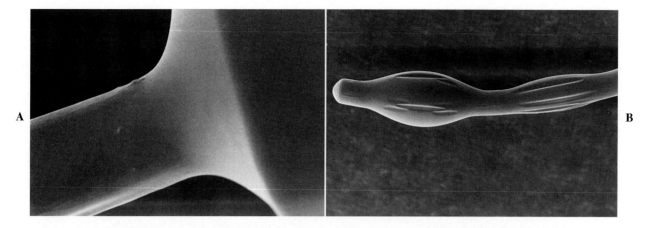

Fig. 4-83. Scanning electron micrographs of a silicone IOL coated with silicone oil. **A,** Haptic-optic junction showing diffuse coating of the oily material over the haptic (left) and optic (right). (×30.) **B,** Micrograph of the peripheral haptic of the same IOL showing droplets of silicone oil also coating the haptic biomaterial. (×100.)

nants (present in Color Plate 4-38 in the form of a Soemmering's ring) often represent origin of cells that migrate posteriorly across the visual axis causing secondary cataract or PCO. Decentration and posterior capsular opacification remain two important problems of modern IOL implantation.

Development of foldable lenses into the twenty-first century is one of fine tuning. Improvement of injectors and insertion techniques is ongoing.[542] For example, there is much effort now being expended to develop even more tissue-friendly optic biomaterials. Color Plates 4-39 and 4-40 and Fig. 4-83, A and B reveal a complication that may occasionally occur in patients with silicone lenses who subsequently require vitreal-retinal surgery using silicone oil.[462,517] Note that the silicone oil adheres to the silicone and, of course, leads to subsequent problems such as difficulty for the surgeon to visualize the interior of the patient's eye, not to mention a decrease in the patient's vision. There is present work in modifying both rigid and soft IOL biomaterials, for example, surface modification such as heparin surface modification (HSM) to change factors such as hydrophilicity and hydrophobicity. Such improvements should not only help address this and other specific iatrogenic complications but should improve general lens biocompatibility and help render lenses more compatible with various preexisting diseases such as uveitis, pseudoexfoliation, pigmentary dispersion syndrome, glaucoma, and diabetes in which unwanted tissue deposits in the IOL optic may be an issue.* There is also work on attaching different type haptic materials with varying mechanical characteristics such as rigidity and memory to the optic to achieve better and more stable fixation of the haptics in the capsular bag.

Pathology of intraocular lenses*

DECENTRATION

Lens malpositions† were very common in the early years of extracapsular surgery with posterior chamber lens implantation (Generation V). (For discussion on decentration and subluxation see page 153.) With modern capsular surgery the incidence of malpositions has markedly decreased in proportion to the continuous and vast improvements of surgical techniques. Decades of clinical and experimental research have shown that the only type of posterior chamber IOL fixation that is satisfactory is in-the-bag fixation of both haptics (see Figs. 4-72, A and B and 4-73) (p. 157).

Asymmetric fixation of haptics causes an almost automatic decentration of the lens optic (Color Plates 4-11–4-21) and, therefore, must be avoided, especially with modern small incision lenses. In the early 1980s, in the early years of posterior chamber IOLs, the most common causes of asymmetric fixation were surgical inexperience and exit of haptics from the capsular bag ("pea-podding") through tears in the anterior capsule following can-opener capsulectomy. By the mid 1980s surgical techniques had improved, but it was not until the development of CCC that a stable anterior capsule was consistently achieved that would allow permanent and stable in-the-bag fixation of both haptics. This has been the greatest and the most important means of reducing the complication of decentration.

INFLAMMATION

Noninfectious causes

Numerous causes of postoperative inflammation following cataract surgery without implantation of IOLs have been documented.[166,702,1020,1021,1024] With the advent of IOL implantation, additional pathogenic factors related to the presence of a foreign body in the eye were introduced and a new terminology emerged. The term *toxic lens*

---

* References 439, 462, 492, 516-518, 527, 529, 530, 532, 540, 601, 607, 627, 629, 630, 631, 633, 677, 687, 691, 708, 709, 712, 713, 715, 730, 736, 742, 743, 749, 754, 755, 769, 774, 791, 798, 799, 812, 817, 818, 821, 826, 827, 831, 832, 846, 867, 869, 873, 874, 878, 889, 890, 893, 899–902, 917, 920–922, 972–974, 995, 1006.

---

* References 1015–1390.
† References 165, 554, 565, 740, 885, 997.

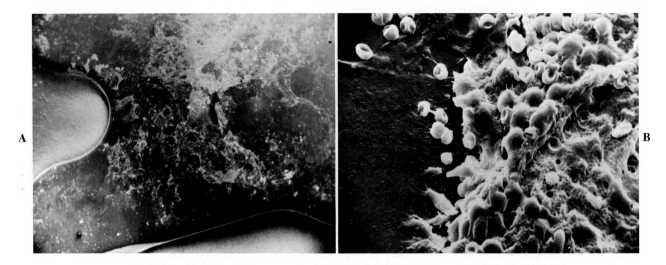

Fig. 4-84. A, Scanning electron micrograph of a rigid Choyce-style anterior chamber IOL removed because of anterior chamber inflammation and hyphema. (×20.) **B,** Higher power scanning electron micrograph of **A.** Inflammatory debris is present on the lens surface and numerous erythrocytes have been deposited on the optic. (×100.) (**A** from Apple DJ, and others: Surv Ophthalmol 29:1, 1984.)

syndrome (Color Plate 4-41) was originally used to denote a sterile postoperative inflammation following IOL implantation. This complication was often associated with hypopyon or vitreous reaction but could be differentiated from infectious endophthalmitis.[1154,1230,1271,1318] Since toxic lens syndrome was first described, many additional causes for this clinical entity have been documented, both infectious and noninfectious. Many of these causes are not related to the IOL itself, but the clinical findings of both types may be indistinguishable.

Toxic lens syndrome has, therefore, lost much of its original meaning and specificity, and in many cases is a misnomer because the inflammation often has nothing to do with the IOL. Even when a lens is involved, it is not clear whether the lens in question is the IOL or remnants of the patient's own crystalline lens.

Inflammation following IOL implantation may be caused by the presence of the lens itself. Contact in chafing of the IOL against sensitive tissue has, from the beginning, been an important pathogenetic factor. The aqueous humor is formed by the nonpigmented ciliary epithelium as a modified ultrafiltrate of blood. It is nearly protein free and acellular.[1069,1070] The composition of the aqueous is maintained by an intact blood-aqueous barrier.[1192,1239] When any portion of this lining is disrupted or manipulated, breakdown of this barrier occurs.* This can cause an anterior segment inflammation and/or a uveitis-glaucoma-hyphema syndrome. The severity or intensity of the breakdown of the blood-aqueous barrier partially determines what clinical signs a patient may have. These signs range from subclinical or symptomatic inflammation to severe uveitis with glaucoma and hyphema (UGH syndrome) (Color Plate 4-42; Figs. 4-84 and 4-85).[267,268] A high incidence of this condition associated with poor-quality, iris-supported and anterior chamber IOLs occurred in the late

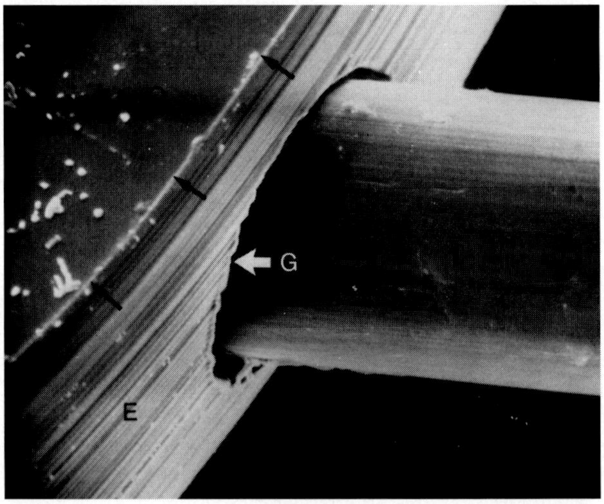

---

* References 737, 808, 846, 1019, 1066, 1077, 1078, 1083, 1084, 1302, 1360.

Fig. 4-85. Higher power scanning electron micrograph of the loop-optic junction of an Azar 91Z lens explanted because of UGH syndrome. The lens optic edges are sharp *(arrows)* and there are numerous parallel lines on the equatorial surface *(E)* of the optic *(O)*, signifying an incomplete polishing process. Note the gap *(G)* between the staking hole in the optic and the polypropylene loop *(L)*, which can form a nidus for accumulation of inflammatory and proteinaceous debris. (×200.)

1970s and early 1980s. Figure 4-84 shows an example of a badly manufactured, poorly polished copy of a Choyce IOL. Figure 4-85 demonstrates the extremely sharp optic edge, which occurred on the Azar 91Z IOL. There is a much lower incidence of UGH syndrome today, but it occasionally occurs. Many thousands of patients have been implanted with poor-quality, iris-supported and anterior chamber IOLs. Although most of these lenses have now been withdrawn from the market, ophthalmologists continue to treat occasional patients with UGH syndrome and other long-term complications caused by these IOLs.

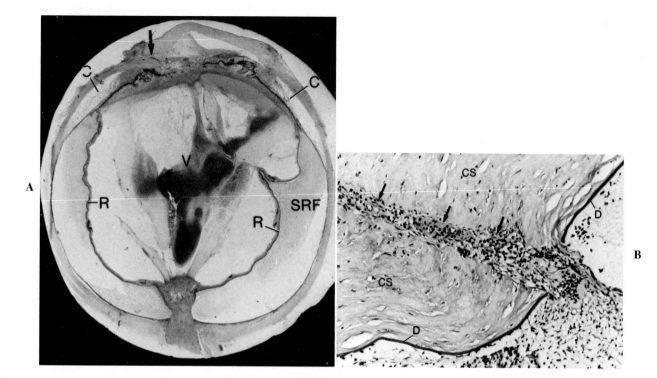

Fig. 4-86. A, Photomicrograph of the eye of a 19-year-old patient 9 months after cataract removal showing the classic features of a bacterial endophthalmitis. Note the surgical wound tract *(tip of the arrow)*. The lens is absent, dense fibrous membranes are present in the ciliary area, and a vitreous abscess *(V)* is present. The deeply stained material represents a dense accumulation of polymorphonuclear neutrophils that have undergone a liquefactive necrosis. There is total detachment of the sensory retina *(R)*, a dense transudate of subretinal fluid *(SRF)* present in all quadrants, and is a hypotonic detachment of the ciliary body and choroid *(C)* from the adjacent sclera. (H&E stain; ×1.) **B,** High-power photomicrograph of a portion of the posterior aspect of the cornea (see **A** and Color Plate 4-43) showing the wound tract *(arrows)*. Descemet's membrane *(D)* is ruptured at this site, and there is an ingrowth of inflammatory cells coursing from within the eye *(lower right)* through the wound tract causing it to gap open. The corneal stroma *(CS)* shows extensive scarring, with loss of the regular parallel structure of the lamellae. The corneal endothelium is totally absent. (PAS stain; ×150.)

Infectious causes

Generalized endophthalmitis. Infectious endophthalmitis (Color Plate 4-43; Figs. 4-86, *A* and *B*, and 4-87) is a possible complication of any intraocular procedure, including cataract removal and IOL implantation° (see also Chap. 3). Because the IOL is a foreign body, and more operative manipulations are required with IOL implantation, one might expect a higher incidence of infectious endophthalmitis in the pseudophakic eye than in the aphakic eye. Most studies, however, show that this is not necessarily the case.[257,406,1092]

Treatment of generalized infectious endophthalmitis depends on prompt recognition of the inflammatory process† and rapid culture of aqueous and/or vitreous aspirate. As a rule, the inflammatory reaction begins within the first few postoperative days, and it typically includes pain, chemosis, hypopyon, and corneal decompensation.[622,1016,1087] Studies by Beyer and coworkers[1044,1045,1128,1271] postulate a benefit from the trend toward extracapsular surgery—an intact posterior capsule creates a barrier effect that may prevent the posterior extension of bacteria.[1128]

Until the late 1970s, IOLs were sterilized with sodium hydroxide, and the sterilized lenses were then stored in a sodium bicarbonate solution.[1108,1111] Two major epidemics have occurred because of contamination of the storage solution. The first epidemic was caused by the organism *Paecilomyces lilacinus* and the second was caused by *Pseudomonas aeruginosa*.[1120,1246,1262,1278] After these two outbreaks, NaOH (wet) sterilization was banned by the FDA and dry sterilization with ethylene oxide was adopted.

Localized endophthalmitis. Microorganisms may become clustered within the lens capsule following accidental trauma causing rupture of the capsule or after planned ECCE, creating a localized, smoldering infection within the capsular sac° (Figs. 4-88 to 4-90). This entity, which

---

° References 702, 1048, 1049, 4164, 1075, 1080, 1087, 1089, 1092, 1102, 1120, 1121, 1124, 1125, 1135, 1147, 1151, 1163, 1166, 1167, 1169, 1178, 1183, 1198, 1216, 1231, 1233, 1237, 1238, 1246, 1266, 1269, 1272, 1283, 1290, 1292, 1304, 1307, 1327, 1333, 1341, 1356, 1359, 1362, 1365, 1372.
† References 1080, 1082, 1087, 1102, 1147, 1218, 1238, 1245, 1253, 1328, 1389.

° References 227, 395, 712, 1022, 1023, 1052, 1055, 1072, 1080, 1089, 1227, 1228, 1268, 1281, 1282, 1287, 1300, 1320, 1328, 1329, 1349, 1350, 1351, 1378, 1390.

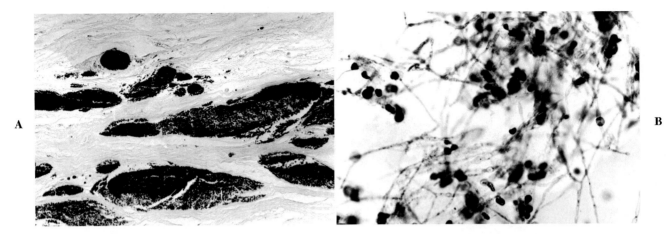

Fig. 4-87. A, Photomicrograph of the cornea of a globe containing an intraocular lens. Complications occurred, including corneal decompensation, corneal ulcer, stromal keratitis, and endophthalmitis. Numerous bacterial colonies (masses of dark-staining punctate structures) are visible within the corneal stroma. (Gram stain; ×175.) **B,** Vitreous aspirate from a case of mycotic endophthalmitis in another eye containing an intraocular lens. The organisms are visible in this photomicrograph. (Potassium hydroxide preparation; ×275.)

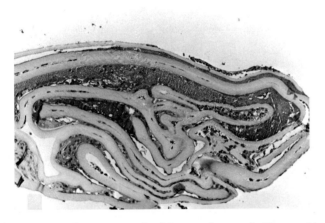

Fig. 4-88. Photomicrograph of the capsular sac of a 60-year-old patient who underwent an ECCE and implantation of a capsule-fixated posterior chamber IOL in November, 1985. Immediate postoperative visual acuity was 20/30, but cell and flare were noted 2 days later. Inflammation increased with formation of keratic precipitates and cells noted in the anterior vitreous. A diagnosis of sterile inflammatory reaction or toxic lens syndrome was considered. A bacterial endophthalmitis was confirmed by a vitreous tap 1 month after implantation when diphtheroids were cultured from the aspirated material. Antibiotics brought only transient improvement, and the IOL and all capsular material were removed. The inflammation slowly subsided and visual acuity returned to 20/30 in the affected eye. As shown in this stain, coccobacilli were identified within the lens capsular sac. (Gram stain; ×40.)

we term *localized end-ophthalmitis*, was first recognized as a cause of persistent postoperative uveitis in the mid 1980s. It has a similar clinical appearance and course as the so-called toxic lens syndrome; therefore, localized endophthalmitis should be considered in the differential diagnosis of otherwise unexplainable postsurgical inflammatory reactions.[1281]

We initially reported on five cases that were clinically diagnosed as toxic lens syndrome, in which patients suffered from postimplantation anterior segment inflammation with keratic precipitates and/or hypopyon.[1022,1281] In all five cases, diagnoses ranging from biomaterial-related inflammation to phacoanaphylaxis (p. 136) were considered. The patients were treated by removal of the IOL and lens capsule, with a careful cleansing to ensure no lens cortical remnants were left in the eye. In three of the five cases, an immediate improvement occurred and the inflammation subsided. In the other two cases, the inflammation diminished but did not subside.

Microscopic examination of such cases reveals organisms sequestered within the residual lens capsule. This localization apparently typically prevents widespread dissemination of the infection and full-blown endophthalmitis.

These cases correlate well with the experimental studies of Beyer and co-workers[1044,1045,1128] in which they note the protective barrier effect of the posterior lens capsule in exogenous bacterial endophthalmitis produced in experiments in nonhuman primate eyes. When the posterior capsule was left intact in these experiments, the infection spread to the vitreous cavity in only 20% of the cases. Of the eyes with a primary posterior capsulotomy, 80% demonstrated a subsequent vitreal infection.

A major reason for the mild clinical course observed in cases of localized endophthalmitis is the low virulence that characterizes the typical pathogen that is isolated in such cases.[1060] Organisms such as *Propionibacterium acnes* and *Staphylococcus epidermidis* generally exhibit minimal virulence. *Propionibacterium acnes* is a bacterium that can originate from several sources including the patient's own skin or conjunctiva or the skin of the surgeon or other operating room personnel.[1062,1224,1327] Like any organism, it may also be transferred as a contaminant to the surface of the IOL during surgery.

Even if the organisms are found in aspirated material following a vitreous tap, confirmation of a *P. acnes*–induced inflammation may be difficult to establish.[1227,1280]

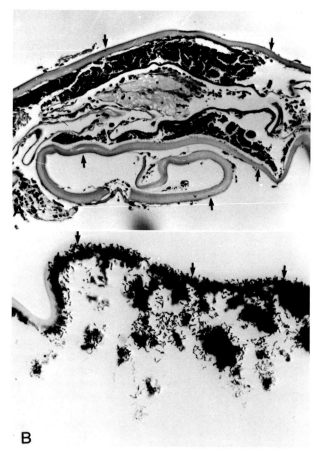

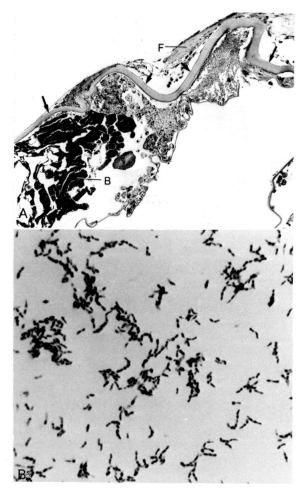

Fig. 4-89. A, Low-power photomicrograph of a removed lens capsular sac showing a dense accumulation of organisms, recognizable as deeply stained granular material. The lighter substance is residual lens cortical material. The capsular sac *(arrows)* is folded and is sectioned in such a way that the organisms and portions of the posterior capsule are sandwiched between folds of the thicker anterior capsule. (H&E stain; ×75.) **B,** Photomicrograph of a lens capsule sac showing gram-positive pleomorphic bacilli. The organisms are localized in the anterior of the capsular sac only and follow the contour of the faintly visible capsular basement membrane *(arrows).* (Gram stain; ×350.)

Fig. 4-90. A, Photomicrograph of the capsular sac removed from the eye of a 71-year-old patient who did well for 6 months with an implanted posterior chamber lens until posterior capsular opacification developed. A Nd-YAG laser capsulotomy was performed. After this procedure the eye developed a severe, diffuse inflammation diagnosed as probable endophthalmitis. The IOL and the lens capsular sac were removed. Note the portion of the lens capsule *(arrows)* and fibrous metaplasia *(F)* of the residual lens cortex. The lightly stained material is residual necrotic lens substance. The deeply stained basophilic material *(B)* at left is gram-positive and represents necrotic organisms. (Gram stain; ×30.) **B,** Culture of the lens capsular sac material grew *Propionibacterium acnes,* a finding that was verified by Gram stain. (Gram stain; ×700.) (**B** courtesy Dr. Francis W Price Jr., Indianapolis, Ind.)

This organism is so ubiquitous in the environment that it is commonly dismissed by microbiology laboratory staff as a contaminant, usually identified only as a diphtheroid. It can take up to 7 days for the organisms to appear on anaerobic culture plates; therefore, the diagnosis may be missed if the cultures are read too early.

Meisler and coworkers[1227] recognized the importance of *P. acnes* as the cause for delayed endophthalmitis after cataract extraction. They reported on a series of six patients with chronic *Propionibacterium* endophthalmitis. In their cases the inflammatory process was more generalized with vitreal involvement, as documented by positive vitreous taps. In contrast, the inflammatory reaction in our cases was localized within the lens capsular sac.[1280,1349]

We have observed a patient who underwent an uneventful ECCE and implantation of a posterior chamber lens in the capsular bag with an excellent postoperative result.[1349] The eye was quiet for several months, and the only complication was gradual development of posterior capsular opac-

ification. A Nd:YAG laser capsulotomy was performed, and a severe, diffuse inflammatory reaction developed quickly after this procedure. This reaction was refractory to intense steroid therapy, and injection of an antibiotic into the vitreous brought little improvement. One month later the IOL along with the entire lens capsular sac was removed.

A culture of this removed material produced *P. acnes.* Microscopic examination revealed dense deposits of gram positive basophilic material that was interpreted as foci of necrotic organisms and nuclear fragments from the bacteria. The organisms were apparently initially confined within the lens capsular sac, producing an asymptomatic or subclinical, low-grade reaction. After release into the vitreous through a Nd:YAG laser–induced opening in the posterior capsule, a generalized endophthalmitis rapidly developed. Other authors[227,1227,1349] have reported similar cases of endophthalmitis that developed in an otherwise quiet eye after a Nd:YAG laser posterior capsulotomy for PCO was performed.

Meisler and coworkers[1227] proposed a hypothesis as to why the infectious process sometimes fails to subside after treatment with seemingly adequate doses of antibiotics. They noted that in an animal model of lens-induced hypersensitivity, sensitization to lens material is most effectively achieved when it is injected in complete Freund's adjuvant (mycobacterial protein). *Propionibacterium* has adjuvant qualities itself and possibly could play a role in promoting hypersensitivity to the lens protein in some patients, thus invoking a cellular reaction characterized by keratic precipitates, hypopyon, and granulomatous inflammation.

There is an interesting historical footnote that supports the synergistic proposal of Meisler and coworkers.[1227] Piest and coworkers[1280] reviewed the 1922 report of Verhoeff and Lemoine,[1366] which is one of the first studies describing the condition now known as phacoanaphylactic endophthalmitis (see p. 136). In discussing the histopathology of their experimental cases, Verhoeff and Lemoine noted,

> In connection with the Gram stain, it may be well to state here that the cataractous lens, after fixation, often in places appears to have undergone transformation into fine granules, some of which are basophilic and stain deeply by the Gram method. Such granules sometimes appear in pus cells, possibly due to precipitation of lens material within the latter, and often closely resemble large cocci.

Perhaps Verhoeff and Lemoine were unknowingly seeing organisms. In this study done 68 years ago, they may have introduced the concept of a synergistic inflammatory reaction between infectious organisms and retained lens substance.

Localized endophthalmitis represents a condition that has undoubtedly occurred for many years but was only recognized in the 1980s in association with ECCE and IOL implantation. Almost all reported cases to date have occurred in instances when polypropylene haptics formed the supporting element of the IOL. This suggests that organisms may stick to this material more than PMMA.[1287] It has probably been diagnosed many times in the past as toxic lens syndrome. Ormerod and coworkers[1268] reported on 18 cases of anaerobic bacterial endophthalmitis. In an editorial in the *American Journal of Ophthalmology*, R.E. Smith[1329] stressed the importance of considering various infectious causes when inflammation occurs after cataract surgery.

Even after the IOL is removed, the infection in such cases may persist. This can lead to cystoid macular edema. When the inflammation does not respond to initial treatment, aggressive diagnostic and therapeutic procedures should be undertaken without delay. Clinically, this entity most closely resembles classic phacoanaphylactic endophthalmitis in that removal of the remaining lens capsular material is required for successful treatment, rather than IOL removal alone.

Regardless of the exact nature of the pathogenesis, removed lens cortical material should always be submitted for pathologic examination so that antibiotic treatment can be quickly initiated, if necessary. In most cases, the causative organisms, for example *P. acnes* or *S. epidermidis*, respond rapidly to antibiotic treatment.[1053,1227,1244,1367]

Crystalline lens-induced inflammation

Inflammation caused by residual lens cortex, phacotoxic reaction, and phacoanaphylactic endophthalmitis is a conditions that in rare instances can complicate an otherwise successful IOL implantation after an ECCE. These may cause an inflammatory process that is refractory to all treatment including removal of the IOL.

Phacoanaphylactic endophthalmitis first reported in 1922[1366] was classically described by Irvine and Irvine[1160,1161] as a sterile granulomatous inflammatory response to retained lens material. This condition is an autoreaction to the patient's own protein derived from residual lens remnants left in the eye after any opening of the capsule, as occurs following ECCE (p. 136). There may be only a transient phacotoxic response, which usually subsides rapidly within days or a few weeks, or a prolonged phacoanaphylactic reaction may develop in some patients.[166]

Rahi and Garner[1284] state that the term *phacoanaphylaxis* is inaccurate, because no IgE is involved in the process. Traumatic or surgical rupture of the lens capsule with escape of the cortical material apparently exposes the normally sequestered lens substance to the immune system.[1306,1379] Before rupture of the capsule, the capsular membrane provides a protective barrier, which prevents a cell-mediated autosensitization to the patient's own protein.[170,920]

Apparently this problem was extremely rare when the majority of IOL implantations took place following ICCE. Since the transition from ICCE to ECCE by many surgeons, phacoanaphylaxis might have been expected to occur again with greater frequency. Thus far this has not been the case, probably because of marked improvements in the ECCE technique. As mentioned on page 00, there is likely an infectious component to this disease. Because adequate sterile techniques are used by most modern surgeons, this would lessen the likelihood of occurrence of this condition. Many clinicopathologic reports have documented various forms of postimplantation uveitis and chronic inflammation, including granulomatous reactions; however, none of these papers discussed phacoanaphylactic endophthalmitis occurring after ECCE with IOL implantation.* Some clinical reports of complications in a large ECCE series do not even mention the disease.[1092] Exceptions to this are the reports of Smith and Weiner,[391] Ishikawa and coworkers,[1164] Awan,[1031] Apple and coworkers,[166,1021] and a section in the Jaffe textbook, *Cataract Surgery and Its Complications*.[702] The diagnosis of phacoanaphylaxis, however, may be difficult, and the true incidence of this condition may be higher than is indicated by the number of published case reports.

Some of the first cases were reported in two independent studies[1021,1380] and in a study by Wohl and associates.[1380] In the case illustrated in Color Plate 4-24, the attending physician did not recognize the cause of the inflammation clinically and removed the modified J-loop posterior

---

* References 1029, 1031, 1050, 1121, 1152, 1215, 1219, 1294, 1316.

chamber IOL. Despite this treatment, the uveitis worsened and the eye was eventually enucleated.

The onset of a phacoanaphylactic reaction typically occurs between 1 and 14 days after traumatic or surgical capsular disruption.[386,1284] Exceptions, however, have been reported in which the reaction occurred as early as several hours postoperatively or as late as several months after lens capsular sac rupture.[1330] Brinkman and Broekhuyse[1166] feel that the clinical response of a rapid phacoanaphylaxis represents a secondary immune response following lens capsular sac rupture in a patient who was already immunologically primed with sensitized lymphocytes to leaking lenticular antigens. The association with localized bacterial endophthalmitis has already been discussed (p. 163). The disease is characterized histologically by a zonal granulomatous inflammatory reaction to the lens capsular remnants.[170,1076,1284] There is a central polymorphonuclear reaction that is surrounded by concentric layers of various inflammatory cells, including epithelioid and giant cells. Foamy macrophages have been seen in eyes with phacoanaphylactic uveitis, which may be similar to the foamy macrophages classically associated with phacolytic glaucoma.[1277] The adjacent iris and ciliary body typically show an infiltration of plasma cells and lymphocytes. The entire inflammatory mass may become encased in granulation tissue and may organize to form dense fibrous tissue.

The uveitis may burn out in some cases with aggressive corticosteroid therapy.[165] Antibiotics to eradicate a possible infectious organism (e.g., *P. acnes*) are often helpful. In rare instances removal of the IOL and thorough cleansing to remove any remaining lens cortical remnants may be required. A report by Mullaney and Condon[1248] discusses the possible role of PMMA in phacoanaphylactic reaction. If unrecognized and thus untreated the disease may lead to any of the sequelae of chronic inflammation, including phthisis bulbi.[1163]

Even in the absence of histopathologic examination, *the main clinical hallmark of both phakoanaphylaxis and localized endophthalmitis is the fact that the inflammation may continue, and may even worsen, despite removal of the IOL.* An understanding that any postoperative uveitis may not only represent a hypersensitivity response to lens protein, as proposed by Verhoeff and Lemoine,[1335] but may also represent a synergistic reaction between bacterial protein and crystalline lens protein, which creates or exacerbates the inflammation, is necessary to lead to decisive therapeutic decisions.

Sympathetic ophthalmia most commonly occurs after accidental trauma.[1046,1207] A search of the literature provides few details in reports of the condition in eyes with IOLs.[379,1031,1050,1076,1099] A sympathetic response, however, can occasionally occur in the opposite eye in association with phacoanaphylactic endophthalmitis.° The histology of sympathetic ophthalmia is discussed in Chapter 7, page 298.

CORNEAL COMPLICATIONS

By the late 1980s the most common reason for corneal transplantation in the United States, at least in cornea re-

ferral centers, was not disease but pseudophakic bullous keratopathy.[1165] Corneal decompensation, pseudophakic corneal edema, and pseudophakic bullous keratopathy (Fig. 4-91; Color Plate 4-44) have been the most common visually disabling conditions of IOL implantation surgery since the introduction of this procedure.

In the early decades of lens implantation, the primary cause of corneal endothelial damage and subsequent decompensation was mechanical in nature. Iris-supported IOLs sometimes dislocated anteriorly, causing endothelial chafing. Some early anterior chamber lens designs had excessive loop flexibility that forced the IOL to vault anteriorly when external pressure was applied to the eye. Lenses that were not correctly sized frequently moved within the eye, and the IOL components intermittently or continuously touched the posterior surface of the cornea.[259] Many intraoperative complications associated with early IOLs were related to the less sophisticated surgical techniques used at that time. Viscoelastic agents (such as Healon), with their tissue protective properties, were not available.

As recently as 1987, pseudophakic bullous keratopathy was still a common problem with many anterior chamber lenses, in particular with some IOLs with small-diameter, closed-loops, which were still being marketed as of the late 1980s (Fig. 4-92). The removal of these lenses and the subsequent widespread use of posterior chamber IOLs has caused the overall rate of corneal decompensation to decrease markedly. Because these lenses are positioned further from the cornea and behind the iris, corneal touch is avoided.

Although the pathogenesis of corneal complications associated with early IOLs often was related to poor lens designs, lens dislocation, intraoperative problems, and overt postoperative inflammation, frequently there was no evidence of direct IOL contact with the corneal endothelium and no preexisting disease to cause a low endothelial cell count.[1059,1110,1118,1352] Why then did corneal decompensation or pseudophakic bullous keratopathy, sometimes associated with cystoid macular edema, occur unexpectedly 5 or more years after implantation in some patients? In most cases the only plausible explanation is that a subclinical, chronic, smoldering inflammation, usually located at the loop fixation sites, was present. A slow release of toxic inflammatory mediators from the foci of cellular infiltrates may gradually damage the corneal endothelium. This process is often insidious; neither the clinician nor the patient is aware the problem exists.

Corneal decompensation and pseudophakic bullous keratopathy can usually be successfully treated with penetrating keratoplasty.[1336,1368] If the eye is not severely damaged by inflammation or cystoid macular edema, good visual results can be achieved by removal or exchange of the offending IOL.

Endothelial cells may be injured by direct contact with surgical instruments or the IOL during surgery° (Figs. 4-93 and 4-94). Intermittent or constant touch of a malpositioned or inappropriately vaulted IOL may cause continued loss of endothelial cells and subsequent corneal decompensation.[1289] Drews[259] described the syndrome of intermit-

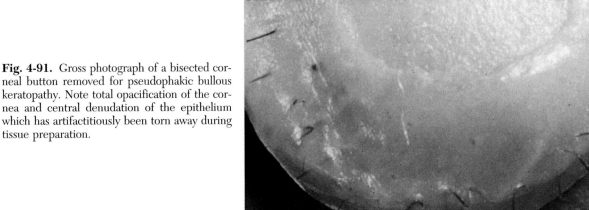

Fig. 4-91. Gross photograph of a bisected corneal button removed for pseudophakic bullous keratopathy. Note total opacification of the cornea and central denudation of the epithelium which has artifactitiously been torn away during tissue preparation.

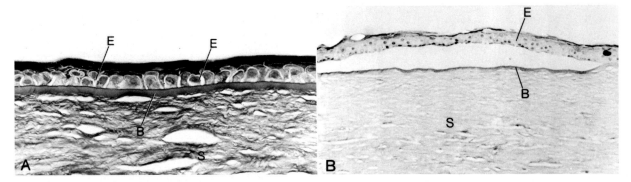

Fig. 4-92. A, Photomicrograph of a cornea from a patient who received a secondary anterior chamber lens implantation in 1981. The patient subsequently developed severe corneal edema that required penetrating keratoplasty. Note the extensive intracellular and intercellular edema *(E)* of the basal layer of the corneal epithelium. Bowman's layer *(B)*, stroma *(S)*. (×200.) **B,** Photomicrograph of a case of pseudophakic bullous keratopathy showing a flat or shallow detachment of the epithelium *(E)* from the underlying Bowman's layer. Stroma *(S)*. (H&E stain; ×150.)

tent touch and described a triad of findings that included ciliary flush, localized corneal changes, and cystoid macular edema.

Cases of late pseudophakic bullous keratopathy and cystoid macular edema often occur inexplicably in the absence of any known cause such as intraoperative trauma, lens instability or decentration, or direct corneal touch by the IOL. These conditions can even occur with well-fixated posterior chamber IOLs that rest far behind the corneal endothelium. These complications can only be explained by assuming a direct toxic effect by mediators derived from foci of chronic smoldering inflammation, either clinical or subclinical.[356] Such inflammation is usually present at loop or haptic fixation sites in the ciliary region. It is known that such inflammatory mediators as prostaglandins can be toxic to the endothelium. Hull and coworkers[1153] and Rao and coworkers[1286] have shown that oxidative free radicals formed by neutrophils and other inflammatory cells may

be toxic to endothelial cells. This inflammatory process is a factor in the high incidence of complications associated with some anterior chamber IOLs.

There are several severe sequelae of corneal decompensation. Decompensated corneas, with or without pseudophakic bullous keratopathy, are clearly more susceptible to serious secondary complications such as severe vascularization and scarring, keratitis and ulceration, descemetocele formation, and melting and perforation* (Fig. 4-95). Severe localized corneal disease can progress to frank endophthalmitis.

Formation of a retrocorneal fibrous membrane is an unusual but potential complication of penetrating keratoplasty, whether it is performed alone or as part of a triple procedure.[1133,1197] One important source for retrocorneal

---

* References 226, 340, 590, 762, 1155, 1271, 1386.

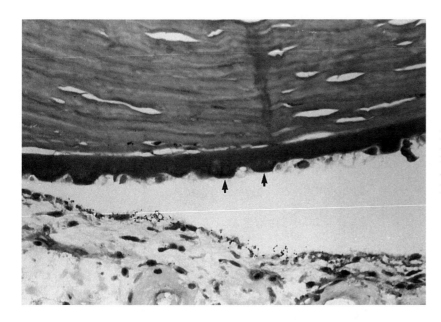

Fig. 4-93. Photomicrograph of the posterior aspect of a cornea with pseudophakic bullous keratopathy showing extensive guttata (*arrows*). Note vaculozation and atrophy of the corneal endothelium. (PAS stain; ×100.)

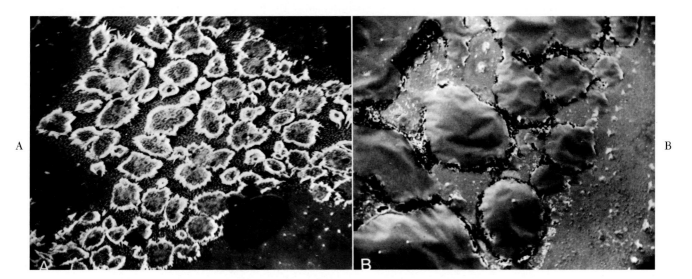

Fig. 4-94. A, Scanning electron micrograph of an IOL optic showing sheets of corneal endothelial cells on the lens surface that were probably scraped off at the time of surgery. The patient developed bullous keratopathy. (×100.) **B,** Scanning electron micrograph of another case of pseudophakic bullous keratopathy showing deposits of corneal endothelial cells upon the Choyce Mark VIII optic, similar to those seen in **A.** Four years postoperatively, penetrating keratoplasty and lens exchange were required. (×200.)

membrane formation is fibrous metaplasia of the corneal endothelium.[1337] Such a metaplastic reaction has been clinically and experimentally documented in several other conditions, including various forms of anterior segment inflammation, cryotherapy, alkali burns, and following accidental or surgical trauma.* The participating endothelial cells are most frequently of host origin but fibrous metaplasia of donor endothelium has also been observed.[1321]

Other sources of retrocorneal membranes (p. 103) include the following: stromal ingrowth through breaks in Descemet's membrane, invasion of conjunctival connective tissue, and fibrous metaplasia and proliferation of iris stromal cells and pigment endothelium.[196,1058,1332,1343,1355]

RETINAL COMPLICATIONS

Achievement of a good result following cataract surgery depends upon the functional status of the sensory retina, both before and after surgery.[1355] Preexisting macular disease discovered after surgery, in particular age-related ("senile") macular degeneration, is one of the most fre-

---

* References 170, 1047, 1177, 1216, 1236, 1288, 1332, 1343.

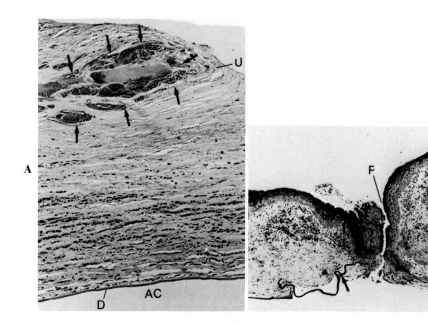

Fig. 4-95. A, Photomicrograph of a cornea from an 84-year-old patient who received a Surgidev Model 10 Leiske anterior chamber lens in January 1983. The patient suffered anterior uveitis, bullous keratopathy, and secondary glaucoma. Severe keratitis, seen here, ensued after the original corneal decompensation. The masses of amorphous material *(arrows)* are gram-positive bacterial colonies. Note the intense infiltration of polymorphonuclear neutrophils situated between the stromal lamellae. The corneal endothelium is totally absent, as is the epithelium that should be present at the upper surface of the cornea. Descemet's membrane *(D)*, anterior chamber *(AC)*, site of diffuse corneal ulceration *(U)*. (H&E stain; ×100.) **B,** Photomicrograph through a cornea from a patient who received a Surgidev Model 10 Leiske anterior chamber lens as a secondary procedure 2 years after an ICCE in 1979. The patient developed corneal decompensation with severe corneal melt (a Mooren-like ulcer) that was nonresponsive to treatment, and the eye was enucleated in June 1983. Note the central perforation *(P)* of the cornea where the epithelium has grown in between the gaps of the wound. There is extensive necrosis and scarring of the corneal stroma, the epithelium is irregular, and there are scattered infiltrates of chronic inflammatory cells within the corneal stroma. Fragments of wrinkled, coiled Descemet's membrane are present, and the endothelium is totally absent. (PAS stain; ×100.)

quent causes of decreased visual acuity (<20/40) in most clinical series. The incidence of postoperative cystoid macular edema has declined markedly with improvements in lens designs and modern surgical techniques, yet an occasional case may occur even after an apparently flawless IOL implantation. Also the incidence of retinal detachment has dropped in recent years. The most important factors in this change are not only the return to ECCE and the use of posterior chamber IOLs but also the overall improvement in surgical technique by most surgeons since the 1980s. As experience with IOLs increases, the number of retinal contraindications to posterior chamber lens implants decreases.[1345]

Pseudophakic cystoid macular edema

Cystoid macular edema[1015,1086] (see Chapter 8, p. 424 for a general discussion of this condition) following cataract extraction was first described by S. R. Irvine[1162] in 1953 and discussed by A. R. Irvine[1157] in 1976 and in 1980.[1158] Both authors felt it was secondary either to postoperative iritis or to vitreous traction to the cataract wound. Using the then-new technique of fluorescein angiography, Gass and Norton[1116,1117] studied patients with cystoid macular edema. This condition, they noted, was a distinct phenome-

non that was different from central serous retinopathy, with which it had been confused previously.[1142]

Cystoid macular edema (Figs. 4-96 to 4-100) is now recognized as a complication of cataract surgery, with or without IOL implantation.* It is not entirely clear whether cystoid macular edema occurs because of (1) an increased permeability of the perifoveolar capillaries, (2) an ischemic tissue injury, (3) a secondary response to intraocular inflammation, or (4) a direct traction on the macula following vitreous shifts. It is possible that a combination of all these factors may be involved.

Obstbaum and Galin[356] reported a connection between anterior segment inflammation associated with prostaglandin release and concurrent corneal decompensation and cystoid macular edema (the corneal-retinal inflammatory syndrome). Several authors have studied the association between inflammatory mediators and other eye diseases, including cystoid macular edema. These include Ambache

---

* References 704, 712, 1015, 1073, 1086, 1093, 1099, 1115–1117, 1137–1139, 1142–1144, 1156, 1158, 1162, 1166, 1179, 1185, 1189, 1191, 1195, 1212, 1232, 1240, 1241, 1243, 1245, 1251, 1296, 1310, 1313, 1315, 1358, 1384.

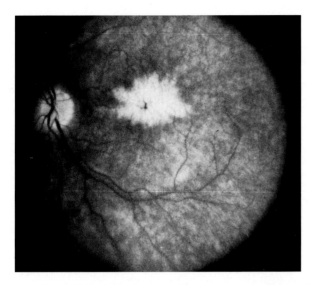

Fig. 4-96. Left fundus of a patient (fluorescein angiogram) with persistent cystoid macular edema after cataract extraction and posterior chamber IOL implantation. The optic nerve is seen at the left. Notice the flower-petal configuration of fluorescein staining in the macular region. The fluorescein leaks into the microcystic spaces that occur primarily in the middle and outer layers of the retina.

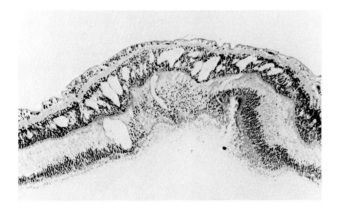

Fig. 4-97. Photomicrograph showing the retina of a postmortem eye. The patient received an anterior chamber IOL and developed clinically evident, persistent cystoid macular edema. Note the multiple spaces in the inner nuclear layer and outer plexiform layer. The fluid within these spaces was washed away during tissue processing. The sensory retina detached artifactitiously from the underlying pigment epithelium (not shown here) and caused distortion and folding of the retina. (H&E stain; ×75.)

and coworkers,[1019] Cole and Unger,[1066,1361] Cunha-Vaz,[1069] Dulaney,[264] Eakins,[1083] Jampol and coworkers,[1309] Miyake and coworkers,[1242] Ozaki,[861] Sears,[1309] Yannuzzi,[1387] and others.[634]

Cataract surgery, particularly that associated with implantation of poorly manufactured IOLs (Fig. 4-100) is obviously not the only cause of cystoid macular edema.[1142] Penetrating keratoplasty and retinal detachment repair are other ocular operations that may cause cystoid macular edema.[170,1142] Many nonsurgical causes of cystoid macular edema include[1099,1115]

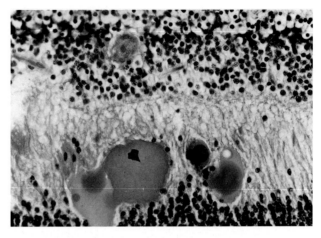

Fig. 4-98. High-power photomicrograph through the outer plexiform retinal layer of a postmortem eye. The patient had an anterior chamber IOL implanted and subsequently developed clinically evident cystoid macular edema. Note the densely stained transudates that are indicative of this condition. (H&E stain; ×200.)

1. retinal vascular diseases such as diabetes mellitus, hypertension, and venous occlusion
2. inflammatory diseases such as uveitis and pars planitis
3. intraocular tumors
4. inherited diseases such as retinitis pigmentosa
5. degenerative phenomena such as age-related macular degeneration
6. drug-induced cystoid macular edema, which occurs with use of epinephrine, tamoxifen, and nicotinic acid

Both ICCE and ECCE are frequently associated with cystoid macular edema whether an IOL is implanted or not. Generally, the edema occurs 4 to 12 weeks postoperatively, although it may not become manifest until months or even years later.[1116,1132] Clinically, the disease appears as a collection of tiny cysts around the fovea, which are sometimes difficult to observe without the high magnification of the direct ophthalmoscope or by use of the slitlamp and contact lens. Fluorescein angiography highlights the cysts, which occur in a flower-petal configuration (Fig. 4-96), and is helpful in identifying vascular leakage sites. The cysts begin to fill with fluorescein early in the course of the angiogram, and they retain the dye well after the initial pass of fluorescein.[1142]

Histologic studies help to explain why the macular area is particularly prone to accumulation of fluid in a flower-petal pattern.[170,1070,1388] The synaptic junctions between the photoreceptors and the next order of neurons, primarily the bipolar cells, are located in the outer plexiform layer of the retina. In the foveal pit, however, the only cells present are the photoreceptor cells; all others are situated in the surrounding perifoveal area. Thus the cell processes of the photoreceptors that form the synapses must angle away from the foveal pit. This region of the outer plexiform layer surrounding the fovea is known as *Henle's fiber layer*. Fluid may collect here, becoming loculated within the spaces between the radiating fibers of this layer. Depending on tissue preservation, fixation, and processing techniques, these spaces may appear empty in histologic sections (Fig. 4-97) or may contain visible deposits that represent pro-

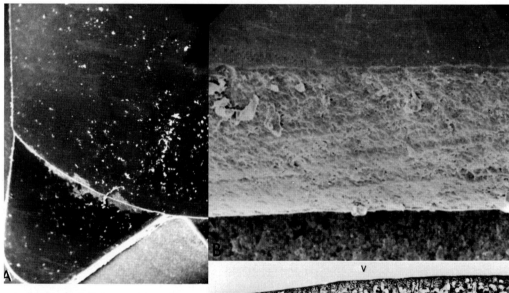

A

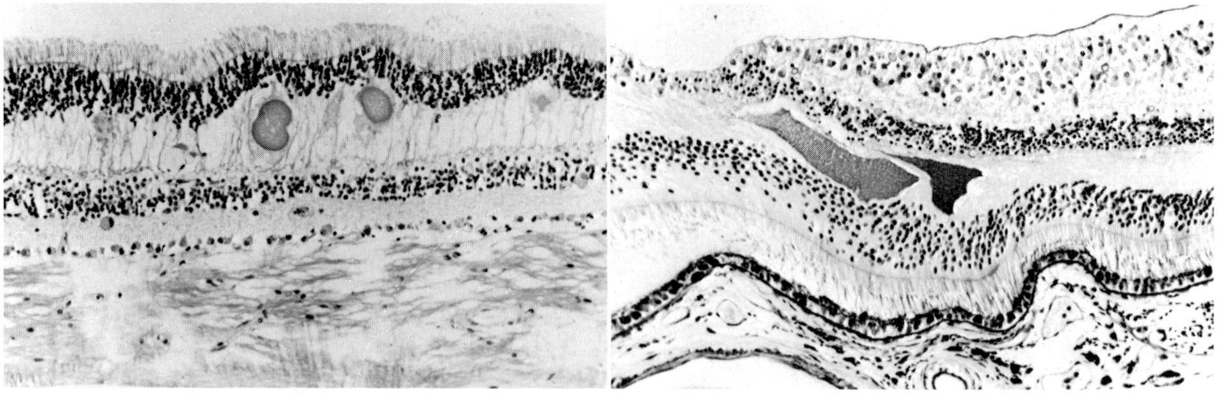

B

Fig. 4-99. A, Photomicrograph of the macular region in the sensory retina from a postmortem eye. The patient received an anterior chamber IOL and subsequently developed clinical cystoid macular edema. This section was cut through the perfoveal region, nasal to the fovea and within the papillomacular bundle. The nerve fiber layer is extremely thick. The two fluid deposits in the outer plexiform layer represent protein-rich serous transudates. (H&E stain; ×150.) **B,** Photomicrograph of the retina of a postmortem eye. The patient had a posterior chamber lens implanted and developed clinically significant cystoid macular edema. Deeply stained transudates are present in the outer plexiform layer. The retina, the underlying pigment epithelium, Bruch's membrane, and the choroid appear to be otherwise normal. (H&E stain; ×75.)

A

B

V

C

RPE

C

Fig. 4-100. A, Scanning electron micrograph of a poorly made, nonlicensed copy of a Choyce anterior chamber lens manufactured by Surgidev Corporation. Such defective copies of Choyce's lens were responsible for numerous cases of UGH syndrome in the late 1970s and early 1980s. This eye was enucleated because of the UGH syndrome. (×15.) **B,** Higher power scanning electron micrograph of the Choyce-like lens copy seen in **A.** Note the extremely rough, sandpaper-like surface of the haptic and the sharp, irregular edges. (×150.) **C,** Photomicrograph of the sensory retina of the same eye seen in **A** and **B.** Note cystoid macular edema that is manifest as a fluid deposit in the outer plexiform layer *(arrows).* The inflammatory component of the UGH syndrome may be partially responsible for the pathogenesis of this condition. Vitreous *(V),* retinal pigment epithelium *(RPE),* choroid *(C).* (×100.) (**B** from Apple DJ and others: Anterior chamber lenses. I. Complications and pathology and a review of designs. II. A laboratory study, J Cataract Refract Surg 13:157, 175, 1987.)

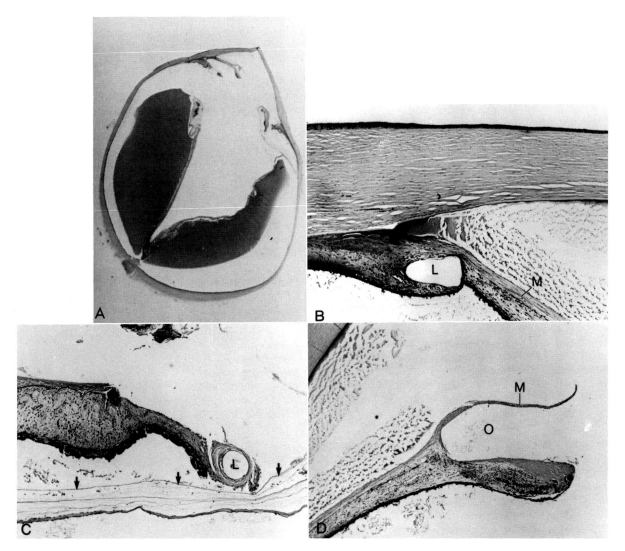

Fig. 4-101. A, Photomicrograph overview of an eye enucleated because of severe problems following implantation of a Shearing-style, J-loop, posterior chamber lens in the anterior chamber. Note the funnel-shaped, total retinal detachment with a serious subretinal transudate present beneath the atrophic retina. The eye became blind and painful and enucleation was required for phthisis bulbi approximately 2 years postoperatively. (H&E stain; ×20.) **B,** Photomicrograph of the anterior segment of the same eye as in **A** showing the loop *(L)* fixation site. The loop eroded deeply into the stroma and muscle of the ciliary body. A dense fibrous membrane *(M)* is present on the anterior surface of the iris and along the loop and covers the lens optic. The anterior chamber *(AC)* contains a dense proteinaceous transudate. (H&E stain; ×20.)

teinaceous transudates (Figs. 4-98, 4-99, and 4-100, *C*; Color Plate 4-45).[170]

Retinal detachment

The influence of the type of cataract extraction and the presence and/or type of IOL on the incidence of retinal detachment (Color Plates 4-46 and 4-47; Fig. 4-101, *A* to *D*) has been debated for years. Studies show that detachments are more common in aphakic eyes regardless of the type of cataract surgery.* Detachments are also more likely

---

* References 395, 463, 699, 918, 1028, 1043, 1063, 1067, 1068, 1071, 1074, 1103, 1104, 1107, 1119, 1130, 1132, 1139, 1145, 1159, 1169, 1170, 1172, 1174–1176, 1196, 1249, 1252, 1258, 1264, 1265, 1274, 1285, 1298, 1299, 1308, 1314, 1317, 1334, 1346, 1354, 1356.

to occur in eyes after vitreous loss, in myopic eyes,[1063] and in the opposite eye of patients with a previous retinal detachment. Among aphakic patients evaluated in a 1981 Iowa study, the estimated incidence of retinal detachment was 1.5%.[1109] This represents a 65% higher risk than for nontraumatic detachment among aphakic individuals. The reported percentage of aphakia found among patients with retinal detachment varies from 7% to 43%.[1028,1043,1258]

Four studies have shown a higher incidence of retinal detachment following ICCE than following ECCE.[218,699,1257,1273] Jaffe and coworkers[699] and Percival and coworkers[1273] reported that ECCE is advantageous because it lowers the relative incidence of aphakic and pseudophakic retinal detachment in highly myopic eyes. In patients who have undergone ICCE and iris-supported

IOL implantation, the reported rate of retinal detachment ranged from 0.6% to 2.4%.[218,702,1081,1107,1381] In his study, Jaffe found that the rate of retinal detachment with ICCE and IOL implantation was lower than with ICCE alone. The incidence of retinal detachment in eyes following ECCE, with or without IOL implantation, has been reported to be between 0.55% and 1.65%.[218,403,1067]

Findings reported from different studies tend to be somewhat contradictory. Binkhorst and coworkers[218] noted a higher detachment rate following ICCE and IOL implantation than with ECCE and IOL implantation. Snider and McReynolds[403] noted that the rate of detachment appeared to increase when a primary posterior capsulotomy was performed. Galin and coworkers[1107] found the incidence of retinal detachment to be identical in both implanted and nonimplanted eyes.

McPherson and coworkers[1225] showed a marked decline in the number of aphakic individuals among a retinal detachment surgery population treated between 1975 and 1982. This decline occurred in spite of the fact that there had been a simultaneous increase in the number of cataract operations performed during the period of this study. These findings imply that significant improvements in cataract surgery techniques, instrumentation, and IOL design occurred during the later stages of this study, most noticeably between 1979 and 1982. The incidence of pseudophakic retinal detachment appears to have decreased steadily during the period of transition from iris-supported IOLs to anterior chamber IOLs to posterior chamber IOLs. This trend parallels the increasing popularity of modern ECCE techniques and serves to confirm the efficacy of ECCE in lowering the incidence of aphakic and pseudophakic retinal detachment.

Tasman[1345,1347] reported a moderate to high incidence of vitreous loss in two series of patients with IOLs and retinal detachment. He suggested that the reported benefit of ECCE compared with ICCE surgery might be offset by the increased difficulty of the former procedure and the potential for a higher rate of vitreous loss. Nevertheless, the clinical experience of many veteran surgeons shows that the rate of vitreous loss with ECCE is lower than that with ICCE.

Although the implantation of modern IOLs does not seem to increase the risk of retinal detachment, in an eye with a retinal detachment the presence of certain styles of IOLs may make surgical reattachment more difficult.[960,1068,1071,1119,1259] Several authors have noted some difficulty in the preoperative observation of a retinal tear; however, in the majority of cases, the hole or tear can be identified, and successful reattachment is usually possible. Despite the reasonable success rate in anatomic reattachment of pseudophakic retinal detachments, the visual results are not as impressive.[1145,1172] In four series of patients with pseudophakic retinal detachment, rates for postoperative visual acuity of 20/50 or better have been reported to range from 26% to 37%.[403,1130]

Some surgeons have suggested that pseudophakic patients might notice symptoms of detachment more quickly than aphakic patients. It has also been postulated that patients with IOLs may have a higher rate of macular detachment. In the majority of reports, these assumptions have not yet been substantiated.[1130,1345,1347]

POSTERIOR CAPSULAR OPACIFICATION

Since the resurgence in popularity of extracapsular surgery, opacification of the posterior capsule has again been recognized as a source of visual compromise* (Color Plates 4-48 and 4-49). Most surgeons agree that the ECCE procedure decreases major postoperative complications, particularly if the posterior capsule is not damaged.[1078,1204,1220,1270] The most common complications attributed to defects in the posterior capsule include cystoid macular edema, alterations in the structure and stability of the vitreous, and retinal detachment.[1273]

The results of cataract extraction and lens implantation usually please most patients. However, in an era when some surgeons advertise perfect visual results after IOL implantation, the new keyword is "refractive cataract surgery." Patients may become upset at having even minimal visual aberrations (such as glare) occur from alterations of the posterior capsule. Their dismay at frank visual loss is, therefore, understandable when significant postoperative PCO occurs.[418] Treatment of PCO by secondary capsulotomy, either surgically† or with the Nd:YAG laser (Color Plate 4-50), is generally successful, to the point of becoming almost trivialized. In reality, it is not a completely innocuous procedure (Color Plate 4-51), and the complications that may occur include IOL damage (Color Plate 4-51), retinal detachment, and cystoid macular edema.[1094,1097] In addition, the cost of a secondary posterior capsulotomy adds a significant economic impact to the total cost of cataract treatment.

According to Sterling and Wood[432] the incidence of late-onset PCO after ECCE and IOL implantation varies from 18.4% to 50% in patients followed postoperatively for as long as 3 to 5 years. Other authors report similar results.‡ A review of their studies suggests that the incidence of this complication is almost the same with ECCE alone as after implantation of either iridocapsular or anterior chamber lenses.

The interval between surgery and opacification varies widely. McDonnell and coworkers[1217] state that up to 50% of all adult patients may develop a secondary membrane within 5 years postoperatively. Wilhelmus and Emery[1376] reported an average opacification time of 26 months after surgery, with a range from 3 months to 4 years.

There is an age-related tendency toward membrane formation, with nearly 100% of pediatric patients developing capsular clouding within 2 years of surgery. In general, the older the human patient, the lower the frequency of capsular opacification. The rate may drop below 10% in patients over the age of 70.[1090,1217,1222,1376]

Causes and cells of origin of posterior capsular opacification

One cause of a usually mild, transient intraoperative and postoperative translucence of the posterior capsule is simple deposition of fibrin, inflammatory cells, and lens epithelial cells during the operation. Rare intracapsular hema-

---

* References 209, 418, 894, 1034, 1205, 1226, 1255, 1256, 1261, 1275, 1277, 1335.
† References 437, 1017, 1106, 1113, 1114, 1140, 1141, 1171, 1187, 1200, 1371.
‡ References 209, 936, 1078, 1203, 1324, 1376.

tomas have been reported.[1129] The cells become sandwiched between the posterior surface of the IOL and the capsule, causing varying amounts of haze. Such cells may be the origin for fibrous membranes that may be dense enough to require surgical or Nd:YAG laser intervention. The most common cause of PCO relates to proliferation and migration into the visual axis of retained lens epithelial cells and their derivatives.* Proliferation of epithelial cells, regeneration of cortical substance, and formation of metaplastic fibrous tissue are all processes that contribute to this complication and its sequelae, as shown in Box 4-5.

Cells having the potential to produce significant visual opacification arise primarily from three sources.[170] The first type, cuboidal epithelial cells that line the anterior capsule and hence the entire anterior surface of the crystalline lens, often transform into fibrous cells that proliferate in situ. These cells typically do not have a propensity for migrating as do cells originating in the equatorial lens bow.

As anterior epithelial cells grow slowly toward the equator, they peel off from the capsule to form the second type of cells, which have an increased level of mitotic activity as they develop in the equatorial lens bow. These germinal cells have an inclination to grow along the posterior capsule, often forming bladder cells during cataract formation or, after ECCE, migrating in clusters to form epithelial pearls posterior to the IOL optic.

Residual cortical fibers from the equatorial lens bow that become dislodged and float freely within the capsule are the third source of lens material that may advance to PCO. These cells may remain localized and organize in the equatorial region to form the outer bulk of a Soemmering's ring, or they may migrate centrally into the visual axis. With time, these cells undergo pseudofibrous metaplasia, which explains why fibrous tissue may be observed both equatorially and posteriorly, at sites far distal to the epithelium of the anterior lens capsule.

Because epithelial pearls have their origin in the peripheral equatorial lens bow, intraoperative polishing of the central posterior capsule, which has no epithelial lining, generally does not help to reduce the incidence of PCO. One exception to this is when extensive posterior-central cell migration has already occurred during the formation of a posterior subcapsular cataract.

Clinical sequelae of retained lens epithelial cells

When epithelial cells migrate and proliferate posteriorly, the resulting opacity usually takes one of two morphologic forms or may be a mixture of both: (1) the formation of clusters of swollen cortical fibers or bladder cells (epithelial pearls), and (2) the formation of a fibrous membrane, usually secondary to fibrous metaplasia of epithelial cells. Box 4-6 lists these problems and other possible complications caused by epithelial remnants remaining after ECCE.

Posterior fibrous lenticular membranes and PCO are usually treatable by either a surgical or a Nd:YAG laser posterior capsulotomy. Experimental studies have been done using the argon laser to debride the posterior capsule of opacification in nonhuman primate eyes.[1219]

Wrinkling of the posterior capsular sac may cause such visual distortions as glare or a Maddox-rod effect. The thicker the membrane, the greater the chance for visual aberrations.[684,1146] Such wrinkles can be caused by the forces exerted (1) by placing a rectangular shape in a naturally round capsular sac, (2) by little or no contact between the posterior capsule and an IOL optic that fits too loosely, or (3) by asymmetrically fixated posterior chamber lens loops. A flaccid capsular sac that is not fully and evenly stretched by the IOL may become folded or corrugated. This effect is increased when cicatrization and contraction of metaplastic epithelial cells, fibrocyte-like cells, or myoepithelial cells exert unequal forces within the capsular sac and the opposite loop in the ciliary region.

Generally both one-piece and three-piece IOLs fabricated from high-molecular-weight PMMA (Perspex CQ) are memory retentive (i.e., have the ability to resume and retain their original shape and curvature after being implanted). The amount of memory retention in a given lens can be controlled by the lens designer and by the manufacturing method used. As the PMMA loops reexpand within the eye, they stretch the capsular sac gently. These loops are more resistant to forces of contraction and are less likely to exhibit extreme loop distortion. This memory-retentive

---

> **Box 4-5.** Retained and newly formed lens cell derivatives after extracapsular cataract extraction.
>
> 1. Epithelium present on the anterior capsule and in the equatorial lens bow and epithelial cells that migrate posteriorly.
> 2. Retained cortical fibers (elongated epithelial cells).
> 3. Bladder cell (Wedl cells; histopathologic correlate of clinical Hirschberg-Elschnig pearls).
> 4. Fibrocyte-like cells derived from metaplasia of lens epithelial cells (pseudofibrous metaplasia).
> 5. Myoepithelial cells (contractile smooth muscle-containing cells derived from transformed lens epithelial cells).

> **Box 4-6.** Clinical problems caused by residual lens epithelial cells after extracapsular extraction.
>
> 1. Posterior capsular opacification (regenerative or secondary cataract).
> 2. Optic decentration or excessive distortion of loops (common following asymmetric loop fixation).
> 3. Phacotoxic or phacoanaphylactic inflammatory reaction to retained crystalline lens remnants (sometimes associated with bacterial infection localized in the lens capsular sac [localized edophthalmitis]).
> 4. Poor view of the peripheral fundus cause by Soemmering's ring.
> 5. Difficulty in achieving long-term success with IOL implantation in children or young adults.
> 6. Difficulty in maintaining consistent, long-term successful optic quality in soft-material IOLs because of optic decentration or surface distortion.

---

* References 209, 464, 689, 711, 1025, 1034, 1065, 1069, 1078, 1090, 1094, 1137, 1203, 1217, 1221, 1222, 1263, 1276, 1301, 1303, 1324, 1340, 1376.

quality is one reason for the increasing use of all-PMMA posterior chamber IOLs.

Proposed methods to reduce posterior capsular opacification

Long before the reintroduction of flexible posterior chamber IOLs in 1977, some investigators and surgeons had made serious attempts to identify the factors that cause opacification after ECCE and IOL implantation.

The hydrodissection technique is a very useful surgical adjunct in enhancing removal of cortex and lens cells (Color Plates 4-24–4-26, 4-52, and 4-53).[458] Information gained from many clinical studies regarding a possible "barrier effect" with modern IOLs (Color Plate 4-54) led to the introduction of many new lens designs and surgical procedures.[994,1373,1374,1385] Leaders in this field include Dr. John Pearce in England and Dr. William Harris and Dr. Richard Lindstrom in the United States, who have long championed a reverse or posteriorly convex lens optic; Dr. Azis Anis, who designed his circular lens optic to maximize contact of the optic with the posterior lens capsule[178]; Dr. William Simcoe, who contributed useful ideas regarding the concept of a barrier effect of IOLs[178]; and Dr. Kenneth Hoffer,[148] who introduced the barrier ridge IOL design that bears his name (Figs. 4-102, 4-103, 4-104). Color Plate 4-54 demonstrates the concept of a "barrier" effect with a modern silicone IOL.

In general, improved results are achieved using posterior chamber IOL designs, but the results vary from surgeon to surgeon. Even with modern IOLs, almost 50% of PCO cases cause sufficient visual disability to require Nd:YAG laser capsulotomies.* It is a puzzle why a surgeon who routinely uses a particular implantation technique and the same lens design achieves excellent visual acuity with no subsequent opacification in some patients, but in other patients severe PCO occurs inexplicably.

This variation in results can be explained partially by recognizing that many factors are involved. Several means of reducing PCO are noted in Box 4-7.

Other methods now being studied include destruction and removal of epithelium by cryosurgery, use of cytostatic and cytotoxic agents to destroy or retard epithelial cells, and attempted development of monoclonal antibodies against lens epithelial cells.[1199] A breakthrough in the management of the anterior capsular epithelium will be extremely important for the success of new surgical procedures and lens designs in the future and for possible

---

* References 209, 1078, 1141, 1203, 1217, 1311, 1324, 1340, 1376.

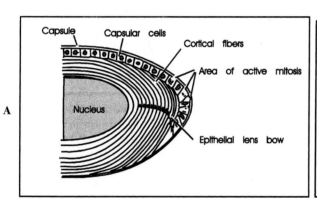
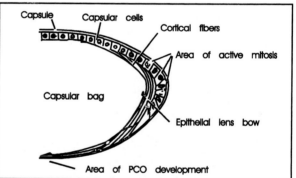

Fig. 4-102. Schematic illustration of a human crystalline lens. **A,** Normal lens, prior to cataract surgery. **B,** Capsular bag after cataract surgery, showing the evacuated capsular bag and the area posteriorly where posterior epithelial migration can occur leading to posterior capsular opacification (PCO). (Courtesy Dr. Gerd Auffarth.)

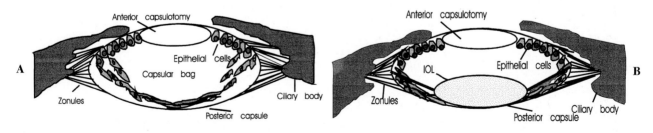

Fig. 4-103. Schematic illustration following extracapsular removal of the cataract. **A,** Schematic illustration showing proliferation of anterior lens epithelial cells and proliferating and migrating equatorial posterior lens epithelial cells. **B,** Schematic illustration demonstrating the barrier effect of an IOL, leading to a "no space–no cells" effect. Note the adhesion of the posterior IOL optic surface from the surface of the posterior capsular capsule. (Courtesy Dr. Gerd Auffarth.)

development of an injectable lens allowing retention of accommodative power.

NEODYMIUM-YTTRIUM-ALUMINUM-GARNET LASER CAPSULOTOMY

The laser era of ophthalmic microsurgery began with the observations of Meyer-Schwickerath[1235] in Germany

---

Box 4-7. Suggested methods of reducing the incidence of posterior capsular opacification (PCO).

1. Atraumatic surgery to minimize intraoperative and postoperative inflammation that may stimulate cellular proliferation.
2. Thorough removal of lens epithelial cells and cortical remnants in the equatorial region during ECCE.
3. Creating radial stretch for 360 degrees on the posterior capsule to create a barrier effect by positioning the IOL optic against the stretched posterior capsule; folds and striae of the posterior capsule are also reduced (best achieved with a capsule-fixated, one-piece, all-PMMA C-loop or with curved loop designs).
4. Complete 360-degree seal between the cut edge of the anterior capsule flap and the subjacent posterior capsule to confine residual cortical material and cells to the equatorial region, thereby retarding migration of cells centrally toward the visual axis.
5. Attaining total contact of the posterior optical surface with the posterior capsule with reverse or biconvex optic IOL designs or various disc-like IOLs (Fig. 4-104 and Color Plate 4-34).

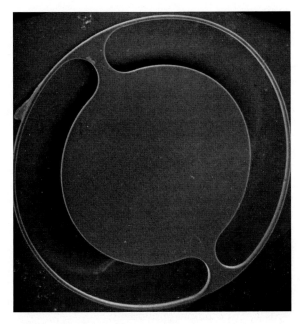

Fig. 4-104. Scanning electron micrograph of a prototype one-piece, all-PMMA, biconvex, posterior chamber lens design with an outer supporting, 10-mm fixation ring, manufactured by Pharmacia Ophthalmics, Inc. The ring makes 360-degree contact with the equator of the lens capsular sac and stretches the posterior capsule to ensure contact between the posterior capsule and the biconvex optic. (×10.)

on solar retinitis, leading to the subsequent development of the first photocoagulator (see Chapter 8). He designed and developed a photocoagulator that focused radiant energy from the sun onto the retina. In 1949 his photocoagulator with a 750-μm spot size was successfully used to produce thermal chorioretinal scars in the treatment of retinal detachment.

For many years, research centered on photocoagulation as a method and mechanism of ophthalmic laser surgery. Most of the surgical applications were for posterior segment problems such as the treatment of retinal detachments, diabetic retinopathy, and other chorioretinal diseases.[1279] Photocoagulators of various wavelengths (e.g., argon, xenon, krypton, ruby) were developed, based on the mechanism of thermal coagulation of pigmented tissues.[170] However, in 1973, Krasnov[1193] in Russia was the first to report on the use of Q-switched ruby laser pulses to cut intraocular tissues. He observed that by using ultrashort pulses of energy over a small focal diameter it was possible to cut tissues by the mechanism of photodisruption.

Simultaneous but independent investigations were being conducted in France by Daniele Aron-Rosa and coworkers[1206,1207] and by Franz Fankhauser[1095,1096] in Switzerland with a 1064 nm neodymium-yttrium-aluminum-garnet (Nd:YAG) laser. The studies of Aron-Rosa led to the development of a mode-locked laser that was suitable for intraocular use, including posterior capsulotomy. Fankhauser and coworkers developed a Q-switched Nd:YAG laser for several intraocular surgical applications in the anterior segment and the posterior segment.[1105,1364] These developments were an important milestone for ophthalmology because for the first time transparent, nonpigmented tissue could be cut using the entirely new mechanism of photodisruption. With the advent of the Nd:YAG laser and photodisruption therapy, ophthalmic surgeons had access to a new method of surgery.[1035,1040–1042]

The Nd:YAG laser produces breakdown of optical tissues through application of extremely short-pulsed, high-energy light in the infrared range.[1229,1357] This laser focally ionizes atoms within tissue to created a plasma, with resultant explosive tissue damage. The plasma has been referred to by laser physicists as the fourth state of matter, the other three states being solid, liquid, and gaseous.

The most important damage mechanisms for ophthalmic applications are the acoustic shock wave effect and the thermal conduction effect. In contrast to argon laser photocoagulation, minimal thermal damage occurs primarily because of the ultrashort duration of the Nd:YAG laser pulse. Typical pulse duration for a mode-locked laser is in picoseconds (10^{-12} seconds) or nanoseconds (10^{-9} seconds) for Q-switched Nd:YAG lasers, compared with milliseconds (10^{-3} seconds) for a typical argon, ruby, or krypton laser. New lasers capable of femtoseconds (10^{-15} seconds) and attoseconds (10^{-18} seconds) pulse duration are currently under investigation.[1269]

There are numerous ophthalmic applications of the Nd:YAG laser. The most common use to date has been posterior capsulotomy in treatment of PCO following ECCE.°

° References 223, 330, 332, 494, 577, 769, 788, 1040, 1042, 1077, 1082, 1100, 1113, 1114, 1127, 1136, 1140, 1141, 1171, 1182, 1186, 1194, 1202, 1208, 1223, 1305, 1326, 1353, 1363, 1369, 1370.

Most surgeons prefer the noninvasive technique of photo-disruption with the Nd:YAG laser rather than knife or needle capsulotomies.* This technique has become the standard procedure for treatment of PCO, particularly for patients with IOLs in place. The Nd:YAG laser treatment is reported to be almost 100% successful in achieving the posterior capsulotomy and 75% to 90% successful in improving vision. Even this noninvasive procedure, however, may provoke complications.

Another application related to cataract surgery is an anterior capsulotomy, either as a primary procedure before ECCE or as a postoperative treatment of the anterior capsule for opacification or membrane formation.† The Nd:YAG laser also is used in goniopuncture, trabeculectomy, and iridotomy in the treatment of glaucoma.[1062] Other applications include pupilloplasty, synechiolysis, vitreolysis, or to cut IOL haptics.[1057,1126,1201] The mechanical effect of the acoustic shock wave produced by the Nd:YAG laser can disrupt vitreous strands in both the posterior and anterior segments.[941] If left untreated, such strands can cause updrawn pupil, vitreoretinal traction, and cystoid macular edema.[1179] The Nd:YAG laser may facilitate repositioning or removal of a decentered IOL by cutting the fibrous adhesions surrounding malpositioned loops.[1250]

The Nd:YAG laser has been used for photodisruption of retrokerato-prosthetic membranes, pseudophakic pigment clusters, and transscleral cyclocoagulation.[755,1035,1088,1375] The mechanical effect of the acoustic shock wave is efficacious for discission of prepupillary membranes of the anterior segment, both capsular and noncapsular. Iridotomy and pupilloplasty are generally successful with the Nd:YAG laser, but iris bleeding may occur because of the lack of thermal effect. In comparison to similar procedures performed with the argon laser, in early clinical investigations the Nd:YAG laser has been reported to be more successful.[1184] For example, patent iridotomies have been created with 1 to 9 Nd:YAG laser pulses representing a cumulative average energy of 0.33 J in the eye compared with 17 to 168 argon laser pulses representing an average cumulative energy of 12 J.[1295] Early investigations seeking to exploit the treatment effect of continuous wave infrared pulses for chorioretinal applications were unsuccessful, possibly because of the deep penetration of Nd:YAG laser pulses, as well as because of the lack of focal hemostatic effect in continuous wave or multimode pulse configurations.[1096] Experiments are now going on to determine whether the Nd:YAG laser or the excimer laser may be useful in phacolysis or in softening the cataractous lens nucleus before removal during ECCE.[562,563,944,947,1039] For the technique of laser phacophotodisruption, a fiberoptic tip is used to fragment the lens nucleus and to permit aspiration of the lens substance through extremely small limbal and anterior capsule incisions.[455]

Photodiscission of the posterior capsule with the Nd:YAG laser eliminates the risks of anesthesia and exogenous endophthalmitis. In comparison to knife or needle capsulotomies, the risks of hemorrhage are minimized; however, in cases of localized endophthalmitis, the inflammatory or-

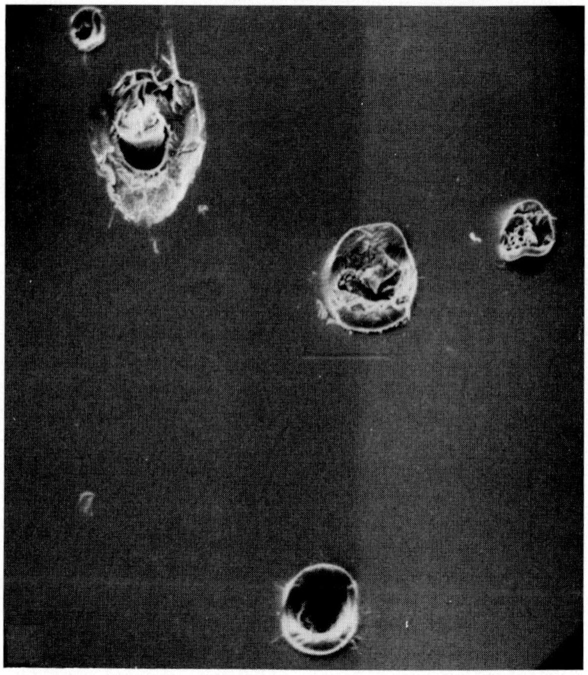

Fig. 4-105. Low-power scanning electron micrograph of an injection-molded, all-PMMA IOL with multiple damage sites on the posterior lens optic caused by the Nd-YAG laser. (×20.)

ganisms are isolated within the capsular sac. Piest and coworkers[1281] described a case in which a more generalized infectious reaction occurred when the laser opened the posterior capsule to allow the organisms to migrate into the vitreous.

There have been some significant operative and postoperative complications following Nd:YAG laser capsulotomy.[1056,1098,1100,1101,1254] Damage to the IOL is the most common (Fig. 4-105; Color Plates 4-50, 4-51, and 4-55) and is seen in up to 30% of photodiscission procedures.* The second most frequent operative complication is rupture of the hyaloid face, reported by Stark and coworkers[1338] to occur in 15% to 22% of cases.

Corneal damage appears to be a rare complication of Nd:YAG therapy because the laser effect is highly localized at the point of focus. Additionally, the IOL optic may block the shock wave anteriorly.† Nevertheless, Stark and coworkers[408] reported 0.3% corneal edema in one series. One study in animals showed damage to the corneal endothelium consisting of focal or diffuse cell loss that was largely irreversible. The damage correlated well with the quantity of power delivered and with the distance between the endothelium and the target tissue. On the other hand, Kraff and coworkers[320] reported no change in endothelial cell density counts in a group of 118 patients who underwent Nd:YAG laser posterior capsulotomy.

The principal concern in a report by Muir and Sherrard[1247] was that the Nd:YAG laser would be used clinically

---

* References 437, 1122, 1123, 1139, 1322, 1137.
† References 185, 427, 1079, 1108, 1112, 1209, 1210, 1291, 1382, 1383.

* References 688, 1030, 1036–1038, 1054, 1056, 1061, 1094, 1098, 1101, 1173, 1181, 1206, 1325, 1331.
† References 341, 348, 905, 906, 956, 1213, 1230, 1234, 1325.

on patients with previously depleted corneal endothelium and that further damage might cause corneal decompensation. While this has not been shown to be a major clinical problem to date, it is clear that a pretreatment inspection of the corneal endothelium with specular microscopy is prudent.

The Nd:YAG laser achieves its effects through photodisruption and plasma formation, rather than through a photocoagulative effect. As a consequence, when such blood vessel-containing tissues as the iris or neovascular membranes are treated, bleeding may occur as an indirect effect from the laser-induced shock wave.

Posterior segment complications of Nd:YAG laser capsulotomy have been reported by several authors Ober and coworkers* and Winslow and Taylor.[1377] These authors described retinal complications in 19 eyes derived from a series of approximately 1100 capsulotomies. Two patients developed full-thickness macular holes, and six others developed cystoid macular edema up to 5 months following the capsulotomy. A retinal flap tear was present in 1 patient, and 10 other patients developed retinal detachment at 1 to 11 months after capsulotomy. This report postulated that these retinal complications were related to the opening of the capsule, rather than to use of the laser. Both the plasma formation and the cone angle of the laser would make direct laser damage to the retina highly unlikely.[1134] In their view, the only possible exception was the formation of a macular hole, which could have been a contrecoup effect from the shock wave. Fastenburg and associates[1097] have reported retinal detachment after Nd:YAG laser posterior capsulotomy, and Howleger[1150] has noted intraocular pressure changes.

REFERENCES

Embryology and anatomy

1. Barnett KC: Lens opacities in the dog as models for human eye disease, Trans Ophthalmol Soc UK 102:346, 1982.
2. Bellows JG: Cataract and anomalies of the lens: growth, structure, composition, metabolism, disorders and treatment of the crystalline lens, St Louis, 1944, The CV Mosby Co.
3. Bellows JG: Cataract and abnormalities of the lens, New York, 1975, Grune & Stratton, Inc.
4. Bochow TW and others: Ultraviolet light exposure and risk of posterior subcapsular cataracts, Arch Ophthalmol 107:369, 1989.
5. Bron AJ and Habgood JO: Morgagnian cataract, Trans Ophthalmol Soc UK 96:265, 1976.
6. Chylack LT Jr: Mechanisms of senile cataract formation, Ophthalmology 91:596, 1984.
7. Cotlier E and Apple DJ: Cataracts induced by the polypeptide antibiotic polymyxin B sulfate, Exp Eye Res 16:69, 1973.
8. Daicker B: Anatomie und Pathologie der menschlichen retinoziliaren Fundusperipherie, Basel, 1972, S Karger, AG.
9. Donaldson DD: Atlas of diseases of the anterior segment of the eye, vol V, The crystalline lens, St Louis, 1976, The CV Mosby Co.
10. Duke-Elder S, editor: System of ophthalmology, vol XI, Diseases of the lens and vitreous: glaucoma and hypotony, St Louis, 1969, The CV Mosby Co.
11. Eshaghian J: Human posterior subcapsular cataracts, Trans Ophthalmol Soc UK 102:365, 1983.
12. Eshaghian J, Rafferty NS, Goossens W: Human cataracta complicata: clinicopathologic correlation, Ophthalmology 88:155, 1981.
13. Eshaghian J and Streeten BW: Human posterior subcapsular cataract: an ultrastructural study of the posteriorly migrating cells, Arch Ophthalmol 98:134, 1980.

14. Fagerholm PPP: The response of the lens to trauma, Trans Ophthalmol Soc UK 102:369, 1982.
15. Flocks M, Litwin CS, and Zimmerman LE: Phacolytic glaucoma: a clinicopathologic study of one hundred thirty-eight cases of glaucoma associated with hypermature cataract, Arch Ophthalmol 78:972, 1974.
16. Font RL and Brownstein S: A light and electron microscopic study of anterior subcapsular cataracts, Am J Ophthalmol 78:972, 1974.
17. Greiner JV and Chylack LT: Posterior subcapsular cataracts: histopathologic study of steroid-associated cataracts, Arch Ophthalmol 97:135, 1979.
18. Haik GM, editor: Symposium on diseases and surgery of the lens: transactions of the New Orleans Academy of Ophthalmology, St. Louis, 1957, The CV Mosby Co.
19. Hamming NA and Apple DJ: Histopathology and ultrastructure of busulfan-induced cataract, Graefes Arch Clin Exp Ophthalmol 200:139, 1976.
20. Hayes BP and Fisher RF: Influence of a prolonged period of low-dosage x-rays on the optic and the ultrastructural appearances of cataract of the human lens, Br J Ophthalmol 63:457, 1979.
21. Jaffe NS: Cataract surgery and its complications, ed 4, St. Louis, 1984, The CV Mosby Co.
22. Kappelhof JP and others: An ultrastructural study of Elschnig's pearls in the pseudophakic eye, Am J Ophthalmol 101:58, 1986.
23. Marshall J, Beaconsfield M and Rothery S: The anatomy and development of the human lens and zonules, Trans Ophthalmol Soc 102:423, 1982.
24. Meyner E: Atlas der Spaltlampenphotographie, Stuttgart, 1976, Ferdinand Enke Verlag.
25. Mimouni F and others: Assessment of gestational age by examination of the anterior vascular capsule of the lens: value in multiple pregnancy (quintuplets), J Pediatr Ophthalmol Strabismus 20:27, 1983.
26. Neetens A and Rubbens MC: Hyperproduction glaucoma, Trans Ophthalmol Soc UK 97:701, 1977.
27. Niesel P: Visible changes of the lens with age, Trans Ophthalmol Soc UK 102:327, 1982.
28. Rohen J: Funktionelle Anatomie des Nervensystems, Stuttgart, 1971, FK Schattauer Verlag, GmbH.
29. Secchi AG: Cataracts in uveitis, Trans Ophthalmol Soc UK 102:390, 1982.
30. Shapiro A, Tso MOM, and Goldberg MF: Argon laser-induced cataract: a clinicopathologic study, Arch Ophthalmol 102:579, 1984.
31. Spemann H: Über den Anteil von Implantät and Wirkskeim an der Orientierung und Beschaffenheit der induzierten Embryonalanlage, Arch Entwicklungsmechan Organ 123:389, 1931.
32. Sperduto RD and Hiller R: The prevalence of nuclear, cortical and posterior subcapsular lens opacities in a general population sample, Ophthalmology 91:815, 1984.
33. Streeten BW and Eshaghian J: Human posterior subcapsular cataract, Arch Ophthalmol 96:1653, 1978.
34. Tripathi RC, Cibis GW, and Tripathi BJ: Pathogenesis of cataracts in patients with Lowe's syndrome, Ophthalmology 93:1046, 1986.
35. Urban RC Jr and Cotlier E: Corticosteroid-induced cataracts, Surv Ophthalmol 31:102, 1986.
36. von Szily A: In Henke F, and Lubarsch O, editors: Handbuch der speziellen pathologischen Anatomie and Histologie, Berlin, 1928, Julius Springer.
37. Vogt A: Vogt's textbook and atlas of slit lamp biomicroscopy, vol 2, Lens and zonule, Bonn-Bad Godesberg, 1979, JP Wayenborgh. (Translated by FC Blodi.)
38. Wedl C: Atlas der pathologischen Histologie des Auges, Leipzig, 1860–1861, Wigand.
39. Zigman S: The role of sunlight in human cataract formation, Surv Ophthalmol 27:317, 1983.

Developmental and congenital anomalies

40. Abbassi V, Lowe CV, and Calcagno PL: Oculo-cerebro-renal syndrome: a review, Am J Dis Child 115:145, 1968.
41. Apple DJ and others: Complications of intraocular lenses: a historical and histopathological review, Surv Ophthalmol 29:1, 1984.
42. Awan KJ: Familial chorioretinal vascular anastomoses and congenital cataracts, J Pediatr Ophthalmol Strabismus 17:384, 1980.

---

*References 168, 1188, 1225, 1260, 1265, 1293.

43. Boniuk M, editor: Rubella and other intraocular viral diseases in infancy, Boston, 1972, Little, Brown & Co.

44. Boniuk M and Zimmerman LE: Ocular pathology in the rubella syndrome, Arch Ophthalmol 77:455, 1967.

45. Cordes FC: Types of congenital and juvenile cataracts. In Haik, GM, editor: Symposium on diseases and surgery of the lens: transactions of the New Orleans Academy of Ophthalmology, St. Louis, 1957, The CV Mosby Co.

46. Cordes FC: Galactosemia cataract: a review, Am J Ophthalmol 50:1151, 1960.

47. Cordes FC and Barber A: Changes in lens of embryo after rubella: microscopic examination of eight week old embryo, Arch Ophthalmol 36:135, 1946.

48. Cruysberg JRM and others: Features of a syndrome with congenital cataract and hypertrophic cardiomyopathy, Am J Ophthalmol 102:740, 1986.

49. Curtin VT, Joyce EE, and Ballin N: Ocular pathology in the oculo-cerebro-renal syndrome of Lowe, Am J Ophthalmol 64:533, 1967.

50. Dark AJ and Streeten BW: Ultrastructural study of cataract in myotonia dystrophica, Am J Ophthalmol 84:666, 1977.

51. Deutman AF and Grizzard WS: Rubella retinopathy and subretinal neovascularization, Am J Ophthalmol 85:82, 1978.

52. Duke-Elder S: Anomalies of the lens. In Duke-Elder S, editor: System of ophthalmology, vol III, Normal and abnormal development, part 2, Congenital deformities, St. Louis, 1963, The CV Mosby Co.

53. François J: Syndromes with congenital cataract, Am J Ophthalmol 52:207, 1961.

54. François J: Syndromes with congenital cataract, Assen, The Netherlands, 1963, Van Gorcum, BV.

55. Frank KE and Purnell EW: Subretinal neovascularization following rubella retinopathy, Am J Ophthalmol 86:462, 1978.

56. Green R and others: Studies of the natural history and prevention of rubella, Am J Dis Child 110:348, 1965.

57. Gregg N: Congenital cataracts following German measles in mother, Trans Ophthalmol Soc Aust 3:35, 1941.

58. Henkind P and Prose P: Anterior polar cataract: electron microscopic evidence of collagen, Am J Ophthalmol 63:768, 1967.

59. Hertzberg R: Rubella and virus induced cataracts, Trans Ophthalmol Soc UK 102:355, 1982.

60. Hittner HM, Kretzer FL, and Mehta RS: Zellweger syndrome: lenticular opacities indicating carrier status and lens abnormalities characteristic of homozygotes, Arch Ophthalmol 99:1977, 1981.

61. Jaffe NS: Cataract surgery and its complications, ed 4, St. Louis, 1984, The CV Mosby Co.

62. Kretzer FA, Hittner HM, and Mehta RS: Ocular manifestations of the Smith-Lemli-Opitz syndrome, Arch Ophthalmol 99:2000, 1981.

63. Krill AE: The retinal disease of rubella, Arch Ophthalmol 77:445, 1967.

64. Krill AE: Retinopathy secondary to rubella, Int Ophthalmol Clin 12(2):89, 1972.

65. Lowe CV, Terrey M, and MacLachlan EA: Organic aciduria, decreased renal ammonia production, hydrophthalmos, and mental retardation: a clinical entity, Am J Dis Child 83:164, 1952.

66. Makley TA Jr: Posterior lenticonus: report of a case with histological findings, Am J Ophthalmol 39:308, 1955.

67. Mann I: The lens. In Mann I: Developmental abnormalities of the eye, London, 1937, Cambridge University Press.

68. Manschot WA: Primary congenital aphakia, Arch Ophthalmol 69:571, 1963.

69. Marshall J, Beaconsfield M, and Rothery S: The anatomy and development of the human lens and zonules, Trans Ophthalmol Soc UK 102:423, 1982.

70. Pallisgaard G and Goldschmidt E: The oculo-cerebro-renal syndrome of Lowe in four generations of one family, Acta Paediatr Scand 60:146, 1971.

71. Parkman PD, Buescher EL, and Artenstein MS: Recovery of rubella virus from army recruits, Proc Soc Exp Biol Med 3:225, 1962.

72. Pinckers A and others: X-linked cataract, Ophthalmic Paediatr Genet 1:169, 1982.

73. Romano A and others: Rate and various aspects of eye infection resulting from congenital rubella, J Pediatr Ophthalmol Strabismus 19:26, 1979.

74. Schiff GM and others: Studies on congenital rubella, Am J Dis Child 110:441, 1965.

75. Streeten BW and others: Lens capsule abnormalities in Alport's syndrome, Arch Ophthalmol 105:1693, 1987.

76. Tripathi RC, Cibis GW, and Tripathi BJ: Lowe's syndrome, Trans Ophthalmol Soc UK 100:132, 1980.

77. Weiss D, Cooper L, and Green R: Infantile glaucoma: a manifestation of congenital rubella, JAMA 195:725, 1966.

78. Weller TH and Neva FA: Propagation in tissue culture of cytopathic agents from patients with rubella-like illness, Proc Soc Exp Biol Med 3:215, 1962.

79. Wolff SM: The ocular manifestations of congenital rubella, Trans Am Ophthalmol Soc 70:577, 1972.

80. Wolff SM: The ocular manifestations of congenital rubella: a prospective study of 328 cases of congenital rubella, J Pediatr Ophthalmol 10:101, 1973.

81. Yanoff M: The retina in rubella. In Tasman W, editor: Retinal diseases in children, New York, 1971, Harper & Row, Publishers.

82. Yanoff M, Schaffer DB, and Scheie HG: Rubella ocular syndrome: clinical significance of viral and pathologic studies, Trans Am Acad Ophthalmol Otolaryngol 72:896, 1968.

83. Zimmerman LE and Font RL: Congenital malformations of the eye, JAMA 196:684, 1966.

84. Zylbermann R and others: Retinal lesions in Alport's syndrome, J Pediatr Ophthalmol Strabismus 17:255, 1980.

Lens displacement syndromes

85. Burian HM and Allen L: Histologic study of the chamber angle of patients with Marfan's syndrome, Arch Ophthalmol 65:323, 1961.

86. Chandler PA: Choice of treatment in dislocation of lens, Arch Ophthalmol 71:765, 1964.

87. Cross HE: Ectopia lentis et pupillae, Am J Ophthalmol 88:381, 1979.

88. Cross HE and Jensen AD: Ocular manifestations in the Marfan syndrome and homocystinuria, Am J Ophthalmol 75:405, 1973.

89. Curtis R: Hereditary luxation of the canine lens, Trans Ophthalmol Soc UK 102:398, 1982.

90. Fagerholm PPP: The response of the lens to trauma, Trans Ophthalmol Soc UK 102:369, 1982.

91. Farnsworth PN and others: Ultrastructural abnormalities in a Marfan's syndrome lens, Arch Ophthalmol 95:1601, 1977.

92. Jarrett WH II: Dislocation of the lens, Arch Ophthalmol 78:289, 1967.

93. Jensen AD and Cross HE: Ocular complications in the Weill-Marchesani syndrome, Am J Ophthalmol 77:261, 1974.

94. Leubbers JA and others: Iris transillumination and variable expression in ectopia lentis pupillae, Am J Ophthalmol 83:647, 1977.

95. von Marchesani O: Brachydaktylie and angeborene Kugellinse als Systemerkrankung, Klin Monatsbl Augenheilkd 103:392, 1939.

96. Maumenee IH: The eye in the Marfan syndrome, Trans Am Ophthalmol Soc 89:684, 1981.

97. McGavic JS: Weill-Marchesani syndrome: brachymorphism and ectopia lentis, Am J Ophthalmol 62:820, 1966.

98. Nelson LB and Maumenee IH: Ectopia lentis, Surv Ophthalmol 29:143, 1982.

99. Ramsey MS and others: The Marfan syndrome: a histopathologic study of ocular findings, Am J Ophthalmol 76:102, 1973.

100. Ramsey MS, Fine BS, and Yanoff M: The ocular histopathology of homocystinuria: a light and electron microscopic study, Am J Ophthalmol 74:377, 1972.

101. Rodman HI: Chronic open-angle glaucoma associated with traumatic dislocation of the lens: a new pathologic concept, Arch Ophthalmol 69:445, 1963.

102. Townes P: Ectopia lentis et pupillae, Arch Ophthalmol 94:1126, 1976.

103. Willi M, Kut L, and Cotlier E: Pupillary-block glaucoma in the Marchesani syndrome, Arch Ophthalmol 90:504, 1973.

Lens-related ocular diseases

Phacolytic glaucoma

104. Flocks M, Litwin CS, and Zimmerman LE: Phacolytic glaucoma: a clinicopathologic study of one hundred thirty-eight cases of glaucoma associated with hypermature cataract, Arch Ophthalmol 54:37, 1955.

105. Goldberg MF: Cytological diagnosis of phacolytic glaucoma utilizing millipore filtration of the aqueous, Br J Ophthalmol 51:847, 1967.

106. Smith ME and Zimmerman LE: Contusive angle recession in phacolytic glaucoma, Arch Ophthalmol 74:799, 1965.

107. Yanoff M and Scheie HG: Cytology of human lens aspirate and its relationship to phacolytic glaucoma and phacoanaphylactic endophthalmitis, Arch Ophthalmol 80:166, 1968.

Phacoanaphylactic endophthalmitis

108. Chishti M and Henkind P: Spontaneous rupture of anterior lens capsule (phacoanaphylactic endophthalmitis), Am J Ophthalmol 69:264, 1970.

109. Eason HA and Zimmerman LE: Sympathetic ophthalmia and bilateral phacoanaphylaxis: a clinicopathologic correlation of the sympathogenic and sympathizing eyes, Arch Ophthalmol 72:9, 1964.

110. Irvine SR and Irvine AR Jr: Lens-induced uveitis and glaucoma. I. Endophthalmitis phacoanaphylactica, Am J Ophthalmol 35:177, 1952.

111. Irvine SR and Irvine AR Jr: Lens-induced uveitis and glaucoma. II. The phacotoxic reaction, Am J Ophthalmol 35:370, 1952.

112. Irvine SR and Irvine AR Jr: Lens-induced uveitis and glaucoma. III. "Phacogenetic glaucoma": lens-induced glaucoma; mature or hypermature cataract; open iridocorneal angle, Am J Ophthalmol 35:489, 1952.

113. Leigh AG: Lens-induced uveitis, Trans Ophthalmol Soc UK 75:51, 1955.

114. Lemoine AN and Macdonald AE: Observations on phacoanaphylactic endophthalmitis, Arch Ophthalmol 53:101, 1924.

115. Perlman EM and Albert DM: Clinically unsuspected phacoanaphylaxis after ocular trauma, Arch Ophthalmol 95:244, 1977.

116. Verhoeff FH and Lemoine AN: Endophthalmitis phacoanaphylactica, Am J Ophthalmol 5:737, 1922.

117. Verhoeff FH and Lemoine AN: Endophthalmitis phacoanaphylactica, Trans Intern Cong Ophthalmol 1:234, 1922.

118. Yanoff M and Scheie, HG: Cytology of human lens aspirate: its relationship to phacolytic glaucoma and phacoanaphylactic endophthalmitis, Arch Ophthalmol 80:166, 1968.

Pseudoexfoliation (glaucoma capsulare) and true exfoliation

119. Aasved H: Study of relatives of persons with fibrillopathia epitheliocapsularis (pseudoexfoliation of the lens capsule), Acta Ophthalmol 53:879, 1975.

120. Aasved H: Prevalence of fibrillopathia epitheliocapsularis (pseudoexfoliation) and capsular glaucoma, Trans Ophthalmol Soc UK 99:293, 1979.

121. Arnesen K, Sunde OA, Schultz-Haudt SD: Histochemical study of deposits of Busacca in eyes with glaucoma simplex and so-called senile exfoliation of the lens capsule, Acta Ophthalmol 41:80, 1963.

122. Ashton N: Discussion of Gifford H: A clinical and pathological study of exfoliation of the lens capsule, Trans Am Ophthalmol Soc 55:215, 1957.

123. Ashton N and others: Electron microscopic study of pseudoexfoliation of the lens capsule. I. Lens capsule and zonular fibers, Invest Ophthalmol 4:141, 1965.

124. Bartholomew RS: Effect of cataract extraction on the intraocular pressure in eyes with pseudoexfoliation of the lens, Trans Ophthalmol Soc UK 99:312, 1979.

125. Bertelsen TI: Fibrillopathia epitheliocapsularis: the so-called senile exfoliation or pseudo-exfoliation of the anterior lens capsule, Acta Ophthalmol 44:737, 1966.

126. Bertelsen TI, Drablös PA, Flood PR: The so-called senile exfoliation (pseudo-exfoliation) of the anterior lens capsule, a product of the lens epithelium: fibrillopathia epithelio-capsularis, Acta Ophthalmol 42:1096, 1964.

127. Broderick JD and Tate GW: Capsular delamination (true exfoliation of the lens): report of a case, Arch Ophthalmol 97:1693, 1979.

128. Brooks AMV and Gillies WE: Fluorescein angiography and fluorophotometry of the iris in pseudoexfoliation of the lens capsule, Br J Ophthalmol 67:249, 1983.

129. Burde RM, Bresnick G and Uhrhammer J: True exfoliation of the lens capsule: an electron microscopic study, Arch Ophthalmol 82:651, 1969.

130. Busacca A: Quoted by Sunde OA: On the so-called senile exfolia-

tion of the anterior lens capsule: a clinical and anatomical study, Acta Ophthalmol Suppl 45:12, 1956.

131. Callahan A and Klien BA: Thermal detachment of the anterior lamella of the anterior lens capsule: a clinical and histopathologic study, Arch Ophthalmol 59:73, 1958.

132. Cashwell LF Jr and others: Idiopathic true exfoliation of the lens capsule, Ophthalmology 96:348, 1989.

133. Dark AJ, Streeten BW and Cornwall CC: Pseudoexfoliative disease of the lens: a study in electron microscopy and histochemistry, Br J Ophthalmol 61:462, 1977.

134. Dickson DH and Ramsey MS: Fibrillopathia epitheliocapsularis: review of the nature and origin of pseudoexfoliative deposits, Trans Ophthalmol Soc UK 99:284, 1979.

135. Eagle RC Jr, Font RL, and Fine BS: The basement membrane exfoliation syndrome, Arch Ophthalmol 97:510, 1979.

136. Gifford H: A clinical and pathological study of exfoliation of lens capsule, Am J Ophthalmol 46:508, 1958.

137. Gillies WE: Effect of lens extraction in pseudoexfoliation of lens capsule, Br J Ophthalmol 57:46, 1973.

138. Gillies WE: Secondary glaucoma associated with pseudoexfoliation of the lens capsule, Trans Ophthalmol Soc UK 98:96, 1978.

139. Johnson DH: Does pigmentation affect the trabecular meshwork? Am J Ophthalmol 107:250, 1989.

140. Layden WE and Shaffer RN: Exfoliation syndrome, Trans Am Ophthalmol Soc 71:128, 1973.

141. Layden WE and Shaffer RN: Exfoliation syndrome, Am J Ophthalmol 78:835, 1974.

142. Prince AM and other: Preclinical diagnosis of pseudoexfoliation syndrome, Arch Ophthalmol 105:1076, 1987.

143. Richardson TM and Epstein DL: Exfoliation glaucoma: a quantitative perfusion and ultrastructural study, Ophthalmology 88:968, 1981.

144. Richter CU, Richardson TM and Grant WM: Pigmentary dispersion syndrome and pigmentary glaucoma: a prospective study of the natural history, Arch Ophthalmol 104:211, 1986.

145. Ringvold A: Ultrastructure of exfoliation material (Busacca deposits), Virchows Arch Pathol Anat 350:95, 1970.

146. Ringvold A: Electron microscopy of the limbal conjunctiva in eyes with pseudoexfoliation syndrome (PE syndrome), Virchows Arch Pathol Anat 355:275, 1972.

147. Ringvold A: On the occurrence of pseudo-exfoliation material in extrabulbar tissue from patients with pseudoexfoliation syndrome of the eye, Acta Ophthalmol 51:411, 1973.

148. Ringvold A: Pseudo-exfoliation material: an amyloid-like substance, Exp Eye Res 17:289, 1973.

149. Roh YB and others: Alteration of microfibrils in the conjunctiva of patients with exfoliation syndrome, Arch Ophthalmol 105:978, 1987.

150. Roth M and Epstein DL: Exfoliation syndrome, Am J Ophthalmol 89:477, 1980.

151. Seland JH and Chaylack LT Jr: Cataracts in the exfoliation syndrome (fibrillopathia epitheliocapsularis), Trans Ophthalmol Soc UK 102:375, 1982.

152. Shakib M, Ashton N and Block R: Electron microscopic studies of pseudoexfoliation of the lens capsule. II. Iris and ciliary body, Invest Ophthalmol 4:154, 1965.

153. Smith RJH: Nature of glaucoma in the pseudoexfoliation syndrome, Trans Ophthalmol Soc UK 99:308, 1979.

154. Streeten BW and others: Pseudoexfoliative fibrillopathy in the conjunctiva: a relation to elastic fibers and elastosis, Ophthalmology 94:1439, 1987.

155. Sunde OA: On the so-called senile exfoliation of the anterior lens capsule: a clinical and anatomical study, Acta Ophthalmol Suppl 45, 1956.

156. Tarkkanen A: Pseudoexfoliation of the lens capsule, Acta Ophthalmol 40(suppl 71):1, 1962.

157. Taylor HR: Pseudoexfoliation: an environmental disease? Trans Ophthalmol Soc UK 99:302, 1979.

158. Theobald GD: Pseudo-exfoliation of the lens capsule: relation to "true" exfoliation of the lens capsule as reported in the literature and role in production of glaucoma capsulocuticulare, Am J Ophthalmol 37:1, 1954.

159. Vogt A: Ein neues Spaltlampenbild des Pupillengebietes: hellblauer Pupillensaumfilz mit Häutchenbildung auf der Linsenvorderkapsel, Klin Monatsbl Augenheilkd 75:1, 1925.

Evolution of IOL implantation

160. Alberti G and others: Glutathione s-transferase m1 genotype and age-related cataracts. lack of association in an Italian population, Invest Ophthalmol Vis Sci 37(6):1167, 1996.

161. Alpar JJ: Glare factor in different intraocular lenses: comparative study in patients with dissimilar binocular implants. In Emery JM, Jacobson AC, editors: Current concepts in cataract surgery. Selected Proceedings of the Seventh Biennial Cataract Surgical Congress, New York, 1982, Appleton-Century-Crofts.

162. Andley UP and others: The role of prostaglandins e2 and f2 alpha in ultraviolet radiation-induced cortical cataracts in vivo, Invest Ophthalmol Vis Sci 37(8):1539, 1996.

163. Apple DJ, Cameron JD and Lindstrom RL: Loop fixation of posterior chamber intraocular lenses, Cataract 2(1):7, 1984.

164. Apple DJ and others: Anterior segment complications and neovascular glaucoma following implantation of a posterior chamber intraocular lens, Ophthalmology 91:403, 1984.

165. Apple DJ and others: Complications of intraocular lenses: a historical and histopathological review, Surv Ophthalmol 29:1, 1984.

166. Apple DJ and others: Phacoanaphylactic endophthalmitis following ECCE and IOL implantation, J Am Intraocul Implant Soc 10:423, 1984. (guest editorial)

167. Apple DJ: Pathology of Intraocular Lenses: Polypropylene vs PMMA. In Jeffe MS (ed): Intraocular lens complications; self-study program. Module II: Proceedings of symposium on IOL complications. Stockholm, Sweden, Pharmacia monograph, Aug 17–24, 1985.

168. Apple DJ and others: A comparison of ciliary sulcus and capsular bag fixation of posterior chamber intraocular lenses, J Am Intraocular Implant Soc 11:44, 1985.

169. Apple DJ, Kincaid MC: Histopathology of intraocular lens explantation, Cataract 2(7):7, 1985.

170. Apple DJ, Rabb MF: Ocular pathology: clinical applications and self-assessment, ed 3, St Louis, 1985, The CV Mosby Co.

171. Apple DJ, Gieser SC, and Isenberg RA: Evolution of intraocular lenses, Salt Lake City, Utah, University of Utah Printing Service, 1985.

172. Apple DJ and others: Posterior chamber intraocular lenses in a series of 75 autopsy eyes. I. Loop location, J Cataract Refract Surg 12:358, 1986.

173. Apple DJ, Olson RJ: Closed-loop anterior chamber lenses, Arch Ophthalmol 105:19, 1987, (letter).

174. Apple DJ and others: Anterior chamber lenses. I. Complications and pathology and a review of designs, J Cataract Refract Surg 13:157, 1987.

175. Apple DJ and others: Anterior chamber lenses. II. A laboratory study, J Cataract Refract Surg 13:175, 1987.

176. Apple DJ: Stableflex lens report, J Cataract Refract Surg 13:456, 1987, (reply to letter to editor by ML Furillo).

177. Apple DJ and others: Visual aberrations caused by optic components of posterior chamber intraocular lenses, J Cataract Refract Surg 13:431, 1987.

178. Apple DJ and others: Intraocular lenses: evolution, designs, complications, and pathology, Baltimore, 1989, The Williams & Wilkins Co.

179. Apple DJ and others: Sutured retropupillary posterior chamber intraocular lenses for exchange or secondary implantation (The Twelfth Annual Binkhorst Lecture, 1988), Ophthalmology 96:1241, 1989.

180. Apple DJ and others: Komplikationen bei Vorderkammerlinsen: eine Analyse von 4000 explantierten IOLs. Abstract. Der Ophthalmologe 90(Suppl I):S113, 1993.

181. Apple DJ, Auffarth GU, and Wesendahl TA: IOL fixation techniques at keratoplasty, Ophthalmology 101:798, 1994, (letter; comment).

182. Apple DJ and others: Sutured retropupillary posterior chamber IOLs, video presented at annual meeting of the American Society of Cataract and Refractive Surgery, Boston, MA, April 9, 1994.

183. Apple DJ and others: Cataract surgery in the developing world, Saudi J Ophthalmol (9)1:2–15, 1995.

184. Apple DJ, Sims J: Harold Ridley and the invention of the intraocular lens, Surv Ophthalmol 40:279, 1996.

185. Aron-Rosa DS: Use of a pulsed neodymium-YAG laser for anterior capsulotomy before extracapsular cataract extraction, J Am Intraocul Implant Soc 7:332, 1981.

186. Assia EI and others: Studies on cataract surgery and intraocular lenses at the Center for Intraocular Lens Research. Ophthalmol Clin North Am 4:251-266, 1991.

187. Assia EI and others: Loop memory of posterior chamber intraocular lenses of various sizes, designs, and loop materials, J Cataract Refract Surg 18:541, 1992.

188. Auffarth G, Wesendahl T, Apple DJ: Surface characteristics of intraocular lens implants: an evaluation using scanning electron microscopy and quantitative three-dimensional noncontacting profilometry (TOPO). J Longterm Effect Med Implants 3(4):321-331, 1993.

189. Auffarth GU and others: Update on complications of anterior chamber intraocular lenses. J Cataract Refract Surg, Special Issue: Best Paper of 1994 ASCRS Meeting: 70-76, 1994.

190. Auffarth GU and others: (Complications after implantation of anterior chamber lenses. an analysis of 4,100 explanted intraocular lenses.) (German), Ophthalmologe 91:512, 1994.

191. Auffarth GU and others: Are there acceptable anterior chamber intraocular lenses for clinical use in the 1990s? an analysis of 4104 explanted anterior chamber intraocular lenses (see comments), Ophthalmology 101:1913, 1994.

192. Auffarth GU and others: Letter (authors' reply to Dr. Drews' letter); Are there acceptable anterior chamber intraocular lenses for clinical use in the 1990s? An analysis of 4104 explanted anterior chamber intraocular lenses, Ophthalmology 102(6):857-859, 1995.

193. Auffarth GU and others: Letter (authors' reply to Dr. Spencer's letter); Are there acceptable anterior chamber intraocular lenses for clinical use in the 1990s? An analysis of 4104 explanted anterior chamber intraocular lenses, Ophthalmology 102(7):1001-1002, 1995.

194. Auffarth GU and others: Update on complications of anterior chamber intraocular lenses, J Cataract Refract Surg 22:1-7, 1995.

195. Ballin N: Iris erosion with the Leiske lens, J Am Intraocul Implant Soc 8:158, 1982, (letter).

196. Barnet RW: Conceptual analysis of IOL implant fixation, Cataract 1(2):25, 1984.

197. Barnet RW: Part III: Conceptual analysis of lens implant fixation, Cataract 1(3):18, 1984.

198. Baron A: Tolérance de l'oeil à la matière plastique: prothèses optiques' cornéennes, prothèses optiques cristalliniennes, Bull Soc Ophthalmol France 9:982, 1953.

199. Bellucci R and others: Secondary implantation of angle-supported anterior chamber and scleral-fixated posterior chamber intraocular lenses, J Cataract Refract Surg 22(2):247, 1996.

200. Binkhorst CD: Iris-supported artificial pseudophakia. A new development in intraocular artificial lens surgery (iris clip lens), Trans Ophthalmol Soc UK 79:569, 1959.

201. Binkhorst CD: Indikation und Implantationstechnik der "Pupillarlinse" oder "Iris-Clip-Linse" bei der Aphakie, Klin Monatsbl Augenheilkd 136:35, 1960.

202. Binkhorst CD: Results of implantation of intraocular lenses in unilateral aphakia; with special reference to the pupillary or iris clip lens—a new method of fixation, Am J Ophthalmol 49:703, 1960.

203. Binkhorst CD: The pupillary (iris clip) lens: an artificial lens for aphakia completely surrounded by the iris (with film and demonstration of patients), Ophthalmologica 141:479, 1961.

204. Binkhorst CD: Use of the pupillary lens (iris clip lens) in aphakia: our experience based on the first fifty implantations, Br J Ophthalmol 46:343, 1962.

205. Binkhorst CD: Eigene Verfahren der Pseudophakie Iris-Clip-Pseudophakos und irido-kapsulärer Pseudophakos, Klin Monatsbl Augenheilkd 151:21, 1967.

206. Binkhorst CD: Iris-clip and irido-capsular lens implants (pseudophakoi): personal techniques of pseudophakia, Br J Ophthalmol 51:767, 1967.

207. Binkhorst CD: Lens implants (pseudophakoi) classified according to method of fixation, Br J Ophthalmol 51:772, 1967.

208. Binkhorst CD: The iridocapsular (two-loop) lens and the iris-clip (four-loop) lens in pseudophakia, Trans Am Acad Ophthalmol Otolaryngol 77:589, 1973.

209. Binkhorst CD: Five hundred planned extracapsular extractions with irido-capsular and iris clip lens implantation in senile cataract, Ophthalmic Surg 8:37, 1977.

210. Binkhorst CD: Corneal and retinal complications after cataract

extraction: the mechanical aspect of endophthalmodonesis, Ophthalmology 87:609, 1980.

211. Binkhorst CD: Extracapsular cataract extraction and lens implantation. In Rosen ES, Haining WM, and Arnott EJ, editors: Intraocular lens implantation, St. Louis, 1984, The CV Mosby Co.

212. Binkhorst CD: About lens implantation. 1. The cataract extraction, Implant 3:11, 1985.

213. Binkhorst CD: About lens implantation. 2. Lens design and classification of lenses, Implant 3:15, 1985.

214. Binkhorst CD: Safe all-in-the-bag pseudophakia with a new lens design (the moustache lens), Doc Ophthalmol 59:57, 1985.

215. Binkhorst CD: The uvea-touch syndrome and how to avoid it: personal thoughts about lens implantation, Acta Ophthalmol 63:609, 1985, (editorial).

216. Binkhorst CD, Kats A and Leonard PAM: Extracapsular pseudophakia: results in 100 two loop iridocapsular lens implantations, Am J Ophthalmol 73:625, 1972.

217. Binkhorst CD and Leonard PAM: Results in 208 iris-clip pseudophakos implantations, Am J Ophthalmol 64:947, 1967.

218. Binkhorst CD and others: Symposium: intraocular lenses. Retinal accidents in pseudophakia—intracapsular vs. extracapsular surgery, Trans Am Acad Ophthalmol Otolaryngol 81:120, 1976.

219. Binkhorst CD and others: Lens injury in children treated with irido-capsular supported intra-ocular lenses, J Am Intraocul Implant Soc 4:34, 1978.

220. Binkhorst RD: The optical design of intraocular lens implants, Ophthalmic Surg 6:17, 1975.

221. Blodi FC: Causes and frequency of enucleation after cataract extraction, Int Ophthalmol Clin 5(1):257, 1965.

222. Blum M and others: Age-related changes of the ciliary sulcus: Implications for implanting sulcus-fixated lenses, J Cataract Refract Surg 23:91, 1997.

223. Brems RN and others: Posterior chamber intraocular lenses in a series of 75 autopsy eyes. III. Correlation of positioning holes and optic edges with the pupillary aperture and visual axis, J Cataract Refract Surg 12:367, 1986.

224. Busin M and others: Complications of sulcus-supported intraocular lenses with iris sutures, implanted during penetrating keratoplasty after intracapsular cataract extraction, Ophthalmology 97:401, 1990.

225. Byron HM: Symposium: intraocular lenses. Anterior segment complications of implant surgery, Ophthalmology 86:621, 1971.

226. Cairns L, Sommer A: Changing indications for cataract surgery, Trans Am Ophthalmol Soc 82:166, 1984.

227. Carlson AN, Koch DD: Endophthalmitis following Nd:YAG laser posterior capsulotomy, Ophthalmic Surg 19:168, 1988.

228. Chirila TV, Thompson DE and Constable IJ: In vitro cytotoxicity of melanized poly(2-hydroxyethyl methacrylate) hydrogels, a novel class of ocular biomaterials, J Biomat Sci, Polymer Edition 3(6): 481, 1992.

229. Chowdhury AM and Bras JF: Posterior dislocation of an intraocular lens implant and its removal, Br J Ophthalmol 61:327, 1977.

230. Choyce DP: The Mark VI, Mark VII and Mark VIII Choyce anterior chamber implants, Proc R Soc Med 58:729, 1965.

231. Choyce DP: Long-term tolerance of Choyce Mk I and Mk VIII anterior chamber implants, Proc R Soc Med 63:310, 1970.

232. Choyce DP: History of intraocular implants, Ann Ophthalmol 5: 1113, 1973.

233. Choyce DP: The Choyce Mark VIII anterior chamber implant: primary and secondary implantation compared, Ophthalmic Surg 8:49, 1977.

234. Choyce DP: The theoretical ideal for an artificial lens implant to correct aphakia, Trans Ophthalmol Soc UK 97:94, 1977.

235. Choyce DP: Complications of the AC implants of the early 1950's and the UGH or Ellingson syndrome of the late 1970's, J Am Intraocul Implant Soc 4:22, 1978.

236. Choyce DP: The evolution of the anterior chamber implant up to, and including, the Choyce Mark IX, Ophthalmology 86:197, 1979.

237. Choyce DP: Anterior chamber lens implantation in children under eighteen years. In Hiles DA, editor: Intraocular lens implants in children, New York, 1980, Grune & Stratton.

238. Choyce DP: Anterior chamber implants: 4-point or 3-point fixation? An illustrative case history, Contact Intraocul Lens Med J 7: 153, 1981.

239. Choyce DP: The Sixth Binkhorst Medal Lecture. Anterior chamber

240. Chylack LT Jr, Leske MC, McCarthy D and others: Lens opacities classification system II (locs II) (see comments), Arch Ophthalmol 107:991, 1989.

241. Chylack LT Jr and others: The lens opacities classification system III. The longitudinal study of cataract study group, Arch Ophthalmol 111:831, 1993.

242. Cohan BE: The broken nylon iris fixation suture, Am J Ophthalmol 93:507, 1982.

243. Cohan BE, Pearch AC and Schwartz S: Broken nylon iris fixation sutures, Am J Ophthalmol 88:982, 1979.

244. Colenbrander A, Woods LV and Stamper RL: Intraocular lens data, Ophthalmology 92:1, 1985.

245. Colenbrander A, Woods LV and Stamper RL: Intraocular lens data, Ophthalmology 93:37, 1986.

246. Colenbrander A, Woods LV and Stamper RL: Intraocular lens data, Ophthalmology 93:1, 1987.

247. Coli AF, Price FW Jr and Whitson WE: Intraocular lens exchange for anterior chamber intraocular lens-induced corneal endothelial damage, Ophthalmology 100:384, 1993.

248. Crawford JB: A histopathologic study of the position of the Shearing intraocular lens in the posterior chamber, Am J Ophthalmol 91:458, 1981.

249. Dahan E: Implantation in the posterior chamber without capsular support, J Cataract Refract Surg 15:339, 1989.

250. Dallas NL: Five-year trial of the Binkhorst iris-clip lens in aphakia, Trans Ophthalmol Soc UK 90:725, 1970.

251. Davis RM, Best D and Gilbert GE: Comparison of intraocular lens fixation techniques performed during penetrating keratoplasty, Am J Ophthalmol 111:743, 1991.

252. de Gottrau P and others: Congenital zonular cataract. clinicopathologic correlation with electron microscopy and review of the literature [review], Arch Ophthalmol 111:235, 1993.

253. Deschatres F and Labrune P: Reflexions apres 256 implants intraoculaires mis en place apres extraction extracapsulaire du cristallin, J Fr Ophthalmol 6:527, 1983.

254. Doane MG, Miller D and Korb D: Applications of high-speed cinematography in the evaluation of intraocular and contact lenses (abstract), Invest Ophthalmol Vis Sci 22(suppl):164, 1982.

255. Donnenfeld ED and others: Soemmering's ring support for posterior chamber intraocular lens implantation during penetrating keratoplasty. Changing trends in bullous keratopathy, Ophthalmology 99:1229, 1992.

256. Drews RC: Intracapsular versus extracapsular cataract extraction. In Wilensky JT, editor: Intraocular lenses. Transactions of the University of Illinois Symposium on intraocular lenses, New York, 1977, Appleton-Century-Crofts.

257. Drews RC: Inflammatory response, endophthalmitis, corneal dystrophy, glaucoma, retinal detachment, dislocation, refractive error, lens removal, and enucleation, Ophthalmology 85:164, 1978.

258. Drews RC: The Pearce tripod posterior chamber intraocular lens: an independent analysis of Pearce's results, J Am Intraocul Implant Soc 6:259, 1980.

259. Drews RC: Intermittent touch syndrome, Arch Ophthalmol 100: 1440, 1982.

260. Drews RC: The Barraquer experience with intraocular lenses: 20 years later, Ophthalmology 89:386, 1982.

261. Duffey RJ and others: Anatomic study of transsclerally sutured intraocular lens implantation, Am J Ophthalmol 108:300, 1989.

262. Duffin RM and Olson RJ: Vaulting characteristics of flexible loop anterior chamber intraocular lenses, Arch Ophthalmol 101:1429, 1983.

263. Duke-Elder S and Abrams D: System of ophthalmology, vol V, Ophthalmic optics and refraction, St. Louis, 1970, The CV Mosby Co.

264. Dulaney DD: IOLs and iris erosion, J Am Intraocul Implant Soc 4:120, 1978, (letter).

265. Dyson C: Retrieval and replacement of an iris plane implant dislocated five years previously into the vitreous cavity, J Am Intraocul Implant Soc 6:284, 1980.

266. Eifrig DE and Doughman DJ: Intraocular lens in laboratory animals, Ophthalmic Surg 8:149, 1977.

267. Ellingson FT: Complications with the Choyce Mark VII anterior

chamber lens implant (uveitis-glaucoma-hyphema), J Am Intraocul Implant Soc 3:199, 1977.

268. Ellingson FT: The uveitis-glaucoma-hyphema syndrome associated with the Mark VIII anterior chamber lens implant, J Am Intraocul Implant Soc 4:50, 1978.

269. Epstein E: The Ridley lens implant, Br J Ophthalmol 43:368, 1957.

270. Fenzl RE and Hahs G: Evaluation of semiflexible and flexible anterior chamber intraocular lenses, J Am Intraocul Implant Soc 9:42, 1983.

271. Finlay JR and Romaine H: Reports on the use of the intraocular acrylic lens (Ridley operation). II. Trans Am Acad Ophthalmol Otolaryngol 58:57, 1954.

272. Fyodorov SN: Long-term results of 2,000 operations of implantation of Fyodorov intraocular lenses performed in the Soviet Union, J Am Intraocul Implant Soc 3:101, 1977.

273. Galand A, Bonhomme L and Collée M: Direct measurement of the capsular bag, J Am Intraocul Implant Soc 10:475, 1984.

274. Galin MA and others: Binkhorst lecture (part 2), experimental cataract surgery—electron microscopy, Ophthalmology 86:608, 1979.

275. Gernet H: The binocular confusion in unilateral aphakia, Ann Ophthalmol 11:617, 1979.

276. Gills JP and Henry J: Posterior chamber lenses—1,000 cases, Contact Intraocul Lens Med J 7:351, 1981.

277. Glasser DB and Bellor J: Necrotizing scleritis of scleral flaps after transscleral suture fixation of an intraocular lens, Am J Ophthalmol 113:529, 1992.

278. Gould HL: Extracapsular pseudophakia—an eight-year study. In Emery JM and Jacobson AC, editors: Current concepts in cataract surgery. Selected proceedings of the Eighth Biennial Cataract Surgical Congress, Norwalk, CT, 1984, Appleton-Century-Crofts.

279. Graziosi P and others: Location and severity of cortical opacities in different regions of the lens in age-related cataract, Invest Ophthalmol Vis Sci 37(8):1698, 1996.

280. Grehn F and Sundmacher R: Fixation of posterior chamber lenses by transscleral sutures: technique and preliminary results, Arch Ophthalmol 107:954, 1989; (letter).

281. Guthoff RF, Singh G and von Domarus D: Vergleich verschiedener Fixationsmethoden bei Binkhorst-4-Schlingenlinsen, Ophthalmologica (Basel) 186:136, 1983.

282. Gwin TD and Apple DJ: A study of posterior chamber intraocular lens fixation and loop configuration: an analysis of 425 eyes obtained postmortem, presented at the American Society of Cataract and Refractive Surgery Meeting, Los Angeles, CA, March 27, 1988.

283. Hansen SO and others: Decentration of flexible loop posterior chamber intraocular lenses in a series of 222 postmortem eyes, Ophthalmology 95:344, 1988.

284. Hansen SO and others: Posterior capsular opacification and intraocular lens decentration. I. Comparison of various posterior chamber lens designs implanted in the rabbit model, J Cataract Refract Surg 14:605, 1988.

285. Helal M and others: Transscleral fixation of posterior chamber intraocular lenses in the absence of capsular support, J Cataract Refract Surg 22:347, 1996.

286. Heslin KB and Guerriero PN: Clinical retrospective study comparing planned extracapsular cataract extraction and phakoemulsification with and without lens implantation, Ann Ophthalmol 16:956, 1984.

287. Hiles DA: Peripheral iris erosions associated with pediatric intraocular lens implants, J Am Intraocul Implant Soc 5:210, 1979.

288. Hirschberg J: The history of ophthalmology, vol 1, Antiquity, Bonn, 1982, JP Wayenborgh Verlag, (translated by FC Blodi).

289. Hirschman H: Intraocular iris clip lens, Am J Ophthalmol 68:1113, 1969, (abstract).

290. Hirschman H: Symposium: intraocular lenses. Complications with the four-loop lens of Binkhorst (the iris-clip lens), Ophthalmology 86:655, 1979.

291. Hoffer KJ: Pathologic examination of a J-loop posterior chamber intraocular lens in the ciliary sulcus, Am J Ophthalmol 92:268, 1981.

292. Holland EJ and others: Penetrating keratoplasty and transscleral fixation of posterior chamber lens, Am J Ophthalmol 114:182, 1992.

293. Hu BV and others: Implantation of posterior chamber lens in the absence of capsular and zonular support, Arch Ophthalmol 106:416, 1988.

294. IOLAB Corporation: History of intraocular lens implants, Covina, Calif, 1982, IOLAB Corp, (monograph).

295. Isaacs R, Ram J, Apple DJ: Cataract blindness in the developing world: Is there a solution? J Agromed 3(4):7–21, 1996.

296. Isaacson WB and Christie B: Mechanical testing of intraocular lenses, J Am Intraocul Implant Soc 7:344, 1981.

297. Isenberg RA and others: Histopathologic and scanning electron microscopic study of one type of intraocular lens, Arch Ophthalmol 104:683, 1986.

298. Jacobi KW and Krey H: Surgical management of intraocular lens dislocation into the vitreous: case report, J Am Intraocul Implant Soc 9:58, 1983.

299. Jaffe NS: The changing scene of intraocular implant lens surgery. The Thirty-first Bedell Lecture, Am J Ophthalmol 88:819, 1979.

300. Jaffe NS: Intracapsular cataract extraction-Binkhorst intraocular lens implantation: a 6-year follow-up. In Emery JM and Jacobson AC, editors: Current concepts in cataract surgery. Selected Proceedings of the Seventh Biennial Cataract Surgical Congress, New York, 1982, Appleton-Century-Crofts.

301. Jaffe NS: The intracapsular-extracapsular controversy, Aust J Ophthalmol 10:115, 1982.

302. Jaffe NS: The current status of intraocular lenses, Geriatr Ophthalmol 1(1):37, 1985.

303. Jaffe NS and others: Comparison of 500 Binkhorst implants with 500 routine intracapsular cataract extractions, Am J Ophthalmol 85:24, 1978.

304. Jaffe NS and others: Dislocation of Binkhorst four-loop lens implant, Ophthalmology 86:207, 1979.

305. Jaffe NS and others: The results of intracapsular cataract extraction with a Binkhorst iris clip lens implant 34 to 40 months after surgery, Ophthalmic Surg 11:489, 1980.

306. Jagger WS and Jacobi KW: An analysis of pseudophakodonesis and iridodonesis, J Am Intraocul Implant Soc 5:203, 1979.

307. Jensen KB and Eisgart F: Experiences with implantations of the semiflexible McGhan/3M, style 70 anterior chamber lens, Acta Ophthalmol 62:300, 1984.

308. Kador PF: Overview of the current attempts toward the medical treatment of cataract, Ophthalmology 90:352, 1983.

309. Karp LA and Scheie HG: Results of 1000 consecutive intracapsular cataract extractions, Ann Ophthalmol 13:1201, 1981.

310. Kaufer G: The results of 1000 intracapsular cataract extractions with the suture-fixated Medallion lens implant, Ophthalmic Surg 12:652, 1981.

311. Kelman CD: Anterior chamber lens design concepts. In Rosen ES, Haining WM and Arnott EJ, editors: Intraocular lens implantation, St. Louis, 1984, The CV Mosby Co.

312. Kincaid MC, Green WR and Iliff WJ: Granulomatous reaction to Choyce style intraocular lens, Ophthalmic Surg 13:292, 1982.

313. Kincaid MC and others: Histopathologic correlative study of Kelman-style flexible anterior chamber intraocular lenses, Am J Ophthalmol 99:159, 1985.

314. Kline OR Jr: Visual results and complications of 500 intraocular lens implantations, J Am Intraocul Implant Soc 4:184, 1978.

315. Koenig SB, Apple DJ and Hyndiuk RA: Penetrating keratoplasty and intraocular lens exchange: open-loop anterior chamber lenses versus sutured posterior chamber lenses, Cornea 13:418, 1994.

316. Koenig SB, Mcdermott ML and Hyndiuk RA: Penetrating keratoplasty and intraocular lens exchange for pseudophakic bullous keratopathy associated with a closed-loop anterior chamber intraocular lens, Am J Ophthalmol 108:43, 1989.

317. Kornmehl EW and others: Penetrating keratoplasty for pseudophakic bullous keratopathy associated with closed-loop anterior chamber intraocular lenses, Ophthalmology 97:407, 1990.

318. Kraff MC and Lieberman HL: Experience with the large circular loop Medallion lens and a critical comparison with the suture Medallion lens: a report of 300 cases, Ophthalmic Surg 8:89, 1977.

319. Kraff MC, Sanders DR and Lieberman HL: 300 primary anterior chamber lens implantations: gonioscopic findings and specular microscopy, J Am Intraocul Implant Soc 5:207, 1979.

320. Kraff MC, Sanders DR and Lieberman HL: Intraocular pressure and the corneal endothelium after neodymium: YAG laser posterior capsulotomy: relative effects of aphakia and pseudophakia, Arch Ophthalmol 103:511, 1985.

321. Kraff MC, Lieberman HL and Sanders DR: Secondary intraocular

lens implantation: rigid/semi-rigid versus flexible lenses, J Cataract Refract Surg 13:21, 1987.

322. Krasnov MM: Extrapupillary iris lens in aphakia, Am J Ophthalmol 78:541, 1974.

323. Krasnov MM: Technique of implantation of extrapupillary iris lens: 8 years of clinical experience, Br J Ophthalmol 61:316, 1977.

324. Kratz RP and others: A comparative analysis of anterior chamber, iris-supported, capsule-fixated, and posterior chamber intraocular lenses following cataract extraction by phacoemulsification, Ophthalmology 88:56, 1981.

325. Kratz RP and others: The Shearing intraocular lens: a report of 1000 cases, J Am Intraocul Implant Soc 7:55, 1981.

326. Kratz RP, Johnson SH, and Olson PF: Comparison of intraocular lenses: anterior chamber, capsule fixated, iris supported and posterior chamber, Ophthalmic Forum 1(3):12, 1983.

327. Krausz E and others: Expression of crystallins, pax6, filensin, cp49, mip, and mp20 in lens-derived cell lines, Invest Ophthalmol Vis Sci 37(10):2120, 1996.

328. Kreter JK, Sall KN, and Keates RH: Report of an incarcerated Lynell anterior chamber intraocular lens, J Cataract Refract Surg 12:300, 1986.

329. Küper J: Komplikationen nach Implantation von Vorderkammer-linsen, Klin Monatsbl Augenheilkd 140:639, 1962.

330. Kupfer C: Bowman lecture. The conquest of cataract: a global challenge, Trans Ophthalmol Soc UK 104:1, 1984.

331. Kwitko ML: Symposium: intraocular lenses. The platinum clip (platina) intraocular lens, Ophthalmology 86:632, 1979.

332. Lang TA and Lindstrom RL: Efficacy of laser interferometry in predicting visual result of YAG laser posterior capsulotomy, J Am Intraocul Implant Soc 11:367, 1985.

333. Leen MM, Ho CC, and Yanoff M: Association between urgically-induced astigmatism and cataract incision size in the early postoperative period, Ophthalmic Surg 24(9):586, 1993.

334. Legler UF and others: Chronic ciliary pain secondary to posterior chamber intraocular lens loop incarceration, Am J Ophthalmol 111:513, 1991; (letter).

335. Leiske LG: Anterior chamber implants. In Rosen ES, Haining WM, Arnott EJ, editors: Intraocular lens implantation, St. Louis, 1984, The CV Mosby Co.

336. Lim ES and others: An analysis of flexible anterior chamber lenses with special reference to the normalized rate of lens explantation, Ophthalmology 98:243, 1991.

337. Lindstrom RL, Harris WS, and Lyle WA: Secondary and exchange posterior chamber lens implantation, J Am Intraocul Implant Soc 8:353, 1982.

338. Lubniewski AJ and others: Histologic study of eyes with transsclerally sutured posterior chamber intraocular lenses, Am J Ophthalmol 110:237, 1990.

339. Malinowski SM and others: Combined pars plana vitrectomy-lensectomy and open-loop anterior chamber lens implantation, Ophthalmology 102:211, 1995.

340. Mamalis N and others: Pathological and scanning electron microscopic evaluation of the 91Z intraocular lens, J Am Intraocul Implant Soc 10:191, 1984.

341. Martin NF and others: Endothelial damage from retrocorneal mode-locked neodymium: YAG laser pulses in monkeys, Ophthalmology 92:1376, 1985.

342. Maynor RC Jr: Lens-induced complications with anterior chamber lens implants: a comparison with iris supported and posterior chamber lenses, J Am Intraocul Implant Soc 9:450, 1983.

343. McCannel MA: An ophthalmologist's reaction to his own intraocular lens implant, Am J Ophthalmol 91:114, 1981, (letter). (Reprinted Ophthalmic Forum 1(3):10, 1983.)

344. McCarty CA and Taylor HR: Recent developments in vision research: light damage in cataract, Invest Ophthalmol Vis Sci 37(9):1720, 1996, (review).

345. McDonnell PJ, Champion R, and Green WR: Location and composition of haptics of posterior chamber intraocular lenses: histopathologic study of postmortem eyes, Ophthalmology 94:136, 1987.

346. McLemore CS: Cadillacs, Volkswagens, and aphakic corrections, Arch Ophthalmol 70:734, 1963, (letter).

347. McLemore CS: Aphakic correction from an aphake's point of view, Arch Ophthalmol 74:443, 1965, (letter).

348. McLeod SD and others: Iris-sutured posterior chamber lens dislo-

cation late after penetrating keratoplasty, Arch Ophthalmol 114(8):1032, 1996, (letter).

349. Menezo JL, Martinez MC, and Cisneros AL: Iris-fixated Worst claw versus sulcus-fixated posterior chamber lenses in the absence of capsular support, J Cataract Refract Surg 22:1476, 1996.

350. Moses L: Complications of rigid anterior chamber implants, Ophthalmology 91:819, 1984.

351. Nadler DJ and Schwartz B: Cataract surgery in the United States 1968–1976: a descriptive epidemiologic study, Ophthalmology 87:10, 1980.

352. Neetens A and Rubbens MC: Complications in primary anterior chamber pseudophakic eyes after intracapsular cataract extraction, Ophthalmologica 187:89, 1983.

353. Neuhann T: Theorie und operationstechnik des kapsulorhexis, Klin Monatsbl Augenheilkd 190:542, 1987.

354. Nordlohne ME: Dislocation and endothelial corneal dystrophy (ECD) in patients fitted with Binkhorst lens implants (1958–1972), Doc Ophthalmol Proc Series 6:15, 1975.

355. Nordlohne ME: The intraocular implant lens: development and results with special reference to the Binkhorst lens, ed 2, Baltimore, 1975, The Williams & Wilkins Co.

356. Obstbaum SA and Galin MA: Cystoid macular edema and ocular inflammation: the corneo-retinal inflammatory syndrome, Trans Ophthalmol Soc UK 99:187, 1979.

357. Ohmi S and Uenoyama K: Decentration associated with asymmetric capsular shrinkage and intraocular lens design in a rabbit model, J Cataract Refract Surg 21:293, 1995.

358. Olson RJ and Kolodner H: The position of the posterior chamber intraocular lens, Arch Ophthalmol 97:715, 1979.

359. Olson RJ, Morgan KS, and Kolodner H: The Shearing-style intraocular lens and the posterior chamber, J Am Intraocul Implant Soc 5:338, 1979.

360. Olson RJ, Morgan KS, and Kolodner H: The Shearing intraocular lens: where does it go and what does it do in the eye? Ophthalmology 87:668, 1980.

361. Olson RJ, Sevel D, and Stevenson D: A histopathologic study of the Choyce VIII intraocular lens, Am J Ophthalmol 92:781, 1981.

362. Park SB and others: Posterior chamber intraocular lenses in a series of 75 autopsy eyes. II. Postimplantation loop configuration, J Cataract Refract Surg 12:363, 1986.

363. Pearce JL: Long-term results of the Binkhorst iris clip lens in senile cataract, Br J Ophthalmol 56:319, 1972.

364. Pearce JL: Experience with 194 posterior chamber lenses in 20 months, Trans Ophthalmol Soc UK 97:258, 1977.

365. Pearce JL: Sixteen months' experience with 140 posterior chamber intraocular lens implants, Br J Ophthalmol 61:310, 1977.

366. Pearce JL: Pearce-style posterior chamber lenses, J Am Intraocul Implant Soc 6:33, 1980.

367. Pearce JL: Current state of posterior chamber intraocular lenses after intracapsular and extracapsular cataract surgery, Trans Ophthalmol Soc UK 101:73, 1981.

368. Pearce JL: The Pearce tripod posterior chamber lenses. In Rosen ES, Haining WM, and Arnott EJ, editors: Intraocular lens implantation, St. Louis, 1984, The CV Mosby Co.

369. Pearce JL and Ghosh T: Surgical and postoperative problems with Binkhorst 2- and 4-loop lenses, Trans Ophthalmol Soc UK 97:84, 1977.

370. Percival SPB and Yousef KM: Treatment of uniocular aphakia: a comparison of iris clip lenses with hard corneal contact lenses, Br J Ophthalmol 60:642, 1976.

371. Persen RD and Farris RL: A CLAO Journal survey of trends in ophthalmology practice, CLAO J 11:251, 1985.

372. Polack FM: Management of anterior segment complications of intraocular lenses, Ophthalmology 87:881, 1980.

373. Rattigan SM and others: Flexible open-loop anterior chamber intraocular lens implantation after posterior capsule complications in extracapsular cataract extraction, J Cataract Refract Surg 22(2):243, 1996, (review).

374. Reidy JJ and others: An analysis of semiflexible, closed-loop anterior chamber intraocular lenses, J Am Intraocul Implant Soc 11:344, 1985.

375. Richburg FA and Sun HS: Size of the crushed cataractous capsule bag, J Am Intraocul Implant Soc 9:333, 1983.

376. Ridley H: Intra-ocular acrylic lenses, Trans Ophthalmol Soc UK 71:617, 1951.

377. Ridley H: Artificial intra-ocular lenses after cataract extraction, St Thomas Hosp Reports 7(series 2):12, 1952.

378. Ridley H: Further observations on intraocular acrylic lenses in cataract surgery, Trans Am Acad Ophthalmol Otolaryngol 57:98, 1953.

379. Ridley H: Intra-ocular acrylic lenses: 10 years' development, Br J Ophthalmol 44:705, 1960.

380. Robinson ML and Overbeek PA: Differential expression of A- and aB-crystallin during murine ocular development, Invest Ophthalmol Vis Sci 37(11):2276, 1996.

381. Rosen ES: Father of the intraocular lens (history in the making), J Cataract Refract Surg 23:4, 1997.

382. Rosen ES: Intracapsular cataract surgery with the Severin (posterior chamber) lens implant, Ophthalmologica (Basel) 187:94, 1983.

383. Rosen ES: IOL implantation with special reference to intracapsular cataract extraction, Cataract 1(4):20, 1984.

384. Rowsey JJ: Peripheral anterior synechiae and intraocular lenses, J Am Intraocul Implant Soc 5:307, 1979.

385. Rowsey JJ and Gaylor JR: Intraocular lens disasters: peripheral anterior synechia, Ophthalmology 87:646, 1980.

386. Roy FH: Fourscore artiphakia, Contact Intraocul Lens Med J 8:41, 1982.

387. Rubin ML: Optics for clinicians, ed 2, Gainesville, Fla, Triad Scientific Publishers, 1974.

388. Serpin G and Lumbroso P: Deplacements postoperatoires de l'implant irido-capulaire (2 anses), Bull Soc Ophthalmol Fr 82:1231, 1982.

389. Severin SL: The Severin posterior chamber lens for intracapsular and extracapsular cataract surgery, Contact Intraocul Lens Med J 6:291, 1980.

390. Severin SL: The Severin posterior chamber lens. In Rosen ES, Haining WM, and Arnott EJ, editors: Intraocular lens implantation, St. Louis, 1984, The CV Mosby Co.

391. Shearing SP: Mechanism of fixation of the Shearing posterior chamber intra-ocular lens, Contact Intraocul Lens Med J 5:74, 1979.

392. Shearing SP: The history of ciliary fixated intraocular lenses, Contact Intraocul Lens Med J 6:295, 1980.

393. Shearing SP: Posterior chamber lens implantation, Int Ophthalmol Clin 22(2):135, 1982.

394. Shearing SP: Five-year postoperative results with J-loop posterior chamber lenses, Cataract 1(1):20 and 33, 1983.

395. Shearing SP: Evolution of the posterior chamber intraocular lenses, J Am Intraocul Implant Soc 10:343, 1984.

396. Shepard DD: Anterior chamber lens implantation today, Int Ophthalmol Clin 22(2):77, 1982.

397. Simcoe CW: Simcoe posterior chamber lens: theory, techniques and results, J Am Intraocul Implant Soc 7:154, 1981.

398. Simcoe CW: Mechanical and design considerations in lens implantation, Int Ophthalmol Clin 22(2):203, 1982.

399. Simcoe CW: Letter to the editor, Ophthalmic Surg 14:434, 1983.

400. Sinskey RM: Posterior chamber lens modification, J Am Intraocul Implant Soc 7:260, 1981, (letter).

401. Sloane AE: Perspectives on management of aphakia after 40 years, Ophthalmic Surg 8:75, 1977.

402. Smith PW and others: Complications of semiflexible, closed-loop anterior chamber intraocular lenses, Arch Ophthalmol 105:52, 1987.

403. Snider NL and McReynolds WU: Results and complications of our first 500 implantations, J Am Intraocul Implant Soc 3:10, 1977.

404. Soong HK and others: Implantation of posterior chamber intraocular lenses in the absence of lens capsule during penetrating keratoplasty, Arch Ophthalmol 107:660, 1989.

405. Stamper RL and Sugar A: The intraocular lens, San Francisco, 1982, American Academy of Ophthalmology Manuals Program, p. 105.

406. Stark WJ and others: The FDA report on intraocular lenses, Ophthalmology 90:311, 1983.

407. Stark WJ and others: Update of intraocular lenses implanted in the United States, Am J Ophthalmol 98:238, 1984, (letter).

408. Stark WJ, Terry AC, Maumenee, AE, editors: Anterior segment surgery: IOLs, lasers, and refractive keratoplasty, Baltimore, 1986, The Williams & Wilkins Co.

409. Stark WJ and others: The role of the food and drug administration in ophthalmology, Arch Ophthalmol 104:1145, 1986.

410. Stark WJ and others: Trends in intraocular lens implantation in the United States, Arch Ophthalmol 104:1769, 1986.

411. Stark WJ and others: Posterior chamber intraocular lens implantation in the absence of capsular support, Arch Ophthalmol 107:1078, 1989.

412. Stark WJ, Sommer A, and Smith RE: Changing trends in intraocular lens implantation, Arch Ophthalmol 107:1441, 1989.

413. Tandon MK and Munton CGF: A review of pseudophakia using angle fixation lenses, Trans Ophthalmol Soc UK 102:24, 1982.

414. Taylor DM, Sachs SW, and Stern AL: Aphakic cystoid macular edema: Longterm clinical observations, Surv Ophthalmol 28(suppl):437, 1984.

415. Taylor VL and others: Morphology of the normal human lens, Invest Ophthalmol Vis Sci 37(7):1396, 1996.

416. Tetz MR and others: Posterior capsular opacification and intraocular lens decentration. II: Experimental findings on a prototype circular intraocular lens design, J Cataract Refract Surg 14:614, 1988.

417. Troutman RC: Artiphakia and aniseikonia, Trans Am Ophthalmol Soc 60:590, 1962.

418. Troutman RC: Artiphakia and aniseikonia, Am J Ophthalmol 56:602, 1963.

419. Van Balen ATM: Four years' experience with Binkhorst lens implantation, Am J Ophthalmol 75:755, 1973.

420. Veress B and Barkman Y: A histomorphological study on the effect of iridocapsular intraocular lens on the iris: a case report, Acta Ophthalmol 60:821, 1982.

421. Vision Research; A National Plan: 1983–1987, US Department of Health and Human Services, Public Health Service, National Institutes of Health, NIH Publication No 82-2469.

422. Wang L and others: Mechanism of calcium-induced disintegrative globulization of rat lens fiber cells, Invest Ophthalmol Vis Sci 37(5):915–922, 1996.

423. Waring GO III: The 50-year epidemic of pseudophakic corneal edema, Arch Ophthalmol 107:657, 1989.

424. Wesendahl TA and others: Textur von IOL-Oberflächen: Ein neues Konzept zur Nachstarprävention. Abstract. Der Ophthalmologe 90(Suppl I):S140, 1993.

425. West S and others: Cigarette smoking and risk for progression of nuclear opacities, Arch Ophthalmol 113:1377, 1995.

426. Williams HW: Cataract extraction operations. 1869, Arch Ophthalmol 114(4):478; discussion: 479, 1996, (classic article).

427. Worst J: Note on fixation of the Binkhorst iris clip lens, Ophthalmologica 163:10, 1971.

428. Worst JGF: Symposium: intraocular lenses. Iris sutures for artificial lens fixation—Perlon vs stainless steel, Trans Am Acad Ophthalmol Otolaryngol 81:102, 1976.

429. Worst JGF, Mosselman CD, and Ludwig HHH: The artificial lens—experience with 2000 lens implantations, J Am Intraocul Implant Soc 3:14, 1977.

430. Worthen DM: FDA study of intraocular lenses, Ophthalmology 90:45, 1983.

431. Worthen DM and others: Interim FDA report on intraocular lenses, Ophthalmology 87:267, 1980.

432. Worthen DM and others: Update report on intraocular lenses, Ophthalmology 88:381, 1981.

433. Zaidman GW and Goldman S: A prospective study on the implantation of anterior chamber intraocular lenses during keratoplasty for pseudophakic and aphakic bullous keratopathy, Ophthalmology 97:757, 1990.

Modern capsular IOLs

434. Allarakhia L, Knoll RL, and Lindstrom RL: Soft intraocular lenses, J Cataract Refract Surg, 13(6):607, 1987, (review).

435. Allarakhia L and Lindstrom RL: Soft intraocular lenses, Ophthalmol 12(3):185, 1988 (review).

436. Allen ED and others: Comparison of a diffractive bifocal and a monofocal intraocular lens, J Cataract Refract Surg 22:446, 1996.

437. Alpar JJ: On-the-table posterior capsulotomy and 1% sodium hyaluronate, J Cataract Refract Surg 12:391, 1986.

438. Alpar JJ: The role of 1% sodium hyaluronate in anterior capsulotomy with the neodymium: YAG laser in patients with diseased cornea, J Cataract Refract Surg 12:658, 1986.

439. Alpar JJ: Diabetes: cataract extraction and intraocular lenses, J Cataract Refract Surg 13:43, 1987.

440. Anonymous: Consultation section. Implanting silicone foldable lenses. J Cataract Refract Surg 18(2):206, 1992.

441. Anonymous: Consultation section: contraindications in use of foldable intraocular lenses, J Cataract Refract Surg 22(2):159, 1996.

442. Anonymous: Consultation section. What would you advise for a patient who has had episodic pupillary capture? J Cataract Refract Surg 22:8, 1996.

443. Anonymous: White paper on cataract surgery, American Academy of Ophthalmology and American Society of Cataract and Refractive Surgery, Ophthalmology 103(7):1152, 1996.

444. Anteby II and Fruchtpery J: Visual outcome following traumatic wound dehiscence after cataract surgery, J Cataract Refract Surg 21:533, 1995.

445. Apple DJ: Utah Center for Intraocular Lens Research. Proceedings of the Research to Prevent Blindness Science Writer's Seminar, Oct 1984.

446. Apple DJ and others: Biocompatibility of implant materials: a review and scanning electron microscopic study, J Am Intraocul Implant Soc 10:53, 1984.

447. Apple DJ: Intraocular lenses: notes from an interested observer Arch Ophthalmol 104:1150, 1986, (special article).

448. Apple DJ and others: A review of the histopathology of intraocular lens fixation, Curr Can Ophthalmic Prac 4:54, 1986.

449. Apple DJ and others: Intercapsular implantation of various posterior chamber IOLs: animal test results, Ophthalmic Pract 5:100, 1987.

450. Apple DJ: Center for Intraocular Lens Research transfers to Medical University of South Carolina, J Cataract Refract Surg 14:481, 1988, (guest editorial).

451. Apple DJ: Pea-podding, Proceedings of The Third International, Implant, Microsurgical & Refractive Keratoplasty Meeting, Fukuoka, Japan, May 26–28, 1989.

452. Apple DJ: Advances in intraocular lens biomechanics, J Cataract Refract Surg 16:543, 1990, (editorial).

453. Apple DJ and others: Preparation and study of human eyes obtained postmortem with the Miyake posterior photographic technique, Ophthalmology 97:810, 1990.

454. Apple DJ and others: Evidence in support of the continuous tear anterior capsulectomy (capsulorhexis technique). In Cangelosi GC, (editor): Advances in cataract surgery, New Orleans Academy of Ophthalmology, Thorofare, New Jersey, 1991, Slack.

455. Apple DJ and others: Posterior chamber intraocular lens (PC IOL): a clinical goal with bifocal and multifocal IOLs, In Maxwell WA, and Nordan LT, (editors): Current concepts of multifocal intraocular lenses, Thorofare, New Jersey, 1991, Slack Inc.

456. Apple DJ: Intraocular lens biocompatibility, J Cataract Refract Surg 18:217, 1992, (editorial; comment).

457. Apple DJ, Legler UF, and Assia EI: (Comparison of various capsulectomy techniques in cataract surgery. an experimental study) (German), Ophthalmologe 89:301, 1992.

458. Apple DJ and others: Posterior capsule opacification, Surv Ophthalmol 37:73, 1992, (review).

459. Apple DJ: Pathological aspects of capsular surgery, European J Imp Refrac Surg 6:223, 1994.

460. Apple DJ, Auffarth GU, and RF Wesendahl TA: Pathophysiology of modern capsular surgery, Steinert (editor): Textbook of modern cataract surgery: technique, complication, & management, Philadelphia, 1995, WB Saunders Company.

461. Apple DJ and others: Verbesserung der befestigung von silikonschiffchenlinsen durch den gebrauch von positionierungslochern in der linsenhaptik, Proceedings of the 10th Annual Deutche Gesellschaft fuer Intraokularlinsen Implantation Meeting, Budapest, Hungary, March 1996.

462. Apple DJ and others: Irreversible silicone oil adhesion to silicone intraocular lenses. A clinicopathologic analysis, Ophthalmology 103:1555, 1996.

463. Arnott EJ: Intraocular implants, Trans Ophthalmol Soc UK 101: 58, 1981.

464. Arnott EJ, Condon R: The totally encircling loop lens—follow-up of 1,800 cases, Cataract 2(8):13, 1985.

465. Arnott EJ, Grindle CFJ, and Krolman GM: Four and one-half year study of the relationship between one-piece encircling loop polymethylmethacrylate lenses and retinal detachment, J Cataract Refract Surg 14:387, 1988.

466. Arnott EJ: Inflammation after lens implantation, J Cataract Refract Surg 18:424, 1992, (letter).

467. Artaria LG, Ziliotti F, and Ziliotti-Mandelli A: (Long-term follow-up of implantation of foldable silicone posterior lenses) (German). Klinische Monatsblatter fur Augenheilkunde 204(5):268, 1994.

468. Ashton N and Boberg-Ans J: Pathology of aphakic eye containing an anterior chamber implant, Br J Ophthalmol 45:543, 1961.

469. Assia EI, Hoggatt JP, and Apple DJ: Experimental nucleus extraction through a capsulorhexis in an eye with pseudoexfoliation syndrome, Am J Ophthalmol 111:645, 1991, (letter).

470. Assia EI and others: Estudio experimental comparando diversas tJcnicas de capsulectomRa anterior. Arch Ophthalmol (Spanish ed) 2:280–285, 1991.

471. Assia EI and others: An experimental study comparing various anterior capsulectomy techniques (see comments), Arch Ophthalmol 109:642, 1991.

472. Assia EI and others: An experimental study comparing various anterior capsulectomy techniques. Arch Ophthalmol (Chinese ed) 109:642–647, 1991.

473. Assia EI and others: The relationship between the stretching capability of the anterior capsule and zonules, Invest Ophthalmol Vis Sci 32:2835, 1991.

474. Assia EI and others: The elastic properties of the lens capsule in capsulorhexis (see comments), Am J Ophthalmol 111:628, 1991.

475. Assia EI and others: Mechanism of radial tear formation and extension after anterior capsulectomy, Ophthalmology 98:432, 1991.

476. Assia EI and others: Studies on cataract surgery and intraocular lenses at the Center for Intraocular Lens Research, Ophthalmol Clin N Am 4:251, 1991.

477. Assia EI and others: A comparison of neodymium: yttrium aluminum garnet and diode laser transscleral cyclophotocoagulation and cyclo-cryotherapy, Invest Ophthalmol Vis Sci 32:2774, 1991.

478. Assia EI and Apple DJ: Side-view analysis of the lens. I. The crystalline lens and the evacuated bag, Arch Ophthalmol 110:89, 1992.

479. Assia EI and Apple DJ: Side-view analysis of the lens. II. Positioning of intraocular lenses, Arch Ophthalmol 110:94, 1992.

480. Assia EI and Apple DJ: Capsulorhexis and corneal magnification, Arch Ophthalmology 110(2):170, 1992, (reply to letter).

481. Assia EI, Blumenthal M, Apple DJ: Hydrodissection and visco extraction of the nucleus in planned extracapsular cataract extraction, Eur J Implant Refract Surg 4:3-8, 1992.

482. Assia EI and others: Removal of viscoelastic materials after experimental cataract surgery in vitro, J Cataract Refract Surg 18:3, 1992.

483. Assia EI and others: Clinicopathologic study of the effect of radial tears and loop fixation on intraocular lens decentration, Ophthalmology 100:153, 1993.

484. Assia EI and others: Photoanalysis of fixation of posterior chamber intraocular lenses, Eur J Implant Refract Surg 1993.

485. Assia EI and others: Clinicopathologic study of ocular trauma in eyes with intraocular lenses, Am J Ophthalmol 117:30, 1994.

486. Assia EI, Levkovichverbin H and Blumenthal M: Management of Descemet's membrane detachment, J Cataract Refract Surg 21: 714, 1995.

487. Assia EI, Legler UFC, Apple DJ: The capsular bag after short- and long-term fixation of intraocular lenses, Ophthalmology 102(8): 1151–1157, 1995.

488. Au YK, Lucius RW and Patel JS: Epikeratophakia to correct traumatic aphakia after penetrating keratoplasty, J Cataract Refract Surg 22:501, 1996.

489. Auer C and Gonvers M: (Silicone one piece intraocular implant and anterior capsule fibrosis) (French). Klinische Monatsblatter fur Augenheilkunde 206(5):293, 1995.

490. Auffarth GU and others: Eine Analyse von Komplikationen bei explantierten Hinterkammerlinsen, Der Ophthalmologe 90(Suppl I):S140, 1993, (abstract).

491. Auffarth GU and others: Eine Kapsulorhexistechnik bei kindlicher Katarakt. Abstract, Der Ophthalmologe 90(Suppl I):S13, 1993.

492. Auffarth GU and others: Zentrierung von Hinterkammerlinsen bei Patienten mit Pseudoexfoliationssyndrom: Befunde in explantierten Autopsieaugen, In Wollensak J, et al, editors: Transactions of the 8th Congress of the German Intraocular Lens Implant Society (DGII) in Berlin, 1994, Springer Verlag, Berlin, Heidelberg, New York, 1994, 530–537.

493. Auffarth GU and others: Häufigkeit und Art von Explantationsgrhnden von einsthckigen und dreisthckigen Hinterkammer-

the Geneva ophthalmological clinic) (French), Klinische Monatsblätter für Augenheilkunde 206(5):296, 1995.

596. Dhaliwal DK and others: Visual significance of glistenings seen in the acrysof intraocular lens, J Cataract Refract Surg 22:452, 1996.

597. Dick B, Kohnen T and Jacobi KW: (Endothelial cell loss after phacoemulsification and 3.5 vs. 5 mm corneal tunnel incision) (German), Ophthalmologe 92(4):476, 1995.

598. Dick HB and others: Long-term endothelial cell loss following phacoemulsification through a temporal clear corneal incision, J Cataract Refract Surg 22:63, 1996.

599. Diestelhorst M and others: Effect of 3.0mm tunnel and 6;0mm corneoscleral incisions on the blood-aqueous barrier, J Cataract Refract Surg 22:1465, 1996.

600. Doren GS, Stern GA and Driebe WT: Indications for and results of intraocular lens explanation, J Cataract Refract Surg 18:79, 1992.

601. Dosso AA and others: Exfoliation syndrome and phacoemulsification, J Cataract Refract Surg 23:122, 1997.

602. Drews RC: Management of patients with intraocular lenses: guidelines for those who do not perform this operation, Trans Ophthalmol Soc UK 97:78, 1977.

603. Drews RC: Quality control and changing indications for lens implantation, Ophthalmology 90:301, 1983.

604. Drews RC: Polypropylene in the human eye, J Am Intraocul Implant Soc 9:137, 1983.

605. Drews RC and Kreiner C: Comparative study of the elasticity and memory of intraocular lens loops, J Cataract Refract Surg 13:525, 1987.

606. Duncker GIW, Westphalen S and Behrendt S: Complications of silicone disc intraocular lenses, J Cataract Refract Surg 21:562, 1995.

607. Eaton AM and others: Condensation on the posterior surface of silicone intraocular lenses during fluid-air exchange [see comments], Ophthalmology 102:733, 1995.

608. Egan CA and others: Prospective study of the SI-40NB foldable silicone intraocular lens, J Cataract Refract Surg 22(2):1272, 1996.

609. Ehrich W and Hoh H: (Intraocular lens materials in the anterior chamber implantation test) (German). Klinische Monatsblatter fur Augenheilkunde 194(2):101, 1989.

610. el-Maghraby A and others: Effect of incision size on early postoperative visual rehabilitation after cataract surgery and intraocular lens implantation, J Cataract Refract Surg 19(4):494, 1993.

611. Epstein E: Modified Ridley lenses, Br J Ophthalmol 43:29, 1959.

612. Eriksen JS and Nielson NV: Visual outcome and complications in 287 intraocular lens implants (Federow) compared with 290 intracapsular cataract extractions, Acta Ophthalmol 61:67, 1983.

613. Ernest PH, Grabow HB, McFarland MS: Advantages and disadvantages of sutureless surgery. In Gills JP, Martin RG, Sanders DR, editors: Sutureless cataract surgery: an evolution toward minimally invasive technique, Thorofare, NJ, 1992, Slack.

614. Ernest PH, Lavery KT, Kiessling LA: Relative strength of scleral corneal and clear corneal incisions constructed in cadaver eyes, J Cataract Refract Surg 20:626, 1994.

615. Erturk H, Ozcetin H: Phakic posterior chamber intraocular lenses for the correction of high myopia, J Cataract Refract Surg 11(5):388, 1995.

616. Evans RB: Peripheral anterior synechia overlying the haptics of posterior chamber lenses. Occurrence and natural history (see comments). Ophthalmology 97:415, 1990.

617. Fagadau WR and others: Posterior chamber intraocular lenses at the Wilmer Institute: a comparative analysis of complications and visual results, Br J Ophthalmol 68:13, 1984.

618. Faulkner GD: Early experience with staar silicone elastic lens implants, J Cataract Refract Surg 12(1):36, 1986.

619. Faulkner GD: Endothelial cell loss after phacoemulsification and insertion of silicone lens implants, J Cataract Refract Surg 13(6):649, 1987.

620. Faulkner GD: Folding and inserting silicone intraocular lens implants, J Cataract Refract Surg 13(6):678, 1987.

621. Faust KJ: Hydrodissection of soft nuclei, J Am Intra Ocu Impl Soc 10:75, 1984.

622. Fechner PU and Fechner MU: Tadini, the man who invented the artificial lens, J Am Intraocul Implant Soc 5:22, 1979.

623. Fechner PU: Intraokularlinsen: Grundlagen und Operationslehre, Stuttgart, Ferdinand Enke Verlag, 1980.

624. Feldman F and Stein H: Delayed glaucoma after implantation of the Choyce intraocular lens, Can J Ophthalmol 14:190, 1979.

625. Fine IH: Cortical cleaving hydrodissection, J Cataract Refract Surg 18:508, 1992.

626. Fine IH: Corneal tunnel incision with a temporal approach, In Fine IH, Fichman RA, Grabow HB, editors: Clear-corneal cataract surgery and topical anesthesia, Thorofare, NJ, 1993, Slack.

627. Fitzsimon JS and Johnson DH: Exfoliation material on intraocular lens implants, Arch Ophthalmol 114:355, 1996.

628. Fogle JA and others: Clinicopathologic observations of a silicone posterior chamber lens in a primate model, J Cataract Refract Surg 12(3):281, 1986.

629. Foster CS, Fong LP and Singh G: Cataract surgery and intraocular lens implantation in patients with uveitis (see comments) Ophthalmology 96:281, 1989.

630. Foster RE and others: Extracapsular cataract extraction and posterior chamber intraocular lens implantation in uveitis patients, Ophthalmology 99:1234, 1992.

631. Francese JE, Pham L and Christ FR: Accelerated hydrolytic and ultraviolet aging studies on si-18nb and si-20nb silicone lenses, J Cataract Refract Surg 18(4):402, 1992.

632. Francese JE and others: Moisture droplet formation on the posterior surface of intraocular lenses during fluid air exchange, J Cataract Refract Surg 21:685, 1995.

633. Freissler K, Kuchle M, and Naumann GOH: Spontaneous dislocation of the lens in pseudoexfoliation syndrome, Arch Ophthalmol 113:1095, 1995.

634. Galin MA and others: Iris-supported lens implantation vs simple cataract extraction: an analysis of data, Trans Ophthalmol Soc UK 97:74, 1977.

635. Galin MA and others: Mechanism of implant inflammation, Trans Ophthalmol Soc UK 100:229, 1980.

636. Gayton JL, van der Karr MA, Sanders V: Combined cataract and glaucoma procedures using temporal cataract surgery, J Cataract Refract Surg 22:1485, 1996.

637. Gelender H: Descemetocele after intraocular lens implantation, Arch Ophthalmol 100:72, 1982.

638. Gerding H, Buchner T and Busse H: Surgical techniques and preliminary results of intraocular lens (iol) implantation, Invest Ophthalmol Vis Sci 37(10):1935, 1996, (letter).

639. Gieser SC and others: Phthisis bulbi after intraocular lens implantation in a child, Can J Ophthalmol 20:184, 1985.

640. Gills JP: Shearing lens insertion after extracapsular cataract extraction with capsular fixation, Contact Intraocul Lens Med J 6:53, 1980.

641. Gills JP and Sanders DR: Use of small incisions to control induced astigmatism and inflammation following cataract surgery, J Cataract Refract Surg 17(Suppl):740, 1991.

642. Gimbel H, Neuhann T: Development, advantages and methods of continuous circular capsulorhexis techniques, J Cataract Refract Surg 16(1):31, 1990.

643. Gimbel HV, Sanders DR, and Raanan MG: Visual and refractive results of multifocal intraocular lenses (see comments), Ophthalmology 98:881, 1991.

644. Gimbel HV: Posterior capsulorhexis with optic capture in pediatric cataract intraocular lens surgery, Ophthalmology 103(11):1871, 1996.

645. Gimbel HV: Endophthalmitis: immediate management using posterior capsulorhexis and anterior vitrectomy through reopened cataract surgery incision, J Cataract Refract Surg 23:27, 1997.

646. Girard LJ and others: Subluxated (ectopic) lenses in adults. Long-term results of pars plana lensectomy-vitrectomy by ultrasonic fragmentation with and without a phacoprosthesis, Ophthalmology 97:462, 1990.

647. Glasser DB and others: Protective effects of viscous solutions in phacoemulsification and traumatic lens implantation, Arch Ophthalmol 107:1047, 1989.

648. Gobel RJ and others: Activation of complement in human serum by some synthetic polymers used for intraocular lenses, Biomaterials 8:285, 1987.

649. Golnik KC, Hund PW, 3rd and Apple DJ: Atonic pupil after cataract surgery (see comments), J Cataract Refract Surg 21:170, 1995, (review).

650. Gonzalez GA and Irvine AR: Posterior dislocation of plate haptic silicone lenses, Arch Ophthalmol 114(6):775, 1996, (letter).

651. Googe JM and others: BSS warning, J Am Intraocul Implant Soc 10:202, 1984, (letter).

652. Gorlin AI and others: Effect of adhered bacteria on the binding of acanthamoeba to hydrogel lenses, Arch Ophthalmol 114(5):576, 1996.

653. Gross RH and Miller KM: Corneal astigmatism after phacoemulsification and lens implantation through unsutured scleral and corneal tunnel incisions, Am J Ophthalmol 121:57, 1996.

654. Gruber E: Contact lens versus intraocular lens in the correction of aphakia, Trans Ophthalmol Soc UK 100:231, 1980.

655. Guthoff R, Abramo F, and Draeger J: (Flexibility of intraocular lens haptics of various geometry and materials) (German), Klinische Monatsblatter fur Augenheilkunde 197(1):27, 1990.

656. Guthoff R and others: Measurement of elastic resisting forces of intraocular haptic loops of varying geometrical designs and material composition, J Cataract Refract Surg 16(5):551, 1990.

657. Guthoff R and others: Forces on intraocular lens haptics induced by capsular fibrosis. An experimental study, Graefes Arch Clin Exper Ophthalmol 228(4):363, 1990.

658. Habal MB: The biologic basis for the clinical application of the silicones. A correlate to their biocompatibility. Arch Surg 119(7):843, 1984, (review).

659. Haefliger E and Parel JM: Accommodation of an endocapsular silicone lens (phaco-ersatz) in the aging rhesus monkey, J Refract Corneal Surg 10(5):550, 1994.

660. Hagan JC III: Insertion of a second intraocular lens following traumatic expulsion of a posterior chamber lens, J Cataract Refract Surg 13:315, 1987.

661. Hall DL: Silicone intraocular lens implants and circular anterior capsulotomy (capsulorhexis), J Louisiana State Med Soc 141(2):20, 1989.

662. Hansen MH and others: Intraocular pressure seven years after extracapsular cataract extraction and sulcus implantation of a posterior chamber intraocular lens, J Cataract Refract Surg 21:676, 1995.

663. Hansen TE, Naeser K, and Nissen JN: Prospective study of intraocular pressure two-and-a-half years after intracapsular cataract extraction and implantation of a semiflexible anterior chamber lens, J Cataract Refract Surg 13:554, 1987.

664. Hansen TE, Naeser K, and Rask KL: A prospective study of intraocular pressure four months after extracapsular cataract extraction with implantation of posterior chamber lenses, J Cataract Refract Surg 13:35, 1987.

665. Hansen TE, Otland N, and Corydon L: Posterior capsule fibrosis and intraocular lens design, J Cataract Refract Surg 14:383, 1988.

666. Hara T and Hara T: Clinical results of endocapsular phacoemulsification and complete in-the-bag intraocular lens fixation, J Cataract Refract Surg 13:279, 1987.

667. Hara T and Hara T: Roundel phacoemulsification technique for in-the-bag intraocular lens fixation, J Cataract Refract Surg 13:441, 1987.

668. Hara T and others: Specular microscopy of the anterior lens capsule after endocapsular lens implantation, J Cataract Refract Surg 14:533, 1988.

669. Hara T, Sakanishi K, and Yamada Y: Efficacy of equator rings in an experimental rabbit study, Arch Ophthalmol 113:1060, 1995.

670. Hardman Lea SJ and others: Pseudophakic accommodation? A study of the stability of capsular bag supported, one piece, rigid tripod, or soft flexible implants, Br J Ophthalmol 74(1):22, 1990.

671. Harris DJ Jr, and Specht CS: Intracapsular lens delivery during attempted extracapsular cataract extraction. Association with capsulorrhexis (see comments), Ophthalmology 98:623, 1991.

672. Hassan TS and others: Implantation of Kelman-style, open-loop anterior chamber lenses during keratoplasty for aphakic and pseudophakic bullous keratopathy. A comparison with iris-sutured posterior chamber lenses, Ophthalmology 98:875, 1991.

673. Hemo I: Intraocular lens implantation in an underdeveloped country, J Cataract Refract Surg 13:414, 1987.

674. Henkind P: No pun intended, intraocular lenses are in, Ophthalmology 90(4):27A, 1983, (editorial).

675. Hennis HL and others: A transcleral cyclophotocoagulation using a semiconductor diode laser in cadaver eyes, Ocular Surgery 22(5):274–278, 1991.

676. Hettlich HJ and others: (Experience with hydrophilic silicone disc intraocular lenses) (German), Fortschritte der Ophthalmologie 88(3):274, 1991.

677. Hettlich HJ and others: Plasma-induced surface modification on silicone intraocular lenses: chemical analysis and in vitro characterization, Biomaterials 12(5):521, 1991.

678. Hettlich HJ and others: In vitro and in vivo evaluation of a hydrophilized silicone intraocular lens, J Cataract Refract Surg 18(2):140, 1992.

679. Heyrman TP and others: Drug uptake and release by a hydrogel intraocular lens and the human crystalline lens, J Cataract Refract Surg 15(2):169, 1989.

680. Hiles DA and Watson BA: Complications of implant surgery in children, J Am Intraocul Implant Soc 5:24, 1979.

681. Hiles DA and Johnson BL: The role of crystalline lens epithelium in postpseudophakos membrane formation, J Ann Intraocul Implant Soc 6:141, 1980.

682. Hiles DA and Hered RW: Modern intraocular lens implants in children with new age limitations, J Cataract Refract Surg 13:493, 1987.

683. Hoffer KJ: Axial dimension of the human cataractous lens Arch Ophthalmol 111:914, 1993, (published erratum appears in Arch Ophthalmol 1993 Dec, 111(12):1626.

684. Holladay JT, Bishop JE, and Lewis JW: Diagnosis and treatment of mysterious light streaks seen by patients following extracapsular cataract extraction, J Am Intraocul Implant Soc 11:21, 1995.

685. Holladay JT and Hoffer KJ: Intraocular lens power calculations for multifocal intraocular lenses (see comments), Am J Ophthalmol 114:405, 1992.

686. Holladay JT: Refractive power calculations for intraocular lenses in the phakic eye, Am J Ophthalmol 116:63, 1993.

687. Holland EJ and others: Penetrating keratoplasty and transscleral fixation of posterior chamber lens, Am J Ophthalmol 114:182, 1992.

688. Hunold W and others: A method to study the interaction between intraocular lens loops and anterior segment vasculature, J Cataract Refract Surg 15:289, 1989.

689. Ibaraki N, Ohara K, and Miyamoto T: Membranous outgrowth suggesting lens epithelial cell proliferation in pseudophakic eyes, Am J Ophthalmol 119:706, 1995.

690. Imkamp E and others: Protective effect of the anterior lens capsule: corneal endothelial cell loss following intercapsular phacoemulsification compared with phacoemulsification with large open capsulotomy (German), Fortschritte der Ophthalmologie 86:15, 1989.

691. Ionides A and others: Posterior capsule opacification following diabetic extracapsular cataract extraction, Eye 8:535, 1994.

692. Irvine AR and Crawford JB: Histopathologic study of lens implants in humans and animals, Ophthalmic Forum 1(3):15, 1983.

693. Isakov I, Madjarov B, and Bartov E: Safe method for cleaning the posterior lens capsule, J Cataract Refract Surg 21:371, 1995.

694. Jacobi KW and Nowak MR: (New materials for intraocular lenses) (German), Fortschritte der Ophthalmologie 86(3):203, 1989, (review).

695. Jacobi PC and Konen W: Effect of age and astigmatism on the amo array multifocal intraocular lens, J Cataract Refract Surg 21:556, 1995.

696. Jaffe GJ and others: Progressive of nonproliferative diabetic retinopathy and visual outcome after extracapsular cataract extraction and intraocular lens implantation (see comments), Am J Ophthalmol 114:448, 1992.

697. Jaffe NS, Clayman HM, and Jaffe MS: A comparison of ICCE-Binkhorst intraocular lens and ECCE-posterior chamber intraocular lens, thirty-four to forty months postoperatively, J Am Intraocul Implant Soc 8:128, 1982.

698. Jaffe NS: Discussion: loss of eyes after intraocular lens implantation, Ophthalmology 90:385, 1983.

699. Jaffe NS, Clayman HM, and Jaffe MS: Retinal detachment in myopic eyes after intracapsular and extracapsular cataract extraction, Am J Ophthalmol 97:48, 1984.

700. Jaffe NS and Clayman HM: Cataract extraction in eyes with congenital colobomata, J Cataract Refract Surg 13:54, 1987.

701. Jaffe NS: New designs of intraocular lenses, Trans N Orl Acad Ophthalmol 36:269, 1988.

702. Jaffe NS, Jaffe MS, and Jaffe GF: Cataract surgery and its complications, ed 5, St. Louis, 1990, The CV Mosby Co.

703. Jaffe NS: History of cataract surgery, Ophthalmology 103(8:suppl):S5, 1996.

704. Jampol LM, Sanders DR, and Kraff MC: Prophylaxis and therapy

of aphakic cystoid macular edema, Surv Ophthalmol 28(suppl):535, 1984.

705. Jensen MK, Crandall AS, Mamalis N, and others: Crystallization on intraocular lens surfaces associated with the use of Healon GV™ (see comments), Arch Ophthalmol 112:1037, 1994.

706. John GR and Stark WJ: Rotation of posterior chamber intraocular lenses for management of lens-associated recurring hyphemas, Arch Ophthalmol 110:963, 1992.

707. John T, Sassari JW, and Eagle RC Jr: The myofibroblastic component of rubeosis iridis, Ophthalmology 90:721, 1983.

708. Jones NP: Cataract surgery in Fuchs' heterochromic uveitis—past, present, and future, J Cataract Refract Surg 22:261, 1996, (review).

709. Joo CK and Kim JH: Compatibility of intraocular lenses with blood and connective tissue cells measured by cellular deposition and inflammatory response in vitro, J Cataract Refract Surg 18(3):240, 1992.

709. Joo CK and Kim JH: Compatibility of intraocular lenses with blood and connective tissue cells measured bu cellular deposition and inflammatory response in vitro, J Cataract Refract Surg 18(3):240, 1992.

710. Juechter KB: Histopathology of capsule-fixed intraocular lenses. In Emery JM, editor: Current concepts in cataract surgery. Selected Proceedings of the Fifth Biennial Cataract Surgical Congress, St. Louis, 1978, The CV Mosby Co.

711. Juechter KB: Histopathology in pseudophakia. In Kwitko ML, and Praeger DL, editors: Pseudophakia: current trends and concepts, Baltimore, 1980, The Williams & Wilkins Co.

712. Junge J: Cystoid macular edema associated with PVP coating of an intraocular lens, J Am Intraocul Implant Soc 6:28, 1980.

713. Kalb IM, Shelton PA, and Barnet RW: Avoiding explantation by locked-lens implantation, Cataract 2(7):27, 1985.

714. Kammann J, Kreiner CF, and Kaden P: (The growth behavior of mouse fibroblasts on intraocular lens surface of various silicone and pmma materials), (German), Ophthalmologe 91(4):521, 1994.

715. Kanellopoulos AJ, Weintraub J, and Rahn EK: Phacoemulsification and silicone foldable intraocular lens implantation in a patient with chronic sarcoid uveitis, J Cataract Refract Surg 21(4):364, 1995, (letter).

716. Kapusta MA, Chen JC, and Lam WC: Outcomes of dropped nucleus during phacoemulsification, Ophthalmology 103(8):1184, 1996.

717. Kassar BS and Varnell ED: Effect of pmma and silicone lens materials on normal rabbit corneal endothelium: an in vitro study, J Am Intra-Ocular Implant Soc 6(4):344, 1980.

718. Keates RH, Pearce JL, and Schneider RT: Clinical results of the multifocal lens, J Cataract Refract Surg 13:557, 1987.

719. Kelman CD: Phaco-emulsification and aspiration: a new technique of cataract removal. A preliminary report, Am J Ophthalmol 64: 23, 1967.

720. Kelman CD: Symposium: phacoemulsification. Summary of personal experience. Trans Am Acad Ophthalmol Otolaryngol 78:35, 1974.

721. Kent DG, Sims JC, and Apple DJ: Pediatric capsulorhexis technique [letter; comment], J Cataract Refract Surg 21:236, 1995.

722. Kershner RM: Keratolenticuloplasty—arcuate keratotomy for cataract surgery and astigmatism, J Cataract Refract Surg 21:274, 1995.

723. Kershner RM: Clear corneal cataract surgery and the correction of myopia, hyperopia and astigmatism, Ophthalmology 104:381, 1997.

724. Kimura W and others: Postoperative decentration of three-piece silicone intraocular lenses, J Cataract Refract Surg 22:1277, 1996.

725. Kirwan JF, Potamitis T, and McDonnell PJ: Spontaneous pseudophakia [letter], Eye 8:146, 1994.

726. Knorz MC and others: Comparison of the optical and visual quality of poly(methyl methacrylate) and silicone intraocular lenses, J Cataract Refract Surg 19(6):766, 1993.

727. Koch DD and others: Pupillary size and responsiveness. Implications for selection of a bifocal intraocular lens, Ophthalmology 98: 1030, 1991.

728. Koch PS, Bradley H, and Swenson N: Visual acuity recovery rates following cataract surgery and implantation of soft intraocular lenses, J Cataract Refract Surg 17(2):143, 1991.

729. Koch DD and Heit LE: Discoloration of silicone intraocular lenses, Arch Ophthalmol 110(3):319, 1992, (letter).

730. Kochounian HH and others: Identification of intraocular lens-adsorbed proteins in mammalian in vitro and in vivo systems, Arch Ophthalmol 112:395, 1994.

731. Kohnen T, Dick B, and Jacobi KW: Comparison of the induced astigmatism after temporal clear corneal tunnel incisions of different sizes, J Cataract Refract Surg 21:417, 1995.

732. Kohnen S, Ferrer A, and Brauweiler P: Visual function in pseudophakic eyes with poly (methyl methacrylate), silicone, and acrylic intraocular lenses, J Cataract Refract Surg 22:1303, 1996.

733. Kohnen, T, Pena-Cuesta R, and Koch DD: Secondary cataract formation following pediatric intraocular lens implantation: 6-month results, Ger J Ophthalmol 5:171, 1996.

734. Kohnen T: The variety of foldable intraocular lens materials, J Cataract Refract Surg 22(2):1255, 1996, (guest editorial).

735. Kohnen T, Magdowski G, Koch DD: Scanning electron microscopic analysis of foldable acrylic and hydrogel intraocular lenses. J Cataract Refract Surg 22:1342, 1996.

736. Kokame GT, Flynn HW Jr, and Blankenship GW: Posterior chamber intraocular lens implantation during diabetic pars plana vitrectomy (see comments) Ophthalmology 96:603, 1989.

737. Kondo T, Yamauchi T, and Nakatsu A: Effect of cataract surgery on aqueous turnover and blood-aqueous barrier, J Cataract Refract Surg 21:706, 1995.

738. Kosmin AS, Wishart PK, and Ridges PJG: Silicone versus poly-(methyl methacrylate) lenses in combined phacoemulsification in trabeculectomy, J Cataract Refract Surg 23:97, 1997.

739. Kostick AMP and others: Analysis of intraocular lens haptic fixation in human cadaver eyes ARVO, Sarasota, FL, May 2–8, 1992, p 1307, (Abstract).

740. Kozaki J and Takahashi F: Theoretical analysis of image defocus with intraocular lens decentration, J Cataract Refract Surg 21:552, 1995.

741. Kraff MC, Sanders DR, and Lieberman HL: Symposium: intraocular lenses. The Medallion suture lens: management of complications, Ophthalmology 86:643, 1979.

742. Kraff MC and others: Membrane formation after implantation of polyvinyl alcohol-coated intraocular lenses, J Am Intraocul Implant Soc 6:129, 1980.

743. Kraff MC and others: Slit-lamp fluorophotometry in intraocular lens patients, Am Acad Ophthalmol 87:877, 1980.

744. Kraff MC: Intraocular lenses: past, present, and future, Paper presented at the Eye Research Seminar, Arlington, VA, May 16, 1982.

745. Kraff MC: IOL update: types of intraocular lenses, Ophthalmic Forum 1(2):50, 1983.

746. Kraff MC, Sanders DR, and Lieberman HL: The results of posterior chamber lens implantation, J Am Intraocul Implant Soc 9:148, 1983.

747. Kreiner CF: Chemical and physical aspects of clinically applied silicones, Dev Ophthalmol 14:11, 1987.

748. Krupin T, Feitl ME, and Bishop KI: Postoperative intraocular pressure rise in open-angle glaucoma patients after cataract or combined cataract-filtration surgery, Ophthalmology 96:579, 1989.

749. Krupsky S and others: Anterior segment complications in diabetic patients following extracapsular cataract extraction and posterior chamber intraocular lens implantation, Ophthal Surg 22:526, 1991.

750. Kulnig W and others: Optical resolution of silicone and polymethylmethacrylate intraocular lenses, J Cataract Refract Surg 13(6):635, 1987.

751. Kulnig W and others: Tissue reaction after silicone and poly(methyl methacrylate) intraocular lens implantation: a light and electron microscopy study in a rabbit model, J Cataract Refract Surg 15(5): 510, 1989, (published erratum appears in J Cataract Refract Surg 1989 Nov; 15(6):719).

752. Kulnig W and Skorpik C. Optical resolution of foldable intraocular lenses. J Cataract Refract Surg 16(2):211–216, 1990.

753. Kurz GH: Histologic findings after successful posterior chamber lens implantation, J Cataract Refract Surg 13:190, 1987.

754. Kusaka S, Kodama T, and Ohashi Y: Condensation of silicone oil on the posterior surface of a silicone intraocular lens during vitrectomy, Am J Ophthalmol 121:574, 1996.

755. Kwasniewska S, Fankhauser F and Klapper RM: Photodisruption of precipitates on the anterior surface of IOL implants, Cataract 2(5):23, 1985.

756. Lam S and others: Atonic pupil after cataract surgery, Ophthalmology 96:589, 1989.

757. Lambert SR and Drack AV: Infantile cataracts, Surv Ophthalmol 40:427, 1996, (review).

758. Landry RA: Unwanted optical effects caused by intraocular lens positioning holes, J Cataract Refract Surg 13:421, 1987.

759. Langston RHS: Intraocular lens implantation, Int Ophthalmol Clin 22(2):22, 1982.

760. Laurell CG and others: Inflammatory response in the rabbit after phacoemulsification and intraocular lens implantation using a 5.2 or 11.0 mm incision, J Cataract Refract Surg 23:126, 1997.

761. Lavery KT and others: Endothelial cell loss after 4 mm cataract surgery, J Cataract Refract Surg 21:305, 1995.

762. Leaming DV: Practice styles and preferences of ASCRS members—1986 survey, J Cataract Refract Surg 13:561, 1987.

763. Leaming DV: Practice styles and preferences of ASCRS members—1987 survey, J Cataract Refract Surg 14:552, 1988.

764. Leaming DV: Practice styles and preferences of ascrs members—1994 survey, J Cataract Refract Surg 21:378, 1995.

765. Legler UF and Apple DJ: Comments on silicone intraocular lens discoloration, Arch Ophthalmol 109:1495, 1991, (letter, comment).

766. Legler UF and others: Prospective experimental study of factors related to posterior chamber intraocular lens decentration, J Cataract Refract Surg 18:449, 1992.

767. Legler UF, Assia El and Apple DJ: (Configuration of the capsular sack after implantation of posterior chamber lenses) (German), Ophthalmologe 90:339, 1993.

768. Leith MM and others: Comparison of the properties of AMVISC and Healon, J Cataract Refract Surg 13:534, 1987.

769. Levin ML and others: Effect of cataract surgery and intraocular lenses on diabetic retinopathy, J Cataract Refract Surg 14:642, 1988.

770. Levy JH and Pisacano AM: Clinical endothelial cell loss following phacoemulsification and silicone or polymethylmethacrylate lens implantation, J Cataract Refract Surg 14:299, 1988.

771. Levy JH and Pisacano AM: Initial clinical studies with silicone intraocular implants, J Cataract Refract Surg 14:294, 1988.

772. Levy JH, Pisacano AM and Anello RD: Displacement of bag-placed hydrogel lenses into the vitreous following neodymium: yag laser capsulotomy, J Cataract Refract Surg 16(5):563, 1990.

773. Levy JH, Pisacano AM, and Chadwick K: Astigmatic changes after cataract surgery with 5.1 mm and 3.5 mm sutureless incisions, J Cataract Refract Surg 20(6):630, 1994.

774. Lichter PR: Intraocular lenses in uveitis patients, Ophthalmology 96:279, 1989, (editorial).

775. Liebert TC and others: Subcutaneous implants of polypropylene filaments, J Biomed Mater Res 10:939, 1976.

776. Lin Z and others: Nd: YAG laser lysis of the fibrinous membrane and remnant substance on the anterior surface of intraocular lens, Yen Ko Hsueh Pao [Eye Science] 11:128, 1995.

777. Lindstrom RL, Allarakhia L, and Knoll RL: Soft intraocular lenses. Trans N Orl Acad Ophthalmol 36:329, 1988.

778. Lindstrom RL: Food and drug administration study update. One-year results from 671 patients with the 3M multifocal intraocular lens, Ophthalmology 100:91, 1993.

779. Liu C and Ophth FRC: Phacoemulsification in a patient with torticollis, J Cataract Refract Surg 21:364, 1995.

780. Lowe KJ and Easty DL: A comparison of 141 polyhemacon (iogel) and 140 poly(methyl methacrylate) intraocular lens implants, Br J Ophthalmol 76(2):88, 1992.

781. Lyle WA: A new phacoemulsification technique for in-the-bag IOL placement, J Am Intraocul Implant Soc 9:461, 1982.

782. Lyle WA and Jin GJ: Phacoemulsification with intraocular lens implantation in high myopia, J Cataract Refract Surg 22(2):238, 1996.

783. Mackool RJ and Gupta A: New soft intraocular lens, J Cataract Refract Surg 14(6):691, 1988, (letter).

784. Mackool RJ and Chhatiawala H: Pediatric cataract surgery and intraocular lens implantation: a new technique for preventing or excising postoperative secondary membranes, J Cataract Refract Surg 17:62, 1991.

785. Mackool RJ and Russell RS: Intracapsular posterior chamber intraocular lens insertion with posterior capsular tears or zonular instability, J Cataract Refract Surg 21:376, 1995.

786. Mackool RJ: Decentration of plate-haptic lenses, J Cataract Refract Surg 22:396, 1996, (letter).

787. Madsen K and others. Histochemical and receptor binding studies of hyaluronic acid and hyaluronic acid binding sites on corneal endothelium, Ophthalmic Prac 7(3):1–8, 1989.

788. Maltzman BA and others: Neodymium: YAG laser capsulotomy of secondary membranes in the pediatric population, J Am Intraocul Implant Soc 11:572, 1985.

789. Mamalis N and others: Comparison of two plate-haptic intraocular lenses in a rabbit model, J Cataract Refract Surg 22:1291, 1996.

790. Mamalis N and others: Neodymium: YAG capsulotomy rates after phacoemulsification with silicone posterior chamber intraocular lenses, J Cataract Refract Surg 22:1296, 1996.

791. Mandal AK: Endocapsular surgery and capsular bag fixation of intraocular lenses in phacolytic glaucoma, J Cataract Refract Surg 22:288, 1996.

792. Marcus DM and others: Pupillary capture of a flexible silicone posterior chamber intraocular lens, Arch Ophthalmol 110(5):609, 1992, (letter).

793. Martin RG and others: Effect of small incision intraocular lens surgery on postoperative inflammation and astigmatism. A study of the amo si-18nb small incision lens, J Cataract Refract Surg 18(1):51, 1992.

794. Martin RG and others: Effect of cataract wound incision size on acute changes in corneal topography, J Cataract Refract Surg 19(Supp): 170, 1993.

795. Martinez Toldos JJ, Artola Roig A, and Chipont Benabent E: Total anterior capsule closure after silicone intraocular lens implantation, J Cataract Refract Surg 22:269, 1996.

796. Masket S: Gull-wing haptic design for posterior chamber intraocular lens, J Cataract Refract Surg 13:410, 1987.

797. Masket S: Keratorefractive aspects of the scleral pocket incision and closure method for cataract surgery, J Cataract Refract Surg 15:70, 1989.

798. Matoba M and others: (Experimental study of the cell response on the intraocular lens surface) (Japanese), Nippon Ganka Gakkai Zasshi 90(11):1333, 1986.

799. Matoba M and others: (Difference of the cellular response between pmma and silicone intraocular lens material) (Japanese), Nippon Ganka Gakkai Zasshi 92(12):2150, 1988.

800. Matsuo K and others: Clinical efficacy of diclofenac sodium on postsurgical inflammation after intraocular lens implantation, J Cataract Refract Surg 21:309, 1995.

801. Mazzocco TR: Early clinical experience with elastic lens implants, Trans Ophthalmol Soc UK 104(Pt 5):578, 1985.

802. Mehta HK: Biodegradation of nylon loops of intraocular implants in children, Trans Ophthalmol Soc UK 99:183, 1979.

803. Menapace R and others: Clinicopathologic findings after in-the-bag implantation of open-loop polymethylmethacrylate and silicone lenses in the rabbit eye, J Cataract Refract Surg 13(6):630, 1987.

804. Menapace R and others: Evaluation of the first 60 cases of poly hema posterior chamber lenses implanted in the sulcus, J Cataract Refract Surg 15(3):264, 1989.

805. Menapace R: (Current state of implantation of flexible intraocular lenses) (German), Fortschritte der Ophthalmologie 88(5):421, 1991, (review).

806. Menapace R and others: Evaluation of the first 100 consecutive phacoflex silicone lenses implanted in the bag through a self-sealing tunnel incision using the prodigy inserter, J Cataract Refract Surg 20(3):299, 1994.

807. Menapace R and others: No-stitch, small incision cataract surgery with flexible intraocular lens implantation, J Cataract Refract Surg 20(5):534, 1994.

808. Menapace R: Evaluation of 35 consecutive SI-30 phacoflex lenses with high-refractive silicone optic implanted in the capsulorhexis bag, J Cataract Refract Surg 21:339, 1995.

809. Menchini U and others: Clinical evaluation of the effect of acetylcholine on the corneal endothelium, J Cataract Refract Surg 15: 421, 1989.

810. Mendivil A: Intraocular lens implantation through 3.2 versus 4.0 mm incisions, J Cataract Refract Surg 22:1461, 1996.

811. Menezo JL, Cisneros A, and Harto M: Extracapsular cataract extraction and implantation of a low power lens for high myopia, J Cataract Refract Surg 14:409, 1988.

812. Michelson JB, Friedlaender MH, and Nozik RA: Lens implant surgery in pars planitis, Ophthalmology 97:1023, 1990.

813. Milauskas AT: Posterior capsule opacification after silicone lens

implantation and its management, J Cataract Refract Surg 13(6): 644, 1987.

814. Milauskas AT: Capsular bag fixation of one-piece silicone lenses, J Cataract Refract Surg 16(5):583, 1990.

815. Milazzo S and others: Long-term follow-up of three-piece, Looped, silicone intraocular lenses, J Cataract Refract Surg 22(suppl 2): 1259, 1996.

816. Milazzo S, Turut P, and Blin H: Alterations to the AcrySof intraocular lens during folding, J Cataract Refract Surg 22:1351, 1996.

817. Miyake K: Fluorophotometric evaluation of the blood-ocular barrier function following cataract surgery and intraocular lens implantation, J Cataract Refract Surg 14:560, 1988.

818. Miyake K and others: Pupillary fibrin membrane. A frequent early complication after posterior chamber lens implantation in Japan (see comments), Ophthalmology 96:1228, 1989.

819. Mondino BJ and Rao H: Effect of intraocular lenses on complement levels in human serum, Acta Ophthalmol 61:76, 1983.

820. Mondino BJ, Rajacich GM, and Summer H: Comparison of complement activation by silicone intraocular lenses and polymethylmethacrylate intraocular lenses with polypropylene loops, Arch Ophthalmol 105(7):989, 1987.

821. Moon J and others: Treatment of postcataract fibrinous membranes with tissue plasminogen activator, Ophthalmology 99:1256, 1992.

822. Moore CR and Steller RT: Early recognition and proper treatment of the VIP syndrome, J Am Intraocul Implant Soc 4:114, 1978.

823. Morrison JC and Van Buskirk EM: Anterior collateral circulation in the primate eye, Ophthalmology 90:707, 1983.

824. Moses L: Pupillary-block glaucoma after Choyce lens implantation, J Am Intraocul Implant Soc 4:50, 1978.

825. Moses L: Kelman anterior chamber lens: a preliminary report, J Am Intraocul Implant Soc 4:54, 1978.

826. Mullaney PB, Wheeler DT, and al-Nahdi T: Dissolution of pseudophakic fibrinous exudate with intraocular streptokinase, Eye 10: 362, 1996.

827. Munden PM and Alward WL: Combined phacoemulsification, posterior chamber intraocular lens implantation, and trabeculectomy with mitomycin c, Am J Ophthalmol 119:20, 1995.

828. Murata T: Capsular bag intraocular lens fixation with retention of the anterior capsule, J Cataract Refract Surg 13:438, 1987.

829. Myers WD and others: Intraocular lens design for the neodymium: YAG laser, J Am Intraocul Implant Soc 11:35, 1985.

830. Nadler DJ, and Schwartz B: Cataract surgery in the United States 1968–1976: a descriptive epidemiologic study, Ophthalmology 87: 10, 1980.

831. Nagamoto T and Hara E: Postoperative membranous proliferation from the anterior capsulotomy margin onto the intraocular lens optic, J Cataract Refract Surg 21:208, 1995.

832. Nasir MA, Toth CA, and Mittra RA: Recombinant hirudin for prevention of experimental postoperative intraocular fibrin, Am J Ophthalmol 121:554, 1996.

833. Neumann AC, McCarty GR, and Osher RH: Complications associated with staar silicone implants, J Cataract Refract Surg 13(6): 653, 1987.

834. Neumann AC and Cobb B: Advantages and limitations of current soft intraocular lenses, J Cataract Refract Surg 15:257, 1989.

835. Neumann AC and others: Refractive evaluation of astigmatic keratotomy procedures, J Cataract Refract Surg 15:25, 1989.

836. Neumann AC and others: Small incisions to control astigmatism during cataract surgery, J Cataract Refract Surg 15:78, 1989.

837. Newland TJ and others: Neodymium: YAG laser damage on silicone intraocular lenses. a comparison of lesions on explanted lenses and experimentally produced lesions, J Cataract Refract Surg 20: 527, 1994.

838. Newman DA and others: Pathologic findings of an explanted silicone intraocular lens, J Cataract Refract Surg 12:292, 1986.

839. Ng EWM, Barrett GD, and Bowman R: In vitro bacterial adherence to hydrogel and poly(methyl methacrylate) intraocular lenses, J Cataract Refract Surg 22:1331, 1996.

840. Nicholson DH: Occult iris erosion: a treatable cause of recurrent hyphema in iris-supported intraocular lenses, Ophthalmology 89: 113, 1982.

841. Nielsen PJ: Prospective evaluation of surgically induced astigmatism and astigmatic ketatotomy effects of various self-sealing small incisions, J Cataract Refract Surg 21:43, 1995.

842. Nishi O: A U-shaped anterior capsulotomy and modified J-loop posterior chamber intraocular lens with new positioning holes, J Cataract Refract Surg 13:317, 1987.

843. Nishi O: Intercapsular cataract surgery with lens epithelial cell removal. I. Without capsulorhexis, J Cataract Refract Surg 15:297, 1989.

844. Nishi O: Intercapsular cataract surgery with lens epithelial cell removal. II. Effect on prevention of fibrinous reaction, J Cataract Refract Surg 15:301, 1989.

845. Nishi O and others: Effects of diclofenac sodium and indomethacin on proliferation and collagen synthesis of lens epithelial cells in vitro, J Cataract Refract Surg 21:461, 1995.

846. Nishi O and others: Effect of indomethacin-coated posterior chamber intraocular lenses on postoperative inflammation and posterior capsule opacification, J Cataract Refract Surg 21:574, 1995.

847. Nishi O and others: Explantation of endocapsular posterior chamber lens after spontaneous posterior dislocation, J Cataract Refract Surg 22:272, 1996.

848. Obstbaum SA: Development of foldable IOL materials, J Cataract Refract Surg 21:233, 1995.

849. Ochi T and others: Intraocular lens implantation and high myopia, J Cataract Refract Surg 14:403, 1988.

850. Oh KT: Proliferation of cells on posterior surface of ubm2f/j lenses following YAG capsulotomy, J Cataract Refract Surg 20(1):108, 1994, (letter).

851. Ohara K and Shimizu H: Finishing of modern posterior chamber intraocular lenses, J Cataract Refract Surg 14:286, 1988.

852. Ohmi S, Uenoyama K, and Apple DJ: Implantation of IOLs with Different Diameters, Acta Soc Ophthalmol Jpn 96:1093, 1992.

853. Ohrloff C, Rothe R, and Spitznas M: Evaluation of endothelial cell function with anterior segment fluorophotometry in pseudophakic patients, J Cataract Refract Surg 13:531, 1987.

854. Olson RJ: Passport system cutting of a chiron c10 ub silicone lens, J Cataract Refract Surg 22(3):282, 1996, (letter).

855. Omar O and others: Scanning electron microscopic characteristics of small-incision intraocular lenses, Ophthalmology 103(7):1124, 1996.

856. Omar O and others: Capsular bag distension with an acrylic intraocular lens, J Cataract Refract Surg 22:1365, 1996.

857. Oshika T, Yoshimura K, and Miyata N: Postsurgical inflammation after phacoemulsification and extracapsular extraction with soft or conventional intraocular lens implantation, J Cataract Refract Surg 18(4):356, 1992.

858. Oshika T and others: Comparative study of intraocular lens implantation through 3.2- and 5.5-mm incisions, Ophthalmology 101: 1183, 1994.

859. Oshika T and others: (Small incision cataract surgery-silicone intraocular lens vs polymethylmethacrylate intraocular lens) (Japanese), Nippon Ganka Gakkai Zasshi 98(4):362, 1994.

860. Oshika T, Shiokawa Y: Effect of folding on the optical quality of soft acrylic intraocular lenses, J Cataract Refract Surg 22:1360, 1996.

861. Oshika T and others: Two year clinical study of a soft acrylic intraocular lens, J Cataract Refract Surg 22:104, 1996.

862. Ota I, Miyake S, and Miyake K: Dislocation of the lens nucleus into the vitreous cavity after standard hydrodissection, Am J Ophthalmol 121(6):706, 1996.

863. Ozaki L: The barrier function of the posterior capsule, J Am Intraocul Implant Soc 10:182, 1984.

864. Packard RB, Garner A, and Arnott EJ: Poly-hema as a material for intraocular lens implantation: a preliminary report, Br J Ophthalmol 65(8):585, 1981.

865. Pallin SL and Walman GB: Posterior chamber intraocular lens implant centration; in or out of "the bag," J Am Intraocul Implant Soc 8:254, 1982.

866. Pallin SL: Comparison of induced astigmatism with phaco-emulsification and extracapsular cataract extraction, J Cataract Refract Surg 13:274, 1987.

867. Pande M, Shah SM, and Spalton DJ: Correlations between aqueous flare and cells and lens surface cytology in eyes with poly(methyl methacrylate) and heparin-surface-modified intraocular lenses, J Cataract Refract Surg 21:326, 1995.

868. Pande M, Spalton DJ, and Marshall J: Continuous curvilinear capsulorhexis and intraocular lens biocompatibility, J Cataract Refract Surg 22:89, 1996.

869. Pande MV, Spalton DJ, and Marshall J: In vivo human lens epithe-

lial cell proliferation on the anterior surface of pmma intraocular lenses, Br J Ophthalmol 80:469, 1996.

870. Park SB and others: In vivo fracture of an extruded polymethylmethacrylate intraocular lens loop, J Cataract Refract Surg 13:194, 1987.

871. Parker JS and others: Combined trabeculectomy, cataract extraction, and foldable lens implantation (see comments), J Cataract Refract Surg 18(6):582, 1992.

872. Patel J and others: Protective effect of the anterior lens capsule during extracapsular cataract extraction. II: Preliminary results of clinical study, Ophthalmology 96:598, 1989.

873. Pavese T and Insler MS: Effects of extracapsular cataract extraction with posterior chamber lens implantation on the development of neovascular glaucoma in diabetics, J Cataract Refract Surg 13:197, 1987.

874. Pavilack MA and others: Peripseudophakic membrane. pathologic features, Arch Ophthalmol 111:240, 1993, (review).

875. Pearson PA and others: Anterior chamber lens implantation after vitreous loss, Br J Ophthalmol 73:596, 1989.

876. Percival P: Prospective study comparing hydrogel with pmma lens implants, Ophthalmic Surg 20(4):255, 1989.

877. Percival SP: Comparing like with like: a prospective study of hydrogel and polymethylmethacrylate lenses, Dev Ophthalmol 18:111, 1989.

878. Percival SP and Pai V: Heparin-modified lenses for eyes at risk for breakdown of the blood-aqueous barrier during cataract surgery, J Cataract Refract Surg 19:760, 1993.

879. Pfister DR: Stress fractures after folding an acrylic intraocular lens, Am J Ophthalmol 121:572, 1996.

880. Pfleger T and others: Long-term course of induced astigmatism after clear corneal incision cataract surgery, J Cataract Refract Surg 22:72, 1996.

881. Pfoff DS and Thom SR: Preliminary report on the effect of hyperbaric oxygen on cystoid macular edema, J Cataract Refract Surg 13:136, 1987.

882. Pham DT, Wollensak J, and Welzl-Hinterkorner E: (Experiences with the p-hema posterior chamber lens) (German), Fortschr Ophthalmol 87(2):144, 1990.

883. Pham DT, Wollensak J, and Wiemer C: (Implantation of folding posterior chamber lenses) (German), Klin Monatsbl Augenheilkd 198(3):181, 1991.

884. Pharmakakis N, Hartmann C, and Bergmann L: (In vitro corneal endothelial damage caused by intraocular lenses of PMMA, silicone and polyhema) (German), Fortschr Ophthalmol 86(4):295, 1989.

885. Phillips P and others: Measurement of intraocular lens decentration and tilt in vivo, J Cataract Refract Surg 14:129, 1988.

886. Portellos M, Orlin SE, and Kozart DM: Electric cataracts, Arch Ophthalmol 114(8):1022, 1996.

887. Pötzsch DK, Pötzsch-Lösch CM: Four year follow-up of the MemoryLens, J Cataract Refract Surg 22:1336, 1996.

888. Powe NR and others: Synthesis of the literature on visual acuity and complications following cataract extraction with intraocular lens implantation: Cataract patient outcome research team (see comments), Arch Ophthalmol 112:239, 1994, (published erratum appears in Arch Ophthalmol 1994 Jul, 112(7):889).

889. Prasad P, Setna PH, and Dunne JA: Accelerated ocular neovascularisation in diabetics following posterior chamber lens implantation, Br J Ophthalmol 74:313, 1990.

890. Probst LE and Holland EJ: Intraocular lens implantation in patients with juvenile rheumatoid arthritis (see comments), Am J Ophthalmol 122(2):161, 1996, (review).

891. Quraishy MM and Casswell AG: May I bend down after my cataract operation, doctor? Eye 10:92, 1996.

892. Ram J and others: Miyake posterior view video technique; a means to reduce the learning curve in phacoemulsification. Ophthalmic Pract 12(5):206–210, 1994.

893. Ram J and others: Postoperative complications of intraocular lens implantation in patients with Fuchs' heterochromic cyclitis, J Cataract Refract Surg 21:548, 1995.

894. Ravalico G and others: Capsulorhexis size and posterior capsule opacification, J Cataract Refract Surg 22:98, 1996.

895. Refojo MF: Current status of biomaterials in ophthalmology, Surv Ophthalmol 26(5):257, 1982, (review).

896. Richards BW and Lesser GR: Complications of positioning holes

897. Riise P: Endophthalmitis phacoanaphylactica in clinical ophthalmology, Am J Ophthalmol 60:911, 1965.

898. Roberts B and Peiffer RL Jr: Experimental evaluation of a synthetic viscoelastic material on intraocular pressure and corneal endothelium, J Cataract Refract Surg 15:321, 1989.

899. Roberts CW and Brennan KM: A comparison of topical diclofenac with prednisolone for postcataract inflammation, Arch Ophthalmol 113:725, 1995.

900. Roberts CW: Pretreatment with topical diclofenac sodium to decrease postoperative inflammation, Ophthalmology 103:636, 1996.

901. Robertson JE Jr: The formation of moisture droplets on the posterior surface of intraocular lenses during fluid/gas exchange procedures, Arch Ophthalmol 110(2):168, 1992, (letter).

902. Rose GE: Fibrinous uveitis and intraocular lens implantation. Surface modification of polymethylmethacrylate during extracapsular cataract surgery, Ophthalmology 99:1242, 1992.

903. Rosner M, Sharir M, and Blumenthal M: Optical aberrations from a well-centered intraocular lens implant, Am J Ophthalmol 101:117, 1986, (letter).

904. Rubin GS, Adamsons IA, and Stark WJ: Comparison of acuity, contrast sensitivity, and disability glare before and after cataract surgery, Arch Ophthalmol 111:56, 1993.

905. Rubsamen PE and others: Primary intraocular lens implantation in the setting of penetrating ocular trauma, Ophthalmology 102:101, 1995.

906. Ruiz RS and Saatci OA: Extracapsular cataract extraction with intraocular lens implantation after scleral buckling surgery, Am J Ophthalmol 111:174, 1991.

907. Rummelt V and others: A 32-year follow-up of the rigid Schreck anterior chamber lens. a clinicopathological correlation, Arch Ophthalmol 108:401, 1990.

908. Sakabe I, Lim SJ, and Apple DJ: (Anatomical evaluation of the anterior capsular zonular free zone in the human crystalline lens [age range, 50 to approximately 100 years]) (Japanese), Nippon Ganka Gakkai Zasshi 99:1119, 1995.

909. Salamon SM: Capsular bag distension, J Cataract Refract Surg 18:537, 1992, (letter; comment).

910. Salamon SM: Second opinion on brevital, J Cataract Refract Surg 22:281, 1996.

911. Salz JJ: Managing complications: imperfect 20/20 vision in a patient with posterior chamber lens implant, Cataract 1(6):30, 1984.

912. Samad A and others: Anterior chamber contamination after uncomplicated phacoemulsification and intraocular lens implantation, Am J Ophthalmol 120:143, 1995.

913. Sanchez E, Artaria L: Evaluation of the first 50 ACR360 acrylic intraocular lens implantations, J Cataract Refract Surg 22:1373, 1996.

914. Sanders DR and others: Breakdown and re-establishment of blood-aqueous barrier with implant surgery, Arch Ophthalmol 100:588, 1982.

915. Sanders DR and others: Quantitative assessment of post-surgical breakdown of the blood-aqueous barrier, Arch Ophthalmol 101:131, 1983.

916. Sawusch MR, and Guyton DL: Optimal astigmatism to enhance depth of focus after cataract surgery, Ophthalmology 98:1025, 1991.

917. Schatz H and others: Severe diabetic retinopathy after cataract surgery (see comments), Am J Ophthalmol 117:314, 1994.

918. Scheie HG, Morse PH, and Aminlari A: Incidence of retinal detachment following cataract extraction, Arch Ophthalmol 89:293, 1973.

919. Schein OD and others: Cataract surgical techniques—preferences and underlying beliefs, Arch Ophthalmol 113:1108, 1995.

920. Schlaegel TF Jr: Uveitis following cataract surgery. In Bellows JG, editor: Cataract and abnormalities of the lens, New York, 1975, Grune & Stratton.

921. Shah SM and Spalton DJ: Natural history of cellular deposits on the anterior intraocular lens surface, J Cataract Refract Surg 21:466, 1995.

922. Shah SM and Spalton DJ: Comparison of the postoperative inflammatory response in the normal eye with heparin-surface-modified and poly(methyl methacrylate) intraocular lenses, J Cataract Refract Surg 21:579, 1995.

923. Shammas HJ: Anterior intraocular lens dislocation after combined cataract extraction and trabeculectomy, J Cataract Refract Surg 22:358, 1996.

924. Sheets JH: A comparable study of intraocular lens cases and cataract removal without lens implantation, Contract intraocul Lens Med J 3:34, 1977.

925. Shepherd JR: Continuous-tear capsulotomy and insertion of a silicone bag lens, J Cataract Refract Surg 15:335, 1989.

926. Shepherd JR: Correction of preexisting astigmatism at the time of small incision cataract surgery, J Cataract Refract Surg 15:55, 1989.

927. Shepherd JR: Induced astigmatism in small incision cataract surgery, J Cataract Refract Surg 15:85, 1989.

928. Shepherd JR: Capsular opacification associated with silicone implants, J Cataract Refract Surg 15(4):448, 1989.

929. Shepherd JR: Small incisions and foldable intraocular lenses, Inter Ophthalmol Clin 34(2):103, 1994, (review).

930. Shimizu H and Sakai H: Physical characteristics of various intraocular lenses, J Cataract Refract Surg 13:151, 1987.

931. Shugar JK: Implantation of AcrySof acrylic intraocular lenses, J Cataract Refract Surg 22:1355, 1996.

932. Shugar JK, Lewis C, Lee A: Implantation of multiple foldable acrylic posterior chamber lenses in the capsular bag for high hyperopia, J Cataract Refract Surg 22:1368, 1996.

933. Siepser SB and Kline OR Jr: Scanning electron microscopy of removed intraocular lenses, J Am Intraocul Implant Soc 9:176, 1983.

934. Simel PJ: Anticoagulation, intraocular bleeding and pupillary paralysis following Choyce intraocular lens implantation, J Am Intraocul Implant Soc 4:117, 1978.

935. Sinskey RM, Karel F, and Dal Ri E: Management of cataracts in children, J Cataract Refract Surg 15:196, 1989.

936. Skelnik DL and others: Neodymium: YAG laser interaction with Alcon IOGEL hydrogel intraocular lenses: an in vitro toxicity assay, J Cataract Refract Surg 13:662, 1987.

937. Skorpik C and others: Evaluation of 50 silicone posterior chamber lens implantations, J Cataract Refract Surg 13(6):640, 1987.

938. Skorpik C, Gottlob I, and Weghaupt H: Comparison of contrast sensitivity between posterior chamber lenses of silicone and PMMA material, Graefes Arch Clin Exp Ophthalmol 227(5):413, 1989.

939. Slusher MM and Seaton AD: Loss of visibility caused by moisture condensation on the posterior surface of a silicone intraocular lens during fluid/gas exchange after posterior vitrectomy, Am J Ophthalmol 118:667, 1994, (letter).

940. Smiddy WE, and Flynn HW, Jr: Management of dislocated posterior chamber intraocular lenses, Ophthalmology 98:889, 1991.

941. Smith R: Histopathological studies of eyes enucleated after failure of intraocular acrylic lens operations, Br J Ophthalmol 40:473, 1956.

942. Smith SG, Snowden F, and Lamprecht EG: Topographical anatomy of the ciliary sulcus, J Cataract Refract Surg 13:543, 1987.

943. Snellingen T and others: The south Asian cataract management study. Part I. The first 662 cataract surgeries: a preliminary report. Br J Ophthalmol 79(11):1029-1035, 1995.

944. Solomon KD and others: Preliminary report of ultrasound and laser energy applications to small incision cataract surgery: SEM and histopathologic analysis, Ophthalmic Prac 6:52, 1988.

945. Solomon KD and others: Protective effect of the anterior lens capsule during extracapsular cataract extraction, I. Experimental animal study, Ophthalmology 96:591, 1989.

946. Solomon KD and others: Complications of intraocular lenses with special reference to an analysis of 2500 explanted intraocular lenses (IOLs). Eur J Implant Refract Surg 3:195-200, 1991.

947. Sperber LTD: Neodymium-yag laser lens ablation in a rabbit model, J Cataract Refract Surg 22:485, 1996.

948. Spigelman AV and others: Visual results following vitreous loss and primary lens implantation, J Cataract Refract Surg 15:201, 1989.

949. Stamper RL, Colenbrander A, and Haugen J-P: Intraocular lens data, Ophthalmology 91:164, 1984.

950. Steinert RF and Wasson PJ: Neodymium: YAG laser anterior vitreolysis for Irvine-Gass cystoid macular edema, J Cataract Refract Surg 15:304, 1989.

951. Steinert RF and others: A prospective, randomized, double-masked comparison of a zonal-progressive multifocal intraocular lens and a monofocal intraocular lens (see comments), Ophthalmology 99:853, 1992.

952. Steinert RF and others: Long-term clinical results of amo phacoflex model SI-18 intraocular lens implantation, J Cataract Refract Surg 21:331, 1995.

953. Steinert RF and Deacon J: Enlargement of incision width during phacoemulsification and folded intraocular lens implant surgery, Ophthalmology 103(2):220, 1996.

954. Steinert RF and others: Hydrogel intracorneal lenses in aphakic eyes, Arch Ophthalmol 114:135, 1996.

955. Stenevi ULF and others: Demonstration of hyaluronic acid binding to corneal endothelial cells in human eye-bank eyes, Eur J Implant Ref Surg 5:228–232, 1993.

956. Straatsma BR and others: Posterior chamber intraocular lens implantation by ophthalmology residents, Ophthalmology 90:327, 1983.

957. Straatsma BR and others: Lens capsule and epithelium in age-related cataract, Am J Ophthalmol 112:283, 1991.

958. Suzuki R and others: Postcataract against-the-rule astigmatism after phacoemulsification procedure. Characteristic changes over time, Doc Ophthalmol 80:157, 1992.

959. Suzuki R and others: Sudden against-the-rule astigmatism 6 months after intraocular lens implantation with the kelman phacoemulsification procedure: 4 of 809 cases, Ophthalmologica 204:71, 1992.

960. Swartz M and others: The use of anterior chamber Na-hyaluronate in a pseudophakic patients requiring intravitreal air during retinal reattachment surgery, Ophthalmic Surg 12:98, 1981.

961. Tablante RT and others: A new technique of congenital cataract surgery with primary posterior chamber intraocular lens implantation, J Cataract Refract Surg 14:149, 1988.

962. Tan AY, Lim AS, Tseng PS: Major blinding complications of intraocular implantation, Ann Acad Med Singapore 22:624, 1993.

963. Tarbet KJ and others: Complications and results of phacoemulsification performed by residents, J Cataract Refract Surg 21:661, 1995.

964. Taylor, DM and others: Pseudophakic bullous keratopathy, Ophthalmology 90:19, 1983.

965. Teichmann KD: Pressurized anterior chamber approach to in-the-bag posterior chamber lens insertion, J Cataract Refract Surg 14:331, 1988.

966. Teichmann KD and others: Wessely-type immune ring following phototherapeutic keratectomy, J Cataract Refract Surg 22:142, 1996.

967. Tielsch JM and others: Preoperative functional expectations and postoperative outcomes among patients undergoing first eye cataract surgery, Arch Ophthalmol 113:1312, 1995.

968. Troutman RC: Correction of unilateral aphakia: the use of intraocular lens implants, Arch Ophthalmol 68:861, 1962.

969. Tsai JC and others: Scanning electron microscopic study of modern silicone intraocular lenses, J Cataract Refract Surg 18:232, 1992.

970. Tsuboi S and others: Effect of continuous circular capsulorhexis and intraocular lens fixation on the blood-aqueous barrier (see comments), Arch Ophthalmol 110:1124, 1992.

971. Tuberville AW and others: Complement activation by nylon-and polypropylene-looped prosthetic intraocular lenses, Invest Ophthalmol Vis Sci 22:727, 1982.

972. Uenoyama K and others: Experimental intraocular lens implantation in the rabbit eye and in the mouse peritoneal space. I. Cellular components observed on the implanted lens surface, J Cataract Refract Surg 14:187, 1988.

973. Uenoyama K and others: Experimental intraocular lens implantation in the rabbit eye and in the mouse peritoneal space. II. Morphological stages of the macrophage on the implanted lens surface, J Cataract Refract Surg 14:192, 1988.

974. Uenoyama K and others: Experimental intraocular lens implantation in the rabbit eye and in the mouse peritoneal space. III: Giant cell formation on the implanted lens surface, J Cataract Refract Surg 14:197, 1988.

975. Unterman SR and others: Collagen shield drug delivery: therapeutic concentrations of tobramycin in the rabbit cornea and aqueous humor, J Cataract Refract Surg 14:500, 1988.

976. Utrata PJ and others: Small incision surgery with the Staar elastimide three-piece posterior chamber intraocular lens, J Cataract Refract Surg 20(4):426, 1994.

977. Vajpayee RB, Angra SK, and Honavar SG: Combined keratoplasty, cataract extraction, and intraocular lens implantation after cor-

neolenticular laceration in children, Am J Ophthalmol 117:507, 1994.

978. Vajpayee RB and others: Capsulotomy for phacoemulsification in hypermature cataracts, J Cataract Refract Surg 21:612, 1995.

979. Van Buskirk EM: Pupillary block after intraocular lens implantation, Am J Ophthalmol 95:55, 1983.

980. Van Heuven WAJ, and Manning ER: From iatrology to iatrogeny, Arch Ophthalmol 97:571, 1979, (letter).

981. Vrabec MP, Syverud JC and Burgess CJ: Forceps-induced scratching of a foldable acrylic intraocular lens, Arch Ophthalmol 114(6):777, 1996, (letter).

982. Walland MJ, Stevens JD, and Steele AD: Repair of Descemet's membrane detachment after intraocular surgery (see comments), J Cataract Refract Surg 21:250, 1995.

983. Wang XH and others: Pediatric cataract surgery and intraocular lens implantation techniques: a laboratory study, J Cataract Refract Surg 20:607, 1994.

984. Waring GO III: Posterior collagenous layer of the cornea: ultrastructural classification of abnormal collagenous tissue posterior to Descemet's membrane in 30 cases, Arch Ophthalmol 100:122, 1982.

985. Wasserman D and others: Anterior capsular tears and loop fixation of posterior chamber intraocular lenses, Ophthalmology 98:425, 1991.

986. Watt RH: Pigment dispersion syndrome associated with silicone posterior chamber intraocular lenses, J Cataract Refract Surg 14:431, 1988.

987. Watt RH: Discoloration of a silicone intraocular lens 6 weeks after surgery, Arch Ophthalmol 109(11):1494, 1991, (letter; comment).

988. Wedrich A, and Menapace R: Effect of acetylcholine on intraocular pressure following small-incision cataract surgery, Ophthalmologica 205:125, 1992.

989. Wedrich A, Menapace R, Stifter S: The influence of the incision length on the early postoperative intraocular pressure following cataract surgery, Int Ophthalmol 18(2):77, 1994.

990. Weghaupt H, Pieh S, Skorpik C: Visual properties of the foldable Array multifocal intraocular lens, J Cataract Refract Surg 22:1313, 1996.

991. Weindler J and others: Bacterial anterior chamber contamination with foldable silicone lens implantation using a forceps and an injector, J Cataract Refract Surg 22(supplement 2):1263, 1996.

992. Welch DB and others: Lens injury following iridotomy with a Q-switched neodymium-YAG laser, Arch Ophthalmol 104:123, 1986.

993. Wenzel MR, Imkamp EM, Apple DJ: Variations in manufacturing quality of diffractive multifocal lenses, J Cataract Refract Surg 18:153, 1992.

994. Wenzel M, Kammann J, and Allmers R: (Biocompatibility of silicone intraocular lenses) (German), Klin Monatsbl Augenheilkd 203(6):408, 1993.

995. Wesendahl TA and others: (Suitability of polyvinylpyrrolidone (pvp) as a substance for hydrogel intraocular lenses) (German), Ophthalmologe 93:22, 1996.

996. Wesendahl TA and others: Eignung von Polyvinylpyrrolidone (PVP) als Material fhr Hydrogelntraocularlinsen, Ophthalmologe 93:22-28, 1996.

997. Wilbrandt TH, and Apple DJ: Posterior chamber intraocular lens decentration: an analysis of 400 eyes obtained postmortem. Presented at the American Society of Cataract and Refractive Surgery Meeting, Los Angeles, CA, March 27, 1988.

998. Wilson DJ, Jaeger MJ, and Green WR: Effects of extracapsular cataract extraction on the lens zonules, Ophthalmology 94:467, 1987.

999. Wilson ME and others: Intraocular lenses for pediatric implantation: biomaterials, designs, and sizing, J Cataract Refract Surg 20:584, 1994.

1000. Wilson ME and others: Comparison of mechanized anterior capsulectomy and manual continuous capsulorhexis in pediatric eyes, J Cataract Refract Surg 20:602, 1994.

1001. Wolter JR, Croasdale RE, Bahn CF: Reactions to an anterior chamber lens—two years after implantation, Ophthalmic Surg 11:794, 1980.

1002. Wolter JR: Pigment in cellular membranes on intraocular lens implants, Ophthalmic Surg 13:726, 1982.

1003. Wolter JR, and Sugar A: Reactive membrane on a foldable silicone lens implant in the posterior chamber of a human eye, Ophthalmic Surgery 20(1):17, 1989.

1004. Wong SK, Koch DD, and Emery JM: Secondary intraocular lens implantation, J Cataract Refract Surg 13:17, 1987.

1005. Yalon M, Blumenthal M, and Goldberg EP: Preliminary study of hydrophilic hydrogel intraocular lens implants in cats, J Am Intra-Ocular Implant Soc 10(3):315, 1984.

1006. Yalon M and others: Polycarbonate intraocular lenses, J Cataract Refract Surg 14:393, 1988.

1007. Yang S and others: Effect of silicone sound speed and intraocular lens thickness on pseudophakic axial length corrections, J Cataract Refract Surg 21(4):442, 1995.

1008. Yeo JH and others: The ultrastructure of an IOL "cocoon membrane," Ophthalmology 90:410, 1983.

1009. Ygge J and others: Cellular reactions on heparin surface-modified versus regular pmma lenses during the first postoperative month. A double-masked and randomized study using specular microphotography, Ophthalmology 97:1216, 1990.

1010. Zehetmayer M and others: (Long-term results of implantation of a plate haptic silicone lens in the capsular sac) (German), Klin Monatsbl Augenheilkd 204(4):220, 1994.

1011. Zelman J: Photophaco fragmentation, J Cataract Refract Surg 13:287, 1987.

1012. Zetterstrom C and others: After-cataract formation in newborn rabbits implanted with intraocular lenses, J Cataract Refract Surg 22:85, 1996.

1013. Zheng YR: (clinical report of transparent silicone intraocular lens implantation) (Chinese), Chung-Hua Yen Ko Tsa Chih 17(1):17, 1981, (author's transl).

1014. Zhou KY: Silicon intraocular lenses in 50 cataract cases, Chin Med J (Engl) 96(3):175, 1983.

Pathology of IOL decentration

1015. Allen A, Jaffe NS: Symposium: intraocular lenses. Cystoid macular edema: a preliminary study, Trans Am Acad Ophthalmol Otolaryngol 81:133, 1976.

1016. Alpar JJ, and Fechner, PU: Fechner's intraocular lenses, New York, 1986, Thieme-Stratton.

1017. Ambache N: Irin, a smooth-muscle contracting substance present in rabbit iris, J Physiol (Lond) 126:65, 1955.

1018. Ambache N: Trigeminomimetic action of iris extracts in rabbits, J Physiol (Lond) 132:49, 1956.

1019. Ambache N, Kavanagh L, and Whiting J: Effect of mechanical stimulation on rabbits' eyes: release of active substances in anterior chamber perfusates, J Physiol (Lond) 176:378, 1965.

1020. Anonymous: Consultation section. How would you manage an eye that developed inflammatory response after uncomplicated phacoemulsification with intraocular lens implantation? J Cataract Refract Surg 21:366, 1995.

1021. Apple DJ and others: Phacoanaphylactic endophthalmitis associated with extracapsular cataract extraction and posterior chamber intraocular lens, Arch Ophthalmol 102:1528, 1984.

1022. Apple DJ, Tetz M, and Hunold W: Lokalisierte Endophthalmitis: eine bisher nicht beschriebene Komplikation der extrakapsulaeren Kataraktextraktion. Bericht der deutsche Gesellschaft fuer Intraokularlinsen Implantation, Giessen, West Germany, March 7, 1987.

1023. Apple DJ, Carlson AN. In Masket S editor: Consultation section: J Cataract Refract Surg 18:413-419, 1992.

1024. Apple DJ, Blotnik C: Postoperative lens deposits, J Cataract Refract Surg 19:441, 1993, (letter).

1025. Aquavella JV: A surgeon's dilemma—when to adopt a new technique, Ophthalmic Surg 19:238, 1988, (editorial).

1026. Aron-Rosa DS and others: Use of the neodymium-YAG laser to open the posterior capsule after lens implant surgery: a preliminary report, J Am Intraocul Implant Soc 6:352, 1980.

1027. Aron-Rosa DS: The 1987 Innovator's lecture: le sens du futur or reading behind the writing on the wall, J Cataract Refract Surg 13:428, 1987.

1028. Ashrafzadeh MT and others: Aphakic and phakic retinal detachment. I. Preoperative findings, Arch Ophthalmol 89:476, 1973.

1029. Ashton N, and Choyce DP: Pathological examination of a human eye containing an anterior chamber acrylic implant, Br J Ophthalmol 43:577, 1959.

1030. Auffarth GU and others: Nd:yag laser damage to silicone intraocular lenses confused with pigment deposits on clinical examination, Am J Ophthalmol 118:526, 1994, (letter).

1031. Awan KJ: Sympathetic uveitis in intraocular implant surgery, J Ocul Ther Surg 3:134, 1984.

1032. Bahn CF, and Sugar A: Endothelial physiology and intraocular lens implantation, J Am Intraocul Implant Soc 7:351, 1981.

1033. Balacco-Gabrieli C and others: Nd-YAG laser in our experience, Ophthalmologica (Basel) 190:112, 1985.

1034. Baller RS: Opacification of the posterior capsule—an alternative to discission, Ophthalmic Surg 8:48, 1977.

1035. Bath PE, McCord RC, and Cox KC: Nd:YAG laser discission of retroprosthetic membrane: a preliminary report, Cornea 2:225, 1983.

1036. Bath PE, Romberger AB, Brown PA: Comparison of Nd:YAG laser damage thresholds for PMMA and silicone intraocular lenses. Invest Ophthalmol Vis Sci 27(5):795, 1986.

1037. Bath PE and others: Quantitative concepts in avoiding intraocular lens damage from the nd:yag laser in posterior capsulotomy, J Cataract Refract Surg 12(3):262, 1986.

1038. Bath PE, Boerner CF, and Dang Y: Pathology and physics of YAG-laser intraocular lens damage, J Cataract Refract Surg 13:47, 1987.

1039. Bath PE and others: Excimer laser lens ablation, Arch Ophthalmol 105:1164, 1987.

1040. Belcher CD III, Mainster MA, and Buzney SM: Current status of neodymium:YAG laser photodisruptors in ophthalmology. I. Ann Ophthalmol 15:997, 1983, (editorial).

1041. Belcher CD III, Mainster MA, and Buzney SM: Current status of neodymium:YAG laser photodisruptors in ophthalmology. II. Ann Ophthalmol 15:1097, 1983, (editorial).

1042. Belcher CD III, Mainster MA, and Buzney SM: Current status of neodymium:YAG laser photodisruptors in ophthalmology. III. Ann Ophthalmol 16:13, 1984, (editorial).

1043. Benson WE, Grand MG, and Okun E: Aphakic retinal detachment: management of the fellow eye, Arch Ophthalmol 93:245, 1975.

1044. Beyer TL and others: Protective barrier effect of the posterior lens capsule in exogenous bacterial endophthalmitis: an experimental pseudophakic primate study, J Am Intraocul Implant Soc 9:293, 1983.

1045. Beyer TL and others: Protective barrier effect of the posterior lens capsule in exogenous bacterial endophthalmitis: an experimental primate study, Invest Ophthalmol Vis Sci 25:108, 1984.

1046. Blodi F: Sympathetic uveitis as an allergic phenomenon, Trans Am Acad Ophthalmol Otolaryngol 63:642, 1959.

1047. Bloomfield SE, Jakobiec FA, and Iwamoto T: Fibrous ingrowth with retrocorneal membrane, Ophthalmology 88:459, 1981.

1048. Bouchard CS and others: Surgical treatment for a case of postoperative pseudallescheria boydii endophthalmitis, Ophthalmic Surgery 22:98, 1991.

1049. Braun M and others: Ochrobactrum anthropi endophthalmitis after uncomplicated cataract surgery, Am J Ophthalmol 122:272, 1996.

1050. Bresnick GH: Eyes containing anterior chamber acrylic implants: pathological complications, Arch Ophthalmol 82:726, 1969.

1051. Brinkman CJJ and Broekhuyse RM: Cell mediated immunity in relation to cataract and cataract surgery, Br J Ophthalmol 63:301, 1979.

1052. Busin M, Cusumano A and Spitzmas M: Intraocular lens removal from eyes with chronic low-grade endophthalmitis, J Cataract Refract Surg 21:679, 1995.

1053. Busin M: Antibiotic irrigation of the capsular bag to resolve low-grade endophthalmitis, J Cataract Refract Surg 22:385, 1996.

1054. Capon M, Mellerio J and Docchio F: Intraocular lens damage from Nd:YAG laser pulses focused in the vitreous. I. Q-switched lasers, J Cataract Refract Surg 14:526, 1988.

1055. Carlson AN, Tetz MR and Apple DJ: Infectious complications of modern cataract surgery and intraocular lens implantation, Infect Dis Clin North Am 3:339, 1989, (review).

1056. Chambless WS: Neodymium:YAG laser posterior capsulotomy results and complications, J Am Intraocul Implant Soc 11:31, 1985.

1057. Charles H, Peyman GA and Pang MP: Management of an extruded footplate of an anterior chamber lens with the Nd:YAG laser, J Cataract Refract Surg 13:313, 1987.

1058. Chen V, Rosner M and Blumenthal M: Protrusion of a posterior chamber lens haptic into the anterior chamber through iris erosion, J Cataract Refract Surg 13:65, 1987.

1059. Cheng H and others: Corneal oedema and endothelial cell loss after iris-clip lens implantation, Trans Ophthalmol Soc UK 97:91, 1977.

1060. Chien AM and others: Propionibacterium acnes endophthalmitis after intracapsular cataract extraction (see comments), Ophthalmology 99:487, 1992.

1061. Chirila TV and others: Laser-induced damage to transparent polymers: chemical effect of short-pulsed (q-switched) nd:YAG laser radiation on ophthalmic acrylic biomaterials. II. Study of monomer release from artificial intraocular lenses, Biomaterials 11(5):313, 1990.

1062. Cinotti DJ and others: Neodymium:YAG laser therapy for pseudophakic pupillary block, J Cataract Refract Surg 12:174, 1986.

1063. Clayman HM and others: Intraocular lenses, axial length, and retinal detachment, Am J Ophthalmol 92:778, 1981.

1064. Clayman HM, Parel JM and Miller D: Bacterial recovery from automated cataract surgical equipment, J Cataract Refract Surg 12:158, 1986.

1065. Cobo LM and others: Pathogenesis of capsular opacification after extracapsular cataract extraction: an animal model, Ophthalmology 91:857, 1984.

1066. Cole DF and Unger WG: Prostaglandins as mediators for the responses of the eye to trauma, Exp Eye Res 17:357, 1973.

1067. Coonan P and others: The incidence of retinal detachment following extracapsular cataract extraction: a ten-year study, Ophthalmology 92:1096, 1985.

1068. Cousins S and others: Pseudophakic retinal detachments in the presence of various IOL types, Ophthalmology 93:1198, 1986.

1069. Cunha-Vaz J: The blood-ocular barriers, Surv Ophthalmol 23:279, 1979.

1070. Cunha-Vaz JG and Travassos A: Breakdown of the blood-retinal barriers and cystoid macular edema, Surv Ophthalmol 28(suppl): 485, 1984.

1071. Curtin VT: Retinal detachment surgery following intraocular lens implantation, Trans Ophthalmol Soc NZ 30:45, 1978.

1072. Cusumano A, Busin M and Spitznas M: Is chronic intraocular inflammation after lens implantation of bacterial origin? Ophthalmology 98:1703, 1991.

1073. Davidorf FH: Pseudophakic cystoid macular edema, Ophthalmic Forum 1(3):26, 1983.

1074. Davison JA: Transverse astigmatic keratotomy combined with phacoemulsification and intraocular lens implantation, J Cataract Refract Surg 15:38, 1989.

1075. Deutsch TA and Goldberg MF: Painless endophthalmitis after cataract surgery, Ophthalmic Surg 15:837, 1984.

1076. de Veer JA: Bilateral endophthalmitis phacoanaphylactica: pathologic study of the lesion in the eye first involved and, in one instance, the secondarily implicated, or "sympathizing," eye, Arch Ophthalmol 49:607, 1953.

1077. Dodick JM: A Q-switched neodymium:YAG laser—clinical experience, Cataract 1(1):25, 1983.

1078. Downing JE: Long-term discission rate after placing posterior chamber lenses with the convex surface posterior, J Cataract Refract Surg 12:651, 1986.

1079. Drews RC: Anterior capsulotomy with the neodymium:YAG laser: results and opinions, J Am Intraocul Implant Soc 11:240, 1985.

1080. Driebe WT Jr and others: Pseudophakic endophthalmitis: diagnosis and management, Ophthalmology 93:442, 1986.

1081. Duffner LR, Wallace WK and Stiles WR: The Miami cooperative community study on the Copeland intraocular lens (pseudophakos), Am J Ophthalmol 82:590, 1976.

1082. Durham DG and Gills JP: Three thousand YAG lasers in posterior capsulotomies: an analysis of complications and comparison to polishing and surgical discissions, Trans Am Ophthalmol Soc 83:218, 1985.

1083. Eakins KE and others: Prostaglandin-like activity in ocular inflammation, Br Med J 3:452, 1972.

1084. Eakins KE: Prostaglandin and non-prostaglandin mediated breakdown of the blood-aqueous barrier. In Bito LZ, Davson H, Fenstermacher JD, editors: The ocular and cerebrospinal fluids (Proceedings of a Fogarty International Center Symposium, Bethesda, MD, May, 1976), Exp Eye Res 25:483, 1977.

1085. Easom HA and Zimmerman LE: Sympathetic ophthalmia and bilateral phacoanaphylaxis: a clinicopathologic correlation of the sympathogenic and sympathizing eyes, Arch Ophthalmol 72:9, 1964.

1086. Easty D, Dallas N and O'Malley R: Aphakic macular oedema following prosthetic lens implantation, Br J Ophthalmol 61:321, 1977.

1087. Eichenbaum DM and others: Pars plana vitrectomy as a primary treatment for acute bacterial endophthalmitis, Am J Ophthalmol 86:167, 1978.

1088. Eifrig DE, Kwasniewska S and Fankhauser F: Letter to the editor and reply, Cataract 2(8):25, 1985.

1089. Elliott RD and Katz HR: Inhibition of pseudophakic endophthalmitis in a rabbit model, Ophthalmic Surg 18:538, 1987.

1090. Emery JM, Wilhelmus KA and Rosenberg S: Complications of phacoemulsification, Ophthalmology 85:141, 1978.

1091. Emery JM and Jacobson AC, editors: Current concepts in cataract surgery. Selected proceedings of the Sixth Biennial Cataract Surgical Congress, St. Louis, 1980, The CV Mosby Co.

1092. Emery JM and McIntyre DJ: Extracapsular cataract surgery, St Louis, 1983, The CV Mosby Co.

1093. Epstein DL: Cystoid macular edema occurring 13 years after cataract extraction, Am J Ophthalmol 83:501, 1977.

1094. Fallor MK, Hoft RH and Fett DR: Intraocular lens damage associated with posterior capsulotomy: a comparison of intraocular lens designs and four different Nd:YAG laser instruments, J Am Intraocul Implant Soc 11:564, 1985.

1095. Fankhauser F, Lörtscher H, and van der Zypen E: Clinical studies on high and low power laser radiation upon some structures of the anterior and posterior segments of the eye. Experiences in the treatment of some pathological conditions of the anterior and posterior segments of the human eye by means of a Nd:YAG laser, driven at various power levels, Int Ophthalmol 5(1):15, 1982.

1096. Fankhauser F and others: The effect of thermal mode Nd:YAG laser radiation on vessels and ocular tissues: experimental and clinical findings, Ophthalmology 92:419, 1985.

1097. Fastenberg DM, Schwartz PL and Lin HZ: Retinal detachment following neodymium: YAG laser capsulotomy, Am J Ophthalmol 97:288, 1984.

1098. Ficker LA, Steele AD and Mo G: Complications of Nd:YAG laser posterior capsulotomy, Trans Ophthalmol Soc UK 104:529, 1985.

1099. Fine BS and Brucker AJ: Macular edema and cystoid macular edema, Am J Ophthalmol 92:466, 1981.

1100. Fishman PH, Peyman GA and Woodhouse M: Alterations in the blood-aqueous barrier of the rabbit eye after neodymium:YAG laser photodisruption, J Am Intraocul Implant Soc 11:364, 1985.

1101. Flohr MJ, Robin AL and Kelley JS: Early complications following Q-switched neodymium:YAG laser posterior capsulotomy, Ophthalmology 92:360, 1985.

1102. Forster RK, Abbott RL and Gelender H: Management of infectious endophthalmitis, Ophthalmology 87:313, 1980.

1103. Foss AJ, Rosen PH and Cooling RJ: Retinal detachment following anterior chamber lens implantation for the correction of ultra-high myopia in phakic eyes, Br J Ophthalmol 77:212, 1993.

1104. Fritch CD and Jungschaffer OH: Phacoemulsification and retinal detachment, Ann Ophthalmol 10:35, 1978.

1105. Gaasterland DE, Rodrigues MM and Thomas G: Threshold for lens damage during Q-switched Nd:YAG laser iridectomy: a study of rhesus monkey eyes, Ophthalmology 92:1616, 1985.

1106. Galand A, Vancauwenberge F and Moosavi J: Posterior capsulorhexis in adult eyes with intact and clear capsules, J Cataract Refract Surg 22:458, 1996.

1107. Galin MA, Poole TA and Obstbaum SA: Retinal detachment in pseudophakia, Am J Ophthalmol 88:49, 1979.

1108. Galin MA and Turkish L: Studies of intraocular lens sterilization: the effect of NaOH on B. subtilis spores, J Am Intraocul Implant Soc 6:18, 1980.

1109. Galin MA and others: Why do implants fail? Trans Ophthalmol Soc UK 101:84, 1981.

1110. Galin MA and others: The long-term effect of an iris-supported lens on the endothelium, Trans Ophthalmol Soc UK 102:410, 1982.

1111. Galin MA and others: Studies of residual alkali on intraocular lenses sterilized with NaOH, J Am Intraocul Implant Soc 9:290, 1983.

1112. Gandham SB and others: Neodymium-yag membranectomy for pupillary membranes on posterior chamber intraocular lenses, Ophthalmology 102:1846, 1995.

1113. Gardner KM and others: Neodymium:YAG laser posterior capsulotomy: the first 100 cases at UCLA, Trans Pac Coast Oto-ophthalmol Soc 65:195, 1984.

1114. Gardner KM, Straatsma BR, Pettit TH: Neodymium:YAG laser posterior capsulotomy: the first 100 cases at UCLA, Ophthalmic Surg 16:24, 1985.

1115. Gass JDM and Norton EWD: Cystoid macular edema and papilledema following cataract extraction: a fluorescein fundoscopic and angiographic study, Arch Ophthalmol 76:646, 1966.

1116. Gass JDM and Norton EWD: Follow-up study of cystoid macular edema following cataract extraction, Trans Am Acad Ophthalmol Otolaryngol 73:665, 1969.

1117. Gass JDM, Anderson DR, Davis EB: A clinical fluorescein angiographic, and electron microscopic correlation of cystoid macular edema, Am J Ophthalmol 100:82, 1985.

1118. Gelender H: Corneal endothelial cell loss, cystoid macular edema, and iris-supported intraocular lenses, Ophthalmology 91:841, 1984.

1119. Gerber M and Shaw EL: Bilateral retinal detachments, pseudophakos, and intraocular hemorrhage: a comparison of implants, Ann Ophthalmol 12:54, 1980.

1120. Gerding DN and others: Treatment of Pseudomonas endophthalmitis associated with prosthetic intraocular lens implantation, Am J Ophthalmol 88:902, 1979.

1121. Gilbert CM and Novak MA: Successful treatment of postoperative Candida endophthalmitis in an eye with an intraocular lens implant, Am J Ophthalmol 97:593, 1984.

1122. Gills JP: Discissions with extracapsular cataract extraction, Contact Intraocul Lens Med J 6:48, 1980.

1123. Gills JP: Polishing of the posterior capsule, Contact Intraocul Lens Med J 7:355, 1981.

1124. Gills JP: Prevention of endophthalmitis by intraocular solution filtration and antibiotics, J Am Intraocul Implant Soc 11:185, 1985.

1125. Gimbel HV and Basti S: Optimal capsulorhexis technique in pediatric eyes, J Cataract Refract Surg 22(1):3, 1996, (letter).

1126. Gorn RA and Steinert RF: Neodymium:YAG laser cutting of intraocular lens haptics, J Am Intraocul Implant Soc 11:568, 1985.

1127. Greenidge KC: Nd:YAG capsulotomy—energy requirements and visual outcome, Cataract 1(4):31, 1984.

1128. Gross KA and Pearce JL: Protective barrier effect of the posterior lens capsule in exogenous bacterial endophthalmitis: a case report, J Cataract Refract Surg 12:413, 1986, (letter).

1129. Hagan JC, Menapace R, and Radax U: Clinical syndrome of endocapsular hematoma—presentation of a collected series and review of the literature, J Cataract Refract Surg 22:379, 1996, (review).

1130. Hagler WS: Pseudophakic retinal detachment, Trans Am Ophthalmol Soc 80:45, 1982.

1131. Haik GM, Waugh RL, and Lyda W: Sympathetic ophthalmia: similarity to bilateral endophthalmitis phacoanaphylactica: new therapeutic methods, Arch Ophthalmol 47:437, 1952.

1132. Haimann MH, Burton TC, and Brown CK: Epidemiology of retinal detachment, Arch Ophthalmol 100:289, 1982.

1133. Hales RH and Spencer WH: Unsuccessful penetrating keratoplasties: correlation of clinical and histologic findings, Arch Ophthalmol 70:805, 1963.

1134. Ham WT Jr and others: The nature of retinal radiation damage: dependence on wavelength, power level and exposure time, Vision Res 20:1105, 1980.

1135. Han DP and others: Spectrum and susceptibilities of microbiologic isolates in the endophthalmitis vitrectomy study, Am J Ophthalmol 122:1, 1996.

1136. Hansen SO and others: Comparative histopathologic study of various lens biomaterials in primates after Nd:YAG laser treatment, J Cataract Refract Surg 13:657, 1987.

1137. Harris WS, Taylor BC, and Winslow RL: Cystoid macular edema following intraocular lens implantation, Ophthalmic Surg 8:134, 1977.

1138. Harris WS: Cystoid macular edema in extracapsular and intracapsular aphakia and pseudophakia. In Kwitko ML and Praeger DL, editors: Pseudophakia: current trends and concepts, Baltimore, 1980, The Williams & Wilkins Co.

1139. Harris WS and Kogan I: Retrospective study of retinal complications with posterior chamber lenses, Contact Intraocul Lens Med J 7:345, 1981.

1140. Harris WS, Herman WK, and Fagadau WR: Management of the posterior capsule before and after the YAG laser, Trans Ophthalmol Soc UK 104:533, 1985.

1141. Harris WS and others: Management of posterior capsule after cataract extraction, CLAO J 11:273, 1985.

1142. Henkind P, editor: The First International Cystoid Macular Edema Symposium, Surv Ophthalmol 28(suppl):431, 1984.

1143. Henry MM, Henry LM, and Henry LM: A possible cause of chronic cystic maculopathy, Ann Ophthalmol 9:455, 1977.

1144. Hitchings RA: Aphakic macular edema: a two-year follow-up study, Br J Ophthalmol 61:628, 1977.

1145. Ho PC and Tolentino FI: Pseudophakic retinal detachment; surgical success rate with various types of IOLs, Ophthalmology 91:847, 1984.

1146. Hockwin O and Lerman S: Clinical evaluation of direct and photosensitized ultraviolet radiation damage to the lens, Ann Ophthalmol 14:220, 1982.

1147. Hoffer KJ: Consultation section: what is your treatment protocol for diagnosed endophthalmitis in an eye with a lens implant? J Am Intraocul Implant Soc 4:236, 1978.

1148. Hoffer KJ: Five years' experience with the ridged laser lens implant. In Emery JM and Jacobson AC, editors: Current concepts in cataract surgery. Selected proceedings of the Eighth Biennial Cataract Surgical Congress, Norwalk, CT, 1984, Appleton-Century-Crofts.

1149. Holladay JT, Bishop JE, and Lewis JW: The optimal size of a posterior capsulotomy, J Am Intraocul Implant Soc 11:18, 1985.

1150. Holweger RR and Marefat B: Intraocular pressure change after neodymium:YAG capsulotomy, J Cataract Refract Surg 23:115, 1997.

1151. Hopen G and others: Intraocular lenses and experimental bacterial endophthalmitis, Am J Ophthalmol 94:402, 1982.

1152. Howard GM and Praeger DL: Histopathologic examination of a globe containing an intraocular implant, Ann Ophthalmol 14:197, 1982.

1153. Hull DS and others: Hydrogen peroxide-mediated corneal endothelial damage: induction by oxygen free radical, Invest Ophthalmol Vis Sci 25:1246, 1984.

1154. Hunter JW: Early postoperative sterile hypopyons, Br J Ophthalmol 62:470, 1978.

1155. Insler MS, Boutros G, and Boulware DW: Corneal ulceration following cataract surgery in-patients with rheumatoid arthritis, J Am Intraocul Implant Soc 11:594, 1985.

1156. Irvine AR and others: Macular edema after cataract extraction, Ann Ophthalmol 3:1234, 1971.

1157. Irvine AR: Cystoid maculopathy, Surv Ophthalmol 21:1, 1976.

1158. Irvine AR: Cystoid maculopathy (cystoid macular edema, Irvine-Gass syndrome). In Fraunfelder FT and Roy FH, editors: Current ocular therapy, Philadelphia, 1980, WB Saunders Co.

1159. Irvine AR: The pathogenesis of aphakic retinal detachment, Ophthalmic Surg 16:101, 1985.

1160. Irvine SR and Irvine AR Jr: Lens-induced uveitis and glaucoma. I. Endophthalmitis phaco-anaphylactica, Am J Ophthalmol 35:177, 1952.

1161. Irvine SR and Irvine AR Jr: Lens-induced uveitis and glaucoma. II. The "phacotoxic" reaction, Am J Ophthalmol 35:370, 1952.

1162. Irvine SR: A newly defined vitreous syndrome following cataract surgery: interpreted according to recent concepts of the structure of the vitreous. The Seventh Francis I Proctor Lecture, Am J Ophthalmol 36:599, 1953.

1163. Isenberg RA and others: Fungal contamination of balanced salt solution, J Am Intraocul Implant Soc 11:485, 1985.

1164. Ishikawa Y, Kawata K, and Ishikawa Y: Three cases of endophthalmitis phacoanaphylactica in the fellow eye after extracapsular lens extraction, J Japan Contact Lens Soc 28:1260, 1977.

1165. Jakobiec FA: I want to say one word to you . . . plastics, Ophthalmology 90(4):29A, 1983, (editorial).

1166. Jansen B and others: Late onset endophthalmitis associated with intraocular lens: a case of molecularly proved s. epidermidis aetiology, Br J Ophthalmol 75:440, 1991.

1167. Javitt JC and others: National outcomes of cataract extraction I. Retinal detachment after inpatient surgery, Ophthalmology 98:895, 1991.

1168. Javitt JC and others: National outcomes of cataract extraction. Increased risk of retinal complications associated with nd:yag laser capsulotomy. The cataract patient outcomes research team (see comments). Ophthalmology 99:1487, 1992.

1169. Javitt JC and others: National outcomes of cataract extraction. Retinal detachment and endophthalmitis after outpatient cataract surgery; cataract patient outcomes research team, Ophthalmology 101: 100, 1994.

1170. Jennette JC, Eifrig DE, Paranjape YB: The inflammatory response to secondary methylmethacrylate challenge in lensimplanted rabbits, J Am Intraocul Implant Soc 8:35, 1982.

1171. Johnson SH, Kratz RP, and Olson PF: Clinical experience with the Nd:YAG laser, J Am Intraocul Implant Soc 10:452, 1984.

1172. Johnston GP and others: Pseudophakic retinal detachment, Mod Probl Ophthalmol 18:499, 1977.

1173. Joo CK and Kim JH: Effect of neodymium:yag laser photodisruption on intraocular lenses in vitro, J Cataract Refract Surg 18(6): 562, 1992.

1174. Jungschaffer OH: Iris clip lens and retinal detachment examination and surgery of three eyes, Arch Ophthalmol 88:594, 1972.

1175. Jungschaffer OH: Retinal detachments after intraocular lens implants, Arch Ophthalmol 95:1203, 1977.

1176. Jungschaffer OH: Retinal detachments and intraocular lenses, Int Ophthalmol Clin 19(3):125, 1979.

1177. Kanai A, Mustakallio AH, and Kaufman HE: Electron microscopic studies of corneal endothelium: the abnormal endothelium associated with retrocorneal membrane, Ann Ophthalmol 4:564, 1972.

1178. Kattan HM and others: Nosocomial endophthalmitis survey. current incidence of infection after intraocular surgery (see comments), Ophthalmology 98:227, 1991.

1179. Katzen LE, Fleischman JA, and Trokel S: YAG laser treatment of cystoid macular edema, Am J Ophthalmol 95:589, 1983.

1180. Kaufman HE and Katz JI: Effect of intraocular lenses on the corneal endothelium, Trans Ophthalmol Soc UK 97:265, 1977.

1181. Keates RH, Sall KN, and Kreter JK: Effect of the Nd:YAG laser on polymethylmethacrylate, HEMA copolymer, and silicone intraocular materials, J Cataract Refract Surg 13:401, 1987.

1182. Kelman CD: A year and a half with the YAG laser, Cataract 1(6): 21, 1984.

1183. Kim JE and others: Endophthalmitis in patients with retained lens fragments after phacoemulsification, Ophthalmology 103:575, 1996.

1184. Klapper RM: Q-switched neodymium:YAG laser iridotomy, Ophthalmology 91:1017, 1984.

1185. Klein RM and Yannuzzi LA: Cystoid macular edema in the first week after cataract extraction, Am J Ophthalmol 81:614, 1976.

1186. Knighton RW, Slomovic AR, and Parrish RK II: Glare measurements before and after neodymium:YAG laser posterior capsulotomy, Am J Ophthalmol 100:708, 1985.

1187. Knolle GE Jr: Knife versus neodymium:YAG laser posterior capsulotomy: a one-year follow-up, J Am Intraocul Implant Soc 11:448, 1985.

1188. Koch DD and others: Axial myopia increases the risk of retinal complications after neodymium:YAG laser posterior capsulotomy, Arch Ophthalmol 107:986, 1989.

1189. Kottow M and Hendrickson P: Iris angiography in cystoid macular edema after cataract extraction, Arch Ophthalmol 93:487, 1975.

1190. Kraff MC, Sanders DR, and Lieberman HL: Endothelial cell loss and trauma during intraocular lens implantation: a specular microscopic study, J Am Intraocul Implant Soc 4:107, 1978.

1191. Kraff MC and others: Factors affecting pseudophakic cystoid macular edema (PCME); posterior capsule status and ultraviolet light, Ophthalmology 91(suppl):113, 1984, (abstract).

1192. Kraff MC and others: Factors affecting pseudophakic cystoid macular edema: five randomized trials, J Am Intraocul Implant Soc 11:380, 1985.

1193. Krasnov MM: Laseropuncture of anterior chamber angle in glaucoma, Am J Ophthalmol 75:674, 1973.

1194. Krauss JM and others: Vitreous changes after neodymium-YAG laser photodisruption, Arch Ophthalmol 104:592, 1986.

1195. Krishnan MM, Lath NK, and Govind A: Aphakic macular edema: some observations on prevention and pathogenesis, Ann Ophthalmol 17:253, 1985.

1196. Kroll P, Busse H, and Berg P: Complications in aphakic eyes after vitreous loss, Ann Ophthalmol 13:983, 1981.

1197. Kurz GH and D'Amico RA: Histopathology of corneal graft failures, Am J Ophthalmol 66:184, 1968.

1198. Lee BL and others: Ovadendron sulphureo-ochraceum endophthalmitis after cataract surgery, Am J Ophthalmol 119:307, 1995.

1199. Legler UF and others: Inhibition of posterior capsule opacification:

the effect of colchicine in a sustained drug delivery system, J Cataract Refract Surg 19:462, 1993.

1200. Leonard PA, Klevering BJ, and de Keizer RJ: Complications of secondary surgical capsulotomy in pseudophakic and aphakic eyes, Ophthalmic Surgery 23:330, 1992.

1201. Levy JH and Pisacano AM: Clinical experience with Nd: YAG laser vitreolysis in the anterior segment, J Cataract Refract Surg 13:548, 1987.

1202. Liesegang TJ, Bourne WM, and Ilstrup DM: Secondary surgical and neodymium: YAG laser discissions, Am J Ophthalmol 100:510, 1985.

1203. Lindstrom RL and Harris WS: Management of the posterior capsule following posterior chamber lens implantation, J Am Intraocul Implant Soc 6:255, 1980.

1204. Little JH: Importance of the posterior capsule. In Emery JM and Jacobson AC, editors: Current concepts in cataract surgery. Selected proceedings of the Sixth Biennial Cataract Surgical Congress, St. Louis, 1980, The CV Mosby Co.

1205. Liu CS and others: A study of human lens cell growth in vitro. A model for posterior capsule opacification, Invest Ophthalmol Vis Sci 37(5):906, 1996.

1206. Loya N and others: Effects of the picosecond neodymium-ylf laser on poly(methyl methacrylate) intraocular lenses during experimental posterior capsulotomy, J Cataract Refract Surg 21:586, 1995.

1207. Lubin JR, Albert DM, and Weinstein M: Sixty-five years of sympathetic ophthalmia: a clinicopathologic review of 105 cases (1913–1978), Ophthalmology 87:109, 1980.

1208. Lynch MG and others: The effect of neodymium: YAG laser capsulotomy on aqueous humor dynamics in the monkey eye, Ophthalmology 93:1270, 1986.

1209. Manchester T: YAG laser anterior capsulotomy, Trans Am Ophthalmol Soc 82:176, 1984.

1210. Manchester T: YAG laser anterior capsulotomy, CLAO J 11:47, 1985.

1211. Manschot WA: Histopathology of eyes containing Binkhorst lenses, Am J Ophthalmol 77:865, 1974.

1212. Martin NF, Green WR, and Martin LW: Retinal phlebitis in the Irvine-Gass syndrome, Am J Ophthalmol 83:377, 1977.

1213. Martin NF and others: Endothelial damage thresholds for retrocorneal Q-switched neodymium: YAG laser pulses in monkeys, Ophthalmology 92:1382, 1985.

1214. Matsuda H and Smelser GK: Endothelial cells in alkali-burned corneas; ultrastructural alterations, Arch Ophthalmol 89:402, 1973.

1215. Mauriello JA Jr, McLean IW, and Wright JD Jr: Loss of eyes after intraocular lens implantation, Ophthalmology 90:378, 1983.

1216. Maxwell DP Jr, Diamond JG, and May DR: Surgical wound defects associated with endophthalmitis, Ophthalmic Surg 25:157, 1994.

1217. McDonnell PJ, Zarbin MA, and Green WR: Posterior capsule opacification in pseudophakic eyes, Ophthalmology 90:1548, 1983.

1218. McDonnell PJ and others: Pathology of intraocular lenses in 33 eyes examined postmortem, Ophthalmology 90:386, 1983.

1219. McDonnell PJ and others: Argon laser debridement of the posterior capsule: a potential treatment for posterior capsule opacification after extracapsular cataract surgery, Ophthalmic Surg 16:549, 1985.

1220. McDonnell PJ, Patel A, and Green WR: Comparison of intracapsular and extracapsular cataract surgery: histopathologic study of eyes obtained postmortem, Ophthalmology 92:1208, 1985.

1221. McDonnell PJ and others: Posterior capsule opacification: an in vitro model, Arch Ophthalmol 103:1378, 1985.

1222. McDonnell PJ, Krause W, and Glaser BM: In vitro inhibition of lens epithelial cell proliferation and migration, Ophthalmic Surg 19:25, 1988.

1223. McIntyre DJ: Safe and efficacious? J Am Intraocul Implant Soc 11:592, 1985, (letter).

1224. McNatt J and others: Anaerobic flora of the normal human conjunctival sac, Arch Ophthalmol 96:1448, 1978.

1225. McPherson AR, O'Malley RE, and Bravo J: Retinal detachment following late posterior capsulotomy, Am J Ophthalmol 95:593, 1983.

1226. McPherson RJE and Govan JAA: Posterior capsule reopacification after neodymium-yag laser capsulotomy, J Cataract Refract Surg 21:351, 1995.

1227. Meisler DM and others: Chronic Propionibacterium endophthal-mitis after extracapsular cataract extraction and intraocular lens implantation, Am J Ophthalmol 102:733, 1986.

1228. Meisler DM and Mandelbaum S: Propionibacterium-associated endophthalmitis after extracapsular cataract extraction. Review of reported cases, Ophthalmology 96:54, 1989.

1229. Melamed S, Ashkenazi I, and Blumenthal M: Nd-YAG laser hyaloidotomy for malignant glaucoma following one-piece 7 mm intraocular lens implantation, Br J Ophthalmol 75:501, 1991.

1230. Meltzer DW: Sterile hypopyon following intraocular lens surgery, Arch Ophthalmol 98:100, 1980.

1231. Menapace R: Delayed iris prolapse with unsutured 5.1 mm clear corneal incisions, J Cataract Refract Surg 21:353, 1995.

1232. Menchini U and others: Cystoid macular oedema after extracapsular cataract extraction and intraocular lens implantation in diabetic patients without retinopathy (see comments), Br J Ophthalmol 77:208, 1993.

1233. Menikoff JA and others: A case-control study of risk factors for postoperative endophthalmitis (see comments), Ophthalmology 98:1761, 1991.

1234. Meyer KT, Pettit TH, and Straatsma BR: Corneal endothelial damage with neodymium: YAG laser, Ophthalmology 91:1022, 1984.

1235. Meyer-Schwickerath G: Light coagulation, St. Louis, 1960, The CV Mosby Co.

1236. Michels RG, Kenyon KR, and Maumenee AE: Retrocorneal fibrous membrane, Invest Ophthalmol 11:822, 1972.

1237. Miller KM, and Glasgow BJ: Bacterial endophthalmitis following sutureless cataract surgery, Arch Ophthalmol 111:377, 1993.

1238. Mirate DJ, Hull DS, and Bobo C: Bacterial endophthalmitis: culture proven failure of combined systemic, periocular, and topical antibiotics, Ann Ophthalmol 13:1341, 1981.

1239. Mitchell PG, Blair NP, and Deutsch TA: Prolonged monitoring of the blood-aqueous barrier with fluorescein-labeled albumin, Invest Ophthalmol 27:415, 1986.

1240. Miyake K: Prostaglandins as a causative factor of the cystoid macular edema after the lens extraction. II. Nippon Ganka Gakkai Zasshi 81:1449, 1977.

1241. Miyake K: Blood-retinal barrier in eyes with long-standing aphakia with apparently normal fundi, Arch Ophthalmol 100:1437, 1982.

1242. Miyake K, Asakura M, and Kobayashi H: Effect of intraocular lens fixation on the blood-aqueous barrier, Am J Ophthalmol 98:451, 1984.

1243. Miyake K and others: Outward transport of fluorescein from the vitreous in aphakic eyes, Br J Ophthalmol 69:428, 1985.

1244. Morrison LK and Waltman SR: Management of pseudophakic bullous keratopathy, Ophthalmic Surg 20:205, 1989, (review).

1245. Moses L: Cystoid macular edema and retinal detachment following cataract surgery, J Am Intraocul Implant Soc 5:326, 1979.

1246. Mosier MA and others: Fungal endophthalmitis following intraocular lens implantation, Am J Ophthalmol 83:1, 1977.

1247. Muir MGK and Sherrard ES: Damage to the corneal endothelium during Nd/YAG photodisruption, Br J Ophthalmol 69:77, 1985.

1248. Mullaney J and Condon PI: Pseudophaco-anaphylactic endophthalmitis—PMMA related? In Tarkkanen A, editor: Pathology of intraocular lens implantation, Acta Ophthalmol 63(suppl 170):34, 1985.

1249. Naeser K and Kobayashi C: Epidemiology of aphakic retinal detachment following intracapsular cataract extraction: a follow-up study with an analysis of risk factors, J Cataract Refract Surg 14:303, 1988.

1250. Nevyas HJ, Keates EU, and Nevyas JY: A YAG laser technique to facilitate removal of posterior chamber intraocular lenses from the capsular bag, J Cataract Refract Surg 13:201, 1987.

1251. Nicholls JVV: Macular edema in association with cataract extraction, Am J Ophthalmol 37:665, 1954.

1252. Ninnpedersen K and Bauer B: Cataract patients in a defined Swedish population, 1986 to 1990-5. Postoperative retinal detachments, Arch Ophthalmol 114:382, 1996.

1253. Nirankari VS and others: Pseudophakic endophthalmitis, Ophthalmic Surg 14:314, 1983.

1254. Nirankari VS and Richards RD: Complications associated with the use of the neodymium: YAG laser, Ophthalmology 92:1371, 1985.

1255. Nishi O: Incidence of posterior capsule opacification in eyes with and without posterior chamber intraocular lenses, J Cataract Refract Surg 12:519, 1986.

1256. Nishi O and Nishi K: Intercapsular cataract surgery with lens epithelial cell removal. Part III: Long-term follow-up of posterior capsular opacification, J Cataract Refract Surg 17:218, 1991.

1257. Nordlohne ME: The intraocular implant lens development and results with special reference to the Binkhorst lens, Doc Ophthalmol 38:1, 1974.

1258. Norton EWD: Retinal detachment in aphakia, Am J Ophthalmol 58:111, 1964.

1259. Norton EWD: Management of retinal detachment in patients with intraocular lens (Copeland model of the Epstein lens), Trans Am Acad Ophthalmol Otolaryngol 81:135, 1976.

1260. Ober RR and others: Rhegmatogenous retinal detachment after neodymium:YAG laser capsulotomy in phakic and pseudophakic eyes, Am J Ophthalmol 101:81, 1986.

1261. Obstbaum SC: Editorial, J Cataract Refract Surg 12:605, 1986.

1262. O'Day DM: Fungal endophthalmitis caused by Paecilomyces lilacinus after intraocular lens implantation, Am J Ophthalmol 83:130, 1977.

1263. O'Donnell FE Jr and Santos B: Posterior capsular-zonular disruption in planned extracapsular surgery, Arch Ophthalmol 103:652, 1985.

1264. Ohrloff C and Dardenne MU: Zur Ablationshäufigkeit nach Hinterkammerlinsenimplantation, Fortschr Ophthalmol 79:189, 1982.

1265. Olson GM and Olson RJ: Prospective study of cataract surgery, capsulotomy, and retinal detachment, J Cataract Refract Surg 21:136, 1995.

1266. Olson JC and others: Results in the treatment of postoperative endophthalmitis, Ophthalmology 90:692, 1983.

1267. Olson RJ and Slappey TE: Corneal endothelial damage induced by intraocular lenses: an in vitro study, J Am Intraocul Implant Soc 5:321, 1979.

1268. Ormerod LD and others: Anaerobic bacterial endophthalmitis, Ophthalmology 94:799, 1987.

1269. Ormerod LD and others: Endophthalmitis caused by the coagulase-negative staphylococci. 2. Factors influencing presentation after cataract surgery, Ophthalmology 100:724, 1993.

1270. Ozaki L: The intraocular lens implantation and the posterior lens capsule, Contact Intraocul Lens Med J 6:418, 1980.

1271. Parelman AG: Sterile uveitis and intraocular lens implantation, J Am Intraocul Implant Soc 5:301, 1979.

1272. Parkkari M, Paivarinta H, and Salminen L: The treatment of endophthalmitis after cataract surgery: review of 26 cases, J Ocul Pharmacol Ther 11:349, 1995.

1273. Percival SPB, Anand V, and Das SK: Prevalence of aphakic detachment, Br J Ophthalmol 67:43, 1983.

1274. Percival SPB: Retinal detachment after lens implantation, Cataract 1(5):15, 1984.

1275. Percival SPB and Setty SS: Analysis of the need for secondary capsulotomy during a five-year follow up, J Cataract Refract Surg 14:379, 1988.

1276. Peiffer RL Jr: Animal models of intraocular lens implantation, J Am Intraocul Implant Soc 10:68, 1984, (letter).

1277. Perlman EM, Albert DM: Clinically unsuspected phacoanaphylaxis after ocular trauma, Arch Ophthalmol 95:244, 1977.

1278. Pettit TH and others: Fungal endophthalmitis following intraocular lens implantation: a surgical epidemic, Arch Ophthalmol 98:1025, 1980.

1279. Peyman GA and others: Early clinical experience with a new generation Q-switched neodymium:YAG laser, J Am Intraocul Implant Soc 11:292, 1985.

1280. Pierce D: Intraocular lens implants: an introduction, Trans Ophthalmol Soc UK 97:64, 1977.

1281. Piest KL and others: Localized endophthalmitis: a newly described cause of the so-called toxic lens syndrome, J Cataract Refract Surg 13:498, 1987.

1282. Posenauer B, Funk J: Chronic postoperative endophthalmitis caused by propionibacterium acnes, Euro J Ophthalmol 2:94, 1992.

1283. Pulido JS and others: Histoplasma capsulatum endophthalmitis after cataract extraction, Ophthalmology 97:217, 1990.

1284. Rahi AHS, Garner A: The lens. In Rahi AHS, Garner A, editors: Immunopathology of the eye, Oxford, 1976, Blackwell Scientific Publications.

1285. Ramsey RC, Cantrill HL, Knobloch WH: Pseudophakic retinal detachment, Can J Ophthalmol 18:262, 1983.

1286. Rao NA and others: Modulation of lens-induced uveitis by superoxide dismutase, Ophthalmic Res 18:41, 1986.

1287. Raskin EM and others: Influence of haptic materials on the adherence of staphylococci to intraocular lenses, Arch Ophthalmol 111:250, 1993.

1288. Ratner BD: Characterization of graft polymers for biomedical applications, J Biomed Mater Res 14:665, 1980.

1289. Richards BW and others: The effects of nonfixated lower lens haptics of Binkhorst lenses on corneal endothelial cell density, Ophthalmic Surg 17:286, 1986.

1290. Richburg FA: Hypopyon and ultrasonic cleaning solution, J Am Intraocul Implant Soc 11:170, 1985, (letter).

1291. Richburg FA: Neodymium:YAG laser for anterior capsulotomy, J Am Intraocul Implant Soc 11:372, 1985.

1292. Richburg FA and others: Sterile hypopyon secondary to ultrasonic cleaning solution, J Cataract Refract Surg 12:248, 1986.

1293. Rickman-Barger L and others: Retinal detachment after neodymium:YAG laser posterior capsulotomy (see comments), Am J Ophthalmol 107:531, 1989.

1294. Riffenburgh RS: Pathology associated with intraocular lens implantation, Trans Pac Coast Otoophthalmol Soc 58:269, 1977.

1295. Robin AL, Pollack IP: A comparison of neodymium:YAG and argon laser iridotomies, Ophthalmology 91:1011, 1984.

1296. Roper DL, Nisbet RM: Effect of hyaluronidase on the incidence of cystoid macular edema, Ann Ophthalmol 10:1673, 1978.

1297. Roper-Hall MJ, Wilson RS: Reduction in endothelial cell density following cataract extraction and intraocular lens implantation, Br J Ophthalmol 66:516, 1982.

1298. Rosen ES: Endophthalmitis following cataract surgery, J Cataract Refract Surg 22:279, 1996.

1299. Ross WH: Pseudophakic retinal detachment, Can J Ophthalmol 19:119, 1984.

1300. Roussel TJ, Culbertson WW, and Jaffe NS: Chronic postoperative endophthalmitis associated with Propionibacterium acnes, Arch Ophthalmol 105:1199, 1987.

1301. Roy FH: After-cataract clinical and pathologic evaluation, Ann Ophthalmol 3:1364, 1971.

1302. Sanders DR and others: Studies on the blood-aqueous barrier after argon laser photocoagulation of the iris, Ophthalmology 90:169, 1983.

1303. Santos BA and others: Lens epithelial inhibition by PMMA optic: implications for lens design, J Cataract Refract Surg 12:23, 1986.

1304. Schanzlin DJ, Goldberg DG, Brown SI: Staphylococcus epidermis endophthalmitis following intraocular lens implantation, Br J Ophthalmol 64:687, 1980.

1305. Schroeder E: A comparison of Q-switched and mode-locked Nd:YAG laser shock waves, Cataract 2(2):28, 1985.

1306. Schumaker A and others: Circulating antilens antibodies following extracapsular lens surgery, J Ocul Ther Surg 4:17, 1985.

1307. Scott IU, Flynn HW, Feuer W: Endophthalmitis after secondary intraocular lens implantation—a case-control study, Ophthalmology 102:1925, 1995.

1308. Scott JD: Retinal dialysis, Trans Ophthalmol Soc UK 97:33, 1977.

1309. Sears ML: Aphakic cystoid macular edema. The pharmacology of ocular trauma, Surv Ophthalmol 28(suppl):525, 1984.

1310. Sebag J, Balazs EA: Pathogenesis of cystoid macular edema: an anatomic consideration of vitreoretinal adhesions, Surv Ophthalmol 28(suppl):493, 1984.

1311. Seelenfreund MH, Sternberg I, Hirsch I: Argon laser treatment of a pupillary membrane in pseudophakia, J Am Intraocul Implant Soc 8:166, 1982.

1312. Severin SL: Late cystoid macular edema in pseudophakia, Am J Ophthalmol 90:223, 1980.

1313. Severin SL: Clinical cystoid macular edema with intracapsular cataract extraction and posterior chamber lens implantation, Ann Ophthalmol 15:631, 1983.

1314. Seward HC, Doran RML: Posterior capsulotomy and retinal detachment following extracapsular lens surgery, Br J Ophthalmol 68:379, 1984.

1315. Shammas HJF, Milkie CF: Cystoid macular edema following the implantation of anterior chamber lenses, J Am Intraocul Implant Soc 4:87, 1978.

1316. Shammas HJ, Milkie CF: Mature cataracts in eyes with unilateral axial myopia, J Cataract Refract Surg 15:308, 1989.

1317. Shepard DD: Retinal detachment with intraocular lenses, J Am Intraocul Implant Soc 4:55, 1978.

1318. Shepard DD: The "toxic lens" syndrome, Contact Intraocul Lens Med J 6:158, 1980.

1319. Sherrard ES, Rycroft PV: Retrocorneal membranes. I. Their origin and structure, Br J Ophthalmol 51:379, 1967.

1320. Sieck EA and others: Contamination of K-Sol corneal storage medium with Propionibacterium acnes, Arch Ophthalmol 107:1023,

1321. Silbert AM, Baum JL: Origin of the retrocorneal membrane in the rabbit, Arch Ophthalmol 97:1141, 1979.

1322. Simcoe CW: Capsular discission behind posterior chamber lens, Contact Intraocul Lens Med J 6:60, 1980.

1323. Singh G: Endophthalmitis after cataract extraction: a retrospective case study, Ann Ophthalmol 13:629, 1981.

1324. Sinskey RM, Cain W Jr: The posterior capsule and phacoemulsification, J Am Intraocul Implant Soc 4:206, 1978.

1325. Sliney DH and others: Intraocular lens damage from Nd:YAG laser pulses focused in the vitreous. II. Mode-locked lasers, J Cataract Refract Surg 14:530, 1988.

1326. Slomovic AR and others: Neodymium:YAG laser posterior capsulotomy; central corneal endothelial cell density, Arch Ophthalmol 104:536, 1986.

1327. Smith LD, Williams BL: The pathogenic anaerobic bacteria, ed 3, Springfield, III, 1984, Charles C Thomas, Publisher.

1328. Smith MA and others: Treatment of experimental methicillin-resistant Staphylococcus epidermis endophthalmitis with intravitreal vancomycin, Ophthalmology 93:1328, 1986.

1329. Smith RE: Inflammation after cataract surgery, Am J Ophthalmol 102:788, 1986, (editorial).

1330. Smith RE, Weiner P: Unusual presentation of phacoanaphylaxis following phacoemulsification, Ophthalmic Surg 7:65, 1976.

1331. Smith SG, Snowden FM: Neodymium:YAG laser damage of intraocular lenses, J Cataract Refract Surg 14:660, 1988.

1332. Snip RC and others: Posterior corneal pigmentation and fibrous proliferation by iris melanocytes, Arch Ophthalmol 99:1232, 1981.

1333. Snyder HP: Intravenous chloramphenicol to prevent postoperative endophthalmitis in cataract surgery—520 consecutive cases, Ann Ophthalmol 10:1041, 1978.

1334. Snyder WB and others: Symposium on intraocular lenses. Retinal detachment and pseudophakia, Ophthalmology 86:229, 1979.

1335. Solomon KD, Legler UFC, Kostick MP: Capsular opacification after cataract surgery, Curr Opin Ophthalmol 3:46-51, 1992.

1336. Speaker MG and others: Penetrating keratoplasty for pseudophakic bullous keratopathy: management of intraocular lens, Ophthalmology 95:1260, 1988.

1337. Stark WJ, Bruner WE, Michels RG: Management of retropseudophakos membranes, J Am Intraocul Implant Soc 6:137, 1980.

1338. Stark WJ and others: Neodymium:YAG lasers: an FDA report, Ophthalmology 92:209, 1985.

1339. Steinert RF, Puliafito CA: The Nd-YAG laser in ophthalmology: principles and clinical applications of photodisruption, Philadelphia, 1985, WB Saunders Co.

1340. Sterling S, Wood TO: Effect of intraocular lens convexity on posterior capsule opacification, J Cataract Refract Surg 12:655, 1986.

1341. Stern WH and others: Epidemic postsurgical Candida parapsilosis endophthalmitis: clinical findings and management of 15 consecutive cases, Ophthalmology 92:1701, 1985.

1342. Sugar J, Mitchelson J, and Kraff FM: Endothelial trauma and cell loss from intraocular lens insertion, Arch Ophthalmol 96:449, 1978.

1343. Swan KC: Fibroblastic ingrowth following cataract extraction, Arch Ophthalmol 89:445, 1973.

1344. Tally FP and others: Susceptibility of anaerobes to cefoxitin and other cephalosporins, Antimicrob Agents Chemother 7:128, 1975.

1345. Tasman W: Are there any retinal contraindications to cataract extraction and posterior chamber lens implants? Arch Ophthalmol 104:1767, 1986, (editorial).

1346. Tasman W and Annesley WH Jr: Retinal detachment in prosthetophakia, Arch Ophthalmol 75:179, 1966.

1347. Tasman WS: Pseudophakic retinal detachment, Trans PA Acad Ophthalmol Otolaryngol 32:139, 1979.

1348. Tasman WS: Pseudophakic retinal detachment, Ophthalmic Forum 1:20, 1983.

1349. Tetz MR and others: A newly described complication of neodymium-YAG laser capsulotomy: exacerbation of an intraocular infection, Arch Ophthalmol 105:1324, 1987.

1350. Tetz MR and others: "Localised endophthalmitis": A complication of extracapsular cataract extraction, Implant Ophthalmol (Singapore) 1(3):93, 1987.

1351. Tetz MR and others: Localized endophthalmitis. Proceedings: International Symposium of the German Ophthalmological Society, Muenster, Germany, Sept 19–21, 1992.

1352. Thorburn DE and Levenson JE: Corneal endothelial damage from previously implanted intraocular lenses, J Am Intraocul Implant Soc 6:236, 1980.

1353. Thornval P and Naeser K: Refraction and anterior chamber depth before and after neodymium-YAG laser treatment for posterior capsule opacification in pseudophakic eyes—a prospective study, J Cataract Refract Surg 21:457, 1995.

1354. Tielsch JM and others: Preoperative functional expectations and postoperative outcomes among patients undergoing first eye cataract surgery, Arch Ophthalmol 113:1312, 1995.

1355. Tornambe PE: Macular hemorrhage during intraocular surgery, Ann Ophthalmol 18:301, 1986.

1356. Townsend-Pico WA and others: Coagulase-negative staphylococcus endophthalmitis after cataract surgery with intraocular vancomycin, Am J Ophthalmol 121(3):318, 1996.

1357. Trokel SL, editor: YAG laser ophthalmic microsurgery, Norwalk, CT, 1983, Appleton-Century-Crofts.

1358. Tso MOM: Animal modeling of cystoid macular edema, Surv Ophthalmol 28(suppl):512, 1984.

1359. Turkalj JW and others: Is the sutureless cataract incision a valve for bacterial inoculation? J Cataract Refract Surg 21:472, 1995.

1360. Unger WG, Perkins ES, and Bass MS: The response of the rabbit eye to laser irradiation of the iris, Exp Eye Res 19:367, 1974.

1361. Unger WG and Bass MS: Prostaglandins and nerve-mediated response of the rabbit eye to argon laser irradiation of the iris, Ophthalmologica 175:153, 1977.

1362. Vafidis GC, Marsh RJ, and Stacey AR: Bacterial contamination of intraocular lens surgery, Br J Ophthalmol 68:520, 1984.

1363. Vallotton WW: How to use the YAG laser—a methodology for the beginner, Cataract 1(6):26, 1984.

1364. Van der Zypen E, Bebie H, and Fankhauser F: Morphological studies about the efficiency of laser beams upon the structures of the angle of the anterior chamber: facts and concepts related to the treatment of the chronic simple glaucoma, Int Ophthalmol 1(2):109, 1979.

1365. Verbraeken H: Treatment of postoperative endophthalmitis, Ophthalmologica 209:165, 1995.

1366. Verhoeff FH and Lemoine AN: Endophthalmitis phacoanaphylactica, Am J Ophthalmol 5:737, 1922.

1367. Wang WLL and others: Susceptibility of Propionibacterium acnes to seventeen antibiotics; Antimicrob Agents Chemother 11:171, 1977.

1368. Waring GO III and others: Results of penetrating keratoplasty in 123 eyes with pseudophakic or aphakic corneal edema, Ophthalmology 90:25, 1983.

1369. Wasserman EL, Axt JC, and Sheets JH: Neodymium: YAG laser posterior capsulotomy, J Am Intraocul Implant Soc 11:245, 1985.

1370. Weiblinger RP: Review of the clinical literature on the use of the Nd:YAG laser for posterior capsulotomy, J Cataract Refract Surg 12:162, 1986.

1371. Weidle EG, Lisch W, and Thiel H-J: Management of the opacified posterior lens capsule: an excision technique for membranous changes, Ophthalmic Surg 17:635, 1986.

1372. Weissgold DJ, Maguire AM, and Brucker AJ: Management of postoperative acremonium endophthalmitis, Ophthalmology 103:749, 1996.

1373. Wesendahl TA and others: (Area of contact of the artificial lens and posterior capsule. systematic study of various haptic parameters (German), Ophthalmologe 91:680, 1994.

1374. Wesendahl TA and others: Verringerung der Nachstarrate durch stärkere Hapikabwinklung von einsthckigen PMMA Hinterkammerlinsen, Der Ophthalmologe 92(Suppl. 1):108, 1995, (abstract).

1375. Wilensky JT, Welch D, and Mirolovich M: Transscleral cyclocoagulation using a neodymium-YAG laser, Ophthalmic Surg 16:95, 1986.

1376. Wilhelmus KR and Emery JM: Posterior capsule opacification following phacoemulsification, Ophthalmic Surg 11:264, 1980.

1377. Winslow RL and Taylor BC: Retinal complications following YAG laser capsulotomy, Ophthalmology 92:785, 1985.

1378. Winward KE and others: Postoperative propionibacterium endophthalmitis. Treatment strategies and long-term results (see comments), Ophthalmology 100:447, 1993.

1379. Wirostko E and Spalter HF: Lens-induced uveitis, Arch Ophthalmol 78:1, 1967.

1380. Wohl LG and others: Pseudophakic phacoanaphylactic endophthalmitis, Ophthalmic Surg 17:234, 1986.

1381. Woodlief NF: Initial observations on the ocular microcirculation in man. I. The anterior segment and extraocular muscles, Arch Ophthalmol 98:1268, 1980.

1382. Woodward PM: Special uses of anterior capsulotomy performed with a nd:YAG laser, Cataract 2(1):1984.

1383. Woodward PM: Anterior capsulotomy using a neodymium:YAG laser, Ann Ophthalmol 16:534, 1984.

1384. Worst JGF: Late CME in the pseudophakic eye, J Am Intraocul Implant Soc 7:158, 1981, (letter).

1385. Yamada K and others: Effect of intraocular lens design on posterior capsule opacification after continuous curvilinear capsulorhexis, J Cataract Refract Surg 21:697, 1995.

1386. Yang HK and Kline OR Jr: Corneal melting with intraocular lenses, Arch Ophthalmol 100:1272, 1982.

1387. Yannuzzi LA, Landau AN and Turtz AI: Incidence of aphakic cystoid macular edema with the use of topical indomethacin, Ophthalmology 88:947, 1981.

1388. Yanoff M and others: Pathology of human cystoid macular edema, Surv Ophthalmol 28(Suppl):505, 1984.

1389. Zaidman GW and Mondino BJ: Postoperative pseudophakic bacterial endophthalmitis, Am J Ophthalmol 93:218, 1982.

1390. Zimmerman PL and others: Chronic nocardia asteroides endophthalmitis after extracapsular cataract extraction (see comments), Arch Ophthalmol 111:837, 1993.

CHAPTER 5

PATHOLOGY OF REFRACTIVE SURGERY

General considerations

Despite the high frequency of refractive errors in the human race, we understand very little about their pathogenesis.[1-14] Patterns of inheritance and genetic transmission of refractive errors are not well defined, although both familial and racial factors play a role. In the United States, about a quarter of the population is myopic,[3,8] and over 70 million have myopia from -1.5 to -7.0 diopters (D). In some regions of the world the prevalence is as high as 70%.[3,8,12] About two thirds of myopes in the United States use spectacles and one third use contact lenses. Although ophthalmic surgery to correct refractive errors has been practiced for more than 110 years, fewer than 1% of myopes elect to have surgery to relieve their handicap.[7] Surgery to correct a refractive error is an elective procedure and many refractive surgical procedures in the past and even today suffer from complication rates that are unacceptably high.

Modern refractive surgery is currently dominated by two procedures.[12] Radial keratotomy (RK) is the most common refractive surgical procedure practiced in the world with some 250,000 procedures annually as of 1994, most all of these in the United States. In the rest of the world, the most frequently performed procedure today is excimer laser photorefractive keratectomy (PRK). Now that the U.S. Food and Drug Administration (FDA) has approved the use of the excimer laser, it is widely predicted that PRK will eventually supersede RK in the United States.

Refractive surgery is currently one of the most rapidly developing fields of ophthalmology. New refractive techniques are constantly being developed and tested.[9] The more established techniques of RK and PRK are now well studied with the publication of well-conducted, scientific, clinical trials. Several promising, newer refractive surgical techniques that are currently in vogue are being evaluated with results published in peer-reviewed journals. Laser in situ keratomileusis and automated lamellar keratoplasty for myopia and hyperopia are current examples of this. As data are collected these and other new techniques are capturing the minds of many refractive surgeons. Only time will tell whether the results of well-conducted, prospective clinical trials, will match the enthusiasm that these newer refractive procedures are generating.

Many promising refractive surgical procedures have not stood the test of time. Epikeratophakia is one example (p. 216). It arrived in 1980 with great promise, was promoted by many highly regarded proponents, and offered predictable and reversible correction of all types of refractive error. By the late 1990s, it is a nonpracticed, "dead" procedure. Predictability of the refractive effect and loss of best corrected visual acuity proved to be unacceptably poor. It was not approved by the FDA. Despite its failure, epikeratophakia taught us many valuable lessons about the response of the cornea to surgery. It showed how the cornea likes to drift back to its original curvature when forced into a new curvature. It showed how loss of stromal keratocytes adversely affects corneal transparency. It taught refractive surgeons to respect the unpredictable and variable nature of corneal wound healing.

Several corneal weakening procedures have also demonstrated unpredictable results. In the Prospective Evaluation of Radial Keratotomy (PERK) study, the weakening of the peripheral cornea has led to progressive hyperopia of at least 1 D in 43% of eyes at 10 years.[10,13] Hexagonal keratotomy caused unsafe levels of irregular astigmatism with loss of best vision in as many as 50% or more of eyes (p. 213). Hyperopic automated lamellar keratoplasty suffers from regression and can also result in the development of iatrogenic keratoconus (p. 215). Weakening procedures that cause the cornea to assume a new shape by producing a controlled ectasia are unlikely to be as stable in the long term as procedures that reshape the cornea by removal of tissue.

New refractive surgical techniques are a major driving force behind the study of the corneal pathophysiology. Computerized corneal topographic analysis has developed in tandem with refractive surgery.[1,2,4,6,14] Radial keratotomy and PRK have both stimulated interest in corneal wound healing. Variations in corneal wound healing have been responsible for most of the unpredictable results after corneal refractive surgical procedures. Generally, the greater the attempted change in refraction, the more effect that corneal wound healing has had on the final refractive and visual outcome. In addition, all current procedures for the correction of hyperopia suffer from regression of effect, which occurs as a direct result of postoperative corneal wound healing. Until more can be done to modulate corneal wound healing, or procedures are developed that are much less affected by corneal wound healing, both the correction of high myopia and hyperopia will remain inaccurate and plagued by regression of effect. Work into corneal wound healing is proceeding in a number of directions at present (pp. 210 and 220). The roles of different subtypes of collagen and molecules such as fibronectin, laminin, glycosaminoglycans, and glycoproteins have been studied. More recently, refractive surgery is stimulating research into how cytokines allow cells to communicate with each other. Understanding corneal wound healing processes and how they are regulated is likely to be the key to achieving controllable and safe refractive surgery in the next century.

Outcome assessment

The two major events that have helped to bring about some standardization of reporting of results of refractive surgery have been the PERK study and the U.S. FDA approval process for excimer laser PRK.[10,13] The PERK study was the first multicenter, prospective study of a standardized refractive surgical technique. New ground was broken and refractive surgery was brought from the realm of random experimentation and andecdotal reporting into the sphere of modern medical science. The PERK study

established repeatable measures of outcome after refractive surgery, which were later built on by the FDA trials of excimer laser PRK. Definitions of success were established for the efficacy of restoration of functional vision without optical aids, the predictability of the refractive outcome and the safe preservation of the patient's best vision. The PERK study and the FDA PRK trials have used an uncorrected visual acuity of 20/40 or better as a measure of good efficacy in refractive surgery. Similarly, a refraction of ±1 D from the intended refraction has been considered good predictability. Decreased safety of a refractive surgical procedure has been defined in terms of the percentage of patients who have lost two lines or more of best spectacle corrected visual acuity following the procedure.

With the burgeoning of new refractive surgical procedures, there have been calls made for standardization of reporting of outcomes.[5,11] Well-conducted prospective trials are required to establish the efficacy, predictability, and safety of any new procedure. Reporting the quality of vision and refractive outcomes need to be standardized. Refractions should be cycloplegic, and a standard Snellen chart, such as that used for the Early Treatment Diabetic Retinopathy Study, should be used. Standardized contrast sensitivity testing is useful, and some measure of patient satisfaction can also be worthwhile. Not infrequently, patients can be unhappy despite good high-contrast visual acuity levels when they have other problems such as disabling glare, poor contrast sensitivity, or poor night vision. Standardization of vector analysis of astigmatism also helps in the comparison of outcomes between different treatments.[4]

Defining success in refractive surgery is continually being refined. One of the many pioneering achievements of the PERK study was to survey the patients to see how satisfied they were. In 328 patients 6 years after RK it was found that there were two measures that predicted high levels of patient satisfaction: not wearing distance glasses and an uncorrected visual acuity of 20/20 or better in the better eye. Having vision of 20/25 to 20/40 without glasses was a poor measure of good outcome with only about one third not wearing distance spectacles. Of those with a refraction ±1.00 D in both eyes, only 39% did not wear distance glasses. In contrast 77% of patients with an unaided visual acuity of 20/20 did not wear glasses, and 85% of patients within ±0.50 D of emmetropia did not wear glasses. The authors concluded that the best criteria for success of a refractive surgical procedure were uncorrected acuity of 20/20 or better and refraction of ±0.50 D. As refractive surgery progresses into the twenty-first century, these are the outcome measures that hopefully will be the most frequently quoted.

Incisional corneal surgery

Incisional keratotomy is one of the oldest and best studied refractive surgical procedures.[15-494] Surveys performed as late as 1994 established that RK was the most common refractive procedure in the United States with approximately 250,000 performed annually.[239-242] It involves near full thickness radial incisions in the cornea, from the peripheral cornea to the paracentral area. A central clear zone or optical zone is left uncut. The incisions gape under the influence of intraocular pressure producing a steepening of the peripheral cornea. A compensatory flattening of the central cornea occurs, shifting the refraction of the eye in the hyperopic direction. The amount of incision gape is positively correlated with the amount of corneal flattening.[350]

About 10% of all ophthalmologists in the United States perform RK.[24] Over 1 million people have undergone RK in the United States alone, making it the most common corneal refractive procedure in history. In comparison, by the mid 1990s, approximately 400,000 people have undergone PRK worldwide. Before the U.S. FDA approval of various excimer lasers in the mid 1990s, only 2,000 to 3,000 PRKs had been performed in the United States.

The principles of incisional keratotomy were first described in 1898 by Dutch ophthalmologist Leendert Jan Lans (Figs. 5-1, *A* and *B* and 5-2, *A* and *B*).[236] These principles were:

- the cornea flattens in the meridian of the incision
- there is more effect with deeper incisions
- healing results in some loss of effect

He also described the phenomenon of coupling. Coupling refers to the rule that when a transverse incision is made in the cornea, a compensatory steepening occurs in the perpendicular meridian. For example, when a transverse (astigmatic) keratotomy is performed, flattening of the cornea occurs in the meridian of the keratotomy and there is a coupled steepening of the opposite meridian.

SATO'S OPERATION (POSTERIOR RADIAL KERATOTOMY)

In the late 1930s, Japanese ophthalmologist Tsutomu Sato observed two patients with keratoconus who developed corneal flattening and a reduction in myopia after a rupture in Descemet's membrane. He subsequently proposed an operation in which incisions were made through the corneal endothelium and Descemet's membrane to treat keratoconus.[392] He then extended his work to the correction of myopia. He designed a sharp angled knife that could be inserted through the limbus and used to make posterior keratotomies from the anterior chamber.[393] Between 1938 and 1943 he operated on 200 patients. For myopia less than 2 D he recommended 45 radial incisions through Descemet's membrane made as deep as possible without perforating back out through the anterior surface of the cornea. For patients with more than 2 D, he recommended an additional 40 anterior radial incisions. Although this procedure was initially described as "proven, safe and efficacious" by Sato,[393] like so many subsequent new operations in the field of refractive surgery, time was to prove him wrong. Some 20 years after the procedure, many of the patients developed the inevitable consequences of corneal

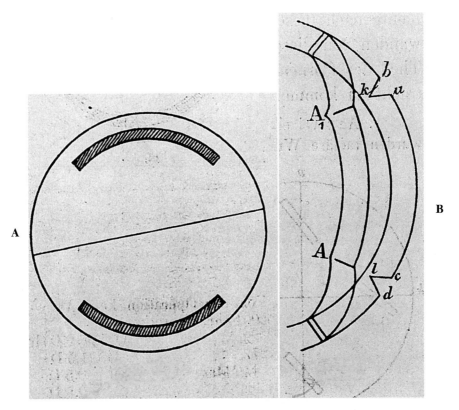

Fig. 5-1. Historic photographs of early attempts at refractive surgery incisions in a rabbit model. **A,** Sketch of an incision reminiscent of modern arcuate astigmatic keratotomy. **B,** Sketch of a section of a cornea showing conceptually the flattening of the cornea that occurs after partial thickness incisions. (From Lans, L: Experientelle Untersuchungen ueber Entstehung von Astigmatismus durch nicht-perforirende Corneawunden, Albrecht von Greafes Arch Ophthalmol 45:17, 1898.)

endothelial cell loss with corneal decompensation and bullous keratopathy.[17-19,48,213,488] More recently, the complication of retrocorneal ridges was described in a 51-year-old man who had undergone Sato's operation at the age of 14 years.[150]

RADIAL KERATOTOMY

In 1960 Svyatoslav Fyodorov of Russia began to experiment with Sato's posterior RK procedure.[457] Fyodorov and his colleague Valerie Durnev performed both laboratory and clinical studies (Fig. 5-3, *A* and *B*). They eliminated the disastrous posterior incisions and observed that 16 anterior corneal incisions produced as much effect as 32 incisions.[127] Fyodorov and Durnev observed that radial corneal

incisions resulted in a flattening of the central cornea and steepening of the peripheral cornea.[151] They also found that decreasing the diameter of the clear zone resulted in an increase in effect.[126]

Fyodorov and Durnev were also the first to develop an algorithm that incorporated surgeon and patient variables in an attempt to improve the predictability of RK.[152,153] Fyodorov tried to introduce RK to the United States in the 1970s but was unsuccessful.[94]

In 1976 Leo Bores from Detroit observed some of the RK procedures being performed on Fyodorov's patients in Moscow. He performed the first RK in the United States in 1978, prompting both interest by the popular press and debate among ophthalmologists.[71,72,75,106] Other ophthal-

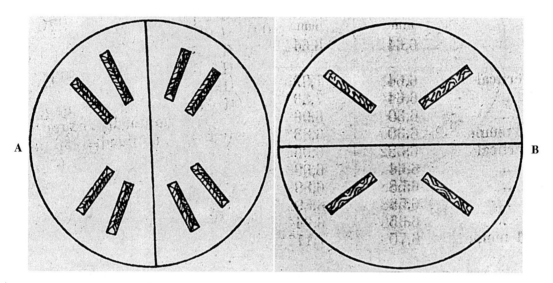

Fig. 5-2. Historic photographs of early attempts at refractive surgery incisions in a rabbit model. **A,** Sketch of radial incisions reminiscent of modern radial keratotomy, in this case 8 incisions. **B,** Sketch of 4 radial incisions reminiscent of modern "mini RK" with 4 incisions. (From Lans, L: Experientelle Untersuchungen ueber Entstehung von Astigmatismus durch nicht-perforirende Corneawunden, Albrecht von Greafes Arch Ophthalmol 45:17, 1898.)

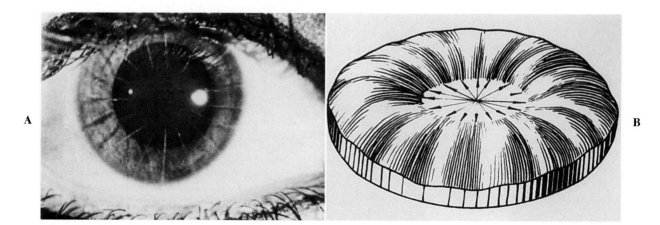

Fig. 5-3. Photographs from early work done in Moscow, representing a rebirth of the original research of procedure of Lans and Sato. **A,** Clinical photograph of a 16-incision radial keratotomy. **B,** Schematic illustration showing concept of corneal flattening following radial keratotomy. (From Fyodorov SN, and Durnev VV: Operation of dosaged dissection of corneal circular ligament in cases of myopia of mild degree, Ann Ophthalmol 11:1185, 1979.)

mologists also conducted clinical and laboratory trials.[°] Organized medicine, including the American Academy of Ophthalmology initially adopted a conservative posture and recommended nonsurgical alternatives such as contact lenses until controlled clinical trials had been performed.[21-25] In the early 1980s the National Eye Institute, in recognition of the need to evaluate the procedure, funded the PERK study.[10,13]

The prospective evaluation of radial keratotomy study

The PERK study involved 793 eyes of 435 patients enrolled at 9 centers in a scientific, prospective, collaborative study.[†] At entry into the study, the mean age of the patients was 33.5 years with a range from 21 to 58. A standardized technique with eight freehand, clear zone–to-limbus, centripetal incisions was used for the correction of myopia between −2.00 and −8.75 D. Repeat operations for undercorrections were performed by making eight additional incisions between the initial eight incisions. Ninety-seven of the 793 eyes (12%) had reoperations. After a 1-year wait to ensure that the procedure was safe, the patients could then have radial keratotomy on the fellow eye. Eighty-two percent elected to have surgery to the second eye.

The patients were treated in 1982 and 1983 and at the time of this writing 374 patients (693 eyes) returned for a 10-year, follow-up examination.[471] The most worrying statistic for all ophthalmologists practicing RK is the significant occurrence of progressive hyperopia that shows no sign of stopping, even after 10 years.[471] A steadily increasing number of PERK study patients are now overcorrected, nearly a quarter of them being 1.00 D or more hyperopic. As of 1995, at least half the patients are now into the presbyopic age group. They will need glasses or contact lenses for both distance and near vision.[77] Another important finding in the PERK study was the decrease in predictability of RK with increasing attempted myopic corrections.

The PERK study today stands as a landmark in refractive surgical clinical research. It was the first clinical refractive surgical study to have a combination of prospective design, standardization of surgical technique, quality control and independent statistical analysis of the results. As a consequence, it produced highly reliable data and set a standard of excellence for all future clinical trials of new refractive surgical techniques to follow.

Modern development of radial keratotomy

The techniques that the PERK study used in 1982 to 1983 are not those used today for modern RK.[454] Perhaps its greatest failure was not to include the age of the patient in the determination of how much surgery to perform. Age is now recognized as an important variable in all modern RK nomograms. Younger patients have less response to the same surgery as older patients.[372] As a result, inclusion of age as a variable in the surgical nomograms has improved

the predictability of modern RK. Three main refinements have occurred with modern RK. Firstly, RK has become a staged procedure. Intentional undercorrection is the aim of the first operation, and subsequent enhancement procedures are used to titrate the effect. Overcorrection is a far worse outcome than undercorrection as the overcorrected patient needs to either exert accommodation or use corrective lenses to be in focus for any distance. There are several ways of enhancing a RK procedure. Either the number of incisions can be increased from four to eight, or the incisions are redeepened after rechecking the pachymetry or the optical zone is decreased. Extending the incisions further toward the limbus is not very effective and may destabilize the cornea leading to progressive hyperopia.[96,146] Overall, modern RK involves more operations, but less surgery is performed with a better end result.

A second refinement has been to reduce the number and length of the incisions. While Russian RK used 16 to 32 incisions (Color Plate 5-1) and the PERK study 8 to 16, most modern RK is performed using only 4 to 8 incisions.[382,415,416] Very little additional refractive effect is obtained by going beyond eight incisions. Going from 8 to 16 incisions also increases the risk of complications such as microperforations and irregular astigmatism. In modern RK nomograms, four incisions produce about 60% of the refractive effect of eight incisions.[92] Some surgeons have also used six-incision RK in selected cases.

The third major improvement has been in instrumentation. More accurate ultrasonic pachymeters have improved the ability of surgeons to know the precise depth to set their diamond knifes. Accurate calibration microscopes for measuring the exact setting of the knife have also improved the accuracy of the incision depth. As a result, more consistency in the depth of the incisions is being achieved, and the more consistent the depth of the incisions the greater the precision of the operation. Other modern refinements include thinner diamond knives and guides to assist in making more controlled, straighter incisions.[54]

American, Russian, and combined (double-pass) techniques

In Russian-style RK the radial incisions are made from the limbus toward the central clear zone (centripetal) with a reverse cutting diamond knife. With this technique there is a significant risk of continuing the incision into the central clear zone. To avoid this often devastating complication, early American exponents of radial keratotomy changed the direction of the incisions. In the so-called American technique the incisions are made from the edge of the central clear zone toward the corneoscleral limbus (centrifugal).[78] Today with modern, thin profile diamond blades, epithelial stripping is rare.[117-119] Although the American-style incision reduces the chance of intrusion into the central clear zone, it is not as effective as the Russian-style incision, which results in a deeper incision than the American-style.[54,70,311,441] In a desire to combine the safety of the American-style incision with the efficacy of the Russian-style incision, the combined or double-pass–style incision was developed.[35,36,92] Special double-edged diamond knives are used, which allow an American-style incision to be performed with the forward edge and a Russian-

---

[°] References 15, 30-34, 45, 56, 57, 59, 61, 70, 105, 111, 118, 119, 129, 133, 147, 185, 191, 192, 206, 207, 212, 221, 231, 285, 290, 293, 294, 297, 314, 317, 318, 329, 330, 367, 368, 370, 371, 375, 378, 381, 394, 395, 400, 407, 408, 414, 415, 419, 420, 425, 447.
[†] References 454, 455, 458, 460, 464, 465, 471.

style incision to be made with the reverse edge (Duo-Tra and Genesis blades).

Results of modern radial keratotomy

The success of less surgery and a staged approach can be seen by comparing the number of overcorrected patients in the PERK study with more modern studies. A comparison of the PERK study with the nomograms developed and taught by Dr. J. Charles Casebeer is valid because about 75% of American RK surgeons employ his nomograms.[229] At 4 years postoperatively in the PERK study, 17% of 435 eyes were more than 1.00 D overcorrected (Color Plate 5-2). In comparison, in the Casebeer-Chiron study,[477] only 1% to 2% were overcorrected at 12 months. Uncorrected visual acuity of 20/40 or better was obtained in 99% in the Casebeer-Chiron study, compared to 74% to 88% in the PERK study. In reflection of the staged approach, the enhancement rate increased from the 12% of the PERK study to 33%. Another modern prospective study that compares the double-pass technique (Duo-Trak) with the Russian-style incision technique is underway in 15 centers in the United States.[110] One-year data are available in eyes that underwent double-pass RK. Postoperative visual acuity of 20/40 or better was achieved in 95% of the double-pass group and 97% of the Russian-style group. Less than 2% of patients lost two lines or more of best corrected visual acuity, and 91% to 93% were within 1.00 D of emmetropia.

Most modern American RK authorities recommend that corneal incisions do not go more peripherally in the cornea than 7.0 to 8.0 mm.[95,253] The smallest central optical zone that is currently recommended is 2.75 to 3.0 mm.[95,253] Modern RK, therefore, consists of the creation of four to eight deep (about 90% depth) radial incisions between a 7.0 to 8.0 mm outer ring and an inner optical zone of 2.75 to 5.5 mm. Radial keratotomy is a corneal weakening procedure, and the unsutured corneal wounds heal slowly, requiring as many as 5 or more years to remodel.[69,331,343] Recently, a technique termed *mini-RK* or minimally invasive RK has been developed to reduce the risks of RK.[253,346] Mini-RK extends the incisions only as far out as the 7.0-mm optical zone. In comparison, conventional RK extends out to the 11.0-mm optical zone. By leaving the most peripheral cornea untouched, it is hoped that as much corneal stability as possible can be preserved. Corneal instability results in long-term refractive instability, resulting in progressive hyperopia, diurnal fluctuation in vision, and a greater potential for traumatic rupture at the site of the keratotomy scars.* In a retrospective evaluation of 100 patients who had undergone mini-RK for myopia between −1.00 D and −6.00 D, Lindstrom reported that 92% of eyes were within 1.00 D of emmetropia and 94% had 20/40 or better uncorrected visual acuity.[253]

Wound healing after radial keratotomy

The refractive outcome of RK is modified by the wound healing response of the cornea (Figs. 5-4 and 5-5; Color Plates 5-3 and 5-4).† Modern RK nomograms take this into account by including age as a variable for estimating the

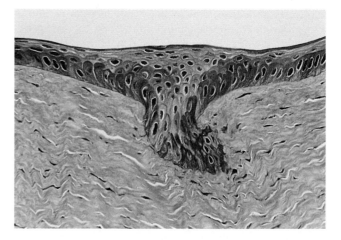

Fig. 5-4. Photomicrograph of an experimental radial keratotomy performed in a rabbit eye with somewhat delayed wound healing with formation of a relatively large epithelial facet that grows into the side of a gaping wound. (H & E stain; ×100.)

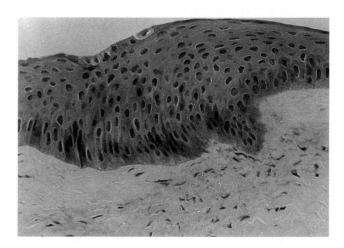

Fig. 5-5. Photomicrograph of radial keratotomy done in a rabbit, showing very poor apposition of the wound with formation of a large thick epithelial facet filling in the defect. (H & E stain; ×100.)

amount of surgery to perform; however, although older patients mount less aggressive corneal wound healing responses than younger patients, there is still some variation in corneal wound healing responses among patients of equivalent chronological age.[209] Unsutured corneal wounds through 90% of the corneal thickness heal slowly. Plugging of the incision with epithelium can persist for at least 7 years postoperatively.[168] Incomplete wound healing leading to a rupture of a RK wound during trephination for penetrating keratoplasty may occur as late as 9 years after the original surgery.[300] Other eyes heal well with the production of a mature scar.[69] The presence of an epithelial plug in the wound has been identified as a cause of poor wound strength in otherwise fully healed RK wounds.[81] Significant variability in wound strength occurs in fully healed RK wounds, depending on both epithelial plugging and the strength of the collagen fibers in the wound.[81]

After creation of a RK wound, the incision gapes produc-

---

* References 68, 69, 88, 125, 140, 168, 299, 343, 347.
† References 37, 154, 307, 341, 366, 418, 443, 451, 491.

ing peripheral corneal steepening and central corneal flattening.[83,84,345] The biomechanics of the cornea act as if tissue has been added in the incisions.[398,399] In reality, however, there is actually a gap between the edges of the incision into which new tissue grows. The first stage of healing of an unsutured corneal wound is epithelial healing.[67,85,205] Epithelial hemidesmosome attachments to its underlying basement membrane are lost in a zone on either side of the incision. Epithelial wound closure is not dependent on mitosis but on migration of cells from the basal layer and deep wing cell layers.[175] The filling of the wound by epithelial cells creates an epithelial plug.[26,199,205] The epithelium begins to synthesize new basement membrane and new anchoring fibrils. Anchoring fibrils, composed of type VII collagen, insert into hemidesmosomes in the basement membrane and then branch out into the underlying stroma. A tight network of anchoring fibrils and stromal collagen fibers holds the epithelium to the stroma.

On either side of the incision, stromal keratocytes transform into myofibroblast-like cells.[156] These cells produce new collagen and glycosaminoglycans, which are essential components in scar formation. On clinical slitlamp examination most patients appear to have healed their incisions within 2 to 3 years; however, others have incompletely healed incisions for up to 9 years.[300] The most consistent finding in human autopsy specimens has been the presence of an epithelial plug indicating incomplete healing.[*] The earliest that complete wound healing has been demonstrated in a human autopsy specimen has been at 5½ years postoperatively.[66] Abnormalities of corneal wound healing have been identified as the most common complication in corneal specimens removed at penetrating keratoplasty following repeated incisional keratotomy procedures.[65] Two factors that influence the rate of RK wound healing have been well established: increasing patient age is associated with slower corneal wound healing, and multiple corneal incisional procedures, especially when the incisions cross each other, have been identified as a factor that produces delayed corneal wound healing.[†] Other factors that are likely to delay epithelial wound healing are the amount of wound gape and the presence of any corneal instability. A wound that gapes more requires deposition of a greater amount of tissue within it to produce a mature scar.[345] Any technique that reduces the amount of wound gape, for example mini-RK, should help to reduce the incidence of wound healing problems.

A hyperopic shift of more than 1.00 D between 6 months and 8½ to 10 years postoperatively may occur in between 43% to 54% of patients.[115,210] Other reports that have studied the stability of refraction after RK have also identified hyperopic shifts.[33,328,397] It remains to be seen whether newer RK techniques utilizing smaller numbers of shorter incisions will reduce the incidence of consecutive hyperopia. If a hyperopic shift continues indefinitely in the more than 1 million Americans who have undergone RK to date, then there will be a serious epidemic of hyperopic, presbyopic, dissatisfied post-RK patients.

Surgical techniques to reduce hyperopia after RK are in a state of development. Hexagonal keratoplasty, hyperopic automated lamellar keratoplasty, and thermokeratoplasty have not been shown to be partially effective for correction of hyperopia after RK.[°] The best recommendation at present is to use sutures to reduce the amount of incision gape.[20] Both interrupted and continuous sutures can be successful in resteepening the central cornea and restoring good uncorrected visual acuity.[20,110,249,251,260]

Other complications of radial keratotomy

The American Academy of Ophthalmology statement on RK for myopia divides the potential complications into three groups[22]:

1. signs and symptoms that occur temporarily as part of the procedure
2. signs and symptoms that persist but do not decrease best corrected visual acuity
3. complications that potentially or actually disrupt visual function

Temporary sequelae includes postoperative pain, foreign body sensation, or aching. Glare and loss of contrast sensitivity can occur.[†] Undercorrection and overcorrection are the most frequent complications of RK, although modern staged techniques as detailed above, have reduced the incidence of overcorrections.[22,248,278] Diurnal fluctuation in vision and variations from one day to the next occur with decreasing severity during the first year but can continue for many years.[‡] The presence of a split or dumbbell shaped central optical zone on corneal topography indicates that the patient is more likely to suffer from diurnal fluctuation of vision.[292] Temporary loss of corneal sensitivity can be associated with deep transverse keratotomies performed for coexisting astigmatism.[412]

Radial keratotomy can increase the asphericity of the cornea and occasionally produce a multifocal cornea.[271,321] This can produce a beneficial increase in the depth of focus, but it can also result in confusing multiple images for some patients.[271] An increase in regular astigmatism and other minor to moderate complications such as epithelial iron lines, map-dot-fingerprint corneal epithelial patterns, epithelial inclusions cysts, a free floating cyst in the anterior chamber blepharoptosis, disruption of binocular vision, and blood in the incisions have been reported.[§] Several laboratory studies have shown variable degrees of endothelial cell damage beneath deep incisions in nonhuman primates.[‖]

Other complications that potentially reduce visual function can also occur after RK.[379] Loss of two or more lines of best corrected visual acuity in the PERK study occurred in between 1% to 3% of patients. Most of this loss is from 20/10 to 20/20. In the PERK study only 0.08% were not correctable to 20/20.[466] Because RK weakens the cornea, blunt trauma to the eye can cause rupture of the incisions with loss of intraocular contents.[¶] The weakening of the

---

* References 58, 66, 114, 199, 304, 305.
† References 65, 116, 167, 263, 279, 342, 372, 374.

° References 44, 93, 100, 195, 253, 427, 472, 492.
† References 27, 38, 76, 91, 165, 188, 230, 287, 435, 436.
‡ References 82, 106, 120, 232, 266, 388, 401, 485.
§ References 16, 33, 90, 123, 247, 325, 337, 369, 397, 423, 478, 484, 494.
‖ References 22, 51, 67, 103, 124, 197, 207, 264, 380, 390, 487, 489, 490.
¶ References 69, 202, 211, 243, 244, 258, 286, 299, 359, 376.

cornea can place the eye at greater risk of perforation from a foreign body. Case reports of this complication are currently used by military medicine authorities to bar the induction into the armed forces of enlistees who have undergone refractive corneal surgery.[331] While there is definite corneal weakening, there have also been case reports of post-RK eyes that have suffered severe blunt trauma without rupture of their corneal incisions.[99]

Although rare, some patients end up requiring penetrating keratoplasty following repeated incisional keratotomy procedures.[190,342] Severe loss of vision following RK is associated with aggressive and repeated incisional procedures to correct residual myopia, astigmatism, keratoconus, and hyperopic overcorrections.[389] Some patients can develop iatrogenic corneal ectasia after repeated procedures for myopic astigmatism.[475] Postoperative descemetocoele has been reported.[42] Radial keratotomy in patients with keratoconus can result in severe complications including corneal perforation, hypopyon, and corneal neovascularization.[125,130,275] Repeated procedures with crossing incisions can result in a persistent epithelial defect, sterile keratitis with vascularization, and corneal perforation.[158,214,410] Persistent epithelial defects can result in viral or bacterial keratitis months or years after the procedure.[121,183,284,385,386] Bilateral simultaneous RK is practiced by some surgeons in the United States. While this is efficient use of patient and surgeon time and may improve the symmetry of the outcome, there have been reports of bilateral microbial keratitis following bilateral procedures.[222,323,426]

Other vision threatening complications include macroperforations (Fig 5-6), cataract, retinal detachment, optic atrophy, bacterial or fungal keratitis, and endophthalmitis.*

The place of modern radial keratotomy

Radial keratotomy has largely been replaced by photorefractive keratectomy (PRK) in most countries other than the United States. This has not happened in the United States because of the long lag period between the first PRK procedure in 1987 and approval of the excimer laser by the U.S. FDA in 1995. During this period, RK gained considerable popularity among American refractive surgeons and reached full maturity as a refractive surgical procedure.[92,229,241,253] It has a well-defined place in the American refractive surgeons' armamentarium. Photorefractive keratectomy on the other hand is still a procedure undergoing refinement and new developments. Many authorities believe that even after the FDA approval for PRK, RK will survive for some time to come. Radial keratotomy future role will largely be limited to the correction of myopia between −1.00 D and −4.00 D. For corrections of −5.00 D or more RK is limited by problems such as undercorrection, variable refractive outcome, and "star burst" type glare due to small central optical zones.[47,406] For corrections less than −4.00 D RK continues to have advantages over PRK. Radial keratotomy requires less expensive equipment and is cheaper to perform. It produces faster visual rehabilitation with significantly less postoperative pain. Recovery after PRK is slower with a larger epithelial defect to heal, and a prolonged postoperative period of

---

* References 40, 129, 136, 159-161, 177, 186, 220, 222, 238, 245, 246, 276, 279, 282, 337, 364, 365, 426.

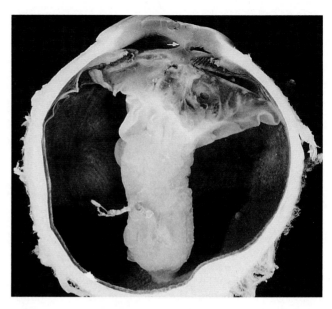

Fig. 5-6. Gross photograph of an eye following traumatic dehiscence of an incision 7 years after RK. Note total funnel shaped retinal detachment and adherent leukoma *(arrows)* between ruptured cornea and mass of intraocular granulation tissue. (Reproduced with permission from Glascow, BJ and others: Am J Ophthalmol 106:703, 1988.)

refractive instability occurs during the process of stromal remodeling. On the other hand there is more long-term fluctuation and volatility of vision and more reoperations with RK than there is with PRK. The long-term outlook for RK is better studied than PRK, but there is a concerning high rate of progressive hyperopia. One final and not to be overlooked appeal of PRK over RK is that of patient acceptance. Many patients find greater appeal in the prospect of having their vision corrected by a laser than with a surgeon wielding a diamond knife. This alone might be appeal enough for RK to be replaced by PRK in the United States, as it has been in most of the rest of the world.

TRANSVERSE (ASTIGMATIC) KERATOTOMY

Incisional surgery of the cornea to correct astigmatism was the first corneal refractive surgical procedure performed. With the start of cataract surgery last century so also began the beginning of surgically induced astigmatism. In the nineteenth century, Schiotz[402] described transverse keratotomy to try to correct a 33-year-old patient who developed 19.5 D of astigmatism following cataract surgery. Schiotz[402] and later Faber[134] performed penetrating transverse keratotomies. The first nonpenetrating corneal incisions for astigmatism were described in 1894 by Bates, an American ophthalmologist.[46,461] In 1898, Dutch ophthalmologist Leendert Jan Lans performed the first systematic laboratory studies of refractive surgery in rabbits. He was the first to describe the corneal phenomenon of coupling: flattening in the meridian perpendicular to the incision produces steepening in the opposite meridian. Coupling occurs during transverse keratotomies for astigmatism.

During the 1970s, surgeons reported on wedge resection techniques to deal with the large amounts of astigmatism that sometimes occurred following 160-degree limbal cataract incisions or penetrating keratoplasty.[41,201,384,437-441] Despite their effectiveness, wedge resections can induce significant irregular astigmatism with prolonged visual rehabilitation.[254] Combinations of tangential and radial incisions, also called trapezoidal keratotomies, can treat large amounts of astigmatism.[250] These procedures have been given various names including "butterfly," "Ruiz," and "bowtie."[195] Trapezoidal keratotomies can correct greater degrees of corneal astigmatism than transverse keratotomy alone, but its refractive effect is not as predictable as simple transverse keratotomy.* Histology of corneas that had undergone crossed combined semiradial and transverse keratotomies (trapezoidal) shows similar histology to that of RK incisions, except that the transverse incisions heal more rapidly than the radial incisions.[113] Epithelial plugging of the incisions is a frequent finding.

The development of modern transverse (astigmatic) keratotomy occurred in the early 1980s, about the time of the introduction and popularization of RK in the United States.[55,354] During this time, straight (nonarcuate) transverse keratotomies were often termed *T cuts*.[95,174,432,446] More recently, transverse keratotomy has been integrated into cataract surgery with the goal of achieving emmetropia for the patient. When a transverse keratotomy is performed the area where the incision is located increases in curvature and a compensatory flattening of the central cornea in the meridian of the incisions then occurs. Corneal coupling causes the opposite meridian to steepen. Transverse keratotomy is effective in reducing idiopathic astigmatism.[431,432] Correction of the patient's preexisting astigmatism has become an integral part of RK.[92,342,469,475]

In the late 1980s, cataract surgeons began to combine transverse keratotomy with phacoemulsification.[112,274,340,409] As a result, cataract surgery has progressed from merely being a procedure to improve vision to being a refractive procedure in itself. Modern cataract surgery now involves not just minimizing surgically induced astigmatism but reducing the patient's preexisting astigmatism as well.

Transverse keratotomy has also been combined with photorefractive keratectomy to correct myopic astigmatism.[255,361] Using the excimer laser to perform incisional transverse keratotomy has not been successful.[403] The combination of transverse keratotomy and compression sutures is currently considered to be a safer treatment of corneal astigmatism following penetrating keratoplasty than previously proposed techniques such as wedge resections.[196,283]

HEXAGONAL KERATOTOMY

Hexagonal keratotomy is an incisional corneal refractive procedure that involves the creation of six incisions in a hexagonal pattern in the midperipheral cornea, in effect defining a "new corneoscleral limbus." The central cornea within the hexagonal pattern then bows anteriorly, creating a steepening of the optic zone.[44] Hexagonal keratotomy has been used to reduce hyperopia, presbyopia, and overcorrected RK patients.

The first description of hexagonal keratotomy was from Akiyama in Japan,[17] and Yamashita and colleagues used anterior hexagonal keratotomy to correct hyperopia after overcorrected RK in rabbits.[492] Mendez[311] reported the first human use of the technique in 1987; several complications of corneal wound healing occurred. Several modifications have been described.*

Hexagonal keratotomy soon became controversial following its arrival in the United States.[144,181,333-335,476] Initially only isolated complications such as globe rupture after blunt trauma and production of irregular astigmatism were described.[288,427] Loss of two or more lines of best corrected visual acuity was reported in 15% of cases in one series and less than 4.0% in another.[19,172] By the mid 1990s combinations of complications including glare, photophobia, polyopia, fluctuation in vision, overcorrection, irregular astigmatism, corneal edema, corneal perforation, bacterial keratitis, cataract, and endophthalmitis occurred in a large number of patients. Most incisional refractive surgeons have now abandoned the procedure.

Lamellar corneal surgery[495-810]

Lamellar refractive procedures involve the use of incisions that are parallel with the anterior surface of the cornea.† These procedures alter the anterior corneal curvature by removing existing tissue, adding new tissue, or creating a controlled corneal ectasia. Because two thirds of the refractive power of the eye is located in the air/tear interface, these procedures are capable of large dioptric corrections. Lamellar corneal refractive procedures are most commonly performed for myopia, particularly higher degrees of myopia. There has also been some reported success with lamellar procedures that reduce hyperopia by steepening the anterior corneal surface.

KERATOMILEUSIS

Myopic cryokeratomileusis

The father of lamellar keratoplasty is Dr. Jose Barraquer of Bogota, Columbia. He described his original keratomileusis technique in 1949 and performed the first case in 1964.‡ First, a 300-μm-thick disc was dissected from the anterior cornea in a freehand fashion using a Paufique knife or corneal dissector.[748,749] He then transported this disc of tissue across Bogota to a separate facility and glued it to a contact lens lathe and froze the tissue to make it rigid. The posterior surface was then reshaped to thin out the center and create a concave lens. He then transported this lens shaped piece of cornea back to the operating room and repositioned it onto the patient's eye with two interrupted sutures. Barraquer's initial results appeared promising with over 80% experiencing a visual improvement.[521] Some problems occurred with epithelial growth into the interface and irregular astigmatism, but only two serious infections occurred in the first 400 cases.[521]

Barraquer developed keratomileusis from these early beginnings and in the process invented most of the techniques used today. He developed the motorized keratome

---

* References 15, 33, 95, 154, 292, 357.

---

* References 44, 97, 144, 163, 170, 172, 203, 204, 326, 327, 338, 362.
† References 498, 533, 630, 631, 660, 731, 789, 803.
‡ References 510-513, 515, 516, 518, 519, 521, 522, 661, 775.

and added a suction ring to fix the keratome to the eye. Lamellar keratotomies performed with a mechanized keratome are more consistent in depth and smoothness than those performed freehand.[534] He also began to use lamellar surgery for correction of hyperopia. He was able to use the cryolathe to thin the midperiphery of the anterior stromal cap, so that when it was placed back onto the eye the anterior corneal surface was made steeper.

Other refractive surgical pioneers adopted Barraquer's keratomileusis technique. These included Ainslie[737] of England in the late 1960s, Fyodorov[595] of Russia in the early 1970s, and Troutman,[771-774] Swinger,[755-761] Kaufman,[594,629] and Nordan[706,707] in the United States. While early results were promising, the main difficulty with myopic keratomileusis is the technical difficulty of the procedure and the steep learning curve. One report documented a series of 61 eyes with preoperative refractions between −4.00 and −8.00 D.[717] After a mean follow-up of 28 months, 61% were within 1.00 D of emmetropia and 72% had 20/40 or better uncorrected visual acuity. After myopic cryokeratomileusis, irregular astigmatism is present in the majority of patients immediately postoperatively and remains the most problematic and common complaint. Reports of its incidence vary from 3.3% to 39%.[519,707,717]

Freezing of the corneal stroma causes a number of adverse effects. Morphological changes include a loss of keratocytes, which can result in corneal haze.[537,723] The frozen tissue needs to be repopulated with keratocytes to maintain its long-term viability. Histologic analyses of human and nonhuman primate corneas following freeze myopic keratomileusis have shown low anterior stromal keratocyte counts and degenerated keratocytes.[526,626,715,806] Other findings include breaks or attenuation of Bowman's layer, porous collagen bundles, irregular epithelial maturation areas of epithelial ingrowth, and subepithelial fibrocellular growth.[526,536,715,781] Corneal sensitivity is reduced in comparison to nonfreeze techniques.[643]

The steep learning curve and complexity of the equipment meant that the majority of surgeons who took up keratomileusis in the 1970s and 1980s did not continue with the technique.

Barraquer-Krumeich-Swinger noncryokeratomileusis

Jose Barraquer was also the first to experiment with non-freeze keratomileusis techniques.[749] Initial refractive results were more variable than freeze myopic keratomileusis because of the poor accuracy of the microkeratome resection. In an attempt to reduce the complexity of the procedure Drs. Barraquer, Krumeich, and Swinger (BKS) developed an improved system that bears their names.[652]

The major advantage of the BKS system is that it does not involve freezing of corneal tissue and, therefore, causes less corneal morphological damage than with in techniques.[809] Despite this, visual rehabilitation was slow, with up to 12 months required to recover best corrected visual acuity, and as many as 30% of eyes lost two or more lines of best corrected visual acuity.[571,581] Significant regression of the refractive correction occurred.[548] In one series only about 5% of high myopes achieved 20/40 uncorrected visual acuity after the BKS procedure.[550] Although results have been variable, patients having the BKS procedure are more comfortable and recover vision more rapidly than in freeze myopic keratomileusis, and, as such, it was considered a major advance.[655,748,749]

Myopic keratomileusis in situ (manual)

Dr. Jose Barraquer and his colleague, Dr. Luis Ruiz, continued to refine keratomileusis in situ.[736,748] In keratomileusis in situ, after the resection of an anterior corneal cap, a refractive cut is made with a second microkeratome pass in the stromal bed. This is in contrast to both classical myopic cryokeratomileusis and the BKS technique in which the removal of tissue takes place in the resected cap. Another difference is that the piece of corneal tissue removed from the stromal bed is a lamellar disc (plano-cut) rather than the lens-shaped resection in keratomileusis and the BKS technique. Early series of manual keratomileusis in situ demonstrated the unpredictability of the refractive results.[500,524]

Myopic automated in situ keratomileusis (myopic automated lamellar keratoplasty)

With manual keratomileusis in situ performed with a hand-driven Barraquer microkeratome proving to be neither precise nor predictable, a new more refined microkeratome was developed, and Dr. Ruiz added an automated geared system to Dr. Barraquer's microkeratome to control the speed of the pass across the cornea (Fig. 5-7).[736] This improved the accuracy of the thickness of the resection of corneal tissue. Use of the Ruiz/Steinway geared microkeratome has increased rapidly in the United States, and the procedure has been successfully marketed as "automated lamellar keratoplasty" (ALK).° The term *automated* refers to the pass of the microkeratome being controlled by the mechanics of the keratome rather than by the surgeon.

° References 495, 499, 509, 650, 667, 745, 746, 750, 801.

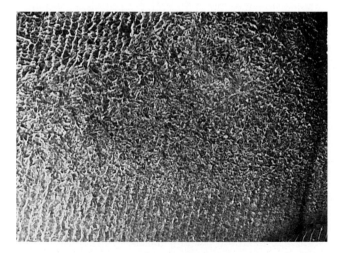

Fig. 5-7. Scanning electron micrograph of a human cornea obtained postmortem following automated lamellar keratoplasty performed experimentally after incubation in organ culture. The anterior corneal flap has been excised to reveal the stromal bed. Note the serrated lines produced by the vibrating metal blade in both the central refractive cut area and the peripheral area. (×10.)

Apart from this change, the procedure is essentially an evolution of Barraquer's keratomileusis. The term *automated in situ keratomileusis* is, therefore, more accurate.[618]

Rozakis[731] describes three theories regarding the mechanism of automated in situ keratomileusis:

1. Positive lenticle theory: small discs are actually positive lenticles, while larger discs are parallel faced. Removal of a small disk, therefore, reduces the central corneal power.
2. Divot theory: the cap or flap falls into the divot created by the resected disc. The cornea flattens in divots up to 5 mm in diameter; greater diameters produce negligible effects.
3. Ridge theory: the keratectomy edge causes corneal flattening. The blade has a downslope of about 25 degrees. The concept here is that the downslope of the cap at the edge of the keratectomy causes abrupt flattening, and, in small keratectomies, the cornea cannot resteepen.

Ricardo and Guimaraes[748] found that it was not necessary to suture the corneal cap, thus reducing suture-induced astigmatism. When placed back onto the bare corneal stroma, the cap adheres to the underlying stroma within a few minutes. This adherence may be enhanced by glycosaminoglycans in the corneal stroma. Keratin sulfate and chondroitin sulfate are so hydrophilic that they act like a tissue glue or the corneal endothelium creates a negative pressure within the stroma that sucks the flap and the posterior stroma together. This theory is supported by micropipette measurements of a high negative pressure within the central corneal stroma.[802] The human corneal stroma has a mean swelling pressure of more than 80 mm Hg because of the hydrophilic nature of its glycosaminoglycans. To prevent the cornea from swelling, the corneal endothelium must constantly pump fluid against this pressure gradient.[659] A second advance was to make an anterior corneal flap rather than resecting a cap by stopping the microkeratome from making a complete passage across the cornea.[566,735]

Several published reports of the results of automated in situ keratomileusis have appeared, and results have been good.[623,664,685,719,731] Some prominent refractive surgeons have spoken out against the increasing popularity of automated in situ keratomileusis and called for a more scientific appraisal of the refractive results.[786,787] They point out that the refractive cut is only 4.5 mm, placing the inflection zone of corneal curvature within the normal pupil under low light conditions as well as creating optical aberrations. There have been reports of other surgical complications. Inadvertent penetration of the anterior chamber due to faulty assembly of the microkeratome can occur.[587] When automated in situ keratomileusis is performed in corneas that have undergone prior surgical procedures, wound healing problems are common.[669] This can lead to loss of the anterior corneal cap or flap.[669] Histologically, the features of caps removed for complications after automated in situ keratomileusis include bullous keratopathy, abnormally thin epithelium, epithelial growth between the cap and the bed, stromal scarring, and stromal inflammation.

Automated lamellar keratoplasty is currently on a wave of popularity among refractive surgeons in the United States. For the most part this has been due to the slow FDA approval process for PRK. With most surgeons limiting RK to the − 1.00 D to − 4.00 D range and PRK only approved for up to − 7.00 D, there has until recently been no other procedure that refractive surgeons in the United States could offer patients with greater degrees of myopia. Automated in situ keratomileusis is no longer the only viable option for correction of high myopia in the United States; the FDA is now allowing use of the more accurate laser in situ keratomileusis (LASIK) procedure.

Despite its problems, automated in situ keratomileusis has certainly helped to pave the way for the development of LASIK. The surgeons who are experienced with the microkeratome used for automated in situ keratomileusis are, not surprisingly, the same surgeons who are taking part in the FDA trials of LASIK. Surgeons outside the United States, who are not controlled by the FDA, have largely abandoned automated in situ keratomileusis in favor of LASIK.

Capless automated in situ keratomileusis (capless automated lamellar keratoplasty)

Hollis and Suarez observed that when a cap was lost following automated in situ keratomileusis, the bed reepithelialized and the myopic refractive change was maintained.[734] Both surgeons have developed nomograms for one-pass correction of myopia, up to − 17.00 D. This procedure is similar in concept to excimer laser PRK, except that the accuracy of the microkeratome is not as good as the laser. It is rarely, if at all, practiced today because it can cause irregular astigmatism and corneal scarring in some eyes.[787]

Hyperopic automated in situ keratomileusis (hyperopic automated lamellar keratoplasty)

Ruiz developed a method of correcting hyperopia using automated in situ keratomileusis.[620,636,670,733] The procedure involves using the microkeratome to make a lamellar cut at a depth of two thirds or more of the corneal thickness. The thin remaining cornea then undergoes a degree of ectasia so that the corneal curvature is steeper. Today most surgeons use a hinged flap technique.

Ruiz and Hollis[545] developed a nomogram that varies with two factors: the diameter of the resection and the depth of the cut. With smaller diameters and deeper cuts, the greater the hyperopic correction.

Several investigative series have been published.[665,719] Some surgeons maintain that hyperopic automated in situ keratomileusis is an excellent procedure for correcting the hyperopia induced by overcorrected RK.[620] Others have opposed this view noting that the deep corneal incisions required to correct more than 3.00 D of hyperopia may risk the development of a progressive myopic shift.[725,787] This shift has been called "iatrogenic keratoconus" by Luiz Ruiz.[725] Regression has also been considerable in hyperopic automated in situ keratomileusis.[725] This is true of all current procedures for the correction of hyperopia.

Homoplastic keratomileusis and automated in situ keratomileusis

A microkeratome can also be used to cut donor and host lenticles for therapeutic lamellar keratoplasty.[718] The primary indication is anterior corneal scarring that is too deep to treat with phototherapeutic keratectomy (Color Plates 5-5 and 5-6). The use of donor tissue to replace the excised corneal scar tissue has led to the use of the term *homoplas-*

tic being applied to both keratomileusis and keratophakia and more recently to automated lamellar keratoplasty.[497,551,568,607,610] A much smoother cut of the cornea can be made with a microkeratome than can be made manually, and this is one of the reasons for the successful visual results of lamellar refractive surgery.[65] In contrast, manually performed lamellar keratoplasty almost always results in some degree of interface haze that limits vision to about the 20/40 level.[720] Radiograph diffraction studies have shown that this does not appear to be the result of changes in the spacing of the collagen fibrils. It may be because of either graft malapposition or the formation of intrastromal, fluid-filled, collagen-free "lakes."[720]

KERATOPHAKIA

Classical cryokeratophakia

Keratophakia (corneal lens) is a technique in which a biconvex lens–shaped piece of tissue is sandwiched into the corneal stroma to steepen the corneal curvature and, thereby, correct hyperopia or aphakia. The procedure was also developed by Jose Barraquer and was the first lamellar refractive surgical procedure ever performed.[517,523] His original procedures involved the use of the cryolathe to shape the donor corneal tissue.[250,522] The technique was adopted in both Russia and the United States in the 1970s.° Even in the largest series with the most experienced surgeons, however, there was considerable variability in the refractive outcome, irregular astigmatism could be induced, and there were technical difficulties.[756,761,764]

As with other cryolathed corneal tissue in keratomileusis and epikeratoplasty, the frozen lenticle is devoid of viable keratocytes and repopulation with host keratocytes is slow.†

In the late 1970s, researchers working with Dr. Herbert Kaufman began the development of preserved precut corneal lenticles for keratophakia.[592-594] They thought that the free availability of precut corneal lenticles would make keratophakia a more viable operation for larger numbers of refractive surgeons. Techniques to allow shaping of keratophakia lenticles without freezing began in the early 1980s, and later the excimer laser was also tried.[596,617,666]

With more advanced microkeratomes, it is no longer necessary to freeze the tissue. In current practice, keratophakia for hyperopia is performed using fresh, unfrozen donor corneal tissue taken from patients who have just undergone myopic automated lamellar keratoplasty.[648] The use of human tissue still makes the refractive outcome quite variable.

Intrastromal corneal implants

Instead of using human corneal tissue in keratophakia, a piece of synthetic tissue can be utilized.[800] Potentially, a piece of synthetic tissue can be machined to a precise thickness far more accurately than human corneal tissue; however, the synthetic tissue must be highly biocompatible, have a high refractive index, and have high oxygen and water permeability to allow sufficient nutrition to the overlying stroma.[526]

The use of hydrogel as a material for keratophakia (intracorneal lens) has been extensively studied in nonhuman models.° Initially, it seemed as if the hydrogel implants would be well tolerated, and some implants survived in monkey corneas as long as 8½ years.[530,710,712] Later, it became apparent that there were significant complications in some eyes.[529,681] While some of these complications were attributed to problems with surgical technique, other complications were not.

Polysulfone lenses have shown some promise, particularly in view of their high refractive index. Animal studies had variable results, with reported complications including interface opacities, lens extrusion, anterior corneal necrosis, refractile particles, and epithelial thinning.[570,576,653,654]

At present there are ongoing trials in the United States and Australia with hydrogel intracorneal lenses for the correction of presbyopia. These lenses are much smaller than previous intracorneal lenses at 2.0 to 2.5 mm in diameter. The small diameter means that the lenses are thinner, allowing easier diffusion of water and oxygen through and around them. The lens corrects presbyopia by increasing the central dioptric power of the cornea by 1.0 to 2.0 D. The patient is able to see around the lens to maintain distance vision. To be successful the patient's brain has to switch from the distance image to the near image and vice versa.

Epikeratoplasty (Epikeratophakia)

The complexity and expense of the cryolathe used for keratomileusis and freeze myopic keratomileusis discouraged many surgeons from continuing with these procedures. To eliminate the cryolathe, Kaufman and Werblin developed preserved corneal lenticles. These lenticles were discs of tissue removed from a donor eye, frozen and then lathed into concave or convex lenses. This was the technique of epikeratophakia—later to be called epikeratoplasty.[495,499] In contrast to keratophakia, in which the preserved corneal lenticle was placed within the anterior corneal stroma, they placed the lenticle onto the deepithelialized anterior corneal surface and the epithelium then grows over the donor lenticle and keratocytes repopulate it. The lenticle was described as a "living contact lens," although it did not contain any living keratocytes and was not immunogenic for the host.[686] It was proposed that epikeratoplasty would allow correction of a wide range of refractive errors, such as high myopia, astigmatism, aphakia, and keratoconus.† The procedure was reversible and far less invasive than keratomileusis or keratophakia. Morgan suggested that epikeratoplasty was a useful procedure in monocular pediatric aphakia; however, problems with significant undercorrection of infants younger than 6 months of age were identified.‡ A significant myopic shift was identified over time in children younger than 1 year of age because of the growth in axial length of the infant eye.[503,681,690] Five-year follow-up of epikeratoplasty in chil-

---

° References 592, 593, 595, 769, 771, 773, 774, 780, 792.

† References 526, 537, 539, 621, 625, 626, 635, 640, 715, 723

° References 528, 532, 534, 538, 541, 542, 668, 674, 702, 711, 743, 788, 791, 798, 799, 810.

† References 543, 552, 553, 555, 556, 558, 578, 583, 608, 609, 611, 614, 616, 621, 622, 629, 632, 633, 656, 657, 676-678, 722, 728, 757, 779, 790.

‡ References 502, 503, 584, 687-690, 692, 694-696, 698, 699, 777, 778.

dren showed successful grafts in 89%, and epikeratoplasty also seemed to have a role in the visual rehabilitation of contact lens intolerant aphakic children.[635,693] Favorable results in the correction of pediatric aphakia and in treatment of children with corneal lacerations and aphakia following trauma were reported.[°]

Epikeratoplasty was also trialed for the correction of adult aphakia.[†] Unfortunately, many aphakic patients may lose some vision, largely because of wound healing complications.[682] In the correction of adult aphakia in the mid 1980s, similar visual acuity results were reported for both epikeratoplasty and secondary anterior chamber intraocular lenses.[508,582]

In the correction of myopia, early results were successful, but some complications occurred.[637,678,682] Promising results were obtained in multicenter trials of epikeratoplasty for the correction of keratoconus.[677,682] Uncorrected visual acuity improved in 99% of cases, and the risk of corneal graft rejection inherent in penetrating keratoplasty was avoided. The safety advantages of an extraocular procedure were appealing, and, if necessary, a penetrating keratoplasty could still be performed at a later date.[590] Despite these successes, surgeons have reported significant complications including interface scarring and folds in Descemet's membrane sufficient to reduce visual acuity to the 20/200 level.[726] Visual results of penetrating keratoplasty are still better than epikeratoplasty; as many as 98% of patients achieve 20/40 or better in corrected visual acuity after penetrating keratoplasty for keratoconus.[770] Management of corneal graft rejection episodes has also improved in the decades since epikeratoplasty for keratoconus was developed.[573,776] Later studies concluded that epikeratoplasty in keratoconus was best reserved for cases with no central corneal scarring, intolerance of contact lenses, corneal curvature flatter than 60 D, in patients with mental retardation, and in patients willing to tolerate both reduced contrast sensitivity and less than 20/20 best corrected visual acuity.[572,617,783]

The complications inherent in using frozen corneal tissue also occurred with epikeratoplasty.[602,603] The lenticles do not contain any living keratocytes, and repopulation with host keratocytes is necessary for the long-term viability of the donor lenticle.[‡] The growth of host epithelium over a denervated corneal surface resulted in a number of epithelial morphological abnormalities.[721] Histology of epikeratoplasty lenticles in nonhuman primates shows keratocyte debris, focal breaks in Bowman's layer,[567,743,807] and irregular epithelial maturation.[526,567,743,807] Significant bends and fractures of Bowman's membrane can occur as well as an increase in the distance between collagen fibrils.[535] Histology of corneas at penetrating keratoplasty can show abnormal morphology in the keratocytes in the underlying host stroma.[§] Human specimens removed because of stromal folding and decreased visual acuity have also shown discontinuities and folds in Bowman's layer.[574,763] The epithelium overlying the removed lenticles was vacuolated with a

thickened basement membrane and reduced numbers of hemidesmosomes.[763] Other complications also reported include scarring in the host Bowman's layer and interface hematomata.[718,752]

While many patients did well after epikeratoplasty, there was significant variability in refractive outcome. Part of this inaccuracy was because of variation in the changes in thickness of the lenticle that occurred with freezing. The rate of visual recovery was relatively slow, as the lenticle needed to be gradually repopulated with host keratocytes. Very few patients attained 20/20 vision as interface opacities and corneal haze were common. After myopic epikeratoplasty there was clinically significant regression between 6 and 12 months.[601] Myopic regression after epikeratoplasty is most likely the result of the period of stromal collagen remodeling, which occurs postoperatively.[628] Clinical complications included interface opacity from epithelial ingrowth in about 7% to 20% of cases.[554,691] Corneal topography after epikeratoplasty for myopia showed that the effective optical zone was smaller than predicted by the lathing measurements.[668] Loss of contrast sensitivity after myopic epikeratoplasty has been reported to be greater than after RK.[563]

A number of variations on the technique were devised in an attempt to improve the procedure. Approaches were devised to avoid freezing the tissue. Lathing the tissue without freezing has been attempted, and others tried the BKS technique (as described earlier) to shape the lenticles.[°] The accuracy of refractive outcome was less predictable than desired, but the rate of visual recovery was greater.[550] Altmann reported using an excimer laser to shape the tissue, but this remained a laboratory technique.[496] Thompson has reported the use of type IV collagen as a synthetic epikeratoplasty lenticle in a monkey model with mixed results.[767,768]

The difficulties of epikeratoplasty were eventually too great for the procedure to survive. The removal rate of epikeratoplasty lenticles was high, and the procedure was unpredictable and unstable because of bending of the epikeratoplasty lenticle.[787] The FDA denied approval for the production of lenticles for the correction of myopia.[574] The U.S. company (Allergan Medical Optics) that prepared the frozen lenticles ceased production. Consequently, epikeratoplasty is no longer or rarely performed today in the United States. Some surgeons continue to use it for selected cases and are investigating the role of various cryoprotective agents.[808]

Laser refractive surgery[811-1464]

PHOTOREFRACTIVE KERATECTOMY

Photoablative lasers

Excimer laser surgery of the cornea for the correction of refractive errors was first described by Trokel and Srinivasan in 1983.[1420-1422] Their report and others[1069,1104,1105,1294,1449] focused on the ability of the excimer laser to remove corneal tissue with great precision, leaving the surrounding tissue undamaged. The excimer laser is a pulsed ultraviolet laser with a wavelength of 193 nm. The photons of the excimer laser are strongly absorbed

---

° References 505, 628, 688, 689, 693, 697.
† References 501, 505, 588, 662, 667, 675, 679, 680, 682, 683, 793-797.
‡ References 535, 569, 628, 631, 686, 743.
§ References 535, 738, 739, 741, 744, 751.

° References 550, 580, 581, 584, 589, 651, 729.

by corneal tissue and penetrate less than the depth of a cell. Excimer laser photons have sufficient energy (6.4 eV) to break molecular bonds. The ablated tissue leaves the cornea as gas molecules traveling as fast as 400 m/sec.[1283]

It was first thought that the excimer laser would be best used as a "laser knife" to make radial or transverse incisions in the cornea.* This approach was not very successful as the excimer laser removes rather than just cuts corneal tissue. In effect, it creates a radial keratectomy rather than RK. Compared with diamond knife incisions, this stimulated an increased wound healing response with more fibroblastic infiltration.[1081] It also proved difficult to precisely control the depth of the incisions.[851] Another application that was envisioned was its use in performing corneal trephination for penetrating keratoplasty. It has been demonstrated that the excimer laser is able to perform trephination with great accuracy.†

In the mid 1980s it was realized that the excimer laser beam could be used to ablate corneal tissue from the central surface layers of the cornea with a large diameter beam.[1038,1185,1223] By using an expanding or contracting diaphragm, more tissue could be removed from the central than the peripheral cornea producing a permanent flattening of the corneal curvature.[1264] This technique is now called photorefractive keratectomy (PRK).‡

To date, the laser that has been almost universally used for PRK is the argon-fluoride excimer laser that has a wavelength of 193 nm. The name "excimer" is a contraction of "excited dimer." High energies are used to bond together the inert gas argon to the highly reactive fluorine and the molecule breaks down rapidly to emit radiation. Other lasers such as solid state lasers with wavelengths in the region of 200 nm are alternatives to the excimer laser§ and are currently undergoing clinical trials. Both excimer and solid-state ultraviolet wavelength lasers produce high energy pulses of radiation that cleave intermolecular bonds and turn the corneal tissue into gas.[1083,1283] This process is termed *photoablation*.

The major advantage of a photoablative laser is its great accuracy of tissue ablation.[1104,1105,1187,1317,1421] Each pulse removes less than a micron of corneal tissue without thermal damage to the underlying tissue.‖ Using computer-controlled algorithms the surgeon can accurately control the depth and diameter of the ablation. The excimer laser can create a much smoother ablation surface in the cornea than any steel or diamond blade.[880,957,1085,1131-1134,1188] Theoretically, the laser can create any anterior radius of curvature in the central cornea by the controlled removal of small amounts of tissue. Little or no damage to the underlying stroma occurs, and there is no significant structural weakening of the cornea.[874] Both controlled flattening of the anterior corneal surface to correct myopia and steepening to correct hyperopia are possible.[858]

There is some discrepancy between most experimentally determined ablation rates and the nominal ablation rate of 0.23 to 0.3 μm per pulse used for clinical procedures. Most experimentally determined ablation rates have been derived from studies on deep keratectomies on autopsy corneas. In these experiments excimer lasers with laser beam energies of 180 mJ/cm^2 were found to ablate 0.4 to 0.5 μm of corneal tissue per pulse.[935,1104,1189,1328,1360] Using this ablation rate in early clinical PRK resulted in insignificant undercorrection.[1243,1451] Through a process of trial and error, a so-called nominal ablation rate of 0.23 to 0.3 μm was determined.[1360] In a recent clinical study Spigelman and associates determined the true ablation rate of anterior corneal stroma by the use of a Scheimpflug camera.[1360] They were able to show that the true ablation rate of in vivo anterior cornea stroma is the same as the nominal ablation rate.

Following successful blind eye studies,* the first sighted human eye was treated in June 1988 by McDonald and colleagues. Trials in Germany and England began soon afterwards.† The first generation excimer lasers use either a diaphragm that expands or contracts with each pulse of the laser. The effect of this is to ablate more tissue in the center of the cornea than in the periphery resulting in a flattening of the corneal curvature. A simple expanding or contracting diaphragm, however, tends to produce an ablation pattern in the cornea that has small steps in it. Recently, newer algorithms and mechanical techniques have been used to create smoother ablation profiles in the cornea. These techniques for shaping the laser beam include multizone ablation algorithms, rotating masks, scanning slit beams, wobbling mirrors, and scanning "flying spot" beams.[1038-1040]

Operative procedure

The procedure is performed under topical anesthesia. Usually the epithelium is mechanically removed, although some surgeons are now removing the epithelium with the laser.[813,1005] Once the epithelium is removed the ablation of the underlying anterior corneal stroma takes about 30 seconds and usually less than 2 minutes.

The amount of tissue ablated depends on the diameter of the optical zone and the degree of refractive correction attempted. Early excimer lasers used optical zones of 4.5 to 5.0 mm. These small optical zones lead to side effects such as glare and halos at night when the pupil is dilated. Most lasers now employ optical zones of 6.0 to 7.0 mm. Deeper ablations are required to effect greater refractive changes. The central ablation depth of a myopic ablation is approximately equal to[1207]

$$\frac{(\text{Number of diopters of myopic correction}) \times (\text{Ablation zone diameter in mm})^2}{3}$$

The formula shows that the larger the optical zone, the greater the ablation depth required for a given correction.

---

* References 829, 830, 843, 851, 921, 1081, 1104, 1188, 1187, 1301.
† References 596, 1062, 1118, 1119, 1143, 1179, 1338, 1408.
‡ References 834, 839, 840, 846, 853-856, 860, 865, 867, 871, 885, 914, 915, 918, 919, 932, 933, 938, 940, 942, 964, 965, 975, 977, 980, 986, 989, 990, 993, 999, 1000, 1003, 1018, 1019, 1031, 1033, 1035, 1044, 1051, 1068, 1069, 1071, 1074, 1086-1093, 1101-1108, 1123, 1127, 1135-1138, 1144, 1146, 1157, 1158-1160, 1167, 1183, 1189, 1198, 1201, 1203, 1205, 1206, 1212, 1213, 1216, 1222-1225, 1240, 1255, 1258, 1274, 1295, 1306-1309, 1318-1366, 1374, 1384, 1387, 1388, 1398, 1409, 1410, 1415, 1420, 1430, 1433, 1435, 1443, 1453-1457, 1460.
§ References 847, 987, 1096, 1097, 1271, 1291, 1292, 1423-1425, 1440.
‖ References 1084, 1188, 1283, 1294, 1360, 1361.

* References 1115, 1116, 1194, 1195, 1389, 1390.
† References 944, 988, 1135, 1136, 1142, 1197, 1237, 1325, 1327, 1342, 1461.

Hyperopic corrections with the excimer laser require even larger optical zones of up to 9 mm. In an attempt to improve centration, some lasers now have active eye trackers that allow the laser beam to follow small amplitude eye movements.[1015,1278,1376] After the procedure, antibiotic eyedrops are instilled, and either a therapeutic soft contact lens or an eye patch is used to protect the bare corneal stroma.

Quite severe postoperative pain can occur,[1367] often peaking at 4 to 6 hours, and sometimes persisting as long as 36 to 48 hours. This may be due to release of prostaglandin E_2 in the cornea.[1207] Nonsteroidal antiinflammatory drugs (NSAIDs) inhibit the enzyme cyclooxygenase, thus blocking production of prostaglandins including prostaglandin E_2.[879,902,1273,1377,1378] Eyedrops with a NSAID, such as diclofenac, have been shown in double-blind clinical trials to reduce postoperative pain.[943,1154,1229,1345] The role of postoperative topical corticosteroid eyedrops in possibly reducing postoperative corneal haze and regression continues to be investigated in clinical trials.[832,962,1156,1399] Topical sodium hyalmonate after PRK has been investigated.[811]

Correction of myopia

Photorefractive keratectomy has been most successful in the treatment of myopia from −1 to −6 D. Despite the inherent accuracy of the laser's ability to ablate the cornea, there is still considerable interpatient variability.[936,947] Some patients mount a weaker than average wound healing response to the anterior keratectomy and end up overcorrected. Other patients mount a stronger than average wound healing response and end up undercorrected. The greater the attempted refractive correction, the more variable the refractive outcome. As the attempted correction goes over −6 D,[897,905,923,971,1034,1300,1339,1344] the percentage of patients within ±1 D of the intended refraction drops below 80% and over −8 D, efficacy and predictability drop to unacceptable levels.

Correction of astigmatism

The excimer laser has met with varied success in the correction of astigmatism. The very first clinical use of the excimer laser was in the correction of astigmatism. In 1985 Theo Seiler in Germany used the excimer laser to make transverse keratectomies, similar in fashion to a diamond blade transverse (astigmatic) keratotomy.[1313,1321,1420] The major problem with this approach is that the excimer laser does not just produce an incision but actually removes tissue. Controlling the depth of the keratectomies is also a problem. Epithelial plugs fill the keratectomies for at least a year, and more recently this approach was shown to be ineffective.[1231,1312] Other surgeons have used the excimer laser to correct the myopic component of the patients' refraction and performed diamond blade transverse keratotomies to correct the astigmatism.[1139,1297]

Correction of astigmatism with the Summit laser has been investigated using an erodible mask positioned between the laser beam and the cornea, but early human trials yielded disappointing results.* To date there are no published results.

A more successful approach to the correction of astigmatism with the excimer laser has been to use toric ablation patterns. The first animal studies and early clinical trials showed promise.[1202] Recent studies show that refractive cylinders can be reduced to half their preoperative value with residual cylinders of about 0.5 D.*

Correction of hyperopia

Correction of hyperopia has tended to be less successful than for myopia.[922,926,1096,1162,1411] To increase the refractive power of the anterior surface of the cornea, tissue must be removed paracentrally while leaving the central cornea unablated. If small treatment zones are employed, the cornea heals in any divot, reforming the original corneal curvature. Significant regression of effect has been common. Large areas of the cornea have to be ablated to achieve a smooth stromal surface. This prolongs the epithelial healing time and increases postoperative pain. Promising early results in the correction of hyperopia were reported by Dausch and colleagues.[925,926] While the results of correction of hyperopia are promising, the number of patients who lost best corrected visual acuity is too high for acceptable safety. The results in the aphakic group from +11.0 to +16.0 D were poor, and the authors did not recommend the use of the excimer laser for correction of aphakia. The patients who lost best corrected visual acuity did so because of decentered ablations.

Complications of PRK

Although some recent studies have reported that as many as 95% to 98% of patients achieve 20/40 or better visual acuity and 93% to 95% within 1 D of intended correction.[1029,1364,1385] Like most refractive surgical procedures, two of the most common postoperative complications are undercorrection and overcorrection. Overcorrection is commonly managed by tapering or discontinuing the topical steroids. This has the effect of removing the steroid inhibition of wound healing to allow myopic regression to occur unhindered. Most patients eventually regress back toward emmetropia and their overcorrection resolves.

Undercorrection is the most common refractive complication of PRK.[1365] This can then be successfully managed by retreatment.[946,954,1126,1363] Many eyes that require retreatment are undercorrected because they exhibited a more vigorous wound healing response than normal. This can be reduced by administration of topical corticosteroids.[699,864,887,954,1161] Corticosteroids, however, have little long-term effect on myopic regression or corneal haze, and patients with significant undercorrections frequently have subepithelial scarring and require a nonrefractive keratectomy with the excimer laser (phototherapeutic keratectomy) to remove the scar tissue.†

Although the combination of NSAID eyedrops and therapeutic soft contact lenses has been effective in making postoperative PRK patients far more comfortable, complications from their use have been reported.[1347,1396] Decentration of the laser photoablation can lead to induction

---

* References 781, 803, 841, 863, 903, 1015, 1024, 1176.

* References 875, 906, 925, 1093, 1266, 1354, 1359, 1391-1393.
† References 948, 991, 992, 1126, 1247, 1363, 1364.

of astigmatism, halo formation, glare, and loss of best corrected visual acuity.[1168] Even with a good refractive and visual result, problems with night vision are common.[1244,1246] Delayed epithelial healing after PRK for greater than 72 hours is unusual but may occur in patients with occult dry eye or other unrecognized ocular surface disorders. Corticosteroid related complications such as ocular hypertension, reactivation of herpes simplex keratitis, and, rarely, a perforated corneal ulcer can occur.[1336] In up to 80% of patients 12 months after PRK, a central intraepithelial iron spot may be found.[1334] Other less commonly reported complications have included blepharoptosis, anisocoria, and subretinal hemorrhages.[1336]

Wound healing after PRK

Early studies in rabbits and monkeys demonstrated that PRK with the excimer laser produced an anterior keratectomy with sufficient smoothness to allow healing without corneal scarring in the majority of cases (Color Plate 5-7).* Despite this success, there was variability in the development of corneal scarring (haze). Deeper ablations tended to produce greater anterior corneal opacity (haze) (Color Plate 5-8) with scarring seen as its histopathological correlate.[1025] Similarly, in the sighted human eye trials, there is a variability in the wound healing response that influences the eventual refractive outcome. Unpredictable corneal wound healing is the "Archilles heel" of PRK with the interaction between the corneal epithelium and the stromal keratocyte thought to be the major reason for this.†

The cornea mounts a wound healing response to any anterior keratectomy, regardless of how it is performed.[830,833,842,1428] After PRK, the cornea has a bare stromal surface with loss of Bowman's layer. While most of the lost stromal tissue has been vaporized, a layer of damaged tissue can be seen as a 100 to 200 nm electron dense layer immediately following PRK.‡ Beneath this layer the stromal appears undisturbed to light microscopy. With the deeper ablations into the cornea required to correct higher levels of myopia, greater degrees of haze or scarring are seen in the subepithelial zone.§ Corneas with haze show histopathological signs of ongoing stromal remodeling.[1025] Corneal haze is associated with regression of the refractive effect, irregular astigmatism, and occasionally the formation of a central zone of corneal steepening known as a "central island."‖ All of these result in loss of uncorrected visual acuity and, if severe enough, loss of best corrected visual acuity.

Over a 2 to 4 day period following PRK, corneal epithelial cells migrate and divide to cover the bare corneal stroma. Repopulation is dependent centripetal migration of new cells derived from libmal stem cells.¶ New base-

ment membrane, hemidesmosomes, and anchoring fibrils are all formed during reepithelialization.[1009] By 7 days after PRK, the epithelium is thickened with focal areas of basement membrane and hemidesmosome formation.[936]

Because the epithelium normally maintains a protective environment for the stromal keratocytes, any loss of the corneal epithelium may cause severe morphological changes to occur in the superficial keratocytes within 30 minutes, and by 24 hours there is a marked decrease in number.* Seven days after PRK, anterior stromal keratocytes undergo fibroblastic transformation and actively repopulate the anterior stroma with a peak density at 4 months. These stromal fibrocytes show increased amounts of rough endoplasmic reticulum, indicative of active protein synthesis. Newly secreted extracellular matrix is seen between the fibrocytes at 3 weeks.[990,1011] The new extracellular matrix consists of new collagen and glycosaminoglycans (Color Plate 5-7). The predominant glycosaminoglycans in the normal adult human cornea are keratin sulfate and dermatin sulfate.[911,912] Hyaluronic acid, a glycosaminoglycan that is normally found only in small quantities in the human and rabbit cornea, can be detected in the subepithelial zone of PRK-treated rabbit corneas.[821,968,1416] It may play a role in an excessive wound healing response.[953] Most studies have found that PRK does not cause significant endothelial alterations.† Corneas with greater amounts of haze at slitlamp examination, show vacuolization at the epithelial-stromal junction, fragmentation of the newly secreted basement membrane, larger numbers of activated fibrocytes in the anterior stroma, and larger amounts of extracellular matrix deposits.[956] Haze typically peaks at about 3 months postoperatively and resolves thereafter.[1336,1364] While clinically termed *haze*, its pathological correlate is subepithelial scar tissue that scatters the incident light.[1148,1288,1289] Over time corneal scar tissue remodels, transparency improves, and the spacing between collagen fibrils approaches normal.‡

Modulation of corneal wound healing after PRK

Early studies in rabbits demonstrated a marked reduction in the intensity of anterior stromal haze with topical corticosteroids, and there is some evidence that topical steroids can reverse myopic regression or maintain a hyperopic shift.§ Other modulators of corneal wound healing have also been studied both experimentally in animals and in clinical trials in humans.[927,961,1151,1296] Topical mitomycin C has been shown in rabbits to reduce the rate of subepithelial haze formation.[1381] Despite this, the complications of antimitotic agents are too potentially sight threatening for their use to become common clinical practice. Other agents that have been used in trials to reduce corneal haze after PRK has been topical interferon-α 2b and neolactoglycosphingolipids.[1221,1261,1262]

The wound healing process after PRK involves cell-to-cell communications between stromal fibroblasts (keratocytes) and the corneal epithelium. Cytokines, including

---

* References 928, 957, 1025, 1042, 1059, 1112, 1173, 1174, 1190, 1196, 1420, 1426.

† References 62, 910, 1011, 1167, 1427, 1429, 1446, 1450, 1459.

‡ References 953, 956, 957, 1014, 1256, 1352.

§ References 889-892, 991, 1045, 1078, 1209, 1395.

‖ References 916, 1109, 1129, 1147-1149, 1150, 1152, 1166, 1245, 1246, 1249, 1284, 1402.

¶ References 821, 835, 852, 956, 976, 978, 985, 997, 1007-1010, 1012-1014, 1043, 1049, 1098, 1112, 1113, 1122, 1171, 1172, 1220, 1227, 1251, 1269, 1370, 1372, 1373, 1375, 1413, 1418, 1444, 1462, 1463.

---

* References 852, 883, 956, 1011, 1041, 1192, 1228, 1379.

† References 812, 815, 983, 1173, 1182, 1267, 1302, 1356, 1414.

‡ References 852, 907-909, 946, 1047, 1174, 1184-1186, 1373.

§ References 954, 969, 991, 992, 1381, 1408, 1428.

growth factors and interleukins, are the mediators of this cell-to-cell signaling. The corneal epithelium signals to the stromal fibroblasts that it has been injured, and the keratocytes respond by migration into the subepithelial area, mitosis, and increased protein synthesis. The keratocytes produce most of the new extracellular matrix materials including collagen and glycosaminoglycans, which are responsible for subepithelial scarring (haze). Corneal epithelial cells and stromal fibroblasts can express a myriad of cytokine receptors, many of which are involved in the process of wound healing.[1130]

The place of PRK in the armamentarium of the refractive surgeon depends on the control of the adverse effects of postoperative corneal wound healing.[1277] Limiting the procedure to low myopia in which results are more predictable and safety acceptable is one option. The development of effective methods to control scar formation determines whether this procedure stands the test of time.

INTRASTROMAL PHOTOREFRACTIVE KERATECTOMY

Because the wound healing response of the cornea is the major cause of variation and unpredictability in the refractive outcome after surface PRK and removal of the corneal epithelium and Bowman's layer often results in considerable postoperative pain, research into new laser techniques for correction of refractive errors without damaging the anterior cornea is ongoing. One method of producing flattening of corneal curvature without removal of either the corneal epithelium or anterior stroma is intrastromal PRK. In this technique a laser is focused in the midcorneal stroma producing minimal damage to the more superficial cornea.° The major attractiveness of intrastromal ablation is the potential of minimizing the wound healing response of the cornea with improvements in refractive predictability. The laser that has shown the most promise for intrastromal PRK is the neodymium:yttrium lithium fluoride (Nd:YLF) laser, with a wavelength of 1053 nm. Tissue removal occurs by plasma-mediated photodisruption at the focal point of the laser, similar to the Nd:YAG laser. Intrastromal PRK with the Nd:YLF laser results in only limited breakdown of the corneal epithelium, making the surgery much less painful than PRK.[1004] Bowman's layer is minimally damaged. In theory, the cornea should maintain long-term clarity with little or no postoperative scarring. The infrared wavelengths of both lasers are only minimally absorbed by corneal tissue. This allows these lasers to be focused and tissue removal by photodisruption can occur at any depth within the transparent corneal tissue.[979,1368] Clinical trials of intrastromal PRK with the picosecond Nd:YLF laser are currently underway in the United States and in Europe.[1236]

LASER THERMAL KERATOPLASTY

Laser thermal keratoplasty (LTK) is a nonincisional treatment for hyperopia.† The concept of thermal keratoplasty is that radial thermal burns placed in the paracentral to midperipheral cornea cause contraction of corneal collagen and steepen the central cornea.[826] It is not a new concept. In 1898 Lans found that superficial thermal burns in the rabbit cornea can induce astigmatism. Terrien was the first to perform thermal keratoplasty in human beings when in 1900 he reported using cauterization to correct astigmatism secondary to Terrien's marginal degeneration. Thermokeratoplasty was then used in the early 1970s to flatten the cone in keratoconic corneas, but regression of the refractive effect over time was common.°

Unfortunately, the thermal injury to the cornea induces a wound healing response. Like all other corneal refractive surgical procedures that do this, interpatient variations in the degree of wound healing reduces the predictability of the refractive outcome. Refraction after LTK shows an initial myopic overshoot followed by gradual regression.[959,1412] Regression continues for at least 2 years, with most patients eventually returning to their preoperative refraction.[900,1305,1412] It is possible that the procedure could then be repeated, but there is a limit to the amount of injury the cornea will stand without adverse results.

PHOTOTHERAPEUTIC KERATECTOMY

The aim of phototherapeutic keratectomy (PTK) is to improve the patient's best corrected visual acuity, either by improving the clarity of the cornea or by reducing irregular astigmatism. It was approved by the U.S. FDA in 1995 and is most effective in the removal of opacities involving the epithelial layer, subepithelial scars, in Bowman's layer, or the most anterior part of the stroma. As such it is an alternative to lamellar keratectomy but does not suffer from the interface opacities of that procedure.†

The application of the excimer laser for removal of experimental anterior corneal pathology was first described in 1985.[1337] Removal of anterior corneal scars or dystrophies with the excimer laser was suggested in 1989 as an alternative to lamellar keratoplasty (Color Plates 5-9 and 5-10).[996,1117] In 1990, in the first case report of removal of a corneal nodule using the excimer laser, the term *phototherapeutic keratectomy (PTK)* was introduced.[1369] The value of masking fluids to allow greater smoothing of the anterior corneal surface and possible reduction in irregular astigmatism was soon realized.[958,967,1100] In two early reports of PTK the causes of anterior stromal opacities included inactive herpes simplex keratitis, recurrent corneal erosion syndrome, stromal dystrophies, and band keratopathy.[988,1342]

Investigators have noted that PTK caused a hyperopic shift and that despite the use of masking fluids, it was difficult to eliminate the irregular astigmatism.[1342] While the excimer laser is very effective in removing anterior stromal scarring, in some cases a wound healing response produced a new scar.[1397] Attempts to improve on the masking of the excimer laser beam to allow better correction of irregular astigmatism have included ablatable gels, which can mold to the corneal surface.[931,945] While the ablatable gel is

° References 979, 982, 1004, 1027, 1028, 1235, 1239, 1358, 1368, 1380, 1371, 1464.

† References 824, 827, 828, 899, 900, 937, 959, 960, 970, 994, 995, 1053, 1060, 1080, 1120, 1170, 1180, 1200, 1217, 1231-1234, 1263, 1293, 1303, 1305, 1310, 1316, 1325, 1341, 1340, 1351, 1401, 1412.

° References 824, 825, 827, 994, 995, 1080.

† References 720, 819, 862, 872, 939, 972, 973, 1055, 1237, 1275, 1285, 1286, 1366, 1407, 1432, 1445.

molding to the corneal surface, a contact lens can be used to mold the external surface of the gel to a smooth regular spherical or aspherical surface. If the ablatable gel has the same ablation rate as the cornea, then a homogeneous, circular excimer laser beam should then theoretically result in a smooth regular corneal surface. The first experiments with a type I collagen gel mold showed that it was possible to find a material with the same ablation rate as the corneal stroma. An alternative approach in the future may be to use a topographic corneal map to plan the amount of tissue to be removed from each part of the cornea.[1001]

Conditions for which good improvements in vision have been reported after PTK include Reis-Buckler's corneal dystrophy, corneal scars due to ulcers, corneal scars resulting from trauma, anterior corneal scars due to trachoma, band keratopathy, familial amyloidosis, shield ulcers from vernal keratoconjunctivitis, and anterior corneal dystrophies including granular, lattice, Schnyder's, Meesman's, and anterior basement membrane dystrophy.* Patients who develop subepithelial scarring following PRK for myopia have also been treated successfully by first removing the scar with a PTK treatment and then repeating the PRK.[1125] Some success has been reported in the treatment of proud nebulae in patients with keratoconus.[1216]

Treatment of anterior stromal opacities caused by prior episodes of herpes simplex keratitis has met with varied success.[955] Reactivation of the herpes simplex keratitis has been reported both clinically and in laboratory studies.[1267,1441,1442]

Phototherapeutic keratectomy can also be a successful treatment for recurrent corneal erosion syndrome.† It appears to be particularly useful in cases that are resistant to conventional medical therapies, especially if the disease involves the visual axis. In a series of 76 cases of recurrent corneal erosion treated with PTK, the authors found that 20 eyes had recurrences, 21 had minor symptoms, and 35 had no symptoms after treatment.[1208] In a corneal graft PTK may induce a graft rejection episode.[950,1054]

Histological examination of corneas removed at penetrating keratoplasty following unsuccessful PTK may reveal epithelial hyperplasia,[1659] loss of Bowman's layer,[1199] loss of normal epithelial basement membrane attachments, sub-epithelial scarring and disorganization of the anterior stroma in the region of the ablation.[856,976,1199,1459,1659]

Unsuccessful PTK with recurrent scarring sufficient to warrant penetrating keratoplasty has been reported after treatment of a number of conditions. These include scarring due to herpes simplex keratitis, herpes zoster keratitis, undercorrected myopic epikeratoplasty, band keratopathy, granular dystrophy, and recurrent lattice dystrophy.[856,1434] Sometimes the scar tissue is resistant to excimer laser ablation, while normal tissue ablates well.[1199] Residual disease is frequently seen in penetrating keratoplasty specimens, indicating that the major reason for failure of PTK is either insufficient ablation of the original pathology or recurrence of the primary disease.[856]

After PTK there is an epithelial defect that must heal

over. The epithelial cells slide into the defect by active contraction of intracellular actin microfilaments and the formation of temporary macromolecular cell-to-cell adhesions. The new basal epithelium synthesizes a new basement membrane and new anchoring fibrils. Production of new extracellular matrix materials, including collagen and glycosaminoglycans, by the stromal fibroblasts can lift up the new basal epithelium and trap the new anchoring fibrils.[1012]

Lamellar surgery and laser surgery combined—laser in situ keratomileusis (LASIK)

HISTORY

Laser in situ keratomileusis (LASIK) is a relatively new corneal refractive procedure, which at the time of writing is generating great enthusiasm among refractive surgeons.[1466] It involves the use of a microkeratome to create an anterior corneal flap and an photoablative laser to impart a refractive correction to the underlying stroma. Early in the development of PRK it became evident to two European ophthalmologists that the efficacy, predictability and safety of surface PRK was not satisfactory for myopia over about −6.00 D. Independently, they each developed separate techniques that moved the site of the excimer laser ablation from the surface of the cornea to the mid corneal stroma. These two new techniques were developed to allow safer and more effective corrections of high myopia. The first of these was Pallikaris' laser in situ keratomileusis[1488] and the second, Buratto's laser intrastromal keratomileusis.[1470,1472]

Peyman and colleagues were the first to report the application of a laser to ablate stromal tissue underneath an anterior corneal cap.[1270,1271] Then in 1990, Pallikaris described the procedure that he named laser in situ keratomileusis.[1488] His first studies were in rabbits, followed by a blind-eye study.[1487] Different types of microkeratomes have been successfully used including a modified BKS-1000 (Barraquer-Krumeich-Swinger), a Draeger microkeratome, and the Chiron Automatic Corneal Shaper.[1468,1489,1491] Most surgeons currently create an anterior corneal flap of between 130 and 160 μm in thickness.

The current enthusiasm for LASIK is based on a number of advantages that the procedure has over both PRK and automated in situ keratomileusis.* Like automated in situ keratomileusis, LASIK can correct myopia as high as −20 to −30 D. But unlike the inaccurate-in-thickness, small-diameter, planodisc refractive cut in automated in situ keratomileusis, the refractive excision in LASIK is made with the accuracy and flexibility of the excimer laser. Any pattern of spherical, spherocylindrical, or hyperopic ablation can be carved into the corneal stroma with the laser. The major advantage that LASIK appears to hold over PRK is the relative absence of a wound healing reaction produced in the cornea (Figs. 5-8, 5-9, *A* and *B*, and 5-10).[1510] By preserving the epithelium and Bowman's layer and shifting the refractive ablation deeper into the cornea, the cornea does not mount an epithelial and subepithelial wound healing response. The laser trauma to the cornea is hidden from the epithelium and postoperative subepithelial haze

---

* References 872, 880, 896, 913, 941, 952, 1023, 1032, 1050, 1070, 1124, 1204, 1242, 1254, 1299, 1304.
† References 924, 998, 1026, 1072, 1252, 1268.

* References 1466, 1475, 1477, 1484-1493, 1498-1506, 1510.

or scarring does not develop. Almost all the surgical trauma is within the midcorneal stroma and the midstroma heals in a slow, nonaggressive fashion (Color Plate 5-11).

The efficacy, predictability, and safety of LASIK are similar to PRK. Results that are similar to those of PRK for

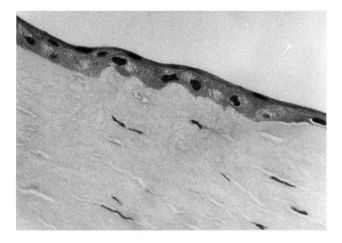

Fig. 5-8. Photomicrograph showing healing of cornea obtained postmortem after incubation in organ and experimental LASIK culture. This is the site of the incision, creating the flap. There is a break in Bowman's layer and basement membrane that has filled in with new extracellular matrix materials. One to two layers of epithelium cover the defect. (H & E stain; ×250.)

myopic corrections between −1 and −6 D are seen with LASIK corrections between −1 and −20 D.[1504,1509]

In stark contrast to PRK patients, patients who have undergone LASIK have little or no postoperative pain. The epithelial defect created by the keratome is small and heals overnight. In contrast, it takes 48 to 72 hours for a post-PRK epithelial defect to heal. The preservation of the corneal epithelium also allows for faster return of vision after LASIK compared to PRK. There is usually a significantly faster stabilization of refraction after LASIK compared to PRK. After PRK continued change in refraction can occur for up to 12 to 18 months.[946]

The disadvantages of LASIK are similar to those of automated in situ keratomileusis. The procedure requires greater surgical skill than PRK and the use of an expensive microkeratome. There are also two surgical maneuvers that involve the central cornea. Unlike PRK it is not a "hands off" procedure. A suction ring must be used to hold the keratome in place as it traverses the cornea. Irregular keratotomies or incomplete flap creation can occur if adequate suction is not achieved. If the keratome is not correctly assembled and the depth determining plate not installed, it is possible to enter the anterior chamber and even deliver the lens from the eye.[587] Like automated in situ keratomileusis, there are complications associated with the anterior corneal flap. Debris from Weck Cell sponges can lodge in the interface (Fig. 5-11, *B*).[1507] Epithelium can grow between the flap and the stromal bed (Fig. 5-11, *A*). The replacement of the flap back onto the cornea can be misa-

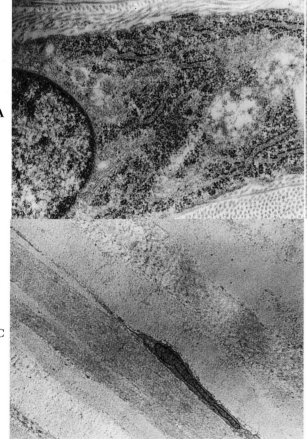

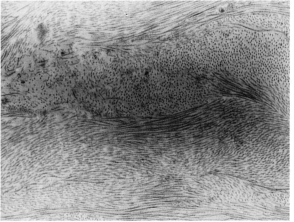

Fig. 5-9. Transmission electron microscopic views of the stromal interface after experimental LASIK. **A,** Anterior stromal keratocyte following 7 days in organ culture. This is at the interface of the stromal flaps. The increased amount of rough surface endoplasmic reticulum indicates upregulation of protein synthesis. (×4000.) **B,** Cornea after 7 days healing in organ culture following LASIK, interface of the anterior corneal flap (top) and the stromal bed (bottom). Note a delicate proliferation of collagen fibers at the interface, which suffices to provide healing and adhesion but does not cause opacification. (×4000.) **C,** Corneal stroma after healing, showing a normal inactive keratocyte and normal collagen lamellae (×1800.)

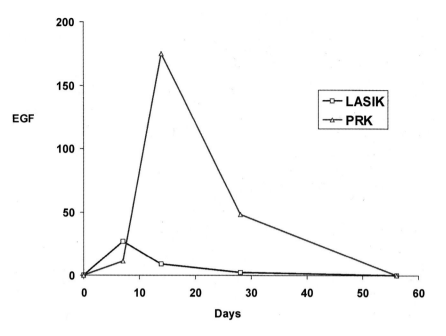

Fig. 5-10. Graph showing activation of cyto-chynes (in the case epithelial growth factor [EGF]) elaborated after PRK and LASIK performed experimentally in human cadaver eyes incubated in organ culture. Note that the level response after PRK very much longer is an indication of protracted wound healing process.

ligned and induce irregular astigmatism. As with automated in situ keratomileusis, the flap can be lifted and replaced again to correct this. Like PRK decentration of the ablation zone can occur.

The interface complications and risks of creating an incomplete flap have led one investigator to comment that LASIK is a procedure that "swaps one set of complications for another."[1466] Most investigators have been enthusiastic, however, especially because of the potential elimination of corneal wound healing as an unpredictable variable that determines the final outcome.

Another potential advantage of LASIK is the ease with which enhancement procedures can be performed. As with automated in situ keratomileusis, LASIK is best enhanced by lifting up the anterior corneal flap and retreating the stromal bed. Healing after LASIK occurs most rapidly at the level of the epithelium, then at Bowman's layer, and finally between the stromal surfaces of the bed and the flap (Fig. 5-8). Because of the slow rate at which the corneal stroma heals, there is very little adherence between the flap and the bed. The surgeon has to only break the adherence at the level of Bowman's layer, and the flap lifts easily off the stromal bed.

Calibration of excimer laser algorithms for LASIK is still in a state of evolution. In PRK much of the ablation is in Bowman's layer, while in LASIK all the ablation takes place in the stroma.[1502]

WOUND HEALING AFTER LASIK

In contrast to PRK, both LASIK (Figs. 5-8, 5-9, *A* and *B*, and 5-10) and automated in situ keratomileusis (ALK) preserve the corneal epithelium and Bowman's layer. After replacement of the anterior cornea flap, a small, nearly complete peripheral circular defect remains in the epithelium. In both LASIK and ALK epithelial coverage of this defect is usually rapid and uneventful. By the next day there is typically no epithelial defect and the patient is free of pain. The cellular processes by which the epithelial defect heals are similar to those described in the section on wound healing after PRK; however, unlike PRK there is no development of subepithelial scarring (haze). One possible reason may be the preservation of Bowman's layer and the corneal epithelium.

The interaction of an injured, healing corneal epithelium with stromal fibroblasts is believed to be the major reason for the development of subepithelial scarring following PRK.[1510] This process is mediated by cell-to-cell communications using cytokines, such as growth factors and interleukins. Because the epithelium is uninjured after LASIK and does not send out injury signaling cytokines to the stromal fibroblasts (Fig. 5-10), LASIK prevents this epithelial cell to fibroblast interaction (Fig. 5-10). The fibroblasts do become activated (Fig. 5-9, *A*) but do not penetrate Bowman's layer. The fibroblasts do not lay down subepithelial new collagen and glycosaminoglycans in the central cornea. The only scarring is in the peripheral defect in Bowman's layer created by the microkeratome.

As is typical of corneal stromal healing in general, the stroma proper is the slowest part of the cornea to heal. The time course for the flap to heal thoroughly to the stromal bed is influenced by patient age and individual variability. Transmission electron microscopy of the interface between the flap and the stromal bed shows the presence of disorganized collagen fibers (Fig. 5-9, *B*). Within 1 week after the procedure, keratocytes in the region of the interface show increased rough surfaced endoplasmic reticulum indicating an increase in the production of new protein by the cells.[1488] Unlike PRK, the stromal after LASIK keratocytes are not influenced by cytokines produced by an actively remodeling corneal epithelium. This difference, plus the physical separation are probably the most important reasons why subepithelial haze and scarring do not develop after LASIK. Bowman's layer is compact acellular collagen and may have a barrier effect to the movement of keratocytes into the subepithelial area.

If the cornea does develop any opacity after LASIK, it

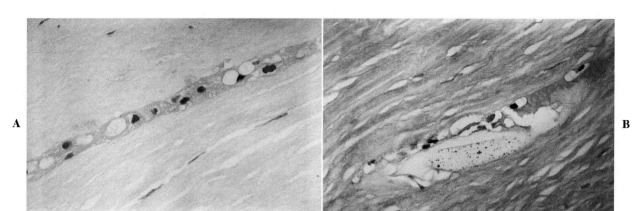

Fig. 5-11. A, Transmission electron micrograph showing epithelial ingrowth between the flap (above) and base. This is a rare and generally innocuous complication of ALK and LASIK. (×4000.) **B,** Photomicrograph of a Weck cell and some epithelial cells trapped between the flap (above) and the stromal bed (below) after a LASIK procedure. This is a rare complication that can be avoided with careful surgical technique. (×4000.)

is typically located within the interface between the flap and the stromal bed. Ingrowth of epithelium occurs between the flap and the bed (Fig. 5-11, *A*). This can be a threat to vision and requires lifting the flap and physical removal of the ingrowing epithelial cells. Sometimes interface haze can occur, although this is usually slight. Some new stromal collagen needs to be laid down in the interface to heal the flap to the underlying stromal bed. The new collagen is almost certainly produced by the activated keratocytes in the region of the interface. Debris from swabs is sometimes seen, although it is seldom visually significant (Fig. 5-11, *B*). There is no damage to corneal endothelium after LASIK.[1476]

At the time of writing, many leading refractive surgeons were expressing enthusiasm about LASIK. The promise of the procedure, which can correct all levels of myopia and possibly hyperopia with safety, is very alluring. The major complications at this time are those related to the production of the flap by the keratome and the accurate replacement of the flap onto the stromal bed. New keratomes are currently under development, and increased surgeon experience with management of anterior corneal flaps can help reduce these complications. Only time will tell whether or not LASIK proves to be the refractive technique of choice.[1509]

Laser intrastromal keratomileusis (Buratto technique) represents an alternative approach. First described by Burrato[1470] in 1992, it is a technique in which an anterior corneal cap (button) is removed with the lamellar keratome and the cap is then placed epithelial surface downward in an antidesiccation chamber. The refractive correction is ablated into the stromal side of the cap, and the cap is sutured back onto the cornea. At the time of writing, the popularity of LASIK was increasing and that of the Burrato technique was waning.

Intrastromal corneal rings[1511-1521]

The Intrastromal Corneal Ring (ICR) is made from polymethylmethacrylate (PMMA) and was developed in the late 1980s as a method for correction of both hyperopia and

myopia.[1514] After insertion of the ring into the peripheral corneal stroma, either flattening or steepening of the central cornea can result. The original mathematical models predicted that with increasing expansion of the ring the central cornea will flatten. With constriction of the ring the central cornea should steepen and smaller diameters of rings create greater steepening or flattening than larger diameters.[1514] Animal and human cadaver eyes showed that the ICR did not affect intraocular pressure and helped to refine the design.[1511,1513] The major advantages of the ICR are that it does not alter the structure of the central cornea and that it is reversible.[1518] In contrast to other procedures for correction of low myopia, the ICR preserves the normal asphericity of the cornea. A normal cornea is more steeply curved in the central than the peripheral areas. Procedures such as RK and PRK flatten the central cornea and thus produce negative corneal asphericity. This can produce significant problems with night vision. The ICR does not appear to have this problem.

The first blind-eye surgeries were performed in 1991, and the results were reported in 1993.[1512,1517,1518] A stable refractive change that corrected about −2.00 D of myopia was obtained. Apart from the alteration of central corneal curvature, the only other side effect reported was the presence of an arcuate epithelial iron line in about half the eyes.[1511] This iron line resolved upon removal of the ICR. Histological examination of a cornea that had had an ICR removed 8 months previously showed minimal morphological changes.[1521] Often there are deposits in the cornea that are associated with the suture holes in the ICR. Scanning and transmission electron microscopy of explanted ICRs has shown that these deposits consist of a disorganized convolution of collagen lamellae.[1519] Within the deposits there is a mixture of amorphous extracellular material, interspersed with cellular processes, collagen fibrils, and proteoglycan molecules.[1519,1520]

In phase I FDA trials there were no problems with implant-associated inflammation or extrusion of the ICR. The ICR had no effect on intraocular pressure, corneal thickness, or endothelial cell counts. The mean reduction in myopia was −2.5 D at the corneal plane. The ICR may prove to be a viable alternative for the correction of low degrees of myopia.[1521] The advantages of low-cost, reversibility, preservation of normal corneal asphericity, and the lack of permanent effect on the central cornea are its greatest assets.

Refractive intraocular lenses[1522-1637]

CLEAR LENS EXTRACTION WITH INTRAOCULAR LENS IMPLANTATION

Although the term *refractive surgery* immediately conjurs up surgery that alters the cornea (keratorefractive surgery), it is not widely appreciated that correction of a high refractive error can be achieved by intraocular lens (IOL) implantation; indeed the stability of refraction after IOL is often better and is less prone to hyperopic or myopic regression (Fig. 5-12).

Removal of the natural lens[1528,1597,1619,1620,1631] has long been a potential alternative to corneal refractive surgery for the correction of high myopia. It was first suggested in Europe in the 18th century and Fukala popularized it in 1890.[1555] In the early 1960s, Barraquer mentioned clear lens extraction when reviewing the indications, contraindications, and complications of the intracapsular procedure.[1531] In the past, clear lens extraction was highly controversial because of high reported complication rates before the era of modern capsular surgery (Chapter 4). Clear lens extraction for high myopia has been practiced in Columbia for more than 25 years.[1529,1614] Rodriguez reported the results of 33 clear lens extractions performed for high myopia between 1972 and 1986.[1614] Intracapsular surgery was performed on 12 eyes, extracapsular in 19, and lens aspiration in 2. There was a high incidence of complications and only 30% had a good result with vision of 20/40 or better. Complications included 60% with ocular motility disturbances, 24% with secondary glaucoma, 30% with retinal detachments, and 36% with lens remnants in

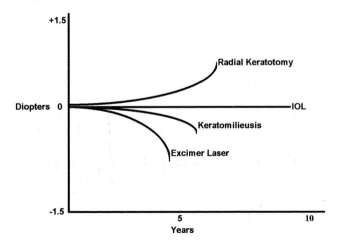

Fig. 5-12. Schematic, conceptual comparison of stability of refractive IOL after various surgical procedures. Note that a refractive IOL shows the least regression and most stability compared with the keratorefractive procedures. For example the PERK staining documented significant hyperopic shift after radial keratotomy (RK).

the visual axis. These results show that the use of intracapsular surgery and older extracapsular techniques yielded quite disastrous results for clear lens extraction in high myopia.

A large series of clear lens extraction for myopia was reported by Barraquer in 1994.[1529] Most cases were done before the era of modern capsular surgery. She reported the results of clear lens extraction in 165 myopic eyes operated on at the Instituto Barraquer de America in Bogota, Columbia, between 1980 and 1990. Intracapsular surgery was performed in 3%, lens aspiration in 59%, and extracapsular surgery in 38%. Fifty-six (35%) of the patients who underwent extracapsular surgery or aspiration required either Nd:YAG laser or surgical posterior capsulotomy for secondary cataracts an average of 25.6 months after surgery. Among the 165 eyes, a retinal detachment developed in 12 (7.3%). Although surgery improved the average uncorrected visual acuity from about 4/200 to 20/200, most patients still had to wear spectacles or contact lenses postoperatively. The reduction in their lens prescriptions significantly reduced the amount of image minification and resulted in an improvement in best corrected visual acuity. The mean patient age in this study was about 30, so the loss of accommodation in the patient represented a real disadvantage.

Arciniegas reported performing clear lens extraction in 114 patients using pars plana lensectomy and vitrectomy with a suction guillotine cutter, combined with a 360-degree silicone exoimplant.[1523] There was a 7% complication rate, including 2.6% for retinal detachment and 4.4% for vitreous hemorrhage.

As noted in Chapter 4, modern cataract surgery underwent several important advances in the 1980s. These include the move into the era of capsular surgery (generation VI, p. 00). Most surgeons have transitioned from intracapsular to extracapsular techniques. The introduction of viscoelastic agents, and the development of continuous curvilinear capsulorhexis, the introduction of hydrodissection, and placement of a posterior chamber IOL in the capsular bag have markedly increased the safety and efficacy of the procedure.[1559]

By the late 1980s small incision cataract surgery using phacoemulsification and foldable lenses began to increase in popularity. The use of phacoemulsification specifically for clear lens extraction was first reported by a Russian ophthalmologist, Dvali, in 1982.[1543,1546] He also utilized cryotherapy to try to reduce the incidence of postoperative aphakic retinal detachment. Verzella was the first to report clear lens extraction with implantation of a low power posterior chamber IOL in the capsular bag.[1623-1627]

Several studies using modern capsular techniques with small-incision phacoemulsification and implantation of a low or minus power posterior chamber IOL have reported much lower incidences of retinal detachment than in Barraquer's study. Lyle and Jin reported the results of clear lens extraction in 31 eyes with high myopia and 6 eyes with high hyperopia.[259] In the eyes with high myopia, 77% achieved 20/40 or better uncorrected visual acuity and 97% attained a corrected visual acuity of 20/40 or better. Sixty-eight percent of eyes were within 1.0 D of emmetropia. None of the 37 eyes developed either retinal detachment or cystoid macular edema in the 20 months of postoperative follow-up.

Colin and Robinet reported an important and illustrative series of clear lens extractions in 52 eyes using phacoemulsification, continuous curvilinear capsulorhexis, and implantation of a low-power IOL in the capsular bag.[1538] Most significantly, they performed thorough retinal examinations and performed prophylactic argon laser treatment of any lesion they deemed might predispose to development of retinal detachment. All patients were 20/100 or better preoperatively and were intolerant of contact lenses. The mean preoperative spherical equivalent was −16.90 ± 3.26 D, and an axial length of more than 29 mm was present in 64.3% of eyes. The target postoperative refraction was −1.00 D. A 6.5-mm round, all PMMA IOL was used. Thirty-one eyes received preoperative, prophylactic, retinal argon laser to areas of lattice degeneration, retinal tears or holes. This treatment was either focal to isolated retinal breaks or circumferential in 12 eyes with widespread lattice degeneration. Following surgery, six eyes had further retinal argon laser treatments. Four eyes (7.6%) had Nd:YAG laser posterior capsulotomies during the 12 months of reported follow-up. In the 16 eyes that had pre- and postoperative corneal specular microscopy, there was a mean cell loss of 66 cells/mm^2 (2.2%). Eighty-eight percent of the patients had a postoperative corrected visual acuity of 20/40 or better compared to 75% preoperatively. No eyes developed retinal detachment, cystoid macular edema, or persistent corneal edema in the first postoperative year. This is in contrast to Barraquer's study, in which four patients (2.4%) developed retinal detachments in the first postoperative year and a further eight (4.8%) developed detachments from 12 to 72 months after surgery. Colin and Robinet's study shows that good results are possible with modern phacoemulsification, capsular surgery, and prophylactic retinal argon laser treatment before and after lensectomy. The study, however, is limited by small numbers and by limited follow-up. Further follow-up will be necessary to confirm this technique's safety and efficacy and to seek further means of improvement.

Clear lens extraction with modern capsular surgery techniques is now clearly part of the advanced surgeon's armamentarium.[1559] This being stated, it must be kept in mind that the most severe potential complication is postoperative retinal detachment.[1560] If one is to proceed with this technique, one should be advised about the magnitude of this complication risk, and it is prudent to look at some statistics of retinal detachment. The yearly incidence of retinal detachment in the general population is between 0.008% and 0.01%.[1564,1632] Myopes in general have about two and one half times the risk of developing a retinal detachment in their lifetime than nonmyopes.[1598] The frequency of retinal detachment increases with increasing myopia such that myopes with refractions over −15 D are at least 60 times more likely to develop a retinal detachment than emmetropes and hyperopes.[1598] Consequently, as is well known, this group of patients is already a high risk group for retinal detachment even before surgery.

Clear lens extraction, certainly as performed in the era before modern capsular surgery (up to about 1990) placed the highly myopic patient at an even greater risk of developing a retinal detachment. The goal and at least partial achievement of capsular surgery is an attempt to minimize this risk. Javitt reported the rate of retinal detachment after cataract surgery in 330,000 patients operated on in 1984 and 57,000 patients operated on in 1986-87.[1571,1573] He found that the rate of retinal detachment within 4 years of cataract extraction is 1.55% for intracapsular surgery and 0.8% to 0.9% for extracapsular surgery. If cataract extraction is accompanied by loss of vitreous, the risk of retinal detachment rises to 5.0% at 4 years.[1573] To compound this risk, high myopes with axial lengths of greater than 25 mm have a three times greater rate of development of retinal detachment following extracapsular cataract surgery than the rest of the population.[1539,1582,1595,1599]

One further risk factor for retinal detachment following clear lens extraction in a high myope is posterior capsulotomy. On average, there is about a 20% rate of posterior capsule opacification after extracapsular surgery, with a greater incidence in younger patients.[1539,1595,1605] High myopes undergoing clear lens extraction are usually younger patients. If a Nd:YAG laser capsulotomy (p. 00) is performed, there is an almost fourfold increase in the rate of retinal detachment.[1572] This complication is now clearly of low incidence now that modern surgical techniques with hydrodissection have helped lower the incidence of PCO from an estimated 50% in the mid 1980s to 10% to 20% by the late 1990s.

As many as half of the retinal detachments that follow clear lens extraction in high myopes occur 18 months or more after surgery.[1529] It is likely that lens extraction alters the physiology of the eye, increasing the rate of vitreous syneresis, and, hence, retinal traction.[1570] High myopes and those with the most formed vitreous, that is, young patients, are the most at risk. Clear lens extraction should only be undertaken with full knowledge of the high risk of retinal detachment in these patients.

If clear lens extraction is to be undertaken in a high myope, then a good quality retinal examination is mandatory.[1528] All retinal breaks that might predispose a patient to a postoperative retinal detachment should be treated preoperatively with retinal argon laser photocoagulation or cryotherapy. Retinal argon laser is effective in forming a strong bond between the neuroretina and the retinal pigment epithelium.[1637] In theory, if all predisposing breaks are treated, then this should prevent postoperative retinal detachments. Several studies, however, have demonstrated that prophylactic retinal photocoagulation or cryotherapy is less than 100% effective.[1561,1586,1618] Kanski reported a series of 701 eyes that received prophylactic photocoagulation or cryotherapy.[1577] During follow-up, the rate of retinal detachment was 4.7% with 8.0% of eyes developing new previously undetected retinal breaks. In addition, both retinal photocoagulation and cryotherapy can lead to complications including uveitis, preretinal membranes, cataract formation, and retinal, vitreous, and choroidal hemorrhages.[1561,1604]

Retinal detachment can also be a complication of other refractive surgical procedures for myopia including RK and keratomileusis.[1552,1563,1596,1613] However, the incidence of retinal detachment after an extraocular refractive surgical procedure is much lower than after an intraocular procedure. At the time of writing, there were no published case reports of retinal detachment following PRK or LASIK.

Retinal detachment is not the only complication that occurs following clear lens extractions in high myopes. Like all intraocular surgery, there is a risk of development of postoperative endophthalmitis. In a series of over 57,000 eyes that underwent extracapsular surgery in 1986 to 1987, the risk of endophthalmitis was about 0.08% or one in 1250 cases.[1571] Calculation of the appropriate power of IOL is not as easy as it is with emmetropes, low hyperopes, and low myopes.[1565,1567,1579,1580,1612] Insertion of an IOL in high myopes gives more accurate refractive corrections and a greater proportion of patients with good uncorrected visual acuity than would be the case if the patient did not have an IOL inserted.[1593] Many myopes prefer to be left undercorrected rather than emmetropic, and low myopic astigmatism gives them the best depth of focus.[1541,1568,1581,1615,1629]

In summary, with clear lens extraction one needs to take into account its complications and the other complications of extracapsular cataract surgery including bullous keratopathy, intraocular lens dislocation, or malposition and cystoid macular edema. If good capsular surgery can be performed, and if these complications can be avoided, the only other significant disadvantage to the patient is the ensuing loss of accommodation.[1559] For young patients, this is an important factor that must be weighed in choosing the type of refractive for each case.

PHAKIC INTRAOCULAR LENSES

Anterior chamber intraocular lenses

European surgeons first tried phakic IOLs in the 1950s and early 1960s.* These lenses were angle-fixated, anterior chamber lenses and of negative power. The lenses they unfortunately used were very poorly designed and manufactured, and the results were very poor, with a very high rate of complications. Many patients lost their vision due to pseudophakic bullous keratopathy, glaucoma, and chronic uveitis. The procedure was considered a failure and abandoned.

By the late 1980s, the options for correction of high myopia were largely limited to epikeratoplasty, classical cryokeratomileusis, clear lens extraction with or without posterior chamber IOL or phakic, negative-power, anterior chamber IOLs. Studies published in the 1990s showed that phakic anterior chamber IOLs were superior to these other options, in that they afforded faster visual recovery and greater refractive predictability.[1526,1527,1537] Several surgeons now consider phakic anterior chamber IOLs to be a good option for phakic IOL implantation.

As noted in detail in Chapter 4, a successful anterior chamber IOL must have the following features:

1. It must be stable in the angle with either three- or four-point fixation.
2. It must not rub on the peripheral cornea as this produces continual loss of peripheral corneal endothelial cells.
3. It must not rub on the iris as this can produce chronic blood-aqueous barrier breakdown and uveitis.
4. There should not be a round closed loop or a haptic with a positioning hole in the anterior chamber angle as this encour-

ages the growth of fibrous tissue and synechia through and around the loop or haptic.

Closed small round loop designs result in formation of peripheral anterior synechiae with loss of peripheral endothelial cells and occlusion of the iridocorneal angle.[1611] Significantly higher rates of complications and IOL explantation occur with closed-loop, anterior chamber IOL designs than with open-loop designs.[1588] Two surgeon variables are also important in the longer term tolerance of an anterior chamber IOL. Firstly, the diameter of the anterior chamber must be well matched to the diameter of the IOL. An undersized IOL moves in the eye and damages the cornea and anterior chamber angle. Oversized IOLs and the haptics erode into the ciliary body over time, cause inflammation, distort the pupil, and adhere to the iris.[1617] Haptic flexibility goes some way toward improving the fit of an anterior chamber IOL, but sizing is still very important. Finally, the surgeon must place the lens accurately with the feet of the haptics in the angle recess against the face of the ciliary body.

The insertion of negative-power, phakic anterior chamber IOLs for high myopia was revived in late 1980s.[1575,1606] Some surgeons implanted closed-loop anterior chamber designs with nonflexible haptics such as the Momose design.[1607] These have not been successful designs because of the high complication rates associated with closed-loop anterior chamber IOLs.[1588,1611] Kelman multiflex designs are among the most successful anterior chamber IOLs, with more than 15 years of implantation history.[1524] French ophthalmologist George Baikoff developed his four-point fixation design from Kelman's multiflex implant.[1525] A high-quality, three-point fixation IOL design that may also function equally well, perhaps with less pupillary ovalley, is now being evaluated (Fig. 5-13). This lens is a variation of Kelman's flexible three-point design but with no positioning hole in the haptics. Baikoff's IOL is very similar in design with Z-shaped haptics and four-point angle fixation.

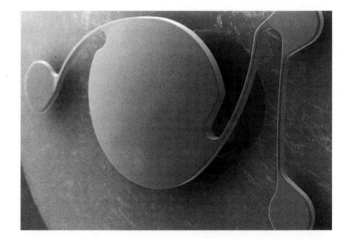

Fig. 5-13. Photograph of one-piece, all PMMA anterior chamber lens, open-loop design developed by Kelman. Kelman, Baikoff, and Clemente have developed several modifications that appear promising. However, the safety and efficacy of phakic anterior chamber IOLs can only be assured after more clinical studies are performed (×10.)

---

* References 1528, 1530-1532, 1535, 1536, 1621, 1622, 1634.

It has a 4.5-mm optic that may be too small when the patient's pupil is widely dilated. As mentioned above, it needs to be carefully sized, but overall it is an easy lens to insert.[1629] His original lens (model ZB) was designed with a 25-degree anterior vault to keep it away from the iris. Later modifications such as the ZB 5M include a 20-degree anterior vault to increase the distance between the corneal endothelium and the IOL. The optic is biconcave with a range of powers from −8.00 to −30.00 D. The earlier models also had quite a thick "shoulder" at the circumference of the optic, which could rub on the cornea and damage the corneal endothelium. The later ZB5M had a thinner profile.[1525,1591] Baikoff's IOL is inserted into the anterior chamber angle under a protective layer of viscoelastic. The patient's pupil is tightly miosed with pilocarpine. As with any angle-fixated anterior chamber IOL, it is important that the pupil is not distorted by the IOL, and it is important to check with gonioscopy that the haptics are correctly positioned in the iridocorneal angle. With the Baikoff IOL the gap between the iris and the IOL is large enough that an iridectomy is not usually performed.

The appropriate power of a phakic anterior chamber IOL to correct a given patient's myopia is approximately equal to the patient's spectacle refraction.[1566] It is rare to use a lens of more than −23 D as this frequently leads to overcorrection.[1525] It is important to avoid overcorrection in any form of refractive surgery for myopia. Aiming for a myopic refraction is often a safe option as almost half of high myopes would prefer to be left at a refraction of −3.00 D rather than have emmetropia.[1581]

Six-month results of Baikoff's IOL in 150 patients from a multicenter study in France were very favorable.[1526] The mean refraction of the patients was reduced from −14.94 ± 4.69 D to a postoperative refraction of −0.22 ± 1.08 D. There was an improvement in spectacle corrected visual acuity from an average of 20/40 to 20/30, although this is probably largely due to a reduction in retinal image minification. In about 2% to 3% of cases, the IOL was exchanged because of incorrect sizing or optical power. Other complications seen in this study included uveitis in 2%, one retinal detachment, and one patient developed a cataract. A third of patients experience halos due to the small size of the optic.

The most serious complication of an anterior chamber IOL is damage and loss of corneal endothelial cells.[1616] Some studies have reported significant endothelial cell loss with the early Baikoff model, the ZB design. Mimouni reported that 1 year after implantation, one third of the 15 patients followed had lost more than 20% of their endothelial cells and 87% had paracentral endothelial cell damage.[1594] Lesroux les Jardin and colleagues reported their results in 21 patients followed for 4 years after implantation of the original Baikoff model ZB IOL.[1587] They found that two eyes (9.5%) had to have their IOL explanted because of significant endothelial cells loss. The remaining 19 eyes (90.5%) had good results without endothelial cell loss. The more advanced Baikoff designs have largely corrected this problem.

Another of the potential complications of anterior chamber IOLs is chronic breakdown of the blood-aqueous barrier. Lesroux les Jardin's study found no evidence of this with the Baikoff IOL.[1578,1587] In the 14 eyes that they examined with a laser flare meter, all had results within normal limits. Using fluorophotometry, Benitez del Castillo and colleagues[1533] found a significantly increased blood-aqueous barrier permeability in 16 eyes with phakic IOLs for up to 6 months after surgery. The same study also found a significant decrease in the light transmittance of the crystalline lens, thus suggesting that these patients should be monitored for eventual development of a cataract.

Retinal detachment has occurred following insertion of a phakic anterior chamber IOL, but the cause and effect is not clear.[1522,1554] The presence of a phakic anterior chamber IOL can make detecting peripheral retinal breaks more difficult. During and following a vitreoretinal procedure the anterior chamber may become shallow, putting the corneal endothelium at risk. Being an intraocular procedure, all the other complications of intraocular surgery previously mentioned can occur.

Iris-fixated intraocular lenses

Another style of phakic IOL that is currently in use for the correction of high myopia is the Worst-Fechner, lobster-claw, iris-fixated lens (Fig. 5-14).[1548,1549,1583,1636] This is sometimes considered to be an anterior chamber lens but is not in the classical definition of the term. Although it is positioned in the anterior chamber, it is fixated to the mid-periphery of the anterior iris. Each haptic has two arms to it that come together like the claws of a lobster. The surgeon incarcerates the iris into the "claws" by pulling the iris tissue between the two arms. In general, it is a more difficult lens to position than angle-fixated anterior chamber IOLs and requires the surgeon to learn a new implantation technique. Kummerich in Germany has developed an insertion device that does address this problem and represents a significant advance.

The theoretical advantage of this lens is that it does not make contact with the iridocorneal angle and, therefore, may not produce the same angle-related complications that the older angle-fixated IOLs did. It may also sit further away from the corneal endothelium than angle-fixated anterior chamber IOLs. It does, however, challenge one of Ridley's original tenants of a successful intraocular lens. Ridley stated that a successful IOL should not move in the eye, nor should parts of the eye move on the IOL. The Worst-Fechner lens is in contact with the iris and can chronically move on the iris tissue. It is also possible to produce distortion of the pupil when fixating the lens on the iris.

The lens is not available in the United States, but there have been several overseas reports of the performance of this lens. One is from Worst's own facility in Holland, where the results of a prospective study of the lens in 35 eyes of 18 patients followed for 6 to 12 months were reported.[584] The preoperative refractions of the patients ranged from −6.00 to −28.00 D. The postoperative spherical equivalent was within 1.00 D of emmetropia in 26 (74.3%) patients. No change in refraction occurred from 1 to 2 months to 12 months and mean corrected vision improved from 20/40 to 20/30. The mean endothelial cell loss was 5.6% at 6 months (range +6.3% to −22.6%) and 8.9% (range +0.77% to −23.5%) at 12 months. No other major complications occurred. A second series from Menezo and colleagues[1592] consisted of 90 highly myopic eyes

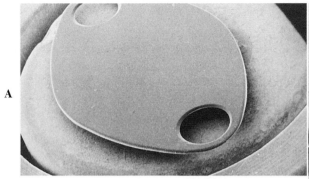

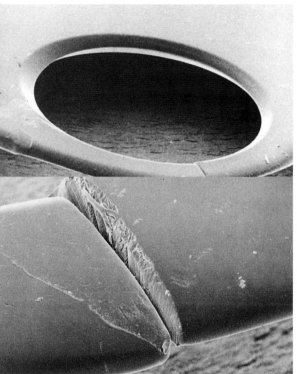

Fig. 5-14. Iris (lobster) claw IOL of Worst, scanning electron micrograph. This lens has been advocated as phakic implantation. **A,** Low power (×10.) **B,** High power view of "claw" (×50.) **C,** Higher power view of tips of "claw" (×100.)

followed after phakic implantation of a Worst-Fechner, lobster-claw IOL. The authors reported that 80% of their patients were within 1.00 D of emmetropia. There was a 3.3% cell loss at 6 months, 7.4% at 1 year, and 7.5% at 2 years. The study was limited in that only 14 of the patients were followed with specular microscopy for 2 years.

As with clear lens extraction and other forms of phakic IOL implantation, implantation of this lens carries with it the potential complications of intraocular surgery including endophthalmitis and retinal detachment. There is also a case report of anterior ischemic neuropathy following implantation of the Worst-Fechner iris-fixated IOL in a 33-year-old high myope, a complication that can occur with almost any intraocular surgical procedure, particularly if viscoelastic is left in the anterior chamber.[1602] This probably occurred as a result of a combination of raised postoperative intraocular pressure and systemic hypotension.

There are two other potential complications of this IOL design. These are the development of cataract and chronic breakdown in the blood-aqueous barrier. These concerns have been well studied by Perez-Santonja and colleagues.[1601] They studied blood-aqueous barrier permeability using fluorophotometry following implantation of the Worst-Fechner, biconcave lobster-claw IOL insertion. They also measured the clarity of the crystalline lens (lens transmittance) to look for any evidence of cataract formation. Fifteen patients were tested preoperatively and then at intervals for 14 months postoperatively. The transmittance of the crystalline lens decreased significantly from a value of 0.971 to 0.962 at 14 months. Fluorophotometry measurements also demonstrated a significant increase in blood-aqueous barrier permeability at all postoperative measurements. These data suggest that the Worst-Fechner

IOL produces chronic breakdown of the blood-aqueous barrier and may also eventually produce cataract in some patients.

We have no personal experience with this IOL except for some explant cases sent to us from South Asia where very poor manufacture was documented. The lenses manufactured in Europe for phakic implantation cannot be compared to these. Although two factors, difficulty of insertion and contact with uveal tissue, pose theoretical concerns, we cannot speak for or against this design. A significantly most worrisome finding, however, is the endothelial cell loss rates found by Worst's group in Holland. The increase in mean endothelial cell loss from 5.6% at 6 months to almost 9% at 12 months signals that one must carefully monitor the IOL for production of ongoing endothelial cell loss. If this were to continue, many of these patients would eventually develop pseudophakic bullous keratopathy and require penetrating keratoplasty. These concerns need to be allayed by long-term follow-up studies.

Posterior chamber intraocular lenses

In addition to implanting tried and true modern capsular posterior chamber IOLs as a refractive procedure after clear lens extraction, researchers are now studying the concept of phakic posterior chamber IOLs. The use of an IOL that occupies the slitlike, almost-potential space of the posterior chamber between the anterior surface of the natural lens and the posterior surface of the iris was first described in Russia in the early 1980s.[1542,1544] An IOL used by Fyodorov is currently being investigated by surgeons in Europe. Various materials such as silicone and collagen hydrogelcopolymers have been used. In general the lens has an anterior concave surface and a posterior convex surface.

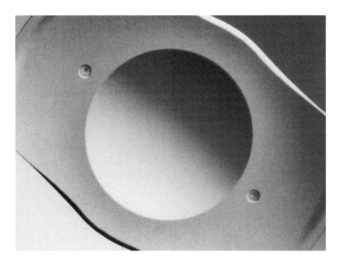

Fig. 5-15. Photograph of plate style posterior chamber IOL designed for phakic implantation manufactured by STAAR surgical. The lens is located between the posterior iris surface and the anterior lens surface.

The shape of the lens is similar to a modern plate-haptic silicone IOL (Fig. 5-15). The term *implantable contact lens* (ICL) has been coined for this IOL, because it is believed to locate itself in the eye with a thin layer of aqueous fluid between the implant and the anterior surface of the natural lens. It is claimed by proponents of the implantable contact lens that the lens is not in contact with the natural lens centrally and, hence, should not cause the natural lens to become cataractous. Certainly, the most attractive feature of the implantable contact lens is that it should be free from the well-described complications of angle-fixated, anterior chamber IOLs.

At the time of writing, this lens was being implanted in early, limited clinical trials, and general questions about the long-term safety and efficacy and the incidence of induced cataract remain unanswered. Also of concern may be the possible development of secondary pigment dispersion from contact between the lens and the posterior pigment epithelium of the iris. There is very little space between the anterior surface of the natural lens and the posterior iris pigment epithelium. There have been anecdotal reports that some patients develop either secondary cataracts or posterior pigment epithelial defects; therefore, it should be documented whether or not this could lead to secondary pigment dispersion and/or pigmentary glaucoma at a later date.

REFERENCES

1. Applegate RA and Howland HC: Magnification and visual acuity in refractive surgery, Arch Ophthalmol 111:1335, 1993.
2. Camp JJ, and others: A computer model for the evaluation of the effect of corneal topography on optical performance, Am J Ophthalmol 109:379, 1990.
3. Curtin BJ: The myopias: basic science and clinical management, New York, 1985, Harper & Row Publishers, Inc.
4. Holladay JT, Cravy TV, and Koch DD: Calculating the surgically induced refractive change following ocular surgery (see comments), J Cataract Refract Surg 18:429, 1992.
5. Koch DD: Refining analysis of refractive surgical outcomes, J Cataract Refract Surg 21:109, 1995, (editorial; comment).
6. McDonnell PJ: Current applications of the Corneal Modeling System, Refract Corneal Surg 7:87, 1991.
7. Schiotz H: Ein Fall von hochgradigem Hornhautastigmatismus nach Starextraction Besserung auf operativem Wege, Archiv fur Augenheilkunde 15:178, 1885.
8. Sperduto RD and others: Prevalence of myopia in the United States, Arch Ophthalmol 101:405, 1983.
9. Van Rij G: The happy patient, J Cataract Refract Surg 23:3, 1997.
10. Waring GO III and others: Results of the prospective evaluation of radial keratotomy (PERK) study one year after study, Ophthalmology 92:177, 1985.
11. Waring GO 3d: Standardized data collection and reporting for refractive surgery, Refract Corneal Surg 8(suppl):1, 1992.
12. Waring GO 3d: Refractive keratotomy for myopia and astigmatism, St. Louis, 1992, Mosby–Year Book, Inc.
13. Waring GO 3d, Lynn MJ, and McDonnell PJ: Results of the prospective evaluation of radial keratotomy (PERK) study 10 years after surgery, Arch Ophthalmol 112:1298, 1994.
14. Wilson SE, Klyce SD, and Husseini ZM: Standardized color-coded maps for corneal topography (see comments), Ophthalmology 100:1723, 1993.

Incisional corneal surgery

15. Agapitos PJ and others: Analysis of astigmatic keratotomy, J Cataract Refract Surg 15:13, 1989.
16. Aguirre Vila-Coro A, Bonafonte S, and Fernandez del Cotero JN: Epithelial inclusion cysts after radial keratotomy, Ann Ophthalmol 20:367, 1988.
17. Akiyama K: Study of surgical treatment for myopia. I. Posterior corneal incisions, Acta Soc Ophthalmol Jpn 56:1142, 1952.
18. Akiyama K: The surgical treatment of myopia. III. Report: anterior and posterior incision, Acta Soc Ophthalmol Jpn 93:797, 1955.
19. Akiyama K and others: Problems arising from Sato's radial keratotomy procedure in Japan, CLAO J 10:179, 1984.
20. Alio J and Ismail M: Management of radial keratotomy overcorrections by corneal sutures (see comments), J Cataract Refract Surg 19:595, 1993.
21. American Academy of Ophthalmology: Radial keratotomy for myopia, Ophthalmology 96:671, 1989.
22. American Academy of Ophthalmology: Ophthalmic procedures assessment. Radial keratotomy for myopia, Ophthalmology 100:1103, 1993.
23. American Medical Association: Diagnostic and therapeutic technology assessment. Radial keratotomy, JAMA 250:420, 1983.
24. American Medical Association: Diagnostic and therapeutic technology assessment. Radial keratotomy for simple myopia, JAMA 260:264, 1988.
25. Anderson JA, Murphy JA, and Gaster RN: Inflammatory cell responses to radial keratotomy, Refract Corneal Surg 5:21, 1989.
26. Applegate RA and Chundru U: Experimental verification of computational methods to calculate magnification in refractive surgery, Arch Ophthalmol 113:571, 1995.
27. Applegate RA and others: Radial keratotomy increases the effects of disability glare: initial results, Ann Ophthalmol 19:293, 1987.
28. Aquavella JV: Major refractive surgical techniques, Ophthalmic Surg 25:573, 1994.
29. Aron-Rosa D and others: Quantitative analysis of corneal excisions using argon fluoride excimer laser (193 nanometers), Bull Soc Ophthalmol Fr 89:1051, 1989.
30. Arrowsmith PN and Marks RG: Visual, refractive, and keratometric results of radial keratotomy. One-year follow-up, Arch Ophthalmol 102:1612, 1984.
31. Arrowsmith PN and Marks RG: Evaluating the predictability of radial keratotomy, Ophthalmology 92:331, 1985.
32. Arrowsmith PN and Marks RG: Visual, refractive, and keratometric results of radial keratotomy. A two-year follow-up, Arch Ophthalmol 105:76, 1987.
33. Arrowsmith PN and Marks RG: Visual, refractive, and keratometric results of radial keratotomy. Five-year follow-up (see comments), Arch Ophthalmol 107:506, 1989.
34. Arrowsmith PN, Sanders DR, and Marks RG: Visual, refractive, and keratometric results of radial keratotomy, Arch Ophthalmol 101:873, 1983.
35. Assil KK: Radial keratotomy: the combined technique, Int Ophthalmol Clin 34:55, 1994.

36. Assil KK and others: A combined incision technique of radial keratotomy. A comparison to centripetal and centrifugal incision techniques in human donor eyes, Ophthalmology 101:746, 1994.

37. Assil KK and Quantock AJ: Wound healing in response to keratorefractive surgery, Surv Ophthalmol 38:289, 1993.

38. Atkin A and others: Radial keratotomy and glare effects on contrast sensitivity, Doc Ophthalmol 62:129, 1986.

39. Avetisov SE and others: Experimental research on the effect of radial keratotomy on the mechanical properties of the corneal, Oftalmol Zh 1:54, 1990.

40. Baldone JA and Franklin RM: Cataract following radial keratotomy, Ann Ophthalmol 15:416, 1983.

41. Barner SS: Surgical induction of corneal astigmatism. An experimental study, Albrecht Von Graefes Arch Klin Exp Ophthalmol 201:213, 1977.

42. Barraquer JI: Transient descemetocele following radial keratotomy, Refract Corneal Surg 5:314, 1989.

43. Bas AM and Nano HD Jr: In situ myopic keratomileusis results in 30 eyes at 15 months, Refract Corneal Surg 7:223, 1991.

44. Basuk WL and others: Complications of hexagonal keratotomy, Am J Ophthalmol 117:37, 1994.

45. Bates AK, Morgan SJ, and Steele AD: Radial keratotomy: a review of 300 cases, Br J Ophthalmol 76:586, 1992.

46. Bates WH: A suggestion of an operation to correct astigmatism, Arch Ophthalmol 9, 1894.

47. Bauerberg J, Sterzovsky M, and Brodsky M: Radial keratotomy in myopia of 6 to 12 diopters using full-length deepening incisions, Refract Corneal Surg 5:150, 1989.

48. Beatty RF and Smith RE: 30-year follow-up of posterior radial keratotomy, Am J Ophthalmol 103:330, 1987.

49. Bechara SJ, Thompson KP, and Waring GO, 3d: Surgical correction of nearsightedness, Br Med J 305:813, 1992.

50. Beldavs RA and others: Bilateral microbial keratitis after radial keratotomy, Arch Ophthalmol 111:440, 1993, (letter).

51. Bergmann L and others: Damage to the corneal endothelium caused by radial keratotomy, Fortschr Ophthalmol 88:368, 1991.

52. Berkeley RG, Sanders DR, and Piccolo MG: Effect of incision direction on radial keratotomy outcome, J Cataract Refract Surg 17:819, 1991.

53. Bettman JW: Radial keratotomy: factors in medicolegal claims, Surv Ophthalmol 30:267, 1986.

54. Binder P: Mastel Byron radial keratotomy guide, J Refract Corneal Surg 10:656, 1994.

55. Binder PS: Astigmatic keratotomy procedures, Cornea 3:229, 1984, (editorial).

56. Binder PS: The status of radial keratotomy in 1984, Arch Ophthalmol 102:1601, 1984.

57. Binder PS: Four-year postoperative evaluation of radial keratotomy, Arch Ophthalmol 103:779, 1985, (editorial).

58. Binder PS: Pathologic findings in cases of refractive corneal surgery, Trans New Orleans Acad Ophthalmol 35:143, 1987.

59. Binder PS: Radial keratotomy in the United States. Where are we six years later? Arch Ophthalmol 105:37, 1987.

60. Binder PS: Barraquer lecture. What we have learned about corneal wound healing from refractive surgery, Refract Corneal Surg 5:98, 1989.

61. Binder PS: Measurement of corneal curvature after corneal transplantation and radial keratotomy using standard and automated keratometry, CLAO J 15:201, 1989.

62. Binder PS: Corneal epithelial and stromal reactions to excimer laser photorefactive keratectomy. III. The excimer laser and radial keratotomy: two vastly different approaches for myopia correction, Arch Ophthalmol 108:1541, 1990, (editorial).

63. Binder PS: Radial keratotomy in the 1990s and the PERK study, JAMA 263:1127, 1990, (editorial; comment).

64. Binder PS: Radial keratotomy and excimer laser photorefractive keratectomy for the correction of myopia, J Refract Corneal Surg 10:443, 1994.

65. Binder PS and Charlton KH: Surgical procedures performed after refractive surgery, Refract Corneal Surg 8:61, 1992.

66. Binder PS and others: An ultrastructural and histochemical study of long-term wound healing after radial keratotomy, Am J Ophthalmol 103:432, 1987.

67. Binder PS and others: Acute morphologic features of radial keratotomy, Arch Ophthalmol 101:1113, 1983.

68. Binder PS and others: Histopathology of traumatic corneal rupture after radial keratotomy, Arch Ophthalmol 106:1584, 1988.

69. Bloom HR, Sands J, and Schneider D: Corneal rupture from blunt trauma 22 months after radial keratotomy, Refract Corneal Surg 6:197, 1990.

70. Bogan SJ and others: Computer-assisted videokeratography of corneal topography after radial keratotomy, Arch Ophthalmol 109:834, 1991.

71. Bores LD: Historical review and clinical results of radial keratotomy, Int Ophthalmol Clin 23:93, 1983.

72. Bores LD: Radial keratotomy. I. A safe, effective way to correct a handicap, Surv Ophthalmol 28:101, 1983.

73. Bores LD: Refractive surgery, J Fla Med Assoc 81:272, 1994, (published erratum appears in J Fla Med Assoc 81(6):407, 1994).

74. Bores LD: Radial keratotomy predictability, Ophthalmology 101:414, 1994, (letter; comment).

75. Bores LD: Myers W, and Cowden J: Radial keratotomy: an analysis of the American experience, Ann Ophthalmol 13:941, 1981.

76. Bourque LB and others: Reported satisfaction, fluctuation of vision, and glare among patients one year after surgery in the Prospective Evaluation of Radial Keratotomy (PERK) Study, Arch Ophthalmol 104:356, 1986.

77. Bourque LB and others: Spectacle and contact lens wearing six years after radial keratotomy in the Prospective Evaluation of Radial Keratotomy Study, Ophthalmology 101:421, 1994.

78. Bourque LB and others: Psychosocial characteristics of candidates for the prospective evaluation of radial keratotomy (PERK) study, Arch Ophthalmol 102:1187, 1984.

79. Bourque LB and Waring GO 3d: Prospective evaluation of radial keratotomy (PERK) study patients, Arch Ophthalmol 103:890, 1985, (letter).

80. Braude LS, McMahon TT, and Sanders DR: Radial keratotomy in an ophthalmology residency program, J Cataract Refract Surg 3:17, 1987.

81. Bryant MR and others: Corneal tensile strength in fully healed radial keratotomy wounds, Invest Ophthalmol Vis Sci 35:3022, 1994.

82. Bullimore MA, Sheedy JE, and Owen D: Diurnal visual changes in radial keratotomy: implications for visual standards. Refractive Surgery Study Group, Optom Vis Sci 71:516, 1994.

83. Busin M and others: Change in corneal curvature with elevation of intraocular pressure after radial keratotomy in the primate eye, CLAO J 14:110, 1988.

84. Busin M and others: The effect of changes in intraocular pressure on corneal curvature after radial keratotomy in the rabbit eye, Ophthalmology 93:331, 1986.

85. Busin M and others: The effect of collagen cross-linkage inhibitors on rabbit corneas after radial keratotomy, Invest Ophthalmol Vis Sci 27:1001, 1986.

86. Buzard KA: Deepening of incision after radial keratotomy using the "tickle" technique, Refract Corneal Surg 6:394, 1990.

87. Buzard KA and others: Quantitative measurement of wound spreading in radial keratotomy, Refract Corneal Surg 8:217, 1992.

88. Campos M, Lee M, and McDonnell PJ: Ocular integrity after refractive surgery: effects of photorefractive keratectomy, phototherapeutic keratectomy, and radial keratotomy, Ophthalmic Surg 23:598, 1992.

89. Carney LG and Kelley CG: Visual losses after myopic epikeratoplasty, Arch Ophthalmol 109:499, 1991.

90. Carroll RP and Lindstrom RL: Blepharoptosis after radial keratotomy, Am J Ophthalmol 102:800, 1986.

91. Cartwright CS and others: Relationship of glare to uncorrected visual acuity and cycloplegic refraction 1 year after radial keratotomy in the prospective evaluation of radial keratotomy (PERK) study, J Am Optom Assoc 59:36, 1988.

92. Casebeer JC, editor: Casebeer incisional keratotomy, Thorofare, NJ, 1995, SLACK Incorporated.

93. Casebeer JC: Side effects and complications. In Casebeer JC, editor: Casebeer incisional keratotomy, Thorofare, NJ, 1995, SLACK, Inc.

94. Casebeer JC: The development of incisional keratotomy. In Casebeer JC, editor: Casebeer incisional keratotomy, Thorofare, NJ, 1995, SLACK, Inc.

95. Casebeer JC: Surgical procedures for correcting myopia and astig-

matism. In Casebeer JC, editor: Casebeer incisional keratotomy, Thorofare, NJ, 1995, SLACK, Inc.

96. Casebeer JC: Corneal anatomy, physiology and wound healing. In Casebeer JC, editor: Casebeer Incisional Keratotomy, Thorofare, NJ, 1995, SLACK, Inc.

97. Casebeer JC and Phillips SG: Hexagonal keratotomy. An historical review and assessment of 46 cases, Ophthalmol Clin North Am 5:727, 1992.

98. Casebeer JC and Shapiro DR: Radial keratotomy in intact epikeratoplasty graft, Refract Corneal Surg 9:133, 1993.

99. Casebeer JC, Shapiro DR, and Phillips S: Severe ocular trauma without corneal rupture after radial keratotomy: case reports, J Refract Corneal Surg 10:31, 1994.

100. Charpentier DY and others: Radial thermokeratoplasty is inadequate for overcorrection following radial keratotomy, J Refract Corneal Surg 10:34, 1994.

101. Chavez S and others: Analysis of astigmatic keratotomy with a 5.0 mm optical clear zone, Am J Ophthalmol 121:65, 1996.

102. Chen TT: Radial keratotomy: eleven-year experiences, Yen Ko Hsueh Pao 8:99, 1992.

103. Chiba K and others: Morphometric analysis of corneal endothelium following radial keratotomy, J Cataract Refract Surg 13:263, 1987.

104. Couvillion JT and others: Radial and astigmatic keratotomy experience by residents and fellows at a teaching institution, J Cataract Refract Surg 23:59, 1997.

105. Cowden JW: Radial keratotomy. A retrospective study of cases observed at the Kresge Eye Institute for six months, Arch Ophthalmol 100:578, 1982.

106. Cowden JW and Bores LD: A clinical investigation of the surgical correction of myopia by the method of Fyodorov, Ophthalmology 88:737, 1981.

107. Cowden JW and Cichocki J: Radial keratotomy in monkeys. A one-year follow-up report, Ophthalmology 89:684, 1982.

108. Cowden JW, Lynn MJ, and Waring GO 3d: Repeated radial keratotomy in the prospective evaluation of radial keratotomy study, Am J Ophthalmol 103:423, 1987.

109. Damiano RE and Forstot SL: Correction of radial keratotomy hyperopia, J Cataract Refract Surg 20:364, 1994, (letter comment).

110. Damiano RE, Forstot SL, and Dukes DK: Surgical correction of hyperopia following radial keratotomy, Refract Corneal Surg 8:75, 1992, (published erratum appears in Refract Corneal Surg 8(4): 314, 1992).

111. Dana MR and others: Dynamic shifts in corneal topography after radial and transverse keratotomy, Ophthalmology 101:1818, 1994.

112. Davison JA: Transverse astigmatic keratotomy combined with phacoemulsification and intraocular lens implantation, J Cataract Refract Surg 15:38, 1989.

113. Deg JK and Binder PS: Wound healing after astigmatic keratotomy in human eyes, Ophthalmology 94:1290, 1987.

114. Deg JK, Zavala EY, and Binder PS: Delayed corneal wound healing following radial keratotomy, Ophthalmology 92:734, 1985.

115. Deitz MR and Sanders DR: Progressive hyperopia with long-term follow-up of radial keratotomy, Arch Ophthalmol 103:782, 1985.

116. Deitz MR, Sanders DR, and Marks RG: Radial keratotomy: an overview of the Kansas City study, Ophthalmology 91:467, 1984.

117. Deitz MR, Sanders DR, and Raanan MG: Progressive hyperopia in radial keratotomy. Long-term follow-up of diamond-knife and metal-blade series, Ophthalmology 93:1284, 1986.

118. Deitz MR, Sanders DR, and Raanan MG: A consecutive series (1982-1985) of radial keratotomies performed with the diamond blade, Am J Ophthalmol 103:417, 1987.

119. Deitz MR and others: Long-term (5- to 12-year) follow-up of metal-blade radial keratotomy procedures, Arch Ophthalmol 112:614, 1994.

120. Diamond S: Present status of radial keratotomy myopia surgery: aerospace considerations, Aviat Space Environ Med 61:732, 1990.

121. Duffey RJ: Bilateral Serratia marcescens keratitis after simultaneous bilateral radial keratotomy, Am J Ophthalmol 119:233, 1995.

122. Duffey WS Jr: Radial keratotomy on trial: new surgical procedures and the antitrust laws. Part 2, Refract Corneal Surg 5:27, 1989.

123. Duling K and Wick B: Binocular vision complications after radial keratotomy, Am J Optom Physiol Opt 65:215, 1988.

124. Dunn S and others: Endothelial cell loss following radial keratotomy in a primate model, Arch Ophthalmol 102:1666, 1984.

125. Durand L and others: Complications of radial keratotomy: eyes with keratoconus and late wound dehiscence, Refract Corneal Surg 8:311, 1992.

126. Durand L, Burillon C, and Mutti P: Correction of severe myopia by refractive lamellar keratoplasty without freezing, J Fr Ophthalmol 14:167, 1991.

127. Durnev VV: Characteristics of surgical correction of myopia after 16 and 32 peripheral anterior radial nonperforating incisions. In Fyodorov SN, editor: Surgery for anomalies in ocular refraction, Moscow, 1981, The Moscow Research Institute for Ocular Microsurgery.

128. Durrie DS, Schumer DJ, and Cavanaugh TB: Photorefractive keratectomy for residual myopia after previous refractive keratotomy, J Refract Corneal Surg 10:S235, 1994.

129. Eghbali F, Yeung KK, and Maloney RK: Topographic determination of corneal asphericity and its lack of effect on the refractive outcome of radial keratotomy, Am J Ophthalmol 119:275, 1995.

130. Ellis W: Radial keratotomy in a patient with keratoconus, J Cataract Refract Surg 18:406, 1992.

131. Epstein RL and Laurence EP: Effect of topical diclofenac solution on discomfort after radial keratotomy, J Cataract Refract Surg 20:378, 1994.

132. Epstein RL and Laurence EP: Relative effectiveness of topical ketorolac and topical diclofenac on discomfort after radial keratotomy, J Cataract Refract Surg 21:156, 1995.

133. Ernst S and others: Radial keratotomy. Optical and functional results after a 5-year postoperative period, J Fr Ophtalmol 16:146, 1993.

134. Faber E: Operative Behandeling von astigmatisme, Nederl Tijdschr v Geneesk 31:495, 1895.

135. Fay AM, Trokel SL, and Myers JA: Pupil diameter and the principal ray, J Cataract Refract Surg 18:348, 1992.

136. Feldman RM and others: Retinal detachment following radial and astigmatic keratotomy, Refract Corneal Surg 7:252, 1991.

137. Feldman ST and others: The effect of increased intraocular pressure on visual acuity and corneal curvature after radial keratotomy, Am J Ophthalmol 108:126, 1989.

138. Fleming JF: Corneal asphericity and visual function after radial keratotomy, Cornea 12:233, 1993.

139. Forstot SL: Radial keratotomy, Int Ophthalmol Clin 28:116, 1988.

140. Forstot SL and Damiano RE: Trauma after radial keratotomy, Ophthalmology 95:833, 1988.

141. Frangie JP and others: Excimer laser keratectomy after radial keratotomy, Am J Ophthalmol 115:634, 1993.

142. Friedberg ML and others: Results of radial and astigmatic keratotomy by beginning refractive surgeons, Ophthalmology 100:746, 1993.

143. Friedberg ML and others: Results of radial and astigmatic keratotomy by beginning refractive surgeons, Ophthalmology 100:746, 1993.

144. Friedlander M: Critique of hexagonal keratotomy raises a ruckus, Refract Corneal Surg 8:408, 1992, (letter; comment).

145. Friedlander MH and Granet NS: Surgical correction of the spherical and aspherical cornea, St. Louis, Storz Ophthalmics, 1992, pp. 64-65, 81-82.

146. Friedlander MH: Radial keratotomy predictability, Ophthalmology 101:411, 1994, (letter; comment).

147. Friedlander MH and others: Videokeratographic evaluation of peripheral redeepening in the cadaver eye, J Cataract Refract Surg 20:490, 1994.

148. Friedlander MH and others: New technique for studying incision depth in experimental radial keratotomy, J Cataract Refract Surg 22(3):294, 1996.

149. Friedman RF, Wolf TC, and Chodosh J: Acanthamoeba infection after radial keratotomy, Brief Reports, Ocular microbiology and immunology group annual meeting 123(3):409, 1996.

150. Fujitani A and others: Retrocorneal ridges after anterior posterior radial keratotomy (Sato's operation) in a patient with retinitis pigmentosa, Ann Ophthalmol 25:392, 1993.

151. Fyodorov SN and Durnev VV: Operation of dosaged dissection of corneal circular ligament in cases of myopia of mild degree, Ann Ophthalmol 11:1185, 1979.

152. Fyodorov SN and others: Calculation method of effectiveness of anterior keratotomy in surgical correction of myopia. In Fyodorov SN, editor: Surgery for anomalies in ocular refraction, Moscow, 1981, The Moscow Research Institute for Ocular Microsurgery.

153. Fyodorov SN, Sarkizova MB, and Kurasova TP: Corneal biomicroscopy following repeated radial keratotomy, Ann Ophthalmol 15: 403, 1983.
154. Ganem S and others: Epithelial and stromal healing after radial keratotomy. Scanning electron microscopy analysis, Ophthalmologie 4:181, 1990.
155. Ganem S and others: Endothelial effects of radial keratotomy in a non-human primate, Ophthalmologie 3:13, 1989.
156. Garana RM and others: Radial keratotomy. II. Role of the myofibroblast in corneal wound contraction, Invest Ophthalmol Vis Sci 33:3271, 1992.
157. Garrett C and others: The use of thiphenamil hydrochloride (Trocinate) to control wound contraction after radial keratotomy, Ophthalmic Surg 18:428, 1987.
158. Geggel HS: Delayed sterile keratitis following radial keratotomy requiring corneal transplantation for visual rehabilitation, Refract Corneal Surg 6:55, 1990.
159. Gelender H, Flynn HW Jr, and Mandelbaum SH: Bacterial endophthalmitis resulting from radial keratotomy, Am J Ophthalmol 93:323, 1982.
160. Gelender H and Gelber EC: Cataract following radial keratotomy, Arch Ophthalmol 101:1229, 1983.
161. Gelisken O, Ozcetin H, and Dogru M: Retinal detachment after radial keratotomy, Bull Soc Belge Ophthalmol 249:63, 1993.
162. Georgaras SP and others: Correction of myopic anisometropia with photorefractive keratectomy in 15 eyes, Refract Corneal Surg 9: S29, 1993.
163. Gilbert ML, Friedlander MH, and Granet N: Corneal steepening in human eye bank eyes by combined hexagonal and transverse keratotomy, Refract Corneal Surg 6:126, 1990.
164. Gills JP and others, editors: Surgical treatment of astigmatism, Thorofare, NJ, 1994, SLACK, Inc.
165. Ginsburg AP and others: Contrast sensitivity under photopic conditions in the Prospective Evaluation of Radial Keratotomy (PERK) Study, Refract Corneal Surg 6:82, 1990.
166. Gipson IK: Cytoplasmic filaments: their role in motility and cell shape, Invest Ophthalmol Vis Sci 16:1081, 1977.
167. Girard LJ and others: Delayed wound healing after radial keratotomy, Am J Ophthalmol 99:485, 1985.
168. Glasgow BJ and others: Traumatic dehiscence of incisions seven years after radial keratotomy, Am J Ophthalmol 106:703, 1988.
169. Grady FJ: Radial keratotomy for astigmatism, Ann Ophthalmol 16: 942, 1984.
170. Grady FJ: Hexagonal keratotomy for corneal steepening, Ophthalmic Surg 19:622, 1988.
171. Grandon SC and Grandon GM: Effects of peripheral redeepening on radial keratotomy surgery, J Cataract Refract Surg 13:268, 1987.
172. Grandon SC and others: Clinical evaluation of hexagonal keratotomy for the treatment of primary hyperopia (see comments), J Cataract Refract Surg 21:140, 1995.
173. Grandon SC and Weber RA: Radial keratotomy in patients with atypical inferior steepening (see comments), J Cataract Refract Surg 20:381, 1994.
174. Grene RB and Lindstrom RL: Astigmatic keratotomy in the refractive patient: the ARC-T study. In Gills JP and others, editors: The surgical treatment of astigmatism, Thorofare, NJ, 1994, SLACK.
175. Grimmett MR, Holland EJ, and Krachmer JH: Therapeutic keratoplasty after radial keratotomy, Am J Ophthalmol 118:108, 1994.
176. Guell JL, Manero F, and Muller A: Transverse ketatotomy to correct high corneal astimatism after cataract surgery, J Cataract Refract Surg 22(3):331, 1996.
177. Gussler JR and others: Infection after radial keratotomy, Am J Ophthalmol 119:798, 1995.
178. Hahn TW, Kim JH, and Lee YC: Excimer laser photorefractive keratectomy to correct residual myopia after radial keratotomy, Refract Corneal Surg 9:S25, 1993.
179. Hanna KD, Jouve FE, and Waring GO 3d: Preliminary computer simulation of the effects of radial keratotomy, Arch Ophthalmol 107:911, 1989.
180. Hanna KD and others: Computer simulation of arcuate keratotomy for astigmatism, Refract Corneal Surg 8:152, 1992.
181. Harr D: Sparring over hexagonal keratotomy (news), Refract Corneal Surg 8:266, 1992.
182. Harris WF, Malan DJ, and Astin CL: Keratoreformation by contact lenses after radial keratotomy: a re-analysis, Ophthalmic Physiol Opt 12:376, 1992.
183. Haruta Y and others: Recurrent herpes simplex virus type 1 corneal epithelial lesions after radial keratotomy in the rabbit, Arch Ophthalmol 105:692, 1987.
184. Haverbeke L: Patient preference—contact lens or radial keratotomy? Refract Corneal Surg 8:315, 1992. (published erratum appears in Refract Corneal Surg 8(6):following 486, 1992.
185. Hecht SD and Jamara RJ: Prospective evaluation of radial keratotomy using the Fyodorov formula: preliminary report, Ann Ophthalmol 14:319, 1982.
186. Heidemann DG, Dunn SP, and Watts JC: Aspergillus keratitis after radial keratotomy, Am J Ophthalmol 120:254, 1995.
187. Helmy SA: Deep lamellar keratotomy after overcorrected excimer laser myopic keratomileusis, J Refract Corneal Surg 10:660, 1994, (letter).
188. Hemenger RP, Tomlinson A, and Caroline PJ: Role of spherical aberration in contrast sensitivity loss with radial keratotomy, Invest Ophthalmol Vis Sci 30:1997, 1989.
189. Hemenger RP, Tomlinson A, and McDonnell PJ: Explanation for good visual acuity in uncorrected residual hyperopia and presbyopia after radial keratotomy, Invest Ophthalmol Vis Sci 31:1644, 1990.
190. Hersh PS, Kalevar V, and Kenyon KR: Penetrating keratoplasty for severe complications of radial keratotomy, Cornea 10:170, 1991.
191. Hoffer KJ and others: UCLA clinical trial of radial keratotomy. Preliminary report, Ophthalmology 88:729, 1981.
192. Hoffer KJ and others: Three years experience with radial keratotomy. The UCLA study, Ophthalmology 90:627, 1983.
193. Holladay JT and others: The relationship of visual acuity, refractive error, and pupil size after radial keratotomy, Arch Ophthalmol 109: 70, 1991.
194. Holladay JT, Cravy TV, and Koch DD: Calculating the surgically induced refractive change following ocular surgery (see comments), J Cataract Refract Surg 18:429, 1992.
195. Hollis S: Astigmatism correction for lamellar keratoplasty. In Rozakis GW editor: Refractive lamellar keratoplasty, Thorofare, NJ, 1994, SLACK, Inc.
196. Hovding G: Transverse keratotomy in postkeratoplasty astigmatism, Acta Ophthalmol (Copenh) 72:464, 1994.
197. Hull DS and others: Radial keratotomy and corneal permeability in Owl Monkey, Acta Ophthalmol (Copenh) 61:240, 1983.
198. Hull DS and others: Radial keratotomy. Effect on cornea and aqueous humor physiology in the rabbit, Arch Ophthalmol 101:479, 1983.
199. Ingraham HJ, Guber D, and Green WR: Radial keratotomy. Clinicopathologic case report, Arch Ophthalmol 103:683, 1985.
200. Insler MS and Semple HC: Delayed microbial keratitis following radial keratotomy, CLAO J 14:163, 1988.
201. Jaffe NS and Clayman HM: The pathophysiology of corneal astigmatism after cataract extraction, Trans Am Acad Ophthalmol Otolaryngol 79:616, 1975.
202. Jean D and Detry-Morel M: Stellar corneal rupture and secondary glaucoma after squash trauma in a keratotomized eye, Bull Soc Belge Ophthalmol 245:109, 1992.
203. Jensen RP: Experience with hexagonal keratotomy, J Cataract Refract Surg 14:580, 1988, (letter).
204. Jensen RP: Hexagonal keratotomy: clinical experience with 483 eyes, Int Ophthalmol Clin 31:69, 1991.
205. Jester JV and others: Radial keratotomy. 1. The wound healing process and measurement of incisional gape in two animal models using in vivo confocal microscopy, Invest Ophthalmol Vis Sci 33: 3255, 1992.
206. Jester JV and others: Radial keratotomy in non-human primate eyes, Am J Ophthalmol 92:153, 1981.
207. Jester JV and others: A statistical analysis of radial keratotomy in human cadaver eyes, Am J Ophthalmol 92:172, 1981.
208. Jester JV, Villasenor RA, and Miyashiro J: Epithelial inclusion cysts following radial keratotomy, Arch Ophthalmol 101:611, 1983.
209. Jester JV and others: Variations in corneal wound healing after radial keratotomy: possible insights into mechanisms of clinical complications and refractive effects, Cornea 11:191, 1992.
210. John ME: High hyperopia after radial keratotomy, J Cataract Refract Surg 19:446, 1993, (letter; comment).

211. John ME, Jr. and Schmitt TE: Traumatic hyphema after radial keratotomy, Ann Ophthalmol 15:930, 1983.

212. Jory WJ: Radial keratotomy: 500 consecutive cases, Eye 3:663, 1989.

213. Kanai A and others: Bullous keratopathy after anterior-posterior radial keratotomy for myopia for myopic astigmatism, Am J Ophthalmol 93:600, 1982.

214. Karr DJ, Grutzmacher RD, and Reeh MJ: Radial keratotomy complicated by sterile keratitis and corneal perforation. Histopathologic case report and review of complications, Ophthalmology 92:1244, 1985.

215. Katz HR and others: Complications of contact lens wear after radial keratotomy in an animal model, Am J Ophthalmol 94:377, 1982.

216. Kaufman HE: Refractive surgery: through the looking glass, Acta Ophthalmol Suppl 192:30, 1989.

217. Keates RH and others: Fibronectin on excimer laser and diamond knife incisions, J Cataract Refract Surg 15:404, 1989.

218. Kelly CG. What is the role of refractive keratotomy in the 1990s? AudioDigest Ophthalmology, 33, 1995, California Medical Association.

219. Kim JW and others: The effect of radial keratotomy (RK) combined with double Ruiz procedure on the corneal curvature, Korean J Ophthalmol 3:55, 1989.

220. Kinota S and others: Changing patterns of infectious keratitis: overview of clinical and histopathologic features of keratitis due to acanthamoeba or atypical mycobacteria, and of infectious crystalline keratopathy, Indian J Ophthalmol 41:3, 1993.

221. Kirn TF: Long-term study evidence accumulating, but radial keratotomy controversy continues (news), JAMA 257:1282, 1987.

222. Kliger CH and Maloney RK: Keratitis as a complication of bilateral, simultaneous radial keratotomy, Am J Ophthalmol 118:680, 1994, (letter; comment).

223. Koch DD: Refining analysis of refractive surgical outcomes, J Cataract Refract Surg 21:109, 1995, (editorial; comment).

224. Koch DD and others: Refractive complications of cataract surgery after radial keratotomy, Am J Ophthalmol 108:676, 1989.

225. Koch JW and others: Corneal wound healing after perforating and non-perforating excimer laser keratectomy. An experimental study, Fortschr Ophthalmol 87:615, 1990.

226. Kohlhaas M and others: Aesthesiometry of the cornea after refractive corneal surgery, Klin Monatsbl Augenheilkd 201:221, 1992.

227. Kohlhaas M and others: Corneal sensitivity after refractive surgery, Eur J Implant Refract Surg 6:319, 1994.

228. Kohlhaas M and others: Corneal reinnervation after keratomileusis in situ and keratomileusis myopia—a comparison, Klin Monatsbl Augenheilkd 206:103, 1995.

229. Kraff MC and others: Changing practice patterns in refractive surgery: results of a survey of the American Society of Cataract and Refractive Surgery, J Cataract Refract Surg 20:172, 1994.

230. Krasnov MM and others: The effect of radial keratotomy on contrast sensitivity, Am J Ophthalmol 105:651, 1988.

231. Kremer FB and Marks RG: Radial keratotomy: prospective evaluation of safety and efficacy, Ophthalmic Surg 14:925, 1983.

232. Kwitko S and others: Diurnal variation of corneal topography after radial keratotomy, Arch Ophthalmol 110:351, 1992.

233. Kwitko S and others: Pharmacologic alteration of corneal topography after radial keratotomy, Ophthalmic Surg 23:738, 1992.

234. Kwitko ML and others: Arcuate keratotomy to correct naturally occurring astigmatism, J Cataract Refract Surg 22:1439, 1996.

235. L'Esperance FA Jr, and others: Human excimer laser corneal surgery: preliminary report, Trans Am Ophthalmol Soc 86:208, 1988.

236. Lans L: Experimentelle Untersuchungen uber Entstehung von Astigmatismus durch nicht-perforirende Corneawunden, Albrecht von Graefes Arch Ophthalmol 45:17, 1898.

237. Larson BC and others: Quantitated trauma following radial keratotomy in rabbits, Ophthalmology 90:660, 1983.

238. Leahey AB and Burkholder TO: Infectious keratitis 1 day after radial keratotomy, Arch Ophthalmol 112:1512, 1994, (letter).

239. Leaming DV: Practice styles and preferences of ASCRS members—1987 survey, J Cataract Refract Surg 14:552, 1988.

240. Leaming DV: Practice styles and preferences of ASCRS members—1988 survey, J Cataract Refract Surg 15:689, 1989.

241. Leaming DV: Practice styles and preferences of ASCRS members—1993 survey. J Cataract Refract Surg 20:459, 1994.

242. Leaming DV: Practice styles and preferences of ASCRS members—1994 survey, J Cataract Refract Surg 21:378, 1995.

243. Lee BL, Manche EE, and Glasgow BJ: Rupture of radial and arcuate keratotomy scars by blunt trauma 91 months after incisional keratotomy, Am J Ophthalmol 120:108, 1995.

244. Leidenix MJ and others: Perforated bacterial corneal ulcer in a radial keratotomy incision secondary to minor trauma, Arch Ophthalmol 112:1513, 1994, (letter).

245. Leroux les Jardins S, Bertrand I, and Massin M: Intraoperative and early postoperative complications in 466 radial keratotomies, Refract Corneal Surg 8:215, 1992.

246. Lin JC, Sheu MM, and Yang IJ: Mycobacterium smegmatis keratitis after radial keratotomy—a case report, Kao Hsiung I Hsueh Ko Hsueh Tsa Chih 10:267, 1994.

247. Linberg JV and others: Ptosis following radial keratotomy. Performed using a rigid eyelid speculum, Ophthalmology 93:1509, 1986.

248. Lindquist TD: Complications of corneal refractive surgery, Int Ophthalmol Clin 32:97, 1992.

249. Lindquist TD, Rubenstein JB, and Lindstrom RL: Correction of hyperopia following radial keratotomy: quantification in human cadaver eyes, Ophthalmic Surg 18:432, 1987.

250. Lindquist TD and others: Trapezoidal astigmatic keratotomy. Quantification in human cadaver eyes, Arch Ophthalmol 104:1534, 1986.

251. Lindquist TD, Williams PA, and Lindstrom RL: Surgical treatment of overcorrection following radial keratotomy: evaluation of clinical effectiveness, Ophthalmic Surg 22:12, 1991.

252. Lindstrom RL: Surgical correction of refractive errors after penetrating keratoplasty, Int Ophthalmol Clin 34:35, 1994.

253. Lindstrom RL: Minimally invasive radial keratotomy: mini-RK, J Cataract Refract Surg 21:27, 1995.

254. Lindstrom RL and Lindquist TD: Surgical correction of postoperative astigmatism, Cornea 7:138, 1988.

255. Lipshitz I, Loewenstein A, and Lazar M: Astigmatic keratotomy followed by photorefractive keratectomy in the treatment of compound myopic astigmatism, J Refract Corneal Surg 10:S282, 1994.

256. Lipshitz I: Refractive and visual results of RK, Ophthalmology 103(8):1164, 1996, (letter).

257. Lopez PF and others: Subregions of differing refractive power within the clear zone after experimental radial keratotomy, Refract Corneal Surg 7:360, 1991.

258. Luttrull JK, Jester JV, and Smith RE: The effect of radial keratotomy on ocular integrity in an animal model, Arch Ophthalmol 100:319, 1982.

259. Lyle WA and Jin GJ: Clear lens extraction for the correction of high refractive error (see comments), J Cataract Refract Surg 20:273, 1994.

260. Lyle WA and Jin JC: Circular and interrupted suture technique for correction of hyperopia following radial keratotomy, Refract Corneal Surg 8:80, 1992.

261. Lynn MJ, Waring GO 3d, and Carter JT: Combining refractive error and uncorrected visual acuity to assess the effectiveness of refractive corneal surgery, Refract Corneal Surg 6:103, 1990.

262. Lynn MJ and others: Symmetry of refractive and visual acuity outcome in the Prospective Evaluation of Radial Keratotomy (PERK) study, Refract Corneal Surg 5:75, 1989.

263. Lynn MJ, Waring GO 3d, and Sperduto RD: Factors affecting outcome and predictability of radial keratotomy in the PERK Study, Arch Ophthalmol 105:42, 1987.

264. MacRae SM, Matsuda M, and Rich LF: The effect of radial keratotomy on the corneal endothelium, Am J Ophthalmol 100:538, 1985.

265. MacRae S and others: The treatment of persistent wound leak after radial keratotomy, Refract Corneal Surg 9:62, 1993.

266. MacRae S and others: Diurnal variation in vision after radial keratotomy, Am J Ophthalmol 107:262, 1989.

267. Mader TH and White LJ: Refractive changes at extreme altitude after radial keratotomy, Am J Ophthalmol 119:733, 1995.

268. Mader TH and others: Refractive changes during 72-hour exposure to high altitude after refractive surgery, Ophthalmology 103(8):1188, 1996.

269. Maguen E and others: Results of excimer laser photorefractive keratectomy for the correction of myopia, Ophthalmology 101:1548, 1994.

270. Maguire LJ: Keratorefractive surgery, success, and the public health, Am J Ophthalmol 117:394, 1994.

271. Maguire LJ and Bourne WM: A multifocal lens effect as a complication of radial keratotomy, Refract Corneal Surg 5:394, 1989.

272. Maloney RK: Effect of corneal hydration and intraocular pressure on keratometric power after experimental radial keratotomy, Ophthalmology 97:927, 1990.

273. Maloney RK, Bogan SJ, and Waring GO 3d: Determination of corneal image-forming properties from corneal topography (see comments), Am J Ophthalmol 115:31, 1993.

274. Maloney WF and others: Astigmatism control for the cataract surgeon: a comprehensive review of surgically tailored astigmatism reduction (STAR), J Cataract Refract Surg 15:45, 1989.

275. Mamalis N and others: Radial keratotomy in a patient with keratoconus, Refract Corneal Surg 7:374, 1991.

276. Mandelbaum S and others: Late development of ulcerative keratitis in radial keratotomy scars, Arch Ophthalmol 104:1156, 1986.

277. Mansour AM, Rowsey JJ, and Munn AR, 3d: Ab interno radial keratotomy, Refract Corneal Surg 7:181, 1991.

278. Marmer RH: Radial keratotomy complications, Ann Ophthalmol 19:409, 1987.

279. Marmer RH: Ocular deviation induced by radial keratotomy, Ann Ophthalmol 19:451, 1987, published erratum appears in Ann Ophthalmol 20(2):60, 1988.

280. Marmer RH: Therapeutic and protective properties of the corneal collagen shield, J Cataract Refract Surg 14:496, 1988.

281. Martin XD and Safran AB: Corneal hypoesthesia, Surv Ophthalmol 33:28, errata 217, 1988.

282. Matoba AY and others: Bacterial keratitis after radial keratotomy, Ophthalmology 96:1171, 1989.

283. McCartney DL and others: Refractive keratoplasty for disabling astigmatism after penetrating keratoplasty, Arch Ophthalmol 105: 954, 1987.

284. McClellan KA and others: Suppurative keratitis: a late complication of radial keratotomy, J Cataract Refract Surg 14:317, 1988.

285. McCluskey DJ, Villasenor R, and McDonnell PJ: Prospective topographic analysis in peripheral arcuate keratotomy for astigmatism, Ophthalmic Surg 21:464, 1990.

286. McDermott ML and others: Corneoscleral rupture ten years after radial keratotomy, Am J Ophthalmol 110:575, 1990.

287. McDonald MB, Haik M, and Kaufman HE: Color vision and contrast sensitivity testing after radial keratotomy, Am J Ophthalmol 103:468, 1987.

288. McDonnell PJ, Lean JS, and Schanzlin DJ: Globe rupture from blunt trauma after hexagonal keratotomy, Am J Ophthalmol 103: 241, 1987.

289. McDonnell PJ and Schanzlin DJ: Early changes in refractive error following radial keratotomy, Arch Ophthalmol 106:212, 1988.

290. McDonnell PJ, Garbus J, and Lopez PF: Topographic analysis and visual acuity after radial keratotomy (see comments), Am J Ophthalmol 106:692, 1988.

291. McDonnell PJ, Caroline PJ, and Salz J: Irregular astigmatism after radial and astigmatic keratotomy, Am J Ophthalmol 107:42, 1989.

292. McDonnell PJ, Fish LA, and Garbus J: Persistence of diurnal fluctuation after radial keratotomy, Refract Corneal Surg 5:89, 1989.

293. McDonnell PJ and Garbus J: Corneal topographic changes after radial keratotomy, Ophthalmology 96:45, 1989.

294. McDonnell PJ, McClusky DJ, and Garbus JJ: Corneal topography and fluctuating visual acuity after radial keratotomy, Ophthalmology 96:665, 1989.

295. McDonnell PJ: Current applications of the Corneal Modeling System, Refract Corneal Surg 7:87, 1991.

296. McDonnell PJ, Garbus JJ, and Salz JJ: Excimer laser myopic photorefractive keratotomy after undercorrected radial keratotomy, Refract Corneal Surg 7:146, 1991.

297. McDonnell PJ and others: Computerized analysis of corneal topography as an aid in fitting contact lenses after radial keratotomy, Ophthalmic Surg 23:55, 1992.

298. McDonnell PJ: Sight-threatening complications after radial keratotomy, Arch Ophthalmol 114(2):211, 1996, (editorial; comment; review).

299. McKnight SJ, Fitz J, and Giangiacomo J: Corneal rupture following radial keratotomy in cats subjected to BB gun injury, Ophthalmic Surg 19:165, 1988.

300. McNeill JI: Corneal incision dehiscence during penetrating keratoplasty nine years after radial keratotomy, J Cataract Refract Surg 19:542, 1993.

301. McNeill JI and Wilkins DL: A purse-string suture for penetrating keratoplasty following radial keratotomy, Refract Corneal Surg 7: 392, 1991.

302. McWhae J and others: Ultrasound biomicroscopy in refractive surgery, J Cataract Refract Surg 20:493, 1994.

303. Melles GR and Binder PS: Effect of radial keratotomy incision direction on wound depth, Refract Corneal Surg 6:394, 1990.

304. Melles GR and Binder PS: Effect of wound location, orientation, direction, and postoperative time on unsutured corneal wound healing morphology in monkeys, Refract Corneal Surg 8:427, 1992.

305. Melles GR, Binder PS, and Anderson JA: Variation in healing throughout the depth of long-term, unsutured, corneal wounds in human autopsy specimens and monkeys, Arch Ophthalmol 112: 100, 1994.

306. Melles GR and others: Scar tissue orientation in unsutured and sutured corneal wound healing, Br J Ophthalmol 79:760, 1995.

307. Melles GR and others: Epithelial-stromal interactions in human keratotomy wound healing, Arch Ophthalmol 113:1124, 1995.

308. Melles GR and others: Three versus four radial keratotomy incisions, J Cataract Refract Surg 18:27, 1992.

309. Melles GR and others: Effect of blade configuration, knife action, and intraocular pressure on keratotomy incision depth and shape, Cornea 12:299, 1993.

310. Mendez AE: Accidental grafting of a donor cornea with radial keratotomy in a keratoconus patient, Refract Corneal Surg 5:198, 1989.

311. Mendez A: Correcao da hipermetropia pela ceratotomia hexagonal. In Guimarares R, editor: Cirugia refractive, Rio de Janeiro, 1987, Pirâmide Livro Médico Editora Ltda.

312. Merlin U and others: Factors that affect keratotomy depth, Refract Corneal Surg 7:356, 1991.

313. Meza J and others: Photorefractive keratectomy after radial keratotomy, J Cataract Refract Surg 20:485, 1994.

314. Miller D and Miller R: Glare sensitivity in simulated radial keratotomy, Arch Ophthalmol 99:1961, 1981.

315. Millin JA and Maguire LJ: Developing entry criteria for studies of severe postkeratoplasty astigmatism, Am J Ophthalmol 112:666, 1991.

316. Molander N and others: Influence of radial keratotomy on endogenous hyaluronan in cornea and aqueous humour, Refract Corneal Surg 9:358, 1993.

317. Momose A and Shen A: Eleven-year experience with radial keratotomy, Yen Ko Hsueh Pao 10:6, 1994.

318. Montard M, Prost F, and Bron A: Indications and motivations of radial keratotomy for the surgical correction of myopial, Bull Soc Ophthalmol Fr 87:119, 1987.

319. Moorhead LC and others: Effects of topical treatment with beta-aminopropionitrile after radial keratotomy in the rabbit, Arch Ophthalmol 102:304, 1984.

320. Moreira H and others: Corneal topographic changes over time after radial keratotomy, Cornea 11:465, 1992.

321. Moreira H and others: Multifocal corneal topographic changes after radial keratotomy, Ophthalmic Surg 23:85, 1992.

322. Moreira H, and others: Multifocal corneal topographic changes with excimer laser photorefractive keratectomy (see comments), Arch Ophthalmol 110:994, 1992.

323. Moreira H and others: Retrospective comparison of simultaneous and non-simultaneous bilateral radial keratotomy, J Refract Corneal Surg 10:545, 1994.

324. Muller-Stolzenburg N and others: Fluorescence behavior of the cornea with 193 nm excimer laser irradiation, Fortschr Ophthalmol 87:653, 1990.

325. Nelson JD and others: Map-fingerprint-dot changes in the corneal epithelial basement membrane following radial keratotomy, Ophthalmology 92:199, 1985.

326. Neumann AC and McCarty GR: Hexagonal keratotomy for correction of low hyperopia: preliminary results of a prospective study, J Cataract Refract Surg 14:265, 1988.

327. Neumann AC and others: Refractive evaluation of astigmatic keratotomy procedures, J Cataract Refract Surg 15:25, 1989.

328. Neumann AC, Osher RH, and Fenzl RE: Radial keratotomy: a comprehensive evaluation, Doc Ophthalmol 56:275, 1984.

329. Nirankari VS and others: Ongoing prospective clinical study of radial keratotomy, Ophthalmology 90:637, 1983.

330. Nirankari VS and others: Prospective clinical study of radial keratotomy, Ophthalmology 89:677, 1982.

331. Nolan BT: Perforation by a foreign body through a pre-existing radial keratotomy wound, Mil Med 156:151, 1991.

332. Nordan LT and others: Photorefractive keratectomy to treat myopia and astigmatism after radial keratotomy and penetrating keratoplasty, J Cataract Refract Surg 21:268, 1995.

333. Nordan LT and Maxwell WA: Refractive surgery and informed consent. Radial keratotomy with small optical zone hexagonal keratotomy, J Cataract Refract Surg 18:420, 1992, (letter).

334. Nordan LT and Maxwell WA: Avoid both radial keratotomy with small optical zones and hexagonal keratotomy [see comments], Refract Corneal Surg 8:331, 1992 (letter).

335. Nordan LT and Maxwell WA: Hexagonal keratotomy, Refract Corneal Surg 9:228, 1993, (letter; comment).

336. Nordan LT and Maxwell WA: Radial keratotomy predictability, Ophthalmology 101:412, 1994, (letter; comment).

337. O'Day DM, Feman SS, and Elliott JH: Visual impairment following radial keratotomy. A cluster of cases, Ophthalmology 93:319, 1986.

338. O'Dell L and Wyzinski P: Hexagonal keratotomy for intraocular lens miscalculation, Can J Ophthalmol 25:355, 1990.

339. Orge Y: The evaluation of pachymetric changes in the central cornea after radial keratotomy, Bull Soc Belge Ophthalmol 234:15, 1989.

340. Osher RH: Paired transverse relaxing keratotomy: a combined technique for reducing astigmatism, J Cataract Refract Surg 15:32, 1989.

341. Palkama A and others: Histochemical analysis of wound healing in radial keratotomy, Acta Ophthalmol Suppl 182:51, 1987.

342. Parmley V and others: Penetrating keratoplasty after radial keratotomy. A report of six patients, Ophthalmology 102:947, 1995.

343. Pearlstein ES and others: Ruptured globe after radial keratotomy, Am J Ophthalmol 106:755, 1988.

344. Percival SP: Radial keratotomy: where did it go wrong? Eye 2:478, 1988.

345. Petroll WM and others: Radial keratotomy. III. Relationship between wound gape and corneal curvature in primate eyes, Invest Ophthalmol Vis Sci 33:3283, 1992.

346. Pinheiro MN Jr and others: Corneal integrity after refractive surgery. Effects of radial keratotomy and mini-radial keratotomy, Ophthalmology 102:297, 1995.

347. Pinsky PM and Datye DV: A microstructurally-based finite element model of the incised human cornea, J Biomech 24:907, 1991.

348. Pinsky PM and Datye DV: Numerical modeling of radial, astigmatic, and hexagonal keratotomy, Refract Corneal Surg 8:164, 1992.

349. Plesner HJ and others: Radial keratotomy for pseudophakic myopia, Acta Ophthalmol (Copenh) 66:120, 1988.

350. Poirier L and others: Effect of peripheral deepening of radial keratotomy incisions, J Refract Corneal Surg 10:621, 1994.

351. Polit F and others: Subepithelial reticular cicatrization following radial keratotomy in a patient with inactive trachoma, Refract Corneal Surg 8:240, 1992.

352. Pouliquen Y, Hanna K, and Saragoussi JJ: The Hanna radial microkeratome: presentation and first experiment, Dev Ophthalmol 14:132, 1987.

353. Powers MK and others: Psychosocial findings in radial keratotomy patients two years after surgery, Ophthalmology 91:1193, 1984.

354. Price FW and others: Astigmatism reduction clinical trial: a multicenter prospective evaluation of the predictability of arcuate keratotomy. Evaluation of surgical nomogram predictability. ARC-T Study Group, Arch Ophthalmol 113:277, 1995, (published erratum appears in Arch Ophthalmol 13(5):577, 1995).

355. Pulaski JP: Transverse incisions for mixed and myopic idiopathic astigmatism, J Cataract Refract Surg 22(3):307, 1996.

356. Rapizzi A and others: Blood staining of the cornea following radial keratotomy, Refract Corneal Surg 7:188, 1991.

357. Rashid ER and Waring GO 3d: Complications of radial and transverse keratotomy, Surv Ophthalmol 34:73, 1989.

358. Rawe IM, Tuft SJ, and Meek KM: Proteoglycan and collagen morphology in superficially scarred rabbit cornea, Histochem J 24:311, 1992.

359. Reichel MB and others: Traumatic wound dehiscence and corneal rupture 3½ years after radial keratotomy, Klin Monatsbl Augenheilkd 206:266, 1995.

360. Ribeiro JC and others: Excimer laser photorefractive keratectomy after radial keratotomy, J Refract Surg 11:165, 1995.

361. Ring CP, Hadden OB, and Morris AT: Transverse keratotomy combined with spherical photorefractive keratectomy for compound myopic astigmatism, J Refract Corneal Surg 10:S217, 1994.

362. Robin JB: Hexagonal keratotomy, (see comments), Refract Corneal Surg 8:486, 1992, (letter; comment).

363. Robin JB: Hyperopic refractive surgery, AudioDigest Ophthalmology, 33, 1995, California Medical Association.

364. Robin JB and others: Mycobacterium chelonei keratitis after radial keratotomy, Am J Ophthalmol 102:72, 1986.

365. Rodriguez A and Camacho H: Retinal detachment after refractive surgery for myopia, Retina 12:S46, 1992.

366. Rosa DS and others: Wound healing following excimer laser radial keratotomy, J Cataract Refract Surg 14:173, 1988.

367. Rowsey JJ: Radial keratotomy: results, complications, and research directions, Trans New Orleans Acad Ophthalmol 35:193, 1987.

368. Rowsey JJ: Radial keratotomy: indications, contraindications, and surgical techniques, Trans New Orleans Acad Ophthalmol 35:121, 1987.

369. Rowsey JJ and Balyeat HD: Radial keratotomy: preliminary report of complications, Ophthalmic Surg 13:27, 1982.

370. Rowsey JJ and Balyeat HD: Preliminary results and complications of radial keratotomy, Am J Ophthalmol 93:437, 1982.

371. Rowsey JJ and others: Prospective evaluation of radial keratotomy. Photokeratoscope corneal topography, Ophthalmology 95:322, 1988.

372. Rowsey JJ and others: Predicting the results of radial keratotomy, Ophthalmology 90:642, 1983.

373. Rowsey JJ and others: Accuracy and reproducibility of KeraScanner analysis in PERK corneal topography. PERK Study Group, Curr Eye Res 8:661, 1989.

374. Rowsey JJ and Rubin ML: Refraction problems after refractive surgery, Surv Ophthalmol 32:414, 1988.

375. Rowsey JJ and others: Corneal topography as a predictor of refractive change in the prospective evaluation of radial keratotomy (PERK) study, Ophthalmic Surg 22:370, 1991.

376. Rylander HG, Welch AJ, and Fremming B: The effect of radial keratotomy in the rupture strength of pig eyes, Ophthalmic Surg 14:744, 1983.

377. Sabates MA and others: Induction of astigmatism by straight transverse corneal incisions, 45 degrees long, at different clear zones in human cadaver eyes, J Refract Corneal Surg 10:327, 1994, (published erratum appears in J Refract Corneal Surg 10(4):479, 1994.

378. Salz J and others: Radial keratotomy in fresh human cadaver eyes, Ophthalmology 88:742, 1981.

379. Salz JJ: Multiple complications following radial keratotomy in an elderly patient: a case report, Ophthalmic Surg 16:579, 1985.

380. Salz JJ and others: Analysis of incision depth following experimental radial keratotomy, Ophthalmology 90:655, 1983.

381. Salz JJ and others: Ten years experience with a conservative approach to radial keratotomy, Refract Corneal Surg 7:12, 1991.

382. Salz JJ and others: Four-incision radial keratotomy for low to moderate myopia, Ophthalmology 93:727, 1986.

383. Sanders DR, Deitz MR, and Gallagher D: Factors affecting predictability of radial keratotomy, Ophthalmology 92:1237, 1985.

384. Sanders N: Wedge resection in host cornea to correct post-keratoplasty astigmatism, Ophthalmic Surg 10:53, 1979.

385. Santos CI: Herpes keratitis after radial keratotomy, Am J Ophthalmol 93:370, 1982, (letter).

386. Santos CR: Herpetic corneal ulcer following radial keratotomy, Ann Ophthalmol 15:82, 1983.

387. Santos VR and others: Relationship between refractive error and visual acuity in the Prospective Evaluation of Radial Keratotomy (PERK) Study, Arch Ophthalmol 105:86, 1987.

388. Santos VR and others: Morning-to-evening change in refraction, corneal curvature, and visual acuity 2 to 4 years after radial keratotomy in the PERK Study (see comments), Ophthalmology 95:1487, 1988.

389. Saragoussi JJ and Pouliquen YJ: Does the progressive increasing effect of radial keratotomy (hyperopic shift) correlate with undetected early keratoconus? J Refract Corneal Surg 10:45, 1994.

390. Saragoussi JJ and others: Ultrastructural changes of the corneal endothelium in experimental radial keratotomy, Bull Soc Ophthalmol Fr 87:245, 1987.

391. Sastry SM and others: Radial keratotomy does not affect intraocular pressure, Refract Corneal Surg 9:459, 1993.

392. Sato T: Treatment of conical corneal incision of Descemet's membrane, Acta Soc Ophthalmol Jpn 43:541, 1939.

393. Sato T, Akiyama K and Shibata H: A new surgical approach to myopia, Am J Ophthalmol 36:823, 1953.

394. Sawelson H and Marks RG: Two-year results of radial keratotomy, Arch Ophthalmol 103:505, 1985.

395. Sawelson H and Marks RG: Three-year results of radial keratotomy, Arch Ophthalmol 105:81, 1987.

396. Sawelson H and Marks RG: Two-year results of reoperations for radial keratotomy, Arch Ophthalmol 106:497, 1988.

397. Sawelson H and Marks RG: Five-year results of radial keratotomy, Refract Corneal Surg 5:8, 1989.

398. Sawusch MR and McDonnell PJ: Computer modeling of wound gape following radial keratotomy, Refract Corneal Surg 8:143, 1992.

399. Sawusch MR, Wan WL, and McDonnell PJ: Tissue addition theory of radial keratotomy: a geometric model, J Cataract Refract Surg 17:448, 1991.

400. Schachar RA: Indications, techniques, and complications of radial keratotomy, Int Ophthalmol Clin 23:119, 1983.

401. Schanzlin DJ and others: Diurnal change in refraction, corneal curvature, visual acuity, and intraocular pressure after radial keratotomy in the PERK Study, Ophthalmology 93:167, 1986.

402. Schiotz H: Ein Fall von hochgradigem Hornhautastigmatismus nach Starextraction Besserung auf operativem Wege, Archiv fur Augenheilkunde 15:178, 1885.

403. Schipper I, Suppelt C, and Senn P: Correction of astigmatism with Excimer laser transverse keratectomy, Acta Ophthalmol (Copenh) 72:39, 1994.

404. Seiler T and Jean B: Photorefractive keratectomy as a second attempt to correct myopia after radial keratotomy, Refract Corneal Surg 8:211, 1992.

405. Shapiro MB and Harrison DA: Radial keratotomy for intolerable myopia after penetrating keratoplasty [see comments], Am J Ophthalmol 115:327, 1993.

406. Shawbitz SD, Damiano RE, and Forstot SL: Radial keratotomy in high myopia: an evaluation of one technique, Ann Ophthalmol 21:375, 1989.

407. Shepard DD: Radial keratotomy: analysis of efficacy and predictability in 1,058 consecutive cases. Part I: Efficacy, J Cataract Refract Surg 12:632, 1986.

408. Shepard DD: Radial keratotomy: analysis of efficacy and predictability in 1,058 consecutive cases. Part II: Predictability, J Cataract Refract Surg 13:32, 1987.

409. Shepard JR: Correction of preexisting astigmatism at the time of small incision cataract surgery, J Cataract Refract Surg 15:55, 1989.

410. Shivitz IA and Arrowsmith PN: Delayed keratitis after radial keratotomy, Arch Ophthalmol 104:1153, 1986.

411. Shivitz IA, Arrowsmith PN, and Russell BM: Contact lenses in the treatment of patients with overcorrected radial keratotomy, Ophthalmology 94:899, 1987.

412. Shivitz IA and Arrowsmith PN: Corneal sensitivity after radial keratotomy, Ophthalmology 95:827, 1988.

413. Simon G and Ren Q: Biomechanical behavior of the cornea and its response to radial keratotomy, J Refract Corneal Surg 10:343, 1994.

414. Singh D, Grewal SP, and Kumar N: Anterior radial keratotomy experience in 600 cases of myopia, Ann Ophthalmol 16:757, 1984.

415. Spigelman AV, Williams PA, and Lindstrom RL: Further studies of four incision radial keratotomy, Refract Corneal Surg 5:292, 1989.

416. Spigelman AV and others: Four incision radial keratotomy, J Cataract Refract Surg 14:125, 1988.

417. Springer M: Court upholds ruling in radial keratotomy suit, Arch Ophthalmol 107:649, 1989.

418. Stainer GA and others: Histopathology of a case of radial keratotomy, Arch Ophthalmol 100:1473, 1982.

419. Stark WJ, Martin NF, and Maumenee AE: Radial keratotomy. II. A risky procedure of unproven longterm success, Surv Ophthalmol 28:101, 106, 1983.

420. Steel D and others: Modification of corneal curvature following radial keratotomy in primates, Ophthalmology 88:747, 1981.

421. Steel DL and Salz JJ: Laboratory evaluation of radial keratotomy, Int Ophthalmol Clin 23:129, 1983.

422. Steinberg EB and Waring GO, 3d: Comparison of two methods of marking the visual axis on the cornea during radial keratotomy, Am J Ophthalmol 96:605, 1983.

423. Steinberg EB and others: Stellate iron lines in the corneal epithelium after radial keratotomy, Am J Ophthalmol 98:416, 1984.

424. Sugar A: Has radial keratotomy finally come of age? Ophthalmology 100:979, 1993, (editorial; comment).

425. Symons SP and Slomovic AR: Visual acuity, refractive and keratometric results of 140 consecutive radial keratotomy procedures, Can J Ophthalmol 29:176, 1994.

426. Szerenyi K and others: Keratitis as a complication of bilateral, simultaneous radial keratotomy (see comments), Am J Ophthalmol 117:462, 1994.

427. Tamura M and others: Complications of a hexagonal keratotomy following radial keratotomy, Arch Ophthalmol 109:1351, 1991, (letter).

428. Teranishi C: A study on the effects of different keratectomies for astigmatism in rabbits' eyes, Hokkaido Igaku Zasshi 63:56, 1988.

429. Thompson V: The surgical correction of myopic and hyperopic astigmatism, Int Ophthalmol Clin 34:87, 1994.

430. Thornton SP and Sanders DR: Graded nonintersecting transverse incisions for correction of idiopathic astigmatism, J Cataract Refract Surg 13:27, 1987.

431. Thornton SP: A comparison of one-stage radial keratotomy with two-stage radial keratotomy in myopia (see comments), Refract Corneal Surg 5:43, 1989.

432. Thornton SP: Astigmatic keratotomy: a review of basic concepts with case reports, J Cataract Refract Surg 16:430, 1990.

433. Thornton SP: Astigmatic keratotomy with corneal relaxing incisions, Int Ophthalmol Clin 34:79, 1994.

434. Thornton SP: Radial and astigmatic keratotomy: The American system of precise, predictable refractive surgery, Thorofare, NJ, 1994, SLACK.

435. Tomlinson A and Caroline P: Effect of radial keratotomy on the contrast sensitivity function, Am J Optom Physiol Opt 65:803, 1988.

436. Trick LR and Hartstein J: Investigation of contrast sensitivity following radial keratotomy, Ann Ophthalmol 19:251, 1987.

437. Troutman RC: Control of corneal astigmatism in cataract and corneal surgery, Trans Pac Coast Otoophthalmol Soc Annu Meet 51:217, 1970.

438. Troutman RC: Microsurgical control of corneal astigmatism in cataract and keratoplasty, Trans Am Acad Ophthalmol Otolaryngol 77:563, 1973.

439. Troutman RC: Corneal wedge resections and relaxing incisions for postkeratoplasty astigmatism, Int Ophthalmol Clin 23:161, 1983.

440. Troutman RC and others: The use and preliminary results of the Troutman surgical keratometer in cataract and corneal surgery, Trans Am Acad Ophthalmol Otolaryngol 83:232, 1977.

441. Troutman RC and Swinger C: Relaxing incision for control of postoperative astigmatism following keratoplasty, Ophthalmic Surg 11:117, 1980.

442. Troutman RC, and Gaster RN: Surgical advances and results of keratoconus, Am J Ophthalmol 90:131, 1980.

443. Updegraff SA, McDonald MB, and Beuerman RW: Freeze-fracture scanning electron microscopy of radial keratotomy incisions, Am J Ophthalmol 117:399, 1994, (letter).

444. Umlas JW and others: Ocular integrity after quantitated trauma in radial keratotomy eyes, Invest Ophthalmol Vis Sci 36(4,suppl): S583, 1995.

445. Utkin VF: Nonpenetrating peripheral radial keratotomy in the treatment of spherical and aspherical myopia, Vestn Oftalmol 21, 1979.

446. van Rij G and Waring GO 3d: Changes in corneal curvature induced by sutures and incisions, Am J Ophthalmol 98:773, 1984.

447. Vaughan ER and Paschall WJ: A statistical analysis of radial keratotomy results, Ann Ophthalmol 17:275, 1985.

448. Vinger PF and others: Ruptured globes following radial and hexagonal keratotomy surgery [see comments], Arch Ophthalmol 114(2): 129, 1996, (review).

449. Vito RP, Shin TJ, and McCarey BE: A mechanical model of the cornea: the effects of physiological and surgical factors on radial keratotomy surgery, Refract Corneal Surg 5:82, 1989.

450. Wang W and others: Excimer laser photorefractive keratectomy

for myopia in China. A report of 750 eyes with a 6-month follow-up, Chin Med J (Engl) 108:601, 1995.

451. Wang ZX: An ultrastructural study of the rabbit cornea after radial keratotomy, Chung Hua Yen Ko Tsa Chih 29:296, 1993.

452. Waring GO III: Radial keratotomy in perspective, Am J Ophthalmol 92:286, 1981.

453. Waring GO III: Radial keratotomy for myopia, South Med J 74:1, 1981 (editorial).

454. Waring GO III:and others: Design features of the prospective evaluation of radial keratotomy (PERK) study, Int Ophthalmol Clin 23:145, 1983.

455. Waring GO III:and others: Rationale for and design of the National Eye Institute Prospective Evaluation of Radial Keratotomy (PERK) Study, Ophthalmology 90:40, 1983.

456. Waring GO III: Making sense of 'keratospeak'. A classification of refractive corneal surgery, Arch Ophthalmol 103:1472, 1985.

457. Waring GO III: Evolution of radial keratotomy for myopia, Trans Ophthalmol Soc U K 104:28, 1985.

458. Waring GO III and others: Results of the prospective evaluation of radial keratotomy (PERK) study one year after surgery, Ophthalmology 92:177, 1985.

459. Waring GO III, Steinberg EB, and Wilson LA: Slit-lamp microscopic appearance of corneal wound healing after radial keratotomy, Am J Ophthalmol 100:218, 1985.

460. Waring GO III and others: Three-year results of the Prospective Evaluation of Radial Keratotomy (PERK) Study, Ophthalmology 94:1339, 1987.

461. Waring GO III: William H. Bates: The originator of astigmatic keratotomy and psycho-ophthalmology, Refract Corneal Surg 5:56, 1989.

462. Waring GO III: Stunning victory for Academy in radial keratotomy antitrust litigation, Refract Corneal Surg 5:140, 1989 (editorial).

463. Waring GO III: Another surprise from radial keratotomy, Refract Corneal Surg 5:6, 1989, (editorial).

464. Waring GO III and others: Results of the Prospective Evaluation of Radial Keratotomy (PERK) Study 4 years after surgery for myopia, JAMA 263:1083, 1990.

465. Waring GO III and others: Results of the Prospective Evaluation of Radial Keratotomy (PERK) Study five years after surgery. The Perk Study Group, Ophthalmology 98:1164, 1991.

466. Waring GO III and others: Stability of refraction during four years after radial keratotomy in the prospective evaluation of radial keratotomy study (see comments), Am J Ophthalmol 111:133, 1991.

467. Waring GO III: Standardized data collection and reporting for refractive surgery, Refract Corneal Surg 8(suppl):1, 1992.

468. Waring GO III: Making sense of keratospeak. IV. Classification of refractive surgery, 1992 (see comments), Arch Ophthalmol 110:1385, 1992.

469. Waring GO III: Refractive keratotomy for myopia and astigmatism, St. Louis, 1992, Mosby–Year Book.

470. Waring GO III: Radial keratotomy predictability Ophthalmology 101:415, 1994, (letter; comment).

471. Waring GO III and others: Results of the prospective evaluation of radial keratotomy (PERK) study 10 years after surgery, Arch Ophthalmol 112:1298, 1994.

472. Waring GO III: Evolution of refractive surgery into the 21st Century (DuPont Guerry III Lecture) Audio-Digest Foundation, Glendale, 1995, California Medical Association.

473. Waring GO, III: Evaluating new refractive surgical procedures: Free market madness versus regulatory rigor mortis, J Refract Surg 11:335, 1995.

474. Waring GO, III: Changing concepts in excimer laser corneal surgery, J Refract Surg 11(Suppl):S224, 1995, (editorial; review).

475. Wellish KL and others: Corneal ectasia as a complication of repeated keratotomy surgery, J Refract Corneal Surg 10:360, 1994.

476. Werblin T: Critique of hexagonal keratotomy raises a ruckus, Refract Corneal Surg 8:408, 1992, (letter, comment).

477. Werblin TP and Stafford GM: The Casebeer system for predictable keratorefractive surgery. One-year evaluation of 205 consecutive eyes (see comments), Ophthalmology 100:1095, 1993.

478. Wharton KR: Corneal stellate iron lines following radial keratotomy, J Am Optom Assoc 60:362, 1989.

479. Wilson DR and Keeney AH: Corrective measures for myopia, Surv Ophthalmol 34:294, 1990.

480. Wilson SE and Klyce SD: Advances in the analysis of corneal topography, Surv Ophthalmol 35:269, 1991.

481. Wilson SE, Klyce SD and Husseini ZM: Standardized color-coded maps for corneal topography (see comments), Ophthalmology 100:1723, 1993.

482. Wray WO, Best ED and Cheng LY: A mechanical model for radial keratotomy: toward a predictive capability, J Biomech Eng 116:56, 1994.

483. Wyzinski P: Daily refractive changes persisting after radial keratotomy, Am J Ophthalmol 108:205, 1989.

484. Wyzinski P and O'Dell L: Subjective and objective findings after radial keratotomy, Ophthalmology 96:1608, 1989.

485. Wyzinski P and O'Dell LW: Diurnal cycle of refraction after radial keratotomy, Ophthalmology 94:120, 1987.

486. Yamaguchi T and others: Corticosteroid therapy after anterior radial keratotomy in primates, Am J Ophthalmol 97:215, 1984.

487. Yamaguchi T and others: Endothelial damage in monkeys after radial keratotomy performed with a diamond blade, Arch Ophthalmol 102:765, 1984.

488. Yamaguchi T and others: Bullous keratopathy after anterior-posterior radial keratotomy for myopia, Am J Ophthalmol 93:600, 1982.

489. Yamaguchi T and others: Histologic and electron microscopic assessment of endothelial damage produced by anterior radial keratotomy in the monkey cornea, Am J Ophthalmol 92:313, 1981.

490. Yamaguchi T and others: Endothelial damage after anterior radial keratotomy. An electron microscopic study of rabbit cornea, Arch Ophthalmol 99:2151, 1981.

491. Yamaguchi T and others: Histologic study of a pair of human corneas after anterior radial keratotomy, Am J Ophthalmol 100:281, 1985.

492. Yamashita T and others: Hexagonal keratotomy reduces hyperopia after radial keratotomy in rabbits, J Refract Surg 2:261, 1986.

493. Young SR, Lundergan MK and Olson RJ: Late complications of combined radial and transverse keratotomy after penetrating keratoplasty associated with atopic keratoconjunctivitis, Refract Corneal Surg 5:194, 1989.

494. Zamora RL, Goldberg MA and Pepose JS: Presumed epithelial cyst in the anterior chamber following refractive keratotomy, J Refract Corneal Surg 10:652, 1994.

Lamellar corneal surgery

495. Ainslie D: The surgical correction of refractive errors by keratomileusis and keratophakia, Ann Ophthalmol 8:349, 1976.

496. Altmann J and others: Corneal lathing using the excimer laser and a computer-controlled positioning system: Part I—Lathing of epikeratoplasty lenticules, Refract Corneal Surg 7:377, 1991.

497. American Academy of Ophthalmology: Keratophakia and keratomileusis: safety and effectiveness, Ophthalmology 99:1332, 1992.

498. Aquavella JV: Major refractive surgical techniques, Ophthalmic Surg 25:573, 1994.

499. Aquavella JV and others: Morphological variations in corneal endothelium following keratophakia and keratomileusis, Ophthalmology 88:721, 1981.

500. Arenas-Archila E and others: Myopic keratomileusis in situ: a preliminary report, J Cataract Refract Surg 17:424, 1991.

501. Arffa RC and others: Epikeratophakia with commercially prepared tissue for the correction of aphakia in adults, Arch Ophthalmol 104:1467, 1986.

502. Arffa RC, Marvelli TL and Morgan KS: Keratometric and refractive results of pediatric epikeratophakia, Arch Ophthalmol 103:1656, 1985.

503. Arffa RC, Marvelli TL and Morgan KS: Long-term follow-up of refractive and keratometric results of pediatric epikeratophakia, Arch Ophthalmol 104:668, 1986.

504. Asbell PA and others: Secondary surgical procedures after epikeratophakia, Ophthalmic Surg 13:555, 1982.

505. Avni I and others: Epikeratophakia after ocular trauma, Am J Ophthalmol 107:268, 1989.

506. Azar DT and others: Reassembly of the corneal epithelial adhesion structures following human epikeratoplasty, Arch Ophthalmol 109:1279, 1991.

507. Azar RF: Secondary implantation, Int Ophthalmol Clin 19:211, 1979.

508. Baikoff G and Joly P: Comparison of minus power anterior cham-

ber intraocular lenses and myopic epikeratoplasty in phakic eyes (see comments), Refract Corneal Surg 6:252, 1990.

509. Barker BA and Swinger CA: Keratophakia and keratomileusis, Int Ophthalmol Clin 28:126, 1988.

510. Barraquer C, Gutierrez AM and Espinosa A: Myopic keratomileusis: short-term results, Refract Corneal Surg 5:307, 1989.

511. Barraquer JI: Queratoplastia refractiva, Estudios Inform Oftal Inst Barraquer 10:2, 1949.

512. Barraquer JI: Method for cutting lamellar grafts in frozen corneas: new orientations for refractive surgery, Arch Soc Am Ophthalmol 1:237, 1958.

513. Barraquer JI: Keratomileusis for the correction of myopia, Ann Inst Barraquer 5:209, 1964.

514. Barraquer JI: Queratomileusis para la correction de la miopia, Arch Soc Am Oftalmol Optom 5:27, 1964.

515. Barraquer JI: Autokeratoplasty with optical carving for the correction of myopia (Keratomileusis) (Spanish), An Med Espec 51:66, 1965.

516. Barraquer JI: Autokeratoplasty with levelins for the correction of myopia. (Keratomileusis). Technic and results (French), Ann Ocul (Paris) 198:401, 1965.

517. Barraquer JI: Modification of refraction by means of intracorneal inclusions, Int Ophthalmol Clin 6:53, 1966.

518. Barraquer JI: Keratomileusis, Int Surg 48:103, 1967.

519. Barraquer JI: Lamellar keratoplasty (special techniques), Ann Ophthalmol 4:437, 1972.

520. Barraquer JI: Keratophakia, Trans Ophthalmol Soc U K 92:499, 1972.

521. Barraquer JI: Keratomileusis for myopia and aphakia, Ophthalmology 88:701, 1981.

522. Barraquer JI: Keratomileusis and keratophakia for the correction of congenital hypermetropia and aphakia, Bull Mem Soc Fr Ophthalmol 95:380, 1983.

523. Barraquer JI: Results of hypermetropic keratomileusis, 1980-1981, Int Ophthalmol Clin 23:25, 1983.

524. Bas AM and Nano HD, Jr. In situ myopic keratomileusis results in 30 eyes at 15 months, Refract Corneal Surg 7:223, 1991.

525. Bas AM and Onnis R: Excimer laser in situ keratomileusis for myopia, J Refract Surg 11:S229, 1995.

526. Baumgartner SD and Binder PS: Refractive keratoplasty. Histopathology of clinical specimens, Ophthalmology 92:1606, 1985.

527. Bechrakis N and others: Recurrent keratoconus, Cornea 13:73, 1994.

528. Beekhuis WH and McCarey BE: Hydration stability of intracorneal hydrogel implants, Invest Ophthalmol Vis Sci 26:1634, 1985.

529. Beekhuis WH and others: Complications of hydrogel intracorneal lenses in monkeys, Arch Ophthalmol 105:116, 1987.

530. Beekhuis WH and others: Hydrogel keratophakia: a microkeratome dissection in the monkey model, Br J Ophthalmol 70:192, 1986.

531. Biermann H and others: Corneal sensibility following epikeratophakia, Klin Monatsbl Augenheilkd 201:18, 1992.

532. Binder PS: Hydrogel implants for the correction of myopia, Curr Eye Res 2:435, 1982.

533. Binder PS: Refractive surgery in the United States, Dev Ophthalmol 18:203, 1989, (review).

534. Binder PS and others: Refractive keratoplasty: microkeratome evaluation, Arch Ophthalmol 100:802, 1982.

535. Binder PS, Baumgartner SD, and Fogle JA: Histopathology of a case of epikeratophakia (aphakic epikeratoplasty), Arch Ophthalmol 103:1357, 1985.

536. Binder PS and others: Refractive keratoplasty: myopic keratomileusis in baboons, Curr Eye Res 3:1187, 1984.

537. Binder PS, Beal JP Jr, and Zavala EY: The histopathology of a case of keratophakia, Arch Ophthalmol 100:101, 1982.

538. Binder PS and others: Hydrogel keratophakia in non-human primates, Curr Eye Res 1:535, 1981.

539. Binder PS and others: Refractive keratoplasty. Keratophakia in a nonhuman primate, Arch Ophthalmol 102:1671, 1984.

540. Binder PS and others: Refractive keratoplasty. Tissue dyes and cryoprotective solutions, Arch Ophthalmol 101:1591, 1983.

541. Binder PS and others: Alloplastic implants for the correction of refractive errors, Ophthalmology 91:806, 1984.

542. Binder PS and others: Hydrophilic lenses for refractive keratoplasty: the use of factory lathed materials, CLAO J 10:105, 1984.

543. Bleckmann H: Epikeratophakia—a new procedure in refractive surgery of the corneal, Klin Monatsbl Augenheilkd 193:345, 1988.

544. Bohm A and others: Corneal reinnervation after lamellar keratoplasty in comparison with epikeratophakia and photorefractive keratectomy, Ophthalmologe 91:632, 1994.

545. Bond WI: Hyperopic ALK results: patients outside the Ruiz nomogram. Best papers of sessions from the ASCRS symposium on cataract, IOL and refractive surgery, Boston, April 1994, p. 25.

546. Bores LD: Refractive surgery, J Fla Med Assoc 81:272, 1994, (published erratum appears in J Fla Med Assoc 81(6):407, 1994).

547. Bornfeld N and others: Ultrastructure of the rabbit corneal stroma after experimental keratomileusis, Arch Ophthalmol 104:253, 1986.

548. Bosc JM and others: Non-freeze myopic keratomileusis. Retrospective study of 27 consecutive operations, J Fr Ophthalmol 13: 10, 1990.

549. Brittain GP and others: The use of a biological adhesive to achieve sutureless epikeratophakia, Eye 3:56, 1989.

550. Buratto L and Ferrari M: Retrospective comparison of freeze and non-freeze myopic epikeratophakia, Refract Corneal Surg 5:94, 1989.

551. Burillon C, Durand L, and Gourraud A: Combined epikeratoplasty and homoplastic keratophakia for correction of aphakia: double curve effect, Refract Corneal Surg 9:214, 1993.

552. Busin M, Bechrakis-Boker I, and Denninger U: Surgical therapy of keratoconus. Epikeratophakia versus penetrating keratoplasty, Fortschr Ophthalmol 88:794, 1991.

553. Busin M and Cusumano A: Modified surgical technique for repeated epikeratophakia surgery in aphakic eyes, Refract Corneal Surg 8:382, 1992.

554. Busin M, Cusumano A, and Spitznas M: Epithelial interface cysts after epikeratophakia, Ophthalmology 100:1225, 1993.

555. Busin M and Nussgens Z: Epikeratophakia, Fortschr Ophthalmol 87 Suppl:S219, 1990.

556. Busin M, Schmidt J, and Koch J: Physiologic analysis of corneal healing after epikeratophakia, Ophthalmology 99:415, 1992.

557. Busin M, Spitznas M, and Hockwin O: Evaluation of functional and morphologic parameters of the cornea after epikeratophakia using prelathed, lyophilized tissue, Ophthalmology 97:330, 1990.

558. Busin M and others: In vivo evaluation of epikeratophakia lenses by means of Scheimpflug photography, Refract Corneal Surg 5: 155, 1989.

559. Camp JJ and others: A computer model for the evaluation of the effect of corneal topography on optical performance, Am J Ophthalmol 109:379, 1990.

560. Campos M and others: Corneal sensitivity after photorefractive keratectomy, Am J Ophthalmol 114:51, 1992.

561. Caporossi A and Manetti C: Epidermal growth factor in topical treatment following epikeratoplasty, Ophthalmologica 205:121, 1992.

562. Carey BE: Synthetic keratophakia. In Brightbill FS, editor: Corneal surgery, St. Louis/Washington, D.C. 1986, CV Mosby Co.

563. Carney LG and Kelley CG: Visual losses after myopic epikeratoplasty, Arch Ophthalmol 109:499, 1991.

564. Casebeer JC: New technologies and the role of incisional keratotomy. In Casebeer JC, editor: Casebeer Incisional Keratotomy, Thorofare, NJ, 1995, SLACK.

565. Casebeer JC and Shapiro DR: Radial keratotomy in intact epikeratoplasty graft, Refract Corneal Surg 9:133, 1993.

566. Casebeer JC and others: Intraoperative pachometry during automated lamellar keratoplasty: a preliminary report, J Refract Corneal Surg 10:41, 1994.

567. Cavallini GM and others: Epikeratophakia: histopathological and cultural study, Int Ophthalmol 16:115, 1992.

568. Chen JQ and Yang B: Homoplastic keratomileusis for aphakic eyes with corneal leucoma, Chung Hua Yen Ko Tsa Chih 30:351, 1994.

569. Chew SJ, Beuerman RW, and Kaufman HE: Real-time confocal microscopy of keratocyte activity in wound healing after cryoablation in rabbit corneas, Scanning 16:269, 1994.

570. Climenhaga H and others: Effect of diameter and depth on the response to solid polysulfone intracorneal lenses in cats, Arch Ophthalmol 106:818, 1988.

571. Colin J and others: The surgical treatment of high myopia: comparison of epikeratoplasty, keratomileusis and minus power anterior chamber lenses (see comments), Refract Corneal Surg 6:245, 1990.

572. Colin J and others: Photorefractive keratectomy following undercorrected myopic epikeratoplasties, J Fr Ophthalmol 15:384, 1992.

573. Coster DJ: The Australian Corneal Graft Registry. 1990 to 1992 report, Aust N Z J Ophthalmol 21:1, 1993, (review).

574. Cusumano A and others: Epikeratophakia for the correction of myopia: lenticule design and related histopathological findings (see comments), Refract Corneal Surg 6:120, 1990.

575. David T and others: Corneal wound healing modulation using basic fibroblast growth factor after excimer laser photorefractive keratectomy, Cornea 14:227, 1995.

576. Deg JK, Binder PS, and Kirkness CM: Unfenestrated polysulfone implants are incompatible with the baboon and human cornea, Invest Ophthalmol Vis Sci 28:276, 1987.

577. Dietze TR and Durrie DS: Indications and treatment of keratoconus using epikeratophakia, Ophthalmology 95:236, 1988.

578. Dingeldein SA and McDonald MB: Epikeratophakia, Int Ophthalmol Clin 28:134, 1988.

579. Dossi F and Bosio P: Myopic keratomileusis: results with a follow-up over one year, J Cataract Refract Surg 13:417, 1987.

580. Durand L, Burillon C, and Mutti P: Correction of severe myopia by refractive lamellar keratoplasty without freezing, J Fr Ophthalmol 14:167, 1991.

581. Durand L, Burillon C, and Resal R: Refractive surgery and the non-freeze BKS set. Reliability of our Lyon methods. Value of our results, Bull Soc Ophthalmol Fr 90:441, 1990.

582. Durrie DS, Habrich DL, and Dietze TR: Secondary intraocular lens implantation vs epikeratophakia for the treatment of aphakia, Am J Ophthalmol 103:384, 1987.

583. Ehrlich MI and Nordan LT: Epikeratophakia for the treatment of hyperopia, J Cataract Refract Surg 15:661, 1989.

584. Elsas FJ: Visual acuity in monocular pediatric aphakia: does epikeratophakia facilitate occlusion therapy in children intolerant of contact lens or spectacle wear? J Pediatr Ophthalmol Strabismus 27:304, 1990.

585. Feldman ST: The effect of epidermal growth factor on corneal wound healing: practical considerations for therapeutic use, Refract Corneal Surg 7:232, 1991, (review).

586. Fiander DC and Tayfour F: Excimer laser in situ keratomileusis in 124 myopic eyes, J Refract Surg 11:S234, 1995.

587. Flores-Tapia IA: Catastrophic keratomileusis: Postoperative complications of intraoperative perforation with lens damage. Best papers of sessions from the ASCRS symposium on cataract, IOL and Refractive Surgery, Boston, April 1994, p. 23.

588. Francis C and Rootman DS: Epikeratophakia for correction of complicated aphakia, Can J Ophthalmol 29:17, 1994.

589. Frantz JM and others: Immunogenicity of epikeratophakia tissue lenses containing living donor keratocytes, Refract Corneal Surg 7:141, 1991.

590. Frantz JM and others: Penetrating keratoplasty after epikeratophakia for keratoconus, Arch Ophthalmol 106:1224, 1988.

591. Frantz JM, McDonald MB, and Kaufman HE: Results of penetrating keratoplasty after epikeratophakia for keratoconus in the nationwide study, Ophthalmology 96:1151, 1989.

592. Friedlander MH and others: Keratophakia using preserved lenticules, Ophthalmology 87:687, 1980.

593. Friedlander MH and others: Update on keratophakia, Ophthalmology 90:365, 1983.

594. Friedlander MH and others: Clinical results of keratophakia and keratomileusis, Ophthalmology 88:716, 1981.

595. Fyodorov SN and Zakharov VD: Surgery of keratomileusis and keratophakia (preliminary report), Vestn Oftalmol 2:19, 1971.

596. Gabay S, Slomovic A, and Jares T: Excimer laser-processed donor corneal lenticules for lamellar keratoplasty, Am J Ophthalmol 107:47, 1989.

597. Gailitis RP and others: Solid state ultraviolet laser (213 nm) ablation of the cornea and synthetic collagen lenticules, Lasers Surg Med 11:556, 1991.

598. Ganem S, Mondon H, and De Felice GP: Local treatment by epidermal growth factor after epikeratoplasty. A double-blind clinical trial, J Fr Ophthalmol 15:443, 1992.

599. Gomes M: Laser in situ keratomileusis for myopia using manual dissection, J Refract Surg 11:S239, 1995.

600. Goodman DF and others: Lamellar keratectomy and repeat epikeratoplasty following failed epikeratoplasty. A clinicopathologic report, Cornea 8:295, 1989.

601. Goosey JD and others: Stability of refraction during two years after myopic epikeratoplasty, Refract Corneal Surg 6:4, 1990.

602. Grabner G: New central, epithelial iron deposit following epikeratophakia in high-grade myopia, Klin Monatsbl Augenheilkd 190:424, 1987.

603. Grabner G: Complications of epikeratophakia in correction of aphakia, myopia, hyperopia and keratoconus, Fortschr Ophthalmol 88:4, 1991.

604. Guimaraes RQ and others: Suturing in lamellar surgery: the BRA-technique, Refract Corneal Surg 8:84, 1992.

605. Guss RB and others: Endothelial cell counts after epikeratophakia surgery, Ann Ophthalmol 15:408, 1983.

606. Hagen KB, Kim EK, and Waring GO 3d: Comparison of excimer laser and microkeratome myopic keratomileusis in human cadaver eyes, Refract Corneal Surg 9:36, 1993.

607. Haimovici R and Culbertson WW: Optical lamellar keratoplasty using the Barraquer microkeratome, Refract Corneal Surg 7:42, 1991.

608. Halliday BL: Epikeratophakia for keratoconus, Eye 4:531, 1990.

609. Halliday BL: Epikeratophakia for aphakia, keratoconus, and myopia see comments, Br J Ophthalmol 74:67, 1990.

610. Hanna KD and others: Lamellar keratoplasty with the Barraquer microkeratome, Refract Corneal Surg 7:177, 1991.

611. Harper RA and Halliday BL: Glare and contrast sensitivity in contact lens corrected aphakia, epikeratophakia and pseudophakia, Eye 3:562, 1989.

612. Helmy SA: Deep lamellar keratotomy after overcorrected excimer laser myopic keratomileusis, J Refract Corneal Surg 10:660, 1994, (letter).

613. Hirano K and others: Long-spacing collagen in the human corneal stroma, Jpn J Ophthalmol 37:148, 1993.

614. Hjortdal JO and Ehlers N: Epikeratophakia for high myopia, Acta Ophthalmol (Copenh) 69:754, 1991.

615. Hoffman CJ and others: Displacement of corneal lenticule after automated lamellar keratoplasty, Am J Ophthalmol 118:109, 1994, (letter).

616. Hoffmann F: Experimental data in keratophakia, Dev Ophthalmol 5:41, 1981.

617. Hoffmann F: Keratomileusis, keratophakia and keratokyphosis, Trans Ophthalmol Soc U K 104:48, 1985.

618. Hoffmann F, Schuler A, and Wachtlin J: Comparison of corneal lenticules produced for keratokyphosis and keratophakia, Ger J Ophthalmol 2:395, 1993.

619. Hofmann RF and Bechara SJ: An independent evaluation of second generation suction microkeratomes, Refract Corneal Surg 8:348, 1992.

620. Hollis S: Hyperopic lamellar keratoplasty. In Rozakis GW, editor: Refractive lamellar keratoplasty, Thorofare, NJ, 1994, SLACK.

621. Hovding G and Bertelsen T: Epikeratophakia for keratoconus. Long-term results using fresh, free-hand made lamellar grafts, Acta Ophthalmol (Copenh) 70:461, 1992.

622. Hovding G, Haugen OH, and Bertelsen T: Epikeratophakia for keratoconus in mentally retarded patients. The use of fresh, free-hand made lamellar grafts, Acta Ophthalmol (Copenh) 70:730, 1992.

623. Ibrahim O and others: Automated in situ keratomileusis for myopia, J Refract Surg 11:431, 1995.

624. Jain S and others: Corneal light scattering after laser in situ keratomileusis and photorefractive keratectomy, Am J Ophthalmol 120:532, 1995.

625. Jakobiec FA and others: Keratophakia and keratomileusis: comparison of pathologic features in penetrating keratoplasty specimens, Ophthalmology 88:1251, 1981.

626. Jester JV and others: Keratophakia and keratomileusis: histopathologic, ultrastructural, and experimental studies, Ophthalmology 91:793, 1984.

627. Katakami C and others: Localization of collagen (I) and collagenase mRNA by in situ hybridization during corneal wound healing after epikeratophakia or alkali-burn, Jpn J Ophthalmol 36:10, 1992.

628. Katakami C and others: Keratocyte activity in wound healing after epikeratophakia in rabbits, Invest Ophthalmol Vis Sci 32:1837, 1991.

629. Kaufman HE: The correction of aphakia. XXXVI Edward Jackson Memorial Lecture, Am J Ophthalmol 89:1, 1980.

630. Kaufman HE: Refractive surgery: through the looking glass, Acta Ophthalmol Suppl 192:30, 1989.

631. Kaufman HE and McDonald MB: Refractive surgery for aphakia and myopia, Trans Ophthalmol Soc U K 104:43, 1985.

632. Kaufman HE and Werblin TP: Epikeratophakia for the treatment of keratoconus, Am J Ophthalmol 93:342, 1982.

633. Keates RH, Lembach RG, and Rabin B: Early results of epikeratophakia, Dev Ophthalmol 14:127, 1987.

634. Keates RH, Watson SA, and Levy SN: Epikeratophakia following previous refractive keratoplasty surgery: two case reports, J Cataract Refract Surg 12:536, 1986.

635. Kelley CG, Keates RH, and Lembach RG: Epikeratophakia for pediatric aphakia, Arch Ophthalmol 104:680, 1986.

636. Kezirian GM and Gremillion CM: Automated lamellar keratoplasty for the correction of hyperopia, J Cataract Refract Surg 21:386, 1995.

637. Kim WJ and Lee JH: Long-term results of myopic epikeratoplasty, J Cataract Refract Surg 19:352, 1993.

638. Kliger C, and Maloney RK: Excimer laser keratomileusis, Part III—Excimer laser myopic keratomileusis at the Jules Stein Eye Institute, Los Angeles. In Salz JJ, McDonnel PJ, and McDonald MB, editors: Corneal laser surgery, St. Louis, 1995, Mosby–Year Book.

639. Koch F and others: Electron microscopic examination of prelathed, lyophilized tissue used for epikeratophakia in humans, Refract Corneal Surg 6:116, 1990.

640. Koch PS and others: Ultrastructure of human lenticles in keratophakia, Arch Ophthalmol 99:1634, 1981.

641. Koenig SB and others: Corneal sensitivity after epikeratophakia, Ophthalmology 90:1213, 1983.

642. Kohlhaas M and others: Aesthesiometry of the cornea after refractive corneal surgery, Klin Monatsbl Augenheilkd 201:221, 1992.

643. Kohlhaas M and others: Corneal reinnervation after keratomileusis in situ and keratomileusis myopia—a comparison, Klin Monatsbl Augenheilkd 206:103, 1995.

644. Kohlhaas M and others: Keratomileusis with a lamellar microkeratome and the excimer laser (German), Ophthalmologe 92:499, 1995.

645. Kratz-Owens K, Huff JW, and Schanzlin DJ: New cryoprotectant for cryorefractive surgery, J Cataract Refract Surg 17:608, 1991.

646. Kratz-Owens KL, Hageman GS, and Schanzlin DJ: An in-vivo technique for monitoring keratocyte migration following lamellar keratoplasty, Refract Corneal Surg 8:230, 1992.

647. Kremer F and Kremer I: Postkeratoplasty myopia treated by keratomileusis, Ann Ophthalmol 25:370, 1993.

648. Kremer FB: Keratophakia—ALK for high hyperopia. In Rozakis GW, editor: Refractive lamellar keratoplasty, Thorofare, NJ, 1994, SLACK, Inc.

649. Kremer FB and Dufek M: Excimer laser in situ keratomileusis, J Refract Surg 11:S244, 1995.

650. Krumeich JH: Indications, techniques, and complications of myopic keratomileusis, Int Ophthalmol Clin 23:75, 1983.

651. Krumeich JH and Knuelle A: Non-freeze epikeratophakia (live epikeratophakia), Fortschr Ophthalmol 87:20, 1990.

652. Krumeich JH and Swinger CA: Nonfreeze epikeratophakia for the correction of myopia, Am J Ophthalmol 103:397, 1987.

653. Lane SL: Polysulfone corneal lenses, J Cataract Refract Surg 12:50, 1986.

654. Lane SS, McCarey BE, and Lindstrom RL: Alloplastic corneal lenses. In Schwab IR, editor: Refractive keratoplasty, New York, 1987, Churchill Livingstone.

655. Laroche L and others: Nonfreeze myopic keratomileusis for myopia in 158 eyes, J Refract Corneal Surg 10:400, 1994.

656. Lawless MA and others: Keratoconus: diagnosis and management: delayed regression of effect in myopic epikeratoplasty vs myopic keratomileusis for high myopia, Refract Corneal Surg 5:161, 1989.

657. Lehtosalo J, Uusitalo RJ, and Mianowizc J: Epikeratophakia for treatment of keratoconus, Acta Ophthalmol Suppl 182:74, 1987.

658. Lerche RC and others: Corneal reinnervation after lamellar refractive corneal surgery (German), Ophthalmologe 92:414, 1995.

659. Liebovitch LS and Weinbaum S: A model of epithelial water transport. The corneal endothelium, Biophys J 35:315, 1981.

660. Lindstrom RL: Seventh annual Lans distinguished refractive surgery lecture, Refract Corneal Surg 9:118, 1993.

661. Littman H: Optic of Barraquer's keratomileusis, Arch Oftal Optom 6:1, 1966.

662. Liu Z, Chen J, and Xuan J: Corneal topography of patients with unsatisfactory visual acuity after epikeratophakia for aphakia, Yen Ko Hsueh Pao 10:81, 1994.

663. Loewenstein A, Lipshitz I, and Lazar M: Photorefractive keratectomy for the treatment of myopia after epikeratoplasty: a case report, J Refract Corneal Surg 10:S285, 1994.

664. Lyle WA and Jin JC: Initial results of automated lamellar keratoplasty for correction of myopia: One year follow-up, J Cataract Refract Surg 22:31, 1996.

665. Maeda N and others: Automated keratoconus screening with corneal topography analysis, Invest Ophthalmol Vis Sci 35:2749, 1994.

666. Maguen E and others: Keratophakia with lyophilized corneal lathed at room temperature: new techniques and experimental surgical results, Ophthalmic Surg 14:759, 1983.

667. Maguire LJ: Corneal topography of patients with excellent Snellen visual acuity after epikeratophakia for aphakia, Am J Ophthalmol 109:162, 1990.

668. Maguire LJ and others: Corneal topography in myopic patients undergoing epikeratophakia, Am J Ophthalmol 103:404, 1987.

669. Mamalis N, Lucius RW, and Casebeer JC: Histopathologic analysis of corneal caps removed after automated lamellar keratoplasty. Best papers of sessions from the ASCRS symposium on cataract, IOL and Refractive Surgery, Boston, April 1994, p. 1.

670. Manche EE, Judge A, and Maloney RK: Lamellar keratoplasty for hyperopia, J Refract Surg 12(1):42, 1996.

671. Manche EE and Maloney RK: Keratomileusis in situ for high myopia, J Cataract Refract Surg 22:1443, 1996.

672. Martel J: Intraepikeratophakia, Ann Ophthalmol 19:287, 1987.

673. Maxwell WA: Myopic keratomileusis: initial results and myopic keratomileusis combined with other procedures, J Cataract Refract Surg 13:518, 1987.

674. McCarey BE and others: Hydrogel keratophakia: a freehand pocket dissection in the monkey model, Br J Ophthalmol 70:187, 1986.

675. McDonald MB and others: The nationwide study of epikeratophakia for aphakia in adults, Am J Ophthalmol 103:358, 1987.

676. McDonald MB and others: The nationwide study of epikeratophakia for myopia, Am J Ophthalmol 103:375, 1987.

677. McDonald MB and others: Epikeratophakia for keratoconus. The nationwide study, Arch Ophthalmol 104:1294, 1986.

678. McDonald MB and others: Epikeratophakia for myopia correction, Ophthalmology 92:1417, 1985.

679. McDonald MB and others: Alloplastic epikeratophakia for the correction of aphakia, Ophthalmic Surg 14:65, 1983.

680. McDonald MB and others: Epikeratophakia: the surgical correction of aphakia. Update: 1982, Ophthalmology 90:668, 1983.

681. McDonald MB and others: Assessment of the long-term corneal response to hydrogel intrastromal lenses implanted in monkey eyes for up to five years, J Cataract Refract Surg 19:213, 1993.

682. McDonald MB and others: A preliminary comparative study of epikeratophakia or penetrating keratoplasty for keratoconus, Am J Ophthalmol 103:467, 1987.

683. McDonnell PJ and Sadun AA: Acquired accommodative esotropia following overcorrection by myopic epikeratophakia, Cornea 9:354, 1990.

684. McWhae J and others: Ultrasound biomicroscopy in refractive surgery, J Cataract Refract Surg 20:493, 1994.

685. Mimouni F, Sammartino A, and Colin J: Automatic in situ keratomileusis, J Fr Ophthalmol 17:278, 1994.

686. Moore MB and others: Fate of lyophilized xenogeneic corneal lenticules in intrastromal implantation and epikeratophakia, Invest Ophthalmol Vis Sci 28:555, 1987.

687. Morgan KS: Visual rehabilitation of aphakic children. IV. Epikeratophakia, Surv Ophthalmol 34:379, 1990.

688. Morgan KS and others: Five year follow-up of epikeratophakia in children, Ophthalmology 93:423, 1986.

689. Morgan KS and others: Surgical and visual results of pediatric epikeratophakia, Metab Pediatr Syst Ophthalmol 7:45, 1983.

690. Morgan KS and others: Preliminary visual results of pediatric epikeratophakia, Arch Ophthalmol 101:1540, 1983.

691. Morgan KS and Beuerman RW: Interface opacities in epikeratophakia, Arch Ophthalmol 104:1505, 1986.

692. Morgan KS and Collins CC: Combined cataract extraction and

epikeratophakia in children, J Pediatr Ophthalmol Strabismus 26: 14, 1989.

693. Morgan KS and others: Epikeratophakia in children with traumatic cataracts, J Pediatr Ophthalmol Strabismus 23:108, 1986.

694. Morgan KS and others: The nationwide study of epikeratophakia for aphakia in children, Am J Ophthalmol 103:366, 1987.

695. Morgan KS and others: The nationwide study of epikeratophakia for aphakia in older children, Ophthalmology 95:526, 1988.

696. Morgan KS and Somers M: Update on epikeratophakia in children, Int Ophthalmol Clin 29:37, 1989.

697. Morgan KS and Stephenson GS: Epikeratophakia in children with corneal lacerations, J Pediatr Ophthalmol Strabismus 22:105, 1985.

698. Morgan KS and others: Epikeratophakia in children, Ophthalmology 91:780, 1984.

699. Morgan KS and others: The use of epikeratophakia grafts in pediatric monocular aphakia, J Pediatr Ophthalmol Strabismus 18:23, 1981.

700. Nagel S, Wiegand W, and Thaer AA: Corneal changes and corneal healing after keratomileusis in situ. In vivo studies using confocal slit-scanning microscopy (German), Ophthalmologe 92:397, 1995.

701. Nascimento EG and others: Nocardial keratitis following myopic keratomileusis, J Refract Surg 11:210, 1995.

702. Neumann AC, McCarty G, and Sanders DR: Delayed regression of effect in myopic epikeratophakia vs myopic keratomileusis for high myopia, Refract Corneal Surg 5:161, 1989.

703. Nichols BD, Lindstrom RL, and Spigelman AV: The surgical management of overcorrection in myopic epikeratophakia, Am J Ophthalmol 105:354, 1988.

704. Nichols BD and others: Epikeratophakia: technique modifications and visual results compared to the national study, J Cataract Refract Surg 15:312, 1989.

705. Nirankari VS and others: Effects of epikeratoplasty on the host cornea. An experimental study, Cornea 9:211, 1990.

706. Nordan LT: Keratomileusis, Int Ophthalmol Clin 31:7, 1991.

707. Nordan LT and Barker BA: Myopic keratomileusis: 74 consecutive non-amblyopic cases with one year of follow-up, J Refract Surg 5:307, 1986.

708. Olsen T and Sperling S: The swelling pressure of the human corneal stroma as determined by a new method, Exp Eye Res 44:481, 1987.

709. Olson PF and others: Measurement of intraocular pressure after epikeratophakia, Arch Ophthalmol 101:1111, 1983.

710. Parks RA and McCarey BE: Hydrogel keratophakia: long-term morphology in the monkey model, CLAO J 17:216, 1991.

711. Parks RA and others: Intrastromal crystalline deposits following hydrogel keratophakia in monkeys, Cornea 12:29, 1993.

712. Peiffer RL, Werblin TP, and Fryczkowski AW: Pathology of corneal hydrogel alloplastic implants, Ophthalmology 92:1294, 1985.

713. Pepose JS and Benevento WJ: Detection of HLA antigens in human epikeratophakia lenticules, Cornea 10:105, 1991.

714. Pico JF, Stamper RL, and McMenemy M: Intraocular pressure and corneal curvature changes on application of limbal-scleral suction fixation ring in rabbits, Cornea 12:25, 1993.

715. Pokorny KS and others: Histopathology of human keratorefractive lenticules, Cornea 9:223, 1990.

716. Polit F and others: Subepithelial reticular cicatrization following radial keratotomy in a patient with inactive trachoma, Refract Corneal Surg 8:240, 1992.

717. Polit F and others: Cryolathe keratomileusis for correction of myopia of 4.00 to 8.00 diopters, Refract Corneal Surg 9:259, 1993.

718. Price FW Jr and Binder PS: Scarring of a recipient cornea following epikeratoplasty, Arch Ophthalmol 105:1556, 1987.

719. Price FW Jr and others: Automated lamellar keratomileusis in situ for myopia, J Refract Surg 12(1):29, 1996.

720. Quantock AJ and others: Remodelling of the corneal stroma after lamellar keratoplasty. A synchrotron x-ray diffraction study, Cornea 13:20, 1994.

721. Rao GN, Ganti S, and Aquavella JV: Specular microscopy of corneal epithelium after epikeratophakia, Am J Ophthalmol 103:392, 1987.

722. Reidy JJ, McDonald MB, and Klyce SD: The corneal topography of epikeratophakia, Refract Corneal Surg 6:26, 1990.

723. Rich LF and others: Keratocyte survival in keratophakia lenticules, Arch Ophthalmol 99:677, 1981.

724. Roat MI and Hiles DA: Epikeratophakia for control of pediatric bullous keratopathy, J Cataract Refract Surg 13:59, 1987.

725. Robin JB: Hyperopic refractive surgery, AudioDigest Ophthalmology, Glendale, 1995, California Medical Association.

726. Rodrigues M and others: Clinical and histopathologic changes in the host cornea after epikeratoplasty for keratoconus (see comments), Am J Ophthalmol 114:161, 1992.

727. Rodriguez A and Camacho H: Retinal detachment after refractive surgery for myopia, Retina 12:S46, 1992.

728. Rostron CK: Epikeratophakia: clinical results and experimental development, Eye 2:56, 1988.

729. Rostron CK, Sandford-Smith JH, and Morton DB: Experimental epikeratophakia using tissue lathed at room temperature, Br J Ophthalmol 72:354, 1988.

730. Rowsey JJ and Rubin ML: Refraction problems after refractive surgery, Surv Ophthalmol 32:414, 1988.

731. Rozakis GW: Theories of myopic lamellar keratoplasty. In Rozakis GW, editor: Refractive lamellar keratoplasty, Thorofare, NJ, 1994, SLACK, Inc.

732. Rozakis GW: Keratomes. In Rozakis GW, editor: Refractive lamellar keratoplasty, Thorofare, NJ, 1994, SLACK, Inc.

733. Rozakis GW and others: Refractive lamellar keratoplasty, Thorofare, NJ, 1994, SLACK, Inc.

734. Rozakis GW, Hollis S, and Suarez R: Future trends. In Rozakis GW, editor: Refractive lamellar keratoplasty, Thorofare, NJ, 1994, SLACK, Inc.

735. Ruiz L, Slade SG, and Updegraff SA: Excimer laser keratomileusis, Part II—Excimer myopic keratomileusis: Bogota experience. In Salz JJ, McDonnell PJ, and McDonald MB, editors: Corneal laser surgery, St. Louis, 1995, Mosby–Year Book.

736. Ruiz LA and Rowsey JJ: In situ keratomileusis, Invest Ophthalmol Vis Sci 29(suppl):392, 1988.

737. Ryan F: Keratomileusis, Nurs Times 66:325, 1970.

738. Sahori A: Long-term follow-up of wound healing following epikeratophakia in rabbits, Nippon Ganka Gakkai Zasshi 94:572, 1990.

739. Sahori A and others: Keratocyte activity in wound healing process following epikeratophakia in rabbits, Nippon Ganka Gakkai Zasshi 93:375, 1989.

740. Sahori A and others: Reepithelialization of keratolens in the wound healing process following epikeratophakia in rabbits, Nippon Ganka Gakkai Zasshi 93:747, 1989.

741. Sahori A and others: The ultrastructural changes in the corneal lens stroma of wound healing process following epikeratophakia in rabbits, Nippon Ganka Gakkai Zasshi 94:469, 1990.

742. Salah T and others: Excimer laser in situ keratomileusis under a corneal flap for myopia of 2 to 20 diopters, Am J Ophthalmol 121:143, 1996.

743. Samples JR and others: Morphology of hydrogel implants used for refractive keratoplasty, Invest Ophthalmol Vis Sci 25:843, 1984.

744. Samples JR and others: Epikeratophakia: clinical evaluation and histopathology of a non-human primate model, Cornea 3:51, 1984.

745. Saragoussi JJ and others: Results of myopic keratomileusis. A retrospective clinical study apropos of 40 cases, J Fr Ophthalmol 11:311, 1988.

746. Sarno EM, Smith RE, and Schanzlin DJ: Comparison of clinical results following radial keratotomy, extended-wear contact lenses, and myopic keratomileusis, Int Ophthalmol Clin 23:167, 1983.

747. Simon G and others: Optics of the corneal epithelium, Refract Corneal Surg 9:42, 1993.

748. Slade SG and Berkeley RG: History of keratomileusis. In Rozakis GW, editor: Refractive lamellar keratoplasty, Thorofare, NJ, 1994, SLACK, Inc.

749. Slade SG and Brint SF: Excimer laser myopic keratomileusis. In Rozakis GW, editor: Refractive lamellar keratoplasty, Thorofare, NJ, 1994, SLACK, Inc.

750. Slade SG and Updegraff SA: Advances in lamellar refractive surgery, Int Ophthalmol Clin 34:147, 1994.

751. Sohn JH, Choi SK and Lee JH: Epithelial healing time and rate of the cornea after myopic epikeratoplasty, Korean J Ophthalmol 9:26, 1995.

752. Stangler RA, Lindquist TD and Lindstrom RL: Interface hematoma after epikeratophakia, Am J Ophthalmol 103:328, 1987.

753. Stern AL and Taylor DM: Particle-free environment for refractive keratoplasty, Ophthalmic Surg 12:360, 1981.

754. Stonecipher KG and others: Refractive corneal surgery with the Draeger rotary microkeratome in human cadaver eyes, J Refract Corneal Surg 10:49, 1994.

869. Burnstein Y, Klapper D, and Hersh PS: Experimental globe rupture after excimer laser photorefractive keratectomy, Arch Ophthalmol 113:1056, 1995.

870. Busin M and Meller D: Corneal epithelial dots following excimer laser photorefractive keratectomy, J Refract Corneal Surg 10:357, 1994.

871. Butuner Z and others: Visual function one year after excimer laser photorefractive keratectomy, J Refract Corneal Surg 10:625, 1994.

872. Cameron JA, Antonios SR, and Badr IA: Excimer laser phototherapeutic keratectomy for shield ulcers and corneal plaques in vernal keratoconjunctivitis, J Refract Surg 11:31, 1995.

873. Campos M and others: Corneal wound healing after excimer laser ablation. Effects of nitrogen gas blower, Ophthalmology 99:893, 1992.

874. Campos M and others: Corneal wound healing after excimer laser ablation in rabbits: expanding versus contracting apertures, Refract Corneal Surg 8:378, 1992.

875. Campos M and others: Photorefractive keratectomy for severe postkeratoplasty astigmatism, Am J Ophthalmol 114:429, 1992.

876. Campos M and others: Corneal sensitivity after photorefractive keratectomy, Am J Ophthalmol 114:51, 1992.

877. Campos M and others: Corneal surface after deepithelialization using a sharp and a dull instrument, Ophthalmic Surg 23:618, 1992.

878. Campos M, Lee M, and McDonnell PJ: Ocular integrity after refractive surgery: effects of photorefractive keratectomy, phototherapeutic keratectomy, and radial keratotomy, Ophthalmic Surg 23:598, 1992.

879. Campos M, Abed HM, and McDonnell PJ: Topical fluorometholone reduces stromal inflammation after photorefractive keratectomy, Ophthalmic Surg 24:654, 1993.

880. Campos M and others: Clinical follow-up of phototherapeutic keratectomy for treatment of corneal opacities (see comments), Am J Ophthalmol 115:433, 1993.

881. Campos M, Trokel SL, and McDonnell PJ: Surface morphology following photorefractive keratectomy, Ophthalmic Surg 24:822, 1993.

882. Campos M and others: Ablation rates and surface ultrastructure of 193 nm excimer laser keratectomies, Invest Ophthalmol Vis Sci 34:2493, 1993.

883. Campos M and others: Keratocyte loss after corneal de-epithelialization in primates and rabbits (see comments), Arch Ophthalmol 112:254, 1994.

884. Campos M and others: Keratocyte loss after different methods of de-epithelialization, Ophthalmology 101:890, 1994.

885. Campos M and McDonnell PJ: Photorefractive keratectomy for astigmatism. In Salz JJ, McDonnell PJ, and McDonald MB, editors: Corneal laser surgery, St. Louis, 1995, Mosby–Year Book.

886. Cantera E, Cantera I, and Olivieri L: Corneal topographic analysis of photorefractive keratectomy in 175 myopic eyes, Refract Corneal Surg 9:S19, 1993.

887. Carones F and others: Efficacy of corticosteroids in reversing regression after myopic photorefractive keratectomy, Refract Corneal Surg 9:S52, 1993.

888. Carones F and others: The corneal endothelium after myopic excimer laser photorefractive keratectomy, Arch Ophthalmol 112:920, 1994.

889. Carr JD, Patel R, and Hersh PS: Management of late corneal haze following photorefractive keratectomy, J Refract Surg 11(Suppl):S309, 1995.

890. Carson CA and Taylor HR: Excimer laser treatment for high and extreme myopia. The Melbourne Excimer Laser and Research Group, Arch Ophthalmol 113:431, 1995.

891. Carter JB, Jones DB, and Wilhelmus KR: Acute hydrops in pellucid marginal corneal degeneration, Am J Ophthalmol 107:167, 1989.

892. Caubet E: Course of subepithelial corneal haze over 18 months after photorefractive keratectomy for myopia Refract Corneal Surg 9:S65, 1993, published erratum appears in Refract Corneal Surg 9(3):236, 1993.

893. Cavanaugh TB and others: Centration of excimer laser photorefractive keratectomy relative to the pupil, J Cataract Refract Surg 19 Suppl:144, 1993.

894. Cavanaugh TB and others: Topographical analysis of the concentration of excimer laser photorefractive keratectomy, J Cataract Refract Surg 19 Suppl:136, 1993.

895. Cennamo G and others: Evaluation of corneal thickness and endothelial cells before and after excimer laser photorefractive keratectomy, J Refract Corneal Surg 10:137, 1994.

896. Cennamo G and others: Phototherapeutic keratectomy in the treatment of Avellino dsytrophy, Ophthalmologica 208:198, 1994.

897. Chan WK and others: Photorefractive keratectomy for myopia of 6 to 12 diopters, J Refract Surg 11:S286, 1995.

898. Chan WK and others: Corneal scarring after photorefractive keratectomy in a penetrating keratoplasty, Am J Ophthalmol 121(5):570, 1996.

899. Chandonnet A and others: CO2 laser annular thermokeratoplasty: a preliminary study, Lasers Surg Med 12:264, 1992.

900. Charpentier DY and others: Intrastromal thermokeratoplasty for correction of spherical hyperopia: a 1-year prospective study (French), J Fr Ophthalmol 18:200, 1995, (review).

901. Chatterjee A and others: Reduction in intraocular pressure after excimer laser photorefractive keratectomy; correlation with pretreatment myopia, Ophthalmology 104:355, 1997.

902. Cherry PM and others: The treatment of pain following photorefractive keratectomy, J Refract Corneal Surg 10:S222, 1994.

903. Cherry PM and others: Treatment of myopic astigmatism with photorefractive keratectomy using an erodible mask, J Refract Corneal Surg 10:S239, 1994.

904. Chew SJ and others: In vivo confocal microscopy of corneal wound healing after excimer laser photorefractive keratectomy, CLAO J 21:273, 1995.

905. Cho YS and others: Multistep photorefractive keratectomy for high myopia, Refract Corneal Surg 9:S37, 1993.

906. Choi YI, Min HK, and Hyun PM: Excimer laser photorefractive keratectomy for astigmatism, Korean J Ophthalmol 7:20, 1993.

907. Cintron C and Kublin CL: Regeneration of corneal tissue, Dev Biol 61:346, 1977.

908. Cintron C and others: Biochemical and ultrastructural changes in collagen during corneal wound healing, J Ultrastruc Res 65:13, 1978.

909. Cintron C and others: Scanning electron microscopy of rabbit corneal scars, Invest Ophthalmol Vis Sci 23:50, 1982.

910. Cintron C: Corneal epithelial and stromal reactions to excimer laser photorefractive keratectomy. II. Unpredictable corneal cicatrization, Arch Ophthalmol 108:1540, 1990, (editorial).

911. Cintron C, Covington HI, and Kublin CL: Morphologic analyses of proteoglycans in rabbit corneal scars, Invest Ophthalmol Vis Sci 31:1789, 1990.

912. Cintron C and others: Biochemical analyses of proteoglycans in rabbit corneal scars, Invest Ophthalmol Vis Sci 31:1975, 1990.

913. Claoue C, Stevens J, and Steele A: Band keratopathy and excimer laser phototherapeutic keratectomy, Eur J Implant Ref Surg 7:260, 1995.

914. Cohen P: Phototorefractive keratectomy—a personal insight, Refract Corneal Surg 9:S121, 1993.

915. Colin J and others: Photorefractive keratectomy following undercorrected myopic epikeratoplasties, J Fr Ophthalmol 15:384, 1992.

916. Colin J, Cochener B, and Gallinaro C: Central steep islands immediately following excimer photorefractive keratectomy for myopia, Refract Corneal Surg 9:395, 1993, (letter).

917. Colin J and others: Myopic photorefractive keratectomy in eyes with atypical inferior corneal steepening, J Cataract Refract Surg 22:1423, 1996.

918. Colliac JP and Shammas HJ: Optics for photorefractive keratectomy, J Cataract Refract Surg 19:356, 1993, (published erratum appears in J Cataract Refract Surg 19(4):569, 1993).

919. Colliac JP, Shammas HJ, and Bart DJ: Photorefractive keratectomy for the correction of myopia and astigmatism [see comments], Am J Ophthalmol 117:369, 1994, (published erratum appears in Am J Ophthalmol 1994 118(1):134, 1994).

920. Costagliola C and others: ArF 193 nm excimer laser corneal surgery as a possible risk factor in cataractogenesis, Exp Eye Res 58:453, 1994.

921. Cotliar AM and others: Excimer laser radial keratotomy, Ophthalmology 92:206, 1985.

922. Dausch D, Klein R, and Schroder E: Excimer laser photorefractive keratectomy for hyperopia, Refract Corneal Surg 9:20, 1993.

923. Dausch D and others: Excimer laser photorefractive keratectomy with tapered transition zone for high myopia. A preliminary report of six cases, J Cataract Refract Surg 19:590, 1993.

924. Dausch D and others: Phototherapeutic keratectomy in recurrent corneal epithelial erosion, Refract Corneal Surg 9:419, 1993.

925. Dausch D and others: Photorefractive keratectomy to correct astigmatism with myopia or hyperopia, J Cataract Refract Surg 20 Suppl:252, 1994.

926. Dausch D and Landesz M: Laser correction of hyperopia: Aesculap-Meditec results from Germany. In Salz JJ, McDonnell PJ, and McDonald MB, editors: Corneal laser surgery, St. Louis, 1995, Mosby–Year Book.

927. David T and others: Corneal wound healing modulation using basic fibroblast growth factor after excimer laser photorefractive keratectomy, Cornea 14:227, 1995.

928. Del Pero RA and others: A refractive and histopathologic study of excimer laser keratectomy in primates, Am J Ophthalmol 109:419, 1990.

929. Delaigue O and others: Quantitative analysis of immunogold labelings of collagen types I, III, IV and VI in healthy and pathological human corneas, Graefes Arch Clin Exp Ophthalmol 233:331, 1995.

930. Demers P and others: Effect of occlusive pressure patching on the rate of epithelial wound healing after photorefractive keratectomy, J Cataract Refract Surg 22(1):59, 1996.

931. DeVore DP and others: Rapidly polymerized collagen gel as a smoothing agent in excimer laser photoablation, J Refract Surg 11:50, 1995.

932. Diamond S: Excimer laser photorefractive keratectomy (PRK) for myopia—present status: aerospace considerations, Aviat Space Environ Med 66:690, 1995.

933. Ditzen K, Anschutz T, and Schroder E: Photorefractive keratectomy to treat low, medium, and high myopia: a multicenter study, J Cataract Refract Surg 20 Suppl:234, 1994.

934. Doane JF and others: Relation of visual symptoms to topographic ablation zone decentration after excimer laser photorefractive keratectomy, Ophthalmology 102:42, 1995.

935. Dougherty PJ, Wellish KL, and Maloney RK: Excimer laser ablation rate and corneal hydration, Am J Ophthalmol 118:169, 1994.

936. Durrie DS, Lesher MP, and Cavanaugh TB: Classification of variable clinical response after photorefractive keratectomy for myopia, J Refract Surg 11:341, 1995.

937. Durrie DS, Schumer DJ, and Cavanaugh TB: Holmium:YAG laser thermokeratoplasty for hyperopia, J Refract Corneal Surg 10:S277, 1994.

938. Durrie DS, Schumer DJ, and Cavanaugh TB: Photorefractive keratectomy for residual myopia after previous refractive keratotomy, J Refract Corneal Surg 10:S235, 1994.

939. Durrie DS, Schumer J, and Cavanaugh T: Phototherapeutic keratectomy: the Summit experience. In Salz JJ, McDonnell PJ, and McDonald MB, editors: Corneal laser surgery, St. Louis, 1995, Mosby–Year Book.

940. Dutt S and others: One-year results of excimer laser photorefractive keratectomy for low to moderate myopia, Arch Ophthalmol 112:1427, 1994.

941. Eggink FA and Beekhuis WH: Granular dystrophy of the cornea. Contact lens fitting after phototherapeutic keratectomy, Cornea 14:217, 1995.

942. Ehlers N and Hjortdal JO: Excimer laser refractive keratectomy for high myopia. 6-month follow-up of patients treated bilaterally, Acta Ophthalmol (Copenh) 70:578, 1992.

943. Eiferman RA and others: Excimer laser photorefractive keratectomy for myopia: six-month results, Refract Corneal Surg 7:344, 1991.

944. Eiferman RA, Hoffman RS, and Sher NA: Topical diclofenac reduces pain following photorefractive keratectomy, Arch Ophthalmol 111:1022, 1993, (letter).

945. Englanoff JS and others: In situ collagen gel mold as an aid in excimer laser superficial keratectomy, Ophthalmology 99:1201, 1992.

946. Epstein D and others: Stability of refraction 18 months after photorefractive keratectomy with excimer laser, Klin Monatsbl Augenheilkd 202:245, 1993.

947. Epstein D and others: Excimer retreatment of regression after photorefractive keratectomy, Am J Ophthalmol 117:456, 1994.

948. Epstein D and others: Twenty-four-month follow-up of excimer laser photorefractive keratectomy for myopia. Refractive and visual acuity results, Ophthalmology 101:1558, 1994.

949. Epstein D and others: Re-operations. Salz JJ, McDonnell PJ, and McDonald MB, editors: Corneal laser surgery, St. Louis, 1995, Mosby–Year Book.

950. Epstein RJ and Robin JB: Corneal graft rejection episode after excimer laser phototherapeutic keratectomy, Arch Ophthalmol 112:157, 1994, (letter; comment).

951. Essepian JP and others: The use of confocal microscopy in evaluating corneal wound healing after excimer laser keratectomy, Scanning 16:300, 1994.

952. Fagerholm P and others: Phototherapeutic keratectomy: long-term results in 166 eyes, Refract Corneal Surg 9:S76, 1993.

953. Fagerholm P, Hamberg-Nystrom H, and Tengroth B: Wound healing and myopic regression following photorefractive keratectomy, Acta Ophthalmol (Copenh) 72:229, 1994.

954. Fagerholm P and others: Effect of postoperative steroids on the refractive outcome of photorefractive keratectomy for myopia with the Summit excimer laser, J Cataract Refract Surg 20 Suppl:212, 1994.

955. Fagerholm P, Ohman L, and Orndahl M: Phototherapeutic keratectomy in herpes simplex keratitis. Clinical results in 20 patients, Acta Ophthalmol (Copenh) 72:457, 1994.

956. Fantes FE and Waring GO 3d: Effect of excimer laser radiant exposure on uniformity of ablated corneal surface, Lasers Surg Med 9:533, 1989.

957. Fantes FE and others: Wound healing after excimer laser keratomileusis (photorefractive keratectomy) in monkeys (see comments), Arch Ophthalmol 108:665, 1990.

958. Fasano AP and others: Excimer laser smoothing of a reproducible model of anterior corneal surface irregularity, Ophthalmology 98:1782, 1991.

959. Feldman ST and others: Regression of effect following radial thermokeratoplasty in humans, Refract Corneal Surg 5:288, 1989.

960. Feldman ST and others: Experimental radial thermokeratoplasty in rabbits, Arch Ophthalmol 108:997, 1990.

961. Feldman ST: The effect of epidermal growth factor on corneal wound healing: practical considerations for therapeutic use, Refract Corneal Surg 7:232, 1991, (review).

962. Ferrari M: Use of topical nonsteroidal anti-inflammatory drugs after photorefractive keratectomy, J Refract Corneal Surg 10:S287, 1994.

963. Fiander DC and Tayfour F: Excimer laser in situ keratomileusis in 124 myopic eyes, J Refract Surg 11:S234, 1995.

964. Fichte CM and Bell AM: Ongoing results of excimer laser photorefractive keratectomy for myopia: subjective patient impressions, J Cataract Refract Surg 20 Suppl:268, 1994.

965. Ficker LA and others: Excimer laser photorefractive keratectomy for myopia: 12 month follow-up, Eye 7:617, 1993.

966. Fields CR, Taylor SM, and Barker FM: Effect of corneal edema upon the smoothness of excimer laser ablation, Optom Vis Sci 71:109, 1994.

967. Fitzsimmons TD and Fagerholm P: Superficial keratectomy with the 193 nm excimer laser: a reproducible model of corneal surface irregularities, Acta Ophthalmol (Copenh) 69:641, 1991.

968. Fitzsimmons TD and others: Hyaluronic acid in the rabbit cornea after excimer laser superficial keratectomy, Invest Ophthalmol Vis Sci 33:3011, 1992.

969. Fitzsimmons TD, Fagerholm P, and Tengroth B: Steroid treatment of myopic regression: acute refractive and topographic changes in excimer photorefractive keratectomy patients, Cornea 12:358, 1993.

970. Fogle JA, Kenyon KR, and Stark WJ: Damage to epithelial basement membrane by thermokeratoplasty, Am J Ophthalmol 83:392, 1977.

971. Forster W: Time-delayed, two-step excimer laser photorefractive keratectomy to correct high myopia, Refract Corneal Surg 9:465, 1993.

972. Forster W and others: Phototherapeutic keratectomy in corneal diseases, Refract Corneal Surg 9:S85, 1993.

973. Forster W, Grewe S, and Busse H: Clinical use of the corneal opacities—therapeutic strategy and case reports, Klin Monatsbl Augenheilkd 202:126, 1993.

974. Forster W, Grewe S, and Busse H: Clinical use of the excimer laser in treatment of surface corneal opacities—therapeutic strategy and case reports, Klin Monatsbl Augenheilkd 202:126, 1993.

975. Forster W and others: 15 months photorefractive keratectomy at the Munster University Eye Clinic, Ophthalmologe 91:646, 1994.

976. Fountain TR and others: Reassembly of corneal epithelial adhesion structures after excimer laser keratectomy in humans, Arch Ophthalmol 112:967, 1994.

977. Frangie JP and others: Excimer laser keratectomy after radial keratotomy, Am J Ophthalmol 115:634, 1993.

978. Frangieh GT and others: Fibronectin and corneal epithelial wound healing in the vitamin A–deficient rat, Arch Ophthalmol 107:567, 1989.

979. Frankhauser F and Kwasniewska S: Neodymium:yttrium-aluminium-garnet laser. In L'Esperance FA, editor: Ophthalmologic lasers, St. Louis, 1989, Mosby–Year Book.

980. Freitas C and others: Effect of photorefractive keratectomy on visual functioning and quality of life, J Refract Surg 11:S327, 1995.

981. Friedman MD and others: OmniMed II: a new system for use with the emphasis erodible mask, J Refract Corneal Surg 10:S267, 1994.

982. Frueh BE, Bille JF, and Brown SI: Intrastromal relaxing incisions in rabbits with a picosecond infrared laser, Lasers Light Ophthalmol 4:165, 1992.

983. Frueh BE and Bohnke M: Endothelial cell morphology after phototherapeutic keratectomy, Ger J Ophthalmol 4:86, 1995.

984. Fulton JC, Cohen EJ, and Rapuano CJ: Bacterial ulcer three days after excimer laser phototherapeutic keratectomy, Arch Ophthalmol 114(5):626, 1996.

985. Fujikawa LS and others: Basement membrane components in healing rabbit corneal epithelial wounds: immunofluorescence and ultrastructural studies, J Cell Biol 98:128, 1984.

986. Fyodorov SN and others: PRK using an absorbing cell delivery system for correction of myopia from 4 to 26 D in 3251 eyes, Refract Corneal Surg 9:S123, 1993.

987. Gailitis RP and others: Solid state ultraviolet laser (213 nm) ablation of the cornea and synthetic collagen lenticules, Lasers Surg Med 11:556, 1991.

988. Gartry DS, Kerr Muir M, and Marshall J: Excimer laser treatment of corneal surface pathology: a laboratory and clinical study (see comments), Br J Ophthalmol 75:258, 1991.

989. Gartry DS, Kerr Muir MG, and Marshall J: Photorefractive keratectomy with an argon fluoride excimer laser: a clinical study, Refract Corneal Surg 7:420, 1991.

990. Gartry DS, Kerr Muir MG, and Marshall J: Excimer laser photorefractive keratectomy. 18-month follow-up, Ophthalmology 99:1209, 1992.

991. Gartry DS and others: The effect of topical corticosteroids on refractive outcome and corneal haze after photorefractive keratectomy: a prospective, randomized, double blind, trial. Arch Ophthalmol 110:944, 1992.

992. Gartry DS, Kerr Muir M, and Marshall J: The effect of topical corticosteroids on refraction and corneal haze following excimer laser treatment of myopia: an update. A prospective, randomized, double-masked study, Eye 7:584, 1993.

993. Gartry DS: Treating myopia with the excimer laser: the present position, Br Med J 310:979, 1995.

994. Gasset AR and others: Thermokeratoplasty, Trans Am Acad Ophthalmol Otolaryngol 77:OP441, 1973.

995. Gasset AR and Kaufman HE: Thermokeratoplasty in the treatment of keratoconus, Am J Ophthalmol 79:226, 1975.

996. Gaster RN and others: Corneal surface ablation by 193 nm excimer laser and wound healing in rabbits, Invest Ophthalmol Vis Sci 30:90, 1989.

997. Gauthier CA and others: Epithelial alterations following photorefractive keratectomy for myopia, J Refract Surg 11:113, 1995.

998. Geggel HS: Successful treatment of recurrent corneal erosion with Nd:YAG anterior stromal puncture (see comments), Am J Ophthalmol 110:404, 1990.

999. Gelvin JB: An introduction to excimer laser photorefractive keratectomy, J Am Optom Assoc 61:842, 1990.

1000. Georgaras SP and others: Correction of myopic anisometropia with photorefractive keratectomy in 15 eyes, Refract Corneal Surg 9:S29, 1993.

1001. Gibralter R and Trokel SL: Correction of irregular astigmatism with the excimer laser, Ophthalmology 101:1310, 1994.

1002. Gimbel HV and Sun R: Effect of contact lens wear on photorefractive keratectomy, CLAO J 19:217, 1993.

1003. Gimbel HV and others: Visual, refractive, and patient satisfaction results following bilateral photorefractive keratectomy for myopia, Refract Corneal Surg 9:S5, 1993.

1004. Gimbel HV and Beldavs RA: Intrastromal photorefractive keratectomy with the Nd:YLF laser, Int Ophthalmol Clin 34:139, 1994.

1005. Gimbel HV and others: Comparison of laser and manual removal of corneal epithelium for photorefractive keratectomy, J Refract Surg 11:36, 1995.

1006. Gipson IK: Cytoplasmic filaments: their role in motility and cell shape, Invest Ophthalmol Vis Sci 16:1081, 1977.

1007. Gipson IK and Kiorpes TC: Epithelial sheet movement: protein and glycoprotein synthesis, Dev Biol 92:259, 1982.

1008. Gipson IK, Spurr-Michaud SJ, and Tisdale AS: Hemidesmosomes and anchoring fibril collagen appear synchronously during development and wound healing, Dev Biol 126:253, 1988.

1009. Gipson IK and others: Reassembly of the anchoring structures of the corneal epithelium during wound repair in the rabbit, Invest Ophthalmol Vis Sci 30:425, 1989.

1010. Gipson IK: The epithelial basement membrane zone of the limbus, Eye 3:132, 1989.

1011. Gipson IK: Corneal epithelial and stromal reactions to excimer laser photorefractive keratectomy. I. Concerns regarding the response of the corneal epithelium to excimer laser ablation, Arch Ophthalmol 108:1539, 1990, (editorial).

1012. Gipson IK: Adhesive mechanisms of the corneal epithelium, Acta Ophthalmol Suppl 13, 1992, (review).

1013. Gipson IK and others: Redistribution of the hemidesmosome components alpha 6 beta 4 integrin and bullous pemphigoid antigens during epithelial wound healing, Exp Cell Res 207:86, 1993.

1014. Gipson IK, Watanabe H, and Zieske JD: Corneal wound healing and fibronectin, Int Ophthalmol Clin 33:149, 1993.

1015. Gobbi PG and others: A simplified method to perform photorefractive keratectomy using an erodible mask, J Refract Corneal Surg 10:S246, 1994.

1016. Gobbi PG and others: Automatic eye tracker for excimer laser photorefractive keratectomy, J Refract Surg 11:S337, 1995.

1017. Gobbi PG and others: Evidence of rarefaction pressure spikes in the eyeball during photorefractive keratectomy: a potential damage mechanism? ARVO abstracts, Invest Ophthalmol Vis Sci 37(3, suppl):S18, 1996.

1018. Goes F: Short term results with excimer laser-photo-refractive keratectomy, Bull Soc Belge Ophtalmol 245:69, 1992.

1019. Goggin M, Algawi K, and O'Keefe M: Astigmatism following photorefractive keratectomy for myopia, J Refract Corneal Surg 10:540, 1994.

1020. Goggin M and others: Regression after photorefractive keratectomy for myopia, J Cataract Refract Surg 22(2):194, 1996.

1021. Goggin M, Kenna P, and Lavery F: Haze following photorefractive and photoastigmatic refractive keratectomy with the Nidek EC5000 and the Summit ExciMed UV200, J Cataract Refract Surg 23:50, 1997.

1022. Goldberg MA, Dorr DA, and Pepose JS: Lack of diurnal variation in vision, refraction, or keratometry after excimer laser photorefractive keratectomy, Brief Reports 123(3):407, 1996.

1023. Goldstein M and others: Phototherapeutic keratectomy in the treatment of corneal scarring from trachoma, J Refract Corneal Surg 10:S290, 1994.

1024. Gomez de Liano MZ and others: Photorefractive keratectomy for myopic astigmatism using the emphasis erodible mask. Spanish User Group, J Refract Surg 11:S343, 1995.

1025. Goodman GL and others: Corneal healing following laser refractive keratectomy, Arch Ophthalmol 107:1799, 1989.

1026. Gyldenkerne GJ and Ehlers N: Excimer laser therapy of recurrent corneal erosions, Ugeskr Laeger 156:5282, 1994.

1027. Habib MS and others: Acute effects of myopic intrastromal ablation of the car cornea with the Nd:YLF picosecond laser, Invest Ophthalmol Vis Sci 35:2026, 1994.

1028. Habib MS and others: Myopic intrastromal photorefractive keratectomy with the neodymium-yttrium lithium fluoride picosecond laser in the cat cornea, Arch Ophthalmol 113:499, 1995.

1029. Hadden OB, Morris AT, and Ring CP: Excimer laser surgery for myopia and myopic astigmatism, A N Z J Ophthalmol 23:183, 1995.

1030. Hahn DW, Ediger MN, and Pettit GH: Dynamics of ablation plume particles generated during excimer laser corneal ablation, Lasers Surg Med 16:384, 1995.

1031. Hahn TW, Kim JH, and Lee YC: Excimer laser photorefractive keratectomy to correct residual myopia after radial keratotomy, Refract Corneal Surg 9:S25, 1993.

1032. Hahn TW, Sah WJ, and Kim JH: Phototherapeutic keratectomy in nine eyes with superficial corneal diseases, Refract Corneal Surg 9:S115, 1993.

1033. Hamberg-Nystrom H and others: Photorefractive keratectomy for low myopia at 5 mm treatment diameter. A comparison of two excimer lasers, Acta Ophthalmol (Copenh) 72:453, 1994.

1034. Hamberg-Nystrom H and others: Photorefractive keratectomy for 1.5 to 18 diopters of myopia, J Refract Surg 11:S265, 1995.

1035. Hamberg-Nystrom H and others: Patient satisfaction following photorefractive keratectomy for myopia, J Refract Surg 11:S335, 1995.

1036. Hamberg-Nystrom H and others: Thirty-six month follow-up of excimer laser photorefractive keratectomy for myopia, Ophthalmic Surg Lasers 27:S418, 1996.

1037. Hamberg-Nystrom H, and others: A comparative study of epithelial hyperplasia after PRK: Summit versus VISX in the same patient, Acta Ophthalmol Copenh 74:228, 1996.

1038. Hanna K and others: A rotating slit delivery system for excimer laser refractive keratectomy, Am J Ophthalmol 103:474, 1987.

1039. Hanna KD and others: Excimer laser keratectomy for myopia with a rotating-slit delivery system, Arch Ophthalmol 106:245, 1988.

1040. Hanna KD and others: Scanning slit delivery system, J Cataract Refract Surg 15:390, 1989.

1041. Hanna KD and others: Corneal stromal wound healing in rabbits after 193-nm excimer laser surface ablation, Arch Ophthalmol 107:895, 1989.

1042. Hanna KD and others: Corneal wound healing in monkeys 18 months after excimer laser photorefractive keratectomy, Refract Corneal Surg 6:340, 1990.

1043. Hanna KD and others: Corneal wound healing in monkeys after repeated excimer laser photorefractive keratectomy (see comments), Arch Ophthalmol 110:1286, 1992.

1044. Hardten DR and Lindstrom RL: Treatment of low, moderate, and high myopia with the 193-nm excimer laser, Klin Monatsbl Augenheilkd 205:259, 1994.

1045. Hardten DR, Sher NA, and Lindstrom RL: Correction of high myopia with the excimer laser: VISX 2015. In: Salz JJ, McDonnell PJ, and McDonald MB, editors: Corneal laser surgery, St. Louis, 1995, Mosby–Year Book.

1046. Harrison JM and others: Forward light scatter at one month after photorefractive keratectomy, J Refract Surg 11:83, 1995.

1047. Hassell JR and others: Proteoglycan changes during restoration of transparency in corneal scars, Arch Biochem Biophys 222:362, 1983.

1048. Haviv D and others: Excimer laser photorefractive keratectomy for myopia, Harefuah 125:1, 1993.

1049. Hayashi K and others: Pathogenesis of corneal epithelial defects: role of plasminogen activator, Curr Eye Res 10:381, 1991.

1050. Heinz P, Wiegand W, and Kroll P: Phototherapeutic keratectomy in recurrences of granular corneal dystrophy after keratoplasty, Klin Monatsbl Augenheilkd 206:184, 1995.

1051. Heitzmann J and others: The correction of high myopia using the excimer laser, Arch Ophthalmol 111:1627, 1993.

1052. Helena MC and others: Effect of 50% ethanol vs. mechanical epithelial debridement on keratocyte loss and inflammatory response after excimer photorefractive keratectomy ARVO, Invest Ophthalmol Vis Sci 36(suppl):24, 1995, (abstract 104-12).

1053. Hennekes R: Holmium: YAG laser thermokeratoplasty for correction of astigmatism, J Refract Surg 11(Suppl):S358, 1995.

1054. Hersh PS, Jordan AJ, and Mayers M: Corneal graft rejection episode after excimer laser phototherapeutic keratectomy (see comments), Arch Ophthalmol 111:735, 1993, (letter).

1055. Hersh PS and others: Phototherapeutic keratectomy: strategies and results in 12 eyes, Refract Corneal Surg 9:S90, 1993.

1056. Hersh PS and Schwartz-Goldstein BH: Corneal topography of phase III excimer laser photorefractive keratectomy. Characterization and clinical effects. Summit Photorefractive Keratectomy Topography Study Group, Ophthalmology 102:963, 1995.

1057. Hersch PS and others: Excimer laser phototherapeutic keratectomy. Surgical strategies and clinical outcomes, Ophthalmology 103(8):1210, 1996.

1058. Hjortdal JO and Ehlers N: Effect of excimer laser keratectomy on the mechanical performance of the human cornea, Acta Ophthalmol Scand 73:18, 1995.

1059. Holme RJ, Fouraker BD, and Schanzlin DJ: A comparison of ablation in the rabbit, Arch Ophthalmol 108:876, 1990.

1060. Horn G and others: New refractive method for laser thermal keratoplasty with the Co: MgF2 laser, J Cataract Refract Surg 16:611, 1990.

1061. Huebscher HJ, Genth U, and Seiler T: Determination of the excimer laser ablation rate of the human cornea using in vivo Scheimpflug videography, Invest Ophthalmol Vis Sci 37(1):42, 1996.

1062. Husinsky W and others: Corneal lathing using the excimer laser and a computer-controlled positioning system: Part II—Variable trephination of corneal buttons, Refract Corneal Surg 7:385, 1991.

1063. Ishikawa T and others: Hypersensitivity following excimer laser ablation through the corneal epithelium, Refract Corneal Surg 8:466, 1992.

1064. Ishikawa T and others: Corneal sensitivity and nerve regeneration after excimer laser ablation, Cornea 13:225, 1994.

1065. Ishikawa T and others: Corneal sensation following excimer laser for photorefractive keratectomy in humans, J Refract Corneal Surg 10:417, 1994.

1066. Ishikawa T and others: Correlation between corneal sensitivity and nerve regeneration following excimer laser ablation, Nippon Ganka Gakkai Zasshi 99:135, 1995.

1067. Jain S and others: Corneal light scattering after laser in situ keratomileusis and photorefractive keratectomy, Am J Ophthalmol 120:532, 1995.

1068. Janakiraman P and Rajendran B: Increasing the number of photorefractive keratectomy procedures from a single excimer laser gas fill, J Refract Surg 11:S319, 1995.

1069. Javitt JC and Chiang YP: The socioeconomic aspects of laser refractive surgery, Arch Ophthalmol 112:1526, 1994.

1070. John ME and others: Excimer laser photoablation of primary familial amyloidosis of the cornea, Refract Corneal Surg 9:S138, 1993.

1071. John ME and others: Photorefractive keratectomy following penetrating keratoplasty, J Refract Corneal Surg 10:S206, 1994.

1072. John ME and others: Excimer laser phototherapeutic keratectomy for treatment of recurrent corneal erosion, J Cataract Refract Surg 20:179, 1994.

1073. Kahle G and others: Wound healing of the cornea of New World monkeys after surface keratectomy: Er:YAG-excimer laser, Fortschr Ophthalmol 88:380, 1991.

1074. Kahle G, Seiler T, and Wollensak J: Report on psychosocial findings and satisfaction among patients 1 year after excimer laser photorefractive keratectomy, Refract Corneal Surg 8:286, 1992.

1075. Kahle G and others: Gas chromatographic and mass spectroscopic analysis of excimer and erbium: yttrium aluminum garnet laser–ablated human cornea, Invest Ophthalmol Vis Sci 33:2180, 1992.

1076. Kalski RS and others: Comparison of 5 mm and 6 mm ablation zones in photorefractive keratectomy for myopia, J Cataract Refract Surg 12:61, 1996.

1077. Kanellopoulos AJ and others: Comparison of corneal sensation following photorefractive keratectomy and laser in situ keratomileusis, J Cataract Refract Surg 23:34, 1997.

1078. Kassar B and Heitzman J: Correction of high myopia with the excimer laser: VISX 2020. In Salz JJ, McDonnell PJ and McDonald MB, editors: Corneal laser surgery, St. Louis, 1995, Mosby–Year Book.

1079. Kaufman HE: Surgical approaches to corneal wound healing, Acta Ophthalmol Suppl 84, 1992.

1080. Keates RH and Dingle J: Thermokeratoplasty for keratoconus, Ophthalmic Surg 6:89, 1975.

1081. Keates RH and others: Fibronectin on excimer laser and diamond knife incisions, J Cataract Refract Surg 15:404, 1989.

1082. Kelly CG: What is the role of refractive keratotomy in the 1990s? AudioDigest Ophthalmology, Glendale, 1995, California Medical Association.

1083. Kermani O and others: Mass spectroscopic analysis of excimer laser ablated material from human corneal tissue, J Cataract Refract Surg 14:638, 1988.

1084. Kermani O and Lubatschowski H: Structure and dynamics of photo-acoustic shock-waves in 193 nm excimer laser photo-ablation of the cornea, Fortschr Ophthalmol 88:748, 1991.

1085. Kerr-Muir MG and others: Ultrastructural comparison of conventional surgical and argon fluoride excimer laser keratectomy, Am J Ophthalmol 103:448, 1987.

1086. Kim JH and others: Photorefractive keratectomy in 202 myopic eyes: one year results, Refract Corneal Surg 9:S11, 1993.

1087. Kim JH and others: Clinical experience of two-step photorefractive keratectomy in 19 eyes with high myopia, Refract Corneal Surg 9:S44, 1993.

1088. Kim JH and others: Excimer laser photorefractive keratectomy for myopia: two-year follow-up, J Cataract Refract Surg 20 Suppl:229, 1994.

1089. Kim JH and others: Some problems after photorefractive keratectomy, J Refract Corneal Surg 10:S226, 1994.

1090. Kim JH and others: Three-year results of photorefractive keratectomy for myopia, J Refract Surg 11:S248, 1995.

1091. Kim KS, Lee JH and Edelhauser HF: Corneal epithelial permeability after excimer laser photorefractive keratectomy, J Cataract Refract Surg 22(1):44, 1996.

1092. Kim WJ, Eui-Sang C, and Lee JH: Effect of optic zone size on the outcome of photorefractive keratectomy for myopia, J Cataract Refract Surg 22:1434, 1996.

1093. Kim YJ and others: Photoastigmatic refractive keratectomy in 168 eyes: six-month results, J Cataract Refract Surg 20:387, 1994.

1094. Klyce SD and Smolek MK: Corneal topography of excimer laser photorefractive keratectomy, J Cataract Refract Surg 19 Suppl:122, 1993.

1095. Knaub J. Excimer laser update: investigating concentric ablation zones for high myopia, Refract Corneal Surg 7:212, 1991.

1096. Koch DD and others: Laser correction of hyperopia: Sunrise holmium laser results. In Salz JJ, McDonnell PJ, and McDonald MB, editors: Corneal laser surgery, St. Louis, 1995, Mosby–Year Book.

1097. Koch DD and others: Alternative lasers and strategies for corneal modification: Laser thermal keratoplasty for correction of astigmatism and myopia. In Salz JJ, McDonnell PJ, and McDonald MB, editors: Corneal laser surgery, St. Louis, 1995, Mosby–Year Book.

1098. Koch JW and others: Corneal wound healing after perforating and non-perforating excimer laser keratectomy. An experimental study, Fortschr Ophthalmol 87:615, 1990.

1099. Kohlhaas M and others: Aesthesiometry of the cornea after refractive corneal surgery, Klin Monatsbl Augenheilkd 201:221, 1992.

1100. Kornmehl EW, Steinert RF, and Puliafito CA: A comparative study of masking fluids for excimer laser phototherapeutic keratectomy, Arch Ophthalmol 109:860, 1991, (published erratum appears in Arch Ophthalmol 109(8):1114, 1991).

1101. Kraff C: Keratorefractive surgery with the excimer laser, J Cataract Refract Surg 20 Suppl:205, 1994, (editorial).

1102. Kraff MC and others: Changing practice patterns in refractive surgery: results of a survey of the American Society of Cataract and Refractive Surgery, J Cataract Refract Surg 20:172, 1994.

1103. Kriegerowski M and others: The ablation behavior of various corneal layers, Fortschr Ophthalmol 87:11, 1990.

1104. Krueger RR and Trokel SL: Quantitation of corneal ablation by ultraviolet laser light, Arch Ophthalmol 103:1741, 1985.

1105. Krueger RR, Trokel SL, and Schubert HD: Interaction of ultraviolet laser light with the cornea, Invest Ophthalmol Vis Sci 26:1455, 1985.

1106. Krueger RR, Sliney DH, and Trokel SL: Photokeratitis from subablative 193-nanometer excimer laser radiation, Refract Corneal Surg 8:274, 1992.

1107. Krueger RR and others: Corneal surface morphology following excimer laser ablation with humidified gases, Arch Ophthalmol 111:1131, 1993.

1108. Krueger RR and others: Photography of shock waves during excimer laser ablation of the cornea. Effect of helium gas on propagation velocity, Cornea 12:330, 1993.

1109. Krueger RR and others: Clinical analysis of excimer laser photorefractive keratectomy using a multiple zone technique for severe myopia, Am J Ophthalmol 119:263, 1995.

1110. Krueger RR, Binder PS, and McDonnel PJ: The effects of excimer laser photoablation on the cornea. In: Salz JJ, editor: Corneal laser surgery, St. Louis, 1995, Mosby Times Mirror.

1111. Krueger RR, Saedy NF, and McDonnell PJ: Clinical analysis of steep central islands after excimer laser photorefractive keratectomy, Arch Ophthalmol 114(4):377, 1996.

1112. Kruse FE and others: Conjunctival transdifferentiation is due to the incomplete removal of limbal basal epithelium, Invest Ophthalmol Vis Sci 31:1903, 1990.

1113. Kruse FE: Stem cells and corneal epithelial regeneration, Eye 8:170, 1994, (review).

1114. Kubota T and others: Lamellar excimer laser keratoplasty: reproducible photoablation of corneal tissue. A laboratory study, Doc Ophthalmol 82:193, 1992.

1115. L'Esperance FA Jr and others: Human excimer laser corneal surgery: preliminary report, Trans Am Ophthalmol Soc 86:208, 1988.

1116. L'Esperance FA Jr, Taylor DM, and Warner JW: Human excimer laser keratectomy. Short-term histopathology, Bull N Y Acad Med 65:557, 1989.

1117. L'Esperance FA Jr, and others: Excimer laser instrumentation and technique for human corneal surgery, Arch Ophthalmol 107:131, 1989.

1118. Lang GK and others: Excimer laser keratoplasty. Part 1: Basic concepts, Ophthalmic Surg 20:262, 1989.

1119. Lang GK and others: Excimer laser keratoplasty. Part 2: Elliptical keratoplasty, Ophthalmic Surg 20:342, 1989.

1120. Lans L: Experimentelle Untersuchungen uber Entstehung von Astigmatismus durch nicht-perforirende Corneawunden, Albrecht von Graefes Arch Ophthalmol 45:17, 1898.

1121. Latvala T and others: Expression of cellular fibronectin and tenascin in the rabbit cornea after excimer laser photorefractive keratectomy: a 12 month study, Br J Ophthalmol 79:65, 1995.

1122. Latvala T, Tervo K, and Tervo T: Reassembly of the alpha 6 beta 4 integrin and laminin in rabbit corneal basement membrane after excimer laser surgery: a 12-month follow-up, CLAO J 21:125, 1995.

1123. Lavery FL: Photorefractive keratectomy in 172 eyes, Refract Corneal Surg 9:S98, 1993.

1124. Lawless MA, Cohen P, and Rogers C: Phototherapeutic keratectomy for Reis-Buckler's dystrophy, Refract Corneal Surg 9:S96, 1993.

1125. Lawless MA, Rogers C, and Cohen P: Excimer laser photorefractive keratectomy: 12 months' follow-up, Med J Aust 159:535, 538, 1993.

1126. Lawless MA, Cohen PR, and Rogers CM: Retreatment of undercorrected photorefractive keratectomy for myopia, J Refract Corneal Surg 10:S174, 1994.

1127. Leroux les Jardins S and others: Results of photorefractive keratectomy on 63 myopic eyes with six months minimum follow-up, J Cataract Refract Surg 20 Suppl:223, 1994.

1128. Lesher MP and others: Phacoemulsification with intraocular lens implantation after excimer photorefractive keratectomy: a case report, J Cataract Refract Surg 20 Suppl:265, 1994.

1129. Levin S and others: Prevalence of central islands after excimer laser refractive surgery, J Cataract Refract Surg 21:21, 1995.

1130. Li DQ and Tseng SC: Three patterns of cytokine expression potentially involved in epithelial-fibroblast interactions of human ocular surface, J Cell Physiol 163:61, 1995.

1131. Liang FQ and others: A new procedure for evaluating smoothness of corneal surface following 193-nanometer excimer laser ablation, Refract Corneal Surg 8:459, 1992.

1132. Liang FQ and others: Surface quality of excimer laser corneal ablation with different frequencies, Cornea 12:500, 1993.

1133. Lin DT, Sutton HF, and Berman M: Corneal topography following excimer photorefractive keratectomy for myopia, J Cataract Refract Surg 19 Suppl:149, 1993.

1134. Lin DT: Corneal topographic analysis after excimer photorefractive keratectomy, Ophthalmology 101:1432, 1994.

1135. Lindstrom RL and others: Use of the 193-NM excimer laser for myopic photorefractive keratectomy in sighted eyes: a multicenter study, Trans Am Ophthalmol Soc 89:155, 1991.

1136. Lindstrom RL and Zabel RW: Myopic excimer laser keratectomy. A preliminary report, Dev Ophthalmol 22:1, 1991.

1137. Lindstrom RL and others: Excimer laser photorefractive keratectomy in high myopia: a multicenter study, Trans Am Ophthalmol Soc 90:277, 1992.

1138. Lindstrom RL, Hardten DR, and Dougherty PJ: Excimer laser photorefractive keratectomy for myopia: a single surgeon best-case analysis, Trans Am Ophthalmol Soc 92:235, 1994.

1139. Lipshitz I, Loewenstein A, and Lazar M: Astigmatic keratotomy followed by photorefractive keratectomy in the treatment of compound myopic astigmatism, J Refract Corneal Surg 10:S282, 1994.

1140. Lipshitz I and others: Late onset corneal haze after photorefractive keratectomy for moderate and high myopia, Ophthalmology 104:369, 1997.

1141. Litwin KL and others: Changes in corneal curvature at different excimer laser ablative depths, Am J Ophthalmol 111:382, 1991, (letter).

1142. Liu JC and others: Myopic excimer laser photorefractive keratectomy: an analysis of clinical correlations, Refract Corneal Surg 6: 321, 1990.

1143. Loertscher H and others: 2d, Noncontact trephination of the cornea using a pulsed hydrogen fluoride laser, Am J Ophthalmol 104: 471, 1987.

1144. Loewenstein A, Lipshitz I, and Lazar M: Photorefractive keratectomy for the treatment of myopia after epikeratoplasty: a case report, J Refract Corneal Surg 10:S285, 1994.

1145. Loewenstein A, Lipshitz I, and Lazar M: Scraping of epithelium for treatment of under-correction and haze after photorefractive keratectomy, J Refract Corneal Surg 10:S274, 1994.

1146. Loewenstein A and others: The effect of spherical photorefractive keratectomy on myopic astigmatism, J Refract Surg 11:S263, 1995.

1147. Lohmann CP and others: Corneal haze after excimer laser refractive surgery: objective measurements and functional implications, Eur J Ophthalmol 1:173, 1991.

1148. Lohmann CP and others: "Haze" in photorefractive keratectomy: origins and consequences. A review. Lasers Light Ophthalmol 4: 15, 1991.

1149. Lohmann CP and others: Corneal opacity after photorefractive keratectomy with an excimer laser. Cause, objective measurement and functional consequences, Ophthalmologe 89:498, 1992.

1150. Lohmann CP and others: Corneal light scattering after excimer laser photorefractive keratectomy: the objective measurements of haze, Refract Corneal Surg 8:114, 1992.

1151. Lohmann CP and Marshall J: Plasmin- and plasminogen-activator inhibitors after excimer laser photorefractive keratectomy: new concept in prevention of postoperative myopic regression and haze, Refract Corneal Surg 9:300, 1993.

1152. Lohmann CP and others: Corneal light scattering and visual performance in myopic individuals with spectacles, contact lenses, or excimer laser photorefractive keratectomy, Am J Ophthalmol 115: 444, 1993.

1153. Lohmann CP and others: Halos—a problem for all myopes? A comparison between spectacles, contact lenses, and photorefractive keratectomy, Refract Corneal Surg 9:S72, 1993.

1154. Loya N and others: Topical diclofenac following excimer laser: effect on corneal sensitivity and wound healing in rabbits, J Refract Corneal Surg 10:423, 1994.

1155. Lubatschowski H and others: ArF-excimer laser-induced secondary radiation in photoablation of biological tissue, Lasers Surg Med 14:168, 1994.

1156. Machat JJ: Double-blind corticosteroid trial in identical twins following photorefractive keratectomy, Refract Corneal Surg 9:S105, 1993.

1157. Machat JJ and Tayfour F: Photorefractive keratectomy for myopia: preliminary results in 147 eyes, Refract Corneal Surg 9:S16, 1993.

1158. Machat JJ and Mintsioulis G: Unilateral vs. simultaneous bilateral photorefractive keratectomy, Can J Ophthalmol 30:181, 1995.

1159. MacInnis B: Excimer laser photorefractive keratectomy, Can J Ophthalmol 30:51, 1995.

1160. MacRobert IJ and Ho SS: Bilateral simultaneous myopic PRK as experienced by an ophthalmologist, Refract Corneal Surg 9:S118, 1993.

1161. MacRobert IJ and Ho SS: The use of corticosteroid/beta-blocker combinations in the management of regression after PRK for high myopia, J Refract Surg 11:S321, 1995.

1162. Macy JI, Nesburn AB, and Salz JJ: Laser correction of hyperopia: VISX blind eye study United States results. In Salz JJ, McDonnell PJ, and McDonald MB, editors: Corneal laser surgery, St. Louis, 1995, Mosby–Year Book.

1163. Maeda N and others: Automated keratoconus screening with corneal topography analysis, Invest Ophthalmol Vis Sci 35:2749, 1994.

1164. Maeda N, Klyce SD, and Smolek MK: Comparison of methods for detecting keratoconus using videokeratography, Arch Ophthalmol 113:870, 1995.

1165. Maguen E and others: Effect of nitrogen flow on recovery of vision after excimer laser photorefractive keratectomy without nitrogen flow, J Refract Corneal Surg 10:321, 1994.

1166. Maguen E and others: Results of excimer laser photorefractive keratectomy for the correction of myopia, Ophthalmology 101: 1548, 1994.

1167. Maguen E and Machat JJ: Complications of photorefractive keratectomy, primarily with the VISX excimer laser. In Salz JJ, McDonnell PJ, and McDonald MB, editors. Corneal laser surgery, St. Louis, 1995, Mosby–Year Book.

1168. Maguire LJ and others: Topography and raytracing analysis of patients with excellent visual acuity 3 months after excimer laser photorefractive keratectomy for myopia, Refract Corneal Surg 7:122, 1991.

1169. Maguire LJ and Bechara S: Epithelial distortions at the ablation zone margin after excimer laser photorefractive keratectomy for myopia, Am J Ophthalmol 117:809, 1994, (letter).

1170. Mainster MA: Ophthalmic applications of infrared lasers—thermal considerations, Invest Ophthalmol Vis Sci 18:414, 1979.

1171. Maldonado BA and Furcht LT: Epidermal growth factor stimulates integrin-mediated cell migration of cultured human corneal epithelial cells on fibronectin and arginine-glycine-aspartic acid peptide, Invest Ophthalmol Vis Sci 36:2120, 1995.

1172. Maldonado BA and Furcht LT: Involvement of integrins with adhesion-promoting, heparin-binding peptides of type IV collagen in cultured human corneal epithelial cells, Invest Ophthalmol Vis Sci 36:364, 1995.

1173. Maldonado MJ and Menezo JL: The corneal endothelium and myopic excimer laser photorefractive keratectomy, Arch Ophthalmol 113:697, 1995, (letter).

1174. Malley DS and others: Immunofluorescence study of corneal wound healing after excimer laser anterior keratectomy in the monkey eye, Arch Ophthalmol 108:1316, 1990.

1175. Maloney RK: Corneal topography and optical zone location in photorefractive keratectomy, Refract Corneal Surg 6:363, 1990.

1176. Maloney RK and others: A prototype erodible mask delivery system for the excimer laser, Ophthalmology 100:542, 1993.

1177. Maloney RK and others: A multicenter trial of photorefractive keratectomy for residual myopia after previous ocular surgery, Ophthalmology 102:1042, 1995.

1178. Maloney RK and others: A prospective multicenter trial of excimer laser phototherapeutic keratotomy for corneal vision loss. The summit phototherapeutic keratectomy study group, Am J Ophthalmol 122(2):149, 1996.

1179. Manabe Y and others: Comparison of wound healing of linear incisions in the rabbit cornea produced by the newly developed excimer laser, a metal blade, and a diamond blade, Nippon Ganka Gakkai Zasshi 96:288, 1992.

1180. Mandelberg AI, Rao GN, and Aquavella JV: Penetrating keratoplasty following thermokeratoplasty, Ophthalmology 87:750, 1980.

1181. Mandell RB: Corneal power correction factor for photorefractive keratectomy, J Refract Corneal Surg 10:125, 1994.

1182. Mardelli PG and others: Corneal endothelial status 12 to 55 months after excimer laser photorefractive keratectomy, Ophthalmology 102:544, 1995.

1183. Markovits AS: Photo-refractive keratectomy (PRK): threat or millennium for military pilots? Aviat Space Environ Med 64:409, 1993.

1184. Marshall GE, Konstas AG, and Lee WR: Immunogold fine structural localization of extracellular matrix components in aged human cornea. I. Types I-IV collagen and laminin, Graefes Arch Clin Exp Ophthalmol 229:157, 1991.

1185. Marshall GE, Konstas AG, and Lee WR: Immunogold fine structural localization of extracellular matrix components in aged human cornea. II. Collagen types V and VI, Graefes Arch Clin Exp Ophthalmol 229:164, 1991.

1186. Marshall GE, Konstas AG, and Lee WR: Collagens in ocular tissues. [Review], Br J Ophthalmol 77:515, 1993.

1187. Marshall J and others: An ultrastructural study of corneal incisions induced by an excimer laser at 193 nm, Ophthalmology 92:749, 1985.

1188. Marshall J and others: A comparative study of corneal incisions induced by diamond and steel knives and two ultraviolet radiations from an excimer laser, Br J Ophthalmol 70:482, 1986.

1189. Marshall J and others: Photoablative reprofiling of the cornea using an excimer laser: Photorefractive keratectomy. Lasers Ophthalmol 1:21, 1986.

1190. Marshall J and others: Long-term healing of the central cornea after photorefractive keratectomy using an excimer laser, Ophthalmology 95:1411, 1988.

1191. Matta CS and others: Excimer retreatment for myopic photorefractive keratectomy failures. Six to 18-month follow-up, Ophthalmology 103:444, 1996.

1192. Matsuda H and Smelser GK: Electron microscopy of corneal wound healing, Exp Eye Res 16:427, 1973.

1193. McCarty CA, Aldred GF, and Taylor HR: Comparison of results of excimer laser correction of all degrees of myopia at 12 months postoperatively. The Melbourne Excimer Laser Group, Am J Ophthalmol 121(4):372, 1996.

1194. McDonald MB and others: Excimer laser ablation in a human eye. Case report (see comments), Arch Ophthalmol 107:641, 1989.

1195. McDonald MB and others: Central photorefractive keratectomy for myopia. The blind eye study, Arch Ophthalmol 108:799, 1990.

1196. McDonald MB and others: One-year refractive results of central photorefractive keratectomy for myopia in the nonhuman primate cornea, Arch Ophthalmol 108:40, 1990.

1197. McDonald MB and others: Central photorefractive keratectomy for myopia. Partially sighted and normally sighted eyes, Ophthalmology 98:1327, 1991.

1198. McDonald MB and Talamo JH: The experience in the United States with the VISX excimer laser. In Salz JJ, McDonnell PJ, and McDonald MB, editors: Corneal Laser Surgery, St. Louis, 1995, Mosby–Year Book.

1199. McDonnell JM, Garbus JJ, and McDonnell PJ: Unsuccessful excimer laser phototherapeutic keratectomy. Clinicopathologic correlation, Arch Ophthalmol 110:977, 1992.

1200. McDonnell PJ: Radial thermokeratoplasty for hyperopia. I. The need for prompt prospective investigation, Refract Corneal Surg 5:50, 1989.

1201. McDonnell PJ, Garbus JJ, and Salz JJ: Excimer laser myopic photorefractive keratectomy after undercorrected radial keratotomy, Refract Corneal Surg 7:146, 1991.

1202. McDonnell PJ and others: Photorefractive keratectomy for astigmatism. Initial clinical results, Arch Ophthalmol 109:1370, 1991.

1203. McDonnell PJ and others: Photorefractive keratectomy to create toric ablations for correction of astigmatism, Arch Ophthalmol 109:710, 1991.

1204. McDonnell PJ and Seiler T: Phototherapeutic keratectomy with excimer laser for Reis-Buckler's corneal dystrophy, Refract Corneal Surg 8:306, 1992.

1205. McDonnell PJ and others: Photorefractive keratectomy for correction of myopic astigmatism, Klin Monatsbl Augenheilkd 202:238, 1993.

1206. McDonnell PJ: Excimer laser corneal surgery: new strategies and old enemies, Invest Ophthalmol Vis Sci 36:4, 1995.

1207. McDonnell PJ: Excimer laser photorefractive keratectomy. The Food and Drug Administration panel speaks, Arch Ophthalmol 113:858, 1995, (editorial).

1208. McWhae J and others: Ultrasound biomicroscopy in refractive surgery, J Cataract Refract Surg 20:493, 1994.

1209. Menezo JL and others: Excimer laser photorefractive keratectomy for high myopia, J Cataract Refract Surg 21:393, 1995.

1210. Mertaniemi P and others: Increased release of immunoreactive calcitonin gene-related peptide (CGRP) in tears after excimer laser keratectomy, Exp Eye Res 60:659, 1995.

1211. Meyer JC and others: Late onset of corneal scar after excimer laser photorefractive keratectomy, Am J Ophthalmol 121(5):529, 1996.

1212. Meza J and others: Photorefractive keratectomy after radial keratotomy, J Cataract Refract Surg 20:485, 1994.

1213. Michelson MA and others: Photorefractive keratectomy: early American experience, Int Ophthalmol Clin 34:97, 1994.

1214. Moller-Pedersen T and others: Quantification of stromal thinning, epithelial thickness, and corneal haze after photorefractive keratectomy using in vivo confocal microscopy, Ophthalmology 104:360, 1997.

1215. Moodaley L and others: Excimer laser superficial keratectomy for proud nebulae in keratoconus, Br J Ophthalmol 78:454, 1994.

1216. Moreira H and others: Multifocal corneal topographic changes with excimer laser photorefractive keratectomy (see comments), Arch Ophthalmol 110:994, 1992.

1217. Moreira H and others: Holmium laser thermokeratoplasty, Ophthalmology 100:752, 1993.

1218. Moreira LB and others: Aerosolization of infectious virus by excimer laser, Am J Ophthalmol 123:297, 1997.

1219. Moretti M: FDA panel gives cautious signal to Summit [news], J Refract Corneal Surg 10:613, 1994.

1220. Morimoto K and others: Role of urokinase type plasminogen activator (u-PA) in corneal epithelial migration, Thromb Haemost 69:387, 1993.

1221. Morlet N and others: Effect of topical interferon-alpha 2b on corneal haze after excimer laser photorefractive keratectomy in rabbits, Refract Corneal Surg 9:443, 1993.

1222. Mortensen J and Ohrstrom A: Excimer laser photorefractive keratectomy for treatment of keratoconus, J Refract Corneal Surg 10:368, 1994.

1223. Munnerlyn CR, Koons SJ, and Marshall J: Photorefractive keratectomy: a technique for laser refractive surgery, J Cataract Refract Surg 14:46, 1988.

1224. Murta JN and others: Photorefractive keratectomy for myopia in 98 eyes, J Refract Corneal Surg 10:S231, 1994.

1225. Nagy ZZ and others: Experience with excimer laser photorefractive keratectomy, Orv Hetil 136:1035, 1995.

1226. Nagy ZZ and others: Ultraviolet-B enhances corneal stromal response to 193-nm excimer laser treatment, Ophthalmology 104:375, 1997.

1227. Nakagawa S, Nishida T, and Manabe R: Actin organization in migrating corneal epithelium of rabbits in situ, Exp Eye Res 41:335, 1985.

1228. Nassaralla BA and others: Prevention of keratocyte loss after corneal deepithelialization in rabbits, Arch Ophthalmol 113:506, 1995.

1229. Nassaralla BA and others: Effect of diclofenac on corneal haze after photorefractive keratectomy in rabbits, Ophthalmology 102:469, 1995.

1230. Nesburn AB and others: Keratoconus detected by videokeratography in candidates for photorefractive keratectomy, J Refract Surg 11:194, 1995.

1231. Neumann AC, Sanders DR, and Salz JJ: Radial thermokeratoplasty for hyperopia. II. Encouraging results from early laboratory and human trials, Refract Corneal Surg 5:50, 1989.

1232. Neumann AC and others: Effect of thermokeratoplasty on corneal curvature, J Cataract Refract Surg 16:727, 1990.

1233. Neumann AC, Fyodorov S, and Sanders DR: Radial thermokeratoplasty for the correction of hyperopia (see comments), Refract Corneal Surg 6:404, 1990.

1234. Neumann AC and others: Hyperopic thermokeratoplasty: clinical evaluation, J Cataract Refract Surg 17:830, 1991.

1235. Niemz MH, Klancnik EG, and Bille JF: Plasma-mediated ablation of corneal tissue at 1053 nm using a Nd:YLF oscillator/regenerative amplifier laser, Lasers Surg Med 11:426, 1991.

1236. Niemz MH and others: Intrastromal ablations for refractive corneal surgery using picosecond infrared laser pulses, Lasers Light Ophthalmol 5:145, 1993.

1237. Niesen U, Thomann U, and Schipper I: Phototherapeutic keratectomy, Klin Monatsbl Augenheilkd 205:187, 1994.

1238. Niizuma T and others: Cooling the cornea to prevent side effects of photorefractive keratectomy, J Refract Corneal Surg 10:S262, 1994.

1239. Nissen M and others: Acute effects of intrastromal ablation with the Nd:YLF picosecond laser on the endothelium of rabbit eyes, Invest Ophthalmol Vis Sci 34:1246, 1993.

1240. Nordan LT and others: Photorefractive keratectomy to treat myopia and astigmatism after radial keratotomy and penetrating keratoplasty, J Cataract Refract Surg 21:268, 1995.

1241. Obata H and others: Histological and ultrastructural study of rabbit cornea ablated by scanning excimer laser system, Jpn J Ophthalmol 38:285, 1994.

1242. O'Brart DP and others: Treatment of band keratopathy by excimer laser phototherapeutic keratectomy: surgical techniques and long term follow up, Br J Ophthalmol 77:702, 1993.

1243. O'Brart DP and others: Excimer laser photorefractive keratectomy for myopia: comparison of 4.00- and 5.00-millimeter ablation zones, J Refract Corneal Surg 10:87, 1994.

1244. O'Brart DP and others: Disturbances in night vision after excimer laser photorefractive keratectomy, Eye 8:46, 1994.

1245. O'Brart DP and others: Discrimination between the origins and functional implications of haze and halo at night after photorefractive keratectomy, J Refract Corneal Surg 10:S281, 1994.

1246. O'Brart DP and others: Night vision after excimer laser photorefractive keratectomy: haze and halos, Eur J Ophthalmol 4:43, 1994.

1247. O'Brart DP and others: The effects of topical corticosteroids and plasmin inhibitors on refractive outcome, haze, and visual performance after photorefractive keratectomy. A prospective, randomized, observer-masked study, Ophthalmology 101:1565, 1994.

1248. O'Brart DP, Muir MG, and Marshall J: Phototherapeutic keratectomy for recurrent corneal erosions, Eye 8:378, 1994.

1249. O'Brart DP and others: The effects of ablation diameter on the outcome of excimer laser photorefractive keratectomy. A prospective, randomized, double-blind study, Arch Ophthalmol 113:438, 1995.

1250. O'Brart DPS and others: Effects of ablation diameter, depth, and edge contour on the outcome of photorefractive keratectomy, J Cataract Refract Surg 12:50, 1996.

1251. Ohashi H and others: Up-regulation of integrin alpha 5 beta 1 expression by interleukin-6 in rabbit corneal epithelial cells, Exp Cell Res 218:418, 1995.

1252. Ohman L, Fagerholm P, and Tengroth B: Treatment of recurrent corneal erosions with the excimer laser, Acta Ophthalmol (Copenh) 72:461, 1994.

1253. Olson RJ: Photorefractive keratoplasty: photorefractive keratomania? Arch Ophthalmol 114(3):338, 1996, (editorial; comment).

1254. Orndahl M and others: Treatment of corneal dystrophies with excimer laser, Acta Ophthalmol (Copenh) 72:235, 1994.

1255. Orssaud C and others: Photorefractive keratectomy in 176 eyes: one year follow-up, J Refract Corneal Surg 10:S199, 1994.

1256. Ozler SA and others: Acute ultrastructural changes of cornea after excimer laser ablation, Invest Ophthalmol Vis Sci 33:540, 1992.

1257. Pallikaris IG and others: A comparative study of neural regeneration following corneal wounds induced by an argon fluoride excimer laser and mechanical methods, Laser Light Ophthalmol 3:89, 1990.

1258. Pallikaris IG and others: Excimer laser photorefractive keratectomy for myopia: clinical results in 96 eyes, Refract Corneal Surg 9:S101, 1993.

1259. Pallikaris IG and Siganos DS: Excimer laser in situ keratomileusis and photorefractive keratectomy for correction of high myopia, J Refract Corneal Surg 10:498, 1994.

1260. Pallikaris IG and others: Rotating brush for fast removal of corneal epithelium, J Cataract Refract Surg 10:439, 1994.

1261. Panjwani N and others: Neutral glycolipids of migrating and non-migrating rabbit corneal epithelium in organ and cell culture, Invest Ophthalmol Vis Sci 31:689, 1990.

1262. Panjwani N and others: Neolactoglycosphingolipids, potential mediators of corneal epithelial cell migration, J Biol Chem 270:14015, 1995.

1263. Parel JM, Ren Q, and Simon G: Noncontact laser photothermal keratoplasty. I: Biophysical principles and laser beam delivery system, J Refract Corneal Surg 10:511, 1994.

1264. Patel S and others: The shape of the corneal apical zone after excimer photorefractive keratectomy, Acta Ophthalmol (Copenh) 72:588, 1994.

1265. Pavlin CJ, Harasiewicz K, and Foster FS: Ultrasound biomicroscopic assessment of the cornea following excimer laser photokeratectomy, J Cataract Refract Surg 20 Suppl:206, 1994.

1266. Pender PM: Photorefractive keratectomy for myopic astigmatism: phase IIA of the Federal Drug Administration study (12 to 18 months follow-up). Excimer Laser Study Group, J Cataract Refract Surg 20 Suppl:262, 1994.

1267. Pepose JS and others: Reactivation of latent herpes simplex virus by excimer laser photokeratectomy, Am J Ophthalmol 114:45, 1992.

1268. Perez-Santonja JJ and others: Short-term corneal endothelial changes after photorefractive keratectomy, J Refract Corneal Surg 10:S194, 1994.

1269. Peters DMP and Mosher DF: Localization of cell surface sites involved in fibronectin fibrillogenesis, J Cell Biol 104:571, 1987.

1270. Peyman GA, Badaro RM, and Khoobchi B: Corneal ablation in rabbits using an infrared (2.9-microns) erbium:YAG laser, Ophthalmology 96:1160, 1989.

1271. Peyman GA and others: Long-term effect of erbium-YAG laser (2.9 microns) on the primate cornea, Int Ophthalmol 15:249, 1991.

1272. Phelan PS, McGhee CN, and Bryce IG: Excimer laser PRK and corticosteroid induced IOP elevation: the tip of an emerging iceberg? Br J Ophthalmol 78:802, 1994, (letter).

1273. Phillips AF and others: Arachidonic acid metabolites after excimer laser corneal surgery, Arch Ophthalmol 111:1273, 1993.

1274. Piebenga LW and others: Excimer photorefractive keratectomy for myopia, Ophthalmology 100:1335, 1993.

1275. Poirier L and others: Results of therapeutic photo-keratectomy using the Excimer laser. Apropos of 12 cases, J Fr Ophthalmol 17: 262, 1994.

1276. Poirier L and others: Energy fluctuations in an excimer laser during photorefractive keratectomy, J Refract Corneal Surg 10:S258, 1994.

1277. Pouliquen Y and others: Is there a future for the Excimer laser in refractive surgery?, Bull Acad Natl Med 174:275, 1990.

1278. Preussner PR and Leukefeld J: Automatic tracking system for laser surgery of the human cornea, Biomed Tech (Berlin) 37:218, 1992.

1279. Probst LE V and Machat JJ: Corneal subepithelial infiltrates following photorefractive keratectomy, J Cataract Refract Surg 22(3):281, 1996, (letter).

1280. Prydal JI and others: Regeneration of subepithelial nerves after excimer laser photokeratectomy in humans examined by confocal microscopy, Invest Ophthalmol Vis Sci 37:S59, 1996, (ARVO abstract 264).

1281. Puliafito CA and others: Excimer laser ablation of the cornea and lens; experimental studies, Ophthalmology 92:741, 1985.

1282. Puliafito CA and others: High-speed photography of excimer laser ablation of the cornea, Arch Ophthalmol 105:1255, 1987.

1283. Puliafito CA, Wong K, and Steinert RF: Quantitative and ultrastructural studies of excimer laser ablation of the cornea at 193 and 248 nanometers, Lasers Surg Med 7:155, 1987.

1284. Rajendran B and Janakiraman P: Multizone photorefractive keratectomy for myopia of 8 to 23 diopters, J Refract Surg 11:S298, 1995.

1285. Rapuano CJ and Laibson PR: Excimer laser phototherapeutic keratectomy, CLAO J 19:235, 1993.

1286. Rapuano CJ and Laibson PR: Excimer laser phototherapeutic keratectomy for anterior corneal pathology, CLAO J 20:253, 1994.

1287. Rask R, Jensen PK, and Ehlers N: Healing velocity of corneal epithelium evaluated by computer. The effect of topical steroid, Acta Ophthalmol Scand 73:162, 1995.

1288. Rawe IM and others: A morphological study of rabbit corneas after laser keratectomy, Eye 6:637, 1992.

1289. Rawe IM and others: Structure of corneal scar tissue: an X-ray diffraction study, Biophys J 67:1743, 1994.

1290. Reinstein DZ and others: Corneal pachymetric topography, Ophthalmology 101:432, 1994.

1291. Ren Q, Simon G, and Parel JM: Ultraviolet solid-state laser (213-nm) photorefractive keratectomy. In vitro study, Ophthalmology 100:1828, 1993.

1292. Ren Q and others: Ultraviolet solid-state laser (213-nm) photorefractive keratectomy. In vivo study, Ophthalmology 101:883, 1994.

1293. Ren Q, Simon G, and Parel JM: Noncontact laser photothermal keratoplasty. III: Histological study in animal eyes, J Refract Corneal Surg 10:529, 1994.

1294. Renard G and others: Excimer laser experimental keratectomy. Ultrastructural study, Cornea 6:269, 1987.

1295. Ribeiro JC and others: Excimer laser photorefractive keratectomy after radial keratotomy, J Refract Surg 11:165, 1995.

1296. Rieck P and others: Basic fibroblast growth factor modulates corneal wound healing after excimer laser keratomileusis in rabbits, Ger J Ophthalmol 3:105, 1994.

1297. Ring CP, Hadden OB, and Morris AT: Transverse keratotomy combined with spherical photorefractive keratectomy for compound myopic astigmatism, J Refract Corneal Surg 10:S217, 1994.

1298. Roberts CW and Koester CJ: Optical zone diameters for photorefractive corneal surgery, Invest Ophthalmol Vis Sci 34:2275, 1993.

1299. Rogers CM, Cohen PR, and Lawless MA: Phototherapeutic keratectomy for Reis Bucklers' corneal dystrophy, Aust N Z J Ophthalmol 21:247, 1993.

1300. Rogers CM, Lawless MA, and Cohen PR: Photorefractive keratectomy for myopia of more than −10 diopters, J Refract Corneal Surg 10:S171, 1994.

1301. Rosa DS and others: Wound healing following excimer laser radial keratotomy, J Cataract Refract Surg 14:173, 1988.

1302. Rosa N and others: Effects on the corneal endothelium six months following photorefractive keratectomy, Ophthalmologica 209:17, 1995.

1303. Rowsey JJ, Stevens SX, and Fouraker BD: Alternative lasers and strategies for corneal modification: intrastromal lasers. In Salz JJ, McDonnel PJ, and McDonald MB, editors: Corneal laser surgery, St. Louis, 1995, Mosby–Year Book.

1304. Sabetti L and others: Measurement of corneal thickness by ultrasound after photorefractive keratectomy in high myopia, J Refract Corneal Surg 10:S211, 1994.

1305. Salazar GJ: Hyperopic thermal keratoplasty procedure in a civilian air traffic controller, Aviat Space Environ Med 65:772, 1994.

1306. Salorio DP and others: Photorefractive keratectomy for myopia: 18-month results in 178 eyes, Refract Corneal Surg 9:S108, 1993.

1307. Salz D and others: One-year results of excimer laser photorefractive keratectomy for myopia, Refract Corneal Surg 8:269, 1992.

1308. Salz JJ and others: A two-year experience with excimer laser photorefractive keratectomy for myopia, Ophthalmology 100:873, 1993.

1309. Salz JJ: Traumatic corneal abrasions following photorefractive keratectomy, J Refract Corneal Surg 10:36, 1994.

1310. Schachar RA: Radial thermokeratoplasty. Int Ophthalmol Clin 31:47, 1991, (review).

1311. Schallhorn SC and others: Preliminary results of photorefractive keratectomy in active-duty United States Navy personnel, Ophthalmology 103:5, 1996.

1312. Schipper I and Senn P: 2 years experience with the Excimer laser photorefractive keratectomy in myopia, Klin Monatsbl Augenheilkd 204:413, 1994.

1313. Schipper I, Suppelt C, and Senn P: Correction of astigmatism with Excimer laser transverse keratectomy, Acta Ophthalmol (Copenh) 72:39, 1994.

1314. Schipper I and others: Intraocular pressure after excimer laser photorefractive keratectomy for myopia, J Cataract Refract Surg 11:366, 1995.

1315. Schipper I, Senn P, and Niesen U: Are we measuring the right intraocular pressure after excimer laser photorefractive laser keratoplasty in myopia?, Klin Monatsbl Augenheilkd 206:322, 1995.

1316. Schirner G and others: Experimental studies on the effect of the Er:glass and Cr:Tm:Ho:YAG laser in thermokeratoplasty (German), Ophthalmologe 91:638, 1994.

1317. Schroder E and others: An ophthalmic excimer laser for corneal surgery, Am J Ophthalmol 103:472, 1987.

1318. Schwartz-Goldstein BH and Hersh PS: Corneal topography of phase III excimer laser photorefractive keratectomy. Optical zone centration analysis. Summit Photorefractive Keratectomy Topography Study Group, Ophthalmology 102:951, 1995.

1319. Scialdone A and others: Randomized study of single vs double exposure in myopic PRK, Refract Corneal Surg 9:S41, 1993.

1320. Seiler T and others: Side effects in excimer corneal surgery. DNA damage as a result of 193 nm excimer laser radiation, Graefes Arch Clin Exp Ophthalmol 226:273, 1988.

1321. Seiler T and others: Excimer laser keratectomy for correction of astigmatism, Am J Ophthalmol 105:117, 1988.

1322. Seiler T Kahle G, and Kriegerowski M: Excimer laser (193 nm) myopic keratomileusis in sighted and blind human eyes (see comments), Refract Corneal Surg 6:165, 1990.

1323. Seiler T and others: Laser keratomileusis for correction of myopia, Fortschr Ophthalmol 87:479, 1990.

1324. Seiler T and others: Ablation rate of human corneal epithelium and Bowman's layer with the excimer laser (193 nm), Refract Corneal Surg 6:99, 1990.

1325. Seiler T, Matallana M, and Bende T: Laser thermokeratoplasty by means of a pulsed holmium: YAG laser for hyperopic correction, Refract Corneal Surg 6:335, 1990.

1326. Seiler T and others: Excimer laser keratomileusis for myopia correction. Results and complications, Klin Monatsbl Augenheilkd 199:153, 1991.

1327. Seiler T and Wollensak J: Myopic photorefractive keratectomy with the excimer laser. One-year follow-up, Ophthalmology 98:1156, 1991.

1328. Seiler T and Wollensak J: Complications of laser keratomileusis with the excimer laser (193 nm), Klin Monatsbl Augenheilkd 200:648, 1992, (published erratum appears in Klin Monatsbl Augenheilkd 201(2):145, 1992.

1329. Seiler T, Hell K, and Wollensak J: Diurnal variation in refraction after excimer laser photorefractive keratectomy, Ger J Ophthalmol 1:19, 1992.

1330. Seiler T and Jean B: Photorefractive keratectomy as a second attempt to correct myopia after radial keratotomy, Refract Corneal Surg 8:211, 1992.

1331. Seiler T and Wollensak J: Results of a prospective evaluation of photorefractive keratectomy at 1 year after surgery, Ger J Ophthalmol 2:135, 1993.

1332. Seiler T, Reckmann W, and Maloney RK: Effective spherical aberration of the cornea as a quantitative descriptor in corneal topography, J Cataract Refract Surg 19 Suppl:155, 1993.

1333. Seiler T and others: Aspheric photorefractive keratectomy with excimer laser, Refract Corneal Surg 9:166, 1993.

1334. Seiler T and Holschbach A: Central corneal iron deposit after photorefractive keratectomy, Ger J Ophthalmol 2:143, 1993.

1335. Seiler T and others: Complications of myopic photorefractive keratectomy with the excimer laser, Ophthalmology 101:153, 1994.

1336. Seiler T, Schmidt-Petersen H, and Wollensak J: Complications after myopic photorefractive keratectomy, primarily with the Summit excimer laser. In Salz JJ, McDonnell PJ, and McDonald MB, editors: Corneal laser surgery, St. Louis, 1995, Mosby–Year Book.

1337. Serdarevic O and others: Excimer laser therapy for experimental *Candida* keratitis, Am J Ophthalmol 99:534, 1985.

1338. Serdarevic ON and others: Excimer laser trephination in penetrating keratoplasty. Morphologic features and wound healing, Ophthalmology 95:493, 1988.

1339. Shahinian L Jr, and Lin DT: Clinical analysis of excimer laser photorefractive keratectomy using a multiple zone technique for severe myopia, Am J Ophthalmol 120:546, 1995, (letter).

1340. Shaw EL and Gasset AR: Thermokeratoplasty (TKP) temperature profile, Invest Ophthalmol 13:181, 1974.

1341. Shaw EL: Pathophysiology and treatment of corneal hydrops, Ophthalmic Surg 7:33, 1976.

1342. Sher NA and others: Clinical use of the 193-nm excimer laser in the treatment of corneal scars (see comments), Arch Ophthalmol 109:491, 1991.

1343. Sher NA and others: The use of the 193-nm excimer laser for myopic photorefractive keratectomy in sighted eyes. A multicenter study [see comments], Arch Ophthalmol 109:1525, 1991.

1344. Sher NA and others: Excimer laser photorefractive keratectomy in high myopia. A multicenter study, Arch Ophthalmol 110:935, 1992.

1345. Sher NA and others: Topical diclofenac in the treatment of ocular pain after excimer photorefractive keratectomy, Refract Corneal Surg 9:425, 1993.

1346. Sher NA and others: 193-nm excimer photorefractive keratectomy in high myopia, Ophthalmology 101:1575, 1994.

1347. Sher NA and others: Role of topical corticosteroids and nonsteroidal antiinflammatory drugs in the etiology of stromal infiltrates after excimer photorefractive keratectomy, J Refract Corneal Surg 10:587, 1994, (letter).

1348. Shieh E and others: Quantitative analysis of wound healing after cylindrical and spherical excimer laser ablations, Ophthalmology 99:1050, 1992.

1349. Shimizu K, Amano S, and Tanaka S: Photorefractive keratectomy for myopia: one-year follow-up in 97 eyes, J Refract Corneal Surg 10:S178, 1994.

1350. Simon G and others: Optics of the corneal epithelium, Refract Corneal Surg 9:42, 1993.

1351. Simon G, Ren Q, and Parel JM: Noncontact laser photothermal keratoplasty. II: Refractive effects and treatment parameters in cadaver eyes, J Refract Corneal Surg 10:519, 1994.

1352. Sinbawy A, McDonnell PJ, and Moreira H: Surface ultrastructure after excimer laser ablation. Expanding vs contracting apertures, Arch Ophthalmol 109:1531, 1991.

1353. Singh D: Photorefractive keratectomy in pediatric patients, J Cataract Refract Surg 21:630, 1995.

1354. Snibson GR and others: One-year evaluation of excimer laser photorefractive keratectomy for myopia and myopic astigmatism. Melbourne Excimer Laser Group, Arch Ophthalmol 113:994, 1995.

1355. Snibson GR and others: Retreatment after excimer laser photorefractive keratectomy. The Melbourne Excimer Laser Group, Am J Ophthalmol 121(3):250, 1996.

1356. Soto-Pedre E and Hernez-Ortega C: The corneal endothelium after myopic excimer laser photorefractive keratectomy, Arch Ophthalmol 113:1356, 1995, (letter).

1357. Spadea L, Sabetti L, and Balestrazzi E: Effect of centering excimer laser PRK on refractive results: a corneal topography study, Refract Corneal Surg 9:S22, 1993.

1358. Spadea L and others: Effect of myopic excimer laser photorefractive keratectomy on the electrophysiologic function of the retina and optic nerve, J Cataract Refractive Surg 22:906, 1996.

1359. Spigelman AV, and others: Treatment of myopic astigmatism with the 193 nm excimer laser utilizing aperture elements, J Cataract Refract Surg 20 Suppl:258, 1994.

1360. Srinivasan R, Dyer PE, and Braren B: Far-ultraviolet laser ablation of the cornea: photoacoustic studies, Lasers Surg Med 6:514, 1987.

1361. Srinivasan R and Sutcliffe E: Dynamics of the ultraviolet laser ablation of corneal tissue, Am J Ophthalmol 103:470, 1987.

1362. Stark WJ and others: Clinical follow-up of 193-nm ArF excimer laser photokeratectomy (see comments), Ophthalmology 99:805, 1992.

1363. Stein HA, Cheskes A, and Stein RM: Retreatment. In Stein HA, Cheskes A, and Stein RM, editors: The excimer: fundamentals and clinical use, Thorofare, NJ, 1995, SLACK, Inc.

1364. Stein HA, Cheskes A, and Stein RM: Photorefractive keratectomy results. In Stein HA, Cheskes A, and Stein RM, editors: The excimer: fundamentals and clinical use, Thorofare, NJ, 1995, SLACK, Inc.

1365. Stein HA, Cheskes A, and Stein RM: Complications and their management. In Stein HA, Cheskes A, and Stein RM, editors: The excimer: fundamentals and clinical use, Thorofare, NJ, 1995, SLACK, Inc.

1366. Stein HA, Cheskes A, and Stein RM: Phototherapeutic keratectomy. In Stein HA, Cheskes A, and Stein RM, editors: The excimer: fundamentals and clinical use, Thorofare, NJ, 1995, SLACK, Inc.

1367. Stein R and others: Photorefractive keratectomy and postoperative pain, Am J Ophthalmol 117:403, 1994.

1368. Steinert RF and Puliafito CA: The Nd:YAG Laser in Ophthalmology, Philadelphia, 1985, WB Saunders Co.

1369. Steinert RF and Puliafito CA: Excimer laser phototherapeutic keratectomy for a corneal nodule, Refract Corneal Surg 6:352, 1990.

1370. Stepp MA, Spurr-Michaud S, and Gipson IK: Integrins in the wounded and unwounded stratified squamous epithelium of the cornea, Invest Ophthalmol Vis Sci 34:1829, 1993.

1371. Stern D and others: Corneal ablation by nanosecond, picosecond, and femtosecond lasers at 532 and 625 nm, Arch Ophthalmol 107:587, 1989.

1372. Stock EL and others: Adhesion complex formation after small keratectomy wounds in the cornea, Invest Ophthalmol Vis Sci 33:304, 1992.

1373. SundarRaj N and others: Healing of excimer laser ablated monkey corneas. An immunohistochemical evaluation, Arch Ophthalmol 108:1604, 1990.

1374. Sutton G and others: Excimer retreatment for scarring and regression after photorefractive keratectomy for myopia, Br J Ophthalmol 79:756, 1995.

1375. Svoboda KK: Embryonic corneal epithelial actin alters distribution in response to laminin, Invest Ophthalmol Vis Sci 33:324, 1992.

1376. Swinger CA and Lai ST: Solid-state photoablative decomposition—the Novatec laser. In Salz JJ, McDonnell PJ, and McDonald MB, editors: Corneal laser surgery, St. Louis, 1995, Mosby–Year Book.

1377. Szerenyi K and others: Topical diclofenac treatment prior to excimer laser photorefractive keratectomy in rabbits, Refract Corneal Surg 9:437, 1993.

1378. Szerenyi KD, Campos M, and McDonnell PJ: Prostaglandin E2 production after lamellar keratectomy and photorefractive keratectomy, J Refract Corneal Surg 10:413, 1994.

1379. Szerenyi KD and others: Keratocyte loss and repopulation of anterior corneal stroma after de-epithelialization, Arch Ophthalmol 112:973, 1994.

1380. Taboada J and others: Intrastromal photorefractive keratectomy with a new optically coupled laser probe, Refract Corneal Surg 8:399, 1992.

1381. Talamo JH and others: Modulation of corneal wound healing after excimer laser keratomileusis using topical mitomycin C and steroids, Arch Ophthalmol 109:1141, 1991.

1382. Talamo JH, Steinert RF, and Puliafito CA: Clinical strategies for excimer laser therapeutic keratectomy, Refract Corneal Surg 8:319, 1992.

1383. Talamo JH, Wagoner MD, and Lee SY: Management of ablation decentration following excimer photorefractive keratectomy, Arch Ophthalmol 113:706, 1995, (letter).

1384. Talley AR and others: Results one year after using the 193-nm excimer laser for photorefractive keratectomy in mild to moderate myopia, Am J Ophthalmol 118:304, 1994.

1385. Talley AR and others: Use of the 193 nm excimer laser for photorefractive keratectomy in low to moderate myopia, J Cataract Refract Surg 20 Suppl:239, 1994.

1386. Tan DT and Tan JT: Will patients with contact lens problems accept excimer laser photorefractive keratectomy? CLAO J 19:174, 1993.

1387. Tavola A and others: Photorefractive keratectomy for myopia: single vs double-zone treatment in 166 eyes, Refract Corneal Surg 9: S48, 1993.

1388. Tavola A and others: The learning curve in myopic photorefractive keratectomy, J Refract Corneal Surg 10:S188, 1994.

1389. Taylor DM and others: Human excimer laser lamellar keratectomy. A clinical study, Ophthalmology 96:654, 1989.

1390. Taylor DM and others: Experimental corneal studies with the excimer laser, J Cataract Refract Surg 15:384, 1989.

1391. Taylor HR and others: Comparison of excimer laser treatment of astigmatism and myopia. The Excimer Laser and Research Group (see comments), Arch Ophthalmol 111:1621, 1993.

1392. Taylor HR, Kelly P, and Alpins NA: Excimer laser correction of myopic astigmatism, J Cataract Refract Surg 20 Suppl:243, 1994.

1393. Taylor HR and Carson CA: Excimer laser treatment for high and extreme myopia, Trans Am Ophthalmol Soc 92:251, 1994.

1394. Taylor HR and others: Predictability of excimer laser treatment of myopia. Melbourne Excimer Laser Group (see comments), Arch Ophthalmol 114(3):248, 1996.

1395. Taylor SM and others: Effect of depth upon the smoothness of excimer laser corneal ablation, Optom Vis Sci 71:104, 1994.

1396. Teal P and others: Corneal subepithelial infiltrates following excimer laser photorefractive keratectomy, J Cataract Refract Surg 21:516, 1995.

1397. Teichmann KD and others: Wessley-type immune ring following phototherapeutic keratectomy, J Cataract Refract Surg 22(1):142, 1996.

1398. Tengroth B and others: Excimer laser photorefractive keratectomy for myopia. Clinical results in sighted eyes, Ophthalmology 100:739, 1993.

1399. Tengroth B and others: Effect of corticosteroids in postoperative care following photorefractive keratectomies, Refract Corneal Surg 9:S61, 1993.

1400. Terrell J and others: The effect of globe fixation on ablation zone centration in photorefractive keratectomy, Am J Ophthalmol 119:612, 1995.

1401. Terrien F: Dystrophie marginale symetrique des deux cornees avec astigmatisme regular consecutif er guerison la cauterisation ignee, Arch Ophthalmol 20:12, 1900.

1402. Tervo T, Mustonen R, and Tarkkanen A: Management of dry eye may reduce haze after excimer laser photorefractive keratectomy, Refract Corneal Surg 9:306, 1993, (letter).

1403. Tervo K, Latvala TM, and Tervo TM: Recovery of corneal innervation following photorefractive keratoablation, Arch Ophthalmol 112:1466, 1994.

1404. Tervo T and others: Tear fluid plasmin activity after excimer laser photorefractive keratectomy, Invest Ophthalmol Vis Sci 35:3045, 1994.

1405. Tervo T and Tuunanen T: Excimer laser and reactivation of herpes simplex keratitis, CLAO J 20:152, 157, 1994.

1406. Tervo TM and others: Release of calcitonin gene-related peptide in tears after excimer laser photorefractive keratectomy, J Refract Surg 11:126, 1995.

1407. Thomann U, Meier-Gibbons F, and Schipper I: Phototherapeutic keratectomy for bullous keratopathy, Br J Ophthalmol 79:335, 1995.

1408. Thompson KP and others: Potential use of lasers for penetrating keratoplasty, J Cataract Refract Surg 15:397, 1989.

1409. Thompson KP and others: Photorefractive keratectomy with the Summit excimer laser: The phase III U.S. results. In Salz JJ, McDonnell PJ, and McDonald MB, editors: Corneal laser surgery, St. Louis, 1995, Mosby–Year Book.

1410. Thompson V, Durrie DS, and Cavanaugh TB: Philosophy and technique for excimer laser phototherapeutic keratectomy, Refract Corneal Surg 9:S81, 1993.

1411. Thompson V: Laser correction of hyperopia: Summit holmium thermal keratoplasty results. In Salz JJ, McDonnell PJ, and Mc-Donald MB, editors: Corneal laser surgery, St. Louis, 1995, Mosby–Year Book.

1412. Thompson VM and others: Holmium:YAG laser thermokeratoplasty for hyperopia and astigmatism: an overview. Refract Corneal Surg 9:S134, 1993, (published erratum appears in Refract Corneal Surg 9(3):236, 1993).

1413. Tisdale AS and others: Development of the anchoring structures of the epithelium in rabbit and human fetal corneas, Invest Ophthalmol Vis Sci 29:727, 1988.

1414. Toda I, Tsubota K, and Itoh S: Endothelial change after excimer laser photorefractive keratectomy, J Refract Corneal Surg 10:379, 1994, (letter).

1415. Tong PP and others: Excimer laser photorefractive keratectomy for myopia: six-month follow-up (see comments), J Cataract Refract Surg 21:150, 1995.

1416. Toole BP: Transitions in extracellular macromolecules during avian ocular development, Prog Clin Biol Res 82:17, 1982, (review).

1417. Trabucchi G and others: Corneal nerve damage and regeneration after excimer laser photokeratectomy in rabbit eyes, Invest Ophthalmol Vis Sci 35:229, 1994.

1418. Trinkaus-Randall V and Gipson IK: Role of calcium and calmodulin in hemidesmosome formation in vitro, J Cell Biol 98:1565, 1984.

1419. Trocme SD and others: Central and peripheral endothelial cell changes after excimer laser photorefractive keratectomy for myopia, Arch Ophthalmol 114(8):925, 1996.

1420. Trokel S: Evolution of excimer laser corneal surgery (see comments), J Cataract Refract Surg 15:373, 1989.

1421. Trokel SL, Srinivasan R, and Braren B: Excimer laser surgery of the cornea, Am J Ophthalmol 96:710, 1983.

1422. Trokel SL: Development of the excimer laser in ophthalmology: a personal perspective, Refract Corneal Surg 6:357, 1990.

1423. Troutman RC and others: A new laser for collagen wounding in corneal and strabismus surgery: a preliminary report, Trans Am Ophthalmol Soc 84:117, 1986.

1424. Troutman RC and others: A new laser for collagen wounding in corneal and strabismus surgery—a preliminary report, Dev Ophthalmol 14:80, 1987.

1425. Tsubota K: Application of erbium: YAG laser in ocular ablation, Ophthalmologica 200:117, 1990.

1426. Tuft SJ, Marshall J, and Rothery S: Stromal remodeling following photorefractive keratectomy, Lasers Ophthalmol 1:177, 1987.

1427. Tuft SJ, Zabel RW, and Marshall J: Corneal repair following keratectomy: a comparison between conventional surgery and laser photoablation, Invest Ophthalmol Vis Sci 30:1769, 1989.

1428. Tuft SJ and others: Assessment of corneal wound repair in vitro, Curr Eye Res 8:713, 1989.

1429. Tuft SJ and others: Photorefractive keratectomy: implications of corneal wound healing, Br J Ophthalmol 77:243, 1993.

1430. Tutton MK and others: Photorefractive keratectomy for myopia: 6-month results in 95 eyes, Refract Corneal Surg 9:S103, 1993.

1431. Tuunanen TH and Tervo TM: Excimer laser phototherapeutic keratectomy for corneal diseases: a follow-up study, CLAO J 21:67, 1995.

1432. Vajpayee RB and others: Overcorrection after excimer laser treatment of myopia and myopic astigmatism, Melbourne Excimer Laser Group (see comments), Arch Ophthalmol 114(3):252, 1996.

1433. van Saarloos PP and Constable IJ: Improved excimer laser photorefractive keratectomy system, Lasers Surg Med 13:189, 1993.

1434. van Setten GB and others: Expression of tenascin and fibronectin in the rabbit cornea after excimer laser surgery, Graefes Arch Clin Exp Ophthalmol 230:178, 1992.

1435. Van Westenbrugge JA and Gimbel HV: A comparison of the Summit and VISX excimer lasers: clinical experience at the Gimbel Eye Centre. In Salz JJ, McDonnell PJ, and McDonald MB, editors: Corneal laser surgery, St. Louis, 1995, Mosby–Year Book.

1436. Vidaurri-Leal JS and others: Excimer photorefractive keratectomy for low myopia and astigmatism with the Coherent-Schwind Keratom, J Cataract Refract Surg 22:1052, 1996.

1437. Virtanen I and others: Integrins as receptors for extracellular matrix proteins in human cornea, Acta Ophthalmol Suppl 18, 1992, (review).

1438. Virtanen T and others: Tear fluid cellular fibronectin levels after photorefractive keratectomy, J Refract Surg 11:106, 1995.

1439. Vogel A, Busch S, and Asiyo-Vogel M: Time resolved measurement

of shock-wave emission and cavitation-bubble generation in intraocular laser surgery with ps- and ns-pulses and related tissue effects, S P I E 312, 1993.

1440. Vogel A and others: Intraocular photodisruption with picosecond and nanosecond laser pulses: tissue effects in cornea, lens, and retina, Invest Ophthalmol Vis Sci 35:3032, 1994.

1441. Vrabec MP, Durrie DS, and Chase DS: Recurrence of herpes simplex after excimer laser keratectomy, Am J Ophthalmol 114:96, 1992, (letter).

1442. Vrabec MP and others: Electron microscopic findings in a cornea with recurrence of herpes simplex keratitis after excimer laser phototherapeutic keratectomy (see comments), CLAO J 20:41, 1994.

1443. Wang W and others: Excimer laser photorefractive keratectomy for myopia in China. A report of 750 eyes with a 6-month follow-up, Chin Med J (Engl) 108:601, 1995.

1444. Wang X and others: Enhancement of fibronectin-induced migration of corneal epithelial cells by cytokines, Invest Ophthalmol Vis Sci 35:4001, 1994.

1445. Ward MA and others: Phototherapeutic keratectomy for the treatment of nodular subepithelial corneal scars in patients with keratoconus who are contact lens intolerant, CLAO J 21:130, 1995.

1446. Waring GO III and others: Wound healing after excimer laser photorefractive keratectomy, Dev Ophthalmol 22:150, 1991.

1447. Waring GO III: Standardized data collection and reporting for refractive surgery, Refract Corneal Surg 8(suppl):1, 1992.

1448. Waring GO III and others: Refractive and visual results of a multicenter trial of excimer laser photorefractive keratectomy. Ophthalmology 99(9S):106, 1992, (abstract).

1449. Waring GO III: Evolution of refractive surgery into the 21st Century (DuPont Guerry III Lecture), Audio-Digest Foundation, Glendale, 1995, California Medical Association.

1450. Waring GO III: The challenge of corneal wound healing after excimer laser refractive corneal surgery, J Refract Surg 11:339, 1995.

1451. Waring GO III and others: Photorefractive keratectomy for myopia using a 4.5-millimeter ablation zone, J Refract Surg 11:170, 1995.

1452. Webber SK, McGhee CN, and Bryce IG: Decentration of photorefractive keratectomy ablation zones after excimer laser surgery for myopia, J Cataract Refract Surg 22(3):299, 1996.

1453. Weinstock SJ: Excimer laser keratectomy: one year results with 100 myopic patients, CLAO J 19:178, 1993.

1454. Weinstock SJ and Machat JJ: Excimer laser keratectomy for the correction of myopia, CLAO J 19:133, 1993.

1455. Weinstock SJ and Weinstock VM: Photorefractive keratectomy for myopia: six month results of 193 eyes, Refract Corneal Surg 9:S142, 1993.

1456. Wetterwald N: 2 years experience in the treatment of myopia with photokeratectomy, Klin Monatsbl Augenheilkd 204:416, 1994.

1457. Wilson SE and others: Changes in corneal topography after excimer laser photorefractive keratectomy for myopia, Ophthalmology 98:1338, 1991.

1458. Wilson SE, Klyce SD, and Husseini ZM: Standardized color-coded maps for corneal topography (see comments), Ophthalmology 100:1723, 1993.

1459. Wu WC, Stark WJ, and Green WR: Corneal wound healing after 193-nm excimer laser keratectomy, Arch Ophthalmol 109:1426, 1991.

1460. Zabel RW, Tuft SJ, and Marshall J: Excimer laser photorefractive keratectomy: endothelial morphology following area ablation of the cornea, Invest Ophthalmol Vis Sci 29:390, 1988.

1461. Zabel RW and others: Myopic excimer laser keratectomy: a preliminary report, Refract Corneal Surg 6:329, 1990.

1462. Zieske JD, Bukusoglu G, and Yankauckas MA: Characterization of a potential marker of corneal epithelial stem cells, Invest Ophthalmol Vis Sci 33:143, 1992.

1463. Zieske JD: Perpetuation of stem cells in the eyes, Eye 8:163, 1994, (review).

1464. Zysset B, and others: Picosecond optical breakdown: tissue effects and reduction of collateral damage, Lasers Surg Med 9:193, 1989, (review).

Lamellar surgery and laser surgery combined

1465. Abad JC and others: Dilute ethanol versus mechanical debridement before photorefractive keratectomy, J Cataract Refract Surg 22:1427, 1996.

1466. Anonymous. LASIK—the ultimate vision correction, Optician 210: 14, 1995, (abstract).

1467. Anschutz T: Laser correction of hyperopia and presbyopia, Int Ophthalmol Clin 34:107, 1994.

1468. Bas AM and Onnis R: Excimer laser in situ keratomileusis for myopia, J Refract Surg 11:S229, 1995.

1469. Brint SF and others: Six-month results of the multicenter phase I study of excimer laser myopic keratomileusis, J Cataract Refract Surg 20:610, 1994.

1470. Buratto L and Ferrari M: Excimer laser intrastromal keratomileusis: case reports, J Cataract Refract Surg 18:37, 1992.

1471. Buratto L, Ferrari M, and Rama P: Excimer laser intrastromal keratomileusis, Am J Ophthalmol 113:291, 1992.

1472. Buratto L, Ferrari M, and Genisi C: Keratomileusis for myopia with the excimer laser (Buratto technique): short-term results, Refract Corneal Surg 9:S130, 1993.

1473. Buratto L, Ferrari M, and Genisi C: Myopic keratomileusis with the excimer laser: one-year follow up, Refract Corneal Surg 9:12, 1993.

1474. Fantes FE and others: Wound healing after excimer laser keratomileusis (photorefractive keratectomy) in monkeys, Arch Ophthalmol 108:665, 1990.

1475. Fiander DC and Tayfour F: Excimer laser in situ keratomileusis in 124 myopic eyes, J Refract Surg 11:S234, 1995.

1476. Frueh BE and Bohnke M: Endothelial cell morphology after phototherapeutic keratectomy, Ger J Ophthalmol 4:86, 1995.

1477. Ganem S and others: Myopic keratomileusis by excimer laser on a lathe, J Refract Corneal Surg 10:575, 1994.

1478. Gomes M: Keratomileusis-in-situ using manual dissection of corneal flap for high myopia, J Refract Corneal Surg 10:S255, 1994.

1479. Gomes M: Laser in situ keratomileusis for myopia using manual dissection, J Refract Surg 11:S239, 1995.

1480. Güell J: Experience with laser in situ keratomileusis, J Cataract Refract Surg 22:1391, 1996, (guest editorial).

1481. Huebscher HJ, Genth U, and Seiler T: Determination of the excimer laser ablation rate of the human cornea using in vivo Scheimpflug videography, Invest Ophthalmol Vis Sci 37:42, 1996.

1482. Jain S and others: Corneal light scattering after laser in situ keratomileusis and photorefractive keratectomy, Am J Ophthalmol 120: 532, 1995.

1483. Kanellopoulos AJ and others: Comparison of corneal sensation following photorefractive keratectomy and laser in situ keratomileusis, J Cataract Refract Surg 23:34, 1997.

1484. Kliger C and Maloney RK: Excimer laser keratomileusis, Part III—excimer laser myopic keratomileusis at the Jules Stein Eye Institute, Los Angeles. In Salz JJ, McDonnell PJ, and McDonald MB editors: Corneal laser surgery, St. Louis, 1995, Mosby–Year Book.

1485. Kohlhaas M and others: Keratomileusis with a lamellar microkeratome and the excimer laser German, Ophthalmologe 92:499, 1995.

1486. Kremer FB and Dufek M: Excimer laser in situ keratomileusis, J Refract Surg 11:S244, 1995.

1487. Kremer I and Blumenthal M: Myopic keratomileusis in situ combined with VISX 20/20 photorefractive keratectomy, J Cataract Refract Surg 21:508, 1995.

1488. Pallikaris IG and others: Laser in situ keratomileusis, Lasers Surg Med 10:463, 1990.

1489. Pallikaris IG and others: A corneal flap technique for laser in situ keratomileusis. Human studies, Arch Ophthalmol 109:1699, 1991.

1490. Pallikaris IG and others: Tecnica de colajo corneal para la queratomileusis in situ mediante laser, Estudios en humanos, Arch Ophthalmol (Ed Espaniola) 3:127, 1992.

1491. Pallikaris IG and Siganos DS: Excimer laser in situ keratomileusis and photorefractive keratectomy for correction of high myopia, J Refract Corneal Surg 10:498, 1994.

1492. Pallikaris IG and Siganos DS: Corneal flap technique for excimer laser in situ keratomileusis to correct moderate and high myopia: two-year follow-up. Best papers of sessions from the ASCRS symposium on cataract, IOL and refractive Surgery, Boston, April 1994, p. 9.

1493. Pallikaris IG and Siganos DS: LASIK complication management, In Talamo JH and Krueger RR, editors, The excimer manual, Boston, 1997, Little, Brown & Co.

1494. Pallikaris IG and Siganos DS: Laser in situ keratomileusis to treat myopia: Early experience, J Cataract Refract Surg 23:39, 1997.

1495. Peyman GA: Excimer laser in situ keratomileusis under a corneal flap for myopia of 2 to 20 diopters, J Cataract Refract Surg 22(3): 281, 1996, (letters).

1496. Pico JF, Stamper RL, and McMenemy M: Intraocular pressure and corneal curvature changes on application of limbal-scleral suction fixation ring in rabbits, Cornea 12:25, 1993.

1497. Rieck P and others: Basic fibroblast growth factor modulates corneal wound healing after excimer laser keratomileusis in rabbits, Ger J Ophthalmol 3:105, 1994.

1498. Rozakis GW and others: Refractive lamellar keratoplasty, Thorofare, NJ, 1994, SLACK, Inc.

1499. Ruiz L, Slade SG, and Updegraff SA: Excimer laser keratomileusis, Part II—excimer myopic keratomileusis: Bogota experience. In Salz JJ, McDonnell PJ, and McDonald MB, editors: Corneal laser surgery, St. Louis, 1995, Mosby–Year Book.

1500. Salah T and others: Excimer laser in situ keratomileusis under a corneal flap for myopia of 2 to 20 diopters, Am J Ophthalmol 121: 143, 1996.

1501. Salah T, Waring GO 3rd, and el-Maghraby A: Excimer laser keratomileusis, Part I—Excimer laser keratomileusis in the corneal bed under a hinged flap: results in Saudi Arabia at the El-Maghraby Eye Hospital. In Salz JJ, McDonnell PJ, and McDonald MB, editors: Corneal laser surgery, St. Louis, 1995, Mosby–Year Book.

1502. Seiler T and others: Ablation rate of human corneal epithelium and Bowman's layer with the excimer laser (193 nm), Refract Corneal Surg 6:99, 1990.

1503. Siganos DS and Pallikaris IG: Laser in situ keratomileusis in partially sighted eyes, Invest Ophthalmol Vis Sci 34:800, 1993.

1504. Slade SG and Brint SF: Excimer laser myopic keratomileusis. In Rozakis GW, editor: Refractive lamellar keratoplasty, Thorofare, NJ, 1994, SLACK, Inc.

1505. Slade SG, Brint SF, and Updegraff SA: Excimer laser keratomileusis, Part II—excimer laser myopic keratomileusis: United States experience, In Salz JJ, McDonnell PJ, and McDonald MB, editors: Corneal laser surgery, St. Louis, 1995, Mosby–Year Book.

1506. Slade SG and Updegraff SA: Advances in lamellar refractive surgery, Int Ophthalmol Clin 34:147, 1994.

1507. Stern AL and Taylor DM: Particle-free environment for refractive keratoplasty, Ophthalmic Surg 12:360, 1981.

1508. Szerenyi KD, Campos M, and McDonnell PJ: Prostaglandin E2 production after lamellar keratectomy and photorefractive keratectomy, J Refract Corneal Surg 10:413, 1994.

1509. Waring GO 3d: Evolution of refractive surgery into the 21st Century (DuPont Guerry III Lecture), Audio-Digest Foundation, Glendale, 1995, California Medical Association.

1510. Waring GO 3d: The challenge of corneal wound healing after excimer laser refractive corneal surgery, J Refract Surg 11:339, 1995.

Intrastromal corneal ring

1511. Assil KK and others: Corneal iron lines associated with the intrastromal corneal ring, Am J Ophthalmol 116:350, 1993.

1512. Assil KK and others: One-year results of the intrastromal corneal ring in nonfunctional human eyes. Intrastromal Corneal Ring Study Group, Arch Ophthalmol 113:159, 1995.

1513. Burris TE and others: Effects of intrastromal corneal ring size and thickness on corneal flattening in human eyes, Refract Corneal Surg 7:46, 1991.

1514. Fleming JF, Wan WL, and Schanzlin DJ: The theory of corneal curvature change with the Intrastromal Corneal Ring, CLAO J 15: 146, 1989.

1515. Kreisberg AL, Bacilious N, and Asbell PA: Intraocular pressure and the intrastromal corneal ring, Refract Corneal Surg 7:303, 1991.

1516. Kuhne F and others: Results of a 2-year animal experiment with reticulated polyethylene oxide intrastromal rings French, J Fr Ophthalmol 17:83, 1994.

1517. Neves R and others: The intrastromal corneal ring—implantation in blind and myopic eyes, Invest Ophthalmol Vis Sci 33:998, 1992.

1518. Nose W and others: Intrastromal corneal ring—one-year results of first implants in humans: a preliminary nonfunctional eye study, Refract Corneal Surg 9:452, 1993.

1519. Quantock AJ, Assil KK, and Schanzlin DJ: Electron microscopic evaluation of intrastromal corneal rings explanted from nonfunctional human eyes, J Refract Corneal Surg 2:142, 1994.

1520. Quantock AJ, Kincaid MC, and Schanzlin DJ: Stromal healing following explantation of an ICR (intrastromal corneal ring) from a nonfunctional human eye, Arch Ophthalmol 113:208, 1995.

1521. Schanzlin DJ and others: One year results of the intrastromal corneal ring implanted in nonfunctional human eyes, Invest Ophthalmol Vis Sci 33:998, 1992.

Refractive intraocular lenses

1522. Alio JL, Ruiz-Moreno JM, and Artola A: Retinal detachment as a potential hazard in surgical correction of severe myopia with phakic anterior chamber lenses (see comments), Am J Ophthalmol 115:145, 1993, (published erratum appears in Am J Ophthalmol 115(6):831, 1993).

1523. Arciniegas A: El tratamiento de miopias elevadas mediante vitrectomia y lensectomia posterior con exoimplante de 360 grados (modificacion del Fukala), Arch S A O O 19:79, 1985.

1524. Auffarth GU, and others: Are there acceptable anterior chamber intraocular lenses for clinical use in the 1990s? An analysis of 4104 explanted anterior chamber intraocular lenses, Ophthalmology 101:1913, 1994.

1525. Baikoff G: Phakic anterior chamber intraocular lenses. [Review], Int Ophthalmol Clin 31:75, 1991, (review).

1526. Baikoff G, and Colin J: Damage to the corneal endothelium using anterior chamber intraocular lenses for myopia, Refract Corneal Surg 6:383, 1990, (letter; comment).

1527. Baikoff G and Joly P: Comparison of minus power anterior chamber intraocular lenses and myopic epikeratoplasty in phakic eyes (see comments), Refract Corneal Surg 6:252, 1990.

1528. Balyeat HD, Parke DW 2d, and Wilkinson CP: Should we consider clear lens extraction for routine refractive surgery? Refract Corneal Surg 9:226, 1993, (letter; comment).

1529. Barraquer C, Cavelier C, and Mejia LF: Incidence of retinal detachment following clear-lens extraction in myopic patients. Retrospective analysis (see comments), Arch Ophthalmol 112:336, 1994.

1530. Barraquer J: Lentes plasticoes de camera anterior, Estudios C Informaciones Oftalmologicas 6:15, 1954.

1531. Barraquer J: La extraccion intracapsular del cristalino: Ponencia oficial del XL Congreso de la Sociedad Histoamerican de Granada, Espana, 1962, Barcelona, 1962, Graficas Typus.

1532. Barraquer JI: Complications de la inclusion segun los diversos tipos de lentes, Annules de Instituto Barraquer 3:588, 1962.

1533. Benitez del Castillo JM and others: Fluorophotometry in phakic eyes with anterior chamber intraocular lens implantation to correct myopia, J Cataract Refract Surg 19:607, 1993.

1534. Binder PS: Refractive surgery in the United States, Dev Ophthalmol 18:203, 1989, (review).

1535. Choyce DP: The correction of high myopia, Refract Corneal Surg 8:242, 1992, (review).

1536. Choyce P: Intraocular Lenses and Implants, London, 1964, H K Lewis.

1537. Colin J and others: The surgical treatment of high myopia: comparison of epikeratoplasty, keratomileusis and minus power anterior chamber lenses (see comments), Refract Corneal Surg 6:245, 1990.

1538. Colin J and Robinet A: Clear lensectomy and implantation of low-power posterior chamber lens for the correction of high myopia (see comments), Ophthalmology 101:107, 1994.

1539. Coonan P and others: The incidence of retinal detachment following extracapsular cataract extraction. A ten-year study, Ophthalmology 92:1096, 1985.

1540. Cunillera C and others: Coreccion de atlas muopias en ojos faquicos mediante la implantacion de lentes de apoyo angular de camara anterior de potencia negativa, Arch Ophthalmol Soc Esp Oftalmol 60:593, 1991.

1541. Datiles MB and Gancayco T: Low myopia with low astigmatic correction gives cataract surgery patients good depth of focus, Ophthalmology 97:922, 1990.

1542. Dvali ML: 150 implants of the "suspended"-modification extrapupillary iris lens (Russian), Vestn Oftalmol 24, 1981.

1543. Dvali ML: Phacoemulsification in correcting high myopia (with prophylactic cryopexy) (Russian), Vestn Oftalmol 40, 1982.

1544. Dvali ML: Correction of high myopia with an extrapupillary iris lens (preliminary report) (Russian), Vestn Oftalmol 29, 1984.

1545. Dvali ML: Intraocular correction of high myopia (Russian), Vestn Oftalmol 102:29, 1986.

1546. Dvali ML, and others: Current possibilities for using a modification of Fukala's operation for correcting high myopia. (Russian), Vestn Oftalmol 101:24, 1985.

1547. Erturk H, Ozcetin H: Phakic posterior chamber lenses for the correction of high myopia, J Cataract Refract Surg 11(5):388, 1995.

1548. Fechner PU, Kania J, and Kienzle S: The value of a zero power intraocular lens, J Cataract Refract Surg 14:436, 1988.

1549. Fechner PU, Van der Heijde GL, and Worst JG: Intraokulare Linse zur Myopiekorrektion des phaken Auges, Klin Monatsbl Augenheilkd 193:29, 1988.

1550. Fechner PU: Intraocular lenses for the correction of myopia in phakic eyes: short-term success and long-term caution, Refract Corneal Surg 6:242, 1990, (editorial).

1551. Fechner PU, Haigis W, Wichmann W: Posterior chamber myopia lenses in phakic eyes (see comments), J Cataract Refract Surg 22(2):178, 1996.

1552. Feldman RM and others: Retinal detachment following radial and astigmatic keratotomy, Refract Corneal Surg 7:252, 1991.

1553. Font T and others: Implantación de lentes intraoculares de Worst-Fechner para correccion de miopia: primeros resultados, Arch Ophthalmol Soc Esp Oftalmol 59:163, 1990.

1554. Foss AJ, Rosen PH, and Cooling RJ: Retinal detachment following anterior chamber lens implantation for the correction of ultra-high myopia in phakic eyes, Br J Ophthalmol 77:212, 1993.

1555. Fukala V: Operative Behandlung der Hochstgradigen Myopice durch Aphakie, Albrecht Von Graefes Arch Klin Exp Ophthalmol 36:230, 1890.

1556. Garcia M, Gonzalez C, and Pascual I: New matrix formulation of spectacle magnification using pupil magnification, I. High myopia corrected with ophthalmic lenses, Ophthalmic Physiol Opt 15:195, 1995.

1557. Garcia M and others: Magnification and visual acuity in highly myopic phakic eyes corrected with an anterior chamber intraocular lens versus by other methods, J Cataract Refract Surg 22:1416, 1996.

1558. Gelisken O, Ozcetin H, and Dogru M: Retinal detachment after radial keratotomy, Bull Soc Belge Ophthalmol 249:63, 1993.

1559. Gimbel HV and Neuhann T: Continuous curvilinear capsulorhexis, J Cataract Refract Surg 17:110, 1991, (letter).

1560. Goldberg MF: Clear lens extraction for axial myopia. An appraisal, Ophthalmology 94:571, 1987, (review).

1561. Govan JA: Prophylactic circumferential cryopexy: a retrospective study of 106 eyes, Br J Ophthalmol 65:364, 1981.

1562. Gris O and others: A clear lens extraction to correct high myopia, J Cataract Refract Surg 22:686, 1996.

1563. Gross KA and Pearce JL: Modern cataract surgery in a highly myopic population, Br J Ophthalmol 71:215, 1987.

1564. Haut J and Massin M: Frequency of incidence of retina detachment in the French population. Percentage of bilateral detachment (French), Arch Ophthalmol Rev Gen Ophthalmol 35:533, 1975.

1565. Hoffer KJ: The Hoffer Q formula: a comparison of theoretic and regression formulas, J Cataract Refract Surg 19:700, 1993.

1566. Holladay JT: Refractive power calculations for intraocular lenses in the phakic eye, Am J Ophthalmol 116:63, 1993.

1567. Holladay JT and others: A three-part system for refining intraocular lens power calculations, J Cataract Refract Surg 14:17, 1988.

1568. Huber C: Myopic astigmatism as a substitute for accommodation in pseudophakia, Dev Ophthalmol 5:17, 1981.

1569. Hyams SW, Neumann E, and Friedman Z: Myopia-aphakia. II. Vitreous and peripheral retina, Br J Ophthalmol 59:483, 1975.

1570. Javitt JC: Clear-lens extraction for high myopia. Is this an idea whose time has come? Arch Ophthalmol 112:321, 1994, (editorial; comment).

1571. Javitt JC and others: National outcomes of cataract extraction. Retinal detachment and endophthalmitis after outpatient cataract surgery. Cataract Patient Outcomes Research Team, Ophthalmology 101:100, 1994.

1572. Javitt JC and others: National outcomes of cataract extraction. Increased risk of retinal complications associated with Nd:YAG laser capsulotomy. The Cataract Patient Outcomes Research Team (see comments), Ophthalmology 99:1487, 1992.

1573. Javitt JC and others: National outcomes of cataract extraction. I.

Retinal detachment after inpatient surgery, Ophthalmology 98:895, 1991.

1574. John ME and others: Clear lens extraction and intraocular lens implantation in a patient with bilateral anterior lenticonus secondary to Alport's syndrome, J Cataract Refract Surg 20:652, 1994.

1575. Joly P, Baikoff G, and Bonnet P: Insertion of a negative implant in the anterior chamber in phakic patients (French), Bull Soc Ophthalmol Fr 89:727, 1989.

1576. Juhas T: The myopic intraocular lens in a phakic eye. Initial experience (Slovak), Cesk Oftalmol 49:368, 1993.

1577. Kanski JJ and Daniel R: Prophylaxis of retinal detachment, Am J Ophthalmol 79:197, 1975.

1578. Kashani AA: Fluorophotometry in myopic phakic eyes with anterior chamber intraocular lenses to correct severe myopia, Am J Ophthalmol 119:381, 1995, (letter; comment).

1579. Kora Y and others: An intraocular lens power calculation for high myopia (Japanese), Nippon Ganka Gakkai Zasshi 99:692, 1995.

1580. Kora Y and others: Modified SRK formula for axial myopia (24.5 mm ≤ axial length < 27.0 mm), Ophthalmic Surg 23:603, 1992.

1581. Kora Y and others: Preferred postoperative refraction after cataract surgery for high myopia, J Cataract Refract Surg 21:35, 1995.

1582. Kraff MC and Sanders DR: Incidence of retinal detachment following posterior chamber intraocular lens surgery, J Cataract Refract Surg 16:477, 1990.

1583. Landesz M and others: Negative implant. A retrospective study, Doc Ophthalmol 83:261, 1993.

1584. Landesz M and others: Correction of high myopia with the Worst myopia claw intraocular lens, J Refract Surg 11:16, 1995.

1585. Lee KH and Jin HL: Long-term results of clear lens extraction for severe myopia, J Cataract Refract Surg 22:1411, 1996.

1586. Le Mesurier R and Chignell AH: Prophylaxis of aphakic retinal detachment, Trans Ophthalmol Soc UK 101:212, 1981.

1587. Leroux les Jardins S and others: Medium-term tolerance of anterior chamber implants in surgical treatment of severe myopia (French), J Fr Ophtalmol 18:45, 1995.

1588. Lim ES and others: An analysis of flexible anterior chamber lenses with special reference to the normalized rate of lens explantation, Ophthalmology 98:243, 1991.

1589. Lyle WA and Jin GJC: Clear lens extraction for the correction of high refractive error, J Cataract Refract Surg 20:273, 1994.

1590. Lyle WA and Jin GJC: Prospective evaluation of early visual and refractive effects with small clear corneal incision for cataract surgery, J Cataract Refract Surg 22:1456, 1996.

1591. Mathys B, Zanen A and Schrooyen M: A new type of negative anterior chamber lens in high myopia Dutch, Bull Soc Belge Ophtalmol 242:19, 1991.

1592. Menezo JL, Cisneros A, and Harto M: Extracapsular cataract extraction and implantation of a low power lens for high myopia, J Cataract Refract Surg 14:409, 1988.

1593. Menezo JL and others: Long-term results of surgical treatment of high myopia with Worst-Fechner intraocular lenses, J Cataract Refract Surg 21:93, 1995.

1594. Mimouni F and others: Damage to the corneal endothelium from anterior chamber intraocular lenses in phakic myopic eyes, Refract Corneal Surg 7:277, 1991.

1595. Nielsen NE and Naeser K: Epidemiology of retinal detachment following extracapsular cataract extraction: a follow-up study with an analysis of risk factors (see comments), J Cataract Refract Surg 19:675, 1993.

1596. O'Day DM, Feman SS, and Elliott JH: Visual impairment following radial keratotomy. A cluster of cases, Ophthalmology 93:319, 1986.

1597. Obstbaum SA: Clear lens extraction for high myopia and high hyperopia (see comments), J Cataract Refract Surg 20:271, 1994, (editorial; comment).

1598. Ogawa A and Tanaka M: The relationship between refractive errors and retinal detachment—analysis of 1,166 retinal detachment cases, Jpn J Ophthalmol 32:310, 1988.

1599. Olsen GM and Olson RJ: Prospective study of cataract surgery, capsulotomy, and retinal detachment, J Cataract Refract Surg 21:136, 1995.

1600. Osher RH: Clear lens extraction, J Cataract Refract Surg 20:674, 1994, (letter; comment).

1601. Perez-Santonja JJ and others: Ischemic optic neuropathy after intraocular lens implantation to correct high myopia in a phakic patient, J Cataract Refract Surg 19:651, 1993.

1602. Perez-Santonja JJ and others: Fluorophotometry in myopic phakic eyes with anterior chamber intraocular lenses to correct severe myopia (see comments), Am J Ophthalmol 118:316, 1994.

1603. Perez-Santonja JJ and others: Chronic subclinical inflammation in phakic eyes with intraocular lenses to correct myopia, J Cataract Refract Surg 22(2):183, 1996.

1604. Pollack A and others: Circumferential argon laser photocoagulation for prevention of retinal detachment, Eye 8:419, 1994.

1605. Powe NR and others: Synthesis of the literature on visual acuity and complications following cataract extraction with intraocular lens implantation, Cataract Patient Outcome Research Team [see comments], Arch Ophthalmol 112:239, 1994, (published erratum appears in Arch Ophthalmol 112:889, 1994).

1606. Praeger DL: Innovations and creativity in contemporary ophthalmology: preliminary experience with the phakic myopic intraocular lens, Ann Ophthalmol 20:456, 1988.

1607. Praeger DL, Momose A, and Muroff LL: Thirty-six month follow-up of a contemporary phakic intraocular lens for the surgical correction of myopia, Ann Ophthalmol 23:6, 1991.

1608. Praeger DL: Five years follow-up in the surgical management of cataracts in high myopia treated with the Kelman phacoemulsification technique, Ophthalmology 86:2024, 1996.

1609. Pruett RC: Refractive surgery: psychophysical considerations in progressive myopia, Ann Acad Med Singapore 18:131, 1989, (review).

1610. Pruett RC: Commentary, Arch Ophthalmol 115:258, 1997.

1611. Reidy JJ and others: An analysis of semiflexible, closed-loop anterior chamber intraocular lenses, J Am Intraocul Implant Soc 11:344, 1985.

1612. Retzlaff JA, Sanders DR, and Kraff MC: Development of the SRK/T intraocular lens implant power calculation formula (see comments), J Cataract Refract Surg 16:333, 1990, (published erratum appears in J Cataract Refract Surg 16:528, 1990).

1613. Rodriguez A and Camacho H: Retinal detachment after refractive surgery for myopia, Retina 12:S46, 1992.

1614. Rodriguez A, Gutierrez E, and Alvira G: Complications of clear lens extraction in axial myopia, Arch Ophthalmol 105:1522, 1987.

1615. Rubin ML: A case for myopia, Surv Ophthalmol 35:307, 1991.

1616. Saragoussi JJ and others: Damage to the corneal endothelium by minus power anterior chamber intraocular lenses, Refract Corneal Surg 7:282, 1991.

1617. Saragoussi JJ, Othenin-Girard P, and Pouliquen YJ: Ocular damage after implantation of oversized minus power anterior chamber intraocular lenses in myopic phakic eyes: case reports, Refract Corneal Surg 9:105, 1993.

1618. Scott JD: Duke-Elder lecture. Prevention and perspective in retinal detachment, Eye 3:491, 1989, (review).

1619. Siganos DS, Siganos CS, and Pallikaris IG: Clear lens extraction and intraocular lens implantation in normally sighted hyperopic eyes, J Refract Corneal Surg 10:117, 1994.

1620. Sinskey RM: Clear lens extraction, J Cataract Refract Surg 20:673, 1994, (letter; comment).

1621. Strampelli B: Soppontabilita di lenti acrliche in camera anteriore nella afachia o nei vizi di refrazione, Ann Oftalmol Clin Oculist Parma 80:75, 1954.

1622. Strampelli B: Complication de l'operation de Strampelli, Anne Therapeutique et Clinique En Ophtalmologique 9:349, 1958.

1623. Verzella F: Microsurgery of the lens in high myopia for optical purposes, Cataract 1:8, 1984.

1624. Verzella F: Microsurgery of the lens in high myopia for optical purposes J Am Intraocul Implant Soc 11:65, 1985, (letter).

1625. Verzella F: High myopia: In the bag refractive implantation, Ophthalmol Forum 3:174, 1985.

1626. Verzella F: Severe myopia: extraction of the crystalline lens and implantation in the posterior chamber for optical purposes (French), Bull Mem Soc Fr Ophtalmol 97:347, 1986.

1627. Verzella F: Refractive microsurgery of the lens in high myopia, Refract Corneal Surg 6:273, 1990.

1628. Verzella F and Calossi A: Multifocal effect of against-the-rule myopic astigmatism in pseudophakic eyes, Refract Corneal Surg 9:58, 1993.

1629. Waring GO 3d: Refractive intraocular lenses, AudioDigest Ophthalmology, Glendale, 1995, California Medical Association.

1630. Waring GO 3d. Phakic intraocular lenses for the correction of myopia—where do we go from here? Refract Corneal Surg 7:275, 1991, (editorial).

1631. Weblin TP: Should we consider clear lens extraction for routine refractive surgery? (see comments), Refract Corneal Surg 8:480, 1992.

1632. Wilkes SR and others: The incidence of retinal detachment in Rochester, Minnesota, 1970-1978, Am J Ophthalmol 94:670, 1982.

1633. Wilmer WH: A case of excessive myopia treated by extraction of the transparent lens, Arch Ophthalmol 115:257, 1997.

1634. Wilson SE: The correction of myopia with phakic intraocular lenses, Am J Ophthalmol 115:249, 1993, (editorial; comment; review).

1635. Wood CA: A system of ophthalmic operations, Chicago, 1911, Cleveland Press.

1636. Worst JG, van der Veen G, and Los LI: Refractive surgery for high myopia. The Worst-Fechner biconcave iris claw lens, Doc Ophthalmol 75:335, 1990.

1637. Yoon YH and Marmor MF: Rapid enhancement of retinal adhesion by laser photocoagulation, Ophthalmology 95:1385, 1988.

Embryology and anatomy of anterior segment compartments; aqueous humor circulation

The forward compartments of the globe, the anterior and posterior chambers, are filled with a continually circulating watery fluid, or aqueous humor.[1-85] The borders of the anterior chamber are the posterior surface of the cornea, the anterior chamber angle recess, the anterior surface of the iris, and the anterior surface of the lens coursing across the pupillary aperture. The anterior chamber volume averages about 0.2 to 0.3 ml.

The anterior chamber is continuous with the posterior chamber through the pupil. The posterior chamber is much smaller, with a volume estimated to be about 0.06 ml. It is lined anteriorly by the posterior surface of the iris, the ciliary processes, zonular fibers, and the anteroequatorial region of the lens.

Posteriorly, the vitreous humor forms the bulk of the volume of the globe and fills the space between the lens, ciliary body, and retina. It consists of a gelatinous substance composed primarily of water and hyaluronic acid admixed with a network of delicate collagen-like fibrils.

The anterior chamber and its bordering structures begin to develop early in gestation. An ingrowth of mesectoderm occurs between the anterior margin of the optic cup and the surface ectoderm. The mesectoderm differentiates into cornea anteriorly (with the exception of the corneal epithelium) and iris stroma posteriorly. The future anterior chamber is the space between these two mesectodermal layers. This cavity remains very narrow and cleft-shaped until the fifth month when it parallels the entire anterior segment of the globe and undergoes a rapid growth. The final differentiation of the definitive filtration apparatus occurs late, shortly before birth.

The fetal angle reveals a characteristic configuration resulting from delicate fibers (iris processes) that course across the reaches of the future angle recess (Fig. 6-1). Near the end of pregnancy a cleavage, or splitting, of the layers of mesectoderm occurs at the angle because of unequal growth of the tissues. This cleavage causes a gradual resorption of a portion of the uveal meshwork, with eventual formation of the definitive deep recess characteristic of the adult globe. The most important malformations caused by faulty differentiation and/or cleavage of the anterior chamber angle mesoderm are congenital glaucoma and the anterior chamber cleavage iridocorneal dysgenesis syndromes (Fig. 2-1).

SECRETION OF AQUEOUS HUMOR

The aqueous humor is secreted by the epithelium of the ciliary processes. It flows through the posterior chamber by way of the narrow space between lens and iris and passes through the pupil into the anterior chamber.[11,16,24] Outflow of the fluid occurs at the angle, through the trabecular meshwork and Schlemm's canal, after which the aqueous humor reaches the systemic circulation through the intrae-piscleral, episcleral, and conjunctival collecting channels (Figs. 6-2 and 6-3).

The structure and function of the richly vascular ciliary processes are greatly reminiscent of the choroid plexus of the brain. Each of the 70 to 80 radially arranged, finger-like processes of the pars plicata ciliaris (Fig. 4-4) contains a network of wide-lumened capillaries within its stroma. The stroma lies immediately adjacent to the characteristic two-layered cuboidal epithelium. The outer layer, derived

from the outer pigmented layer of the embryonic optic cup, is pigmented. The inner layer develops from the inner embryonic layer of the optic cup and remains unpigmented. The latter epithelium possesses numerous mitochondria and other specialized cell organelles, which are largely responsible for the production of aqueous humor. The secretory process is not merely a filtration or dialysis but represents an active transport system in which a low-protein aqueous is produced. The aqueous passes through

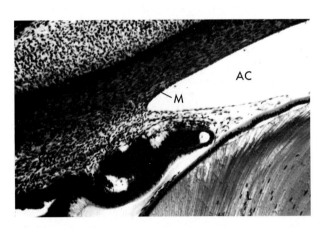

Fig. 6-1. Fetal anterior chamber angle. Same specimen as Fig. 1-8. *M.* Mesodermal tissue bridging the fetal anterior chamber recess; *AC,* anterior chamber; *C,* cornea; *I,* iris epithelium; *CM,* ciliary muscle; *L,* lens. (H & E stain; ×125.)

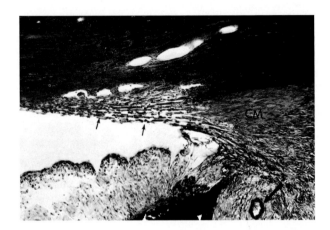

Fig. 6-3. Anterior chamber angle stained by the trichrome technique. The intrascleral aqueous outflow channels are prominent. *Small arrows,* Trabecular meshwork; *large arrow,* major iris circle; *CM,* ciliary muscle. (Masson trichrome stain; ×75.)

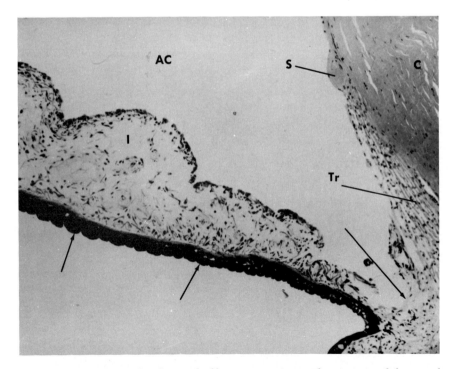

Fig. 6-2. Normal anterior chamber angle filtration structures. The junction of the peripheral cornea *(C)* and iris stroma *(I)* forms the anterior chamber angle recess *(arrow). AC,* Anterior chamber; *S,* Schwalbe's line, the posterior terminus of Descemet's membrane (in this section Schwalbe's line exhibits a bulbous enlargement, which is a normal anatomic variant). *Tr,* trabecular meshwork; *small arrows,* iris pigment epithelium. (H & E stain; ×100.)

the blood-aqueous barrier, the nature of which is not yet entirely clear. The ciliary body capillary endothelial cells are tightly interconnected by intercellular bridges of the zonula occludens type, which may contribute to the barrier. The lining epithelial cells of the ciliary processes are also bound together by tight junctions. These probably have the greatest effect on the permeability of this barrier.

OUTFLOW OF AQUEOUS HUMOR

The anterior chamber angle recess is bounded by the root of the iris, the anterior fourth of the ciliary body, and the corneoscleral junction (Figs. 6-2 and 6-3). The scleral spur or roll is an important landmark that forms a 360-degree ring and delimits the posterior aspect of the filtration apparatus.[1] In cross section it appears as a lip-like protrusion of scleral collagen, which forms the posterior margin of the trabecular meshwork. It is best localized in histologic sections by examination of the ciliary muscle. The muscle is triangular in sagittal sections, and its most anterior point, the apex of the triangle, is always attached to, or "points toward," the scleral spur (Fig. 6-3). This fact enables the pathologist to locate the spur and differentiate between an anterior synechia and a recessed angle, even in severely deformed globes in which the cleft forming the recess may have sealed and is, therefore, not so obvious (p. 265).

The trabecular meshwork and the canal of Schlemm° fill a concavity in the posterior sclera at the corneoscleral junction, the inner scleral sulcus. The meshwork inserts posteriorly into the scleral spur (Figs. 6-2 and 6-3). The anterior termination of the trabecular meshwork is at Schwalbe's line, which is the peripheral termination of Descemet's membrane. Sometimes the membrane tapers and gradually disappears at this point (Fig. 6-3); in other cases Schwalbe's line is prominent because of a bulbous termination or thickening of the membrane (Fig. 6-2). The latter is gonioscopically recognizable as a white line. Such a thickening can be considered a normal anatomic variant; similar thickenings may also occur in pathologic states, for example, posterior embryotoxon (Figs. 2-20, *B*, 2-37, and 2-38; p. 27).

The trabecular meshwork consists of two parts, the more external corneosclera meshwork and an internal component in continuity with the uveal trait posteriorly, the uveal meshwork.

The meshwork is a sponge-like, porous tissue with walls composed of an endothelial lining supported by collagen and elastic tissue.[23,25,31,70,71] It also contains a ground substance composed primarily of hyaluronic acid.[84,85] The center of each pore wall consists of long spacing and normal collagen. The endothelium, a continuation of the corneal epithelium, forms the outer lining of each pore wall. The aqueous humor must pass through this network to reach Schlemm's canal and the collecting channels. The pores gradually decrease in size toward Schlemm's canal, with the largest ones lining the anterior chamber angle.[75,76] The juxtacanalicular pores are the smallest and offer the greatest resistance to aqueous outflow. The facility of aqueous

outflow, and hence the intraocular pressure, depends primarily on the outflow resistance at this level.

The aqueous passes through Schlemm's canal and enters endothelial-lined collecting channels in the intrascleral and episcleral vascular plexus (Fig. 6-3). By slitlamp examination one can observe a lamellar flow of fluid in some of the collecting channels that reach the surface of the sclera (the aqueous veins of Ascher), in which blood and aqueous flow side by side in columns before mixing.[5] The collecting channels flow into the anterior ciliary veins and into the veins of the extraocular muscles.[5,24]

The intraocular pressure depends on a balance between aqueous formation and outflow. The aqueous turnover time is approximately 80 minutes. The maintenance of an adequate outflow facility is of utmost importance in the maintenance of a median pressure. Most modes of modern medical and surgical therapy are geared toward either preserving adequate outflow facility° or decreasing aqueous formation.

Definition and classification of glaucoma

The maintenance of a relatively constant intraocular pressure (between approximately 10 and 20 mm Hg as measured by tonometry) (1) is required for maintenance of the spheric form of the globe, (2) makes possible regular corneal curvature required for refraction of incoming light, and (3) promotes, by way of pressure transmitted through the vitreous, a constant apposition between retina, pigment epithelium, and choroid. Short-term, mild variations from this normal state, such as transient ocular hypertension or temporary hypotony, may be tolerated, but long-term, severe increases or decreases in pressure may lead to irreversible intraocular damage.[1–85]

Glaucoma is often mistakenly considered to be a discrete disease entity. In reality it is a syndrome; there are many different forms of glaucoma with different causes, clinical courses, and treatments. What most of these glaucomas have in common is a complete clinical picture characterized by increased intraocular pressure, excavation and degeneration of the optic disc, and typical nerve fiber bundle damage, producing defects in the field of vision. Most cases of glaucoma result from an impaired outflow of aqueous; hypersecretion glaucoma is unusual.[7] Unfortunately, the term *primary* or *essential glaucoma* admits ignorance of the basic cause.[17,30,34,35]

Glaucoma is the leading cause of permanent blindness among the one-half million legally blind people in the United States. It affects 14% (1 in 7) of blind people, 0.5% to 1% of the population, 2% of all people over 35 years old and 3% of all people age 65 and older have glaucoma. Primary open-angle glaucoma occurs in white patients, with a prevalence of 0.9% in ages 40 to 49 and a prevalence of 2.2% in patients 80 and older. It has an even higher prevalence in blacks ranging from 1.2% in ages 40 to 49 to 11.5% in patients 80 years or older.[69,81]

Ocular hypertension is defined as an intraocular pressure increased above the "normal range" that does not produce clinically detectable tissue change or ocular functional impairment. Affected patients can be carefully observed with-

---

° References 5, 24, 25, 31, 45, 66, 70, 71, 73–76, 83.

° References 2, 3, 29, 39, 41, 43, 47, 53, 56, 58, 59, 61, 63, 72, 77, 80.

out treatment or with minimal treatment as long as such changes do not occur.

On the other hand, some patients with pressures within the "normal range" may have tissue damage and functional loss, presumably because of an increased susceptibility of the ocular tissues. Although pressures are "normal" in this condition, the term *low tension glaucoma* is entrenched in clinical usage.[10,18,19,40]

Hypotony is defined as a decrease in intraocular pressure resulting from decreased secretion of aqueous humor or from a fistulous tract leading to loss of aqueous from the eye. Causes or associated diseases include intraocular inflammation, retinal and choroidal detachment, accidental and surgical penetration of the globe, and phthisis bulbi.

The anatomy of the tissues involved in the histopathology of glaucoma and its sequelae, that is, the ciliary epithelium (from which the aqueous fluid is secreted), the anterior chamber angle outflow channels, and the retina and optic nerve, have been considered here and in Chapters 8 and 10. Degeneration and atrophy of the retina and optic nerve are the ultimate reason for visual loss caused by increased intraocular tension. Quigley,[249] Quigley and coworkers,[286–291] and Radius and Maumenee[293] have studied the connective tissue structure of the lamina cribrosa, its mechanical effect on nerve bundles, and its compressive effect on vasculature.

The clinical features of the various types of glaucoma are well known, and most of the diseases listed in the following outline that may lead to elevated intraocular pressure are described in other chapters. This discussion is confined to selected illustrations of salient anterior segment changes that occur in several types of glaucoma. The histopathologic changes in the eye resulting from increased intraocular pressure are emphasized here because a knowledge of these is useful for understanding the mechanisms of visual loss.

The following outline, modified from a classification of the late Dr. Charles Phelps, Department of Ophthalmology, University of Iowa, classifies glaucoma into three major categories: angle-closure glaucoma, open-angle glaucoma, and congenital glaucoma.

I. Angle-closure glaucoma
  A. With pupillary block
    1. Primary
    2. Secondary
      a. Phacomorphic: resulting from swollen lens, spherophakia
      b. Traumatic, postsurgical, or postinflammatory (posterior synechiae, seclusion or occlusion of pupil, leukoma adherens, iris bombé, subluxation of lens, epithelial ingrowth over pupil)
      c. Interstitial keratitis
      d. Tumor
      e. Any retrolental mass exerting pressure anteriorly (retrolental fibroplasia, persistent hyperplastic primary vitreous)
  B. Without pupillary block
    1. Hyperopia
    2. Primary plateau iris
    3. Resulting from peripheral anterior synechiae caused by various factors

      a. Previous pupillary block
      b. Persistent flat anterior chamber (usually after surgical or nonsurgical trauma)
      c. Malignant glaucoma (aqueous sequestered in vitreous)
      d. Ciliary body swelling (after scleral buckling operation, after panretinal photocoagulation, or spontaneous)
      e. Anterior segment hemorrhage, inflammation, exudation (anterior uveitis)
      f. Neovascular glaucoma, rubeosis iridis
      g. Tumors
      h. Iridocorneal endothelial (ICE) syndrome: essential iris atrophy, Chandler's syndrome, iris nevus (Cogan-Reese) syndrome
      i. Endothelialization of the anterior chamber angle
      j. Epithelial ingrowth and anterior chamber cysts
      k. Retinopathy of prematurity
      l. Spherophakia
II. Open-angle glaucoma
  A. Primary
    1. Primary open-angle glaucoma (higher incidence seen in diabetes mellitus and high myopia)
    2. Ocular hypertension
    3. Low tension glaucoma
  B. Secondary
    1. Induced by corticosteroids
    2. Resulting from inflammation: uveitis, endophthalmitis, Fuchs' heterochromic iridocyclitis, glaucomatocyclitic crisis (Posner-Schlossman syndrome), interstitial keratitis, phacoanaphylaxis
    3. Phacolytic glaucoma
    4. Pseudoexfoliation of lens capsule (glaucoma capsular) associated with Sampaolesi's line
    5. Traumatic
      a. Contusion angle deformity, angle recession with tears into ciliary body or iris
      b. Blood in angle (hemolytic or ghost cell)
      c. Wound track or scar tissue in angle
      d. Siderosis
    6. Induced by alpha chymotrypsin
    7. Associated with tumors
    8. Epithelial ingrowth
    9. Neovascular glaucoma
    10. Elevated episcleral venous pressure
    11. Hypersecretion (rare)
    12. Pigmentary glaucoma (Krukenberg spindle, Sampaolesi's line)
    13. After congenital cataract surgery
III. Congenital (infantile) glaucoma and glaucoma associated with congenital malformations
  A. Primary
  B. Secondary (associated with other anomalies)
    1. Gross malformations of globe, such as microphthalmia, trisomy 13, sclerocornea, microcornea, spherophakia.
    2. Aniridia
    3. Colobomas
    4. Sturge-Weber syndrome
    5. Neurofibromatosis
    6. Anterior chamber angle cleavage syndromes: Axenfeld's anomaly, Rieger's anomaly, Peter's anomaly

7. Rubella
8. Persistent hyperplastic primary vitreous
9. Retinopathy of prematurity
10. Lens displacement syndromes
11. Lowe's syndrome
12. Pierre Robin syndrome
13. Retinoblastoma
14. Juvenile xanthogranuloma

Angle-closure glaucoma[86,107]

WITH PUPILLARY BLOCK

Angle-closure glaucoma with pupillary block is occasionally "primary." This form of primary angle-closure glaucoma often results from pupillary block in a shallow anterior segment. Particularly, small hyperopic eyes are especially vulnerable. Affected patients typically have a shallow anterior chamber angle. The sudden rise of pressure results from apposition of the peripheral iris to the trabecular meshwork following the pupillary block.

Secondary angle-closure glaucoma with pupillary block occurs most commonly following trauma (Figs. 4-11, *A* and 6-4–6-6) and intraocular inflammation. The pupillary block may also be induced by a swollen lens (phacomorphic glaucoma) or by a subluxated or dislocated lens that becomes apposed or adherent to the pupillary border of the iris. Occlusion of the pupil signifies pupillary block by formation of a membrane across the pupillary aperture; seclusion of the pupil is created by posterior synechiae (Fig. 6-6, *o* and *s*). The synechiae usually consist of adherences of the pupillary margin of the iris to the lens or lens remnants, but when the lens is absent, the iris can adhere to other structures such as a cyclitic membrane or the anterior face of the vitreous.

Iris bombé (Figs. 6-4–6-6) is a sequela of glaucoma with pupillary block, and peripheral anterior synechiae invariably occur in late states (Figs. 6-6 and 6-7).

WITHOUT PUPILLARY BLOCK

Secondary angle-closure glaucoma without pupillary block is characterized by apposition of the peripheral iris

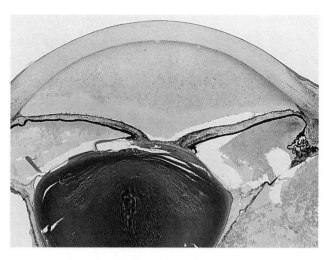

Fig. 6-5. Photomicrograph of the anterior segment of a globe with uveitis and formation of posterior synechiae between the pupillary margin of the iris and the anterior surface of the lens. In this case both occlusion and seclusion of the pupil have occured and iris bombé is present. (H & E stain; ×30.)

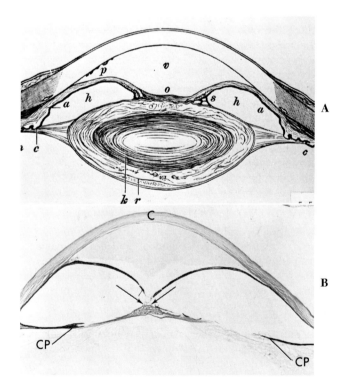

Fig. 6-6. A, Fuchs' classic schematic illustration of the microscopic anatomy of angle closure with pupillary block, iris bombé, and occlusion (*o*) and seclusion (*s*) of the pupil. **B,** Membranous cataract associated with closed-angle pupillary block glaucoma and iris bombé. A few tiny remnants of lens capsule adhere to the pupillary margin of the atrophic iris (*arrows*). The iris-lens adhesions create a seclusion of the pupil (posterior synechiae for 360 degrees). The anterior face of the vitreous also contributes to the membrane coursing between the atrophic ciliary processes (*CP*). The vitreous face is incorporated into the mass of lens remnants that block the pupil. Broad peripheral anterior synechiae have formed as a result of long-standing anterior bulging of the iris. *C*, Cornea. (H & E stain; ×12.) (**A** from Fuchs E: Lehrbuch der Augenheilkunde, Vienna, 1889, Franz Deuticke.)

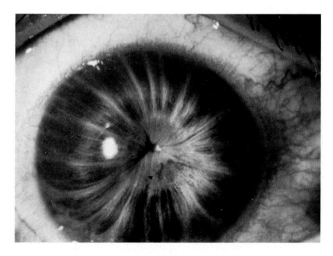

Fig. 6-4. Iris bombé (forward bowing of the iris with seclusion of the pupil).

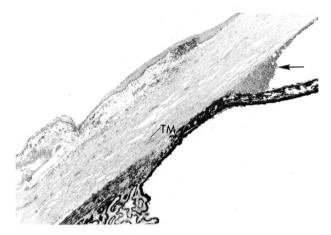

Fig. 6-7. Many diverse insults and diseases often terminate in the formation of peripheral anterior synechiae. In this example, the iridocorneal adhesion is a result of hyphema and organization of the blood in the anterior chamber. *Arrow,* Residual blood in the anterior chamber; *TM,* site of the markedly sclerotic trabecular meshwork, which is now far removed from any continuity with the anterior chamber. (H & E stain; ×30.)

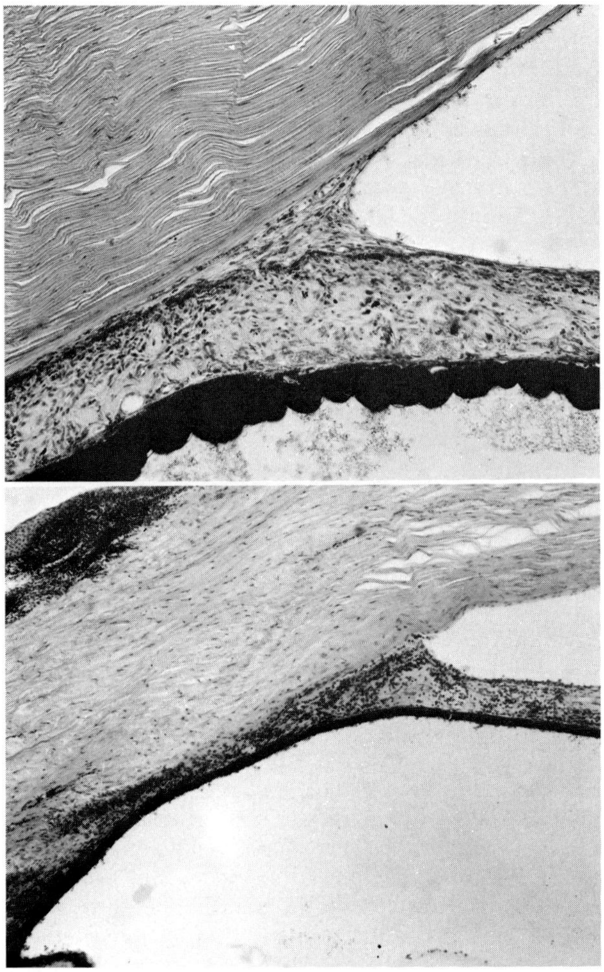

Fig. 6-8. Peripheral anterior synechiae. **A,** Adhesion caused by a fibrovascular membrane on the anterior iris surface. (H & E stain; ×16.) **B,** Secondary to organization of inflammatory debris. Note residual lymphocytes. (H & E stain; ×20.)

to the trabecular meshwork and formation of peripheral anterior synechiae. The histopathologic appearance is easily appreciated in most cases (Figs. 6-7 and 6-8). In equivocal cases, particularly those involving a globe badly damaged by trauma or other causes, it is imperative that one accurately determine the site of the normal angle recess. The recess is immediately adjacent to the scleral spur (Figs. 6-2 and 6-3). Even in greatly distorted globes, the scleral spur can usually be found by locating the site where the ciliary muscles insert into the collagenous fibers of the spur. The angle is abnormal if the angle recess is deviated from the site of the scleral spur.

IRIDOCORNEAL ENDOTHELIAL SYNDROME

The iridocorneal endothelial (ICE) syndrome[108–157] (Figs. 6-9 and 6-10) is a nonfamilial, unilateral ocular disease characterized by corneal endothelial proliferation, iris stromal abnormalities, and angle-closure glaucoma in about 50% of cases. The disease occurs mainly in young to middle-aged women.

The ICE syndrome actually encompasses a wide spectrum of pathologic changes, which have been variously categorized as essential iris atrophy, the iris nevus (Cogan-Reese) syndrome, and Chandler's syndrome.° Although each of the three entities may be distinct in its pure form, the clinical findings often overlap; therefore, they probably represent different subgroups of the same disease process (Table 6-1).[55]

The common pathogenesis of the three entities appears to be fundamental abnormality of the corneal endothelium.† In the early stages of the ICE syndrome, patients often complain of a visual disturbance. They describe this disturbance as halos around lights or blurred vision. Slit-lamp biomicroscopy of most eyes reveals a subtle abnor-

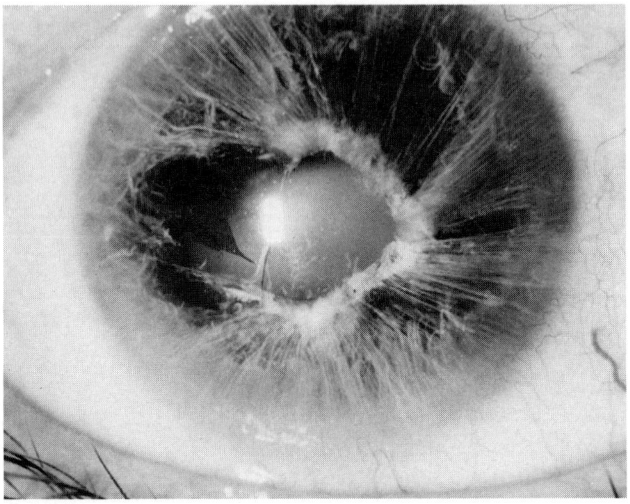

° References 108, 109, 112, 113, 115, 117, 120, 123, 124, 127, 129, 130, 136, 138, 141–143, 145–147, 151, 154–156, 175.
† References 110–112, 116, 118–120, 125, 131, 135, 139, 148, 152, 153.

Fig. 6-9. Clinical photograph of an eye with advanced iris atrophy.

mality at the posterior aspect of the cornea. Chandler[116] described this as having "a fine hammered silver appearance similar to Fuchs' dystrophy but less coarse." Corneal dystrophy and edema are most pronounced in Chandler's syndrome.

Ultrastructural studies of the corneal endothelium have shown extensive loss of endothelial cells associated with thickening and proliferation of Descemet's membrane. Although with this type of cellular dystrophy one would expect an increased permeability, Bourne and Brubaker[113] demonstrated a decreased permeability to fluorescein. Because the corneal epithelium depends on the aqueous humor for its supply of glucose, they suggested that epithelial nutrition and metabolism may be impaired in the ICE syndrome.

The differentiation of the three entities rests primarily on changes observed in the iris.[118] In its purest form, essential iris atrophy (Fig. 6-10, *A*) shows peripheral anterior synechiae with displacement of the pupil toward the synechiae. There is mild to moderate ectropion uveae, atrophy of the iris stroma, through-and-through hole formation (on the side opposite the synechiae), and relatively normal-appearing stroma between areas of atrophy (Fig. 6-10, *A*). As the synechiae forms, a secondary glaucoma often develops. As the intraocular pressure increases, corneal edema develops. A fully developed essential iris atrophy (Fig. 6-10, *A*) may resemble multiple atypical colobomas of the iris (p. 26), extreme persistence and hyperplasia of the pupillary membrane (p. 29; Fig. 2-25) and iridoschisis. The latter is a bilateral condition of the elderly that does not affect the pupil but may cause glaucoma due to synechia formation. Each must be considered in the differential diagnosis of iris stromal disorders, but they are usually easily distinguished by their various subtle clinical features and clinical history.

In the iris nevus syndrome (Cogan-Reese), the most prominent feature is an effacement of the normal pattern of the iris surface, which appears matted or smudged with a velvety, whorl-like iris surface and loss of crypts. Heterochromia, ectopion uvae, and peripheral anterior synechiae as well as secondary closed-angle glaucoma may occur. Histologically a diffuse or nodular iris nevus is present.[115,126] There is endothelialization of the anterior chamber angle and iris surface.[116,119,121,122,136,157] A diffuse nevus of the anterior iris, which occasionally becomes a full-thickness stromal nevus, is present. These features can occur with or without associated iris nodules. The iris changes in Chandler's syndrome, probably the most common variant, fall in the range between those of the other two entities. In general, the glaucoma is less severe than in the other two variants.

Histopathologic examination of eyes affected by the ICE syndrome shows an abnormal basement membrane, similar in appearance to Descemet's membrane, covered by endothelium growing on the surface of the trabecular meshwork

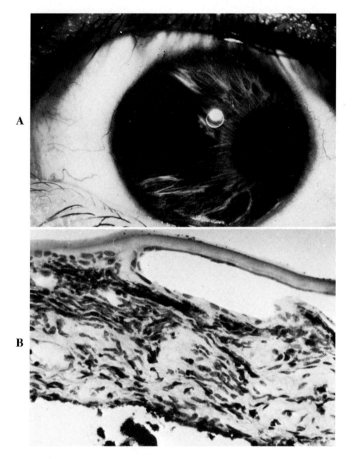

Fig. 6-10. A, Essential iris atrophy (Chandler's syndrome), iris nevus syndrome of Cogan and Reese, iridocorneal endothelial (ICE) syndrome, external photograph. The pupil is displaced, and the iris stroma has undergone significant atrophy, particularly toward the left in the figure. Secondary glaucoma is a frequent complication. (Compare with Fig. 2-25.) **B,** Photomicrograph of the iris in a case of ICE syndrome, showing overgrowth of the basement membrane on the anterior iris surface. (H & E stain; ×200.)

Table 6-1. Clinical subgrouping of the ICE syndrome

Groups	Alternative terms	Corneal abnormality	Peripheral anterior synechiae	Atrophy, corectopia, or both	Nodular or diffuse pigmented lesions, or both
Essential iris atrophy	Progressive essential iris atrophy	Variable	Present	Marked, with holes	Absent
Chandler's syndrome	None	Marked	Present	Mild, with no holes	Absent
Iris nevus syndrome	Cogan-Reese syndrome, iris nodule syndrome	Variable	Present	Mild to marked	Present

Modified by Dr. Stephen C. Gieser from Shields MB: Surv Ophthalmol 24:3, 1979.

and peripheral iris (Fig. 6-10, *B*).[117,118–120,123,132–134,140] This membrane is often deep to the synechiae, indicating that the corneal endothelium proliferation may be primary, because it precedes the formation of anterior synechiae.

Campbell, Shields, and Smith[115] have suggested that the ICE syndrome begins as a corneal-endothelial degeneration, which somehow prompts the growth of an abnormal endothelial membrane over the anterior chamber angle and onto the iris. This membrane then contracts, producing the peripheral anterior synechiae and pupillary distortion with subsequent iris thinning. The protracted clinical course of the disease, including a slow evolution toward angle-closure glaucoma, often occurs over several years.

Rodriguez notes that ICE syndrome and posterior polymorphous corneal dystrophy (Table 3-2, p. 88) share similar characteristics. Both show endothelial degeneration and endothelialization of the anterior chamber angle, iridocorneal adhesions, corneal edema, and glaucoma. They differ in that posterior polymorphous dystrophy in inherited and progresses much more slowly.

Open-angle glaucoma

PRIMARY OPEN-ANGLE GLAUCOMA

Primary open-angle glaucoma competes with cataract, diabetic retinopathy, macular disease, and ocular trauma as the leading cause of blindness in the United States today, affecting up to 1% to 2% of the adult population.[152–229] It is usually bilateral, although the onset of glaucoma in each eye is usually not simultaneous. It is often inherited as an autosomal-recessive trait, and a family history of open-angle glaucoma is commonly elicited. Gonioscopically the angle appears open. One tell-tale side of early retinal damage is the presence of splinter hemorrhages on the optic nerve.

The classic morphologic description of sclerosis of the trabecular meshwork in such eyes is not sufficiently specific or meaningful to indicate the exact pathogenetic mechanisms responsible for this common condition. By the time affected eyes become blind and painful and are enucleated, the histopathologic picture is indeed that of a sclerotic, or fibrotic, trabecular meshwork in which the pores are obliterated by dense fibrous tissue. Many types of glaucoma create this picture; for example, Fig. 6-16, *B* illustrates a sclerotic trabecular meshwork following traumatic angle recession. Such changes are, therefore, nonspecific, and the pathogenesis of chronic simple glaucoma remains obscure.

SECONDARY OPEN-ANGLE GLAUCOMA

Obstruction of aqueous outflow in most cases of secondary open-angle glaucoma is usually a result of blockage of the trabecular meshwork by particulate matter such as inflammatory cells or blood (hemolytic/ghost cell glaucoma) (Fig. 6-11), tumor cells (Fig. 6-12), macrophages or lens material in lens-induced glaucoma (Fig. 4-41), particulate matter in pseudoexfoliation (Fig. 4-44), or zonular fragments (in α-chymotrypsin-induced glaucoma).* Growth of scar tissue or endothelium or epithelium can also cause obstruction.[167,207,221] Any condition that causes an increased episcleral venous pressure, for example, an intraoc-

---

* References 164, 170, 172–174, 189, 194, 196, 199, 222, 226, 227.

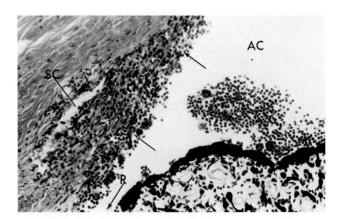

Fig. 6-11. Secondary open-angle glaucoma in an eye with a corneal ulcer and hypopyon is induced by blockage of the trabecular meshwork *(arrows)* with myriad acute inflammatory cells (polys). Inflammatory conditions may create secondary glaucoma in this way or may lead to closed-angle glaucoma as a result of peripheral anterior synechiae. *AC*, Anterior chamber, *SC*, Schlemm's canal; *R*, angle recess. (H & E stain; ×430.)

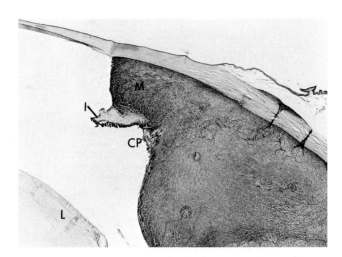

Fig. 6-12. Malignant melanoma of the choroid and ciliary body with invasion of anterior segment. The melanotic tumor *(M)* has permeated the anterior chamber, and the aqueous filtration structures have been totally destroyed, producing a secondary glaucoma. The iris *(I)* and ciliary processes *(CP)* are displaced by the tumor. *L*, Lens. (H & E stain, ×15.)

ular tumor or Sturge-Weber syndrome (p. 513), can cause a secondary glaucoma (Figs. 6-13 and 9-59).[200]

Pigmentary glaucoma, tumor-induced glaucoma, and posttraumatic glaucoma are secondary open-angle glaucomas that warrant special mention.

Pigmentary glaucoma

Pigment is commonly seen in the trabecular meshwork of eyes with normal intraocular pressure. It increases with advancing age and is also seen in such conditions such as post–blunt trauma, after anterior segment surgery, or following iridocyclitis. The pigment also may be found in the angle structures of eyes with various forms of open-angle glaucoma, including pigmentary glaucoma and exfoliation

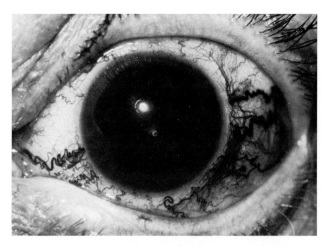

Fig. 6-13. Dilated episcleral vessels indicative of increased episcleral venous pressure, which may lead to elevated intraocular pressure.

syndrome (Figs. 6-17 and 6-18; Color Plates 6-3–6-7).*
Pigment dispersion syndrome (PDS) is a disorder in which pigment granules released from ruptured iris pigment epithelial cells are deposited on structures throughout the anterior segment. The classic triad of clinical features consists of (1) a vertical band of pigment on the corneal endothelium (Krukenberg spindle) (Fig. 3-33, Color Plate 6-1), (2) slitlike, radial, midperipheral iris transillumination defects (p. 80; Color Plate 6-2), and (3) dense homogeneous pigment deposition on the trabecular meshwork.

The entity known as pigmentary glaucoma was first identified by Sugar and Barbour (1949). It typically occurs in young (20–45 years), myopic men. It is characteristically bilateral, with clinically evident loss of pigment from peripheral portions of the iris. Pigment granules circulating in the aqueous humor may be mistaken for inflammatory cells. The anterior chamber is usually deep, and there may be iridodonesis. It is uncertain whether the pigment initiates aqueous outflow obstruction or merely enhances a preexisting outflow abnormality. Some patients with all of the findings just noted never develop glaucoma, while in others pressure rise has been detected as many as 20 years after pigment dispersion was first noted clinically. In some individuals, the amount of pigment in the angle decreases over a period of years, and this is accompanied by a decrease in the severity of the glaucoma. Some of the pigment granules carried to the trabecular meshwork are phagocytized by the trabecular endothelium (Fig. 6-17). Other granules either pass through the angle or become entrapped within the meshwork (Fig. 6-18). Iris pigment does not seem to initiate an inflammatory response; however, nonfixed macrophages play a role in pigment clearance. The pigment is deposited more heavily inferiorly and lies predominately within the meshwork in front of Schlemm's canal. Heavy amounts may appear as a uniform broad, dark brown or black band in the entire circumference of the angle. Mechanical abrasion of pigment granules from the posterior iris has been demonstrated.

---

* References 161, 165, 169, 171, 178, 180, 181, 183, 185, 193, 198, 202–204, 206, 209, 212, 216, 217–219.

There are two major forms of pigmentary dispersion: (1) a primary or natural disease based on anatomic considerations and (2) a secondary, iatrogenic form following cataract intraocular lens (IOL) surgery.

In primary pigmentary glaucoma, the iris, which is in a constant state of fluctuating miosis and mydriasis, causes the pigment-dislodging abrasion.[171] The zonules insert on the anterior lens surface (Fig. 10-16) not only in single strands, but also in thick aggregates or packets. These packets tend to be regularly distributed, approximately one packet per ciliary process. The zonular anatomy is such that if a normal iris makes contact with the zonules between dilation and constriction, radial slits are rubbed into its posterior aspect. The defects extend from the iris periphery to the mid-iris (Color Plate 6-2). The radial disposition of the zonules under the periphery of the iris explains the configuration of the pigment epithelial loss and its position in the outer half of the iris. In myopic eyes a wide ciliary body ring surrounds the lens and the peripheral iris rests in a posteriorly convex position. It is, therefore, more prone to contact the zonules.[178]

Pigmentary glaucoma is seen less frequently in the elderly because with aging the gradual enlargement of the lens lifts the peripheral iris anteriorly away from the zonules. Histologically, the posterior layer of iris pigment epithelium, mainly at the junction of middle and peripheral thirds of the iris, atrophies in foci that correspond to the clinically observed peripheral foci of increased iris transillumination.

Secondary pigment dispersion after IOL implantation, a complication caused by iris chafing and erosion, was recognized clinically by Harold Ridley in the early 1950s, shortly after his first IOL implantation. In histopathological studies as early as 1974, Manschot discussed this problem in relation to chafing from iris support IOLs. Nevertheless, only recently has this complication been widely recognized. A minimum of 20 cases with secondary pigmentary glaucoma have now been reported in the literature. Mechanical chafing by components of an IOL against the posterior iris pigment epithelium can induce the same findings as seen with idiopathic pigmentary glaucoma. This fact lends support to Campbell's hypothesis[171] that pigmentary glaucoma is caused by mechanical contacts of zonules against the posterior iris surface. Studies on the trabecular meshwork in eyes enucleated for IOL complications have shown that the dense deposits of pigment found within trabecular tissues in pseudophakic pigmentary dispersion syndrome are indistinguishable from the deposits seen in idiopathic pigmentary dispersion. Patients with uvea-fixated, posterior chamber IOLs may be at risk to develop pigment dispersion (Figs. 6-17 and 6-18; Color Plates 6-3 to 6-6). In patients in whom any component of a posterior chamber IOL is in contact with the iris epithelium, pigment granules can be released and collect in the trabecular meshwork. Iris or ciliary body defects caused by mechanical chafing from ciliary region–fixated IOL loops can be documented by transillumination biomicroscopy and histopathological examination. In concurrent but independent reports, our laboratory and Johnson, Kratz, and Olson documented by histopathological and clinical studies, respectively, that long-term complications caused by uveal chafing of posterior chamber IOL loops may occur more often than has been

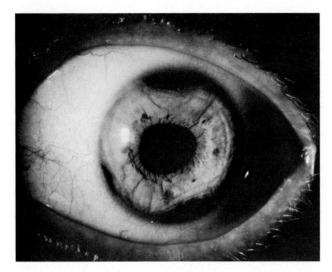

Fig. 6-14. Multiple iridodialysis caused by blunt trauma. (From Meyner E: Atlas der Spaltlampenphotographie, Stuttgart, 1972, Ferdinand Enke Verlag.)

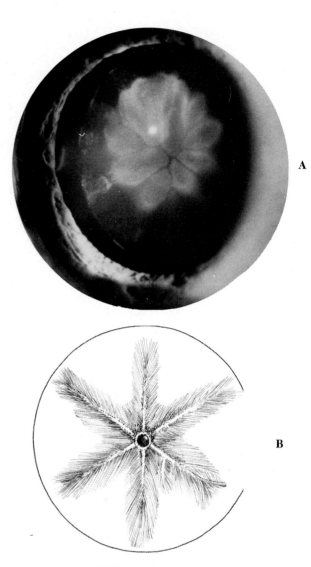

Fig. 6-15. Cataract following contusion injury. **A,** Flower-petal or rosette appearance. **B,** Schematic illustration. The rosette is formed by swelling of damaged lens fibers. (**A** courtesy Dr. Ernst Martin Meyner, formerly of University of Tübingen, Tübingen, West Germany; **B** drawn by Dr. Steven Vermillion, University of Iowa.)

previously recognized. Contact commonly occurs either peripherally at the bend of the loop curve or more centrally toward the loop-optic junction at sites where the loop may make contact with the posterior iris surface (Figs. 6-17 and 6-18). Lenses that have a 10-degree angulation of the loops from the plane of the optic reduce, but do not eliminate, the incidence of this complication. The only fixation procedure that totally avoids direct contact of some IOL component with uveal ocular tissues is in-the-bag implantation of posterior chamber IOLs (see Fig. 4-71, site 6). Another important advantage of capsular fixation for posterior chamber IOLs is that the entire length of both loops, as well as the lens optic, is situated as far as possible posterior to the cornea and uveal tissue, approximating the anatomical position of the natural lens.

Although we have some understanding of the pathogenesis of pigment dispersion, we still do not know why some patients with the syndrome develop glaucoma and others remain clinically entirely normal. With age the signs and symptoms of pigmentary dispersion may actually decrease in some individuals, possibly as a result of normal growth of the lens and an increase in physiological pupillary dilation. High intraocular pressure (IOP) often occurs when pigment is released into the aqueous humor, such as following exercise or pupillary dilation. Loss of accommodation may also be a factor. Symptoms may include halos and intermittent visual blurring. An individual with pigment dispersion syndrome may or may not ever develop elevated IOP. Various studies have suggested that the risk of an individual with this syndrome developing glaucoma is approximately 25% to 50%. Pigmentary glaucoma is characterized by wide fluctuations in IOP. Treatment is the same as that for primary open-angle glaucoma. Response to medications is good. Laser trabeculoplasty and standard filtering procedures generally give good results.

Malignant melanoma-induced glaucoma

Yanoff has documented the various mechanisms producing secondary glaucoma in eyes with uveal malignant mela-

noma (Fig. 6-12).[222,226,227] Melanoma cells may seal the anterior chamber and block the angle producing a secondary open-angle glaucoma. A ring melanoma (a tumor largely confined to the iris root and ciliary body that involves these structures circumferentially for 360 degrees) may invade the anterior chamber angle structure and block the open angle. A third type of secondary open-angle glaucoma is melanomalytic glaucoma.[227] This occurs after necrosis of tumor cells with liberation of melanin pigment. This pigment is phagocytized by macrophages, which may then migrate to and obstruct the outflow channels. In addition to a secondary open-angle glaucoma, melanoma may induce a secondary closed angle form. A large posterior tumor may cause anterior displacement of the lens-iris diaphragm, resulting in posterior synechiae and iris bombé (Figs. 6-4 to 6-6). This may then induce secondary peripheral anterior synechiae. Iris neovascularization, a noninfre-

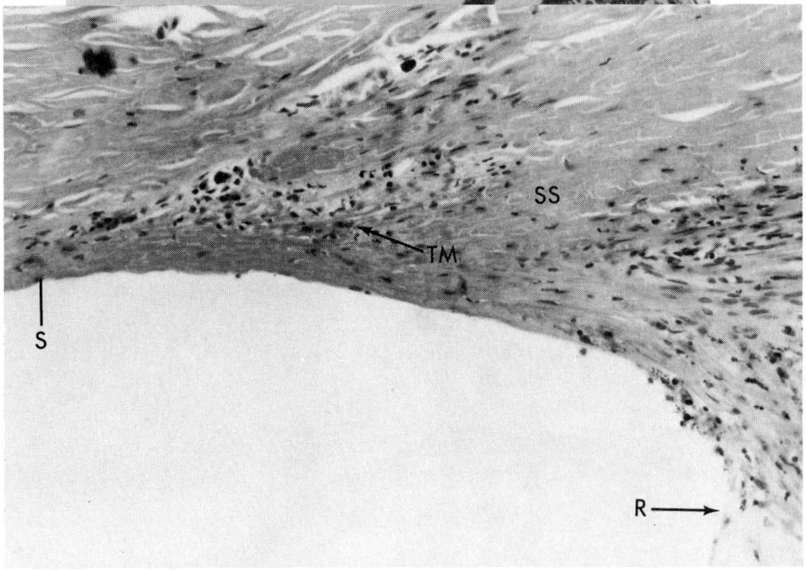

Fig. 6-16. A, Secondary open-angle glaucoma caused by blunt trauma and creation of a contusion deformity of the angle. The angle is recessed in this condition. *R,* Approximate original site of angle recess; *C,* deepest extent of plane of cleavage, which creates a new recess more posteriorly; *SC,* Schlemm's canal and adjacent trabecular meshwork; *AC,* anterior chamber; *I,* iris; *S,* Schwalbe's line. (H & E stain; ×120.) **B,** Old contusion angle deformity with angle recession. Schwalbe's line *(S)* is the anterior terminus of the markedly sclerotic (fibrotic) trabecular meshwork *(TM).* Normally, the angle recess is immediately adjacent to the scleral spur *(SS),* but in this condition the abnormal recess *(R)* is displaced posteriorly (to the right). (H & E stain; ×300.)

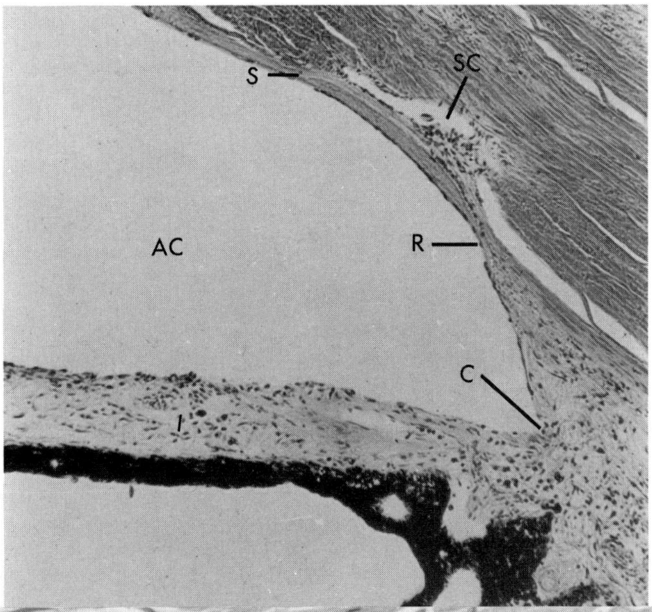

quent sequela of advanced intraocular tumors, may also lead to peripheral anterior synechiae.

Posttraumatic open-angle glaucoma

Posttraumatic open-angle glaucoma occasionally results from blunt trauma and recession of the angle (contusion angle deformity)* (Chapter 3, p. 102). Actual symptomatic glaucoma develops only in a small percentage of such cases,

however. Increased intraocular pressure may be manifest within a short period following the trauma, although it is not unusual for the glaucoma to become evident after a delay of many years. Such cases are often associated with iridodialysis with hemorrhage (Fig. 6-14), secondary cataract (Fig. 6-15), or lens dislocation (Fig. 4-38), which might explain the glaucoma. In cases in which these cannot be implicated, the mechanism of this type of secondary glaucoma is not always easily explained. The trabecular meshwork may incur mechanical damage following the initial injury. Histopathologic examination of globes enucleated

---

* References 158, 167, 168, 177, 187, 188, 195, 208, 213, 224, 228.

after complications of angle recession deformity glaucoma usually shows end-stage sclerosis of the trabecular meshwork (Fig. 6-16). The presence of a Descemet-like basement membrane lining the anterior chamber border of the meshwork has been microscopically confirmed in a few cases. This membrane could be partially responsible for decreased outflow and glaucoma in some cases.

CONGENITAL AND INFANTILE GLAUCOMA

Primary congenital glaucoma is a bilateral condition usually inherited in an autosomal-recessive fashion.[230-261] It occurs in 1:5000 to 1:10,000 live births. The majority of affected patients are boys.

Several theories attempt to define the pathogenesis of congenital glaucoma:[230-236,238-245,248-261]

1. Faulty cleavage of the differentiating mesectoderm occurs during anterior chamber angle embryogenesis (Fig. 6-19).
2. Abnormally situated persistent fetal iris processes (Fig. 2-37) block aqueous humor outflow.
3. A membrane or sheath (Barkan's membrane) covers the anterior chamber angle and retards aqueous humor outflow.

The term *congenital glaucoma*, in the strictest sense, should be used only in cases with glaucoma-inducing anomalies present at birth, although the actual increase in

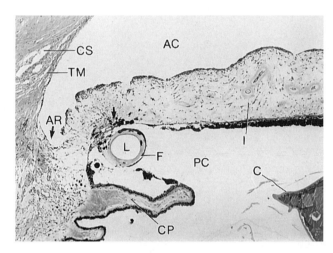

Fig. 6-17. Photomicrograph of the anterior segment of an eye with atrogenic, IOL-induced pigmentary dispersion and pigmentary glaucoma. Note that the lens haptic or loop *(L)* is fixated in the ciliary sulcus and is surrounded by a fibrous capsule *(F)*. Note the chaffing of the posterior iris pigment epithelium by the lens loop *(arrow)*. *AC*, anterior chamber; *CS*, canal of Schlemm; *TM*, trabecular meshwork; *AR*, angle recess; *PC*, posterior chamber; *CP*, ciliary processes; *LC*, lens capsule. (H & E; ×100.)

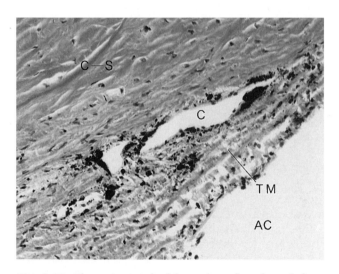

Fig. 6-18. Photomicrograph of the angle outflow channels from a patient with IOL-induced secondary pigmentary dispersion and glaucoma. Note that the trabecular meshwork *(TM)* and surrounding structures are permeated with dispersed pigment that has migrated from the posterior pigment epithelium of the iris. *C*, canal of Schlemn; *C-S*, corneal scleral junction; *AC*, anterior chamber. (H & E ×180.)

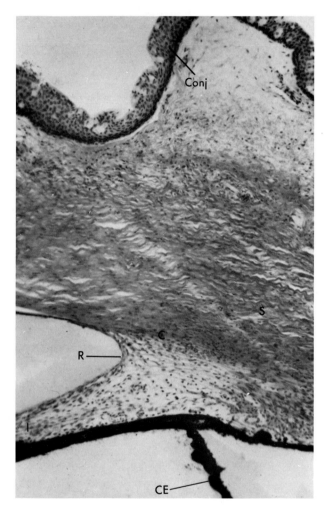

Fig. 6-19. Anterior chamber angle from globe of an infant who died from trisomy 13. Note the severely malformed angle and almost total lack of development of the filtration apparatus. Cleavage of the iris *(I)* from the posterior surface of the cornea *(C)* is incomplete. There is no evidence of differentiation of the trabecular meshwork or Schlemm's canal. In addition to maldevelopment of the angle filtration structures, hypoplasia of the ciliary body has occurred, with a lack of formation of folded ciliary processes. *R*, Angle recess; *CE*, maldeveloped inner layer or ciliary epithelium at the junction with the iris epithelium; *S*, sclera; *Conj*, limbal conjunctiva. (H & E stain; ×115.) (From Apple DJ: In Goldberg MF, editor: Genetic and metabolic eye disease, Boston, 1974, Little, Brown & Co.)

intraocular pressure may occur later. Detailed discussions of the pathogenesis, clinical manifestations, and histopathologic appearance of primary congenital glaucoma are beyond the scope of this chapter. Many of the diseases listed on page 264, which cause secondary congenital or infantile glaucoma, are described in other chapters.

Sequelae of glaucoma

An understanding of the mechanisms leading to persistent visual loss or complete blindness caused by untreated progressive glaucoma requires a knowledge of the tissue effects induced by elevated intraocular pressure.[262–302]

ENLARGEMENT OF THE GLOBE

Figures 6-20 to 6-23 illustrate the typical defects of progressive congenital or infantile glaucoma. The outer tunics of the eye (cornea and sclera) are stretched and thinned, a characteristic of buphthalmos, or ox eye. Enlargement of the globe or focal ectasia or staphyloma formation may even occur in the mature sclera if the intraocular pressure is sufficiently increased for long. This happens most commonly at the limbus, creating an intercalary staphyloma; however, staphylomas are far more common in infants, because the immature sclera is more elastic and, therefore, more susceptible to stretching. Haab's stria (see p. 73) are sequela of cornea stretching.

The globe illustrated in Figure 6-23 had been subjected to numerous goniotomies, and very little remains of the outflow channels and mesodermal processes that were originally responsible for increased intraocular tension. As in most cases of congenital glaucoma, the angle separating the cornea and iris appears wide and the anterior chamber is very deep.

A common complication of buphthalmos in children is rupture of the suspensory ligaments of the lens and lens subluxation. This rupture follows marked enlargement of the eyes and is caused by mechanical traction on the zonules as the distance between the ciliary processes increases. In Fig. 6-23 the lens (which is extremely cataractous) is displaced toward the ciliary body on the right.

An end-stage, blind eye with absolute glaucoma, normal in size or enlarged, and exhibiting atrophy and thinning of all three tunics is termed an *atrophia bulbi*. This differs from the shrunken, thickened globe called a *phthisis bulbi*.

Trabecular meshwork

By the time most eyes with glaucoma are submitted to the pathology laboratory, the trabecular meshwork is largely composed of dense fibrous tissue and has the "sclerotic" appearance seen in Fig. 6-16. Disappearance of Schlemm's canal is a late sequela.

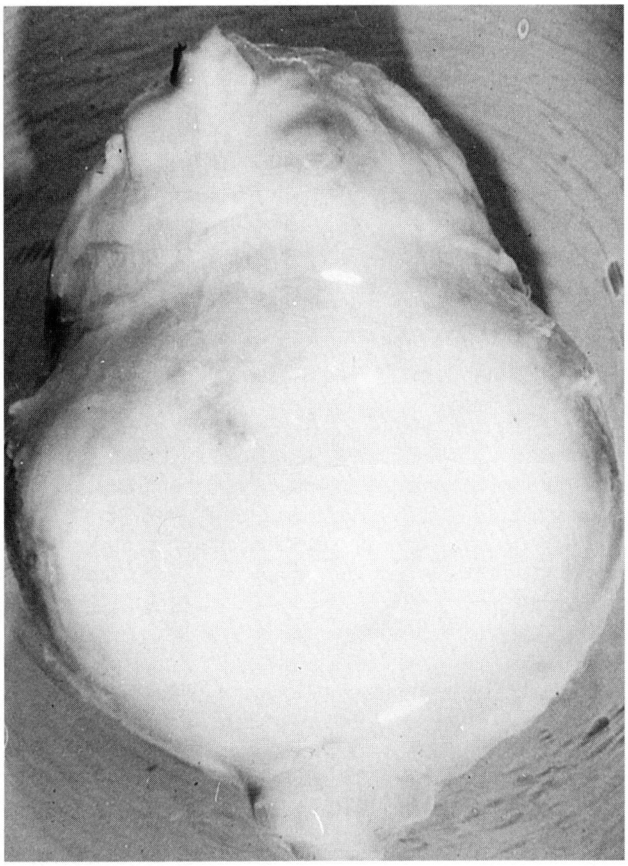

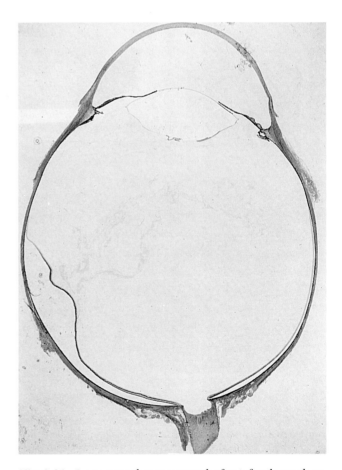

Fig. 6-20. Gross photograph of an eye enucleated from a young child with advanced buphthalmos.

Fig. 6-21. Low power photomicrograph of an infantile eye showing buphthalmos, with marked stretching and anterior bowing of the cornea and glaucomatous excavation of the optic nerve head. (H & E stain; ×1.)

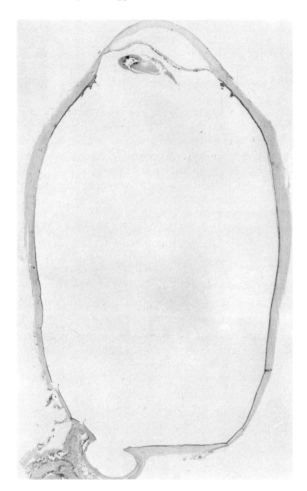

Fig. 6-22. Buphthalmos. The eye is 35 mm long, the sclera is thinned, the lens is cataractous as a result of zonular rupture, and the nerve head is deeply cupped. (H & E stain; ×15.)

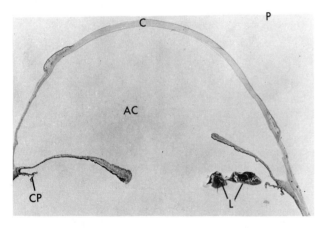

Fig. 6-23. Buphthalmos caused by infantile glaucoma in a patient with Axenfeld's anomaly. Note thinning of cornea (*C*) and sclera. The patient underwent several goniotomies. As with most congenital glaucomas, the angle is wide open, and the anterior chamber (*AC*) is remarkably deep. Because of the massive enlargement of the eye, the zonules have stretched and ruptured, forcing a displacement of the lens (*L*) toward the ciliary region on the right. The secondary cataract results from rupture of the lens capsule and partial extrusion of lens cortex. *CP*. Ciliary process. (H & E stain; ×5.)

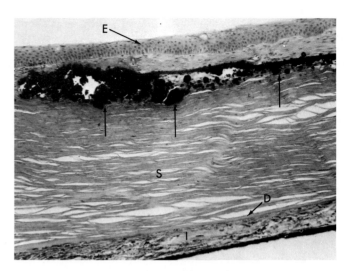

Fig. 6-24. Band keratopathy and degenerative pannus resulting from long-standing closed-angle glaucoma. *Arrows,* Deposits of densely staining calcium in the region of Bowman's layer. The fibrovascular (degenerative) pannus is situated between Bowman's layer and the epithelium (*E*). The iris (*I*) is adherent to the posterior corneal surface, forming a total anterior synechia. *D*, Descemet's membrane; *S*, corneal stroma. (H & E stain; ×180.)

Cornea

Acute or long-standing persistent pressure elevations may initiate corneal edema (Fig. 3-19). Corneal edema is manifest as a hydropic swelling of the corneal epithelium. Both intracellular and intercellular epithelial edema is visible by histopathologic examination. Stromal edema is more difficult to appreciate in microscopic sections because of tissue preparation artifacts, which often mimic stromal edema.

Stromal edema is particularly common in congenital glaucoma (hydrops).[237] Haab's striae (p. 73) represent breaks in Descemet's membrane that are frequently associated with increased intraocular pressure and corneal edema. These most commonly course in a horizontal direction, in contrast to the injuries to Descemet's membrane during forceps delivery, where they usually course in a diagonal direction.

Long-standing glaucoma is commonly associated with many other nonspecific degenerative changes in the cornea as a result of chronic edema. Endothelial changes, bullous keratopathy (Fig. 3-20), rupture of blebs, band keratopathy (Figs. 3-19 and 3-26), degenerative pannus, and corneal vascularization and scarring (Figs. 3-24, 3-27, and 6-20) may occur.[280]

Lens

Cataracts resulting from all forms of glaucoma show histopathologic changes identical to those described in Chapter 4. Glaukomflecken are multiple, white, punctate opacities appearing in the subcapsular cortex (Fig. 6-25). They tend to follow the lines of the sutures. These lesions, which occasionally occur after sudden acute rises in pressure, represent a vacuolation in the anterior subcapsular cortex, with focal necrosis of the affected fibers and adjacent epithelium.

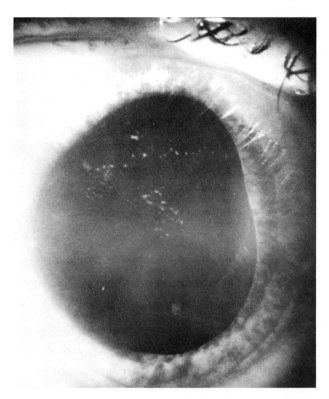

Fig. 6-25. Glaukomflecken. Punctate foci of necrosis of the anterior epithelium and subepithelial cortex.

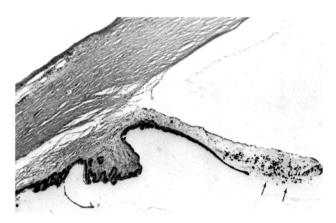

Fig. 6-26. Iris necrosis caused by long-standing glaucoma, involving hyalinization of the iris stroma, atrophy of the pigment epithelium, and formation of pigment clumps near the pupillary margin. (H & E stain; ×12.)

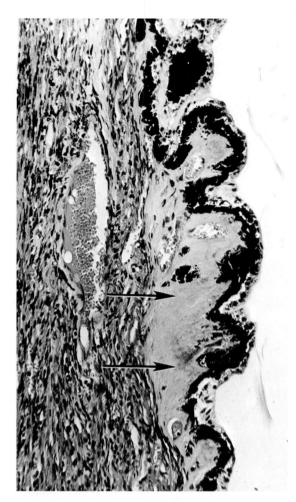

Fig. 6-27. Marked atrophy, blunting, and hyalinization of the stroma of the ciliary processes as a result of long-standing glaucoma. The ciliary muscle (cellular tissue at left) is intact, but the stroma between this muscle and the epithelial layers on the right is significantly hyalinized (*arrows*). (H & E stain; ×75.)

Iris and ciliary body

Following acute increases in intraocular pressure, the iris and ciliary body stroma may undergo necrosis (Fig. 6-26). The smooth muscles of the iris are particularly affected, and iris movements are impaired. A segmental iris atrophy may occur after acute or long-standing chronic glaucoma because of compromise in the iris blood supply from the major arterial circle induced by the increased pressure.

The appearance of the stroma of the ciliary body is char-

acteristic in long-standing glaucoma. The ciliary processes become atrophied, are shortened and blunted, and become hyalinized (Fig. 6-27). Cellularity and vascularity of the ciliary stroma decrease significantly. This diffuse stromal hyalinization is not diagnostic of glaucoma; it also occurs as a normal aging process. It should not be mistaken for tissue changes after treatment.[298] Also it should not be confused with the specific ciliary body change that occurs in diabetes mellitus. In the latter there is a diffuse thickening of the ciliary body basement membrane (Fig. 8-31) rather than a stromal hyalinization.

Unsuccessfully treated eyes with irreversible acute or chronic glaucoma often progress to an end-stage neovascular glaucoma, characterized by rubeosis iridis and ectropin uveal (Figs. 8-27 and 8-29). This is often a result of venous stasis retinopathy (occlusion of the central retinal vein), which eventually is caused by the increased intraocular pressure that retards venous outflow from the eye.

Retina

The innermost portion of the retina is most susceptible to intraocular pressure increases.[263] Nerve fiber layer hem-

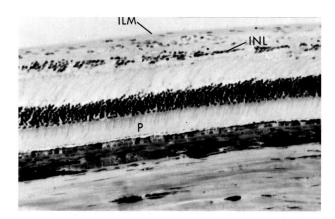

Fig. 6-28. Retinal atrophy caused by long-standing glaucoma. The outer retina (photoreceptor cell layer, *P*) is intact. The ganglion cell layer and nerve fiber layer are totally absent, and the inner nuclear layer *(INL)* is greatly attenuated. Therefore, the inner nuclear layer and the internal limiting membrane *(ILM)* are separated only by a narrow band of tissue composed primarily of glia. (H & E stain; ×150.)

orrhages may occur.[265,266] The hallmark of retinal atrophy in glaucoma is degeneration and eventual disappearance of ganglion cells and their axons, which form the nerve fiber layer (Fig. 6-28). In long-standing cases, the vessels of the inner half of the retina eventually become attenuated. Also, there may be ultimate dropout of cells in the inner nuclear layer and in the ganglion cells, the so-called transsynaptic atrophy.[300] The histopathologic appearance of glaucomatous retinal atrophy (Fig. 6-28) is similar to that seen in occlusion of the central retinal artery (Fig. 8-43) in which the inner layers of the retina are selectively destroyed by the ischemic process.[43] The photoreception situated in the outermost retinal layer is not lost in substantial numbers. Paripapillary chorioretinal atrophy, manifested by irregular hypo- and/or hyperpigmentation and exposure of large choroidal vessels and sclera may occur.

Optic Nerve

In acute glaucoma a papilledema (p. 537) may develop in early stages. It probably results from an obstruction of venous return at the optic disc caused by the increased pressure.[279]

The clinical and histopathologic appearance of the deeply cupped or excavated optic nerve head is illustrated in Figs. 6-29 to 6-35 and Color Plates 6-6 and 6-7.° The destruction of retinal nerve fiber layer axons as they pass from the retina into the optic nerve probably results from a combination of forces. The mechanical force of the intraocular pressure on the fibers as they course around the margin of the cup may interfere with normal axoplasmic flow within each fiber and may produce axonal necrosis. A compromise in the vascular supply to the optic nerve occurring in progressive glaucoma also leads to an ischemic necrosis of nerve fibers.

Hayreh[269–272] has shown that anterior ischemic optic

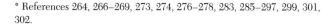

° References 264, 266–269, 273, 274, 276–278, 283, 285–297, 299, 301, 302.

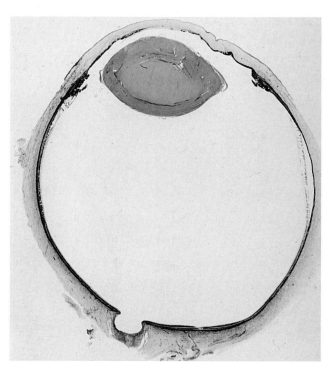

Fig. 6-29. Photomicrograph of an eye with secondary closed angle glaucoma. Note complete peripheral anterior synechiae and deep excavation of the optic cup. (H & E stain; ×1.)

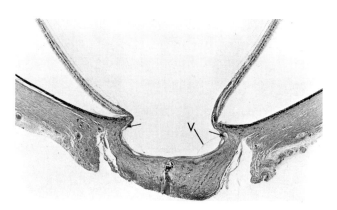

Fig. 6-30. Glaucomatous cupping of the optic nerve head. The overhanging ridges at the disc margins are prominent. The exiting central vessels *(arrows)* are situated under the lips of the ridge. This explains why the exiting vessels appear at the base of the cup, disappear from view by ophthalmoscopy as they course under the ridge, and reappear as they emerge around the lip of the cup into the retina. *V,* Vitreous fibril near the base of the cup. (See also Color Plate 6-1.) (H & E stain; ×30.)

neuropathy, glaucoma, and low-tension glaucoma are manifestations of ischemia of the optic nerve head and retrolaminar optic nerve caused by interference with posterior ciliary artery circulation. This is a result of an imbalance between perfusion pressure in the posterior ciliary arteries and intraocular pressure. If the process is sudden, it produces anterior ischemic optic neuropathy with infarction of the optic nerve head and retrolaminar region (p. 547). If it is chronic (as in glaucoma and low-tension glaucoma),

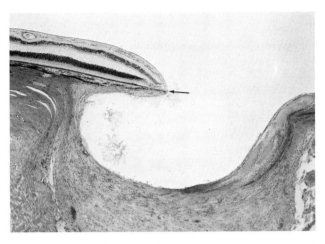

Fig. 6-31. Glaucomatous excavation. *Arrow,* An unusually prominent overhanging ridge. (H & E stain; ×40.)

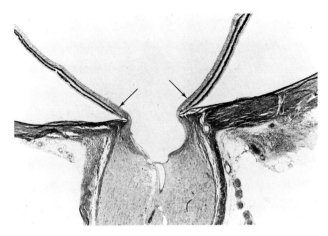

Fig. 6-33. Glaucomatous optic atrophy with extreme pathologic excavation of the nerve head. Note the virtual absence of retinal nerve fibers as they course around the edge of the disc. *Arrows,* Absence of retinal ganglion cells. (H & E stain; ×20.)

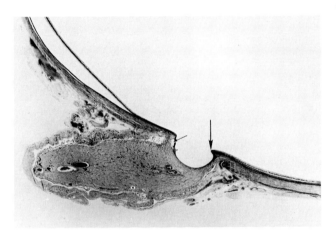

Fig. 6-32. Glaucomatous optic atrophy, showing marked degeneration of the axons of the nerve fiber layer as they pass around the exposed margin of the disc *(large arrow).* Note the posterior bowing of the lamina cribrosa and the location of the central vessel *(small arrow)* under the ridge of the cup. (See also Color Plate 6-2.) (H & E stain; ×15.)

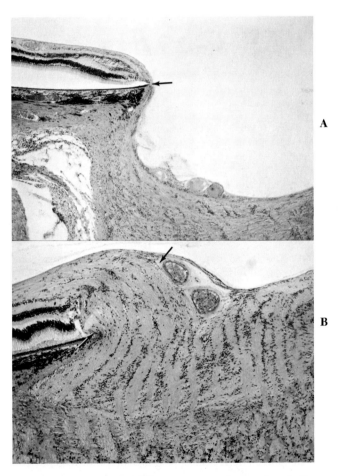

A

B

Fig. 6-34. Comparison of glaucomatous and normal optic disc. **A,** Absence of retinal nerve fiber layer at disc margin *(arrow).* (H & E stain; ×40.) **B,** Normal nerve head with normal quota of nerve fibers passing from the retina around the margin *(arrows)* into the nerve. (H & E stain; ×40.)

it produces slow degeneration of neural tissue in the optic nerve head and retrobulbar region, resulting in cupping of the optic disc, cavernous degeneration of the retrolaminar optic nerve, or both.

The major histopathologic criteria of optic atrophy, as described in Chapter 9, are present in glaucomatous optic atrophy. These include gliosis, loss of nerve fibers, demyelination, and decrease in diameter of the nerve. They are nonspecific changes that indicate atrophy but do not necessarily provide clues to the pathogenesis of the disease. A more specific diagnosis of glaucomatous optic atrophy requires observation of the typical pathologic excavation of the cup or, when present, identification of the cavernous spaces of Schnabel.

Schnabel's cavernous optic atrophy (Fig. 6-35) is a specific type of atrophy with large cavernous spaces within the nerve parenchyma.[262,279,294–296,302] In most cases it signifies previous episodes of acute severe increases in intraocu-

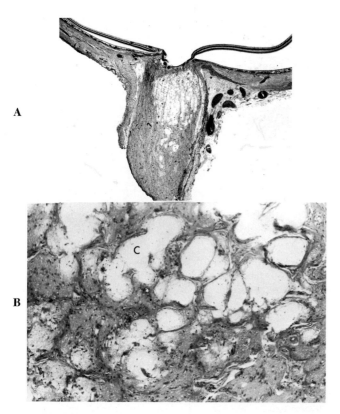

Fig. 6-35. Cavernous atrophy of the optic nerve (Schnabel's atrophy). **A,** The cystoid spaces resemble Swiss cheese in the nerve parenchyma. (H & E stain; ×5.) **B,** High-power photomicrograph of the optic nerve parenchyma showing the formation of numerous large spaces (cavernous spaces, *C*), which have replaced the normal nerve tissue. These spaces contain hyaluronic acid and therefore appear to represent a permeation of vitreous into the optic nerve parenchyma. (H & E stain; ×420.) (**A** from Naumann GOH and Apple DJ: In Doerr W, Seifert G, and Uehlinger E, editors: Handbuch der speziellen pathologischen Anatomie, Band Auge, Berlin, 1980 Springer-Verlag.)

lar tension. It also occurs in anterior ischemic optic neuropathy (pp. 544–545), for example, giant cell arteritis (p. 545). Mucopolysaccharide stains reveal hyaluronic acid in the large spaces within the nerve substance. Hyaluronic acid from the vitreous human is apparently forced into the optic nerve during the episodes of pressure elevation. It is not clear whether the large cavities form as a result of the permeation of hyaluronic acid into the solid nerve parenchyma or as a result of previous atrophy with secondary absorption of vitreous humor. A report by Shields and Eagle demonstrating that therapeutically injected silicone oil can penetrate the nerve substance and produce a pseudo-Schnabel's atrophy supports the permeation theory.

An appreciation of the appearance of the various physiologic variations in the "normal" disc and an awareness of these anomalies is required to distinguish an otherwise healthy eye from a glaucomatous eye. These anomalies are considered in Chapter 2.

Following is a list of various congenital anomalies of the optic disc that may mimic or disguise glaucomatous optic atrophy with cupping.

1. Congenital deep cup (genetic influences)
2. Anomalous embryonic hyaloid glial-vascular remnants
   a. Congenital deep cup due to extensive resorption of Bergmeister's papilla
   b. Epipapillary membranes (remnants of Bergmeister's papilla) producing a deceptively shallow optic cup
   c. Vascular loops mimicking optociliary shunt vessels
3. Myopia, usually with conus
4. Coloboma of the optic nerve
5. Morning glory syndrome
6. Tilted disc syndrome
7. Congenital optic pit

REFERENCES

General

1. Allen L, Burian HM, and Braley AE: The anterior border ring of Schwalbe and the pectinate ligament, Arch Ophthalmol 53:799, 1955.
2. Acott TS and others: Trabecular repopulation by anterior trabecular meshwork cells after laser trabeculoplasty (see comments), Am J Ophthalmol 107:1, 1989.
3. Allingham RR and others: Probe placement and power levels in contact transscleral neodymium:yag cyclophotocoagulation, Arch Ophthalmol 108:738, 1990.
4. Anderson D: Pathology of the glaucomas, Br J Ophthalmol 56:146, 1972.
5. Ascher KW: Aqueous veins, Am J Ophthalmol 25:31, 1942.
6. Barkan O: Glaucoma: classification, causes, and surgical control, Am J Ophthalmol 21:1099, 1938.
7. Becker B, Keaky GR, and Christensen RE: Hypersecretion glaucoma, Arch Ophthalmol 56:180, 1956.
8. Becker SC: Clinical gonioscopy: a text and stereoscopic atlas, St. Louis, 1972, The CV Mosby Co.
9. Bellows JC, editor: Glaucoma: contemporary international concepts, New York, 1980, Masson Publishing USA, Inc.
10. Bennett SR and others: An autosomal dominant form of low-tension glaucoma, Am J Ophthalmol 108:238, 1989.
11. Brubaker RF: Flow of aqueous humor in humans, Invest Ophthalmol Vis Sci 32:3145, 1991.
12. Chandler PA and Grant WM: Lectures on glaucoma, Philadelphia, 1965, Lea & Febiger.
13. Chandler PA and Grant WM: Glaucoma, ed 2, Philadelphia, 1980, Lea & Febiger.
14. Clark WB, editor: Symposium on glaucoma: transactions of the New Orleans Academy of Ophthalmology, St. Louis, 1959, The CV Mosby Co.
15. Congdon N and others: Issues in the epidemiology and population-based screening of primary angle-closure glaucoma, Surv Ophthalmol 36:411, 1992.
16. de Kater AW, Melamed S, and Epstein DL: Pattern of aqueous humor outflow in glaucomatous and nonglaucomatous human eyes: a tracer study using cationized ferritin, Arch Ophthalmol 107:572, 1989.
17. Dielemans I and others: The prevalence of primary open-angle glaucoma in a population-based study in the Netherlands, The Rotterdam Study, Ophthalmol 101:1851, 1994.
18. Drance SM: Low-pressure glaucoma. Enigma and opportunity, Arch Ophthalmol 103:1131, 1985.
19. Drance SM: Low-pressure glaucoma. Enigma and opportunity, Arch Ophthalmol 103:1131, 1985.
20. Duke-Elder S, editor: System of ophthalmology, vol XI, Diseases of the lens and vitreous: glaucoma and hypotony, St. Louis, 1969, The CV Mosby Co.
21. Fine BS, Yanoff M: Ocular histology. A text and atlas, ed 2, Hagerstown, 1979, Harper & Row.
22. Fuchs E: Lehrbuch der Augenheilkunde, Vienna, 1889, Franz Deuticke.
23. Garron LK: The fine structure of the normal trabecular apparatus in man. In Newell FW, editor: Transactions of the fourth conference on glaucoma, New York, 1959, Josiah Macy, Jr Foundation.
24. Goldmann H: Abfluss des Kammerwassers beim Menschen, Ophthalmologica 3:146, 1946.

25. Grierson I and Rabi AHS: Microfilaments in the cells of the human trabecular meshwork, Br J Ophthalmol 63:3, 1979.
26. Halasa AH: The basic aspects of the glaucomas, Springfield, Ill, 1972, Charles C Thomas, Publisher.
27. Halberg GP, editor: Glaucoma update, Birmingham, Ala, 1980, Inter-Optics Publications, Inc.
28. Heilmann K and Richardson KT, editors: Glaucoma: conceptions of a disease—pathogenesis, diagnosis, therapy, Philadelphia, 1978, WB Saunders Co.
29. Higginbotham EJ: Is laser sclerostomy surgery ready for prime time, Arch Ophthalmol 113:1243, 1995.
30. Hiller R, Kahn HA: Blindness from glaucoma, Am J Ophthalmol 80:62, 1975.
31. Holmberg A: Ultrastructure of the normal trabecular apparatus in man. In Newell FW, editor: Transactions of the fourth conference on glaucoma, New York, 1959, Josiah Macy, Jr Foundation.
32. Jampol LM and Miller NR: Carotid artery disease and glaucoma, Br J Ophthalmol 62:324, 1978.
33. Jonas JB and Dichtl A: Evaluation of the retinal nerve fiber layer, Surv Ophthalmol 40:369, 1996, (review).
34. Kahn HA and Moorehead HB: Statistics on blindness in the model reporting area, 1969–70, US Department of Health, Education and Welfare, Public Service Publication No. (NIH) 73-427, Washington, DC, 1973, US Government Printing Office.
35. Klein BEK and others: Prevalence of glaucoma, Ophthalmol 99:1499, 1992.
36. Knies M: Über das Glaucom, Graefes Arch Ophthalmol 22:163, 1876.
37. Kolker AE and Hetherington J Jr: Becker-Shaffer's diagnosis and therapy of the glaucomas, ed 5, St. Louis, 1983, The CV Mosby Co.
38. Lambrou FH, Vela MA, and Woods W: Obstruction of the trabecular meshwork by retinal rod outer segments, Arch Ophthalmol 107:742, 1989.
39. L'Esperance FA Jr and Mittl RN: Carbon dioxide laser trabeculotomy for the treatment of neovascular glaucoma, Trans Am Ophthalmol Soc 80:262, 1982.
40. Levene RZ: Low tension glaucoma: a critical review and new material, Surv Ophthalmol 24:621, 1980.
41. Lichter PR: Argon laser trabeculoplasty, Trans Am Ophthalmol Soc 80:288, 1982.
42. Lichter PR and Anderson DR, editors: Discussions on glaucoma: proceedings of the 1975-1976 symposia on open and closed angle glaucoma, sponsored by the National Society for the Prevention of Blindness, London, 1977, Grune & Stratton, Inc.
43. Luntz MH and Berlin MS: Combined trabeculectomy and cataract extraction: advantages of a modified technique and review of current literature, Trans Ophthalmol Soc UK 100:533, 1980.
44. Maumenee AE: Classification of glaucoma. In Clark WB, editor: Symposium on glaucoma: transactions of the New Orleans Academy of Ophthalmology, St. Louis, 1959, The CV Mosby Co.
45. McMenamin PG, Lee WR, and Aitken DAN: Age-related changes in the human outflow apparatus, Ophthalmology 93:194, 1986.
46. Meyner E: Atlas der Spaltlampenphotographie, Stuttgart, 1976, Ferdinand Enke Verlag.
47. Murray SB and Jay JL: Trabeculectomy: its role in the management of glaucoma, Trans Ophthalmol Soc UK 99:492, 1979.
48. Naumann GOH and Apple DJ: Pathology of the eye, New York, 1985, Springer-Verlag. (Translation, modification, and update of Pathologie des Auges by DJ Apple.)
49. Nesterov A, Bunin A, and Katsnelson L: Intraocular pressure: physiology and pathology, Moscow, 1978, Mir Publishers. (Revised from the 1974 edition; translated by A Aksenov.)
50. New Orleans Academy of Ophthalmology: Symposium on glaucoma: transactions of the New Orleans Academy of Ophthalmology, St. Louis, 1967, The CV Mosby Co.
51. New Orleans Academy of Ophthalmology: Symposium on glaucoma: transactions of the New Orleans Academy of Ophthalmology, St. Louis, 1975, The CV Mosby Co.
52. New Orleans Academy of Ophthalmology: Symposium on glaucoma: transactions of the New Orleans Academy of Ophthalmology, St. Louis, 1981, The CV Mosby Co.
53. Noureddin BN and others: Advanced uncontrolled glaucoma. Nd:YAG cyclophotocoagulation or tube surgery, Ophthalmol 99:430, 1992.
54. Phelps CD and Podos SM: Glaucoma. In Goldberg MF, editor: Genetic and metabolic eye disease, Boston, 1974, Little, Brown & Co.
55. Portney GA: Glaucoma guidebook, Philadelphia, 1977, Lea & Febiger.
56. Rabowsky JH and others: The use of bioerodible polymers and daunorubicin in glaucoma filtration surgery, Ophthalmol 103:800, 1996.
57. Ritch R, Shields MB, and Krupin T: The glaucomas, St. Louis, 1996, Mosby–Year Book, Inc.
58. Rodrigues MM and others: Histopathology of 150 trabeculectomy specimens in glaucoma, Trans Ophthalmol Soc UK 96:245, 1976.
59. Rubin B and others: Histopathologic study of the molteno glaucoma implant in three patients, Am J Ophthalmol 110:371, 1990.
60. Schumer RA and Podos SM: The nerve of glaucoma!, Arch Ophthalmol 112:37, 1994.
61. Schwartz LW and others: Argon laser iridotomy in the treatment of patients with primary angle-closure or pupillary block glaucoma: a clinicopathologic study, Ophthalmology 85:294, 1978.
62. Shaffer RN: Stereoscopic manual of gonioscopy, St. Louis, 1962, The CV Mosby Co.
63. Shields MB and others: Clinical and histopathologic observations concerning hypotony after trabeculectomy with adjunctive mitomycin C, Am J Ophthalmol 116:673, 1993.
64. Smith R: Clinical glaucoma, London, 1965, Cassell, Ltd.
65. Sommer A and others: The nerve fiber layer in the diagnosis of glaucoma, Arch Ophthalmol 95:149, 1977.
66. Sommers I: Histology and histopathology of the eye, New York, 1949, Grune & Stratton, Inc.
67. Sugar HS: Surgical anatomy of glaucoma, Surv Ophthalmol 13:143, 1968.
68. Tielsch JM and others: Diabetes, intraocular pressure, and primary open-angle glaucoma in the Baltimore Eye Study, Ophthalmol 102:48, 1995.
69. Tielsch JM and others: Racial variations in the prevalence of primary open-angle glaucoma, JAMA 266:369, 1991.
70. Theobald GD: Further studies on the canal of Schlemm: its anastomoses and anatomic relations, Am J Ophthalmol 39:65, 1955.
71. Theobald GD: Histology of tissues surrounding the angle of the anterior chamber. In Clark WB, editor: Symposium on glaucoma: transactions of the New Orleans Academy of Ophthalmology, St. Louis, 1959, The CV Mosby Co.
72. Tomey KF and Al-Rajhi AA: Neodymium:yag laser iridotomy in the initial management of phacomorphic glaucoma, Ophthalmol 99:660, 1992.
73. Tripathi BJ and Tripathi RC: Neural crest origin of human trabecular meshwork and its implications for the pathogenesis of glaucoma, Am J Ophthalmol 107:583, 1989.
74. Tripathi BJ and Tripathi RC: Neural crest origin of human trabecular meshwork and its implications for the pathogenesis of glaucoma (see comments), Am J Ophthalmol 107:583, 1989.
75. Tripathi R: Ultrastructure of Schlemm's canal in relation to aqueous outflow, Exp Eye Res 7:335, 1968.
76. Tripathi R: Aqueous outflow pathway in normal and glaucomatous eyes, Br J Ophthalmol 56:157, 1972.
77. Van Buskirk EM: Patholphysiology of laser trabeculoplasty, Surv Ophthalmol 33:264, 1989, (review).
78. von Graefe, A: Vorlumlautaufige Notiz umlautuber das Wesen des Glaucoms, Graefes Arch Ophthalmol 1:371, 1854.
79. Weber A: Die Ursache des Glaucoms, Graefes Arch Ophthalmol 23:1, 1877.
80. Weinreb RN and others: Immediate intraocular pressure response to argon laser trabeculoplasty, Am J Ophthalmol 95:279, 1983.
81. Wilensky J: Racial influences in glaucoma, Ann Ophthalmol 9:1545, 1977.
82. Wilhelmus KR, Grierson I, and Watson PG: Histopathologic and clinical associations of scleritis and glaucoma, Am J Ophthalmol 91:697, 1981.
83. Yue BYJT: The extracellular matrix and its modulation in the trabecular meshwork, Surv Ophthalmol 40:379, 1996, (review).
84. Zimmerman LE: Demonstration of hyaluronidase-sensitive acid mucopolysaccharide in trabecula and iris in routine paraffin sections of adult human eyes, Am J Ophthalmol 44:1, 1957.
85. Zimmerman LE: Application of histochemical methods for the demonstration of acid mucopolysaccharides to ophthalmic pathology, Trans Am Acad Ophthalmol Otolaryngol 62:697, 1958.

205. Mohan V and Eagling EM: Peripheral retinal cryotherapy as a treatment for neovascular glaucoma, Trans Ophthalmol Soc UK 98:93, 1978.

206. Murphy CG and others: Juxtacanalicular tissue in pigmentary and primary open-angle glaucoma, Arch Ophthalmol 110:1779, 1992.

207. Mullaney PB and others: Congenital hereditary endothelial dystrophy associated with glaucoma, Ophthalmol 102:186, 1995.

208. d'Ombrain A: Traumatic or "concussion" chronic glaucoma, Br J Ophthalmol 33:495, 1949.

209. Netland PA and others: Elastosis of the lamina cribrosa in pseudoexfoliation syndrome with glaucoma, Ophthalmol 102:878, 1995.

210. Pederson JE and Anderson DR: The mode of progressive disc cupping in ocular hypertension and glaucoma, Arch Ophthalmol 98:490, 1980.

211. Phelps CD and Watzke RC: Hemolytic glaucoma, Am J Ophthalmol 80:690, 1975.

212. Richardson TM, Hutchinson BT, and Grant WM: The outflow tract in pigmentary glaucoma, Arch Ophthalmol 95:1015, 1977.

213. Rodman H: Chronic open angle glaucoma associated with traumatic dislocation of the lens: a new pathogenic concept, Arch Ophthalmol 69:445, 1963.

214. Rohen JW: Why is intraocular pressure elevated in chronic simple glaucoma? Anatomical considerations, Ophthalmol 90:758, 1983.

215. Schulzer M and others: Biostatistical evidence for two distinct chronic open angle glaucoma populations, Br J Ophthalmol 74:196, 1990.

216. Shimizu R, Hara K, and Futa R: Fine structure of trabecular meshwork and iris in pigmentary glaucoma, Graefes Arch Clin Exp Ophthalmol 215:171, 1981.

217. Sugar HS: Pigmentary glaucoma: a 25 year review, Am J Ophthalmol 67:499, 1966.

218. Sugar HS and Barbour FA: Pigmentary glaucoma: a rare clinical entity, Am J Ophthalmol 32:90, 1949.

219. Sugar S: Pigmentary glaucoma and the glaucoma associated with the exfoliation-pseudoexfoliation syndrome update: Robert N Shaffer lecture, Ophthalmology 91:307, 1984.

220. Susanna R and others: Disc hemorrhages in patient with elevated intraocular pressure. Occurrence with and without field changes, Arch Ophthalmol 97:284, 1979.

221. Ueno H and others: Trabecular and retrocorneal proliferation of melanocytes and secondary glaucoma, Am J Ophthalmol 88:592, 1979.

222. Van Buskirk EM and Leure-duPree AE: Pathophysiology and electron microscopy of melanomalytic glaucoma, Am J Ophthalmol 85:160, 1978.

223. Weiss DI: Vascular insufficiency (neovascular) glaucoma: an integrating pathogenetic concept, Trans Ophthalmol Soc UK 97:280, 1977.

224. Wolf SM and Zimmerman LE: Chronic secondary glaucoma associated with retrodisplacement of iris root and deepening of the anterior chamber angle secondary to contusion, Am J Ophthalmol 54:547, 1962.

225. Worthen D: Scanning electron microscopy after alpha-chymotrypsin perfusion in man, Am J Ophthalmol 73:637, 1972.

226. Yanoff M: Glaucoma mechanism in ocular malignant melanomas, Am J Ophthalmol 70:898, 1970.

227. Yanoff M: Mechanisms of glaucoma in eyes with uveal malignant melanomas, Ophthalmol Clin 12(1):51, 1972.

228. Zimmerman LE: Acute secondary open angle glaucoma ten years after contusion—phacolytic glaucoma and contusion deformity, Surv Ophthalmol 8:26, 1963.

229. Zimmerman LE: Secondary open angle glaucoma, Arch Ophthalmol 69:421, 1963.

Congenital and infantile glaucoma

230. Allen L, Burian HM, and Braley AE: A new concept of the development of the anterior chamber angle, Arch Ophthalmol 53:783, 1955.

231. Anderson DR: The development of the trabecular meshwork and its abnormality in primary infantile glaucoma, Trans Am Ophthalmol Soc 79:458, 1981.

232. Anderson JR: Hydrophthalmia or congenital glaucoma: its causes, treatment and cure, London, 1939, Cambridge University Press.

233. Barkan O: Operation for congenital glaucoma, Am J Ophthalmol 25:552, 1942.

234. Barkan O: Pathogenesis of congenital glaucoma: gonioscopic and anatomic observations of the anterior chamber in the normal eye and in congenital glaucoma, Am J Ophthalmol 40:1, 1955.

235. Barkan O: Goniotomy for glaucoma associated with nevus flammeus, Am J Ophthalmol 43:545, 1957.

236. Broughton WL, Fine BS, and Zimmerman LE: Congenital glaucoma associated with chromosomal defect: a histologic study, Arch Ophthalmol 99:481, 1981.

237. Cibis GW, Tripathi RC: The differential diagnosis of Descemet's tears (Haab's striae) and posterior polymorphous dystrophy bands. A clinicopathologic study, Ophthalmol 89:614, 1982.

238. DeLuise VP, Anderson DR: Primary infantile glaucoma (congenital glaucoma), Surv Ophthalmol 28:1, 1983, (review).

239. Hoskins HD Jr, Shaffer RN, and Hetherington J: Anatomical classification of the developmental glaucomas, Arch Ophthalmol 102:1331, 1984.

240. Jerndal T: Congenital glaucoma due to dominant goniodysgenesis. A new concept of the heredity of glaucoma, Am J Hum Genet 35:645, 1983.

241. Joos KM and others: Experimental endoscopic goniotomy. A potential treatment for primary infantile glaucoma, Ophthalmol 100:1066, 1993.

242. Kwitko ML: Glaucoma in infants and children, New York, 1973, Appleton-Century-Crofts.

243. Maul E and others: The outflow pathway in congenital glaucoma, Am J Ophthalmol 89:667, 1980.

244. Maumenee AE: The pathogenesis of congenital glaucoma: a new theory, Trans Am Ophthalmol Soc 56:507, 1958.

245. Maumenee AE: Further observations on the pathogenesis of congenital glaucoma, Am J Ophthalmol 55:1163, 1963.

246. Merin S and Morin D: Heredity of congenital glaucoma, Br J Ophthalmol 56:414, 1972.

247. Mullaney PB and others: Congenital hereditary endothelial dystrophy associated with glaucoma, Ophthalmol 102:186, 1995.

248. Phelps CD: The pathogenesis of glaucoma in Sturge-Weber syndrome, Ophthalmology 85:276, 1978.

249. Quigley HA: The pathogenesis of reversible cupping in congenital glaucoma, Am J Ophthalmol 84:358, 1977.

250. Richards JE and others: Mapping of a gene for autosomal dominant juvenile-onset open-angle glaucoma to chromosome 1q, Am J Hum Genet 54:62, 1994.

251. Scheie HG: Symposium—congenital glaucoma: diagnosis, clinical course, and treatment other than goniotomy, Trans Am Acad Ophthalmol Otolaryngol 59:309, 1955.

252. Shaffer RN: Pathogenesis of congenital glaucoma: gonioscopic and microscopic anatomy, Trans Am Acad Ophthalmol Otolaryngol 59:297, 1955.

253. Shaffer RN: New concepts in infantile glaucoma, Trans Ophthalmol Soc UK 87:581, 1967.

254. Shaffer RN and Weiss DI: Congenital and pediatric glaucomas, St. Louis, 1970, The CV Mosby Co.

255. Stambolian D and others: Congenital glaucoma associated with a chromosomal abnormality, Am J Ophthalmol 106:625, 1988.

256. Tawara A and Inomata H: Developmental immaturity of the trabecular meshwork in congenital glaucoma, Am J Ophthalmol 92:508, 1981.

257. Tawara A and Inomata H: Developmental immaturity of the trabecular meshwork in juvenile glaucoma, Am J Ophthalmol 98:82, 1984.

258. Tawara A, Inomata H: Distribution and characterization of sulfated proteoglycans in the trabecular tissue of goniodysgenetic glaucoma, Am J Ophthalmol 117:741, 1994.

259. Toulement PJ and others: Association of congenital microcoria with myopia and glaucoma. A study of 23 patients with congenital microcornea, Ophthalmol 102:186, 1995.

260. Walton DS: Primary congenital open angle glaucoma: a study of the anterior segment abnormalities, Trans Am Ophthalmol Soc 77:746, 1979.

261. Worst JGF: The pathogenesis of congenital glaucoma, Springfield, Ill, 1966, Charles C Thomas, Publisher.

Sequelae of glaucoma

262. Brownstein SD and others: Nonglaucomatous cavernous degeneration of the optic nerve: report of two cases, Arch Ophthalmol 98:354, 1980.

263. Caprioli J: Correlation of visual function with optic nerve and nerve

Table 7-1. Relationship of each intraocular epithelial structure with its basement membrane and stroma

Ocular epithelial structure	Basement membrane	Stroma
Corneal epithelium	Corneal epithelial basement membrane (not to be confused with Bowman's layer)	Corneal stroma
Conjunctival epithelium	Conjunctival basement membrane	Conjunctival substantia propria
Corneal endothelium	Descemet's membrane	Corneal stroma
Lens epithelium	Lens capsule	Zonules
Iris pigment epithelium	Basement membrane not prominent	Iris stroma
Ciliary epithelium	Ciliary basement membrane	Ciliary muscles and connective tissue stoma
Retinal pigment epithelium	Inner portion of Bruch's membrane	Bruch's membrane and choroid
Sensory retina	Internal limiting membrane	Vitreous

Table 7-2. Stromal and epithelial components of the uvea

	Iris	Ciliary body	Choroid
Stromal part			
Mesodermal (mesectodermal) layer	1. Stroma a. Vessels b. Connective tissue 2. Chromatophores 3. Dilator and sphincter muscles (derived from the outer epithelial layer of the optic cup)	1. Stroma a. Vessels b. Connective tissue 2. Ciliary muscle Chromatophores°	1. Lamina suprachoroidea 2. Lamina vasculosa a. Large vessels (Haller's layer)
Epithelial part			
Neuroectodermal layer (pars iridica, pars ciliaris, and pars optica retinae) of the embryonic cup	1. Outer layer: pigmented 2. Inner layer: pigmented	1. Outer layer: pigmented 2. Inner layer: nonpigmented	1. Outer layer: pigmented epithelium of the retina 2. Inner layer: sensory retina

° The chromatophores in all parts of the uvea become situated in the stroma following a migration during fetal life from the neural crest. These pigment cells are therefore of neuroectodermal origin rather than from the epithelial optic cup itself.

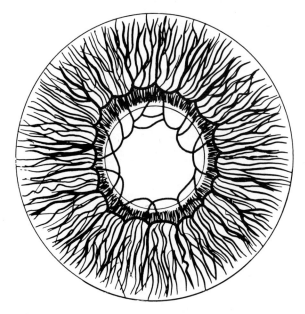

Fig. 7-1. Schematic drawing of fetal iris vasculature. The partially regressed arcades of the pupillary membrane arise at the collarette.

bleached preparations (Fig. 7-2, *B*). In some forms of albinism (Chapter 2) a relative or absolute decrease in pigmentation of the iris epithelium occurs so that the inner and outer layers of iris epithelium are visible without bleaching.

The smooth muscles of the iris, the dilator and sphincter, are also derived from the iris epithelium. This derivation of muscles from ectoderm contrasts with almost all other muscles of the body, which develop from the mesoderm. One other muscle that develops from ectoderm is the erector pili muscle of the pilosebaceous apparatus. The dilator muscle consists of a thin, radially arranged layer of muscle fibers that courses along the entire length of the iris immediately adjacent to and merging with the most anterior of the two epithelial layers (Fig. 7-2). The sphincter muscle is located within the stroma at the pupillary margin.

During histologic examination of an embryonic eye, one often sees a circumscribed cystic space situated between the two epithelial layers at the anterior optic cup margin (Fig. 4-2). This marginal sinus of von Szily is probably at least partly an artifact of preparation, because it is rarely seen in specimens that are embedded in plastic media rather than in paraffin. The former technique produces less artifact. Such a separation of the layers of epithelium, however, can occur in vivo and provides a basis for the pathogenesis of some forms of acquired cysts of the pupillary margin of the iris (Fig. 7-3).[27]

The stroma of the iris is divided into (1) a central pupil-

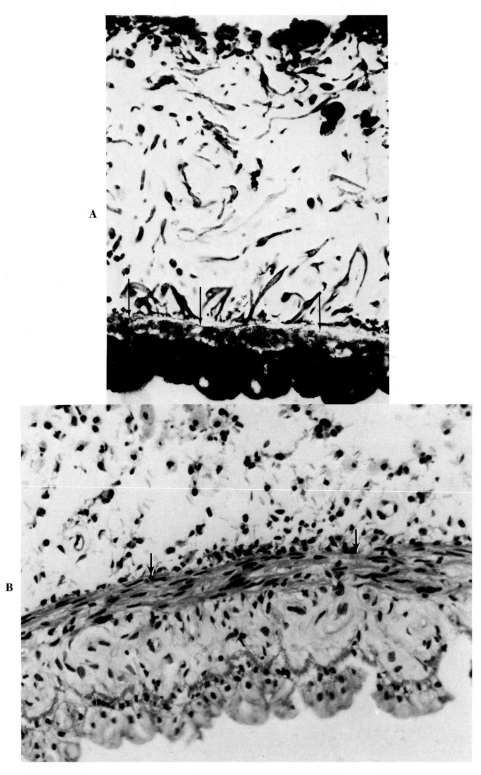

Fig. 7-2. A, Normal iris of a black adult. The dendritic melanocytes are elongated, branching pigmented cells in the stroma. They may undergo the process of neoplasia and form nevi or malignant melanomas. The number of stromal melanocytes determines iris color. The degree of pigmentation of the iris epithelium is usually constant, except in some forms of albinism. The melanin pigment within the iris pigment epithelium *(below)* arises in situ in the optic cup. *Arrows,* Dilator muscle. (H & E stain; ×275.) **B,** Bleach preparations of posterior iris showing sphincter muscle *(arrows)* and two-layered iris epithelium below. (H & E stain bleached; ×375.)

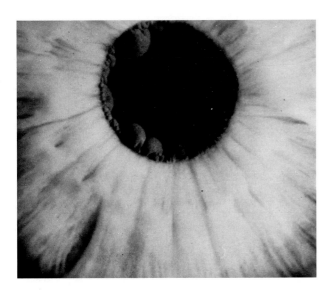

Fig. 7-3. Iris cysts at the pupillary margin. Compare with Fig. 4-4. (From Meyner E: Atlas der Spaltlampenphotographie, Stuttgart, 1976, Ferdinand Enke Verlag.)

lary zone and (2) a peripheral ciliary zone. The latter is further subdivided into the midpheriphery and the iris root. Faulty development of the peripheral iris stroma may result in iridocorneal dysgenesis (anterior cleavage syndromes) described in Chapter 2. Dystrophies of the iris (ICE syndrome) are discussed in Chapter 6. The collarette separates the pupillary zone and the ciliary zone (Figs. 2-23, 2-26, 7-1, and 7-2). This is the site of the minor arterial circle of the iris, where the embryonic iris vessels insert to form the pupillary membrane. The major iris circle is situated within the ciliary body near the iris root (Fig. 5-3). It is the site of a major anastomotic plexus of the vessels of the anterior and posterior ciliary systems. The stroma of the iris is supplied by vessels from the major and minor iris circles.

By the eighth month of gestation most of the pupillary membrane and tunica vasculosa lentis is resorbed. In the ninth month and shortly after birth one often finds remnants of the pupillary membrane. Most are of little clinical significance (Figs. 2-26, 4-2, and 7-1). The configuration of the anterior iris surface, which is characterized by formation of deep crypts (Fuchs' crypts), is partially determined by the type and degree of resorption of these embryonic vessels. Disease affecting the embryonic vasculature of the iris and lens are described in Chapter 2, page 28.

The color of the iris depends on both the number and pigment content of the stromal chromatophores or melanocytes (Fig. 7-2, *A*; Table 7-2).[18,35] These melanocytes originate in the embryonic neural crest and, following migration into the iris stroma, develop into star-shaped or dendritic melanocytes (Fig. 7-2, *A*). The neural crest is defined as a cluster of cells that in embryonic life lies directly adjacent to the embryonic neural tube. Cells that originate in the neural crest include stromal chromatophores of the iris and mesectoderm, which contributes to the uveal stroma, pigment cells in other parts of the uvea, dendrite-shaped pigment cells of the conjunctival stroma, and melanocytes

of the skin (Fig. 7-4). The development of stromal dendritic melanocytes from neural crest cells differs from that of the cells of the pigmented epithelia, which are characterized by in situ origin within the optic cup. This difference in embryonic origin is important in the understanding of the pathogenesis of the pigmented tumors of the eye. Neoplasia of the pigment epithelium (iris, ciliary body, and retinal pigment epithelium) is seldom observed, while neoplasia of the stromal, dendritic (neural crest) melanocytes of the uvea is relatively common (nevi, melanosis, melanocytoma, and malignant melanoma).

The migration of chromatophores from the neural crest into the uvea is one of the last phases in uveal development. The chromatophore cells show star-shaped, branched, protoplasmic processes. Pigment consisting of very fine round granules is regularly distributed throughout the entire cell body (Fig. 7-2, *A*). Pigmentation of these cells is not completed until after birth. For this reason a blue iris is usually seen in white newborns and only later does the iris of a brown-eyed person become fully pigmented. In contrast, the pigment epithelium of the iris becomes pigmented early in gestation; it shows a similar degree of pigmentation in the various races. The pigment epithelium does not contribute greatly to variability in normal iris color. A noteworthy exception is seen in albinism (Chapter 2) in which extreme variations in the number of pigment cells and/or amount of epithelial pigment can be observed.

CILIARY BODY

The ciliary epithelium is derived from the two-layered, light-insensitive pars ciliaris retinae, or pars caeca retinae, which is situated between the future iris epithelium and the epithelium of the future peripheral sensory retina (Figs. 1-9 and 1-11). The first trace of the ciliary processes occurs in the form of folds or convolutions of the epithelium. The adjacent mesodermal or mesectodermal tissue becomes richly vascularized, and the ciliary muscles begin to differentiate.[21]

The ciliary body is divided into two parts, both of which we separate from the sclera by a potential space, the suprachoroidal space, which can open pathological conditions.

1. The corona ciliaris, or pars plicata, is characterized by 70 to 80 meridionally directed folds or processes with intermediate valleys (Figs. 1-1, 4-2, 4-27, and 8-10; Color Plate 2-2). The zonular fibers insert onto and between these processes (Figs. 4-2 and 4-3). In sagittal sections the pars plicata is triangular in shape, and its stroma contains a rich vascular plexus, which provides a source of blood for aqueous secretion. The aqueous humor is actively secreted by the ciliary epithelium (Chapter 6). The ciliary muscle is the muscle of accommodation. In sagittal histologic section the ciliary muscle appears roughly triangular, with an anterior apex pointing directly into the scleral spur where it inserts. It consists of three portions: the outer longitudinal or meridional muscle of Brücke, the intermediate radial or oblique muscle, and the inner circular fibers of Müller.
2. The orbicularis ciliaris, or pars plana, is situated immediately posterior to the ciliary processes, between them and the ora serrata (Fig. 4-4).

The inner, nonpigmented epithelial layers contribute to the formation of aqueous humor. The outer pigmented layer of ciliary epithelium is continuous with the pigment

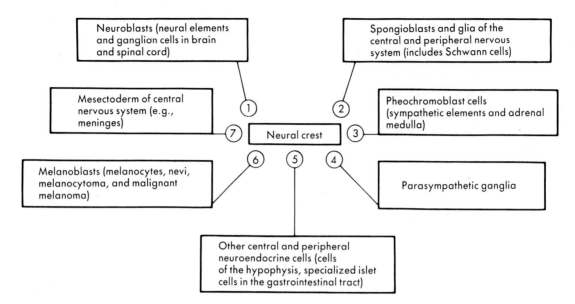

Fig. 7-4. Cell differentiation from the neural crest.

epithelium of the iris anteriorly and with the retinal pigment epithelium posteriorly (Fig. 1-11). Its basement membrane, particularly at the pars plicata, is commonly thickened in diabetes mellitus, a characteristic ocular histopathologic sign of this disease (Fig. 8-31).

The epithelial layers of the ciliary body in older persons often are characterized by formation of flat or protruding excrescences. Epithelial hyperplasia, for example, Fuchs' adenoma, commonly occurs as a benign aging process (Fig. 7-70). The most important tumors of the ciliary epithelium, adenoma and medulloepithelioma, are described on page 330. Typical cysts of the pars plana are so common that they may almost be considered physiologic (Fig. 8-65). They represent a reopening of the original space between the two layers of the embryonic optic cup and often are filled with hyaluronic acid produced by the epithelial layers.

CHOROID

The choroid (Figs. 7-5, 8-3 to 8-5, and 8-8) is approximately 0.2 mm thick and is composed of delicate connective tissue and vessels admixed with chromatophores. The embryologic origin and morphology of the melanocytes are similar to those of the iris (pp. 6-9). Hematopoesis within the choroid is a normal finding in premature infants and even in some full-term infants for the first few months of life. The ciliary vessels and nerves also traverse this structure (Figs. 1-2, 1-3, 7-5, and 7-6). The choroid's main function is to provide a vascular supply to the globe, in particular to the retinal pigment epithelium and the sensory retinal photoreceptors.[28,37] The choroid has four main layers:

1. Choriocapillaris (lamina vasculosa), including the outer layer of Bruch's membrane
2. Medium-sized vessels (Sattler's layer)
3. Large vessels (Haller's layer)
4. Lamina suprachoroidea

The choriocapillaris consists of a rich capillary network, the largest capillaries in the body that receives most of its

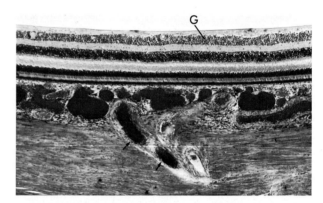

Fig. 7-5. Retina, choroid, and sclera in the macular region. *G*, Multilayered ganglion cell layer; *arrows*, posterior ciliary arteries, which penetrate the sclera and nourish the choroid. (H & E stain; ×150.) (From Naumann GOH and Apple DJ: In Doerr W, Seifert G, and Uehlinger E, editors: Handbuch der speziellen pathologischen Anatomie, Band Auge, Berlin, 1980, Springer-Verlag.)

blood supply from the branches of the ciliary vessels external to it, the medium-sized vessels of Sattler, and the outermost large vessels of Haller. Diffusion of nutrients from the choriocapillaris is directly responsible for nutrition of the pigment epithelium and outer layers of the retina.

The choriocapillaris is not a freely anastomotic organ as previously believed. It is divided into nonoverlapping lobules in a manner similar to that seen in the liver. Hence destruction of segments of choriocapillaris, for example, vascular infarcts or iatrogenic damage by photocoagulation treatment, is not always compensated for by anastomotic flow from adjacent areas. For this reason ischemia and infarcts of the choroid may be seen clinically.

By light microscopy Bruch's membrane can be differentiated into two components. The inner layer is mostly derived from the pigment epithelium and represents the basement membrane of this structure. The outer layer is

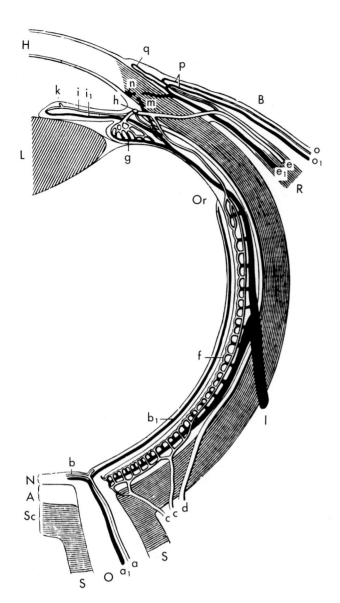

Fig. 7-6. Leber's classic schema of the vascular supply to the globe. *a, a₁*, and *b,* Central retinal vessels; *c,* short posterior ciliary vessels; *d,* long posterior ciliary vessels; *e, e₁,* anterior ciliary vessels; *f,* choriocapillaris; *h,* major iris circle; *k,* minor iris circle; *l,* vortex vein. (From Axenfeld T: Lehbuch und Atlas der Augenheilkunde, Jena, 1912, Gustav Fischer.)

VASCULAR SUPPLY OF THE UVEA

The uveal vessels are derived from the ciliary branches of the ophthalmic artery (Fig. 7-6). The main trunk of the ophthalmic artery divides into two relatively independent systems: (1) the retinal vascular system, which supplies a large portion of the optic nerve and the inner aspect of the sensory retina, and (2) the ciliary vascular system. Rarely do anastomoses occur between these two systems.

The very first anlage of the choroidal vascular system consists of a network forming a plexus around the optic vesicle and cup. The primitive choroid and choriocapillaris develop a close anastomotic communication with the long and short ciliary arteries, with the embryonic hyaloid artery in the region of the embryonic intraocular fissure, and with the major and minor circles of the iris (Fig. 2-23).

Branches of the anterior and posterior ciliary arteries supply the entire uvea. The seven anterior ciliary arteries, which enter the globe by way of the extraocular muscles (two from each rectus muscle except for the lateral rectus, from which there is only one), and the two horizontally located long posterior ciliary arteries (Figs. 1-2 and 1-3) form a plexus of channels that converge at the major iris circle (Fig. 7-6). The two long ciliary arteries pass through the sclera nasally and temporally to the optic nerve and course forward in the suprachoroid until merging with the anterior vessels in the major iris circle. The major iris circle and to a lesser extent the minor iris circle supply the ciliary body and iris (Fig. 7-3).

The 6 to 20 short posterior ciliary arteries are situated in a circle around the optic nerve forming the so-called circle of Zinn-Haller.* They immediately enter the uvea and divide into smaller channels, forming the vessels of the choroid and choriocapillaris.[9,28,37]

The venous outflow of the eye occurs through the four to seven vortex veins, which pass through obliquely coursing scleral canals or scleral emissaria into the ophthalmic vein (Fig. 1-3). The vortex veins are important in cases of malignant melanoma of the choroid, because these channels are the main site of exit of the tumor from the globe (Figs. 7-60 and 7-61). Emissarial extension of a tumor usually reflects a worsening prognosis, so they should be carefully examined in cases of intraocular melanoma.

Uveitis

Several congenital malformations affecting the uvea are considered in Chapter 2. This chapter discusses uveitis and uveal tumors.[41-403]

Uveitis is defined as an inflammation of any or all portions of the middle vascular tunic of the eye, for example, iritis, iridocyclitis, pars planitis, choroiditis, or panuveitis.† A simple involvement of a uveal tissue may occur without

---

* The existence of the circle of Zinn-Haller is doubted by some authors. At most it is usually incompletely developed, occurring only in segments around the optic nerve. A complete ring of vessels rarely, if ever, can be demonstrated.
† References 48, 49, 54, 57, 59, 66, 71, 74, 75, 77, 79, 80, 87-90, 99, 104, 105, 107, 112, 114, 116, 117, 120, 126, 127, 130-132, 137, 139, 145, 147-148, 150-155, 157, 162, 164, 167, 168, 170, 174-178, 180-182, 184, 190, 191, 195, 196, 201, 208-210, 214, 215, 218-220, 222, 223, 227-233, 236, 237, 242, 245-247, 249, 252-254, 257, 258, 261, 263, 264, 267, 269-271, 273, 275, 276, 278-281, 283-285, 287, 288, 290-294.

more closely related to the capillary endothelium of the choriocapillaris and is formed in part by the inner basement membrane of the choriocapillaris.

The lamina suprachoroidea is composed of delicate connective tissue and elastic fibrils situated between the vascular portion of the choroid and the adjacent sclera, within the slitlike potential space between the two structures. The major nerves and vessels that traverse the sclera in this area and enter the globe pass through the suprachoroid (Figs. 7-5 and 7-6). The lamina suprachoroidea probably also serves a protective function as a junctional point where the choroid and sclera may slide on one another during movement or distortion of the globe.

involvement of adjacent structures. On the other hand the inflammation is not always confined to the uvea, and adjacent structures or cavities can be involved; therefore a chorioretinitis, a keratoiritis, or an endophthalmitis with inflammation of the vitreous and other structures still broadly falls into the category of "uveitis."

A list of the major forms of uveitis follows. Groups A and B are classified according to origin and pathogenesis, and group C is classified according to a specific type of inflammatory reaction (granulomatous inflammation). We consider the latter as a single group because each often has a specific, recognizable clinical picture, and all are characterized by a granulomatous inflammatory reaction.

A. Exogenous, usually after perforating wounds with secondary infection
   1. Infections: bacterial, viral, or fungal
      a. Acute suppurative uveitis or keratouveitis
      b. Endophthalmitis and panophthalmitis
   2. Lens-induced uveitis (phacoanaphylactic uveitis) and sympathetic ophthalmia (These forms of uveitis are listed here because of their common association with perforating wounds. Because they show a granulomatous inflammatory response and not infectious processes, however, they are classified under section C and are discussed with those forms in the text.)

B. Endogenous (originates within the eye or from contiguous structures or is blood-borne)
   1. Hypersensitivity uveitis; common forms of nonspecific, nonsuppurative, nongranulomatous acute and chronic uveitis
      a. Idiopathic
      b. Collagen diseases
      c. Rheumatoid arthritis
      d. Reiter's syndrome
      e. Crohn's Disease
      f. Behçet's Disease
      g. Reaction to viruses (e.g., herpes simplex, Epstein-Barr virus and measles virus [subacute sclerosing panencephalitis])
      h. Pars planitis
      i. Glaucomatocyclitic crisis
      j. Uveal effusion
      k. Fuchs' heterochromic uveitis
      l. Iatrogenic, for example, intraocular lens-induced uveitis and uveitis, glaucoma, hyphema (UGH) syndrome
   2. Infectious (bacterial, viral, or fungal)
      a. Acute suppurative uveitis
      b. Endophthalmitis and panophthalmitis
   3. Necrosis of intraocular tumors

C. Specific forms (usually a granulomatous inflammation)
   1. Sarcoidosis
   2. Juvenile xanthogranuloma
   3. Histiocytosis X
   4. Presumed histoplasmic chorioretinitis
   5. Toxoplasmic retinochoroiditis
   6. Sympathetic ophthalmia
   7. Lens-induced endophthalmitis
   8. Nematode endophthalmitis
   9. Miscellaneous, for example, infectious granulomatous uveitis (tuberculous, leprotic, fungal syphilitic, etc.)
   10. Foreign body granulomas
   11. Iatrogenic, for example, intraocular lens-induced uveitis

EXOGENOUS AND ENDOGENOUS UVEITIS

Exogenous uveitis generally results from introduction of foreign material or infectious agents into the globe after perforating wounds.[30] Uveal inflammation caused by disturbances within the eye or within contiguous structures or by metastatic spread of infection from other portions of the body is termed *endogenous uveitus*.[89,121]

Most cases of endogenous uveitis that begin within the eye involve a nonsuppurative inflammation and are believed to represent an allergic response to foreign antigens. Some cases may be induced by a virus, causing an acute or chronic uveitis characterized by infiltration of mononuclear inflammatory cells (Figs. 7-7 and 7-8; Color Plate 7-1).

A suppurative infectious uveitis beginning primarily within the eye is much less common. The histologic hallmark of suppurative inflammation is an infiltration of polymononuclear neutrophils and extensive tissue necrosis and purulent exudation (see Chapter 3, p. 65). It almost always represents an influx of organisms from elsewhere in the body. Such metastatic intraocular inflammation is unusual today because of antibiotic therapy.

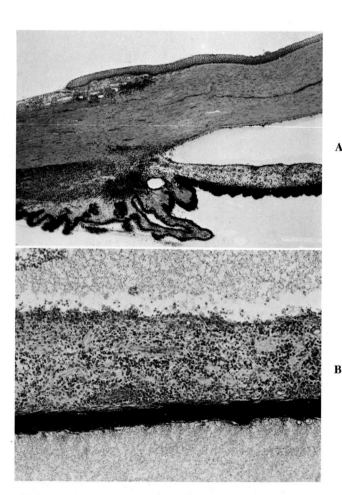

A

B

Fig. 7-7. Nongranulomatous iridocyclitis. **A,** Inflammatory infiltrates are located in iris, ciliary body, peripheral cornea, and subconjunctivally. (H & E stain; ×10.) **B,** Note intense fibrin deposition in anterior and posterior chambers. (H & E stain; ×125.)

Endophthalmitis (Figs. 7-9 to 7-11) is usually a sequela of trauma or injury.° Endophthalmitis arises only occasionally after an endogenous uveitis. Pseudophakic endophthalmitis is considered in Chapter 4. It is a severe, acute, purulent inflammation of all tissues within the eye except the sclera. By definition it always involves the vitreous cavity, often forming a vitreous abscess. Modern therapeutic regimens include intravitreal injection of antibiotics and diagnostic and therapeutic vitrectomy. Panophthalmitis is an extension of an endophthalmitis with involvement of sclera and adjacent orbital tissue.

The signs and symptoms of nonsupurrative nongranulo-

° References 41, 42, 50, 51, 52, 61, 72, 83, 92-94, 98, 111, 115, 119, 123, 133, 163, 173, 187-189, 203, 212, 213, 224, 225, 235, 238-240, 274, 297

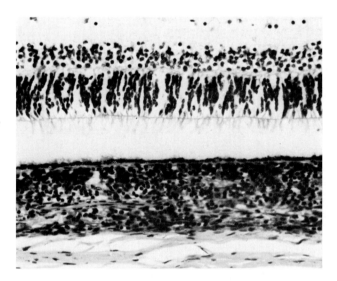

Fig. 7-8. Chronic nongranulomatous choroiditis, with a monotonous infiltrate of lymphocytes. Compare with the granulomatous type shown in Fig. 7-19. (H & E stain; ×250.)

matous and granulomatous iritis or iridocyclitis (pain, ciliary flush, miosis, flare and cells, hypopyon, and keratic precipitates) are well known. In most cases, however, the cellular response is nonspecific, microorganisms are rarely demonstrated, and microscopic examination of the inflamed uveal tissue usually fails to provide clues as to cause.

Mononuclear cells (particularly lymphocytes and plasma cells) are characteristic of chronic nonsuppurative and nongranulomatous uveitis. Plasma cell infiltrates are common, particularly in hypersensitivity uveitis in which the antibody-forming function of this cell presumably plays a role in the pathogenesis of the disease.

A close association with the HLA-B27 antigen has been noted.

Careful evaluation of the plasma cell infiltrate helps determine the longevity of a lesion under study. Chronic, long-standing lesions are characterized by relatively greater numbers of plasmacytoid cells or Russell bodies (Fig. 3-5) within the affected uveal tissue.

GRANULOMATOUS UVEITIS

Some types of uveitis have specific and often pathognomonic, clinical, and/or histopathologic appearances and, therefore, warrant special mention. Most of these forms are examples of granulomatous uveitis (see outline, section C, on p. 290).

Histopathologic recognition of chronic granulomatous uveitis is particularly useful because the pathologist can determine a specific diagnosis in a greater percentage of cases than is possible for the nongranulomatous type (Figs. 3-6, 3-7, and 7-12 to 7-15). Special staining techniques identify infectious organisms (such as those causing tuberculous, fungal, leprotic, or syphilitic uveitis) that evoke a granulomatous response. In several noninfectious granulomatous diseases the general appearance of the involved area is sufficiently characteristic.

Sarcoidosis, juvenile xanthogranuloma, histiocytosis X, sympathetic ophthalmia, and the Vogt-Koyanagi-Harada syndrome are described in this chapter. Histoplasmosis,

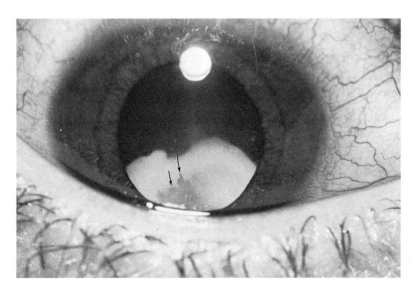

Fig. 7-9. Exogenous endophthalmitis resulting from an intraocular foreign body (wood, *arrows*). The white intraocular mass represents a massive inflammatory response to the foreign material.

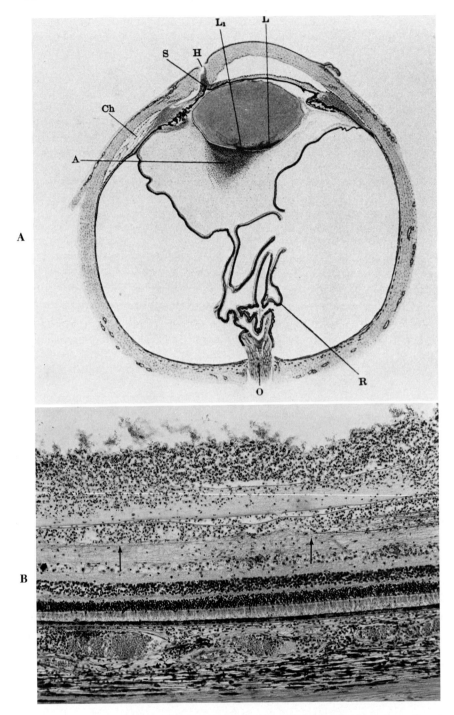

Fig. 7-10. A, Schematic drawing of endophthalmitis with beginning formation of a vitreous abscess *(A)* caused by corneal perforation *(H).* **B,** Acute endophthalmitis. Photomicrograph of inflamed vitreous, retina, and choroid. *Arrows,* Vitreal retinal junction. There is secondary membrane formation in the vitreous. (H & E stain; ×180.) (**A** from Greef R: In Orth J: Lehrbuch der speziellen pathologischen Anatomie, Berlin, 1902, Hirschwald.)

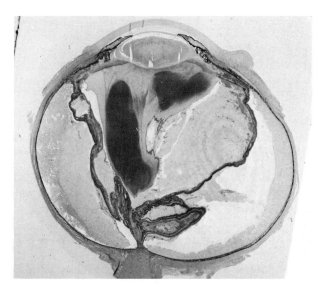

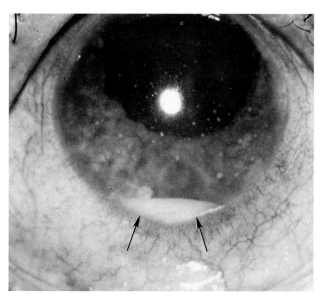

Fig. 7-11. Photomicrograph through an eye with acute purulent endophthalmitis showing a loculated vitreous abscess. The margins of the abscess are defined by the posterior border of the lens and the retina, which shows a total funnel-shaped detachment. (H & E stain; ×1.)

Fig. 7-12. Granulomatous anterior uveitis with keratic precipitates and hypopyon *(arrows).*

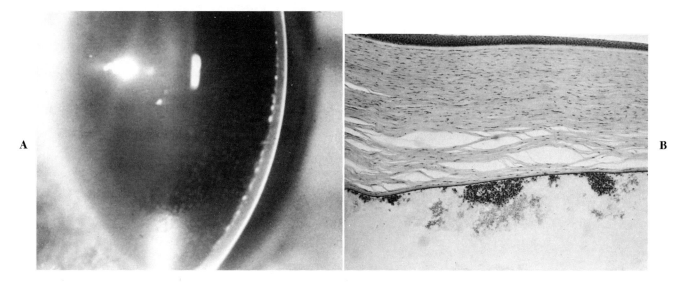

Fig. 7-13. Granulomatous anterior uveitis. **A,** Slitlamp view of keratic precipitates on the posterior corneal surface. **B,** Photomicrograph of keratitic precipitates. (H & E stain; ×100.)

toxoplasmosis and cytomegalic inclusion retinitis are considered in Chapter 8. Nematode endophthalmitis and lens-induced (phacoanaphylactic) uveitis are considered in Chapters 7 and 4, respectively.

Sarcoidosis

Sarcoidosis (Boeck-Schaumann disease) is a disease of unknown cause, which affects both sexes equally but most often affects blacks.° Sarcoid granulomas most commonly

affect the lungs, lymph nodes, liver, the subcutaneous layers of the skin, and the eyes (Fig. 7-15). The pulmonary lesion varies from a hilar adenopathy to diffuse mottling of the entire lung. Skin granulomas are responsible for the presence of maculopapular eruptions. Intraosseous granulomas occasionally lead to radiolucencies and subsequent formation of cystic spaces within bones. Elevation of serum calcium levels sometimes accompanies the bone involvement. In rare instances the granulomas may infiltrate the meninges.

Subconjunctival nodules provide an easily accessible biopsy site for tissue diagnosis (p. 571). They are most often

---

° References 64, 68, 91, 106, 128, 140, 149, 172, 194, 250, 266.

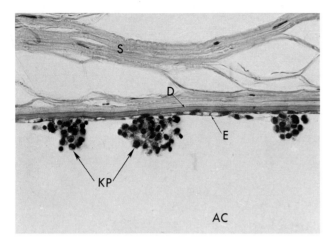

Fig. 7-14. Granulomatous anterior uveitis. Keratic precipitates *(KP)* are on the posterior corneal endothelium *(E)*. The cell clusters are composed of epithelioid cells admixed with a few lymphocytes and polymorphonuclear cells. Similar epithelioid cell clusters in different locations have received different eponyms, for example, Koeppe or Busacca nodules on the iris and Dalén-Fuchs' nodules, which are seen beneath the pigment epithelium in sympathetic ophthalmia. *S*, Corneal stroma; *D*, Descemet's membrane; *AC*, anterior chamber. (H & E stain; ×325.)

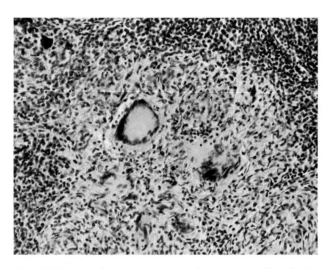

Fig. 7-15. Sarcoid noncaseating granuloma. Giant cells and pale-staining epithelioid cells are surrounded by deeply staining lymphocytes (far periphery). (H & E stain; ×325.)

positive when a clinical lesion is seen. It is necessary to take multiple sections through a biopsy not to miss a small lesion. According to Duke-Elder and Perkins,[11] the salivary and lacrimal glands are affected in as many as 10% of cases. This association sometimes leads to symptoms of Sjögren's syndrome. This syndrome, sometimes designated the Gougerot-Sjögren syndrome, is not a specific disease with a single cause but is a symptom complex characterized by dry eyes (keratoconjunctivitis sicca). Sjögren's syndrome should be distinguished from Mikulicz's syndrome, a symmetric enlargement of the lacrimal and salivary glands caused by a wide variety of inflammatory processes, includ-

ing sarcoidosis, tuberculosis, or other bacterial infections. Mikulicz's syndrome does not necessarily lead to dry eye.

Secretion of the lacrimal, salivary, and conjunctival mucous glands fails, probably as a result of an autoimmune dacryosialoadenitis. Although most cases are associated with rheumatoid arthritis or other collagen diseases, sarcoidosis is causative in a minority of cases.

A bilateral anterior uveitis is the most common intraocular manifestation of sarcoidosis. Mutton-fat keratic precipitates are the most characteristic anterior segment findings. The uveitis is usually isolated and unassociated with salivary gland involvement. Such an association (known as uveoparotitis, or Heerfordt's disease) does occur, however. This syndrome consists of a chronic bilateral, painless swelling of the parotid gland associated with typical granulomatous uveitis. The cornea may be affected with interstitial keratitis and band keratopathy, especially if hypercalcemia is present (see Chapter 3).

Posterior uveitis (chorioretinitis) occurs less commonly than iritis or iridocyclitis. The fundus lesions occur frequently in the absence of anterior uveitis or systemic involvement. As many as a third of cases with fundus involvement show other evidence of central nervous system involvement, such as papillitis, leptomeningitis, and encephalitis (p. 541).

Sarcoid chorioretinitis has two distinctive features:

1. Sheathing of retinal vessels, usually veins, occurs because of infiltration of granulomas about the retinal vascular wall. This vasculitis and perivasculitis is characteristic although not pathognomonic. The granulomatous infiltrates occasionally may lead to small-vessel occlusions, and in exceptional cases secondary retinal neovascularization and proliferative retinopathy may occur. Indeed, "sea fans," patches of neovascularization similar to those seen in sickle retinopathy (Fig. 8-34), may develop. Presumably, the microvascular occlusion resulting from granulomatous cellular infiltration creates a state of relative retinal hypoxia, which stimulates a compensatory neovascular process (p. 374).

2. The "candle-wax" lesion (taches de bougie) is probably the most characteristic lesion of fundus sarcoidosis. These yellow-white, waxy patches represent foci of granulomatous chorioretinitis.

Retinal hemorrhage resulting from inflammatory vasculitis, from papillitis or papilledema, or, exceptionally, from the neovascular retinopathy may lead to decreased visual function.

The histopathologic hallmark of sarcoidosis, the noncaseating granuloma (Figs. 3-7, 7-15, 11-14), is usually easy to distinguish from the caseating granuloma of tuberculosis. The granulomatous nodules show a distinctive appearance no matter what tissue is involved. They are composed of epithelioid cells and giant cells, with varying degrees of infiltration of lymphocytes and mononuclear cells (see discussion of the morphology of granulomatous inflammation, p. 62). Star-shaped, eosinophilic asteroid bodies and laminated Schaumann bodies composed of calcium oxalate are sometimes found in the inflammatory lesions.

Juvenile xanthogranuloma

Juvenile xanthogranuloma, or nevoxanthoendothelioma, is a benign dermatologic disease that usually affects infants

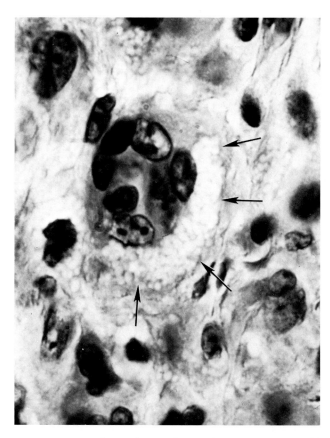

Fig. 7-16. Juvenile xanthogranuloma. This section reveals diffuse accumulation of epithelioid cells, which are generally elongated and contain a vesicular nucleus within a pale cytoplasm. Touton giant cells are characterized by deposition of lipid *(arrows, empty spaces)* that is nonstaining when processed through paraffin and stained with the hematoxylin and eosin technique. The lipid is deposited about the circumference of the cell between the rows of central nuclei and the cytoplasmic border. (H & E stain; ×1000.)

and children.* The typical raised orange skin lesions occur singly or in crops and may regress spontaneously. They are characterized by proliferation of lipid-laden histiocytes and giant cells. A similar pathologic reaction may occur on the iris. The inflammatory infiltrate on the iris is occasionally mistaken for a neoplasm, and it sometimes induces anterior segment bleeding. This condition is probably the most common cause of spontaneous hyphema in children. Trauma and bleeding from the iris neovascularization, which may be associated with retinoblastoma, need to be considered in the differential diagram of infantile-childhood hyphema. The Touton giant cell is usually abundant in the skin and iris lesions (Fig. 7-16).

Langerhan's cell histiocytosis X

The term *histiocytosis X*, first proposed by Lichtenstein[123] in 1952, refers to a spectrum of diseases of unclear cause, characterized by an abnormal proliferation of

histiocytes (Table 7-3). There has been a recent reorganization of these histiocytic syndromes into three groups based primarily on pathologic features.* The first of these three groups includes the Langerhans' cell histiocytoses. Included under this category are Letterer-Siwe, Hand-Schüller-Christian syndrome, and eosinophilic granuloma. Until recently, these three diseases were referred to singly as histiocytosis X. Now they are termed *Langerhans' cell histiocytosis X.* The second category is a distinct group that includes histiocytes that are *not* Langerhans' cells. Included in this group is juvenile xanthogranuloma.[61,82] The final group encompasses malignant disorders of histiocytes, including histiocytic lymphoma and acute monocytic leukemia.[101]

Langerhans' cells are bone marrow–derived cells characterized by a dendritic pattern, clear cytoplasm, and ultrastructurally by Birbeck granules. By cell surface markers, they belong to the monocyte/macrophage group. These cells may be detected in tissue sections by monoclonal antibodies directed against cell surface antigens including T_4 and T_6 markers, class II histocompatibility antigens, and an intracytoplasmic marker, the S-100 protein.[92,137] The widespread location of the histiocytic system in the human body explains the numerous clinical manifestations of this disease.

Letterer-Siwe disease, sometimes termed *acute differentiated histiocytosis* and the hallmark of the disease being a *moderate* degree of cellular differentiation, is typically much more "malignant" than the former two entities both in the cytologic and in the clinical sense.[157] Some authors consider eosinophilic granuloma and Hand-Schüller-Christian disease as variants of the same disease process, that is, proliferative histiocytic diseases with *well-differentiated* cells. Highly disseminated forms of Hand-Schüller-Christian disease, however, may occur, which may clinically resemble Letterer-Siwe disease (Fig. 7-17). Therefore, because Langerhans' cell histiocytosis X may exhibit such a wide variety of clinical manifestations, it does not always fit precisely into one of the three previously mentioned categories.

Eosinophilic granuloma of bone (Color Plate 7-2), the most "benign" disease in this group, may occur over a wide age range, from the preschool years to adulthood.[119] Most cases are diagnosed before the age of 10; but onset well into adult life is not unusual; therefore, these patients are on the average slightly older than those in the other two categories. The hallmark of the disease consists of bone infiltrates, which may be unifocal or multifocal. They most commonly affect the skull, ribs, vertebrae, pelvis, scapula, and proximal long bones. These lesions may be visible or palpable and may be associated with pain or tenderness.[117-119] So-called extraosseous forms of eosinophilic granuloma, most commonly affecting the gastrointestinal tract and lung, have also been described.

Unifocal eosinophilic granuloma behaves almost invariably as a benign lesion and responds readily to excision or radiation therapy. With multifocal disease, there is clear overlap in symptoms with Hand-Schüller-Christian

---

* References 58, 63, 76, 78, 108, 125, 129, 179, 183, 205, 207, 251, 255, 256, 259, 282, 295, 300, 301

* References 45, 47, 53, 60, 62, 81, 95, 96, 110, 118, 122, 124, 138, 158-161, 165, 169, 185, 193, 197, 212, 234, 243, 268, 286, 289.

Table 7-3. Langerhan's cell histiocytoses (histiocytosis X)

	Age of onset	Clinical presentation	Tissues involved	Cell differentiate	Prognosis	Therapy
Eosinophilic granuloma	Preschool years to adulthood	Exophthalmos of periorbital lesions	Usually bony infiltrates most common in skull, ribs, vertebrae, pelvis, scapula, and proximal long bones	Well differentiated	Excellent	Excision or radiation
Hand-Schuller-Christian disease	Usually before age 4	Exophthalmos or periorbital lesion; diabetes insipidus; signs and symptoms of visceral involvement as in Letterer-Siwe disease	Bony lesions as in eosinophilic granuloma and visceral involvement as in Letterer-Siwe disease	Well differentiated	Intermediate	Excision or radiation for bony lesions; radiation for diabetes insipidus; chemotherapy for visceral involvement
Letterer-Siwe disease (acute differentiated histiocytosis)	Usually before age 2; may be congenital	Signs and symptoms of visceral involvement of skin, lungs, lymph nodes, liver, spleen, bone marrow, and gingival mucosa	No bony lesions but visceral involvement of skin, lungs, lymph nodes, liver, spleen bone marrow, and gingival mucosa	Moderate degree of differentiation	Poor	Aggressive chemotherapy

Courtesy Dr. Kevin Miller, University of Utah Medical Center, Salt Lake City.

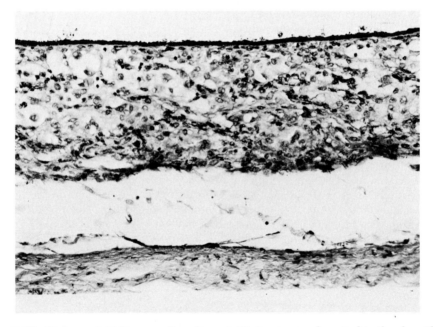

Fig. 7-17. Histiocytosis X (Letterer-Siwe disease). Histiocytes are deposited in the choroid, so this layer is several times normal thickness. Both the nuclei and cytoplasm of the histiocytes, which have almost completely replaced the choroidal melanocytes, are poorly stained, presenting a foamy appearance. The sensory retina has been artifactitiously removed, but the retinal pigment epithelium remains at the top. The sclera *(below)* was separated from choroid during processing. (H & E stain; ×200.) (From Mittelman D, Apple DJ, and Goldberg MF: Am J Ophthalmol 75: 261, 1973.)

disease, and the two entities may be difficult to separate by either clinical or histologic criteria.

Hand-Schüller-Christian disease connotes an intermediate form between eosinophilic granuloma and Letterer-Siwe disease.[39] It includes a combination of the bony lesions that are more typically associated with eosinophilic granuloma and some of the visceral and soft tissue lesions that are the hallmarks of Letterer-Siwe disease. The classic clinical triad of Hand-Schüller-Christian disease includes bony lesions in the skull, exophthalmos, and diabetes insipidus. Actually, the full triad occurs in only a small percentage of patients. This disease manifests itself during childhood, usually occurring before the age of 4.

This is a slightly older age group than that seen in Letterer-Siwe disease, which typically occurs in infancy. As one might expect, Hand-Schüller-Christian disease often has a clinical course intermediate in character between that of eosinophilic granuloma and Letterer-Siwe disease.

Letterer-Siwe disease. Letterer-Siwe disease (acute differentiated histiocytosis), the most severe form of histiocytosis X, is usually seen in children under 2 years of age (Fig. 7-17). In addition, congenital forms have been described. The disease is rapidly progressive, often fatal, and is characterized by widespread tissue involvement with cellular infiltration. Most commonly involved are the skin, lungs, lymph nodes, liver, spleen, bone marrow, and gingival mucosa. The disease is not uniformly fatal, however. In one series, a mortality rate of 70% in children under the age of 6 months was reported. In general, the younger the child at the onset of the disease, the worse the prognosis. The bony involvement typically seen in eosinophilic granuloma is less prominent. These patients may develop liver, lung, or bone marrow dysfunction, all of which are poor prognostic signs. Most deaths are secondary to hepatic or lung failure or complications, such as bleeding or infection.

The widespread effects of all three forms of Langerhan's histiocytosis sometimes lead to infiltration of ocular and periocular structures (Table 7-4).[93,147,150] Several studies have shown that the incidence of orbital involvement is about 20%. In addition, only about half of these cases develop proptosis. The most commonly seen signs of eye involvement include unilateral and bilateral proptosis and, less frequently, papilledema with optic atrophy.

Exophthalmos is usually caused by lytic lesions of the orbital bones but rarely may be the result of involvement of the orbital soft tissues. On rare occasions the globe may have infiltrates, such as the choroidal infiltrates seen in Letterer-Siwe disease. In addition, secondary open-angle glaucoma, bilateral perforating corneal ulcers, nystagmus, secondary intracranial palsies, posterior scleritis, eyelid infiltration, and secondary infection all have been reported.

When confronted with a questionable case of Langerhans' cell histiocytosis X, appropriate studies include a chest radiograph, bone scan, bone marrow biopsy, and/or liver function tests. In addition, appropriate consultations should be made. Orbital radiographs may reveal evidence of a lytic lesion that frequently shows a narrow zone of sclerosis. The gold standard of diagnosis is still a detailed histopathologic examination of appropriate biopsy specimens.

Single bony lesions and even cases with multifocal le-

Table 7-4. Ocular or periocular manifestations of Langerhan's histiocytosis

1. *Anterior chamber*: Cells and flare caused by anterior uveitis; hypopyon; spontaneous hemorrhage
2. *Choroid*: Extramedullary hematopoiesis (rare); infiltration by histiocytic cells leading to a rather diffuse flat thickening
3. *Conjunctiva*: Chemosis; dilated vessels
4. *Cornea*: Bullous keratopathy; endothelial atrophy; infiltration; pannus; perforation; scarring; ulcer; vascularization
5. *Eyelids*: Edema; infiltration; rash; xanthoma, especially in patients with icterus
6. *Globe*: Exophthalmos; luxation
7. *Iris or ciliary body*: Cellular infiltration with possible secondarily increased intraocular pressure; infiltration; iridocyclitis or cyclitis with possible formation of a cyclitic membrane; nodular lesions mimicking tumors or juvenile xanthogranuloma; pigmentary changes, including heterochromia; secondary atrophy; uveitis or iridocyclitis with potential for synechiae formation
8. *Lens*: Cataract
9. *Optic nerve*: Atrophy and gliosis; infiltration of surrounding meninges; papilledema
10. *Orbit*: Infiltrates; periorbital bone lesions
11. *Retina*: Degeneration; detachment and retinal folds; edema; histiocytic infiltration
12. *Sclera*: Episcleritis; scleritis
13. *Vitreous*: Histiocytic infiltration, often leading to liquefaction
14. *Other*: Glaucoma; nystagmus; phthisis bulbi; poor pupillary dilatation with mydriatics; visual loss

sions affecting bone carry excellent prognosis.[119] Spontaneous clearing may actually occur in some cases. When therapy is required, lesions are often best treated with curettage and/or local low-dose irradiation.[46,61,72,88,174]

The most common ophthalmic complications of Langerhans' cell histiocytosis X include localized orbital and periorbital lesions with or without exophthalmos. These complications can be treated much like other localized lesions. Low-dose radiation therapy with 300 to 600 rads and/or curettage is often effective.

The optimum treatment regimen for disseminated Langerhans' cell histiocytosis X (usually connoting severe forms of the Hand-Schüller-Christian disease variant and Letterer-Siwe disease) has not been established. The variable clinical presentation or course of the disease and the fact that it sometimes undergoes spontaneous remission have made evaluation of therapy difficult. This has been further complicated by the fact that histiocytosis X has been found to respond to a wide variety of therapeutic modalities. These include steroids, vinca alkaloids (vincristine or vinblastine), alkylating agents, antimetabolites, antibiotics, radiation, and thymic extract.[19]

Diabetes insipidus is a classic complication and local radiation therapy may be beneficial in preventing its progression. This treatment is most effective in patients with at least partial urinary-concentrating ability. Low doses of 800 to 1200 rad delivered to the hypothalmic-pituitary region are probably sufficient for treatment. Vasopressin is important in the management of patients who retain some degree of pituitary dysfunction. Intrathecal methotrexate has also been used to treat diabetes insipidus, but the results have been disappointing.

Some patients have been shown to have decreased levels of human growth hormone associated with impaired linear growth. Therapy with human growth hormone is, therefore, indicated in selected patients.

Infections are common in patients with Langerhans' cell histiocytosis X, because of both the nature of the disease and its treatment. Otitis media is a frequent complication and may result in loss of hearing. The physician should watch for and be prepared to treat these infections; however, prophylactic antibiotics are not useful because they predispose the patient to opportunistic infections.

Sympathetic ophthalmia

Sympathetic ophthalmia[81,84,302-356] (Color Plates 7-3 and 7-4) is a bilateral diffused, granulomatous T-cell-mediated inflammation of the uveal tract, which generally occurs after a perforating wound involving uveal prolapse in the injured (exciting) eye. Unilateral sympathetic ophthalmia has been reported, but it is probable that many such cases actually represent a subclinical inflammation in the other eye or a mild inflammation in the opposite eye that may have been missed clinically. Sympathetic ophthalmia not associated with ocular perforation is an extreme rarity, but has been observed after noninvasive therapeutic procedures, for example, transscleral cryopexy.

This type of uveitis most commonly follows accidental trauma in which the iris or ciliary body tissue is incarcerated in the wound (Fig. 3-57, A). Roughly half to three fourths of cases result from accidental trauma; the remainder are postsurgical. Although sympathetic ophthalmia has been reported after modern surgical techniques such as retinal procedures and vitrectomy, the number of cases following surgery is clearly decreasing in incidence because of better surgical techniques developed in recent years.[303,330,342] In unusual instances sympathetic ophthalmia may be caused by perforation of a corneal ulcer or rupture of a corneoscleral ulcer or corneoscleral staphyloma. In the past a particularly high incidence of sympathetic ophthalmia occurred after certain glaucoma procedures, particularly iridencleisis or other filtering operations. Although corneoscleral perforation with prolapse of uveal tissue into the wound is usually considered a prerequisite to the development of sympathetic ophthalmia, fortunately this complication occurs in only a small percentage of such cases.

The classic theory of pathogenesis of sympathetic ophthalmia states that this disease is caused by a hypersensitivity to uveal pigment liberated during injury to the exciting eye, which acts as an antigen leading to an autoimmune reaction against the affected patient's own uveal pigment. This induces a granulomatous uveitis, not only in the exciting eye but also in the opposite, noninjured (sympathizing) eye.

The pathogenesis of sympathetic ophthalmia is under current investigation. New studies have indicated that sympathetic ophthalmia may actually be an autoimmune disease in which the patient reacts to a protein on the membrane of the outer segment of retinal photoreceptors.* The wound in sympathetic ophthalmia, which is often followed by uveal prolapse, is believed by some authorities to be an important mechanism by which the retinal **S** antigen is introduced into the lymphatic system. Because the eye contains no lymphatics, an uninjured eye theoretically cannot introduce the retinal antigen in such a way as to activate this immune system.

Sympathetic ophthalmia occurs most commonly in men, presumably because of their greater exposure to injury. The incidence of the disease has greatly decreased in recent years, probably because of improved treatment of injured eyes and the use of corticosteroids. Duke-Elder and Perkins[11] stated that the interval between injury and the onset of inflammation may vary from extremes of 5 days to 42 years. They noted, however, that onset of inflammation is rare within 2 weeks and that 65% of cases occur between 2 weeks and 2 months, 80% within 3 months, and 90% within a year.[353] The most dangerous time is considered to be the fourth to the eighth week after injury. Development after 3 months is, therefore, unusual but may occur. In some cases of late-onset sympathetic ophthalmia, it is probable that the patient may have had a mild inflammation that was clinically undetected in early stages.

The usual clinical picture is that of a bilateral granulomatous uveitis. Accompanying systemic signs such as poliosis, vitiligo (see Vogt-Koyanagi-Harada syndrome, p. 299), and central nervous system alterations may occur. When the anterior segment is involved, mutton-fat keratic precipitates are sometimes deposited on the cornea, and flare and cells form in the anterior chamber. The clinical picture is, therefore, similar to that of other forms of granulomatous inflammation. The history of injury, the determination of the interval of time between the injury and the onset of inflammation, the bilaterality of the disease, and a lack of findings to support other causes of granulomatous uveitis all distinguish sympathetic uveitis from other diseases.

In untreated persons the disease is progressive, leading to phthisis bulbi in the majority of cases. Improved techniques of wound closure, corticosteroid therapy, and immunosuppressive therapy and rapid removal of blind, perforated globes that may predispose to a sympathetic ophthalmia in the fellow eye have greatly improved the prognosis in recent years. Evisceration rather than enucleation of the traumatized eye does not prevent a contralateral sympathetic response.

Two thirds of patients with sympathetic ophthalmia have been shown to achieve visual acuity of 20/60 or better. Major complications include cataracts, glaucoma, exudative retinal detachments, corneoretinal scarring, and inflammation of the optic nerve. The cataracts can easily be removed when the disease is quiescent, but the glaucoma is extremely difficult to treat. The disease waxes and wanes, and relapses may occur even after years.

Sympathetic ophthalmia must be considered when evaluating the differential diagnosis of a diffuse choroidal thickening. Other conditions that increase the width of the choroid in a similar manner include other forms of uveitis such as the Vogt-Koyanagi-Harada syndrome (p. 299) and phacoanaphylactic uveitis. Tumors to be considered in this differential diagnosis include the diffuse, flat malignant melanoma of the choroid (p 310; Figs. 7-49 and 7-50), carcinoma metastatic to the choroid (p. 328), and benign or malignant lymphoid (or leukemic) lesions that may infil-

---

* References 328, 336, 343, 344, 346, 347, 356.

trate the choroid. The true nature of each condition can usually be determined by correlation of the history and clinical findings with the histopathologic appearance.

The histopathologic appearance of the sympathizing eye is identical to that of the exciting eye, with the notable exception that the wound track is identifiable only in the exciting eye. Predictably, the wound in most cases consists of a corneal or scleral perforation with uveal incarceration in the wound. The uveitis is recognizable as a granulomatous inflammatory process that leads to diffuse thickening of any or all components of the uvea (Figs. 7-18 and 7-19). A panuveitis is not uncommon in severe cases.

The choroid contains epithelial cells, varying numbers of giant cells, mononuclear cells, lymphocytes (predominantly T-lymphocytes), eosinophils, and plasma cells. The choriocapillaris is typically spared of inflammatory infiltrates (Fig. 7-19, *A*). Although the epithelioid and giant cell components of the inflammatory infiltrate indicate a granulomatous reaction, discrete nodular granulomas such as those often seen in sarcoidosis, tuberculosis, or tuberculoid leprosy do not commonly appear. Thus the cellular infiltrate is considered more diffuse in nature and is designated a diffuse granulomatous inflammation (Fig. 7-18). The epithelioid component is easily distinguished from the nonspecific mononuclear infiltrate in tissue sections (Fig. 7-19, *C*). Actually, in many cases the lymphocytic infiltrate predominates, especially early in the course of the disease. In such cases, the epithelioid component is sometimes scarcely visible. In other instances, eosinophils are prominent. The latter finding suggests a role of this cell in the allergic process.

In most patients with sympathetic ophthalmia, clumps of dispersed melanin pigment are deposited within the inflammatory infiltrate. Most of the pigment is phagocytosed by epithelioid cells and giant cells. This finding partially accounts for the early, classic theory of the pathogenesis of sympathetic ophthalmia: that the inflammatory response represents an immune reaction to uveal pigment. As noted previously, this theory is now being questioned.

In contrast to the findings in tuberculosis, the sensory retina in the majority of eyes with sympathetic ophthalmia remains free of inflammation (Fig. 7-18); however, recent studies have indicated that the retina may be at least minimally involved in 25% to 30% of cases. In addition, when the granulomatous reaction is especially severe, the choriocapillaris may also be obliterated by the inflammatory infiltration.

Recent experimental models of sympathetic ophthalmia, created by injection of variable doses of retinal **S** antigen into guinea pigs, may explain the differences seen histopathologically in various cases.[343,344] Small doses of the injected antigen produce only a chronic lymphocytic inflammation at or near the posterior pole, correlating with the early stages seen clinically. Medium-sized doses produce a typical picture of granulomatous inflammation of the choroid. Large doses also produce an acute necrotizing inflammation containing polymorphonuclear neutrophils that may also involve the choriocapillaris and retina and may become admixed with the background granulomatous inflammation of the choroid. Large doses of antigen are thought to activate an immune complex mechanism and the cell-mediated mechanism activated by smaller doses.

When the iris and ciliary body are extensively involved or incarcerated in the wound and the inflammatory infiltrate is particularly massive in the anterior segment around the lens, differentiation of phacoanaphylactic uveitis from sympathetic uveitis is difficult.[304,314] In fact, these two conditions sometimes exist simultaneously (Chapter 4). In such cases the presence or absence of choroidal involvement is the major means of documenting sympathetic ophthalmia. Diffuse granulomatous thickening of the choroid is not a feature of uncomplicated phacoanaphylactic uveitis.

As with any granulomatous uveitis, mutton-fat keratic precipitates may occur. These are nodules or clusters of epithelioid cells (Figs. 3-6, 7-13, and 7-14). The Dalén-Fuchs' nodule (Fig. 7-19, *B*) also is composed of aggregates of cells that lie immediately beneath the retinal pigment epithelium. There are two theories as to the origin of these nodules: they probably represent infiltrates of epithelioid cells and monocytes but may also in part represent clusters of proliferated retinal pigment epithelial cells or a combination of the two.[230,246] In microscopic sections, these mounds of cells resemble a pile of cannon balls that elevate the overlying pigment epithelium and lead to varying degrees of degeneration and hypopigmentation of the affected pigment epithelium. Dalén-Fuchs' nodules are characteristic, although not diagnostic, of sympathetic ophthalmia. They may occur in other forms of granulomatous intraocular inflammation, particularly those that typically involve and destroy the sensory retina (as in tuberculosis).

Vogt-Koyanagi-Harada syndrome (uveomeningoencephalitis)

The Vogt-Koyanagi-Harada (VKH) syndrome (Figs. 7-20 and 7-21) combines two diseases previously believed to be separate entities: (1) the Vogt-Koyanagi syndrome, which connotes a severe granulomatous bilateral iridocycli-

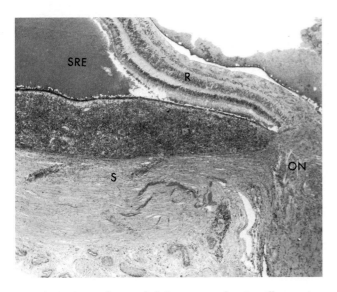

Fig. 7-18. Sympathetic ophthalmia: view of peripapillary region. The choroid has been diffusely thickened by the granulomatous infiltrate. *R,* Detached but noninflamed retina; *ON,* optic nerve. *SRE,* subretinal exudate; *S,* sclera (H & E stain; ×25.)

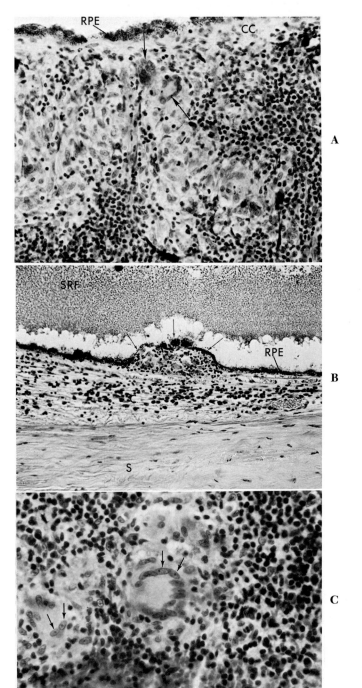

Fig. 7-19. Sympathetic ophthalmia. **A,** Section of choroid with overlying retinal pigment epithelium *(RPE).* The sensory retina is artifactitiously detached. Two distinct cellular patterns occur within the choroidal infiltrate. Major portions in the center and toward the left consist primarily of epithelioid cells, palestaining cells with vesicular oval nuclei that contain nucleoli. Because these cells are arranged in a syncytium, individual cell borders are not visible and the cells appear to merge with one another. Two giant cells *(arrows)* are within the central infiltrate of epithelioid cells. The second cellular pattern consists of lymphocytic infiltrates surrounding the central granulomatous focus. The lymphocytes are recognized as small round cells with hyperchromatic (deeply staining) nuclei. There is sparing of the choriocapillaris *(CC),* which appears as an uninvolved zone between the pigment epithelium and inflamed choroid. (H & E stain; ×160.) **B,** Dalén-Fuchs' nodule (demarcated by *arrows*) from a patient with sympathetic ophthalmia. This lesion consists of a piling up of epithelioidlike cells and proliferative pigment epithelial cells (sometimes likened to a pile of cannon balls) immediately subjacent to the overlying retinal pigment epithelium *(RPE).* The sensory retina is detached by a serous subretinal fluid *(SRF).* The choroid *(C)* contains a diffuse infiltrate of chronic inflammatory cells, which signifies a diffuse form of chronic granulomatous inflammation. *S,* Sclera. (H & E stain; ×150.) **C,** Langhans type of giant cell, characterized by a margination of nuclei *(arrows)* about the periphery of the cell, is seen within the granulomatous choroidal infiltrate. A giant cell probably represents the fusion of several epithelioid cells. The central focus of epithelioid-giant cell reaction is ringed by lymphocytes.

tis associated with posterior uveitis, meningoencephalitis, and other signs, including poliosis, alopecia, and vitiligo, and (2) Harada's disease, which in general shows fewer changes of the skin but similar eye and central nervous system changes, including posterior uveitis with exudative retinal detachment and meningoencephalitis.* Because of this overlap, many thought that these two conditions represent clinical variations of a single disease entity.

* References 43, 44, 55, 65, 69, 70, 85, 97, 102, 103, 121, 134-136, 143, 156, 171, 198-200, 206, 211, 216, 221, 241, 244, 248, 260, 265, 272, 277, 296, 298, 299.

The VKH syndrome is most common in Orientals, blacks, American Indians, and other dark-skinned races. It comprises only 1% to 4% of uveitis cases in the United States but up to 7% of those in Japan. Age of onset is generally in the range of 20 to 40 years, and the incidence is the same for both sexes. The VKH syndrome is predominantly a sporadic disease; only two affected families have been reported. The HLA-Bw22J has been positive in 40% of Japanese patients.

The clinical picture is marked by extreme variability. In most cases, the disease is heralded by an acute onset of the ocular inflammatory symptoms, closely followed by

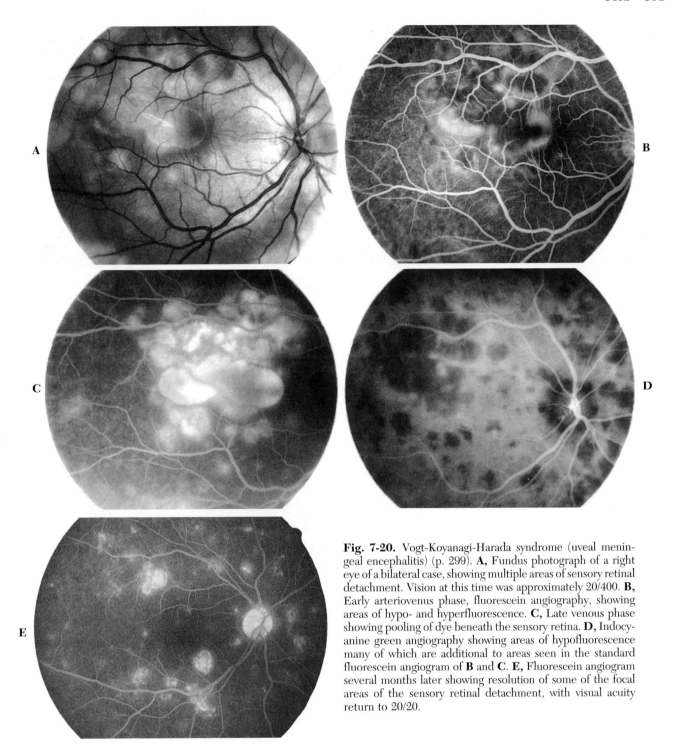

Fig. 7-20. Vogt-Koyanagi-Harada syndrome (uveal meningeal encephalitis) (p. 299). **A,** Fundus photograph of a right eye of a bilateral case, showing multiple areas of sensory retinal detachment. Vision at this time was approximately 20/400. **B,** Early arteriovenus phase, fluorescein angiography, showing areas of hypo- and hyperfluorescence. **C,** Late venous phase showing pooling of dye beneath the sensory retina. **D,** Indocyanine green angiography showing areas of hypofluorescence many of which are additional to areas seen in the standard fluorescein angiogram of **B** and **C**. **E,** Fluorescein angiogram several months later showing resolution of some of the focal areas of the sensory retinal detachment, with visual acuity return to 20/20.

neurologic signs and symptoms. The skin lesions may appear later, but this is variable. In most instances, the uveitis is bilateral; the most common signs are the features of anterior uveitis, including cell and flare, keratic precipitates, and iris nodules. Increased intraocular pressure may occur.

Posterior uveitis with vitreous cells may also be present. Extensive retinal detachments occur. These often begin in the macular region and progress inferiorly. These detachments are often bullous, with shifting fluid. Optic disc edema and hyperemia, retinal edema, and optic neuritis

may also be seen. Late ocular signs include anterior and posterior synechiae, glaucoma, cataract, and the so-called sunset glow fundus with marked decrease in pigmentation.

Fluorescein angiography is the only ancillary study that is likely to be of any benefit in establishing the diagnosis. Early in the disease, multiple hyperfluorescent dots at the level of the retinal pigment epithelium are present. These are associated with slowly expanding areas of staining of the subretinal fluid. The capillaries of the optic nerve head may also leak. Window defects are seen in late stages. Retinal vessels generally remain normal. The neurologic signs,

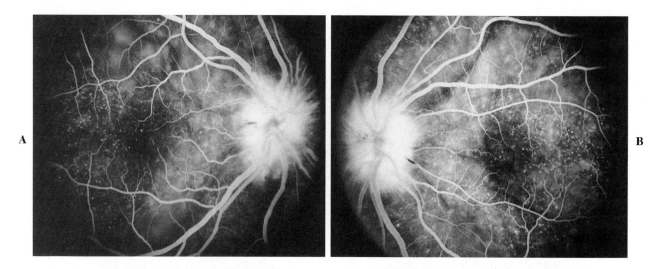

Fig. 7-21. Vogt-Koyanagi-Harada syndrome, bilateral case, fluorescein angiograms, late venous phase. There is leakage of the optic disc at the optic nerve head, with typical pinpoints of hyperfluorescence and pooling of dye beneath the sensory retina. **A,** Right eye. **B,** Left eye.

Table 7-5. Comparison of the Vogt-Koyanagi-Harada syndrome with sympathetic ophthalmia

	VKH syndrome	Sympathetic ophthalmia
Age	20–40 years	All ages
Race	Asian, blacks and other dark skinned persons	Mostly whites
Sex	Equal	Male predominance
History of trauma	None	Always
Uveitis	Granulomatous or nongranulomatous	Granulomatous
Phacoanaphylaxis	Absent	Up to 46%
Neurologic findings	Common	Rare
Dermatologic findings	Common	Rare
Genetic markers	HLA-Bw22J	HLA-A11
Histopathologic findings		
Choriocapillaris sparing	Absent	Present
Predominant cellular infiltrate	Plasma cells	Lymphocytes, epitheliod cells
Choroidal involvement	Patchy	Diffuse
Retinal pigment epithelial migration into retina	Present	Absent
Increased inflammation in black persons	Absent	Present

Courtesy Dr. Randall Johnston, University of Utah Medical Center, Salt Lake City.

which result from the meningoencephalitis, include headache, personality changes and confusion, cranial nerve palsies, and evidence of chronic meningitis with increased white blood cells in the cerebrospinal fluid. The dermatologic signs of poliosis (whitening of the hair, eyelashes, and eyebrows), alopecia, and vitiligo are characteristic of the Vogt-Koyanagi variation of the VKH syndrome.

Histopathologically, the uveal infiltrates, particularly in the posterior segment, may be difficult to differentiate from the picture seen in sympathetic ophthalmia (p. 298; Table 7-5). The uveitis may be both granulomatous or nongranulomatous, and Dalén-Fuchs' nodules may be present. In general, infiltration of plasma cells is more prominent than in sympathetic ophthalmia, and the choriocapillaris is generally involved in contrast to most cases of sympathetic ophthalmia. Focal areas of retinal pigment epithelial migration into the retina and active chorioretinitis are also present.

The cause of the VKH syndrome is unknown, but theo-

ries of pathogenesis include viral infection, immunologic response to pigment of the uvea or of the retinal pigment epithelium, or hypersensitivity to other unknown substances.

ANTERIOR SEGMENT ISCHEMIA SYNDROME

Although the anterior segment ischemia syndrome may occur in association with various forms of uveitis, it is sometimes manifested in instances that do not involve a true "inflammatory process."[359-403] The sequelae of this disease, however, forms a clinical and pathologic picture similar to that seen after primary inflammation of the uvea and are, therefore, described here. Although the cause differs from that of classic uveitis, both have in common a secondary breakdown of the blood-aqueous barrier with release of cells and protein into the anterior segment, leading to destruction of tissue and many of the sequelae listed on page 303.[360,369,372,373,392]

The term *anterior segment ischemia* connotes that an

ischemic (either hypoxic or anoxic) insult to this portion of the eye has lead to secondary complications. This occurs when all or a portion of the vascular supply to the area is disrupted.[390,391,403] The two basic types are (1) that resulting from various types of vascular disease (reviewed by Knox[385,386]) and (2) that which is iatrogenic, usually a result of surgical intervention, which may disrupt the anterior or posterior ciliary circulation. Following is an outline of the pathogenesis of anterior segment ischemia:[*]

A. Vascular disease
  1. Diffuse arteriosclerosis or arteritis
    a. Carotid artery occlusion: poor collateral circulation resulting in decreased total blood flow
    b. Ophthalmic artery occlusion: interruption of vascular supply
    c. Aortic arch syndromes: decreased blood flow to the head and upper extremities, possibly a result of diffuse arteriosclerosis or an arteritis, for example, Takayasu's disease[362,370,392,394]
    d. Diabetes mellitus: predisposition caused by circulation impaired by microvascular disease and arteriosclerosis
  2. Carotid-cavernous fistulae: decreased total blood flow resulting from venous stasis and shunting[396]
  3. Acute angle-closure glaucoma: increased intraocular pressure higher than the capillary filling pressure, resulting in a decrease or cessation of blood flow
B. Iatrogenic disruption of the vascular supply
  1. Strabismus surgery: major disruption of anterior ciliary circulation because of multiple disinsertions of the recti muscle[364,365,384,402]
  2. Retinal detachment surgery
    a. Scleral buckling: compromise of the posterior ciliary arteries because of direct compression
    b. Temporary tenotomization: disruption of the anterior ciliary arteries if muscles are temporarily disinserted for greater exposure
    c. Scleral resection: possible disruption of posterior ciliary artery or arteries
    d. Diathermy or cryotherapy: coagulation or direct destruction of the posterior ciliary artery or arteries
  3. Hyperviscosity syndrome: predisposition to intravascular thrombosis and decreased blood flow as a result of increased viscosity and, consequently, possible development of anterior segment ischemia after surgery (for example, hemoglobin SC and chronic lymphocytic leukemia disease)[277,291,302]
  4. Pharmacologic origin: intravenous perfusion of alkylating agents (for instance, nitrogen mustard) in an attempt to treat intracranial malignancies, causing ischemic changes
  5. Radiation: possible ischemic or necrotic changes when administered in or around the orbit[389]
  6. Intraocular lens implantation[361]: compression and/or erosion into the major arterial circle or vascular plexus of the ciliary muscle by footplates or hoops of intraocular lenses implanted at the limbus or in the ciliary sulcus

The most important iatrogenic causes of ischemia of the anterior segment are muscle removal in strabismus surgery

and surgery for retinal detachment.[*] The actual degree of vascular compromise necessary for ischemia or necrosis to occur is still uncertain; however, studies have shown that certain factors predispose one to anterior segment ischemia. Advanced age is one factor, probably because of the diffuse arteriosclerosis in some members of this age group. This fact reduces the number of simultaneous muscle disinsertions that can be safely performed in the elderly. Disease states that increase the viscosity of the blood and thus cause decreased peripheral blood flow and stasis (such as hemoglobin SC disease and chronic lymphocytic leukemia) similarly predispose one to ischemia of the anterior segment.[367,383,395]

A chronic anterior segment ischemia following posterior chamber lens implantation has been reported by Apple and coworkers.[361] The ischemia resulted from deep erosion of a lens loop into the iridociliary sulcus with partial bisection of the ciliary body and pressure on the major arterial circle and the rich plexus of vessels within the ciliary muscle.

Clinical signs of anterior segment ischemia are related to breakdown of the blood-aqueous barrier with outpouring of cells and exudate into the anterior chamber. This causes a reaction resembling or identical to that of an anterior uveitis. The changes include chemosis, striate keratopathy with folds in Descemet's membrane, corneal edema, and corneal vascularization. Aqueous flare with cells, hypopyon, hyphema, and a poorly reactive eccentric pupil may ensue. Other complications are segmental iris atrophy, anterior subcapsular and/or cortical cataract formation (complicated cataract), posterior and/or peripheral anterior synechiae, and rubeosis iridis. Intraocular pressure changes varying from hypotony to glaucoma may occur. A small percentage of cases progress to phthisis bulbi. The frequency and severity of these assorted clinical manifestations can be highly variable. Many of these signs are more typical of acute, massive ischemia, whereas ocular neovascularization and neovascular glaucoma are considered responses to chronic ischemia.

Iris fluorescein angiography can demonstrate distinct areas of ischemia and can be a useful diagnostic or confirmatory test in patients with suspected anterior segment ischemia.[368,380]

The most prominent and consistent histopathologic changes in anterior segment ischemia include segmental necrosis and atrophy of the iris and ciliary body, which occur as sequelae to the early inflammatory process.[361,364,365,402] The necrosis is manifest as a loss of iris structure with dispersion of the iris and ciliary body pigment epithelium. The necrotic and atrophic changes are often localized to the area of greatest surgical manipulation in iatrogenically induced anterior segment ischemia.

SEQUELAE OF UVEITIS

The major sequelae of uveitis are

A. Cornea
  1. Endothelial degeneration and corneal edema
  2. Bullous keratopathy
  3. Degenerative pannus

---

[*] Courtesy Drs. Katherine Loftfield and James Reidy, University of Utah Medical Center, Salt Lake City.

[*] References 364, 365, 369, 371, 376-378, 383, 384, 388, 397, 400, 402.

4. Band keratopathy
5. Corneal ulceration, keratitis
6. Scarring and vascularization
B. Anterior chamber and pupil
  1. Angle closure and glaucoma caused by peripheral anterior synechiae
  2. Secondary open-angle glaucoma after organization of inflammatory debris (hypopyon) or blood, with formation of retrocorneal fibrous membrane
  3. Glaucoma secondary to occlusion and seclusion of the pupil with iris bombé
C. Iris and lens
  1. Iris atrophy
  2. Pupillary membranes
  3. Rubeosis iridis and ectropion uveae
  4. Secondary cataract
D. Ciliary body
  1. Degeneration and hypotony, often with retinal and choroidal detachment and macular edema
  2. Cyclitic membrane (proliferation of ciliary epithelium, organization of inflammatory residue or blood between the ciliary processes)
E. Vitreous
  1. Liquefaction, shrinkage, posterior detachment
  2. Fibrous organization
  3. Neovascularization
F. Reactive proliferation of the retinal pigment epithelium, ultimate phthisis bulbi

The major corneal changes are illustrated individually in Chapter 3.

Incompletely treated anterior uveitis can lead to formation of peripheral anterior synechiae through various mechanisms. They may result from anterior bowing of the lens-iris diaphragm by retrolental space-occupying tissue or debris; from pupillary block; from iridocorneal adhesions caused by fibrinous exudate or cells in the anterior chamber; or from rubeosis iridis, anterior chamber hemorrhage, or both. Rubeosis iridis and ectropion uveae are described and illustrated in Chapter 8.

Occlusion and seclusion of the pupil (Figs. 7-4 and 7-5) with iris bombé resulting from uveitis are common in ineffectively treated cases. The formation of a pupillary membrane (occlusion) or posterior synechiae (seclusion) is usually caused by organization of the inflammatory mass or blood. Not infrequently, occlusion and seclusion of the pupil occur simultaneously. The pupillary membrane seen in acquired occlusion of the pupil differs from the congenital pupillary membrane (p. 28) in that the former may arise at sites along the iris other than the collarette.

Secondary cataract following uveitis shows the histopathologic features described in Chapter 5. The main changes include liquefaction of the cortex with posterior migration of the lens epithelium and posterior subcapsular cataract and occasional formation of an anterior subcapsular cataract. The latter is often a fibrous metaplasia of the anterior lens epithelium caused by irritation from an anterior uveitis or posterior synechiae.

Long-standing uveitis leads to a degeneration or "hyalinization" of the ciliary body stroma. This can result in a decrease in aqueous formation, hypotony, macular edema, and choroidal detachment.

Ciliary epithelium and retinal pigment epithelium need little stimulation to commence proliferation or reactive hyperplasia. Intraocular inflammatory processes and irritation caused by other nonspecific insults, such as penetrating or perforating trauma, often stimulate aimless ciliary epithelial and retinal pigment epithelial overgrowth. Such extensive proliferation of the ciliary epithelium contributes to the formation of a cyclitic membrane. A cyclitic membrane is formed by a combination of factors, including proliferation and fibrous metaplasia of the ciliary epithelium, organization of inflammatory residue after uveitis or endophthalmitis, organization of blood in the retrolental region, and/or condensation and fibrosis of the anterior vitreous face.[67] Contraction or shrinkage of a cyclitic membrane may cause retinal or choroidal detachment.

Proliferation and degenerative changes of the retinal pigment epithelium occur similarly to that seen in the ciliary epithelium. Eyes showing such degenerative changes often contain abundant drusen. The pigment epithelium also undergoes fibrous and osseous metaplasia, changes that indicate a progression toward phthisis bulbi.

PHTHISIS BULBI

With the exception of eyes enucleated because of intraocular tumors, most globes received in the ocular pathology laboratory are removed because of blindness, pain and disfigurement created by injury, glaucoma, or intraocular inflammation. Such eyes are usually designated as "phthisic" by the contributing surgeon. This term is useful and acceptable for a clinical designation that connotes an end-stage eye. Microscopically, however, the term *phthisis bulbi* should be reserved for cases in which the specific histopathologic criteria described next are met. Hogan and Zimmerman[629] classify end-stage eyes into three categories:

1. Atrophy of the eyeball without shrinkage (for example, postglaucomatous atrophy)
2. Atrophy of the eyeball with shrinkage
3. Atrophy of the eyeball with disorganization (phthisis bulbi)

In atrophy without shrinkage, the internal architecture of the globe is relatively well preserved; that is, the various tissues are in normal or near-normal locations. The tissue disorganization typical of phthisis bulbi is notably absent; however, the various ocular tissues, particularly the retina and optic nerve, have undergone diffuse atrophy. In most cases the eye is of normal size, but the globe is frequently enlarged because of glaucoma (Fig. 7-16). Indeed, most such eyes are atrophic because of long-standing glaucoma (absolute glaucoma).

In atrophy with shrinkage, the globe is small and soft. Again, the intraocular tissues show atrophy, but the tissue relationships are relatively intact. This type of atrophy is sometimes difficult to distinguish from phthisis bulbi but can generally be differentiated by the lack of scleral thickening, absence of intraocular bone formation, and a lack of general disorganization of intraocular tissues, all of which are characteristic findings of a phthisic globe.

Phthisis bulbi most commonly occurs in eyes disrupted by trauma or intraocular inflammation. Following the rare occurrence of spontaneous regression of a retinoblastoma (Chapter 9), the affected globe sometimes becomes phthisic.

Four tissue changes are indicative of phthisis bulbi (Figs. 7-22 to 7-24).

1. The globe is small and soft. The eye typically measures less than 20 mm in diameter (compared with a normal adult measurement of 24 to 25 mm). Hypotony is evident in tissue sections as a partial separation of the choroid and ciliary body stroma from the adjacent sclera (Fig. 7-20).

2. The sclera shows marked thickening and is wrinkled or indented because of loss of the normal supportive intraocular pressure. Scleral thickening is presumably caused by secondary scarring. The cornea is typically flattened, shrunken, and opaque, and many of the degenerative corneal changes described in Chapter 3 may be evident. If, as is often the case, the phthisis is a result of perforating injury, the myriad changes indicative of perforation is evident in the region of the wound track (p. 99).

3. Generalized disorganization of intraocular contents

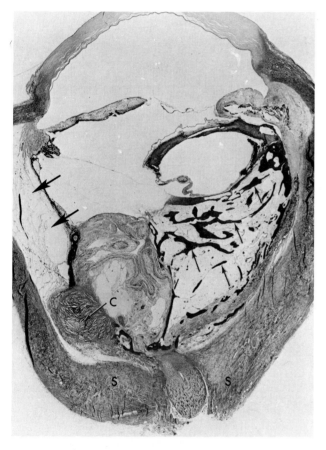

Fig. 7-22. Phthisis bulbi caused by previous blunt trauma. Several features characterize an end-stage phthisic eye: (1) The globe is small and soft. Hypotony is indicated by extensive choroidal and ciliary body detachment *(large arrows)*. (2) The sclera *(S)* is typically wrinkled and thickened. (3) The intraocular contents are greatly disorganized. A cyclitic membrane (only partially formed in this specimen) is often present. (4) Intraocular bone forms as a result of osseous metaplasia of the retinal pigment epithelium. *Small arrows,* Numerous bone spicules. The retina is totally detached and thrown into folds adjacent to the optic nerve. *C,* Large cluster of cholesterol clefts beneath the retina. These lipid deposits signify previous hemorrhage with degeneration and organization of old blood. (H & E stain; ×6.)

differentiates a phthisic eye from an atrophic eye. Diffuse intraocular scarring and detachment of the sensory retina is a universal finding. The lens, if not previously extruded or resorbed, may be displaced and commonly shows calcareous degeneration. Following trauma, extravasated blood is a common finding (Fig. 7-22). Most phthisic eyes contain a cyclitic membrane. As a consequence of perforating trauma, the densely scarred cyclitic membrane typically communicates with scar tissue within the wound track.[50]

4. Intraocular bone formation is a characteristic finding of phthisis bulbi (Figs. 7-22 to 7-24). The formation of a cyclitic membrane and the laying down of bone, which are so typical of this condition, are related to the propensity of the ciliary epithelium and retinal pigment epithelium to undergo a reactive hyperplasia. These epithelia are also capable of undergoing eventual fibrous and/or osseous metaplasia. Metaplasia is a transformation of one type of tissue into another, such as transformation of cuboidal pigment epithelium into fibrous tissue (collagen-forming fibroblasts and fibrocytes) or into bone. A reactive hyperplasia and subsequent fibrous metaplasia of the ciliary body epithelium contribute to the formation of a fibrous band across the retrolental space, creating the cyclitic membrane.

On many occasions we have noticed students' tendency to confuse intraocular *bone*, which represents a degenerative process occurring in phthisic eyes, with intraocular *cartilage* seen in trisomy 13 (p. 45) and in neuroepithelial tumors of the ciliary body (medulloepitheliomas, p. 330). The microscopic appearance of bone (Figs. 7-22 to 7-24) is easily distinguished from that of hyaline cartilage (Fig. 7-25). The former is recognized by the distinct appearance of the calcified spicules that often line fat-laden marrow spaces.

Trauma, intraocular inflammation, or necrosis of intraocular tissues stimulate such reactive processes in the retinal pigment epithelium. In addition to hyperplasia and hypertrophy of the epithelium, an important step in the differentiation of bone is drusen formation. Drusen are composed of basement membrane-like materials that accumulate as degenerative and secretory products of the pigment epithelium. These nodular excrescences on Bruch's membrane may enlarge enormously and are eventually transformed into osteoid. Subsequent calcification and osteoblastic and osteoclastic molding of the osteoid into a spicular configuration creates bone (Figs. 7-22 to 7-24). The maturation of the bone may proceed to such a degree that fatty marrow spaces containing blood precursors develop between the spicules.

Although the bone in phthisis bulbi is situated within the subretinal space and appears to arise from the choroid, it is probably derived from the abnormally proliferating pigment epithelium. This sequence of (1) pigment epithelial hyperplasia, (2) fibrous and osseous metaplasia, (3) drusen formation, (4) deposition of osteoid, and (5) ultimate formation of true cancellous bone is an interesting phenomenon in which the neuroectodermal pigment epithelium (arising from the outer layer of the optic cup) is transformed into a "mesodermal" structure (bone). Such a "crossing" of germ layers is an unusual occurrence.

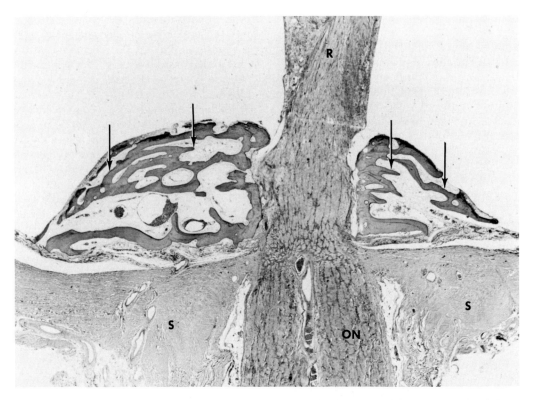

Fig. 7-23. Phthisis bulbi, posterior segment, showing total detachment of the sensory retina *(R)* in which the retina extends upward from the optic nerve *(ON)*. Bone is present on either side of the optic disc. It is recognizable by the densely staining bone spicules *(arrows)* intertwining around bone marrow spaces that contain fat and fibrovascular tissue. *S,* Sclera. (H & E stain; ×35.)

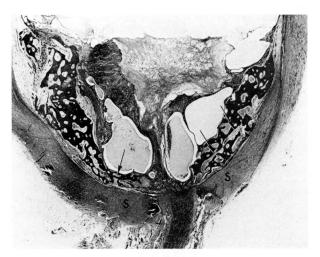

Fig. 7-24. Photomicrograph of a phthisic globe resulting from an old case of uveitis. *S,* Greatly thickened sclera. The optic nerve is reduced in diameter because of advanced atrophy. Osseous metaplasia of the retinal pigment epithelium has led to formation of bone along the entire posterior third of the globe *(arrows).* The dark-staining areas of bone are calcified spicules; the light intervening areas are marrow spaces. (H & E stain; ×10.)

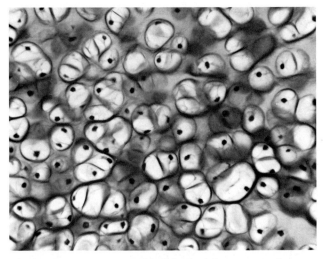

Fig. 7-25. Photomicrograph of cartilage from a case of trisomy 13. The chondrocyte-containing lacunae embedded within a chondroitin sulfate-rich matrix is easily differentiated from the spicular pattern of bone (Figs. 7-22 to 7-24). (H & E stain; ×350.)

Uveal tumors

Melanocytic tumors are the most common neoplasms that affect the eye.[404-1182] A knowledge of basic terminology and cellular classification is useful to describe the clinicopathologic features of these tumors.

TERMINOLOGY AND CLASSIFICATION

Intraocular melanin and melanin-containing cells

Intraocular melanin-containing cells are classified into two distinct groups (Fig. 7-2): the pigmented epithelia and uveal (dendritic) melanocytes.

The pigmented epithelia of the retina, ciliary body, and iris are derived from the neuroepithelium of the embryonic optic cup (Figs. 2-9 and 2-11). The melanin pigment forms in situ in the outer layer of the cup during the first few weeks of gestation. The concentration of intracellular melanin is approximately equal between white and black persons. Except for the neuroepithelial tumors of the ciliary body such as the medulloepithelioma (p. 330), these cells rarely undergo neoplastic differentiation. The retinal and ciliary body epithelial, however, commonly undergo non-neoplastic proliferation or reactive hyperplasia in response to a wide variety of insults.

Uveal, or dendritic, melanocytes are elongated or star-shaped cells with long dendrite-like cell processes emanating from the cell body. They reside in the stromal component of the uvea. (The differences and interrelationships between the stromal and epithelial components of ocular tissues are defined in Tables 7-1 and 7-2.) The dendritic cells differ in many respects from the melanin-containing epithelial cells. Embryologically, the former probably originate from the neural crest, a structure that consists of a row of cells localized along either side of the midline of the embryo adjacent to the neural tube (pp. 7 and 284; Fig. 7-4).

Uveal pigment is typically finer and more delicate than its retinal counterpart. The pigment concentration within stromal melanocytes varies considerably among individuals and is, therefore, the most important factor responsible for variations in iris color.

The most important and clinically relevant difference between the pigment epithelial cell and the dendritic melanocyte is the potential for new growth. Whereas the pigmented epithelia of the eye rarely undergo neoplastic growth, the dendritic melanocyte is considered the cell of origin for most intraocular pigmented growths, including nevi, melanocytomas, and malignant melanoma. (Melanocytomas are considered in detail in Chapter 10.)

In the older literature it was believed that malignant melanomas were derived from mesenchymal (mesodermal) cells in the uvea. They were, therefore, designated "melanosarcoma."[576]

Because melanocytes are derived from embryonic neural crest primordia, a pigmented neoplasm of the eye might, therefore, be considered to be neurogenic in nature. Indeed, Theobald[937] postulated a Schwann cell origin for uveal melanomas. Schwann cell tumors of the peripheral nervous system are also probably derived from the neural crest (Fig. 7-4). Schwannomas, neurofibromas (p. 509), and fascicular uveal melanomas (Fig. 7-56) have certain basic similarities in histopathologic appearance that support this hypothesis.

Melanocytic tumors

One of the major hindrances in diagnosing melanocytic neoplasms of the uvea is the lack of a widely accepted, unifying terminology.[414-417] When does an unquestionable nevus become a "suspicious" nevus, an "early" melanoma, or a nevus "with some characteristics of melanoma"?[426] With the exception of obvious nevi as defined below and of obvious full-blown malignant melanomas, assigning each case a specific slot with a specific nomenclature is extremely difficult. For example, a small lesion with many of the clinical criteria of a nevus may have a cell type typical of a malignant melanoma.

These tumors represent biologic entities that cannot be tossed arbitrarily into a computer to obtain a prognosis. One can only observe and analyze a given case, using all known diagnostic modalities, and then proceed according to common sense. Such an approach covers the spectrum of recommended treatment modalities ranging from observation to performing enucleation.

Pigmented uveal tumors can be conceptualized as being located at a given locus on a spectrum or growth curve at the time of diagnosis (Fig. 7-32).[414-416] The clinician's task is (1) to attempt to identify as closely as possible the approximate site on the curve in each case and (2) to strive to prevent the growth of the tumor to a point at which the prognosis clearly worsens.

Based on general clinical and laboratory experience suggesting that most choroidal melanomas arise from preexisting nevi, Apple and Blodi[414-417] proposed the following division of melanocytic neoplasms into two major categories.[407,739,989,990,998] This categorization is primarily based on what these authors believed to be three of the most important prognostic factors that influence the behavior and course of uveal melanocytic neoplasms: size, cell type, and extrascleral extension.

I. Obvious and unquestionable nevi and melanocytoma
II. Malignant melanoma
  A. Phase A tumors
    1. In the majority of cases are relatively small
    2. Are composed largely of cells that one classifies toward the benign end of the spectrum (according to the Callender classification[461,462] on p. 320 or the McLean classification[713,715])
    3. Have not extended or metastasized beyond the eye
    4. In general are stationary or slow growing, at least in their initial stages
  B. Phase B tumors
    1. Tend to be large
    2. Are usually composed of more malignant cell types
    3. May show evidence of extension and more rapid growth

This classification of uveal melanocytic tumors has certain features that may (1) provide a reasonable, practical approach for the clinician in defining the status, prognosis, and possible treatment of such tumors and (2) enable the practitioner to avoid many of the numerous semantic problems regarding terminology and the plethora of statistics now in the literature, which, although helpful to the specialist and statistician in ocular oncology, are often confusing to the practicing clinician who is trying to evaluate a given case.

Although much confusion and controversy regarding terminology remains to be resolved, our interpretation of the literature indicates that the Apple-Blodi classification is generally consistent with the findings of other authors.[414–417] The "tumor doubling time" concept of Collins, Loeffler, Tivey and Marquardt[705] is consistent with this classification.

Several authors have recently observed that "uveal melanomas vary greatly in their cytologic makeup, growth characteristics, and potential for spontaneous dissemination."[*] They reported that "tumors that measure less than 8 mm in greatest diameter and 2 mm in elevation, those that are composed exclusively of bland spindle cells and devoid of epithelioid cells, and those that exhibit no mitotic activity are often frankly benign."[711] This latter subgroup falls into group A of the Apple-Blodi classification of malignant melanomas. On the other hand, Zimmerman and associates also determined that "larger melanomas that have a considerable component of loosely cohesive epithelioid cells and a great supply of large, thin-walled blood vessels are the ones that are most vulnerable."[1001,1005] Tumors such as these are categorized as group B melanomas in the Apple-Blodi clinical guide to prognosis.

Other reports—those of Barr, McLean, and Zimmerman,[431] Davidorf and Lang,[505,506] Gas,[588–591] Kersten,[654] Blodi,[967] Shammas and Blodi,[853] Thomas, Green, and Maumenee,[940] Warren,[967] and many others (reviewed by Apple and Blodi[414–417])—have generated statistics regarding prognosis in relation to the previously mentioned major factors. We believe their findings are essentially in general agreement with this clinical classification.

OBVIOUS AND UNQUESTIONABLE NEVI AND MELANOCYTOMA

This group comprises the vast majority of uveal melanocytic neoplasms (Figs. 7-26 and 7-30). (Melanocytoma is described in Chapter 10, p. 550.) Fortunately, nevi are easily diagnosed by an experienced clinician and have an excellent prognosis. The diagnosis is clear cut for this type of tumor; almost no possibility of malignancy exists, and treatment is certainly not required.

Iris tumors

Iris freckles (increased pigmentation of the anterior stroma without an increase number of melanocytes), localized nevi (Fig. 7-26), and even suspected malignant melanomas (Figs. 7-27 to 7-29) that do not encroach into the anterior chamber angle or communicate with the ciliary body are easily recognized clinically and can often simply be followed or can be easily excised. In children they should be differentiated from juvenile xanthogranuloma of the iris (p. 294).[623,835] Most benign nevi and malignant melanomas of the iris are composed of relatively slow-growing, spindle-type cells (p. 309, Fig. 7-29).[†] and offer

---

[*] References 435, 493, 504, 624, 711, 713, 714.

[†] References 404, 410, 415, 416, 423, 481, 482, 496, 526, 529, 535, 543, 552, 598, 600, 611, 613, 620, 622, 635–640, 650, 653, 664, 680, 724, 733, 735, 750, 762, 778, 794, 799, 805, 818, 824, 827, 848, 859, 872, 887, 891, 892, 899, 903, 904, 921, 922, 923, 925, 932, 938, 941, 948, 985, 995.

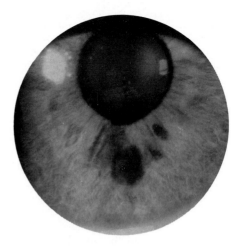

Fig. 7-26. Iris nevus at the 6 o'clock position.

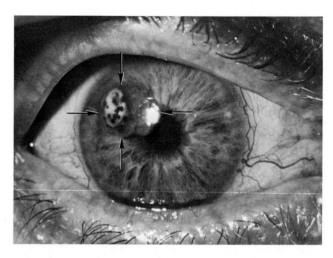

Fig. 7-27. Malignant melanoma of the iris (demarcated by *arrows*). There is no evident involvement of the iris root or ciliary body. Local excision was sufficient, and histopathologic analysis confirmed a spindle A cell type. Such anteriorly located uveal melanomas typically demonstrate a more benign cell type than do melanomas arising in the choroid or ciliary body. (Courtesy Dr. John Hattenhauer.)

an excellent prognosis. Some show the histological patterns of melanocytoma (p. 307), in which the cell type is also benign. With few exceptions, iris nevi have a very low malignancy potential.[922,991] Most iris nevi reveal a discrete mass or nodule, but a diffuse pattern occurs in the iris-nevus syndrome (Chapter 6, p. 266) and may occur with congenital ocular melanosis (Chapter 2, p. 42).[410,747]

Iris melanomas usually arise from preexisting nevi and may present in many ways, as a discrete or diffuse mass, as an iritis, as a hyphema, associated with glaucoma, and as a heterochromia. Although malignant melanoma is said to be the most common tumor, the behavior of the vast majority is generally very benign, metastases are rare, and this condition is probably overdiagnosed. The mortality rate is less than 5%.[637,653]

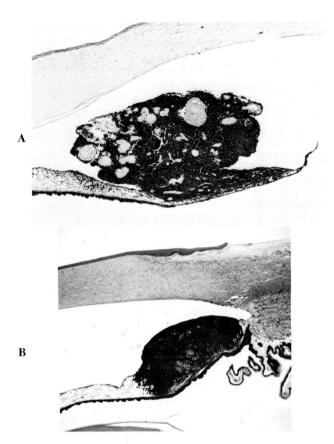

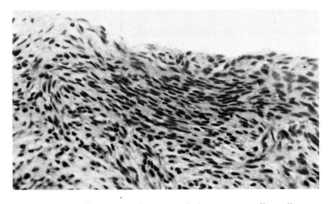

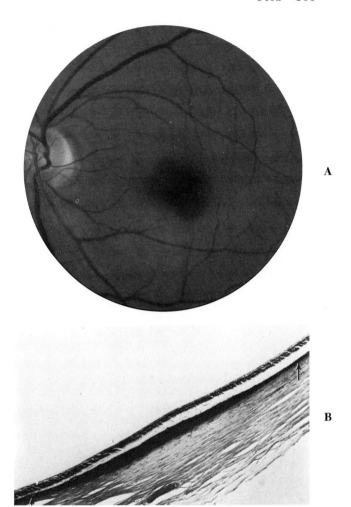

Fig. 7-28. Malignant melanoma of the iris. **A,** This elevated tumor is near the pupillary margin. (H & E stain; ×35.) **B,** This tumor encroaches on the angle but does not involve the filtration structures or ciliary body. (H & E stain; ×15.)

Fig. 7-29. Malignant melanoma of the iris, spindle cell type. These elongated spindle-shaped cells are distinguished from spindle B cells by their slightly smaller size and by the absence of nucleoli (compare with Figs. 7-53 and 7-55). (H & E stain; ×200.) (Courtesy Dr. John Hattenhauer.)

Fig. 7-30. Choroidal nevi. **A,** Benign, nonelevated nevus. **B,** Slight, fusiform elevation of the deeply pigmented growth. *Arrows,* Approximate margins of the nevus. (H & E stain; ×25.)

Choroidal nevi

Ciliary body and choroidal nevi are common, occurring in one third of the population. The vast majority occur in the posterior region. The clinical characteristics of choroi-

dal nevi (Fig. 7-30, Color Plate 7-5) have been described in detail by Ganley and Comstock.[*] The lesion often looks slate gray, can be oval to circular in configuration, and may have definite, but not always sharp, borders that may at times appear feathery. Diffuse nevi can occur in association with congenital ocular melanomas (Chapter 2). Bilateral diffuse melanocytic proliferation, consisting of multiple, slightly elevated uveal nevi, may be associated with systematic malignant tumors.

The underlying choriocapillaris is usually obscured. The nevi may vary in size from 0.5 to 6.0 disc diameters; the most common size range is 0.5 to 1.5 disc diameters. They are usually flat or only minimally elevated. When compared with choroidal malignant melanomas, nevi often exhibit a greater quantity of pigmentation. Because they are usually relatively avascular, fluorescein angiographic examination of nevi exhibits hypofluorescence. Furthermore, except for drusen formation, the overlying retina and pigment epithelium tend to be less affected by a choroidal nevus, and

---

[*] References 580, 604, 696, 727-736, 738, 740, 784, 820, 876, 909, 928, 929.

scotomas are less common than in malignant melanomas. In choroidal malignant melanomas the overlying retina frequently exhibits significant degeneration leading to noticeable loss of visual field.[514]

These generalizations, although true in the majority of instances, are merely textbook descriptions of choroidal nevi set up as guidelines for differentiating benign from malignant uveal melanocytic neoplasms. These rules have many exceptions. In equivocal cases, there is no substitute for a careful clinical follow-up.

Ganley and Comstock[580] determined that choroidal nevi are found in a range of 1% to 6% of the general population. They also concluded from their study and from the literature that uveal malignant melanoma occurs at an annual incidence between 0.5 and 1.3 per 100,000 white population over the age of 30. From these figures it is evident that very few (on the order of 1 of 5000) persons with nevi will develop a malignant melanoma. A *minimal* possibility of malignant transformation, therefore, may exist, but for practical purposes it is too minuscule to warrant a "short-interval" follow-up by a busy practitioner. We suggest that the ophthalmologist (1) avoid statements that cause concern to the patient (perhaps let him know he has a "freckle in the eye" or the equivalent) and (2) simply look at the eye by refraction or tonometry at each routine ophthalmologic examination.

In the past many nevi have probably been included in prognostic studies of uveal "malignant melanoma" when actually they should have been excluded. For example, if one is testing a given treatment modality such as radiation, photocoagulation, or local excision, one would undoubtedly achieve excellent results in such cases, results that are misleading as far as the problem of treating actual malignant melanomas is concerned.

Most choroidal nevi are of the spindle cell type ("spindle cell nevus cell" of McLean, Zimmerman, and Evans[713]) (Fig. 7-30, *B*). The balloon cell nevus represents an uncommon variant in which large, plump cells with a foamy cytoplasm predominate. The melanocytoma, which is also considered a nevus, is composed of cells that are histogenetically related to those implicated in uveal nevi and malignant melanomas. Although the melanocytoma is most commonly recognized as a tumor involving the optic nerve (p. 550), it may affect any portion of the uvea, that is, any site of uveal melanocytes—even within scleral emissaria or on the episclera. The distinct cytologic appearance of melanocytoma is easily differentiated from the spindle-shaped cells seen in most nevi (Fig. 10-33, *B*). One of the few cases of malignant transformation of a melanocytoma has been recorded by Apple and associates,[413,495] who also reviewed the literature on this subject.

Angiomatous lesions (Fig. 7-31) and pigment epithelial proliferative hyperplastic or hamartomatous lesions and congenital hypertrophy of the pigment epithelium may resemble choroidal nevi.* The latter are usually flat, sharply bordered, intensely dark lesions of variable size. The pig-

---

* References 437, 446, 455, 467, 468, 489, 497, 517, 527, 542, 565, 572, 573, 581, 585, 596, 607, 665, 672, 683, 693, 695, 708, 709, 752, 785, 796, 797, 801, 807, 808, 815, 822, 837, 841, 882, 938, 942, 943, 947, 956, 957, 980, 982.

mented foci also block choroidal fluorescence in a manner similar to many choroidal nevi.

In the *rare* instance of significant growth of these pigmented lesions, they would then move into category II of the Apple-Blodi classification and should be so considered.

MALIGNANT MELANOMA

To further understand the concept of staging of uveal malignant melanomas[380] proposed by Apple and Blodi,[414-417,444] an understanding of a basic growth curve, characteristic for many *general tumors* and intraocular pigmented tumors, is useful.[380,414-417,444]

A general rule of oncology states that the growth rates and, therefore, the potential for morbidity and mortality for most tumors, can be categorized into two phases (Fig. 7-32):

1. An early lag or pre–rapid growth phase (phase A: left, flat portion of the curve)
2. An accelerated phase (phase B: right exponentially, ascending portion of the curve), which usually implies a poorer prognosis

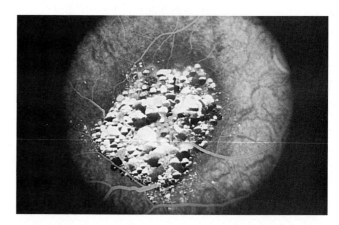

Fig. 7-31. Retinal cavenous hemangioma. Fluorescein angiogram (same case as Color Plate 7-6, *B*) showing leakage of tumor vessels. Note that each individual cavernous saccule is composed of a *hypo*fluorescent cellular component and a *hyper*fluorescent serum element, due to layering of the blood in the lesion. (Courtesy of Dr. William F. Mieler, Milwaukee, WI.)

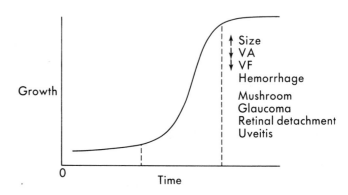

Fig. 7-32. Growth patterns of malignant melanoma. *VA,* Visual acuity; *VF,* visual field.

This growth curve concept has been verified clinically and experimentally in many tumors and is demonstrated in the work of Collins, Loeffler, and Tivey,[493] who developed a method to measure growth rates of human tumors by measuring the increase in diameter of the shadows of pulmonary metastases in radiographs. The growth rate is expressed in terms of "doubling time," that is, the time necessary for a tumor nodule to double its volume. The diameter of the mass can be plotted arithmetically, and one finds a curve similar to that of the fast phase component of Fig. 7-32. This concept of tumor doubling implies that increase in tumor size and growth rate is at first very small but eventually may reach a point where tumor enlargement increases greatly.[426,493] For example, Collins and coworkers[493] followed a tumor that, after 24 doublings, reached a diameter of no more than 2.5 mm, but after 6 further doublings quickly increased to 10 mm in diameter, and after another 6 doublings massively enlarged to 40 mm in diameter. These data correspond directly to the general configuration of the exponential curve illustrated in Fig. 7-32.

The characteristics that make each tumor different (benign, malignant, slow-growing, fulminating) are represented graphically by simple variations in (1) the length of time (that is, the doubling time of each type of tumor) of each respective phase on the curve (abscissa), (2) the height (ordinate) and slope of each point on the curve of each phase, and (3) the locus on each curve where the "rapid growth" phase begins (Fig. 7-32). We believe that the growth patterns of uveal melanocytic neoplasms correspond to this general curve. Manschot and van Peperzeel[700] have also analyzed the behavior of uveal malignant melanomas in relation to tumor doubling times.

Variations of this curve occur, thereby illustrating the wide variability in rate of tumor growth.* In a given patient, a lesion may continue to show the static or slow growth characteristic of a nevus or phase A malignant melanoma, and phase B is *never attained*. On the other hand, a frank malignant melanoma may appear to arise spontaneously or de novo in the phase of rapid growth without clinical evidence of the antecedent slow growth that characterizes many nevi or small melanomas.[574] An infinite combination of intermediate phases between these two extremes is clearly possible and accounts for differences in course and prognosis for each affected patient.

These tumors do not grow uniformly because their cells are so heterogeneous. Moreover, the growth process proceeds at different rates in different people, a fact perhaps related to the patient's immune status. Eventually the lesion reaches a point where it is capable of rapid growth and metastasis. Once this occurs, symptoms appear and the tumor is diagnosed. If surgical intervention occurs at this point in the tumor's natural history, the surgeon gets the blame for what happens even though the result is due to the biologic change in the tumor. Simply stated, at the point where we institute treatment, metastasis either has or has not occurred. If it has not, the eye is enucleated, and the patient is cured. Very often, however, the tumor already has metastasized and treating it with enucleation

or anything else does not affect the outcome. An option would be to treat every eye that is diagnosed with a nevus or small melanoma before it has had a chance to metastasize. If you enucleate these eyes, you certainly would prevent the increase in mortality 2 years after surgery; you also would be enucleating eyes that should not be enucleated!

Category I includes all nevi that pose little or no diagnostic problems to most clinicians. How do we clinically identify the phases of growth of category II uveal melanomas? By implication, category II, phase A, begins with any lesion that raises doubt as to possible malignancy (in particular, a beginning elevation of the tumor or minor changes in the overlying pigment epithelium). The mortality of this phase is low (10%–15% over 6 years). By definition this phase extends to a point at which significant changes indicate growth acceleration; that is, more advanced changes can be observed clinically and histopathologically and usually produce symptoms (Fig. 7-32; Table 7-6). When these latter changes occur rapidly or with increasing intensity, they represent the best clinical evidence that a tumor is entering or has reached phase II-B, in which the chances for survival diminish considerably (40%–50% or greater mortality over 6 years). Following are factors that may indicate progression of uveal malignant melanomas.[416]

1. Changes in size, shape, and elevation
2. Development of collar-button appearance
3. Decrease in visual acuity
4. Visual field changes
5. Retinal detachment
6. Deposition of orange pigment
7. Degeneration of the overlying retina
8. Secondary glaucoma
9. Intraocular hemorrhage
10. Inflammation and necrosis
11. Rubeosis iridis[466]
12. Heterochromia iridium
13. Fluorescein angiographic changes
14. Echographic changes
15. Radioactive phosphorus (^{32}P)

Unfortunately, two of the most reliable variables for assessing prognosis—cell type and small scleral extensions—cannot be evaluated clinically. Deep scleral extensions can be diagnosed by using the standardized A-scan echography.

The mushroom-shaped melanoma (Fig. 7-45, *A*) demonstrates what we consider to have been a shift toward the right on the curve (Fig. 7-32). The lesion was carefully followed for 11 years as a relatively flat or sessile, nongrowing, moderately pigmented, fundus lesion (phase II-A). It suddenly showed evidence of accelerated growth and developed the characteristic mushroom or collar-button (pp. 216 and 217) appearance over a 7-month period (phase II-B).

This biphasic subdivision of melanocytic neoplasms has been helpful because it leads to the practical conclusion that we are dealing essentially with two basic entities with striking prognostic and therapeutic implications. Exceptions to these general concepts occur that no one can predict because, as mentioned previously, a tumor is a biologic variable, a product of nature, not a product of a computer. Small tumors (apparent phase A lesions as viewed clinically) can lead to metastases. This is the chance one must

---

* References 459, 500, 518, 536, 574, 614.

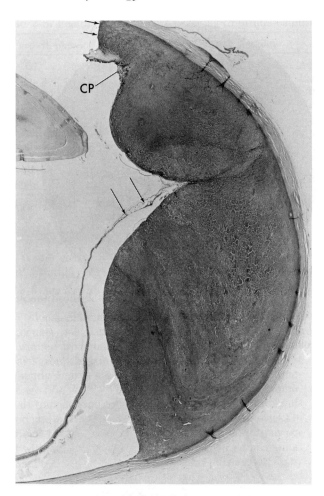

Fig. 7-35. Sparsely pigmented malignant melanoma of the ciliary body and choroid, with separation of the iris root from the sclera and invasion of the anterior chamber *(small arrows)*. *CP,* Ciliary processes; *large arrows,* areas of cystoid retinal degeneration overlying the tumor. (H & E stain; ×5.)

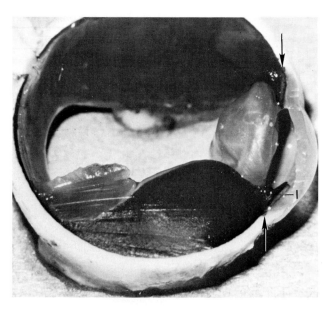

Fig. 7-36. Gross photograph of a globe with choroidal malignant melanoma extending anteriorly into the ciliary body with encroachment on the anterior chamber angle filtration structures *(arrows)*. In such cases, secondary glaucoma may result from (1) direct tumor cell invasion and plugging of the trabecular meshwork or (2) anterior displacement of the iris *(I),* leading to angle closure.

and retinal vessels into cystoid spaces within the degenerate retina, producing the characteristic angiographic picture of dye within multiloculated intraretinal cystoid spaces (see Fig. 7-41).[454,722,723] When the overlying retina is completely destroyed, dye sometimes leaks into the vitreous. Although degeneration of the overlying retina is unusual in nevi, similar changes are commonly seen in slowly growing hemangiomas. Second, in almost all malignant melanomas, some exudative serous detachment of the retina occurs at the tumor margin. Fluorescein stains the subretinal fluid during the later stages of the study. The majority of choroidal nevi do not exhibit exudative detachment.

Relatively unpigmented uveal malignant melanomas are the rule rather than the exception (Fig. 7-35; Color Plates 7-7 and 7-10). Most choroidal melanomas are light brown to gray (Color Plates 7-12 to 7-14 and 7-16). Melanomas are less commonly jet black (Figs. 7-36 to 7-38). Although a deep pigmentation is more characteristic of melanocytoma, not all melanocytomas are jet black. Although these pigmentation generalizations often provide clues to the diagnosis, the absolute diagnosis cannot be established solely on the basis of color.

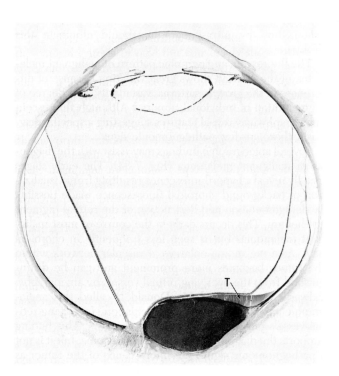

Fig. 7-37. Heavily pigmented malignant melanoma of the choroid. Most melanomas arise near the posterior pole. Those affecting the macula are generally diagnosed earlier because the patient complains of visual difficulties. *T,* Transudate in the subretinal space adjacent to the tumor. (H & E stain; ×4.)

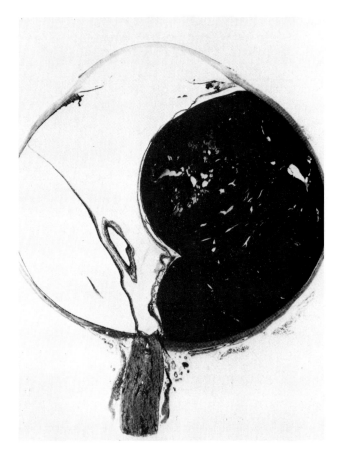

Fig. 7-38. Large choroidal malignant melanoma. Large vascular channels are present within the heavily pigmented mass. (H & E stain; ×4.)

The degree of pigmentation often varies within different sites of a single tumor (Fig. 7-39); therefore, such cases may involve two or more distinct populations of cells: heavily pigmented cells and relatively amelanotic cells. Such differences indicate a pattern of growth in which different clones of tumor cells predominate during varying periods of the growth of the tumor, a phenomenon that has been observed in tissue culture studies.[633] For example, during the early period of growth a mass may be composed of highly pigmented tumor cells. As tumor growth continues, a second population composed primarily of amelanotic tumor cells may appear. Such variation in cell lines presumably results from spontaneous mutation of the actively proliferating cells. This concept is of more than academic significance because a similar type of tumor cell mutation could also be responsible for transformation of a relatively benign malignant melanoma into one that exhibits more malignant behavior. For example, we have seen choroidal tumors containing varying cell populations ranging from plum, polyhedral "melanocytoma-type" cells to spindle B cells to epithelioid cells, all within a single mass. Just as a clone of amelanotic tumor cells might replace a line of heavily pigmented cells, a clone of highly malignant epithelioid cells could be expected to replace a population of spindle cells.

Most choroidal malignant melanomas originate in the region of the posterior pole. Peripapillary melanomas

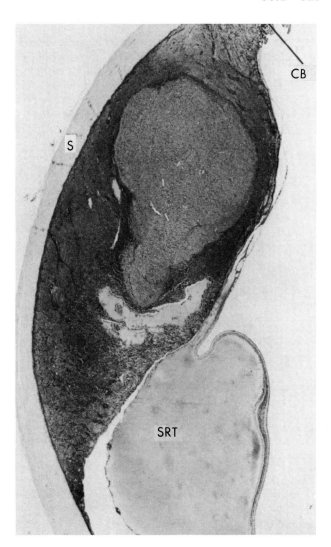

Fig. 7-39. Malignant melanoma of the choroid with serous detachment of the retina posterior to the main neoplasm. The central core of the neoplasm is relatively unpigmented, compared with the heavy pigmentation of the more peripheral tumor cells. *CB,* Ciliary body, which shows early invasion by the tumor; *SRT,* subretinal transudate; *S,* adjacent sclera. (H & E stain; ×12.)

(Figs. 7-40 and 7-42) may encircle the optic nerve or also grow over the optic nerve head in an epipapillary manner.[515,516,684,855] The differential diagnosis of pigmented masses on or adjacent to the disc is sometimes difficult. Epipapillary or peripapillary choroidal nevi and melanocytomas (Chapter 10), metastatic tumors, osteomas and hyperplastic, hamartomatous, or neoplastic lesions of the pigment epithelium may mimic a malignant melanoma.° Pigment epithelial neoplasia is extremely uncommon, but adenocarcinoma of the retinal pigment epithelium has been reported.

The collar-button or mushroom-shaped malignant mela-

° References 437, 446, 455, 456, 467, 468, 489, 497, 498, 512, 517, 527, 541, 542, 564, 566, 572, 573, 581, 585, 592, 596, 607, 608, 651, 660, 665, 672, 683, 693, 695, 708, 709, 749, 752, 785, 796, 797, 801, 807, 808, 815, 822, 837, 841, 858, 864, 882, 918, 942, 943, 945–947, 956, 957, 978, 980, 982.

noma of the choroid (Figs. 7-43 to 7-46; Color Plate 7-16) has a clinical and pathologic appearance highly characteristic of choroidal malignant melanoma. In the early stages of growth of a malignant melanoma, the tumor is relatively sessile and confined to the choroid. As the tumor grows, Bruch's membrane, the pigment epithelium, and the sensory retina are elevated by the surface of the tumor. Bruch's

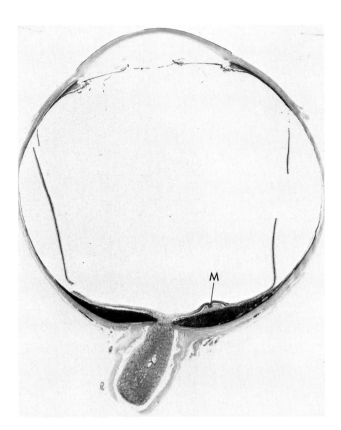

Fig. 7-42. Flat malignant melanoma of the choroid encircling the optic nerve. This tumor involved the macula *(M)* and caused a significant visual disturbance. (H & E stain; ×4.)

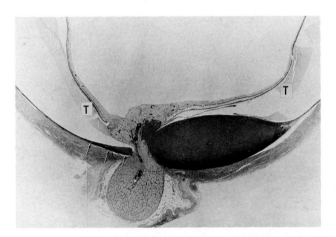

Fig. 7-40. Peripapillary choroidal malignant melanoma encircling the optic nerve head. *Arrows,* Focus of the tumor on the side of the disc opposite the main tumor mass. Degeneration of the overlying retina has occurred (see also Fig. 7-39). The clinical observation of a scotoma corresponding to the retinal field overlying the tumor is sometimes a major differential point in distinguishing malignant melanoma from a benign nevus. *T,* Serous transudate in the subretinal space. Although the tumor directly overlies the optic nerve head, there is no deep invasion of the optic nerve itself. Such peripapillary melanomas must be distinguished from nevi, melanocytomas, and benign or malignant growths of the retinal pigment epithelium that may occur in a similar location. (H & E stain; ×20.)

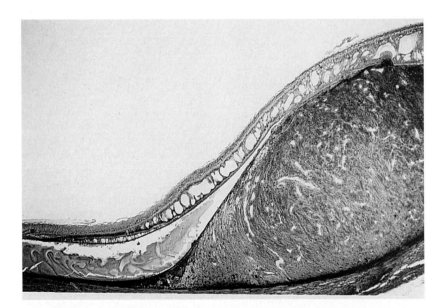

Fig. 7-41. Photomicrograph of a choroidal malignant melanoma with severe microcystoid change in the adjacent and overlying sensory retina. Note also a nonrhegmatogenous exudative retinal detachment (arrows) adjacent to the mass (H & E stain; ×80.)

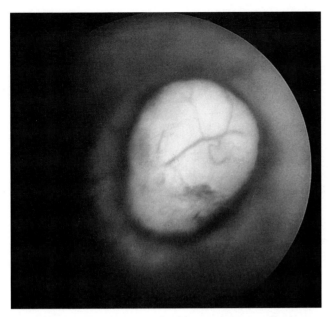

Fig. 7-43. Fundus photograph of an amelanotic, collar-button (mushroom) choroidal malignant melanoma (see also Figs. 7-43 and 7-46). The focus of the camera is on the apex of the lesion, well anterior to the sensory retina.

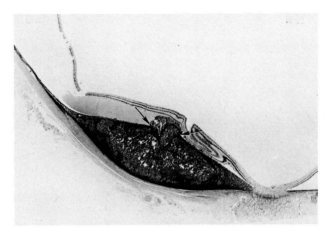

Fig. 7-44. Choroidal malignant melanoma with sudden rupture of a previously flat tumor through Bruch's membrane *(arrows)*. This appears to be the earliest manifestation of what eventually forms the mushroom or collar-button type of melanoma seen in Fig. 7-45. Since Bruch's membrane is a relatively tough, durable barrier, such a tumor breakthrough would presumably imply a significant degree of aggressiveness by the neoplasm. (H & E stain; ×40.)

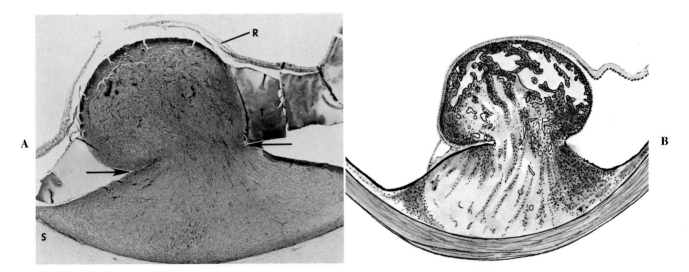

Fig. 7-45. A, Malignant melanoma of the choroid, mushroom type. The margins of the ruptured Bruch's membrane are situated at the points of indentation of the tumor *(arrows)*. It is believed that these margins create a constricting "purse-string" or "tourniquet" effect in which the vessels of the inner aspect of the tumor become congested and engorged with blood because of restriction of outflow. *R,* Overlying retina, which has undergone significant cystic degeneration; *T,* subretinal transudate on either side of the tumor; *S,* sclera. (H & E stain; ×35.) **B,** Schematic illustration of a mushroom melanoma. (**B,** redrawn by Dr Steven Vermillion, University of Iowa, from Ginsburg S: In Henke F and Lubarsch O: Handbuch der speziellen pathologischen Anatomie und Histologie, vol 1, Berlin, 1928, Springer-Verlag.)

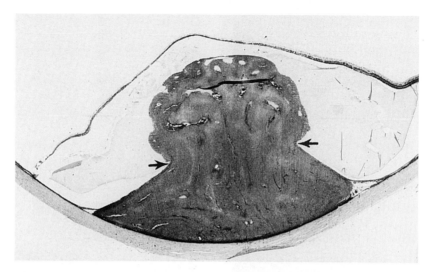

Fig. 7-46. Photomicrograph of a mushroom (collar-button) choroidal malignant melanoma. The arrows connote the site of break through Bruch's membrane. Note the engorged tumor stromal vessels near the apex of the tumor. (H & E stain; ×35.)

membrane may eventually rupture as a result of pressure from the underlying neoplasm (Fig. 7-44). When rupture occurs, this relatively tough barrier, which in early stages served to impede the growth and degree of elevation of the tumor, is eliminated. The tumor is then free to commence growth through the rupture site. As the tumor permeates the gap, it assumes the configuration of a dome-like protuberance projecting toward the vitreous. A "collar-button" or "purse-string" constriction occurs at the site of the rupture of Bruch's membrane. The resultant bottleneck and subsequent impedance of outflow of blood from the apex of the tumor lead to vasodilatation of the tumor vessels at the apex of the mass.[983]

Tumors that exhibit sufficient growth to induce rupture of Bruch's membrane often (but by no means invariably) reveal evidence of extension or show cytologic changes characteristic of more aggressive forms of malignant melanoma; therefore, the mushroom shape suggests a more aggressive or accelerated growth pattern. Because nevi and other choroidal tumors rarely show this pattern of growth, the mushroom-shaped tumor is considered highly suggestive of malignant melanoma. We have seen only a few instances in which metastatic tumor to the choroid has assumed this configuration.

Most choroidal malignant melanomas form discrete, localized masses (Figs. 7-35–7-39, 7-45, 7-49, and 7-60; Color Plates 7-6–7-16). Such intrachoroidal masses or tumors may produce folds (wrinkles or striae) in the fundus, particularly at the base of the tumor.

Occasionally, however, a tumor may grow in a diffuse rather than a discrete manner, involving a large surface area of the choroid but creating only minimal elevation of the overlying retina and pigment epithelium (Figs. 7-47, 7-48, and 7-52, *A*). This type of tumor is given a specific designation: diffuse flat malignant melanoma.* The pattern of growth is noteworthy in that it has the poorest prognosis

---

* References 425, 433, 450, 477, 562, 595, 616, 678, 817, 821, 839, 866.

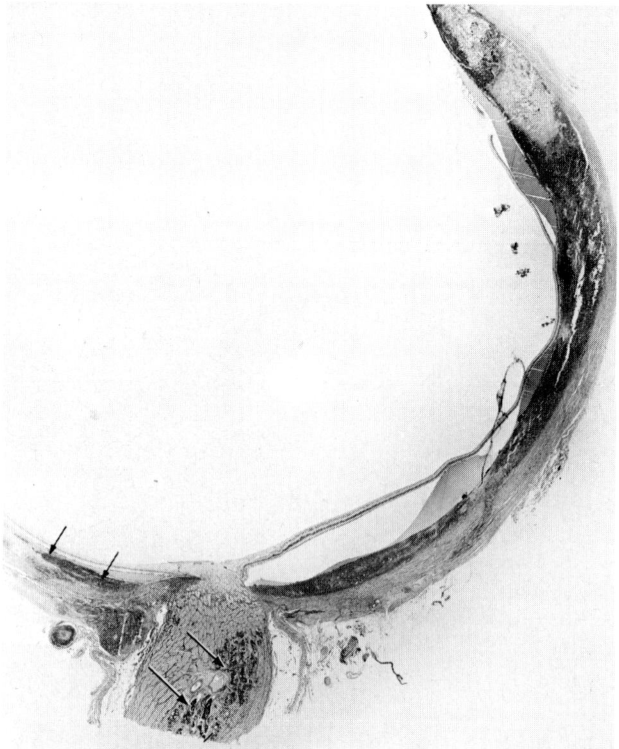

Fig. 7-47. Diffuse flat malignant melanoma of the choroid, the most ominous form of uveal malignant melanoma. Note the invasion of the optic nerve *(arrows)* by tumor infiltrates. The tumor occupies the entire right hemisphere of the globe and a portion to the left of the optic nerve *(small arrows)*. The retina is elevated minimally to moderately; such tumors are often diagnosed at a relatively late stage. Many of these tumors contain an epithelioid cell component. When faced with the differential diagnosis of a diffusely thickened choroid, one must also consider metastatic carcinoma, sympathetic ophthalmia, and lymphoid hyperplasia or neoplasia. (H & E stain; ×7.)

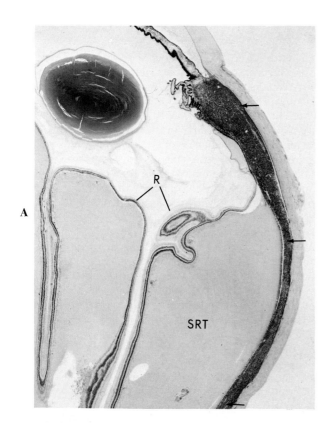

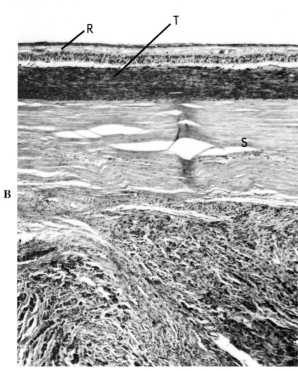

A

B

Fig. 7-48. Diffuse flat malignant melanoma of choroid and ciliary body. **A,** The length of the uveal thickening is demarcated by arrows. A total retinal detachment overlies the tumor. *R,* Retina; *SRT,* subretinal transudate. (H & E stain; ×7.) **B,** High-power photomicrograph showing minimal choroidal thickening by the tumor *(T)* but massive extension of tumor *(below,* deeply staining cells) outside of the sclera. *R,* Retina; *S,* sclera. (H & E stain; ×85.) (**A** from Naumann GOH and Apple DJ: In Doerr W, Seifert G, and Uehlinger E, editors: Handbuch der speziellen pathologischen Anatomie, Band Auge, Berlin, 1980, Springer-Verlag.)

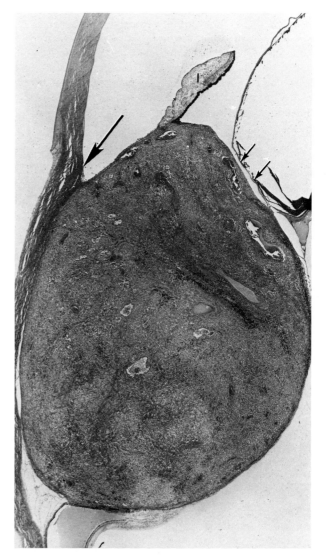

Fig. 7-49. Large malignant melanoma of the ciliary body and anterior choroid. The iris *(I)* has been displaced away from its root or insertion at the scleral spur. *Large arrow,* Site of the original angle recess; *small arrows,* compression of the adjacent lens by the tumor. (H & E stain; ×14.)

of all uveal melanomas (see list on p. 311). The cause of the poor prognosis is often the delay in diagnosis resulting from the minimal elevation of the tumor. The overlying retina frequently is uninvolved for a long period, and few visual symptoms are experienced. Also, it is probable that the large surface area of choroid involved by the tumor provides a higher statistical risk of vascular invasion. Such tumors necessarily are closely adjacent to several emissarial channels, thereby increasing the probability of extraocular extension and subsequent metastasis.

Malignant melanomas arising from the ciliary body (Figs. 7-49, 7-50, 7-51, *D*, 7-52, *C*; Color Plates 7-17 to 7-19) have a more favorable prognosis than do diffuse flat melanomas. Cytologically they are probably similar to melanomas of the posterior choroid, and one would expect a similar behavior; however, we have noticed that ciliary body melanomas are often "hidden" from easy viewing by the ophthalmologist and also may not cause early visual symptoms. For this reason they are sometimes detected at a later stage than posterior pole melanomas.[960] The latter cause early loss of visual function and are easily detected by ophthalmoscopy. Anteriorly located tumor masses can even show extrabulbar extension in the absence of visual difficulties (Fig. 7-50; Color Plate 7-19). Figures 7-51 and 7-52 illustrate most of the previously described growth patterns of uveal melanoma. The following list correlates the relative prognosis (from best to worst) of uveal malignant melanoma with tumor location:

1. Malignant melanoma of the iris (no ciliary body involvement)
2. Small- to medium-sized melanoma of the choroid, often recognized early because of early decreased visual function caused by posterior pole lesions
3. Malignant melanoma of the ciliary body, especially if diagnosed late as a result of a "hidden" location without early visual loss
4. Diffuse flat choroidal malignant melanoma

Histopathologic classification

Microscopic identification of the major cell types in a uveal melanocytic neoplasm can be useful in assigning a prognosis in a specific case.° Although the major cell types of uveal malignant melanoma have long been recognized (Fig. 7-53; Color Plate 7-20), the Callender classification of 1931 provided the first data, derived from a large series of cases, that have proved useful in estimating the prognosis of these tumors.[435,461,462,693] Following is the classification of cell types ranked from best to poorest prognosis:

1. Spindle A
2. Spindle B
3. Fascicular
4. Mixed spindle cell and epithelioid
5. Epithelioid
6. Necrotic

The spindle cell group consists of cells with slender, elongated, spindle-shaped nuclei. McLean, Zimmerman, and Evans[713] have introduced the term *spindle cell nevus*

° References 436, 461, 462, 492, 576, 577, 578, 579, 594, 629, 634, 658, 663, 713-716, 736, 766, 767, 783, 795, 809, 830, 896, 936, 974, 975, 1000, 1001, 1009.

cell to categorize the extremely benign appearing cells seen in many nevi. The spindle A cell (5% of cases) as defined by Callender (Fig. 7-54) is devoid of a nucleolus. The spindle B (39% of cases) (Fig. 7-55; Color Plate 7-20) is slightly larger than the spindle A cell and contains a prominent nucleolus. The cytoplasmic borders of individual spindle cells are poorly visualized, and the cells tend to merge into a syncytium. These characteristics contrast sharply with those of the more malignant epithelioid cells, in which the large, irregular, polygonal cells, as seen in tissue sections, are often distinctly separated from each other.

A small tumor composed entirely of spindle A cells or spindle cell nevus cells may be regarded as little more than a nevus; however, such tumors can rarely progress toward a more malignant form.[523]

Most malignant melanomas of the iris are composed of spindle cells that are devoid of nucleoli (Fig. 7-29). These either represent spindle A cells (classified strictly in terms of cellular morphology) or spindle cell nevus cells according to the newer terminology.[713] This cell type, along with the fact that the iris tumors are more quickly recognized and excised, accounts for the relatively good prognosis of these tumors. Most choroidal nevi also contain these benign spindle cells.

According to classic survival figures published in 1962 by Hogan and Zimmerman,[629] the 5-year survival rate of patients with spindle A uveal malignant melanoma is 95%. Patients with a spindle B malignant melanoma have a postenucleation 5-year survival rate of 84%. These figures, which take into account only the cell type of the tumor, are modified in individual cases by variation in size of the tumor, rapidity of diagnosis, and presence or absence of epibulbar extension. When all spindle cell melanomas are considered as a group, it is estimated that approximately 75% of affected patients are cured, that is, survive at least 15 years after enucleation. Data concerning prognosis and mortalities in relation to new treatment modalities are still being collected and analyzed.

The fascicular type of uveal malignant melanoma (6% of cases) refers to a tissue pattern rather than a specific cell type. The tumor cells are arranged in parallel rows, bundles, or palisades (Fig. 7-56). They are sometimes arranged in rows around vessels. Such an arrangement is reminiscent of the pattern seen in neurilemoma. It is partially for this reason that the "schwannian" derivation of this category of tumor was postulated.[671] Most fascicular melanomas are composed of spindle A or B cells; therefore, the fascicular melanoma is assigned the same prognosis as tumors composed of similar spindle cells arranged in a random, nonpalisading arrangement.

As a rule, the epithelioid cell (3% of cases) (Figs. 7-57 and 7-58) is larger than the spindle-shaped cells and exhibits a great deal of variation in size and shape (pleomorphism). There is abundant evidence of cellular anaplasia, with formation of numerous abnormal mitotic figures and extensive nuclear hyperchromatism. The cytoplasmic borders are often irregular and polygonal. Although the cells of spindle cell melanomas are arranged in a tightly packed syncytium, epithelioid cells are often noncohesive and the cytoplasmic borders are usually easily observed. This type represents the most extreme degree of cellular anaplasia of uveal malignant melanoma. The epithelioid cell is best

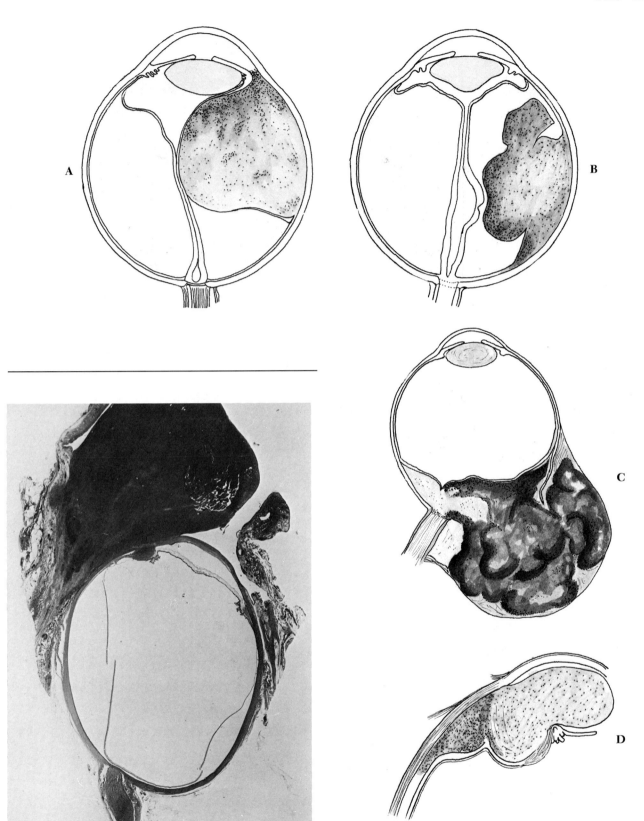

Fig. 7-50. Small primary malignant melanoma of the ciliary body, with massive episcleral extension and development of a conjunctival and eyelid mass that was diagnosed as a primary conjunctival melanoma. (H & E stain; ×1.) (Courtesy Dr. Heinrich Witschel, Freiburg, West Germany.)

Fig. 7-51. Composite drawings of basic growth patterns of uveal melanomas. **A,** Nodular mass. **B,** Mushroom or collar-button type. **C,** Extension through sclera. **D,** Iris-ciliary body melanoma. (Redrawn by Dr. Steven Vermillion, University of Iowa, from Fuchs' E: Das Sarcom des Uvealtractus, Vienna, 1882, Wilhelm Braumüller.)

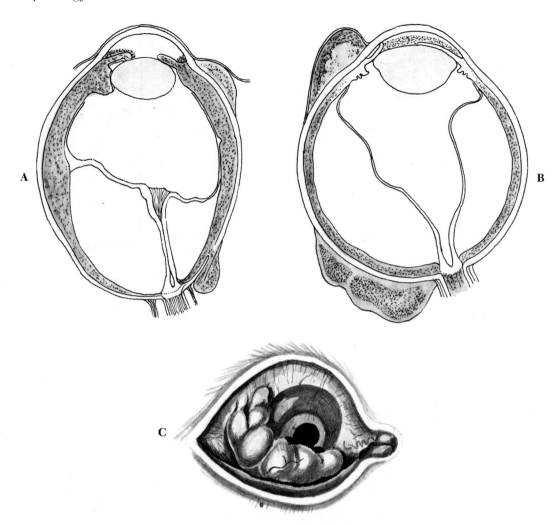

Fig. 7-52. Fuchs' drawings of diffuse flat melanoma. **A** and **B,** Extension into episclera and limbal conjunctiva. **C,** Clinical appearance of **B.** (Redrawn by Dr. Steven Vermillion, University of Iowa, from Fuchs' E: Das Sarcom des Uvealtractus, 1882, Wilhelm Braumüller.)

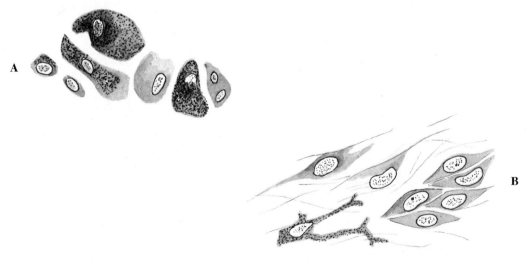

Fig. 7-53. Fuchs' interpretation of cell types in uveal melanomas. **A,** Epithelioid cells. **B,** *Right,* spindle cells; *left,* one normal pigmented dendritic melanocyte. (Redrawn by Dr. Steven Vermillion, University of Iowa, from Fuchs' E: Das Sarcom des Uvealtractus, Vienna, 1882, Wilhelm Braumüller.)

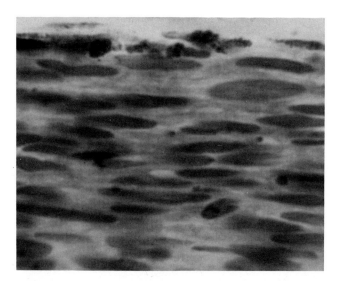

Fig. 7-54. Spindle A melanoma cells. The cells are in a syncytium, oriented in a parallel manner. Each cell contains elongated nuclei with rare or absent nucleoli. (H & E stain; ×400.)

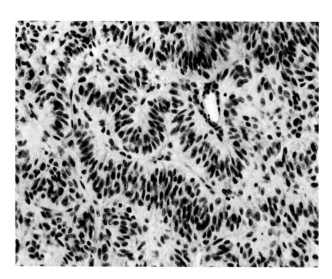

Fig. 7-56. Fasicular type of malignant melanoma of uvea. The spindle-shaped nuclei are arranged in rows forming palisades. (H & E stain; ×340.)

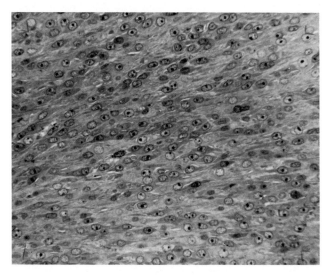

Fig. 7-55. Malignant melanoma of the uvea, spindle B cell type. The nucleoli are prominent in this section and appear as numerous deeply staining dots within the pale-staining tumor cell nuclei. Individual cell borders are difficult to distinguish; the cells are therefore arranged in a syncytium. (Mallory blue stain; ×350.) (From Apple DJ and others: Arch Ophthalmol 90:97, 1973. Copyright 1973, American Medical Association.)

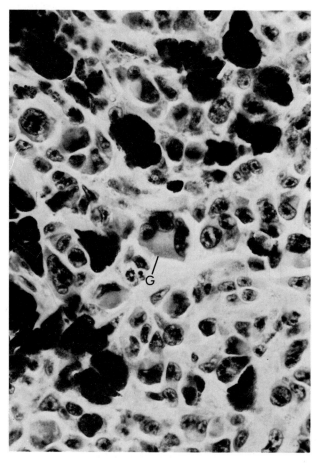

Fig. 7-57. Malignant melanoma of the choroid, epithelioid cell type. The large, multinucleated giant cell *(G)* is distinct and clearly distinguishes this cell type from the spindle cell variety. (H & E stain; ×400.)

recognized in histopathologic sections by identification of large multinucleated giant cells. The prognosis of an eye affected with a pure epithelioid cell type (which, fortunately, is unusual) is very poor; the 5-year survival rate is usually less than 30%.

The mixed cell type (45% of cases) involves a combination of both spindle and epithelioid cells. As would be expected, it usually has an intermediate prognosis between the more favorable life expectancy of the pure spindle forms and the more ominous prognosis of pure epithelioid tumors. As a group, patients with tumors of the mixed cell

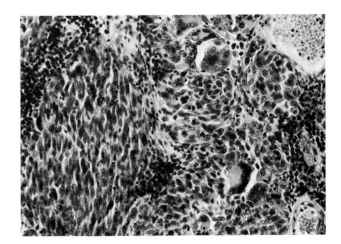

Fig. 7-58. Malignant melanoma, mixed cell type. The anaplastic epithelioid cells *(right)*, particularly the tumor giant cells, contrast with the vertically coursing bundle of spindle B cells *(left)*. (H & E stain; ×375.)

type show a 50% mortality after 5 years, but the prognosis is even more grim as the relative percentage of epithelioid cells within the tumor increases. For example, a patient with a tumor composed of 95% spindle B cells and 5% epithelioid cells is expected to have a better prognosis than one with a tumor composed of 5% spindle B cells and 95% epithelioid cells.

An epithelioid cell component is frequently seen in the diffuse flat malignant melanoma of the choroid (p. 317). As noted previously, this type of malignant melanoma usually behaves aggressively, a behavior commensurate with this cell type.[847]

The necrotic cell type (7% of cases), as defined by the Callender classification, signifies a microscopic pattern in which the tumor cells become so necrotic that they defy histologic classification into the other definitive groups (Fig. 7-59).[806,833] Massive tumor cell necrosis results from outgrowth of the tumor blood supply, from intraocular inflammation, or from an autoimmune mechanism. Both retinoblastomas and malignant melanomas have been shown to produce antigens that can cause a cutaneous hypersensitivity reaction.* The necrotic process itself may initiate an intense intraocular inflammatory response. Such cases involve a definite hazard of mistakenly considering the clinical diagnosis to be uveitis or endophthalmitis rather than a malignant neoplasm. Patients with these tumors have prognoses similar to those with malignant melanomas of the mixed cell type.

Uveal melanoma cells are S-100 protein, HMB-45 and K167 positive. Lymphocytes in melanomas are predominately T-supressor/cytotoxic cells (see Chapter 1, p. 6).[491,558,647,918,973]

As mentioned previously, evidence indicates that differentiation of a uveal malignant melanoma may proceed through a spectrum of changes in which a tumor that originally exhibited a relatively benign appearance evolves to-

* References 470, 473, 475, 476, 490, 499, 507, 524, 530, 545-547, 664, 677, 707, 727, 748, 761, 766, 788, 789, 924, 965.

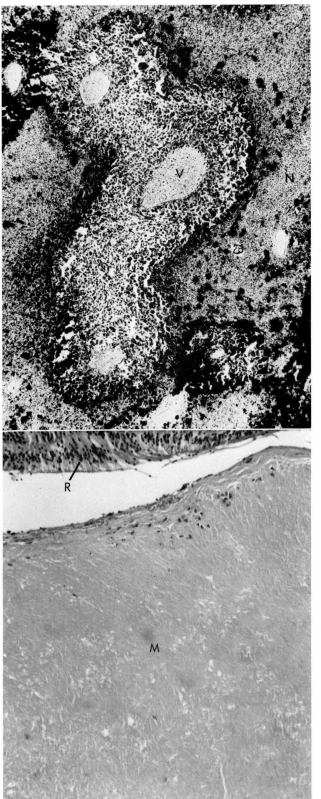

Fig. 7-59. Malignant melanoma, necrotic cell type. **A,** Partial necrosis *(N)* of tumor in areas distally located from tumor vessels *(V)*. Cells are viable in immediate perivascular region. (H & E stain; ×140.) **B,** Total necrosis of choroidal melanoma *(M)*. Complete loss of cell outlines and stainability (coagulation necrosis). *R,* Retina. (H & E stain; ×170.)

ward one with a more malignant course (Fig. 7-32). For example, a pigmented growth containing primarily spindle cells may develop. As the mass grows, more malignant clones of cells appear as a result of spontaneous mutation. Further tumor growth is then characterized by an increased number of cells comprising a more malignant cell type. Evidence for such a theory is manifold. For example, local recurrences in the orbit or metastatic foci in the liver and other organs usually are predominantly epithelioid cells. This is true even when the intraocular primary mass was composed predominantly of spindle B cells or was of the mixed cell type.

Transformation of a spindle cell primary tumor seen in an enucleated eye into the more malignant form observed in a focus of recurrence or metastasis can be explained by assuming that a mutation has taken place. The modified, more dangerous cell type produced has led to overgrowth.

In addition, a definite correlation exists between tumor size, cell type, and behavior.* Very large masses, many of which exhibit a more malignant cellular differentiation, are responsible for significantly greater mortality than smaller masses (Fig. 7-32; Table 7-6). Smaller tumors that are enucleated before the process of malignant transformation has occurred usually show spindle rather than epithelioid cell differentiation.

Spontaneous mutation of tumor cells in a single tumor has been demonstrated in tissue culture studies and is further supported by the existence of intraocular melanomas in which clearly different cell types exist within a single tumor.[633] Figure 7-39, which shows both amelanotic and hyperpigmented tumor cells localized within discrete zones of the tumor, illustrates this concept. Just as a clone of amelanotic tumor cells might replace a line of highly pigmented cells, a clone of highly malignant epithelioid cells could be expected to supersede a population of spindle cells. The spectrum of progression of a given tumor, therefore, appears to follow the course defined by the Callender classification and by the curve in Fig. 7-32.

Clinical observation of an apparently benign or slow-growing melanotic lesion of the choroid should include consideration of the potential of each tumor to evolve toward a more malignant cell type and therefore, malignant behavior (Fig. 7-32; Table 7-6; p. 310). In most cases, enucleation can be deferred as long as the lesion remains stationary. One should consider treatment when certain changes indicate a more malignant, aggressive behavior. These signs include many of the items listed in Fig. 7-32, for instance, changes in size and shape of the tumor, decrease in visual acuity and/or changes in the visual field, detachment of the retina adjacent to the margin of the tumor, deposition of orange pigment (presumed lipofuscin) on the surface of the tumor, degeneration of the overlying retina, formation of the mushroom or collar-button appearance as a result of rupture of Bruch's membrane, rubeosis iridis, secondary glaucoma, and intraocular inflammation and hemorrhage.

* References 415, 416, 427, 428, 432, 435, 472, 500, 505, 528, 556, 559, 649, 710, 725, 745, 759, 766, 790, 791, 848, 853, 897, 967, 969, 972, 1009.

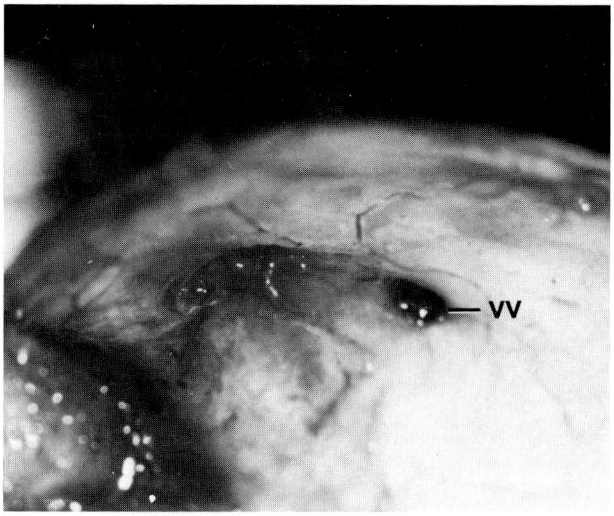

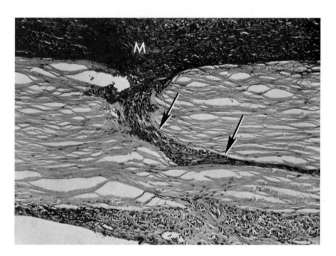

Fig. 7-60. Gross photograph of the external posterior aspect of an enucleated globe with malignant melanoma of the choroid. The pigmented tumor has extended through a vortex vein *(VV)*. The optic nerve is at lower left.

Fig. 7-61. Advanced emissarial growth *(arrows)* of malignant melanoma cells with episcleral deposits (cells at bottom of photograph). *M,* Main choroidal tumor mass. (H & E stain; ×95.)

Extension and metastasis (Color Plates 7-17, 7-19, 7-21 and 7-22)

The vortex veins and other vessels and nerves that penetrate the sclera and provide a route for tumor extension are termed the *scleral emissaria.** The vortex veins are important routes of exit of choroidal malignant melanoma from the globe (Figs. 1-3 and 7-60 to 7-64; Color Plates 1-1 and 7-19). There are four or more vortex veins; logically, the larger the surface area of the tumor, the greater the opportunity for invasion of an adjacent transscleral channel (hence, the high invasive potential of the diffuse flat melanoma). Invasion of an emissarial channel and

* References 405, 415, 416, 464, 471, 478, 520, 525, 599, 655, 675, 727, 760, 854, 875, 917.

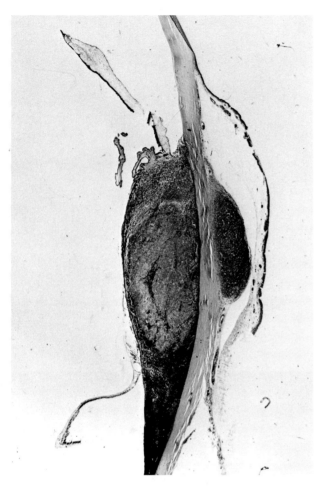

Fig. 7-62. Malignant melanoma of the choroid and ciliary body with extrabulbar extension. (H & E stain; ×8.)

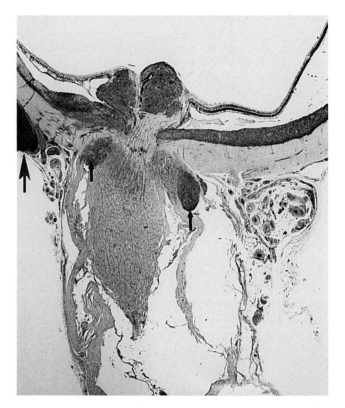

Fig. 7-63. Photomicrograph of an enucleated eye with an epiperipapillary choroidal malignant melanoma. Note that the tumor has already extended extrasclerally behind the globe (left, *large arrow*) and into the optic nerve meningeal sheathing (*small arrows*). It is sometimes difficult to distinguish a highly malignant lesion such as this from an epipapillary melanocytoma. (H & E stain; ×35.)

deposition of the tumor on the outer surface of the sclera can significantly affect prognosis. Survival is difficult to predict accurately in cases in which extension has occurred because other factors such as tumor size and cell type strongly influence the behavior pattern of the tumor. The probability of tumor recurrence, hematogenous metastasis, and death, however, is significantly increased in cases in which emissarial extension has occurred.

Flat diffuse melanomas and tumors arising from the ciliary body sometimes extend into the anterior segment (Figs. 7-48 and 7-52). Dilated episcleral or conjunctival vessels caused by an intraocular tumor can lead to a mistaken diagnosis of conjunctivitis. Permeation into the anterior chamber angle outflow channels and deposition of tumor nodules within the subconjunctival stroma at or near the limbus occasionally occur (Fig. 7-35, 7-36, 7-49, 7-50, and 7-62; Color Plate 7-20). Melanomas of the peripheral choroid and ciliary body are sometimes missed and are first detected after invasion of the subconjunctival stroma. In observing pigmented foci in the subconjunctival stroma just posterior to the limbus, one should rule out the possibility of an Axenfeld nerve loop (p. 60; Fig. 3-1) or a staphyloma caused by other factors that may mimic a hyperpigmented neoplasm.[520] Careful examination of the peripheral fundus

with scleral depression may help identify a primary intraocular mass.

In contrast to the retinoblastoma, in which optic nerve invasion is common, uveal malignant melanoma only rarely invades deeply into the nerve (Fig. 7-47).[913] The extraocular tumor may be locally confined to the epibulbar surface or may infiltrate and fill the orbit (rarely leading to proptosis). According to Hogan and Zimmerman,[629] about 45% of all patients with uveal melanoma die of metastasis within 5 years after enucleation. We have not observed such a high mortality in our patients at the Medical University of South Carolina. This difference probably reflects the fact that the Armed Forces Institute of Pathology functions as a referral center and as such receives enucleated specimens from more advanced and complicated cases than the ones we see in our medical centers.

The liver (Fig. 7-65; Color Plate 7-22) is by far the most common site of metastasis of the uveal melanoma.[521,522,523,548,765] Liver enlargement may be noticed before enucleation (rare), within months following the diagnosis of the primary neoplasm, or many decades after enucleation.[576] Immunologic factors may play an important role in prevention of metastases.* Liver metastasis is most

---

* References 470, 473, 475, 476, 490, 499, 507, 524, 530, 545, 546, 547, 664, 677, 707, 748, 788, 789, 924, 965.

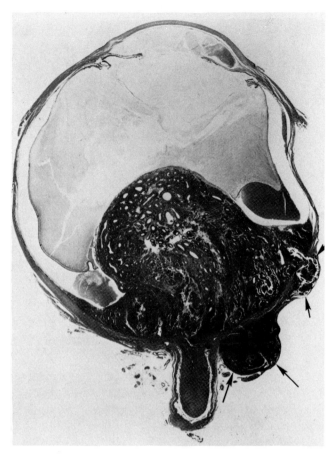

Fig. 7-64. Large malignant melanoma of the choroid, with extraocular extension. *Arrows,* Two episcleral deposits. The tumor has directly permeated the sclera at the site of the smaller deposit *(right).* (H & E stain; ×2.)

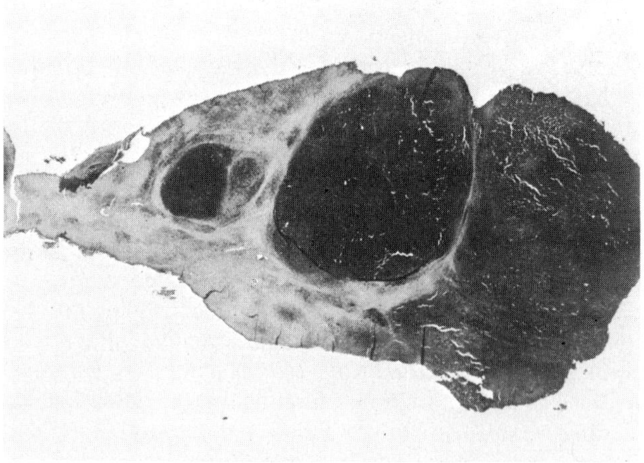

Fig. 7-65. Photomicrograph of a section of liver containing numerous nodules of malignant melanoma cells in a 34-year-old woman. The liver weighed more than 5000 g (a normal liver weighs less than 1500 g). These deposits metastasized from a primary tumor in the choroid. The intervening clear areas between the pigmented tumor deposits consist of fibrotic liver parenchyma. Three deeply pigmented tumor deposits are situated within paler-staining areas of degenerate, fibrotic liver parenchyma. The metastatic foci are of the epithelioid cell type. The liver is the organ most commonly involved by distant metastasis of uveal malignant melanoma. (H & E stain; ×3.)

commonly encountered in cases in which the primary intraocular mass was composed of epithelioid cells or showed a mixed cell type.

One cannot assign a prognosis to a given case of uveal malignant melanoma based solely on single factors such as cell type. Four major criteria must be assessed to estimate prognosis in a specific case: (1) cell typing according to the Callender classification, (2) location of the tumor within the uvea, (3) size of the tumor, and (4) presence or extent of extraocular extension and/or metastasis.

Treatment

Several authors have hypothesized that enucleation of uveal malignant melanoma may be harmful and may actually promote metastasis.* Many of the arguments related to this issue are reasonable but, to date, are based to a great extent on retrospective data and circumstantial evidence. This question can be resolved only by performing a randomized prospective study, a difficult task.

The main thrust of their data is that distant metastasis is rare before enucleation, while a distinct increase in metastatic disease and mortality occurs in the years immediately

following enucleation. It may be true that enucleation accelerates the metastatic process. On the other hand, an understanding of the patterns of growth of melanomas outlined in this chapter could provide an equally feasible explanation of the postenucleation peak in the death rate. One cannot ignore the fact that any postenucleation peak in tumor-related death might simply reflect the fact that (1) the tumor has entered the more "malignant" phase of growth (as described in detail in this chapter); (2) the resultant clinical symptoms were recognized only after advancement to this phase (Fig. 7-32; Table 7-6; p. 312), indicating a relative delay in the clinical diagnosis; (3) the eye was enucleated at this later, poor prognosis stage; and (4) death occurred later, *independent of the therapy.* Regardless of the current controversy, the choice of treatment of a uveal melanoma depends on many factors, including location, size, and cell type of the tumor (p. 311).

Solitary iris tumors (Fig. 7-26) can usually be completely excised by a simple iridectomy, if indeed they require therapy at all. Such tumors are relatively slow growing, are characterized by a relatively benign cell type, and are diagnosed during early stages of growth. It is important to differentiate a localized iris melanoma from a melanoma on the iris that extends into the angle. Many such tumors actually arise from the ciliary body and involve the iris secondarily. These tumors, therefore, exhibit the more malignant course associated with ciliary body malignant melanomas (p. 310). For example, Color Plate 7-17 illustrates a malignant melanoma of the ciliary body and iris. If a simple iridectomy were performed in this case, residual tumor could remain in the eye; however, such a tumor could be locally excised by an iridocyclectomy.[449,567,569,799,804] A suc-

---

* Reference 496, 503, 867, 868, 893, 999, 1002-1008.

cessful, complete excision with this procedure obviates further surgery or enucleation.

Enucleation is still a widely used treatment for choroidal melanoma. Unfortunately, many otherwise normal globes are lost in enucleation; however, largely because of the efforts of Zimmerman and colleagues, unnecessary enucleations are now much less common. Malignant melanocytic tumors are now being watched or treated locally with success, leading to a great reduction in morbidity. Local forms of treatment would be highly desirable in many cases, particularly when the mass is small. Several articles provide up-to-date information concerning alternative (nonenucleation) forms of treatment of uveal malignant melanoma.*

Local treatment by transscleral diathermy, radiation, including cobalt or iodine radiation and chemotherapy and charged-particle (helium ion and proton) therapy, photocoagulation and photodynamics therapy, transpupillary thermotherapy, are now considered rational but still experimental approaches.† The efficacy of these therapeutic modalities requires further evaluation. In particular, clinicopathologic confirmation of the degree of tumor destruction by these physical energy modalities must be obtained. Such forms of treatment have one major disadvantage: histopathologic confirmation of the nature of the tumor and the efficacy of treatment cannot be established. One cannot determine the cell type or assess the degree of emissarial tumor extension as long as the tumor remains in situ.[355] Furthermore, some experimental evidence has shown that photocoagulation may only partially destroy a choroidal malignant melanoma.‡

Peyman's, Kara's, and Foulds's recent experiences indicate that local surgical resection of choroidal tumors may be feasible (Fig. 7-66).§ If future experiments and clinical trials support this conclusion, a major breakthrough will be accomplished. One major advantage is the fact that the excised tumor mass could be histologically studied and the completeness of the excision evaluated. The implications of local surgical excision of choroidal melanomas by full-thickness, eye-wall resection for cosmesis and retention of vision are obvious. The clearest indication of this technique is in the treatment of monocular patients with intraocular malignant melanoma.

The concept that uveal melanomas may enter various phases of growth (Fig. 7-32) indicates that it is no longer sufficient to determine a single unqualified diagnosis of malignant melanoma of the uvea without an attempt to classify the lesion according to its particular growth phase. In essence, one is basically dealing with two tumors, one with a mortality no higher than 10% to 15%, the second with a mortality of 40% to 50% or greater. If we can arrest or eradicate the tumor before the latter stage is reached, the prognosis is favorable. If the tumor has reached (or we allow it to reach) the second phase of the curve, we are faced with a much more vicious neoplasm.

The 10% to 15% death rate that occurs in small phase

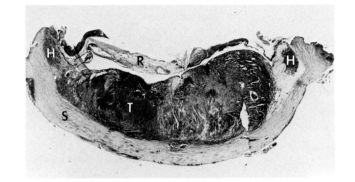

Fig. 7-66. Photomicrograph of a local excision of choroidal malignant melanoma. *T,* Main tumor mass; *R,* overlying retina destroyed by photocoagulation; *H,* small foci of hemorrhage adjacent to the margins of excision; *S,* sclera. (H & E stain; × 100.) (From Peyman GA and Apple DJ: Arch Ophthalmol 92:216, 1974. Copyright 1974, American Medical Association.)

A tumors probably results from the unfortunate fact that (1) a small percentage of "small" melanomas may contain epithelioid cells (an indication of transition into the rapid growth phase that is clinically impossible to detect) or that (2) a hidden posterior extrascleral extension without detectable symptoms may occur. This is the risk that one takes when one simply observes a tumor or uses a local treatment that does not reach the posterior aspect of the tumor. For this reason, advocates of early enucleation press their conviction to treat early, that is, to salvage the additional 10% to 15% of patients who will theoretically succumb if one does not intervene.

In instances in which the more aggressive growth phase has not yet commenced, the most important and difficult question is whether the visual loss caused by treatment of the melanoma to keep it from advancing is tolerable to a given patient. There is no simple answer. A blanket statement concluding that *all* small melanomas should be left alone, that *all* should be enucleated, or that *all* degrees of "in-between treatment" should be carried out is impossible. Many patients would agree to the loss of an eye or a decreased visual acuity if a reasonable hope existed that the mortality could be held to that expected from phase II-A lesions (less than 10%–15% over 6 years.) In practice, we have found that many patients who have good or reasonably good vision in the opposite eye accept this course when the options are carefully explained. On the other hand, some patients undoubtedly would prefer to take a chance with the tumor (with the possible higher mortality of [40%–50% or greater over 6 years] of phase II-B lesions) if treatment is accompanied by any visual loss, particularly patients in whom the visual acuity of the opposite eye is compromised.

METASTASIS OF TUMORS TO THE EYE

Metastasis of tumors to the choroid from distant primary sources must be included in the differential diagnosis of malignant melanoma.[1011-1086] Carcinoma of the breast and bronchogenic carcinoma are among the most common malignancies in women and men, respectively, and these are the malignant tumors that most frequently metastasize to

---

* References 449, 567, 569, 648, 729, 730, 771, 772.
† References 474, 479, 483, 494, 508, 509, 575, 593, 605, 606, 615, 654, 656, 657, 685-688, 691, 694, 701, 703, 742, 763, 811, 823, 838, 844, 846, 863, 865, 890, 914, 915, 919, 1010.
‡ References 420, 422, 501, 531, 630, 690-692, 720, 721, 895, 954, 955.
§ References 449, 729, 730, 771-777, 900, 979.

the eye.° Because of its rich vascular supply, the uvea is the usual site of involvement.† Increased cigarette smoking in women is rapidly altering these statistics. The rate of bronchogenic carcinoma in women has now equaled or surpassed that of breast carcinoma in some states. The diagnosis of cutaneous malignant melanoma to the uvea is sometimes difficult to make sure the primary lesion may not be obvious.[1034,1044,1047]

Metastatic infiltrates in the choroid are often relatively flat (Color Plate 7-23), the area of involvement is broad or diffuse, and multiple infiltrates are not unusual. In contrast, most malignant melanomas tend to be more localized and discrete and to show a greater tendency to elevate toward the vitreous cavity. Minimally elevated metastatic tumors must be considered in the differential diagnosis of a diffusely thickened uvea. Other conditions that cause diffuse uveal thickening include diffuse flat melanoma (p. 310), sympathetic ophthalmia (p. 298), lymphoid hyperplasia, reticular cell sarcoma, leukemia, and diseases that cause uveal effusion.‡

Occasionally an eye is enucleated and, after pathological study of the specimen, a metastatic tumor is discovered despite an absence of any clinical confirmation of a primary neoplasm elsewhere in the body. Histopathologic examination of the intraocular deposits of tumor can assist in determining the tissue origin in such cases. A bronchogenic carcinoma is suggested if a squamous cell differentiation is observed or if the tumor within the choroid has the appearance of the so-called oat cell carcinoma. An adenocarcinoma (Fig. 7-67, A) within the choroid in a woman suggests a carcinoma in the breast. Figures 7-67, B, and 7-68 and Color Plate 7-24 show relatively rare examples of adenocarcinoma that originate in the lung. A clear cell carcinoma suggests a renal cell carcinoma (hypernephroma) and should prompt a urologic workup.[742,1056] Color Plates 7-25 through 7-28 show metastatic thyroid and amyloid-cyst carcinomas to the choroid.

Although metastasis to the retina and optic nerve is much rarer than metastasis to the highly vascular uvea, it sometimes occurs.[679,1057,1066] Plasma cell myeloma may cause fundus alterations (Fig. 7-69). Leukemic infiltrates to the choroid and retina occasionally occur (Color Plates 7-29 and 7-30). About 30% of autopsy eyes from fatal leukemic cases show ocular involvement, mainly leukemic infiltrates in the choroid. Also 42% of newly diagnosed cases of acute leukemia show ocular findings, especially intraretinal hemorrhages, white-centered hemorrhages, and cotton-wool spots.

NEUROEPITHELIAL TUMORS OF THE CILIARY BODY

The ciliary body is composed of (1) the bilayered epithelial lining derived from the pars ciliaris retinae of the two-layered optic cup (Figs. 1-9, B, and 1-11, B) and (2) the stroma, which is composed of mesodermal structures (primarily smooth muscle) and uveal melanocytes derived from the neural crest. Tumors of the ciliary body may arise either within the stroma or from the epithelium that borders the posterior chamber and vitreous.[1087-1182] Tumors originating within the stroma include the melanocytic tumors (nevi, melanocytoma, and malignant melanoma) and leiomyomas, some which probably represent unclassified neural crest tumors.

Epithelial tumors of the ciliary body occur in children and adults. In infants and children they often appear as a white retropupillary mass, causing a leukokoria. (See Chapter 9, p. 492, for a discussion of the differential diagnosis of leukokoria.) These childhood tumors were formerly designated "diktyomas"; they are now classified as medulloepitheliomas.

Consideration of neuroepithelial tumors of the ciliary body would be equally appropriate in the chapter on the retina because the epithelial layers (that is, the outer pigmented layer and the inner nonpigmented layer from which the tumors often originate) are derived from the embryonic optic cup, are, therefore, "retinal" in derivation and sometimes arise from the retina.[1087,1117] This portion of the optic cup is called the pars ciliaris or pars caeca retinae (Fig. 1-11). This category of tumors, however, is discussed in detail in this chapter because ciliary body masses are sometimes considered in the differential diagnosis of malignant melanoma of the ciliary body.

Apart from the relatively rare neuroepithelial tumors of the ciliary body described here, the retinal pigment epithelium and the pigmented epithelia of the ciliary body and iris are not prone to neoplasia.[794] Benign reactive proliferation or hyperplasia of these layers, however, occurs frequently as a response to many stimuli, such as trauma or intraocular inflammation. Proliferative and degenerative changes of the retinal pigment epithelium are responsible for the formation of drusen or for laying down of bone in phthisic eyes (p. 304). Proliferation of ciliary body epithelium frequently contributes to the formation of a cyclitic membrane. This typically occurs in uveitis or as a sequela of trauma. It consists of fronds of ciliary epithelium interspersed with amorphous, eosinophilic ground substance composed of basement membrane material, collagen, and mucopolysaccharides (Fig. 7-70).

The ciliary epithelium often undergoes a more localized hyperplasia, forming a circumscribed nodular enlargement of the ciliary body. Such a growth may follow trauma or other forms of irritation or may be a spontaneous growth caused by unknown factors. Such lesions, seen in up to one quarter of the adult population, are sometimes designated "Fuchs' adenoma" (Fig. 7-62; Color Plate 7-31).° Fuchs' adenoma is proliferation rather than neoplastic lesion.

In 1908 Fuchs'[776-1113] adopted the term *diktyoma* to describe a group of ciliary body tumors occurring in infancy and childhood. He chose this term because the microscopic arrangement of the tumor cells was such that interlacing rows or cords of epithelial cells created the appearance of a lacework or network (Greek *diktyon*, net) (Fig. 7-63). This term is not widely accepted today, and tumors of this type are now considered neuroepithelial tumors of the cili-

---

° References 1018, 1019, 1026, 1041, 1046, 1050.

† References 409, 488, 1011, 1012, 1013, 1015, 1023, 1025, 1027, 1028-1033, 1036-1040, 1042, 1043, 1048, 1050-1052, 1083, 1085.

‡ References 411, 430, 457, 480, 485, 511, 513, 597, 670, 689, 764, 769, 786, 813, 828, 829, 850, 926, 959, 961, 992, 996, 1017, 1035, 1045, 1049, 1053, 1080, 1081, 1084, 1086.

° References 1090, 1092, 1103, 1113, 1119, 1180.

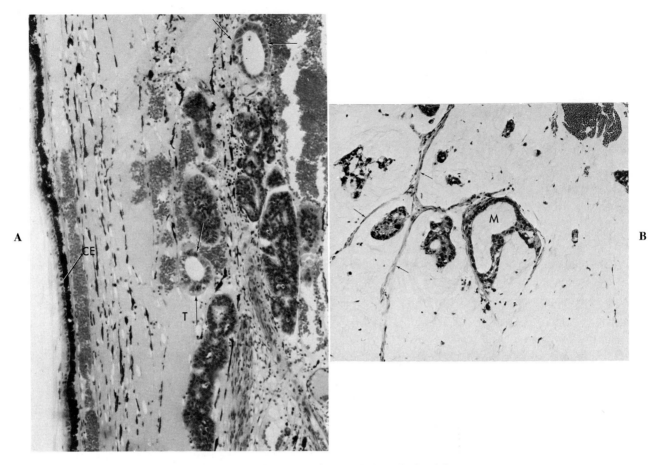

Fig. 7-67. A, Photomicrograph of the ciliary body and choroid of a globe containing metastatic adenocarcinoma from the breast. The tumor cells demonstrate formation of glandlike structures *(arrows).* The cells are arranged around a central lumen. Because breast tumor is a common form of tumor in the female and lung carcinoma is relatively common in males, it follows that these two tumors are the types that most frequently metastasize to the uvea. *CE,* Bilayered ciliary epithelium; *T,* transudate (edema fluid) within the stroma. (H & E stain; ×200.) **B,** High-power photomicrograph through the choroid of the eye of an 81-year-old man with metastatic mucin-secreting adenocarcinoma from the lung. The tumor cell nests are arranged in solid cords and in glandular patterns. Outpouring of mucin *(M)* is extensive within the gland lumen and throughout the major bulk of the tumor. The mucin is poorly stained by the hematoxylin and eosin technique and appears as a white matrix with a delicate fibrillar background. *Arrows,* Collagenous fibrils in the choroid, which are separated by the epithelial and mucinous components of the tumor. (H & E stain; ×350.) (See also Fig. 7-68 and Color Plate 7-24.) (Courtesy Dr. John Hattenhauer.)

ary body. The most widely accepted classification of these tumors is that of Zimmerman.[816]

A. Congenital
   1. Glioneuroma
   2. Medulloepithelioma
      a. Benign
      b. Malignant
   3. Teratoid medulloepthelioma
      a. Benign
      b. Malignant
B. Acquired
   1. Pseudoadenomatous hyperplasia
   2. Adenoma
      a. Solid
      b. Papillary
      c. Pleomorphic

   3. Adenocarcinoma
      a. Solid
      b. Papillary
      c. Pleomorphic

Medulloepithelioma

The tumor that usually appears in the pediatric age group, formerly called the diktyoma, is designated the medulloepithelioma.* The prefix *medullo* signifies an origin from cells resembling the medullary epithelium that lines the neural tube. This same cell line, following evagination from the brain, forms the primitive bilayered optic cup during normal ocular development (p. 7).

The tumor is unilateral and may be well-circumscribed

---

* In exceptional cases, this tumor occurs in adults.

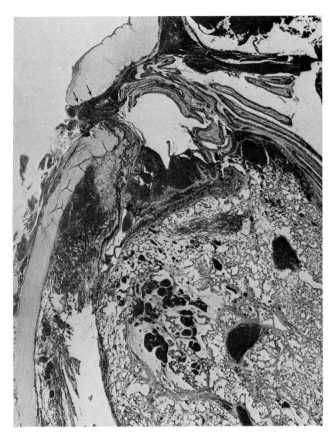

Fig. 7-68. Metastatic adenocarcinoma filling the globe. The glandular acini are arranged in a Swiss cheese pattern. A dense cataract prevented visual observation of the tumor. An operative expulsive hemorrhage occurred through a corneal cataract incision *(arrows)*. Note the multiple folds of detached retina. (H & E stain; ×17.) (Courtesy Dr. John Hattenhauer.)

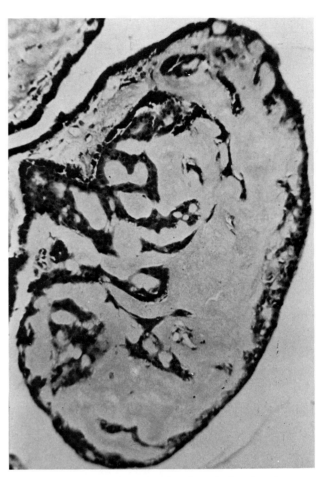

Fig. 7-70. Fuchs" adenoma of the ciliary body. The ciliary epithelium has proliferated with deposition of amorphous ground substance between cells. (H & E stain; ×50.)

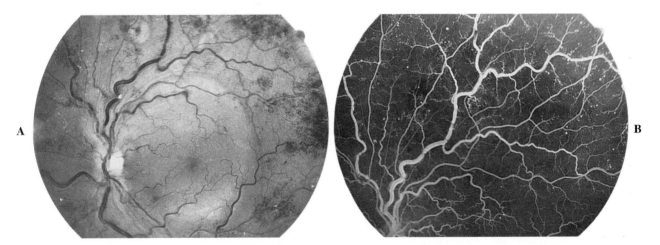

Fig. 7-69. Fundus appearance of multiple myeloma. **A,** Fundus photograph showing a large sensory retinal detachment, with engorgement of retinal venules, attenuation of retinal arteries, and scattered intraretinal hemorrhages throughout the fundus periphery. **B,** Fluorescein angiogram, venous phase, showing venous dilatation, tortuosity and multiple microaneurysms in the periphery.

or infiltrate the area around the lens. Most cases present at birth with a papillary reflex or leukocoria, glaucoma may occur, and most tumors grow slowly and are only locally aggressive.

The medulloepithelioma consists of two cellular components: epithelial cords and a fibrillar matrix.° Rows of epithelial cells (Fig. 7-71, Color Plate 7-32) are arranged in convoluted patterns showing various sizes and shapes. Sometimes the cells are arranged in a circular pattern around a lumen, forming a rosette-like structure or a structure that resembles an embryonic neural tube (Fig. 7-71, *B*). More commonly, however, the epithelial cells are arranged in elongated, interlacing cords. Occasionally a bilayered, crescent-shaped structure forms that closely resembles an embryonic optic cup (Fig. 7-71, *B*). Both pigmented

and nonpigmented epithelial cells may be present, indicating that this growth represents an attempt to differentiate into the pigmented and nonpigmented layers characterizing the normal embryonic optic cup epithelium. In the more malignant tumors some of the cells are very poorly differentiated and may resemble retinoblastoma cells. Special stains that may be positive include neuron-specific enolase, vimentin, and S-100 protein.

Like most other epithelial neoplasms, the medulloepithelioma forms a tumor stroma, or matrix, which occasionally is extensive and sometimes forms the bulk of the mass. It is composed of loose, delicate fibrils with abundant ground substance, which strongly resembles embryonic mesenchyme or myxoid tissue (Fig. 7-71). It has long been known that this interstitial material resembles embryonic vitreous. Special staining techniques have demonstrated the presence of hyaluronic acid within the stroma, and it is now clear that this component of the tumor is an attempt by the tumor cells to form embryonic vitreous. Just as the

---

° References 1088, 1091, 1095, 1100, 1102, 1110, 1112, 1113, 1114, 1119, 1125, 1134–1136, 1143, 1144, 1151, 1152, 1169, 1175.

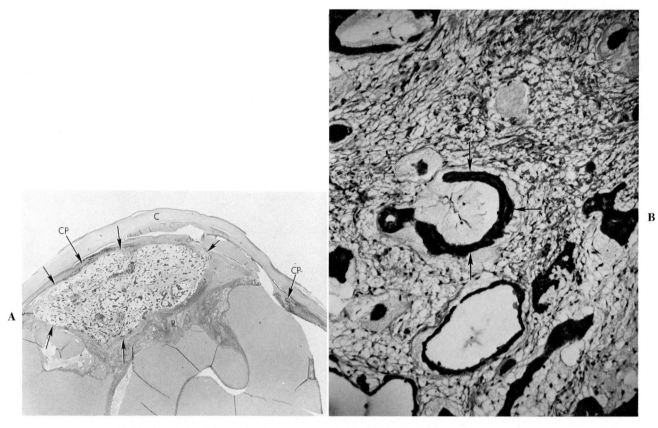

Fig. 7-71. Medulloepithelioma of the ciliary body in a child. **A,** The tumor mass *(arrows)* may induce a leukokoria and mimic a retinoblastoma. The tumor is composed of cords of deeply staining epithelium and a loose background stroma. *C,* Cornea; *CP,* ciliary processes; *R,* totally detached retina adherent to the posterior aspect of the tumor. (H & E stain; ×10.) **B,** Medulloepitheliomas have two components. The epithelial component is composed of rows or cords of cuboidal cells resembling those found in the embryonic eye. Note the formation of tubular or rosettelike structures, which some authors interpret as representing an attempt to form a neural tube. A differentiation of the epithelial component of the tumor toward a structure resembling an embryonic, two-layered, crescent-shaped optic cup *(arrows)* is also apparent. The second component is an interstitial fibrillar matrix composed of elongated spindle-shaped cells with delicate fibrils. This tumor stroma contains a ground substance that has been shown to contain hyaluronic acid. The formation of the stroma represents an attempt by the tumor to form embryonic vitreous. (H & E stain; ×35.)

fibrillar component of the normal primary vitreous humor is derived from the epithelium of the optic cup, the fibrillar matrix of a medulloepithelioma is derived from enoplastic cells that stem from the same cell line as those forming the optic cup.

The *teratoid* medulloepithelioma exhibits epithelial and stromal growth identical to that of the simple medulloepithelioma.[1097,1115,1118,1176–1179] A teratoid medulloepithelioma, however, is further distinguished by the presence of one or more heteroplastic elements (abnormally positioned tissues that are not normally present in the globe; cells that one would not generally expect to form from the optic anlage) in addition to the simple epithelial and stromal components. Because this tumor is composed of embryonic cells that are presumably capable of differentiating toward several cell lines (that is, exhibit pluripotentiality), it should not be surprising that differentiation toward various bizarre, heteroplastic elements is possible. The most frequently observed heteroplastic element formed by this tumor is hyaline cartilage (Fig. 7-72). This tumor, therefore, shares with trisomy 13 cartilage within the ciliary body. Cartilage formed within the ciliary body coloboma in trisomy 13 (Fig. 2-57) is an example of a *dysplastic growth*; the cartilage seen within a teratoid medulloepithelioma is formed from *neoplastic growth*. Other heteroplastic elements occasionally seen in a medulloepithelioma are brain tissue and rhabdomyoblastic cells. In rare instances the rhabdomyoblastic component may predominate, and the microscopic pattern is that of a rhabdomyosarcoma.[817–1182]

Most medulloepitheliomas are relatively benign or are only locally invasive. Even when malignant differentiation occurs, metastasis to distant organs is unusual but does occur.[1097,1135,1148]

Adenoma and adenocarcinoma

Acquired neuroepithelial tumors of the ciliary body (Fig. 7-73, *A*), usually seen in adults, are characterized by tumor

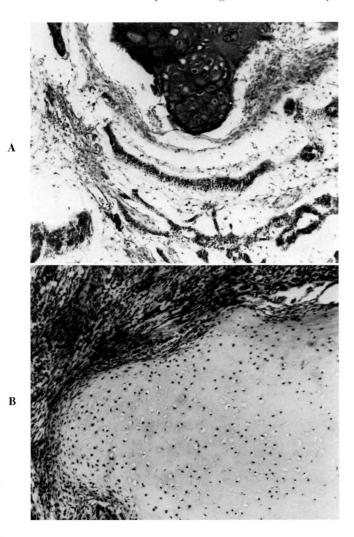

Fig. 7-72. Medulloepithelioma with cartilage within the ciliary body tumor. **A,** Cartilage *(above)*, epithelial cords, and stroma *(below)*. (H & E stain; ×300.) **B,** Higher power micrograph of cartilage. (H & E stain; ×350.)

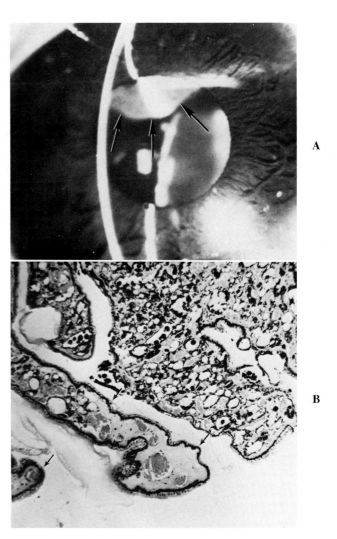

Fig. 7-73. A, Slitlamp appearance of an adenoma of the ciliary epithelium in a 20-year-old man. *Arrows,* Inferior margin of the moderately pigmented, well-circumscribed ciliary body mass. **B,** Benign pigment epithelial adenoma of the ciliary process in a young adult, same cases as **A.** *Arrows,* Normal ciliary processes. The tumor (above) is composed of tiny, pigmented cuboidal cells arranged in an adenomatous manner around a lumen. (H & E stain; ×175.) (**A** courtesy Dr. James Bizzell.)

cell differentiation, which approximates that of the normal, mature, cuboidal ciliary epithelium.[767,772,819] The immature, embryonic neuroepithelial cells that characterize the congenital or infantile medulloepithelioma are usually absent. In keeping with the fact that the normal ciliary epithelium is composed of a pigmented and a nonpigmented layer, these acquired tumors may show a similar variation in pigmentation. The simple terms *adenoma* and *carcinoma* satisfactorily describe these tumors. Embryonic differentiation of tumor cells rarely occurs in the adult form; the term *adult medulloepithelioma*, therefore, rarely applies and should be used only when embryonic tissue is noticed. Most tumors of this type are benign adenomas (Fig. 7-73, *B*). Even cases in which mitotic activity is great and which are, therefore, classified as carcinomas show little propensity to metastasize; however, local invasion in untreated cases can lead to loss of the eye. When the mass is sufficiently small and localized, local excision, such as iridocyclectomy, is considered the treatment of choice (Fig. 7-73). If the tumor is fully excised, the eye is saved. If the tumor is incompletely excised or is found to be highly malignant (including an unsuspected ciliary body malignant melanoma), subsequent enucleation may be indicated.

REFERENCES

General References

1. Bedford MA: A colour atlas of ocular tumours, London, 1979, Wolfe Medical Publications, Ltd.
2. Blodi FC, Allen L, and Braley AE: Stereoscopic manual of the ocular fundus in local and systemic disease, vol 1, St. Louis, 1964, The CV Mosby Co.
3. Blodi FC, Allen L, and Frazier O: Stereoscopic manual of the ocular fundus in local and systemic disease, vol 2, St. Louis, 1970, The CV Mosby Co.
4. Brovkina AF and Chichua AG: Value of fluorescein iridography in diagnosis of tumors of the iridociliary zone, Br J Ophthalmol 63: 157, 1979.
5. Capo H, Palmer E, and Nicholson DH: Congenital cysts of the iris stroma, Am J Ophthalmol 116:228, 1993.
6. Coburn A and others: Spontaneous intrastromal iris cyst. A case report with immunohistochemical and ultrastructural observations, Ophthalmology 92:1691, 1985.
7. Coster DJ: Teacher Collins Prize Essay, 1979: Inflammatory disease of the outer eye, Trans Ophthalmol Soc 99:163, 1979.
8. Daicker B: Anatomie and Pathologie der menschilichen Retinoziliaren Fundusperipherie, Basel, 1972, S Karger, AC.
9. Deutman AF: Choriocapillaris filling patterns in health and disease, Trans Ophthalmol Soc UK 100:553, 1980.
10. Donaldson D: Atlas of external diseases of the eye, vol IV. Anterior chamber, iris, and ciliary body, St. Louis, 1973, The CV Mosby Co.
11. Duke-Elder S and Perkins ES: System of ophthalmology, vol IX. Diseases of the uveal tract, St. Louis, 1966, The CV Mosby Co.
12. Easty D: Manifestations of immunodeficiency diseases in ophthalmology, Trans Ophthalmol Soc UK 97:8, 1977.
13. Fine BS: Free-floating pigmented cyst in the anterior chamber, Am J Ophthalmol 67:493, 1969.
14. Fuchs" E: Das Sarcoin des Uvealtractus, Vienna, 1882, Wilhelm Braumüller.
15. Gartner S and Henkind P: Neovascularization of the iris (rubeosis iridis), Surv Ophthalmol 22:291, 1978.
16. Ginsburg D: Die Uvea. In Henke F, and Lubarsch O, editors: Handbuch der speziellen pathologischen Anatomic and Histologie, Berlin, 1928, Julius Springer.
17. Greef L: Dic pathologische Anatomie des Auges. In Orth J: Lehrbuch der speziellen pathologischen Anatomic, Berlin, 1902, Hirschwald.
18. Imesch PD and others: Melanocytes and iris color—electron microscopic findings, Arch Ophthalmol 114:443, 1996.
19. Jakobiec FA: Ocular and adnexal tumors, Amsterdam, The Netherlands, 1978, Kugler Publications, BV.
20. Kaufman H: The uvea, Arch Ophthalmol 75:407, 1966.
21. Khalil AK and others: Ultrastructural age-related changes on the posterior iris surface. A possible relationship to the pathogenesis of exfoliation, Arch Ophthalmol 114:721, 1996.
22. Kottow MH: Anterior segment fluorescein angiography, Baltimore, 1978, The Williams & Wilkins Co.
23. Leber T: In Axenfeld T: Lehrbuch und Atlas der Augenheilkunde, Jena, 1912, Gustav Fischer.
24. McGovern VJ: Malignant melanoma: clinical and histological diagnosis, New York, 1976, John Wiley & Sons, Inc.
25. Meyncr E: Atlas der Spaltlampenphotographic, Stuttgart, 1976, Ferdinand Enke Verlag.
26. Morrison JC and Van Buskirk EM: Ciliary process microvasculature of the primate eye, Am J Ophthalmol 97:372, 1984.
27. Oeller J: Atlas scltener ophthalmoskopischer Befunde, Wiesbaden, 1903, JF Bergmann.
28. Perry HD, Hatfield RV, and Tso MOM: Fluorescin pattern of the choriocapillaris in the neonatal rhesus monkey, Am J Ophthalmol 81:197, 1977.
29. Peyman GA, Apple DJ, and Sanders DR, editors: Intraocular tumors, New York, 1977, Appleton-Century-Crofts.
30. Reese AB: Tumors of the eye, ed 3, New York, 1976, Harper & Row, Publishers.
31. Rummelt V, Rummelt C, and Naumann GOH: Congenital nonpigmented epithelial iris cyst after amniocentesis, Ophthalmology 100: 776, 1993.
32. Schlaegel T: The uvea, Arch Ophthalmol 84:391, 1970.
33. Swan K: Iris pigment nodules complicating miotic therapy, Am J Ophthalmol 37:886, 1954.
34. Waeltermann JM, Hettinger ME, and Cibis GW: Congenital cysts of the iris stroma, Am J Ophthalmol 100:549, 1985.
35. Wilkerson CL and others: Melanocytes and iris color—light microscopic findings, Arch Ophthalmol 114:437, 1996.
36. Yanoff M and Zimmerman IE: Pseudomelanoma of anterior chamber caused by implantation of iris pigment epithelium, Arch Ophthalmol 74:302, 1965.
37. Yoneya S and Tso MOM: Angio-architecture of the human choroid, Arch Ophthalmol 105:681, 1987.
38. Young LHY and others: Photodynamic therapy of pigmented choroidal melanomas using a liposomal preparation of benzoporphyrin derivative, Arch Ophthalmol 114:186, 1996.
39. Zimmerman LE and Sobin LH: Histological typing of tumors of the eye and its adnexa, Geneva, 1980, World Health Organization.
40. Zografos L and others: Cobalt-60 treatment of choroidal hemangiomas, Am J Ophthalmol 121:190, 1996.

Uveitis

41. Affeldt JC and others: Microbial endophthalmitis resulting from ocular trauma, Ophthalmology 94:407, 1987.
42. Afran SI, Budenz DL, and Albert DM: Does enucleation in the presence of endophthalmitis increase the risk of postoperative meningitis? Ophthalmology 94:235, 1987.
43. Albert DM, Norlund JJ, and Lerner AB: Ocular abnormalities occurring with vitiligo, Ophthalmology 86:1145, 1979.
44. Albert DM and others: Vitiligo and disorders of the retinal pigment epithelium, Br J Ophthalmol 67:153, 1983.
45. Almanaseer IY, Kosova L, and Pellettiere EV: Composite lymphoma with immunoblastic features and Langerhans' cell granulomatosis (histiocytosis X), Am J Clin Pathol 85:111, 1986.
46. Alward WLM and Ossoinig KC: Pigment dispersion secondary to cysts of the iris pigment epithelium, Arch Ophthalmol 113:1574, 1995.
47. Apple DJ and Miller K: Letterer-Siwe disease. In Fraunfelder FT and Roy FH, editors: Current ocular therapy, ed 2, Philadelphia, 1984, WB Saunders Co.
48. Aronson SB and Elliott JH: Ocular inflammation, St. Louis, 1972, The CV Mosby Co.
49. Aronson SB and others, editors: Clinical methods in uveitis: the Fourth Sloan Symposium on Uveitis, St. Louis, 1963, The CV Mosby Co.

50. Avendaño J, Tanishima T, and Kuwabara T: Ocular cryptococcosis, Am J Ophthalmol 86:110, 1978.

51. Axelrod AJ, Peyman GA, and Apple DJ: Intravitreal injection of amphotericin B. I. Evaluation of toxicity, Am J Ophthalmol 76:578, 1973.

52. Axelrod AJ, Peyman GA, and Apple DJ: Intravitreal amphotericin B toxicity, Am J Ophthalmol 78:875, 1974, (letter to the editor).

53. Basset F, Nezelof C, and Ferrans VJ: The histiocytosis. Pathol Ann 27, 1982.

54. Beckingsale, AB, Guss RB, and Rosenthal AR: Acute uveitis associated with HLA B27 positive tissue type: a comparative study in two populations, Trans Ophthalmol Soc UK 102:168, 1982.

55. Beniz J and others: Variations in clinical features of the Vogt-Koyanagi-Harada syndrome, Retina 11:275, 1991.

56. Berger BB and Reeser F: Retinal pigment epithelial detachments in posterior scleritis, Am J Ophthalmol 90:604, 1980.

57. Berger BB, Tessler HH, and Kottow MH: Anterior segment ischemia in Fuchs'" heterochromic cyclitis, Arch Ophthalmol 98:499, 1980.

58. Blank H, Eglick P, and Beerman H: Nevoxanthoendothelioma with ocular involvement, Pediatrics 4:349, 1949.

59. Bloch-Michel E: Physiopathology of Fuchs'" heterochromic cyclitis, Trans Ophthalmol Soc UK 101:384, 1981.

60. Blodi FC: Histiocytosis X in an adult, Trans Am Acad Ophthalmol Otolaryngol 68:1012, 1964.

61. Blodi FC and Hervoust F: Syphilitic chorioretinitis: a histologic study, Arch Ophthalmol 78:294, 1968.

62. Bray PT: Histiocytosis X: In Deeley TJ, editor: Modern radiotherapy and oncology: malignant diseases in children, London, 1974, Butterworth & Co, Publishers, Ltd.

63. Bruner WE, Stark WJ, and Green WR: Presumed juvenile xanthogranuloma of the iris and ciliary body in an adult, Arch Ophthalmol 100:457, 1982.

64. Campo RV and Aaberg TM: Choroidal granuloma in sarcoidosis, Am J Ophthalmol 97:419, 1984.

65. Carlson MR and Kerman BM: Hemorrhagic macular detachment in the Vogt-Koyanagi-Harada syndrome, Am J Ophthalmol 84:632, 1977.

66. Carroll DM and Franklin RM: Vitreous biopsy in uveitis of unknown cause, Retina 1:245, 1981.

67. Chan CC and others: Immunohistochemistry and electron microscopy of cyclitic membrane: report of a case, Arch Ophthalmol 104:1040, 1986.

68. Chan CC and others: Immunohistopathology of ocular sarcoidosis: report of a case and discussion of immunopathogenesis, Arch Ophthalmol 105:1398, 1987.

69. Chan CC and others: Immunopathologic study of Vogt-Koyanagi-Harada syndrome, Am J Ophthalmol 105:607, 1988.

70. Chan CC and others: Anti-retinal auto-antibodies in Vogt-Koyanagi-Harada syndrome, Behcet's disease, and sympathetic ophthalmia, Ophthalmology 92:1025, 1985.

71. Chandler JW and Gillette TE: Immunologic defense mechanisms of the ocular surface, Ophthalmology 90:585, 1983.

72. Chapman-Smith JS: Cryptococcal chorioretinitis: a case report, Br J Ophthalmol 61:411, 1977.

73. Cherry PMH, Faulkner JD: A case of subacute sclerosing panencephalitis with exophthalmos, Ann Ophthalmol 7:1579, 1976.

74. Char DH: Immunology of uveitis and ocular tumors, New York, 1978, Grune & Stratton, Inc.

75. Chester GH, Blach RK, and Cleary PE: Inflammations in the region of the vitreous base: pars planitis, Trans Ophthalmol Soc UK 96:151, 1976.

76. Cleasby G: Nevoxanthoendothelioma of iris, Arch Ophthalmol 66:26, 1961.

77. Cogan DG: Immunosuppression and eye disease, Am J Ophthalmol 83:777, 1979.

78. Cogan DG, Kuwabara T, and Parke D: Epibulbar nevoxanthoendothelioma, Arch Ophthalmol 59:717, 1958.

79. Colvard DM, Robertson DM, and O'Duffy JD: The ocular manifestations of Behcet's disease, Arch Ophthalmol 95:1813, 1977.

80. Corwin JM and Weiter JJ: Immunology of chorioretinal disorders, Surv Ophthalmol 25:287, 1981.

81. Crocker AC: The histiocytosis syndromes. In Gellis SS and Kagan BM: Current pediatric therapy 10, Philadelphia, 1982, WB Saunders Co.

82. Croxatto JO and others: Sympathetic ophthalmia after pars plana vitrectomy-lensectomy for endogenous bacterial endophthalmitis, Am J Ophthalmol 91:312, 1981.

83. Cutler JE and others: Metastatic coccidioidal endophthalmitis, Arch Ophthalmol 96:689, 1978.

84. Dalén A: Zur Kenntnis der sogenannten Choroiditis Sympathica, Mitt Augenklin Carol Medchir Inst Stockholm 6:3, 1904.

85. Davis JL and others: HLA associations and ancestry in Vogt-Koyanagi-Harada disease and sympathetic ophthalmia, Ophthalmology 97:1137, 1990.

86. De Abrew MT and others: T-lymphocyte subsets in the aqueous humor and peripheral blood of patients with acute untreated uveitis, Am J Ophthalmol 98:62, 1984.

87. Demeler U: Value of fluorescein angiography of the iris in uveitis, Trans Ophthalmol Soc UK 101:380, 1981.

88. Derhaag PJFM and others: A familial study of the inheritance of HLA-B27 positive acute anterior uveitis, Am J Ophthalmol 105:603, 1988.

89. Dias PLR: Postinflammatory and malignant protein patterns in aqueous humor, Br J Ophthalmol 63:161, 1979.

90. Dinning WJ: Management of chronic uveitis, Trans Ophthalmol Soc UK 96:158, 1976.

91. Doxanas MT, Kelley JS, and Prout TE: Sarcoidosis with neovascularization of the optic nerve head, Am J Ophthalmol 90:347, 1980.

92. Driebe WT Jr and others: Pseudophakic endophthalmitis: diagnosis and management, Ophthalmology 93:442, 1986.

93. Edwards JE and others: Ocular manifestations of *Candida* septicemia: review of seventy-six cases of hematogenous *Candida* endophthalmitis, Medicine 53:47, 1974.

94. Engel JM and others: Diagnostic vitrectomy, Retina 1:121, 1981.

95. Enriquez P and others: Histiocytosis X: a clinical study, Mayo Clin Proc 42:88, 1967.

96. Epstein DL and Grant WM: Secondary open-angle glaucoma in histiocytosis X, Am J Ophthalmol 84:332, 1977.

97. Fine B and Gilligan J: The Vogt-Koyanagi syndrome, a variant of sympathetic ophthalmia: report of two cases, Am J Ophthalmol 43:433, 1957.

98. Fish LA and others: *Propionibacterium acnes* lens abscess after traumatic implantation of intralenticular cilia, Am J Ophthalmol 105:423, 1988.

99. Fisher RF: The lens in uveitis, Trans Ophthalmol Soc UK 101:317, 1981.

100. Font RL and others: Ocular involvement in Whipple's disease: light and electron microscopic observations, Arch Ophthalmol 96:1431, 1978.

101. Font RL, Jenis EH, and Tuck KD: Measles maculopathy associated with subacute sclerosing panencephalitis, Arch Ophthalmol 96:168, 1973.

102. Forster DJ and others: Echographic features of the Vogt-Koyanagi-Harada syndrome, Arch Ophthalmol 108:1421, 1990.

103. Forster DJ and others: Incidence and management of glaucoma in Vogt-Koyanagi-Harada syndrome, Ophthalmology 100:613, 1993.

104. Foster CS, Fong LP, and Singh G: Cataract surgery and intraocular lens implantation in patients with uveitis, Ophthalmology 96:281, 1989.

105. Foster CS and Barrett F: Cataract development and cataract surgery in patient with juvenile rheumatoid arthritis-associated iridocyclitis, Ophthalmology 100:809, 1993.

106. Frank KW and Weiss H: Unusual clinical and histopathological findings in ocular sarcoidosis, Br J Ophthalmol 67:8, 1983.

107. Friedlaender MH: Allergy and immunology of the eye, New York, 1979, Harper & Row, Publishers.

108. Gass J: Management of juvenile xanthogranuloma of iris, Arch Ophthalmol 71:344, 1964.

109. Gibbs CJ: Virus-induced subacute degenerative diseases of the central nervous system, Ophthalmology 87:1208, 1980.

110. Giller RH and others: Xanthoma disseminatum: an unusual histiocytosis syndrome, Am J Pediat Hematol Oncol 10:252, 1988.

111. Glasgow BJ and others: Bilateral endogenous fusarium endophthalmitis associated with acquired immunodeficiency syndrome [clinical conference], Arch Ophthalmol 114:873, 1996.

112. Golden B and Givioset M: Uveitis: immunologic and allergic phenomena, Springfield, III, 1973, Charles C Thomas, Publisher.

113. Googe JM Jr and others: Choroiditis in infantile periarteritis nodosa, Arch Ophthalmol 103:81, 1985.

114. Green WR and Koo BS: Behçet's disease. A report of the ocular histology of one case, Surv Ophthalmol 12:324, 1967.

115. Green MT and others: Endogenous *Clostridium* panophthalmitis, Ophthalmology 94:435, 1987.

116. Green WR, Kincaid MC, and Fogle JA: Uveal effusion syndrome, Trans Ophthalmol Soc UK 101:368, 1981.

117. Green WR and others: Pars planitis, Trans Ophthalmol Soc UK 101:361, 1981.

118. Greenberger JS and others: Results of treatment of 127 patients with systemic histiocytosis (Letterer-Siwe syndrome, Schuller-Christian syndrome and multifocal eosinophilic granuloma), Medicine 60:311, 1981.

119. Greenwald MJ, Wohl LG, and Sell CH: Metastatic bacterial endophthalmitis: a contemporary reappraisal, Surv Ophthalmol 31: 81, 1986.

120. Guyton J and Woods A: Etiology of uveitis: a clinical study of five-hundred and sixty-two cases, Arch Ophthalmol 26:982, 1941.

121. Harada Y: Beiträge zur klinischen Kenntnis von nichteitriger Choroiditis, Nippon Canka Zasshi 30:356, 1926.

122. Harrist TJ and others: Histiocytosis-X: *In situ* characterization of cutaneous infiltrates with monoclonal antibodies, Am J Clin Pathol 79:294, 1983.

123. Haslett RS and others: Candida endophthalmitis in job syndrome, Arch Ophthalmol 114:617, 1996, (letter).

124. Heath P: The ocular features of a case of acute reticuloendotheliosis (Letterer-Siwe type), Trans Am Ophthalmol Soc 57:290-302, 1959.

125. Helwig E and Hackney V: Juvenile xanthogranuloma (nevoxanthoendothelioma), Am J Pathol 30:625, 1954.

126. Hogan MJ, Thygeson P, and Kimura SJ: Uveitis in association with rheumatism, Trans Am Ophthalmol Soc 54:93, 1956.

127. Holland GN and others: Ocular disorders associated with a new severe acquired cellular immunodeficiency syndrome, Am J Ophthalmol 93,393, 1982.

128. Hoover DL, Khan JA, and Giangiacomo J: Pediatric ocular sarcoidosis, Surv Ophthalmol 30:215, 1985.

129. Howard G: Spontaneous hyphema in infancy and childhood, Arch Ophthalmol 68:615, 1962.

130. Howe JW, Narang HK, and Codd AA: Herpes simplex virus uveitis and optic neuropathy: an experimental investigation, Trans Ophthalmol Soc UK 99:111, 1979.

131. Howes EL and Cruse VK: The structural basis of altered vascular permeability following intraocular inflammation, Arch Ophthalmol 96:1668, 1978.

132. Howes JF: New treatments for anterior uveitis, Ophthalmology 103:1163, 1996, (letter).

133. Hunt KE and Glasgow BJ: Aspergillus endophthalmitis—an unrecognized endemic disease in orthotopic liver transplantation, Ophthalmology 103:757, 1996.

134. Ibanez HE and others: Magnetic resonance imaging findings in Vogt-Koyanagi-Harada syndrome, Retina 14:164, 1994.

135. Ikui H and Hiyama H: Clinical and experimental studies on idiopathic uveitis. (2) Histopathology of Harada's disease. Report of case, Acta Societ Ophthalmol Japonicae 60:1687, 1956.

136. Islam SMM and others: HLA class II genes in Vogt-Koyanagi-Harada disease, Invest Ophthalmol Vis Sci 35:3890, 1994.

137. Jain IS and others: Fuchs''' heterochromic cyclitis: some observations on clinical picture and on cataract surgery, Ann Ophthalmol 15:640, 1983.

138. Jakobiec FA and Nelson D: Lymphomatous, plasmacytic, histiocytic, and hematopoietic tumors of the orbit. In Duane TD, editor: Clinical ophthalmology, vol 5, Philadelphia, 1988, JB Lippincott Co.

139. James DG, Friedmann AI, and Graham E: Uveitis: a series of 368 patients, Trans Ophthalmol Soc UK 96:108, 1976.

140. James DG, Neville E, and Langley, DA: Ocular sarcoidosis, Trans Ophthalmol Soc UK 96:133, 1976.

141. John T, Sassani JW, and Eagle RC Jr: The myofibroblastic component of rubeosis iridis, Ophthalmology 90:721, 1983.

142. Johnston HM, Wise GA, and Henry JG: Visual deterioration as presentation of subacute sclerosing panencephalitis, Arch Dis Child 55:899, 1980.

143. Kahn M and others: Immunocytologic findings in a case of Vogt-Koyanagi-Harada syndrome, Ophthalmology 100:1191, 1993.

144. Kampik A, Patrinely JR, and Green WR: Morphologic and clinical features of retrocorneal melanin pigmentation and pigmented pupillary membranes: review of 225 cases, Surv Ophthalmol 27:161, 1982.

145. Kanski JJ: Clinical and immunological study of anterior uveitis in juvenile chronic polyarthritis, Trans Ophthalmol Soc UK 96:123, 1976.

146. Kanski JJ: Anterior uveitis in juvenile rheumatoid arthritis, Arch Ophthalmol 95:1794, 1977.

147. Kanski JJ: Care of children with anterior uveitis, Trans Ophthalmol Soc UK 101:387, 1981.

148. Kanski JJ and Shun-Shin GA: Systemic uveitis syndromes in childhood: an analysis of 340 cases, Ophthalmology 91:1247, 1984.

149. Karma A, Huhti E, and Poukkula A: Course and outcome of ocular sarcoidosis, Am J Ophthalmol 106:467, 1988.

150. Karma A and others: Diagnosis and clinical characteristics of ocular lyme borreliosis, Am J Ophthalmol 119(2):127, 1994.

151. Kijlstra A, Linssen A, Ockhuizen T: Association of Gm allotypes with the occurrence of ankylosing spondylitis in HLA-B27-positive anterior uveitis, Am J Ophthalmol 98:732, 1984.

152. Kimura SJ and Hogan MJ: Chronic cyclitis, Arch Ophthalmol 71: 193, 1964.

153. Kimura SJ, Hogan MJ, and Thygeson P: Uveitis in children, Arch Ophthalmol 51:80, 1954.

154. Kimura SJ, Thygeson P, and Hogan MJ: Signs and symptoms of uveitis. II. Classification of the posterior manifestations of uveitis, Am J Ophthalmol 47:171, 1959.

155. Knox DL and King J Jr: Retinal arteritis, iridocyclitis, and giardiasis, Ophthalmology 89:1303, 1982.

156. Koyanagi Y: Dysakusis, Alopecia and Poliosis bei schwerer Uveitis nicht traumatischen Ursprungs, Klin Monatsbl Augenheilkd 82:194, 1929.

157. Kraus-Mackiw E and O'Connor GR, editors: Uveitis: pathophysiology and therapy, New York, 1983, Thieme-Stratton, Inc.

157a. Laatikainen L: Vascular changes in the iris in chronic anterior uveitis, Br J Ophthalmol 63:145, 1979.

158. Lahav M and Albert D: Unusual ocular involvement in acute disseminated histiocytosis X, Arch Ophthalmol 91:455, 1974.

159. Lahey ME: Histiocytosis. In Spittell JA Jr: Clinical medicine, vol V, Philadelphia, 1986, Harper & Row, Publishers.

160. Lahey ME: Histiocytosis X. In Spittell JA Jr: Clinical medicine, vol VI, Hagerstown, Md, 1979, Harper & Row, Publishers.

161. Lahey ME: Prognostic factors in histiocytosis X, Am J Pediat Hematol Oncol 3:57, 1981.

162. Lamberts DW and Foster CS: Chronic unilateral external ocular inflammation, Surv Ophthalmol 24:157, 1979.

163. Lance SE, Friberg TR, and Kowalski RP: *Aspergillus flavus* endophthalmitis and retinitis in an intravenous drug abuser: a therapeutic success, Ophthalmology 95:947, 1988.

164. Lee DA and others: The clinical diagnosis of Reiter's syndrome: ophthalmic and non-ophthalmic aspects, Ophthalmology 93:350, 1986.

165. Lichtenstein L: Histiocytosis X: integration of eosinophilic granuloma of bone, "Letterer-Siwe disease," and "Schueller-Christian disease" as related manifestations of a single nosologic entity, Arch Pathol 56:84, 1953.

166. Liesegang TJ: Clinical features and prognosis in Fuchs''' uveitis syndrome, Arch Ophthalmol 100:1622, 1982.

167. Loewenfeld I and Thompson H: Fuchs''' heterochromic cyclitis: a critical review of the literature. I. Clinical characteristics of the syndrome, Surv Ophthalmol 17:294, 1973.

168. Loewenfeld I and Thompson H: Fuchs''' heterochromic cyclitis: a critical review of the literature. II. Etiology and mechanisms, Surv Ophthalmol 18:2, 1973.

169. Lucaya J: Histiocytosis X, Am J Dis Child 121:289, 1971.

170. Malinowski SM, Pulido JS, Folk JC: Long-term visual outcome and complications associated with pars planitis, Ophthalmology 100:818, 1993.

171. Manger CC and Ober RR: Retinal arteriovenous anastomoses in the Vogt-Koyanagi-Harada syndrome, Am J Ophthalmol 89:186, 1980.

172. Marcus DF, Bovino JA, and Burton TC: Sarcoid granuloma of the choroid, Ophthalmology 89:1326, 1982.

173. Margo CE, Mames RN, and Guy JR: Endogenous *Klebsiella* endophthalmitis. Report of two cases and review of the literature, Ophthalmology 101:1298, 1994.

174. Mark DB and McCulley JG: Reiter's keratitis, Arch Ophthalmol 100:781, 1982.

175. Martenet A-C: Role of viruses in uveitis, Trans Ophthalmol Soc UK 101:308, 1981.

176. Martenet A-C: Uveitis in connective tissue disorders, Trans Ophthalmol Soc UK 101:376, 1981.

177. Martin DF and others: The role of chorioretinal biopsy in the management of posterior uveitis, Ophthalmology 100:705, 1993.

178. Matoba AY: Ocular disease associated with Epstein-Barr virus infection, Surv Ophthalmol 35:145, 1990, (review).

179. Maumence AE: Ocular lesion of nevoxanthoendothelioma, Trans Am Acad Ophthalmol Otolaryngol 60:401, 1956.

180. Maumenee AE: Clinical entities in "uveitis": an approach to the study of intraocular inflammation, Am J Ophthalmol 69:1, 1970.

181. Maumenee AE: Clinical entities in "uveitis": an approach to the study of intraocular inflammation, Trans Am Acad Ophthalmol Otolaryngol 74:173, 1970.

182. Maumenee AE: Symposium—then and now: uveitis, Trans Ophthalmol Soc UK 100:9, 1980.

183. Maumenee AE and Longfellow D: Treatment of intraocular JXC, Am J Ophthalmol 49:1, 1960.

184. McCarron MJ and Albert DM: Iridocyclitis and an iris mass associated with secondary syphilis, Ophthalmology 91:1264, 1984.

185. McMillan EM and others: Analysis of histiocytosis X infiltrates with monoclonal antibodies directed against cells of histiocytic, lymphoid, and myeloid lineage, Clin Immunol Immunopathol 38: 295, 1986.

186. Meadow WL, Tipple MA, and Rippon JW: Endophthalmitis caused by *Petriellidium boydii*, Am J Dis Child 135:378, 1981.

187. Meisler DM and Mandelbaum S: *Propionibacterium*-associated endophthalmitis after extracapsular cataract extraction: review of reported cases, Ophthalmology 96:54, 1989.

188. Meisler DM and others: Chronic *Propionibacterium* endophthalmitis after extracapsular cataract extraction and intraocular lens implantation, Am J Ophthalmol 102:733, 1986.

189. Meisler DM and others: Endophthalmitis associated with sequestered intraocular *Propionibacterium acnes*, Am J Ophthalmol 104: 428, 1987.

190. Merriam JC, Chylack LT Jr, and Albert DM: Early onset pauciarticular juvenile rheumatoid arthritis: a histopathologic study, Arch Ophthalmol 101:1085, 1983.

191. Michelson JB, and Chisari FV: Behçet's disease, Surv Ophthalmol 26:190, 1982.

192. Michelson JB and others: Ocular reticulum cell sarcoma: presentation as retinal detachment with demonstration of monoclonal immunoglobulin light chains on the vitreous cells, Arch Ophthalmol 99:1409, 1981.

193. Mittelman D, Apple DJ, and Goldberg MF: Ocular involvement of Letterer-Siwe disease, Am J Ophthalmol 75:261, 1973.

194. Mizuno K and Takahashi J: Sarcoid cyclitis, Ophthalmology 93: 511, 1986.

195. Mishima H and others: Plasminogen activator activity levels in patients with Behçet's syndrome, Arch Ophthalmol 103:935, 1985.

196. Mochizuki M and others: Uveitis associated with human T-cell lymphotropic virus type 1, Am J Ophthalmol 114:123, 1992.

197. Moore AT, Pritchard J, Taylor DSI: Histiocytosis X: an ophthalmological review, Br J Ophthalmol 69:7, 1985.

198. Moorthy RS and others: Subretinal neovascular membranes in Vogt-Koyanagi-Harada syndrome, Am J Ophthalmol 116:164, 1993.

199. Moorthy RS, Inomata H, and Rao NA: Vogt-Koyanagi-Harada syndrome, Surv Ophthalmol 39,265, 1995, (major review).

200. Moorthy RS and others: Incidence and management of cataracts in Vogt-Koyanagi-Harada syndrome, Am J Ophthalmol 118:197, 1994.

201. Motoaki D and Uji Y: A case of uveitis associated with idiopathic retroperitoneal fibrosis, Am J Ophthalmol 117:358, 1994.

202. Narose K and others: Immunologic analysis of cerebrospinal fluid lymphocytes in Vogt-Koyanagi-Harada disease, Invest Ophthalmol Vis Sci 31:1210, 1990.

203. Naumann G, Ortbauer R, and Witzenhausen R: *Candida albicans*—Endophthalmitis nach Kataraktextraktion, Ophthalmologica 162:160, 1971.

204. Nelson DA and others: Retinal lesions in subacute sclerosing panencephalitis, Arch Ophthalmol 84:613, 1970.

205. Newell FW: Nevoxanthoendothelioma with ocular involvement: a report of two cases, Arch Ophthalmol 58:321, 1957.

206. Numaga J and others: Analysis of human leukocyte antigen HLA-DR β amino acid sequence in Vogt-Koyanagi-Harada syndrome, Invest Ophthalmol Vis Sci 32:1958, 1991.

207. Oberman HA: Idiopathic histiocytosis: a correlative review of eosinophilic granuloma, Hand-Schuller-Christian disease and Letterer-Siwe disease, J Pediatr Ophthalmol 5:86, 1968.

208. O'Connor GR: Factors related to the initiation and recurrence of uveitis, Am J Ophthalmol 96:577, 1983.

209. O'Connor GR: Heterochromic iridocyclitis, Trans Ophthalmol Soc UK 104:219.

210. Ohno S and others: Close association of HLA-Bw51 with Behçet's disease, Arch Ophthalmol 100:1455, 1982.

211. Olmo S: Immunological aspects of Behçet's and Vogt-Koyanagi-Harada's diseases, Trans Ophthalmol Soc UK 101:335, 1981.

212. Ormerod LD and others: Anaerobic bacterial endophthalmitis, Ophthalmology 94:799, 1987.

213. Ormerod LD and others: The intraocular environment and experimental anaerobic bacterial endophthalmitis, Arch Ophthalmol 105: 1571, 1987.

214. Palestine AG and others: Histopathology of the subretinal fibrosis and uveitis syndrome, Ophthalmology 92:838, 1985.

215. Parver LM and Font RL: Malignant lymphoma of the retina and brain: initial diagnosis by cytologic examination of vitreous aspirate, Arch Ophthalmol 97:1505, 1979.

216. Pattison EM: Uveomeningoencephalitic syndrome (Vogt-Koyanagi-Harada), Arch Neurol 122:197, 1965.

217. Pearlstone AD and Flom L: Letterer-Siwe's disease, J Pediatr Ophthalmol 7:103, 1970.

218. Pederson JE and others: Pathology of pars planitis, Am J Ophthalmol 86:762, 1978.

219. Perkins ES: Uveitis and toxoplasmosis, Boston, 1961, Little, Brown & Co.

220. Perkins ES: Symposium on uveitis: epidemiology of uveitis, Trans Ophthalmol Soc UK 96:105, 1976.

221. Perry HD and Font RL: Clinical and histopathologic observations in severe Vogt-Koyanagi-Harada syndrome, Am J Ophthalmol 83: 242, 1977.

222. Perry HD, Yanoff M, and Scheie HG: Fuchs" heterochromic iridocyclitis, Arch Ophthalmol 93:337, 1975.

223. Petrelli EA, McKinley M, and Troncale FJ: Ocular manifestations of inflammatory bowel disease, Ann Ophthalmol 14:356, 1982.

224. Peyman GA and Sanders DR: Advances in uveal surgery and the treatment of endophthalmitis, Englewood Cliffs, NJ, 1975, Prentice-Hall, Inc.

225. Peyman GA and others: Biopsy of human scleral-chorioretinal tissue, Invest Ophthalmol 14:707, 1975.

226. Rahi AHS and Garner A: Immunopathology of the eye, Philadelphia, 1976, JB Lippincott Co.

227. Rahi AHS, Kanski JJ, and Fielder A: Immunoglobulins and antinuclear antibodies in aqueous humour from patients with juvenile "rheumatoid" arthritis (Still's disease), Trans Ophthalmol Soc UK 97:217, 1977.

228. Rahi AHS and others: Immunological investigations in uveitis, Trans Ophthalmol Soc UK 96:113, 1976.

229. Rahi and others: Immunological investigations in post-traumatic granulomatous and non-granulomatous uveitis, Br J Ophthalmol 62:722, 1978.

230. Raju VK and Green WR: Reticulum cell sarcoma of the uvea, Ann Ophthalmol 14:555, 1982.

231. Rao NA, Marak GE, and Hidayat AA: Necrotizing scleritis: clinicopathologic study of 41 cases, Ophthalmology 92:1542, 1985.

232. Rao NA, Wacker WB, and Marak GE: Experimental allergic uveitis: clinicopathologic features associated with varying doses of S antigen, Arch Ophthalmol 97:1954, 1979.

233. Reese AB: Tumors of the eye, ed 2, New York, 1976, Harper & Row, Publishers.

234. Richter MP and D'Angio GJ: The role of radiation therapy in the management of children with histiocytosis X, Am J Pediatr Hematol Oncol 3:161, 1981.

235. Rodenbiker HT and Ganley JP: Ocular coccidioidomycosis, Surv Ophthalmol 24:263, 1980.

236. Rodrigues A and others: Posterior segment ocular manifestations

in patients with HLA-B27 associated uveitis, Ophthalmology 101: 1267, 1994.

237. Rothova A and others: Iris nodules in Fuchs''' heterochromic uveitis, Am J Ophthalmol 118:338, 1994.

238. Rosenberg LF and Siegfried CJ: Enophthalmitis associated with a releasable suture [letter], Arch Ophthalmol 114:767, 1996.

239. Roussel TJ, Culberston WW, and Jaffe NS: Chronic postoperative endophthalmitis associated with *Propionibacterium acnes*, Arch Ophthalmol 105:1199, 1987.

240. Roussel TJ and others: Postoperative mycobacterial endophthalmitis, Am J Ophthalmol 107:403, 1989.

241. Rubsamen PE and Gass JDM: Vogt-Koyanagi-Harada syndrome. Clinical course, therapy, and long-term visual outcome, Arch Ophthalmol 109, 682, 1991.

242. Ruby AJ and Jampol LM: Crohn's disease and retinal vascular disease, Am J Ophthalmol 110:349, 1990.

243. Rupp RH and Holloman KR: Histiocytosis X affecting the uveal tract, Arch Ophthalmol 84:468, 1970.

244. Rutzen AR and others: Simultaneous onset of Vogt-Koyanagi-Harada syndrome in monozygotic twin, Am J Ophthalmol 119:239, 1995.

245. Saari M, Vuorre I, and Nieminen H: Fuchs'' heterochromic cyclitis: a simultaneous bilateral fluorescein angiographic study of the iris, Br J Ophthalmol 62:715, 1978.

246. Sabates R, Smith T, and Apple DJ: Histopathology of juvenile rheumatoid arthritis, Ann Ophthalmol 11:733, 1979.

247. Saga T and others: Ocular involvement by a peripheral T-cell lymphoma, Arch Ophthalmol 102:399, 1984.

248. Sakamoto T, Murata T, and Inomata H: Class II major histocompatibility complex on melanocytes of Vogt-Koyanagi-Harada disease, Arch Ophthalmol 109:1270, 1991.

249. Salmon JF and others: Granulomatous uveitis in Crohn's disease: a clinicopathologic case report, Arch Ophthalmol 107:718, 1989.

250. Sanders MD and Shilling JS: Retinal choroidal and optic disc involvement in sarcoidosis, Trans Ophthalmol Soc UK 96:140, 1976.

251. Sanders TE: Intraocular juvenile xanthogranuloma (nevoxanthogranuloma): a survey of 20 cases, Trans Am Ophthalmol Soc 58: 59, 1960.

252. Schlaegel TF Jr: Essentials of uveitis, Boston, 1969, Little, Brown & Co.

253. Schlaegel TF Jr: Bacterial and protozoal uveitis, Trans Ophthalmol Soc UK 101:312, 1981.

254. Schwab IR: The epidemiologic association of Fuchs''' heterochromic iridocyclitis and ocular toxoplasmosis, Am J Ophthalmol 111:356, 1991.

255. Schwartz LW, Rodrigues MM, and Hallett JW: Juvenile xanthogranuloma diagnosed by paracentesis, Am J Ophthalmol 77:243, 1974.

256. Schwartz TL and others: Congenital macronodular juvenile xanthogranuloma of the eyelid, Ophthalmology 98:1230, 1991.

257. Secchi AG: Cataracts in uveitis, Trans Ophthalmol Soc UK 102: 390, 1982.

258. Sheppard RD and others: Measles virus matrix protein synthesized in a subacute sclerosing panencephalitis cell line, Science 228:1219, 1985.

259. Shields CL, Shields JA, and Buchanon HW: Solitary orbital involvement with juvenile xanthogranuloma, Arch Ophthalmol 108:1587, 1990.

260. Shimizu K: Harada's, Behçet's, Vogt-Koyanagi syndromes—are they clinical entities? Trans Am Acad Ophthalmol Otolaryngol 77: 281, 1973.

261. Simon JW and Friedman AH: Ocular reticulum cell sarcoma, Br J Ophthalmol 64:793, 1980.

262. Sims DG: Histiocytosis X: follow-up of 43 cases, Arch Dis Childhood 52:433, 1977.

263. Sloas HA and others: Update of ocular reticulum cell sarcoma, Arch Ophthalmol 99:1048, 1981.

264. Smolin G and O'Connor GR: Ocular immunology, Philadelphia, 1981, Lea & Febiger.

265. Snyder DA and Tessler HH: Vogt-Koyanagi-Harada syndrome, Am J Ophthalmol 90:69, 1980.

266. Spalton DJ: Fundus changes in sarcoidosis: review of 33 patients with histological confirmation, Trans Ophthalmol Soc UK 99:167, 1979.

267. Staal SP and others: A survey of Epstein-Barr virus DNA in

lymphoid tissue. Frequent detection in Hodgkin's disease, Am J Clin Pathol 91:1, 1989.

268. Starling KA: Chemotherapy of histiocytosis, Am J Pediatr Hematol Oncol 3:157, 1981.

269. Stevens G Jr and others: Iris lymphocytic infiltration in patients with clinically quiescent uveitis, Am J Ophthalmol 104:508, 1987.

270. Swartz M and Schumann GB: Acute leukemic infiltration of the vitreous diagnosed by pars plana aspiration, Am J Ophthalmol 90: 326, 1980.

271. Tabbut BR, Tessler HH, and Williams D: Fuchs''' heterochromic iridocyclitis in blacks, Arch Ophthalmol 106:1688, 1988.

272. Tagawa Y and others: HLA and Vogt-Koyanagi-Harada syndrome, N Eng J Med 295:173, 1976.

273. Tarkkanen A and Laatikainen L: Late ocular manifestations in neonatal herpes simplex infection, Br J Ophthalmol 61:608, 1977.

274. Topilow HW and others: Bilateral multifocal intraocular cysticercosis, Ophthalmology 88:1166, 1981.

275. Vogiatzis KV: Bilateral blindness due to necrotizing scleritis in a case of Wegener's granulomatosis, Ann Ophthalmol 15:185, 1983.

276. Wagoner MD and others: Ocular pathology for clinicians. 3. Intraocular reticulum cell sarcoma, Ophthalmology 87:724, 1980.

277. Wagoner MD and others: New observations on vitiligo and ocular disease, Am J Ophthalmol 96:16, 1983.

278. Wakefield D and others: Distribution of lymphocytes and cell adhesion molecules in iris biopsy specimens from patients with uveitis, Arch Ophthalmol 110:121, 1992.

279. Walton RC, Wilsion J, and Chan CC: Metastatic choroidal abscess in the acquired immunodeficiency syndrome, Arch Ophthalmol 114:880, 1996, (letter).

280. Watanabe K, Ohashi Y: Natural killer cell activity in patients with Behçet's disease, Am J Ophthalmol

281. Watson PG: The diagnosis and management of scleritis, Ophthalmology 87:716, 1980.

282. Wertz FD and others: Juvenile xanthogranuloma of the optic nerve, disc, retina, and choroid, Ophthalmology 89:1331, 1982.

283. Whitcup SM and others: Expression of cell adhesion molecules in posterior uveitis, Arch Ophthalmol 110:662, 1992.

284. Wilhelmus KR, Watson PG, and Vasavada AR: Uveitis, associated with scleritis, Trans Ophthalmol Soc UK 101:351, 1981.

285. Witmer R: Clinical implications of aqueous humor studies in uveitis, Am J Ophthalmol 86:39, 1978.

286. Woda BA and Sullivan JL: Reactive histiocytic disorders, Am J Clin Pathol 99:459, 1993.

287. Wolf MD, Lichter PR, and Ragsdale CG: Prognostic factors in the uveitis of juvenile rheumatoid arthritis, Ophthalmology 94:1242, 1987.

288. Wong KW and others: Ocular involvement associated with chronic Epstein-Barr virus disease, Arch Ophthalmol 105:788, 1987.

289. Wood CM and others: Globe luxation in histiocytosis X, Br J Ophthalmol 72:631, 1988.

290. Woodlief NF: Initial observations on the ocular microcirculation in man. I. The anterior segment and extraocular muscles, Arch Ophthalmol 98:1268, 1980.

291. Woods AC: Endogenous uveitis, Baltimore, 1956, The Williams & Wilkins Co.

292. Woods AC: Endogenous inflammations of the uveal tract, Baltimore, 1961, The Williams & Wilkins Co.

293. Yamaguchi K and others: Immunosuppressive acidic protein in Behçet's disease. Am J Ophthalmol 105:213, 1988.

294. Yanoff M and Allman MI: Congenital herpes simplex virus, type 2, bilateral endophthalmitis, Trans Am Ophthalmol Soc 75:325, 1977.

295. Yanoff M and Perry HD: Juvenile xanthogranulomatous of the corneoscleral limbus, Arch Ophthalmol 113:915, 1995.

296. Yokoyama MM and others: Humoral and cellular immunity studies in patients with Vogt-Koyanagi-Harada syndrome and pars planitis, Invest Ophthalmol 20:364, 1981.

297. Zakka KA, Foos RY, and Brown WJ: Intraocular coccidioidomycosis, Surv Ophthalmol 22:313, 1978.

298. Zhao M, Jiang Y, and Abrahams IW: Association of HLA antigens with Vogt-Koyanagi-Harada syndrome in a Han Chinese population, Arch Ophthalmol 109:1270, 1991.

299. Zhao M, Jiang Y and Abrahams IW: Association of HLA antigens with Vogt-Koyanagi-Harada syndrome in a Han Chinese population, Arch Ophthalmol 109:368, 1991.

300. Zimmerman JE: Ocular lesions of juvenile xanthogranuloma, Am J Ophthalmol 60:1011, 1965.
301. Zimmerman LE: Ocular lesions of juvenile xanthogranuloma: nevo-xanthoendothelioma, Trans Am Acad Ophthalmol Otolaryngol 69: 412, 1965.

Sympathetic ophthalmia

302. Albert DM and Diaz-Rohena R: A historical review of sympathetic ophthalmia and its epidemiology, Surv Ophthalmol 34:1, 1989.
303. Allen JC: Sympathetic ophthalmia: a disappearing disease, JAMA 209:1090, 1969.
304. Blodi FC: Sympathetic uveitis as an allergic phenomenon; with a study of its association with phaco-anaphylactic uveitis and a report on the pathological findings in sympathizing eyes, Trans Am Acad Ophthalmol Otolaryngol 63:642, 1959.
305. Blodi FC: Sympathetic uveitis. In Freeman HM, editor: Ocular trauma, New York, 1979, Appleton-Century-Crofts.
306. Brauninger G and Polack F: Sympathetic ophthalmitis, Am J Ophthalmol 72:967, 1971.
307. Chan C-C and others: Granulomas in sympathetic ophthalmia and sarcoidosis: immunohistochemical study, Arch Ophthalmol 103: 198, 1985.
308. Chan C-C and others: Immunohistochemistry and electron microscopy of choroidal infiltrate and Dalen-Fuchs" nodules in sympathetic ophthalmia, Ophthalmology 92:580, 1985.
309. Chan C-C and others: Sympathetic ophthalmia: immunopathological findings, Ophthalmology 93:690, 1986.
310. Chan C-C and others: Immunopathologic study of Vogt-Koyanagi-Harada syndrome, Am J Ophthalmol 105:607, 1988.
311. Davis JL and others: HLA associations and ancestry in Vogt-Koyanagi-Harada disease and sympathetic ophthalmia, Ophthalmology 97:1137, 1990.
312. DeVoe AG: Sympathetic ophthalmia: a case treated by prolonged use of corticotropin and adrenal steroids, Trans Am Ophthalmol Soc 58:75, 1960.
313. Dreyer WB Jr and others: Sympathetic ophthalmia, Am J Ophthalmol 92:816, 1981.
314. Easom H and Zimmerman LE: Sympathetic ophthalmia and bilateral phacoanaphylaxis: a clinicopathologic correlation of the sympathogenic and sympathizing eyes, Arch Ophthalmol 72:9, 1964.
315. Elschnig A: Studien zur sympathischen Ophthalmie. II. Die antigenc Wirkung des Augenpigmentes, Arch Ophthalmol 76:509, 1910.
316. Elschnig A: Zur frage der sympathischen Ophthalmie, Klin Monatsbl Augenheilkd 80:289, 1928.
317. Font RL and others: Light and electron microscopic study of Dalén-Fuchs" nodules in sympathetic ophthalmia, Ophthalmology 90:66, 1983.
318. Friedenwald J: Notes on the allergy theory of sympathetic ophthalmia, Am J Ophthalmol 17:1003, 1934.
319. Fries PD and others: Sympathetic ophthalmia complicating helium ion irradiation of a choroidal melanoma, Arch Ophthalmol 105: 1561, 1987.
320. Fuchs" E: Über sympathisierende Entzündung, Graefes Arch Ophthalmol 38:95, 1892.
321. Fuchs" E: Über sympathisierende Entzündung (Nebst. Bermerkungen über seröse traumatische Iritis). Graefes Arch Ophthalmol 61:365, 1905.
322. Gass JDM: Sympathetic ophthalmia following vitrectomy, Am J Ophthalmol 93:552, 1982.
323. Green W and others: Sympathetic uveitis following evisceration, Trans Am Acad Ophthalmol Otolaryngol 76:625, 1972.
324. Greeves R: A contribution to the microscopical anatomy of the sympathizing eye, Br J Ophthalmol 32:545, 1948.
325. Hirose S and others: Uveitis induced in primates by interphotoreceptor retinoid-binding protein, Arch Ophthalmol 104:1698, 1986.
326. Inomata H: Necrotic change of choroidal melanocytes in sympathetic ophthalmia, Arch Ophthalmol 106:239, 1988.
327. Ishikawa T and Ikui H: The fine structure of the Dalén-Fuchs" nodule in sympathetic ophthalmia. I. Changes of the pigment epithelial cells within the Dalén-Fuchs" nodule, Jpn J Ophthalmol 16:254, 1972.
328. Jakobiec FA and others: Human sympathetic ophthalmia: an analysis of the inflammatory infiltrate by hybridoma-monoclonal antibodies, immunochemistry, and correlative electron microscopy, Ophthalmology 90:76, 1983.
329. Kay ML, Yanoff M, and Katowitz JA: Development of sympathetic uveitis in spite of corticosteroid therapy, Ophthalmology 78:90, 1974.
330. Kinyoun JL, Bensinger RE, and Chuang EL: Thirty-year history of sympathetic ophthalmia, Ophthalmology 90:59, 1983.
331. Lewis ML, Gass JDM, and Spencer WH: Sympathetic uveitis after trauma and vitrectomy, Arch Ophthalmol 96:263, 1978.
332. Liddy BSL, and Stuwart J: Sympathetic ophthalmia in Canada, Can J Ophthalmol 7:175, 1972.
333. Lubin JR and Albert DM: Early enucleation in sympathetic ophthalmia, Oc Inflam Ther 1:47, 1983.
334. Lubin JR, Albert DM, and Weinstein M: Sixty-five years of sympathetic ophthalmia: a clinicopathologic review of 105 cases (1913-1978), Ophthalmology 87:109, 1980.
335. Makley TA and Azar A: Sympathetic ophthalmia, Arch Ophthalmol 96:257, 1978.
336. Marak GE Jr: Recent advances in sympathetic ophthalmia, Surv Ophthalmol 24:1241, 1979.
337. Marak GE Jr, Font RL, and Zimmerman LE: Histologic variations related to race in sympathetic ophthalmia, Am J Ophthalmol 78: 935, 1974.
338. Marak GE Jr and Ikui H: Pigmentation associated histopathological variations in sympathetic ophthalmia, Br J Ophthalmol 64:220, 1980.
339. Mueller-Hermelink HK, Krause-Maciw E, and Daus W: Early stage of human sympathetic ophthalmia: histologic and immunopathologic findings, Arch Ophthalmol 102:1353, 1984.
340. Perry HD and Font RL: Clinical and histopathologic observations in severe Vogt-Koyanagi-Harada syndrome, Am J Ophthalmol 83: 242, 1977.
341. Pietruschka G and Schill J: Clinical importance and incidence of sympathetic ophthalmia, Klin Monatsbl Augenheilkd 162:451, 1973.
342. Puliafito CA and others: Sympathetic uveitis, Ophthalmology 87: 355, 1980.
343. Rao NA, Wacker WB, and Marak GE Jr: Experimental allergic uveitis: clinicopathologic features associated with varying doses of S antigen, Arch Ophthalmol 97:1954, 1979.
344. Rao NA and Wong VG: Aetiology of sympathetic ophthalmitis, Trans Ophthalmol Soc UK 101:357, 1981.
345. Rao NA, Xu S, and Font RL: Sympathetic ophthalmia: an immunohistochemical study of epithelioid and giant cells, Ophthalmology 92:1660, 1985.
346. Rao NA and others: The role of the penetrating wound in the development of sympathetic ophthalmia: experimental observations, Arch Ophthalmol 101:102, 1983.
347. Reynard M and others: Histocompatibility antigens in sympathetic ophthalmia, Am J Ophthalmol 95:216, 1983.
348. Reynard M, Riffenburgh RS, and Maes EF: Effect of corticosteroid treatment and enucleation on the visual prognosis of sympathetic ophthalmia, Am J Ophthalmol 96:290, 1983.
349. Schlaegel TF Jr: Uveitis of suspected viral original. In Duane TD Jr, editor: Clinical ophthalmology, vol 4, New York, 1976, Harper & Row, Publishers.
350. Shah DN and others: Inflammatory cellular kinetics in sympathetic ophthalmia. A study of 29 traumatized (exciting) eyes, Ocular Immunol 1:255, 1993.
351. Schreck E: Weitere Beiträge zur Frage der Klinik, Microbiologie und pathologischen Anatomie der sympathischen Ophthalmic, Arch Ophthalmol 149:656, 1949.
352. Sharp DC and others: Sympathetic ophthalmia: histopathologic and fluorescein angiographic correlation, Arch Ophthalmol 102: 232, 1984.
353. Stafford WR: Sympathetic ophthalmia: report of a case occurring ten and one half days after injury, Arch Ophthalmol 74:521, 1965.
354. Thies O: Gedankenüber den Ausbruch der sympathischen Ophthalmie, Klin Monatsbl Augenheilkd 112:185, 1947.
355. Wang WJ: Clinical and histopathological report of sympathetic ophthalmia after retinal surgery, Br J Ophthalmol 67:150, 1983.
356. Wong VG, Anderson R, and O'Brien PJ: Sympathetic ophthalmia and lymphocytic transformation, Am J Ophthalmol 72:960, 1971.
357. Woods AC: Allergy in its relation to sympathetic ophthalmia, NY State J Med 36:67, 1936.

479. Char DH and others: Failure of choroidal melanoma to respond to helium ion therapy, Arch Ophthalmol 10:236, 1983.

480. Char DH and others: Primary intraocular lymphoma (ocular reticulum cell sarcoma): diagnosis and management, Ophthalmology 95: 625, 1988.

481. Char DH and others: Iris melanomas—diagnostic problems, Ophthalmology 103:251, 1996.

482. Char DH and others: Iris melanomas with increased intraocular pressure, Arch Ophthalmol 107:548, 1989.

483. Char DH and others: Failure of pre-enucleation radiation to decrease uveal melanoma mortality, Am J Ophthalmol 106:21, 1988.

484. Charles NC and Steiner GC: Ganciclovir intraocular implant—a clinicopathologic study, Ophthalmology 103:416, 1996.

485. Cheung MK and others: Diagnosis of reactive lymphoid hyperplasia by chorioretinal biopsy, Am J Ophthalmol 118:457, 1994.

486. Chess J and others: Uveal melanoma presenting after cataract extraction with intraocular lens implantation, Ophthalmology 92:827, 1985.

487. Christensen GR and Linder MW: Bilateral rhegmatogenous retinal detachment associated with unilateral choroidal melanoma, Ann Ophthalmol 15:252, 1983.

488. Cibis GW and others: Bilateral choroidal neonatal neuroblastoma, Am J Ophthalmol 109:445, 1990.

489. Cleary PE, Gregor Z, and Bird AC: Retinal vascular changes in congenital hypertrophy of the retinal pigment epithelium, Br J Ophthalmol 60:499, 1976.

490. Cochran AJ: Immunological mechanisms in malignant melanoma of the skin, Trans Ophthalmol Soc UK 97:385, 1977.

491. Cochran AJ and others: Detection of cytoplasmic S-100 protein in primary and metastatic intraocular melanomas, Invest Ophthalmol Vis Sci 24:1153, 1983.

492. Coleman K and others: Prognostic value of morphometric features and the callender classification in uveal melanomas, Ophthalmology 103:1634, 1996.

493. Collins VP, Loeffler RK, and Tivey H: Observations on growth rates of human tumors, Am J Radiol 76:988, 1956.

494. Constable IJ: Proton irradiation therapy for ocular melanoma, Trans Ophthalmol Soc UK 97:430, 1977.

495. Craythorn JM, Apple DJ, and Bohart WA: Malignant melanoma arising from a melanocytoma of the optic disc and juxtapapillary choroid Can J Ophthalmol 19:320, 1984.

496. Croxatto JO and Malbran ES: Unusual ciliary body tumor: mesectodermal leiomyoma, Ophthalmology 89:1208, 1982.

497. Croxatto JO, D'Alessandro C, and Lombardi A: Benign fibrous tumor of the choroid, Arch Ophthalmol 107:1793, 1989.

498. Cunha SL: Osseous choristoma of the choroid. A familial disease, Arch Ophthalmol 102:1052, 1984.

499. Currie G: Is there a role for immunotherapy in the treatment of human cancer? Trans Ophthalmol Soc UK 97:442, 1977.

500. Curtin VT and Cavender JC: The natural course of selected malignant melanomas of the choroid and ciliary body, Mod Probl Ophthalmol 12:523, 1974.

501. Curtin VT and Norton EWD: Pathological changes in malignant melanomas after photocoagulation, Arch Ophthalmol 70:150, 1963.

502. Daicker B: Melanosis retinae et papillae durch transretinal in den Glasköorper cingebrochenen malignes Aderhautmelanom, Ophthalmologica 166:460, 1963.

503. Davidorf FH: The melanoma controversy: a comparison of choroidal, cutaneous, and iris melanomas, Surv Ophthalmol 25:373, 1981.

504. Davidorf FH, editor: Choroidal melanoma: diagnosis and treatment (with round-table discussion), Ophthalmic Forum 1(4):3, 1983.

505. Davidorf FH and Lang JR: Small malignant melanomas of the choroid, Am J Ophthalmol 78:788, 1974.

506. Davidorf FH and Lang JR: The natural history of malignant melanoma of the choroid: small vs large tumors, Trans Am Acad Ophthalmol Otolaryngol 79:310, 1975.

507. Davidorf FH and Lang JR: Lymphocytic infiltration in choroidal melanoma and its prognostic significance, Trans Ophthalmol Soc UK 97:394, 1977.

508. Davidorf FH, Makley TA, and Lang JR: Radiotherapy of malignant melanoma of the choroid, Trans Am Acad Ophthalmol Otolaryngol 81:OP 849, 1976.

509. Davidorf FH and others: Conservative management of malignant melanoma. II. Transscleral diathermy as a method for malignant melanomas of the choroid, Arch Ophthalmol 83:273, 1970.

510. Davidorf FH and others: Incidence of misdiagnosed and unsuspected choroidal melanomas: a 50-year experience, Arch Ophthalmol 101:410, 1983.

511. Del Canizo C and others: Discrepancies between morphologic, cytochemical and immunologic characteristics in acute myeloblastic leukemia, Am J Clin Pathol 88:38, 1987.

512. DePotter P and others: Magnetic resonance imaging in choroidal osteoma, Retina 11:221, 1991.

513. Desroches G and others: Reactive lymphoid hyperplasia of the uvea. A case with ultrasonographic and computed tomographic studies, Arch Ophthalmol 101:725, 1983.

514. Deutsch TA and Jampol LM: Large druse-like lesions on the surface of choroidal nevi, Ophthalmology 92:73, 1985.

515. deVeer J: Juxtapapillary malignant melanoma of the choroid and so-called malignant melanoma of the optic disc, Arch Ophthalmol 51:147, 1954.

516. deVeer J: Melanotic tumors of the optic nerve head, Arch Ophthalmol 65:536, 1961.

517. Diaz-Llopis M and Menezo JL: Congenital hypertrophy of the retinal pigment epithelium in familial adenomatous polyposis, Arch Ophthalmol 106:412, 1988.

518. Diener-West M and others: A review of mortality from choroidal melanoma, Arch Ophthalmol 110:245, 1992.

519. Donaldson DD: Atlas of external diseases of the eye, vol IV, Anterior chamber, iris, and ciliary body, St. Louis, 1973, The CV Mosby Co.

520. Donoso LA, Shields JA, and Nagy RM: Epibulbar lesions simulating extraocular extension of uveal melanomas, Ann Ophthalmol 14: 1120, 1982.

521. Donoso LA and others: Metastatic choroidal melanoma: hepatic binding protein reactivity toward a liver-metastasizing clone, Arch Ophthalmol 101:787, 1983.

522. Donoso LA and others: Metastatic uveal melanoma: hepatic metastasis identified by hybridoma-secreted monoclonal antibody Mab8-1H, Arch Ophthalmol 103:799, 1985.

523. Donoso LA and others: Metastatic uveal melanoma: pretherapy serum liver enzyme and liver scan abnormalities, Arch Ophthalmol 103:796, 1985.

524. Donoso LA and others: Antigenic and cellular heterogeneity of primary uveal malignant melanomas, Arch Ophthalmol 104:106, 1986.

525. Duffin RM and others: Small malignant melanoma of the choroid with extraocular extension, Arch Ophthalmol 99:1827, 1981.

526. Duke JR and Dunn SN: Primary tumors of the iris, Arch Ophthalmol 59:204, 1958.

527. Duke JR and Maumenee AE: An unusual tumor of the retinal pigment epithelium, Am J Ophthalmol 47:311, 1959.

528. Dunphy EB: Management of intraocular malignancy, Am J Ophthalmol 44:313, 1957.

529. Dunphy EB and others: Melanocytic tumor of the anterior uvea, Am J Ophthalmol 86:680, 1978.

530. Durie FH and others: Analysis of lymphocytic infiltration in uveal melanoma, Invest Ophthalmol Vis Sci 31:2106, 1990.

531. Duvall J and Lucas DR: Argon laser and xenon arc coagulation of malignant choroidal melanomata: histological findings in 6 cases, Br J Ophthalmol 65:464, 1981.

532. Eagle RC Jr and Shields JA: Pseudoretinitis pigmentosa secondary to preretinal malignant melanoma cells, Retina 2:51, 1982.

533. Edwards WC, Layden WE, and MacDonald RJ Jr: Fluorescein angiography of malignant melanoma of the choroid, Am J Ophthalmol 68:797, 1969.

534. Egan KM and others: Epidemiologic aspects of uveal melanoma, Surv Ophthalmol 32:239, 1988.

535. Eiferman RA and Rodrigues MM: Squamous epithelial implantation cyst of the iris, Ophthalmology 88:1281, 1981.

536. Eisinger M and others: Growth regulation of human melanocytes: mitogenic factors in extracts of melanoma, astrocytoma, and fibroblast cell lines, Science 299:984, 1985.

537. El Baba F and Blumenkranz M: Malignant melanoma at the site of penetrating ocular trauma, Arch Ophthalmol 104:405, 1986.

538. El Baba F and others: Choroidal melanoma with pigment dispersion in vitreous and melanomalytic glaucoma, Ophthalmology 95: 370, 1988.

539. Erie JC, Robertson DM: Serous detachments of the macula associated with presumed small choroidal melanomas, Am J Ophthalmol 102:176, 1986.

540. Erie JC and others: Presumed small-choroidal melanomas with serous macular detachments with and without surface laser photocoagulation treatment, Am J Ophthalmol 109(3):259, 1990.

541. Eting E, Savir H: An atypical fulminant course of choroidal osteoma in two siblings, Am J Ophthalmol 113:52, 1992.

542. Fair JR: Tumors of the retinal pigment epithelium, Am J Ophthalmol 45:495, 1958.

543. Farber MG, Smith ME, and Gans LA: Astrocytoma of the ciliary body, Arch Ophthalmol 105:536, 1987.

544. Federman JL: The fenestrations of the choriocapillaris in the presence of choroidal melanoma, Trans Am Ophthalmol Soc 80:498, 1982.

545. Federman JL, Felberg NT, and Shields JA: Effect of local treatment on antibody levels in malignant melanoma of the choroid, Trans Ophthalmol Soc UK 97:436, 1977.

546. Federman JL, Lewis MG, and Clark WH: Tumor-associated antibodies to ocular and cutaneous malignant melanomas: negative interaction with normal choroidal melanocytes, J Natl Cancer Inst 52:587, 1974.

547. Federman JL and others: Tumor-associated antibodies in the serum of ocular melanoma patients, Trans Am Acad Ophthalmol Otolaryngol 78:784, 1974.

548. Felberg NT and others: Gamma-glutamyl transpeptidase in the prognosis of patients with uveal malignant melanoma, Am J Ophthalmol 95:467, 1983.

549. Ferry AP: Lesions mistaken for malignant melanoma of the posterior uvea: a clinicopathologic analysis of 100 cases with ophthalmoscopically visible lesions, Arch Ophthalmol 72:463, 1964.

550. Ferry AP: Lesions mistaken for malignant melanoma of the iris, Arch Ophthalmol 74:918, 1965.

551. Ferry AP, editor: Ocular and adnexal tumors, Int Ophthalmol Clin 12(1), 1972.

552. Fischer R, Henkind P, and Gartner S: Microcysts of the human iris pigment epithelium, Br J Ophthalmol 63:750, 1979.

553. Fishman GA: The value of fluorescein angiography in the differential diagnosis of choroidal melanomas. In Peyman GA, Apple DJ, and Sanders DR, editors: Intraocular tumors, New York, 1977, Appleton-Century-Crofts.

554. Fishman GA, Apple DJ, and Goldberg MF: Retinal and pigment epithelial alterations over choroidal malignant melanomas, Ann Ophthalmol 7:487, 1975.

555. Flindall RJ and Gass JDM: A histopathologic fluorescein angiographic correlated study of malignant melanomas of the choroid, Can J Ophthalmol 6:258, 1971.

556. Flocks M, Gerende JH, and Zimmerman LE: The size and shape of malignant melanomas of the choroid and histologic characteristics: a statistical study of 210 tumors, Trans Am Acad Ophthalmol Otolaryngol 59:740, 1955.

557. Folberg R and others: Fine-needle aspirates of uveal melanomas and prognosis, Am J Ophthalmol 100:654, 1985.

558. Folberg R and others: An antimelanoma monoclonal antibody and the histopathology of uveal melanomas, Arch Ophthalmol 103:275, 1985.

559. Foldberg R and others: Comparison of direct and microslide pathology measurements of uveal melanomas, Invest Ophthalmol Vis Sci 86:1788, 1985.

560. Foldberg R and others: The morphologic characteristics of tumor blood vessels as a marker of tumor progression in primary human uveal melanoma: a matched case-control study, Hum Pathol 23:1298, 1992.

561. Foldberg R and others: The prognostic value of tumor blood vessel morphology in primary uveal melanoma, Ophthalmology 100:1389, 1993.

562. Font RL, Spaulding AC, and Zimmerman LE: Diffuse malignant melanoma of the uveal tract: a clinicopathologic report of 54 cases, Trans Am Acad Ophthalmol Otolaryngol 72:877, 1968.

563. Font RL, Zimmerman LE, and Armaly MF: The nature of the orange pigment over a choroidal melanoma: histochemical and electron microscopic observations, Arch Ophthalmol 91:359, 1974.

564. Font RL, Zimmerman LE, and Fine BS: Adenoma of the retinal pigment epithelium: histochemical and electron microscopic observations, Am J Ophthalmol 73:544, 1972.

565. Font RL and others: Combined hamartoma of sensory retina and retinal pigment epithelium, Retina 9:302, 1989.

566. Font RL, Zimmerman LE, and Fine BS: Adenoma of the retinal pigment epithelium: histochemical and electron microscopic observations, Am J Ophthalmol 73:544, 1972.

567. Forrest AW, Keyser RB, and Spencer WH: Iridocyclectomy for melanomas of the ciliary body: a follow-up study of pathology and surgical morbidity, Ophthalmology 85:1237, 1978.

568. Foss AJE and others: Estrogen and progesterone receptor analysis in ocular melanomas, Ophthalmology 102:431, 1995.

569. Foulds WS: Experience of local excision of uveal melanomas, Trans Ophthalmol Soc UK 97:412, 1977.

570. Francois J: Malignant melanomata of the choroid, Br J Ophthalmol 47:736, 1963.

571. Fraser DJ and Font RL: Ocular inflammation and hemorrhage as initial manifestations of uveal malignant melanoma: incidence and prognosis, Arch Ophthalmol 97:1311, 1979.

572. Frayer WC: Reactivity of the retinal pigment epithelium: an experimental and histopathologic study, Trans Am Ophthalmol Soc 64:586, 1966.

573. Frayer WC: Neoplasms and related lesions of the retinal pigment epithelium, Ophthalmol Clin 12(1):63, 1972.

574. Friberg TR, Fineberg E, and McQuaig S: Extremely rapid growth of a primary choroidal melanoma, Arch Ophthalmol 101:1375, 1983.

575. Fries PD and others: Sympathetic ophthalmia complicating helium ion irradiation of a choroidal melanoma, Arch Ophthalmol 105:1561, 1987.

576. Fuchs" E: Das Sarcom des Uvealtractus, Vienna, 1882, Wilhelm Braumüller.

577. Gallagher RP and others: Risk factors for ocular melanoma. Western Canada melanoma study, J Natl Cancer Inst 74:775, 1985.

578. Gamel JW and McLean JW: Quantitative analysis of the Callender classification of uveal melanoma cells, Arch Ophthalmol 95:686, 1977.

579. Gamel JW, McCurdy JB, and McLean IW: A comparison of prognostic covariates for uveal melanoma, Invest Ophthalmol Vis Sci 33:1919, 1992.

580. Ganley JP and Comstock GW: Benign nevi and malignant melanomas of the choroid, Am J Ophthalmol 76:19, 1973.

581. Garner A: Tumors of the retinal pigment epithelium, Br J Ophthalmol 54:715, 1970.

582. Gartner S: Malignant melanoma of the choroid and von Recklinghausen's disease, Am J Ophthalmol 23:73, 1940.

583. Gass JDM: Hemorrhage into the vitreous, a presenting manifestation of malignant melanoma of the choroid, Arch Ophthalmol 69:778, 1963.

584. Gass JDM: Fluorescein angiography: an aid in the differential diagnosis of intraocular tumors, Int Ophthalmol Clin 12(1):85, 1972.

585. Gass JDM: An unusual hamartoma of the pigment epithelium and retina simulating choroidal melanoma and retinoblastoma, Trans Am Ophthalmol Soc 71:171, 1973.

586. Gass JDM: Iris abscess simulating malignant melanoma, Arch Ophthalmol 90:299, 1973.

587. Gass JDM: Differential diagnosis of intraocular tumors: a stereoscopic presentation, St. Louis, 1974, The CV Mosby Co.

588. Gass JDM: Differential diagnosis of benign and malignant melanomas of the choroid, Trans Ophthalmol Soc UK 97:358, 1977.

589. Gass JDM: Problems in the differential diagnosis of choroidal nevi and malignant melanomas, Am J Ophthalmol 83:299, 1977.

590. Gass JDM: Changing concepts of natural course and management of uveal melanomas. In Nicholson DH, editor: Ocular pathology update, New York, 1980, Masson Publishing USA, Inc.

591. Gass JDM: Observation of suspected choroidal and ciliary body melanomas for evidence of growth prior to enucleation, Ophthalmology 87:523, 1980.

592. Gass JDM and others: Choroidal osteoma, Arch Ophthalmol 96:428, 1978.

593. Gass JDM: Comparison of prognosis after enucleation vs cobalt 60 irradiation of melanomas, Arch Ophthalmol 103:916, 1985.

594. Gass JDM: Comparison of uveal melanoma growth rates with mitotic index and mortality, Arch Ophthalmol 103:924, 1985.

595. Gass JDM and others: Bilateral diffuse uveal melanocytic proliferation in patients with occult carcinoma, Arch Ophthalmol 108:527, 1990.

596. Gass JDM: Focal congenital anomalies of the retinal pigment epithelium, Eye 3:1, 1989.

597. Gass JDM and others: Multifocal pigment epithelial detachments by reticulum cell sarcoma: a characteristic funduscopic picture, Retina 4:135, 1984.

598. Geisse LJ and Robertson DM: Iris melanomas, Am J Ophthalmol 99:638, 1985.

599. Gherardi G, Scherini P, and Ambrosi S: Occult thyroid metastasis from untreated uveal melanoma, Arch Ophthalmol 103:689, 1985.

600. Gieser SC and others: Hemangiopericytoma of the ciliary body, Arch Ophthalmol 106:1269, 1988.

601. Gilbert CM and others: Nonsimultaneous primary choroidal and cutaneous melanomas: report of a case, Ophthalmology 94:1169, 1987.

602. Goldberg B, Kara GB, and Previte LR: The use of radioactive phosphorus (^{32}P) in the diagnosis of ocular tumors, Am J Ophthalmol 90:817, 1980.

603. Gonder JR, Shields JA, and Albert DM: Malignant melanoma of the choroid associated with oculodermal melanocytosis, Ophthalmology 88:372, 1981.

604. Gonder and others: Visual loss associated with choroidal nevi, Ophthalmology 89:961, 1982.

605. Goodman DF and others: Uveal melanoma necrosis after helium ion therapy, Am J Ophthalmol 101:643, 1986.

606. Gragoudas ES and others: Proton beam irradiation of uveal melanomas: results of a 5 1/2 year study, Arch Ophthalmol 100:928, 1982.

607. Graham GG: Juxtapapillary retinal pigment epithelial tumor, Arch Ophthalmol 85:299, 1971.

608. Grand MG and others: Choroidal osteoma: treatment of associated subretinal neovascular membranes, Retina 4:84, 1984.

609. Greer CH and others: An Australian choroidal melanoma survey, Aust J Ophthalmol 9:255, 1981.

610. Griffin CA, Long PP, and Schachat AP: Trisomy 6p in an ocular melanoma, Cancer Genet Cytogenet 32:129, 1988.

611. Grossniklaus HE and others: Iris melanoma seeding through a trabeculectomy site, Arch Ophthalmol 108:1287, 1990.

612. Grossniklaus HE and others: Iris melanoma seeding through a trabeculectomy site, Arch Ophthalmol 108:1287, 1990.

613. Grossniklaus HE: Fine-needle aspiration biopsy of the iris, Arch Ophthalmol 110:969, 1992.

614. Gunderson T and others: Choroidal melanocytic tumor observed for 41 years before enucleation, Arch Ophthalmol 96:2089, 1978.

615. Guyer DR and others: Radiation maculopathy after proton beam irradiation for choroidal melanoma, Ophthalmology 99:1278, 1992.

616. Haas BD and others: Diffuse choroidal melanocytoma in a child: a lesion extending the spectrum of melanocytic hamartomas, Ophthalmology 93:1632, 1986.

617. Hagler WS, Jarrett WH, and Killian JH: The use of the ^{32}P test in the management of malignant melanoma of the choroid: a five-year follow-up study, Trans Am Acad Ophthalmol Otolaryngol 83:OP 49, 1977.

618. Haim T and others: Oculodermal melanocytosis (nevus of Ota) and orbital malignant melanoma, Ann Ophthalmol 14:1132, 1982.

619. Halasa A: Malignant melanoma in a case of bilateral nevus of Ota, Arch Ophthalmol 84:176, 1970.

620. Hale P, Allen R, and Straatsma B: Benign melanomas (nevi) of the choroid and ciliary body, Arch Ophthalmol 74:532, 1965.

621. Hall WC, O'Day DM, and Glick AD: Melanotic neuroectodermal tumor of infancy: an ophthalmic appearance, Arch Ophthalmol 97:922, 1979.

622. Harbour JW, Augsburger JJ, and Eagle RC: Initial management and follow-up of melanocytic iris tumors, Ophthalmology 102:1987, 1995.

623. Harley RD, Romayananda N, and Chan GH: Juvenile xanthogranuloma, J Pediatr Ophthalmol Strabismus 19:33, 1982.

624. Hayreh S: Choroidal melanomata: fluorescence angiographic and histopathological study, Br J Ophthalmol 54:145, 1970.

625. Hayreh S: Choroidal tumors: role of fluorescein fundus angiography in their diagnosis. In Blodi FC, editor: Current concepts in ophthalmology, vol IV, St. Louis, 1974, The CV Mosby Co.

626. Henkind P and Roth M: Breast carcinoma and concurrent uveal melanoma, Am J Ophthalmol 71:198, 1971.

627. Hodes BL and Choromokos E: Standardized A-scan echographic diagnosis of choroidal malignant melanomas, Arch Ophthalmol 95:593, 1977.

628. Hogan MJ: Clinical aspects, management, and prognosis of melanomas of the uvea and optic nerve. In Boniuk M, editor: Ocular and adnexal tumors: new and controversial aspects, St. Louis, 1964, The CV Mosby Co.

629. Hogan MJ and Zimmerman LE: Ophthalmic pathology: an atlas and textbook, ed 2, Philadelphia, 1962, WB Saunders Co.

630. Hopping W, Meyer-Schwickerath G, and Lund O: Light coagulation in intraocular melanomas. In Boniuk M, editor: Ocular and adnexal tumors: new and controversial aspects, St. Louis 1964, The CV Mosby Co.

631. Horsman DE and White VA: Cytogenetic analysis of uveal melanoma. Consistent occurrence of monosomy 3 and trisomy 8q, Cancer 71:811, 1993.

632. Hoskins JC and Kearney CJ: A case of a negative ^{32}P test in a histologically proven choroidal hemangioma, Arch Ophthalmol 96:438, 1977.

633. Irvine A, Mannagh J, and Arya D: Change in cell type of human choroidal malignant melanoma in tissue culture, Am J Ophthalmol 80:417, 1975.

634. Iwamoto T, Jones I, and Howard G: Ultrastructural comparison of spindle A, spindle B, and epithelioid-type cells in uveal malignant melanoma, Invest Ophthalmol 11:873, 1972.

635. Iwamoto T, Reese A, and Mund M: Tapioca melanoma of the iris. II. Electron microscopy of the melanoma cells compared with normal iris melanocytes, Am J Ophthalmol 74:851, 1972.

636. Jakobiec FA and Iwamoto T: Mesectodermal leiomyoma of the ciliary body associated with a nevus, Arch Ophthalmol 96:692, 1978.

637. Jakobiec FA, Moorman LT, and Jones IS: Benign epithelial cell nevi of the iris, Arch Ophthalmol 97:917, 1979.

638. Jakobiec FA and Silbert G: Are most iris "melanomas" really nevi? A clinicopathologic study of 189 lesions, Arch Ophthalmol 99:2117, 1981.

639. Jakobiec FA and others: Balloon cell melanomas of the ciliary body, Arch Ophthalmol 97:1687, 1979.

640. Jakobiec FA and others: Solitary iris nevus associated with peripheral anterior synechia and iris endothelialization, Am J Ophthalmol 83:884, 1977.

641. Jarrett W and others: Clinical experience with presumed hemangioma of the choroid, as an aid in differential diagnosis, Trans Am Acad Ophthalmol Otolaryngol 81:OP 862, 1976.

642. Jensen OA: Malignant melanomas of the uvea in Denmark, 1943–1952, Acta Ophthalmol Suppl 75, 1963.

643. Jensen OA: Effect of dietetic factors on the growth of malignant melanomas, Trans Ophthalmol Soc UK 97:402, 1977.

644. Jensen OA and Andersen SR: Spontaneous regression of a malignant melanoma of the choroid, Acta Ophthalmol 52:173, 1974.

645. Johnson MW and others: Malignant melanoma of the iris in xeroderma pigmentosum, Arch Ophthalmol 107:402, 1989.

646. Jürgens I and others: Presumed melanocytoma of the macula, Arch Ophthalmol 112:305, 1994.

647. Kan-Mitchell J and others: S100 immunopheno-types of uveal melanomas, Invest Ophthalmol Vis Sci 31:1492, 1990.

648. Kara GB: Excision of uveal melanomas: a 15-year experience, Ophthalmology 86:997, 1979.

649. Kath R and others: Prognosis and treatment of disseminated uveal melanoma, Cancer 72:2219, 1993.

650. Katz NR and others: Ultrasound biomicroscopy in the management of malignant melanoma of the iris, Arch Ophthalmol 113, 1462, 1995.

651. Katz RS and Gass JDM: Multiple choroidal osteomas developing in association with recurrent orbital inflammatory pseudotumor, Arch Ophthalmol 101:1724, 1983.

652. Keeney AH, Waddell WJ, and Perraut TC: Carcinogenesis and nicotine in malignant melanoma of the choroid, Trans Am Ophthalmol Soc 80:131, 1982.

653. Kersten RC, Tse DT, and Anderson R: Iris melanoma: nevus or malignancy? Surv Ophthalmol 29:423, 1985.

654. Kersten RC: Management of choroidal malignant melanoma at Iowa, Ophthalmologica 189:24, 1984.

655. Kersten RC and others: The role of orbital exenteration in choroidal melanoma with extra scleral extension, Ophthalmology 92:436, 1985.

656. Kiehl H, Kirsch I, and Lommatzsch P: Survival after treatment for malignant choroidal melanoma. Comparison between conservative therapy (106 ru/106Rh application) and enucleation with and without postoperative irradiation on the orbit, Klin Monatsbl Augenbeilkd 184:2, 1984.

657. Kincaid MC and others: Complications after proton beam therapy for uveal malignant melanoma. A clinical and histopathologic study of five cases, Ophthalmology 95:982, 1988.

658. Kirk H and Petty R: Malignant melanoma of the choroid: a correlation of clinical and histological findings, Arch Ophthalmol 56:843, 1956.

659. Kishore K and others: P53 gene and cell cycling in uveal melanoma, Am J Ophthalmol 121:561, 1996.

660. Kline LB and others: Bilateral choroidal osteomas associated with fatal systemic illness, Am J Ophthalmol 93:192, 1982.

661. Kolodny NH and others: Characterization of human uveal melanoma cells by phosphorus 31 nuclear magnetic resonance spectroscopy, Am J Ophthalmol 100:38, 1995.

662. Kolodny NH and others: Magnetic resonance imaging and spectroscopy of intraocular tumors, Surv Ophthalmol 33:502, 1989.

663. Kroll A and Kuwabara T: Electron microscopy of uveal melanoma: a comparison of spindle and epithelioid cells, Arch Ophthalmol 73:378, 1965.

664. Ksander BR and others: Studies of tumor-infiltrating lymphocytes from a human choroidal melanoma, Invest Ophthalmol Vis Sci 32:3198, 1991.

665. Kurz G and Zimmerman LE: Vagaries of the retinal pigment epithelium, Int Ophthalmol Clin 2:441, 1962.

666. Lahav M and Gutman I: Subretinal pigment cells in malignant melanoma of the choroid, Am J Ophthalmol 86:239, 1978.

667. LaHey E and others: Immune deposits in iris biopsy specimens from patients with Fuchs'" heterochromic iridocyclitis, Am J Ophthalmol 113:75, 1992.

668. Lambert SR and others: Spontaneous regression of a choroidal melanoma, Arch Ophthalmol 104:732, 1986.

669. Lamping KA and others: Melanotic neuroectodermal tumor of infancy (retinal anlage tumor), Ophthalmology 92:143, 1985.

670. Lang GK and others: Ocular reticulum cell sarcoma. Clinicopathologic correlation of a case with multifocal lesions, Retina 5:79, 1985.

671. Lanning R and Shields JA: Comparison of radioactive phosphorus (^{32}P) uptake test in comparable sized choroidal melanomas and hemangiomas, Am J Ophthalmol 87:769, 1979.

672. Laqua H and Wessing A: Congenital retino-pigment epithelial malformation, previously described as hamartoma, Am J Ophthalmol 87:34, 1979.

673. Laties AM, Lerner AB: Iris colour and relationship of tyrosinase activity to adrenergic innervation, Nature 255:152, 1975.

674. Leopold I: Symposium: the diagnosis and management of intraocular melanomas, Trans Am Acad Ophthalmol Otolaryngol 62:517, 1958.

675. Levine RA, Putterman AM, and Korcy MS: Recurrent orbital malignant melanoma after the evisceration of an unsuspected choroidal melanoma, Am J Ophthalmol 89:571, 1980.

676. Gass JDM and others: Multifocal pigment epithelial detachments by reticulum cell sarcoma: a characteristic funduscopic picture, Retina 4:135, 1984.

677. Lewis M: Tumor specific antibodies in human malignant melanoma and their relationship to the extent of the disease, Br Med J 3:547, 1969.

678. Leys AM, Dierick HG, and Sciot RM: Early lesions of bilateral diffuse melanocytic proliferation, Arch Ophthalmol 109:1590, 1991.

679. Leys AM and others: Metastatic carcinoma to the retina. Clinicopathologic findings in two cases, Arch Ophthalmol 108:1448, 1990.

680. Li Z-Y, Tso MOM, and Sugar J: Leiomyoepithelioma of iris pigment epithelium, Arch Ophthalmol 105:819, 1987.

681. Litricin O: Unsuspected uveal melanomas, Am J Ophthalmol 76:734, 1973.

682. Liu LHS and Ni C: Hematoporphyrin phototherapy for experimental intraocular malignant melanoma, Arch Ophthalmol 101:901, 1983.

683. Lloyd WC 3rd and others: Congenital hypertrophy of the retinal pigment epithelium; electron microscopic and morphometric observations, Ophthalmology 97:1052, 1990.

684. Loeffler KU and Tecklenborg H: Melanocytoma-like growth of a juxtapapillary malignant melanoma, Retina 12, 29, 1992.

685. Logani S and others: Single-dose compared with fractionated-dose radiation of the OM431 choroidal melanoma cell line, Am J Ophthalmol 120:5-06, 1995.

686. Lommatzsch PK: Treatment of choroidal melanomas with ^{106}Ru/^{106}Rh beta-ray applicators, Trans Ophthalmol Soc UK 97:428, 1977.

687. Lommatzsch PK: Beta-irradiation of choroidal melanoma with ^{106}Ru/^{106}Rh applicators: 16 years experience, Arch Ophthalmol 101:713, 1983.

688. Long R, Galin M, and Rotman M: Conservative treatment of intraocular melanomas, Trans Am Acad Ophthalmol Otolaryngol 75:84, 1971.

689. Lopez JS and others: Immunohistochemistry findings in primary intraocular lymphoma, Am J Ophthalmol 112:472, 1991.

690. Lund O: Histological studies on light-coagulated melanoblastoma of the choroid, Graefes Arch Ophthalmol 164:433, 1962.

691. Lund O: Changes in choroidal tumors after light coagulation (and diathermy coagulation): a histopathological investigation of 43 cases, Arch Ophthalmol 75:458, 1966.

692. Lund O: Lichtcoagulation von malignene Melanoblastomen der Choroidea: klinische und histopathologische Untersuchungen, Mod Probl Ophthalmol 7:45, 1968.

693. Lyons LA and others: A genetic study of Gardner syndrome and congenital hypertrophy of the retinal pigment epithelium, Am J Hum Genet 42:290, 1988.

694. MacFaul PA: Local radiotherapy in the treatment of malignant melanoma of the choroid, Trans Ophthalmol Soc UK 97:421, 1977.

695. Machemer R: Die primäre retinale Pigmentepithelhyperplasie, Graefes Arch Ophthalmol 167:284, 1964.

696. MacIlwaine WA, Anderson B, and Klintworth CK: Enlargement of a histologically documented choroidal nevus, Am J Ophthalmol 87:480, 1979.

697. MacLean A and Maumenee AE: Hemangioma of the choroid, Trans Am Ophthalmol Soc 57:171, 1959.

698. Magauran RG, Gray B, Small KW: Chromosome 9 abnormality in choroidal melanoma, Am J Ophthalmol 117:109, 1994.

699. Makley R and Teed R: Unsuspected intraocular malignant melanomas, Arch Ophthalmol 60:475, 1958.

700. Manschot WA and van Peperzeel HA: Choroidal melanoma: enucleation or observation? A new approach, Arch Ophthalmol 98:71, 1980.

701. Manschot WA and van Strik R: Is irradiation a justifiable treatment of choroidal melanoma? Analysis of published results, Br J Ophthalmol 71:348, 1987.

702. Margo CE and McLean IW: Malignant melanoma of the choroid and ciliary body in black patients, Arch Ophthalmol 102:7, 1984.

703. Margo C and Pautler SE: Granulomatous uveitis after treatment of a choroidal melanoma with proton-beam irradiation, Retina 10:140, 1990.

704. Margo CE and others: Bilateral melanocytic uveal tumors associated with systemic non-ocular malignancy. Malignant melanomas or benign paraneoplastic syndrome? Retina 7:137, 1987.

705. Marquardt R: Mitosehäufigkeit und Wachstumsgeschwindigkeit: Zwei Parameter fur die Prognose maligner Melanome der Chorioidea, Fortschr Ophthalmol 80:312, 1983.

706. Mauriello JA, Zimmerman LE, and Rothstein TB: Intrachoroidal hemorrhage mistaken for malignant melanoma, Ann Ophthalmol 15:282, 1983.

707. McConnell I: Immune response to tumour antigens, Trans Ophthalmol Soc UK 97:381, 1977.

708. McDonald HR and others: Clinicopathologic results of vitreous surgery for epiretinal membranes in patients with combined retinal and retinal pigment epithelial hartomas, Am J Ophthalmol 100:806, 1985.

709. McLean EB: Hamartoma of the retinal pigment epithelium, Am J Ophthalmol 82:227, 1976.

710. McLean IW, Foster WD, and Zimmerman LE: Prognostic factors in small malignant melanomas of choroid and ciliary body, Arch Ophthalmol 95:48, 1977.

711. McLean IW, Foster WD, and Zimmerman LE: Uveal melanoma: location, size, cell type, and enucleation as risk factors in metastasis, Hum Pathol 13:123, 1982.

712. McLean IW and Shields JA: Prognostic value of ^{32}P uptake in posterior uveal melanomas, Ophthalmology 87:543, 1980.

713. McLean IW, Zimmerman LE, and Evans RM: Reappraisal of Callender's spindle A type of malignant melanoma of choroid and ciliary body, Am J Ophthalmol 86:557, 1978.

714. McLean IW and others: Inferred natural history of uveal melanoma, Invest Ophthalmol Vis Sci 19:760, 1980.

715. McLean IW and others: Modifications of Callender's classification of uveal melanoma at the Armed Forces Institute of Pathology, Am J Ophthalmol 96:502, 1983.

716. McMahon RT, Tso MOM, and McLean IW: Histologic localization of sodium fluorescein in choroidal malignant melanomas, Am J Ophthalmol 83:836, 1977.

717. Meyer-Schwickerath G: Light coagulation, St. Louis, 1960, The CV Mosby Co (Translated by SM Drance).

718. Meyer-Schwickerath G: The preservation of vision by treatment of intraocular tumors with light photocoagulation, Arch Ophthalmol 66:458, 1961.

719. Medlock RD and others: Enlargement of circumscribed choroidal hemangiomas, Retina 11:385, 1991.

720. Meyer-Schwickerath G and Vogel M: Malignant melanoma of the choroid treated with photocoagulation: a ten-year follow-up, Mod Probl Ophthalmol 12:544, 1974.

721. Meyer-Schwickerath G and Vogel M: Treatment of malignant melanomas of the choroid by photocoagulation, Trans Ophthalmol Soc UK 97:416, 1977.

722. Michael JC, DeVenecia G: Retinal trypsin digest study of cystoid macular edema associated with peripheral choroidal melanoma, Am J Ophthalmol 119:152, 1995.

723. Michael JC, de Venecia G: Retinal trypsin digest study of cystoid macular edema associated with choroidal melanoma, Am J Ophthalmol 119:152, 1995.

724. Michelson JB and Shields JA: Relationship of iris nevi to malignant melanoma of the uvea, Am J Ophthalmol 83:694, 1977.

725. Milares T: Structural differences in intraocular tumors and their metastases, Ophthalmologica 98:271, 1940.

726. Mims JL and Shields JA: Follow-up studies of suspicious choroidal nevi, Ophthalmology 85:929, 1978.

727. Mooy CM and others: Ki-67 immunostaining in uveal melanoma. The effect of pre-enucleation radiotherapy, Ophthalmology 97:1275, 1990.

728. Morgan CM and Gragoudas ES: Limited choroidal hemorrhage mistaken for a choroidal melanoma, Ophthalmology 94:41, 1987.

729. Müller H: Die particlle Ausschneidung von Iris and Ciliarkörper, Doc Ophthalmol 26:679, 1969.

730. Müller H and others: Die operative Behandlung von Tumoren des Kaminerwinkels und des Ciliarkörpers, Doc Ophthalmol 200:500, 1966.

731. Murray PI and others: Immunohistochemical analysis of iris biopsy specimens from patients with Fuchs'" heterochromic cyclitis, Am J Ophthalmol 109:394, 1990.

732. Naidoff MA, Kenyon KR, and Green WR: Iris hemangioma and abnormal retinal vasculature in a case of diffuse congenital hemangiomatosis, Am J Ophthalmol 72:633, 1971.

733. Nakazawa MM and Tamai M: Iris melanocytoma with secondary glaucoma, Am J Ophthalmol 97:797, 1984 (letter to the editor).

734. Nakhleh RE and others: Morphologic diversity in malignant melanomas, Am J Clin Pathol 93:731, 1990.

735. Naumann G: Pigmentierte Naevi der Aderhaut und des Ciliarkörpers, Adv Ophthalmol 23:187, 1970.

736. Naumann C and Apple DJ: Spezielle Pathologische Anatomie (das Auge), Berlin, 1980, Springer-Verlag.

737. Naumann G, Hellner K, and Naumann LK: Pigmented nevi of the choroid: clinical study of secondary changes in the overlying tissues, Trans Am Acad Ophthalmol Otolaryngol 75:110, 1971.

738. Naumann G and Ruprecht KW: Xanthom der Iris, Ophthalmologica 164:293, 1972.

739. Naumann G, Yanoff M, and Zimmerman LE: Histogenesis of malignant melanoma of the uvea, Arch Ophthalmol 76:784, 1966.

740. Naumann G, Zimmerman LE, and Yanoff M: Visual field defect associated with choroidal nevus, Am J Ophthalmol 62:914, 1966.

741. Nelson CC, Hertzberg BS, and Klintworth GK: A histopathologic study of 716 unselected eyes in patients with cancer at the time of death, Am J Ophthalmol 95:788, 1983.

742. Newman and others: Conservative management of malignant melanoma. I. Irradiation as a method of treatment for malignant melanoma of the choroid, Arch Ophthalmol 83:21, 1970.

743. Newton FH: Malignant melanoma of the choroid: report of a case with clinical history of 36 years and follow-up of 32 years, Arch Ophthalmol 73:198, 1965.

744. Ni C and Albert DM, editors: Ocular tumors and other ocular pathology: a Chinese-American collaborative study, Int Ophthalmol Clin 22(3), 1982.

745. Nicholson DH and others: Echographic and histologic tumor height measurements in uveal melanoma, Am J Ophthalmol 100:454, 1985.

746. Nik NA, Glero WB, and Zimmerman LE: Malignant melanoma of the choroid in the nevus of Ota of a black patient, Arch Ophthalmol 100:1641, 1982.

747. Nik NA and others: Diffuse iris nevus manifested by unilateral open angle glaucoma, Arch Ophthalmol 99:125, 1981.

748. Nitta T and others: Predominant expression of T cell receptor V7 in tumor-infiltrating lymphocytes of uveal melanoma, Science 249:672, 1980.

749. Noble KG: Bilateral choroidal osteoma in three siblings, Am J Ophthalmol 109:656, 1990.

750. Noor Sunba MS, Rahi AHS, and Morgan G: Tumors of the anterior uvea. I. Metastasizing malignant melanoma of the iris, Arch Ophthalmol 98:125, 1981.

751. Nordmann J and Brini A: von Recklinghausen's disease and melanoma of the uvea, Br J Ophthalmol 54:641, 1970.

752. Norris JL and Cleasby GW: An unusual case of congenital hypertrophy of the retinal pigment epithelium, Arch Ophthalmol 94:1910, 1976.

753. Noyes WD: Cutaneous melanoma and its relation to melanoma of the uveal tract, Surv Ophthalmol 23:443, 1978.

754. Oosterhuis JA and van Waveren CW: Fluorescein photography in malignant melanoma, Ophthalmologica 156:101, 1968.

755. Oosterhuis JA, Went LN, and Lynch HT: Primary choroidal and cutaneous melanomas, bilateral choroidal melanomas, and familial occurrence of melanomas, Br J Ophthalmol 66:230, 1982.

756. Osborn EI, Walker JP, and Weitzer JJ: Bilateral choroidal melanomas: a case report, Ann Ophthalmol 1043:1624, 1986.

757. Ossoinig KC and Blodi FC: Preoperative differential diagnosis of tumors with echography. III. Diagnosis of intraocular tumors. In Blodi FC, editor: Current concepts in Ophthalmology, vol IV, St. Louis, 1974, The CV Mosby Co.

758. Ossoinig KC and Till P: Methods and results of ultrasonography in diagnosing intraocular tumors. In Gitter KA and others, editors: Ophthalmic ultrasound, St. Louis, 1969, The CV Mosby Co.

759. Pach and others: Prognostic factors in choroidal and ciliary body melanoma with extrascleral extension, Am J Ophthalmol 101:325, 1986.

760. Pach JM and Robertson DM: Metastasis from untreated uveal melanomas, Arch Ophthalmol 104:1624, 1986.

761. Packard RBS: Pattern of mortality in choroidal malignant melanoma, Br J Ophthalmol 64:565, 1980.

762. Paridaens D and others: Familial aggressive Nevi of the iris in childhood, Arch Ophthalmol 109:1552, 1991.

763. Parks SS, Walsh SM, and Gragoudas ES: Visual-field deficits associated with proton beam irradiation for parapapillary choroidal melanoma, Ophthalmology 103:110, 1990.

764. Parver LM and Font RI: Malignant lymphoma of the retina and brain. Initial diagnosis by cytologic examination of vitreous aspirate, Arch Ophthalmol 97:1505, 1979.

765. Pascal SG and others: An investigation into the association between liver damage and metastatic uveal melanoma, Am J Ophthalmol 100:448, 1985.

766. Paul EV, Parnell BL, and Fraker M: Prognosis of malignant melanomas of the choroid and ciliary body, Int Ophthalmol Clin 2:387, 1962.

767. Pe'er J and others: Mean of the ten largest nucleoli, microcirculation architecture, and prognosis of ciliochoroidal melanomas, Ophthalmology 101:1227, 1994.

768. Perry HD, Hsieh RC, and Evans RM: Malignant melanoma of the choroid associated with spontaneous expulsive choroidal hemorrhage, Am J Ophthalmol 84:205, 1977.

769. Peterson K and others: The clinical spectrum of ocular lymphoma, Cancer 72:843, 1993.

770. Pettit TH and others: Fluorescein angiography of choroidal melanomas, Arch Ophthalmol 83:27, 1970.

771. Peyman GA: Eye wall resection, Ophthalmic Forum 1:38, 1983.

772. Peyman GA and Apple DJ: Local excision of choroidal malignant melanoma by full-thickness eye wall resection, Arch Ophthalmol 92:216, 1974.

773. Peyman GA, Apple DJ, and Sanders DR, editors: Intraocular tumors, New York, 1977, Appleton-Century-Crofts.

774. Peyman GA and Dodich NA: Full thickness eye wall resection: an experimental approach for treatment of choroidal melanoma. I. Dacron graft, Invest Ophthalmol 11:115, 1972.

775. Peyman GA and Sanders DR: Advances in uveal surgery: vitreous surgery and the treatment of endophthalmitis, New York, 1975, Appleton-Century-Crofts.

776. Peyman GA and others: Biopsy of human scleral-chorioretinal tissue, Invest Ophthalmol 14:707, 1975.

777. Peyman GA and others: Ten years experience with eye wall resection for uveal malignant melanomas, Ophthalmology 91:1720, 1984.

778. Pineda R II and others: Ciliary body neurilemoma; unusual clinical findings intimating the diagnosis, Ophthalmology 102:918, 1995.

779. Pitta CG and others: Solitary choroidal hemangioma, Am J Ophthalmol 88:698, 1979.

780. Pitts RE, Awan KJ, and Yanoff M: Choroidal melanoma with massive retinal fibrosis and spontaneous regression of retinal detachment, Surv Ophthalmol 20:273, 1976.

781. Pizzuto D, deLuise V, and Zimmerman N: Choroidal malignant melanoma appearing as acute panophthalmitis, Am J Ophthalmol 101:249, 1986.

782. Pomeranz GA, Bunt AH, and Kalina RE: Multifocal choroidal melanoma in ocular melanocytosis, Arch Ophthalmol 99:857, 1981.

783. Prause JU and Jensen OA: Scanning electron microscopy of frozen-cracked, dry-cracked and enzyme-digested tissue of human malignant choroidal melanomas, Albrecht Von Graefes Arch Ophthalmol Klin Exp Ophthal 212:217, 1980.

784. Pro M, Shields JA, and Tomer TL: Serous detachment of the macula associated with presumed choroidal nevi, Arch Ophthalmol 96:1374, 1979.

785. Purcell JJ and Shields JA: Hypertrophy with hyperpigmentation of the retinal pigment epithelium, Arch Ophthalmol 93:1122, 1975.

786. Qualman SJ and others: Intraocular lymphomas, Cancer 52:878, 1983.

787. Radnót M and Antal M: Vessels of intraocular malignant melanomas, Am J Ophthalmol 88:472, 1979.

788. Rahi AHS: Autoimmune reactions in uveal melanoma, Br J Ophthalmol 55:793, 1971.

789. Rahi AHS: Immunologic aspects of malignant melanoma of the choroid, Trans Ophthalmol Soc UK 93:79, 1973.

790. Rahi AHS and Agrawal PK: Prognostic parameters in choroidal melanomata, Trans Ophthalmol Soc UK 97:368, 1977.

791. Rajpal S, Moore R, and Karakousis CP: Survival in metastatic ocular melanoma, Cancer 52:334, 1983.

792. Rawles ME: Origin of pigment cells from neural crest in mouse embryo, Physiol Zool 20:248, 1947.

793. Rednam KRV and others: Uveal melanoma in association with multiple malignancies: a case report and review, Retina 1:100, 1981.

794. Reese AB: Spontaneous cysts of the ciliary body simulating neoplasms, Am J Ophthalmol 33:1739, 1950.

795. Reese AB: Tumors of the eye and adnexa. In Reese AB: Atlas of tumor pathology, section X, fascicle 38, Washington, DC, 1956, Armed Forces Institute of Pathology.

796. Reese AB: The role of the pigment epithelium in ocular pathology, Am J Ophthalmol 50:1066, 1960.

797. Reese AB: Hyperplasia and neoplasia of the pigment epithelium. In Boniuk M, editor: Ocular and adnexal tumors: new and controversial aspects, St. Louis, 1964, The CV Mosby Co.

798. Reese AB: Congenital melanomas, Am J Ophthalmol 77:798, 1973.

799. Reese AB and Cleasby GW: The treatment of iris melanoma, Am J Ophthalmol 47:118, 1959.

800. Reese AB and Howard GM: Flat uveal melanomas, Am J Ophthalmol 64:1021, 1967.

801. Reese AB and Jones IS: Benign melanomas of the retinal pigment epithelium, Am J Ophthalmol 42:208, 1948.

802. Reese AB and Jones IS: The differential diagnosis of malignant melanoma of the choroid, Arch Ophthalmol 58:477, 1957.

803. Reese AB and Jones IS: Hematomas under the retinal pigment epithelium, Trans Am Ophthalmol Soc 59:43, 1961.

804. Reese AB, Jones IS, and Cooper WC: Surgery for tumors of the iris and ciliary body, Am J Ophthalmol 66:173, 1968.

805. Reese AB, Mund ML, and Iwamoto T: Tapioca melanoma of the iris: clinical and light microscopy studies, Am J Ophthalmol 74:840, 1972.

806. Reese AB and others: Necrosis of malignant melanoma of the choroid, Am J Ophthalmol 69:91, 1970.

807. Reynolds WD and Goldstein BG: Retinal pigment epithelial hamartoma, Ophthalmology 90:117, 1983.

808. Regillo CD and others: Histopathologic findings in congenital grouped pigmentation of the retina, Ophthalmology 100:400, 1993.

809. Riley FC: Balloon cell melanoma of the choroid, Arch Ophthalmol 92:131, 1974.

810. Rini FJ and others: The treatment of advanced choroidal melanoma with massive orbital extension, Am J Ophthalmol 104:634, 1987.

811. Robertson DM: A rationale for comparing radiation to enucleation in the management of choroidal melanoma, Am J Ophthalmol 108:448, 1989.

812. Robertson DM and Campbell RJ: Errors in the diagnosis of malignant melanoma of the choroid, Am J Ophthalmol 87:269, 1979.

813. Rockwood EJ, Zakov ZN, and Bay JW: Combined malignant lymphoma of the eye and CNS (reticulum-cell sarcoma), J Neurosurg 61:369, 1984.

814. Rohrbach JM and others: Simultaneous bilateral diffuse melanocytic uveal hyperplasia, Am J Ophthalmol 110:49, 1990.

815. Romania A and others: Congenital hypertrophy of the retinal pigment epithelium in familial adenomatous polyposis, Ophthalmology 96:879, 1989.

816. Rones B and Linger HT: Early malignant melanoma of the choroid, Am J Ophthalmol 38:163, 1954.

817. Rones B and Zimmerman LE: The production of heterochromia and glaucoma by diffuse malignant melanoma of the iris, Trans Am Acad Ophthalmol Otolaryngol 61:447, 1957.

818. Rones B and Zimmerman LE: The prognosis of primary tumors of the iris treated by iridectomy, Arch Ophthalmol 60:193, 1958.

819. Rootman J and Gallagher RP: Color as a risk factor in iris melanoma, Am J Ophthalmol 98:558, 1984.

820. Rosen ES and Garner A: Benign melanoma of the choroid, Br J Ophthalmol 53:621, 1969.

821. Rosenbaum PS, Boniuk M, and Font RL: Diffuse uveal melanoma in a 5-year-old child, Am J Ophthalmol 106:601, 1988.

822. Roseman RL and others: Solitary hypopigmented nevus of the retinal pigmented epithelium in the macula, Arch Ophthalmol 110:1358, 1992.

823. Rotman M and others: Radiation therapy of choroidal melanoma, Trans Ophthalmol Soc UK 97:431, 1977.

824. Roy PE: Diffuse nonpigmented iris melanoma in a child, J Pediatr Ophthalmol 4:30, 1967.

825. Royds JA and others: Enolase isoenzymes in uveal melanomas: a possible parameter of malignancy, Br J Ophthalmol 67:244, 1983.

826. Rummelt V, Microcirculation architecture of melanocytic nevi and malignant melanomas of the ciliary body and coroid. A comparative histopathologic and ultrastructural study, Ophthalmology 101:718, 1994.

827. Rummelt V and others: Surgical management of melanocytoma of the ciliary body with extrascleral-extension, Am J Ophthalmol 117:169, 1994.

828. Ryan SJ, Zimmerman LE, and King FM: Reactive lymphoid hyperplasia: an unusual form of intraocular pseudotumor, Trans Am Acad Ophthalmol Otolaryngol 76:652, 1972.

829. Ryan SJ Jr, Frank RN, and Green WR: Bilateral inflammatory pseudotumors of the ciliary body, Am J Ophthalmol 72:586, 1971.

830. Sakamoto T and others: Histologic findings and prognosis of uveal malignant melanoma in Japanese patients, Am J Ophthalmol 121:276, 1996.

831. Sahel JA and others: Melanoma arising de novo over a 16-month period, Arch Ophthalmol 106:381, 1988.

832. Sahel JA and others: Idiopathic retina ghosts mimicking a choroidal melanoma, Retina 8:282, 1988.

833. Samuels B: Anatomic and clinical manifestations of necrosis in 84 cases of choroidal sarcoma, Arch Ophthalmol 11:998, 1934.

834. Sanborn GF, Augsburger JJ, and Shields JA: Treatment of circumscribed choroidal hemangiomas, Ophthalmology 89:1374, 1982.

835. Sanders TE: Intraocular juvenile xantho-granuloma (nevoxanthoendothelioma), Am J Ophthalmol 53:455, 1962.

836. Sanke RF and others: Local recurrence of choroidal malignant melanoma following enucleation, Br J Ophthalmol 65:846, 1981.

837. Santos A and others: Congenital hypertrophy of the retinal pigment epithelium associated with familial adenomatous polyposis, Retina 14:6, 1994.

838. Saornil MA and others: Histopathology of proton beam—irradiated vs enucleated uveal melanomas, Arch Ophthalmol 110:1112, 1992.

839. Sassani JW, Weinstein JM, and Graham WP: Massively invasive diffuse choroidal melanoma, Arch Ophthalmol 103:945, 1985.

840. Sassani JW and Blankenship G: Disciform choroidal melanoma, Retina 14:177, 1994.

841. Schachat AP and others: Combined hamartomas of the retina and pigment epithelium, Ophthalmology 91:1609, 1984.

842. Scheie HG and Yanoff M: Pseudomelanoma of ciliary body, report of a patient, Arch Ophthalmol 77:81, 1967.

843. Scheie HG and Yanoff M: Iris nevus (Cogan-Reese) syndrome, Arch Ophthalmol 93:963, 1975.

844. Schmidt-Erfurth U and others: Photodynamic therapy of experimental choroidal melanoma using lipoprotein-delivered benzoporphyrin, Ophthalmology 101:89, 1994.

845. Seddon JM and others: Uveal melanomas presenting during pregnancy and the investigation of oestrogen receptors in melanomas, Br J Ophthalmol 66:695, 1982.

846. Seddon JM and others: Comparison of survival rates for patients with uveal melanoma after treatment with proton beam irradiation or enucleation, Am J Ophthalmol 99:282, 1985.

847. Seddon JM and others: Death from uveal melanoma: number of epithelioid cells and inverse SD of nucleolar area as prognostic factors, Arch Ophthalmol 105:801, 1987.

848. Seddon JM and others: A prognostic factor study of disease-free interval and survival following enucleation for uveal melanoma, Arch Ophthalmol 101:1894, 1983.

849. Seddon JM and others: Host factors. UV radiation and risk of uveal melanoma, Arch Ophthalmol 108:1274, 1990.

850. Selwa AFA and others: Uveal involvement in systemic angiotropic large cell lymphoma. Microscopic and immunohistochemical studies, Ophthalmology 100:961, 1993.

851. Seregard S and others: Two cases of primary bilateral malignant melanoma of the choroid, Br J Ophthalmol 72:244, 1988.

852. Shahabuddin S and Kumar S: Quantitation of angiogenesis factor in bovine retina tumor extracts by means of radioimmunoassay, Br J Ophthalmol 67:286, 1983.

853. Shammas HF and Blodi FC: Prognostic factors in choroidal and ciliary body melanomas, Arch Ophthalmol 95:63, 1977.

854. Shammas HF and Blodi FC: Orbital extension of choroidal and ciliary body melanomas, Arch Ophthalmol 95:2002, 1977.

855. Shammas HF and Blodi FC: Peripapillary choroidal melanomas, Arch Ophthalmol 96:440, 1978.

856. Shammas HF and Watzke RC: Bilateral choroidal melanomas, Arch Ophthalmol 95:617, 1977.

857. Shammas HF and Wood LW: Choroidal melanoma and retinal tear, Arch Ophthalmol 95:1825, 1977.

858. Shields CL, Shields JA, and Augsburger JJ: Choroidal osteoma, Surv Ophthalmol 33:17, 1988.

859. Shields CL and others: Differentiation of adenoma of the iris pigment epithelium from iris cyst and melanoma, Am J Ophthalmol 100:678, 1985.

860. Shields CL and others: Prevalence and mechanisms of secondary intraocular pressure elevation in eyes with intraocular tumors, Ophthalmology 94:839, 1987.

861. Shields CL and others: Uveal melanoma and pregnancy. A report of 16 cases, Ophthalmology 98:1667, 1991.

862. Shields CL and others: Uveal melanoma in teenagers and children. A report of 40 cases, Ophthalmology 98:1662, 1991.

863. Shields CL and others: Enucleation after plaque radiotherapy for posterior uveal melanoma. Histopathologic findings, Ophthalmology 97:1665, 1990.

864. Shields CL and others: Choroidal osteoma (major review), Surv Ophthalmol 33:17, 1988.

865. Shields CL and others: Transpupillary thermotherapy in the management of choroidal melanoma, Ophthalmology 103:1642, 1996.

866. Shields C and others: Diffuse choroidal melanoma. Clinical features of predictive metastasis, Arch Ophthalmol 114:956, 1996.

867. Shields JA: Concepts and philosophies in the management of malignant melanomas of the choroid. In Peyman CA, Apple DJ, and Sanders DR, editors: Intraocular tumors, New York, 1977, Appleton-Century-Crofts.

868. Shields JA: Current approaches to the diagnosis and management of choroidal melanomas, Surv Ophthalmol 21:443, 1977.

869. Shields JA: Modern methods in the diagnosis of uveal melanomas, Trans Ophthalmol Soc UK 97:407, 1977.

870. Shields JA: The differential diagnosis of malignant melanoma of the choroid. In Peyman GA, Apple DJ, and Sanders DR, editors: Intraocular tumors, New York, 1977, Appleton-Century-Crofts.

871. Shields JA: The management of small malignant melanomas of the choroid. In Brockhurst R, editor: Controversy in ophthalmology, Philadelphia, 1977, WB Saunders Co.

872. Shields JA: Primary cysts of the iris, Trans Am Ophthalmol Soc 79:771, 1981.

873. Shields JA: Diagnosis and management of intraocular tumors, St. Louis, 1983, The CV Mosby Co.

874. Shields JA, Annesley WH Jr, and Totino JA: Nonfluorescent malignant melanoma of the choroid diagnosed with the radioactive phosphorus uptake test, Am J Ophthalmol 79:634, 1975.

875. Shields JA, Augsburger JJ, and Dougherty MJ: Orbital recurrence of choroidal melanoma 20 years after enucleation, Am J Ophthalmol 97:767, 1984.

876. Shields JA and Font RL: Melanocytoma of the choroid clinically simulating a malignant melanoma, Arch Ophthalmol 87:396, 1972.

877. Shields JA and others: Multilobed uveal melanoma masquerading as postoperative choroidal detachment, Br J Ophthalmol 60:386, 1976.

878. Shields JA and Joffe L: Choroidal melanoma clinically simulating a retinal angioma, Am J Ophthalmol 85:67, 1978.

879. Shields JA and McDonald PR: Improvements in the diagnosis of posterior uveal melanomas, Arch Ophthalmol 93:259, 1974.

880. Shields JA, McDonald PR, and Sarin LK: Problems and improvements in the diagnosis of posterior uveal melanomas. In Croll M and others, editors: Nuclear ophthalmology, New York, 1976, John Wiley & Sons, Inc.

881. Shields JA, Sanborn GE, and Augsburger JJ: The differential diagnosis of malignant melanoma of the iris: a clinical study of 200 patients, Ophthalmology 90:716, 1983.

882. Shields JA and Tso MOM: Congenital grouped pigmentation of the retina: histopathologic description and report of a case, Arch Ophthalmol 93:1149, 1975.

883. Shields JA and Zimmerman LE: Lesions simulating malignant melanoma of the posterior uvea, Arch Ophthalmol 89:466, 1973.

884. Shields JA and others: Lipofuscin pigment over benign and malignant choroidal tumors, Trans Am Acad Ophthalmol Otolaryngol 81:871, 1976.

885. Shields JA and others: Fluorescein angiography and ^{32}P studies in photocoagulated choroidal melanomas. In L Esperance FA Jr, editor: Current diagnosis and management of chorioretinal diseases, St. Louis, 1977, The CV Mosby Co.

886. Shields JA and others: The diagnosis of uveal melanoma in eyes with opaque media, Am J Ophthalmol 82:95, 1977.

887. Shields JA and others: Melanocytoma of the ciliary body and iris, Am J Ophthalmol 89:632, 1980.

888. Shields JA and others: The differential diagnosis of posterior uveal melanoma, Ophthalmology 87:518, 1980.

889. Shields JA and others: Benign peripheral nerve tumor of the choroid, Ophthalmology 88:1322, 1981.

890. Shields JA and others: Cobalt plaque therapy of posterior uveal melanomas, Ophthalmology 89:1201, 1982.

891. Shields JA and others: Adenoma of the iris-pigment epithelium, Ophthalmology 890:735, 1983.

892. Shields JA and others: Epithelioid cell nevus of the iris, Arch Ophthalmol 103:235, 1985.

893. Shields JA and others: Management of posterior uveal melanoma, Surv Ophthalmol 36(3):161, 1991.

894. Shields JA and others: Observations on seven cases of intraocular leiomyoma. The 1993 Byron Demorest Lecture, Arch Ophthalmol 112:521, 1994.

895. Shields JA and others: Comparison of xenon arc and argon laser

photocoagulation in the treatment of choroidal melanoma, Am J Ophthalmol 109:647, 1990.

896. Shields JA and others: Melanotic Schwannoma of the choroid. Immunohistochemistry and electron microscopic observation, Ophthalmology 101:843, 1994.

897. Shields JA and others: Risk factors for growth and metastasis of small choroidal melanocytic lesions, Ophthalmology 102:1351, 1995.

898. Shields JA, Annesley WH Jr, and Spaeth GL: Necrotic melanocytoma of iris with secondary glaucoma, Am J Ophthalmol 84:826, 1977.

899. Shields JA, Sanborn GE, and Augsburger JJ: The differential diagnosis of malignant melanoma of the iris. A clinical study of 200 patients, Ophthalmology 90:716, 1983.

900. Shields JA and others: Partial lamellar sclerouvectomy for ciliary body and choroidal tumors, Ophthalmology 98:971, 1991.

901. Shields JA and others: Progressive enlargement of a circumscribed choroidal hemangioma, Arch Ophthalmol 110:1276, 1992.

902. Shields JA and others: Adenocarcinoma of retinal pigment epithelium arising from a juxtapapillary histoplasmosis scar, Arch Ophthalmol 112:650, 1994.

903. Shields MB and Klintworth GK: Anterior uveal melanomas and intraocular pressure, Ophthalmology 87:503, 1980.

904. Shields MB and Proia AD: Neovascular glaucoma associated with an iris melanoma. A clinicopathologic report, Arch Ophthalmol 105:672, 1987.

905. Sigelman and others: Amelanotic small flat lesions of the choroid, Arch Ophthalmol 96:1805, 1978.

906. Singh AD and others: Familial uveal melanoma—clinical observations on 56 patients, Arch Ophthalmol 114:392, 1996.

907. Singh AD and others: Familial uveal melanoma: absence of constitutional cytogenic abnormalities in 14 cases, Arch Ophthalmol 114:502, 1996 (letter, comment).

908. Singh AD and others: Bilateral primary uveal melanoma—bad luck or bad genes, Ophthalmology 103:256, 1996.

909. Slusher MM and Weaver RG: Presumed choroidal nevus and sensory retinal detachment, Br J Ophthalmol 61:414, 1977.

910. Smith L and Irvine A: Diagnostic significance of orange pigment accumulation over choroidal tumors, Am J Ophthalmol 76:212, 1973.

911. Sneed SR and others: Choroidal detachment associated with malignant choroidal tumors, Ophthalmology 98:963, 1991.

912. Snip RC and others: Choroidal nevus with subretinal pigment epithelial neovascular membrane and a positive p-32 test, Ophthalmic Surg 9:35, 1993.

913. Spencer W: Optic nerve extension of intraocular neoplasms, Am J Ophthalmol 80:465, 1975.

914. Stallard H: Malignant melanoma of the choroid treated with radioactive applicators, Trans Ophthalmol Soc UK 79:373, 1959.

915. Stallard H: Radiotherapy for malignant melanoma of the choroid, Br J Ophthalmol 50:147, 1966.

916. Stallard H: Malignant melanoblastoma of the choroid, Mod Probl Ophthalmol 7:16, 1968.

917. Starr H and Zimmerman LE: Extrascleral extension and orbital recurrence of malignant melanomas of the choroid and ciliary body, Int Ophthalmol Clin 2:369, 1962.

918. Steuhl KP and others: Significance, specificity, and ultrastructural localization of HMB-45 antigen in pigmented ocular tumors, Ophthalmology 100:208, 1993.

919. Straatsma BR and others: Enucleative versus plaque irradiation for choroidal melnoma, Ophthalmology 100:208, 1993.

920. Strickland D and Lee JAH: Melanomas of the eye: stability of rates, Am J Epidemiol 113:700, 1981.

921. Sugar HS and Nathan LE: Congenital epithelial cysts of the iris stroma, Ann Ophthalmol 14:483, 1982.

922. Sunba MSN, Rahi AHS, and Morgan G: Tumors of the anterior uvea. I. Metastasizing malignant melanoma of the iris, Arch Ophthalmol 98:82, 1980.

923. Sunba MSN, Rahi AHS, and Morgan G: Tumours of the anterior uvea. II. Intranuclear cytoplasmic inclusions in malignant melanoma of the iris, Br J Ophthalmol 64:453, 1980.

924. Sunba MSN and others: Lymphoproliferative response as an index of cellular immunity in malignant melanoma of the uvea and its correlation with the histological features of the tumour, Br J Ophthalmol 64:576, 1980.

925. Sunba MSN and others: Tumours of the anterior uvea. III. Oxytalan fibres in the differential diagnosis of leiomyoma and malignant melanoma of the iris, Br J Ophthalmol 64:867, 1980.

926. Tabbara KF and Beckstead JH: Acute promonocytic leukemia with ocular involvement, Arch Ophthalmol 98:1055, 1980.

927. Takagi T, Ueno Y, and Matsuya N: Mesectodermal leiomyoma of the ciliary body: an ultrastructural study, Arch Ophthalmol 103:1711, 1985.

928. Tamler E: A clinical study of choroidal nevi: a follow-up report, Arch Ophthalmol 84:29, 1970.

929. Tamler E and Maumenee AE: A clinical study of choroidal nevi, Arch Ophthalmol 62:196, 1959.

930. Tasman W: Familial intraocular melanoma, Trans Am Acad Ophthalmol Otolaryngol 74:955, 1970.

931. Taylor MR and others: Lack of association between intraocular melanoma and cutaneous dysplastic nevi, Am J Ophthalmol 98:478, 1984.

932. Teichmann KD, Karcioglu ZA: Melanocytoma of the iris with rapidly developing secondary glaucoma, Surv Ophthalmol 40:136, 1995 (review).

933. ten Berge PJM and others: Integrin expression in uveal melanoma differs cutaneous melanoma, Invest Ophthalmol Vis Sci 34:3635, 1993.

934. Terner I, Leopold I, and Eisenberg I: The radioactive phosphorus (^{32}P) uptake test in ophthalmology: a review of the literature and analysis of results in 262 cases of ocular and adnexal pathology, Arch Ophthalmol 55:52, 1956.

935. Territo C and others: Natural course of melanocytic tumors of the iris, Ophthalmology 95:1251, 1988.

936. The Collaborative Ocular Melanoma Study Group: Accuracy of diagnosis of choroidal melanoma differs from cutaneous melanoma study, Arch Ophthalmol 108:1268, 1990.

937. Theobald G: Neurogenic origin of choroidal sarcoma, Arch Ophthalmol 18:971, 1937.

938. Theobald C, Floyd G, and Kirk H: Hyperplasia of the retinal pigment epithelium, Am J Ophthalmol 45:235, 1958.

939. Thomas G, Krohmer J, and Storaasli F: Detection of intraocular tumors with radioactive phosphorus: a preliminary report with special reference to differentiation of the cause of retinal separation, Arch Ophthalmol 49:276, 1952.

940. Thomas JV, Green WR, and Maumenee AE: Small choroidal melanoma: a long-term follow-up study, Arch Ophthalmol 97:861, 1979.

941. Ticho BH and others: Bilateral diffuse iris nodular nevi; clinical and histopathologic characterization, Ophthalmology 102:419, 1995.

942. Traboulsi EI and others: A clinicopathologic study of the eyes in a familial adenomatous polyposis with extracolonic manifestations (Gardner's syndrome), Am J Ophthalmol 110:550, 1990.

943. Traboulsi EI and others: Congenital hypertrophy of the retinal pigment epithelium predicts colorectal polyposis in Gardner's syndrome, Arch Ophthalmol 108:525, 1990.

944. Trediei T and Fenton R: Hematoma beneath the retinal pigment epithelium, Arch Ophthalmol 72:796, 1964.

945. Trimble SN and Schatz H: Choroidal osteoma after intraocular inflammation, Am J Ophthalmol 96:759, 1983.

946. Trimble SN, Schatz H, and Schneider GB: Spontaneous decalcification of choroidal osteoma, Ophthalmology 95:631, 1988.

947. Tso MOM and Albert DM: Pathological condition of the retinal pigment epithelium: neoplasms and nodular non-neoplastic lesions, Arch Ophthalmol 88:27, 1972.

948. Tso MOM and others: Nodular adenomatosis of iris pigment epithelium, Am J Ophthalmol 100:87, 1985.

949. Tucker M and others: Sunlight exposure as risk factor for intraocular malignant melanoma, N Engl J Med 313:789, 1985.

950. Turner BJ and others: Other cancers in uveal melanoma patients and their families, Am J Ophthalmol 107:601, 1989.

951. Van Rens GH and others: Uveal malignant melanoma and levodopa therapy in Parkinson's disease, Ophthalmology 89:1464, 1982.

952. Vannas M: On the diagnosis of intraocular tumors and foreign bodies by means of anterior pupillary transillumination, Acta Ophthalmol 26:125, 1948.

953. Verhoeff F: Sarcoma of the choroid with destructive hemorrhage, Arch Ophthalmol, 32:241, 1904.

954. Vogel M: Histopathologic observations of photocoagulated malignant melanomas of the choroid, Am J Ophthalmol 74:466, 1972.

955. Vogel M: Treatment of malignant choroidal melanoma with photocoagulation: evaluation of ten-year follow-up data, Am J Ophthalmol 74:1, 1972.

956. Vogel M and Wessing A: Die Proliferation des juxtapapillären retinalen Pigmentepithels, Klin Monatsbl Augenheilkd 162:736, 1973.

957. Vogel M, Zimmerman LE, and Gass JDM: Proliferation of the juxtapapillary retinal pigment epithelium simulating malignant melanoma, Doc Ophthalmol 26:461, 1969.

958. Völcker HE and Naumann GOH: Multicentric primary malignant melanomas of the choroid: two separate malignant melanomas of the choroid and two uveal naevi in one eye, Br J Ophthalmol 62:408, 1978.

959. Völcker HE, Naumann GOH: "Primary" reticulum cell sarcoma of the retina, Dev Ophthal 2:114, 1981.

960. Wagoner MD and Albert DM: The incidence of metastases from untreated ciliary body and choroidal melanoma, Arch Ophthalmol 100:939, 1982.

961. Wagoner MD and others: Intraocular reticulum cell sarcoma, Ophthalmology 87:724, 1980.

962. Wallow HL and Tso MOM: Proliferation of the retinal pigment epithelium over malignant choroidal tumors: a light and electron microscopic study, Am J Ophthalmol 73:914, 1972.

963. Waltman DD and others: Choroid neovascularization associated with choroidal nevi, Am J Ophthalmol 85:704, 1978.

964. Wang C-L, Brucker AJ: Vitreous hemorrhage secondary to juxtapapillary vascular hamartoma of the retina, Retina 4:44, 1984.

965. Wang MX and others: An ocular melanoma-associated antigen. Molecular characterization, Arch Ophthalmol 110:399, 1992.

966. Wang WJ and others: Choroidal melanoma associated with rhegmatogenous retinal detachment, Ophthalmic Surg 15:302, 1984.

967. Warren R: Prognosis of malignant melanomas of the choroid and ciliary body. In Blodi FC, editor: Current concepts in ophthalmology, vol IV, St. Louis, 1974, The CV Mosby Co.

968. Watson PC: A patient with malignant melanoma treated with a phenylalanine/tyrosine free diet, Trans Ophthalmol Soc UK 97:406, 1977.

969. Weinhaus RS and others: Prognostic factor study of survival after enucleation for juxtapapillary melanomas, Arch Ophthalmol 103:1673, 1985.

970. Weiter JJ and others: Retinal pigment epithelial lipofuscin and melanin and choroidal melanin in human eyes, Invest Ophthalmol Vis Sci 27:145, 1986.

971. Westbury G: Chemotherapy in the treatment of malignant melanomas, Trans Ophthalmol Soc UK 97:455, 1977.

972. Westerveld-Brandon E and Zeeman W: The prognosis of melanoblastomata of the choroid, Ophthalmologica 134:20, 1957.

973. Whelchel JC and others: Immunohistochemistry of infiltrating lymphocytes in uveal malignant melanoma, Invest Ophthalmol Vis Sci 34:2603, 1993.

974. Wilder H and Callender G: Malignant melanoma of the choroid: further studies of prognosis by histologic type and fiber content, Am J Ophthalmol 22:851, 1939.

975. Wilder H and Paul E: Malignant melanoma of the choroid and ciliary body: a study of 2533 cases, Milit Surg 109:370, 1951.

976. Wilhelm JL and Zakov ZN: Choroidal malignant melanoma with liver metastasis before enucleation, Ann Ophthalmol 14:789, 1982.

977. Wilkes SR and others: Incidence of uveal malignant melanoma in the resident population of Rochester and Olmstead County, Minnesota, Am J Ophthalmol 87:639, 1979.

978. Williams AT and others: Osseous choristoma of the choroid simulating a choroidal melanoma, Arch Ophthalmol 96:1874, 1978.

979. Winter F: Surgical excision of tumors of the ciliary body and iris, Arch Ophthalmol 70:19, 1963.

980. Wirz K, Lee WR, and Coaker T: Progressive changes in congenital hypertrophy of the retinal pigment epithelium. An electron microscopic study, Graefes Arch Clin Exp Ophthalmol 219:214, 1982.

981. Wiznia RA and others: Malignant melanoma of the choroid in neurofibromatosis, Am J Ophthalmol 87:639, 1979.

982. Wolter J: Proliferating pigment epithelium, producing a simple organoid structure in the subretinal space of a human eye, Arch Ophthalmol 77:651, 1967.

983. Wolter J, Schut A, and Martonyi D: Hemangioma-like clinical appearance of a collar-button melanoma caused by the strangulation effect of Bruch's membrane, Am J Ophthalmol 76:730, 1973.

984. Wright D: Prognosis in cutaneous and ocular malignant melanomas: a study of 222 cases, J Pathol 61:507, 1949.

985. Yanoff M and Zimmerman LE: Pseudomelanoma of anterior chamber caused by implantation of iris pigment epithelium, Arch Ophthalmol 74:302, 1965.

986. Yanoff M: Melanoma and the incidence of neoplastic disease, N Eng J Med 273:284, 1965 (letter to the editor).

987. Yanoff M and Scheie HG: Melanomalytic glaucoma: report of patient, Arch Ophthalmol 84:471, 1970.

988. Yanoff M: Glaucoma mechanisms in ocular malignant melanomas, Am J Ophthalmol 70:898, 1970.

989. Yanoff M and Zimmerman LE: Histogenesis of malignant melanoma of the uvea. II. Relationship of uveal nevi to malignant melanomas, Cancer 20:493, 1967.

990. Yanoff M and Zimmerman LE: Histogenesis of malignant melanoma of the uvea. III. The relationship of congenital ocular melanocytosis and neurofibromatosis to uveal melanomas, Arch Ophthalmol 77:331, 1967.

991. Zakka KA, Foos RY, and Sulit H: Metastatic tapioca melanoma, Br J Ophthalmol 63:744, 1979.

992. Zakka KA and others: Leukemic iris infiltration, Am J Ophthalmol 89:204, 1980.

993. Zakka KA and others: Malignant melanoma analysis of an autopsy population, Ophthalmology 87:549, 1980.

994. Zakov ZN, Smith TR, and Albert DM: False-positive ^{32}P uptake tests, Arch Ophthalmol 96:2240, 1978.

995. Zimmerman LE: Clinical pathology of iris tumors, Am J Clin Pathol 39:214, 1963.

996. Zimmerman LE: Lymphoid tumors. In Boniuk M, editor: Ocular and adnexal tumors: new and controversial aspects, St. Louis, 1964, The CV Mosby Co.

997. Zimmerman LE: Macular lesions mistaken for malignant melanoma of the choroid, Trans Am Acad Ophthalmol Otolaryngol 69:623, 1965.

998. Zimmerman LE: Melanocytes, melanocytic nevi, and melanocytomas, Invest Ophthalmol 4:11, 1965.

999. Zimmerman LE: Changing concepts concerning the malignancy of ocular tumors, Arch Ophthalmol 78:166, 1967.

1000. Zimmerman LE: Histopathological considerations in the management of tumors of the iris and ciliary body, An Inst Barraquer 10:27, 1971-1972.

1001. Zimmerman LE: Problems in the diagnosis of malignant melanomas of the choroid and ciliary body, Am J Ophthalmol 75:917, 1973.

1002. Zimmerman LE: Melanocytic tumours of interest to the ophthalmologist, Ophthalmology 87:497, 1980.

1003. Zimmerman LE: Metastatic disease from uveal melanomas: a review of current concepts with comments concerning future research and prevention, Trans Ophthalmol Soc UK 100:34, 1980.

1004. Zimmerman LE and McLean IW: Do growth and onset of symptoms of uveal melanomas indicate subclinical metastasis? Ophthalmology 91:685, 1984.

1005. Zimmerman LE and McLean LW: An evaluation of enucleation in the management of uveal melanoma, Am J Ophthalmol 87:741, 1979.

1006. Zimmerman LE and McLean LW: Metastatic disease from untreated uveal melanomas, Am J Ophthalmol 85:524, 1979.

1007. Zimmerman LE, McLean LW, and Foster WD: Does enucleation of the eye containing a malignant melanoma prevent or accelerate the dissemination of tumour cells? Br J Ophthalmol 62:420, 1978.

1008. Zimmerman LE, McLean LW, and Foster WD: Statistical analysis of follow-up data concerning uveal melanomas, and the influence of enucleation, Ophthalmology 87:557, 1980.

1009. Zimmerman LE, Paul E, and Parnell B: Evaluation of prognostic factors in intraocular melanoma. Cited in symposium: the diagnosis and management of intraocular melanoma, Trans Am Acad Ophthalmol Otolaryngol 62:517, 1958.

1010. Zinn KM and others: Proton-beam irradiated epithelial cell melanoma of the ciliary body, Ophthalmology 88:1315, 1981.

Metastasis of tumors to the eye

1011. Albert DM and others: Bilateral metastatic choroidal melanoma, nevi, and cavernous degeneration. Involvement of the optic nerve-head, Arch Ophthalmol 87:39, 1972.

1012. Albert DM, Rubenstein RA, and Scheie HG: Tumor metastasis to the eye, Am J Ophthalmol 63:723, 1967.

1013. Albert DM, Ryan LM, and Borden EC: Metastatic ocular and cutaneous melanoma: a comparison of patient characteristics and prognostics, Arch Ophthalmol 114:107, 1996 (letter).

1014. Bardenstein DS and others: Metastatic ciliary body carcinoid tumor, Arch Ophthalmol 108:1590, 1990.

1015. Block HR and Gartner S: The incidence of ocular metastatic carcinoma, Arch Ophthalmol 85:673, 1971.

1016. Bowman CB and others: Cutaneous malignant melanoma with diffuse intraocular metastases, Arch Ophthalmol 112:1213, 1994.

1017. Britt JM, Karr DJ, and Kalina RE: Leukemic iris infiltration in recurrent acute leukemia, Arch Ophthalmol 109:1456, 1991.

1018. Bullock JD and Yanes B: Ophthalmic manifestations of metastatic breast cancer, Ophthalmology 87:961, 1980.

1019. Buys R and others: Simultaneous ocular and orbital involvement from metastatic bronchogenic carcinoma, Ann Ophthalmol 14: 1165, 1982.

1020. Char DH and others: Ocular metastases from systemic melanoma, Am J Ophthalmol 90:702, 1980.

1021. Char DH and Christensen M: Immune complexes and carcinoembryonic antigen levels in metastatic choroidal tumors, Am J Ophthalmol 89:628, 1980.

1022. Coupland SE and others: Metastatic choroidal melanoma to the contralateral orbit 40 years after enucleation, Arch Ophthalmol 114:751, 1996 (review).

1023. Davis D and Robertson D: Fluorescein angiography of metastatic choroidal tumors, Arch Ophthalmol 89:97, 1973.

1024. DeBustros S and others: Intraocular metastases from cutaneous malignant melanoma, Arch Ophthalmol 103:937, 1985.

1025. Denslow GT and Kielar RA: Metastatic adenocarcinoma to the anterior uvea and increased carcinoembryonic antigen levels, Am J Ophthalmol 85:363, 1991.

1026. DeRivas P and others: Metastatic bronchogenic carcinoma of the iris and ciliary body, Arch Ophthalmol 109:470, 1991.

1027. Endo EG, Walton DS, and Albert DM: Neonatal hepatoblastoma metastatic to the choroid and iris, Arch Ophthalmol 114:757, 1996 (review).

1028. Eting E and Savir H: An atypical fulminant course of choroidal osteoma in two siblings, Am J Ophthalmol 113:52, 1992.

1029. Fan JT and others: Clinical features and treatment of seven patients with carcinoid tumor metastatic to the eye and orbit, Am J Ophthalmol 119:211, 1995.

1030. Ferry AP: The biological behavior and pathological features of carcinoma metastatic to the eye and orbit, Trans Am Ophthalmol Soc 71:373, 1973.

1031. Ferry AP and Font RL: Carcinoma metastatic to the eye and orbit. I. A clinicopathologic study of 227 cases, Arch Ophthalmol 92:276, 1974.

1032. Ferry AP and Font RI: Carcinoma metastatic to the eye and orbit, Arch Ophthalmol 93:472, 1975.

1033. Fidler IJ and Hart IR: Biological diversity in metastatic neoplasms: origins and implications, Science 217:998, 1982.

1034. Fishman M, Tomaszewski M, and Kuwabara T: Malignant melanoma of the skin metastatic to the eye, Arch Ophthalmol 94:1309, 1976.

1035. Font RI, Mackay B, and Tang R: Acuite monocytic leukemia recurring as bilateral perilimbal infiltrates. Immunohistochemical and ultrastructural confirmation, Ophthalmology 92:1681, 1985.

1036. Frank KW and others: Anterior segment metastases from an ovarian chonocarcinoma, Am J Ophthalmol 87:778, 1979.

1037. Freeman TR and Friedman AH: Mestatic carcinoma of the iris, Am J Ophthalmol 80:947, 1975.

1038. George DP and Zamber RW: Chondrosarcoma metastatic to the eye, Arch Ophthalmol 114:349, 1996.

1039. Gitter K and others: Fluorescein angiography of metastatic choroid tumors, Arch Ophthalmol 89:97, 1973.

1040. Godtfredsen E: On the frequency of secondary carcinomas in the choroid, Acta Ophthalmol 22:304, 1944.

1041. Greer C: Choroidal carcinoma metastatic from the male breast, Br J Ophthalmol 38:312, 1954.

1042. Greer C: Metastatic carcinoma of the iris, Br J Ophthalmol 38: 699, 1954.

1043. Greer J Jr: Metastatic carcinoma of the eye, Am J Ophthalmol 33: 1015, 1950.

1044. Greven CM and others: Cutaneous malignant melanoma metastatic to the choroid, Arc Ophthalmol 109:547, 1991.

1045. Guyer DR and others: Leukemic retinopathy, Ophthalmology 96: 860, 1989.

1046. Harbour JW and others: Uveal metastasis from carcinoid tumor. Clinical observations in nine cases, Ophthalmology 101:1084, 1994.

1047. Hirst LW, Reich J, and Galbraith JEK: Primary cutaneous malignant melanoma metastatic to the iris, Br J Ophthalmol 63:165, 1979.

1048. Jaeger EA and others: Effect of radiation therapy on metastatic choroidal tumors, Trans Am Acad Ophthalmol Otolaryngol 75:94, 1971.

1049. Jakobiec FA and others: Multifocal static creamy choroidal infiltrates. An early sign of lymphoid neoplasia, Ophthalmology 94:397, 1987.

1050. Kaiser-Kupfer MA: Role of the ophthalmologist in the therapy of breast carcinoma, Trans Ophthalmol Soc UK 98:184, 1978.

1051. Keltner JL and others: Mycosis fungoides: intraocular and central nervous system involvement, Arch Ophthalmol 95:645, 1977.

1052. Khaliland MK and Lorenzetti DWC: Eye manifestations in medullary carcinoma of the thyroid, Br J Ophthalmol 64:789, 1980.

1053. Kincaid MC and Green WR: Ocular and orbital involvement in leukemia, Surv Ophthalmol 27:211, 1983.

1054. Kincaid MC and Green WR: Ocular and orbital involvement in leukemia, Surv Ophthalmol 27:211, 1983 (review).

1055. Kincaid MC, Green WR, and Kelley JS: Acute ocular leukemia, Am J Ophthalmol 87:698, 1979.

1056. Kindermann WR and others: Metastatic renal cell carcinoma to the eye and adnexae: a report of three cases and review of the literature, Ophthalmology 88:1347, 1981.

1057. Klein R, Nicholson DH, and Luxenberg MN: Retinal metastasis from squamous cell carcinoma of the lung, Am J Ophthalmol 83: 358, 1977.

1058. Leonardy NJ and others: Analysis of 135 autopsy eyes for ocular involvement in leukemia, Am J Ophthalmol 109:436, 1990.

1059. Manor RS and others: Visual fields in metastatic choroidal carcinoma, Br J Ophthalmol 62:122, 1978.

1060. Mewis L and Young SE: Breast carcinoma metastatic to the choroid, Ophthalmology 89:147, 1982.

1061. Michelson JB, Feldberg NT, and Shields JA: Evaluation of metastatic cancer to the eye, Arch Ophthalmol 95:692, 1977.

1062. Nelson CC, Hertzberg BS, and Klintworth GK: A histopathologic study of the 716 unselected eyes in patients with cancer at the time of death, Am J Ophthalmol 95:788, 1983.

1063. Perry HD and Mallen FJ: Iris involvement in granulocytic sarcoma, Am J Ophthalmol 87:530, 1979.

1064. Piro P and others: Diagnostic vitrectomy in metastatic breast carcinoma in the vitreous, Retina 2:182, 1982.

1065. Reynard M and Font RL: Two cases of uveal metastasis from breast carcinoma in men, Am J Ophthalmol 95:208, 1983.

1066. Robertson DM and others: Metastatic tumor to the retina and vitreous cavity from primary melanoma of the skin; treatment with systemic and subconjunctival chemotherapy, Ophthalmology 88: 1296, 1981.

1067. Rodrigues M and Shields JA: Iris metastasis from a bronchial carcinoid tumor, Arch Ophthalmol 96:77, 1978.

1068. Rootman J and others: Congenital fibrosarcoma metastatic to the choroid, Am J Ophthalmol 87:632, 1979.

1069. Rubenstein RA and others: Thrombocytopenia, anemia, and retinal hemorrhage, Am J Ophthalmol 65:435, 1968.

1070. Saga T and others: Ocular involvement by a peripheral T-cell lymphoma, Arch Ophthalmol 102:399, 1984.

1071. Schachat AP and others: Ophthalmic manifestations of leukemia, Arch Ophthalmol 107:697, 1989.

1072. Shields JA: Metastatic tumors to and from the eye. In Croll M and others, editors: Nuclear ophthalmology, New York, 1976, John Wiley & Sons, Inc.

1073. Shields CL and others: Differentiation of adenoma of the iris pigment epithelium from iris cyst and melanoma, Am J Ophthalmol 100:678, 1985.

1074. Slamovits TL, Mondzelewski JP, and Kennerdell JS: Thyroid carcinoma metastatic to the globe, Br J Ophthalmol 63:169, 1979.

1075. Stephens RF and Shields JA: Diagnosis and management of cancer metastatic to the uvea: a study of 70 cases, Ophthalmology 86:1336, 1980.

1076. Tabbara KF and Beckstead JH: Acute promonocytic leukemia with ocular involvement, Arch Ophthalmol 98:1055, 1980.

1077. Usher C: Cases of metastatic carcinoma of the choroid and iris, Br J Ophthalmol 7:10, 1923.

1078. Weiner MA and Harris MB: Leukemia in children—a review, J Pediatr Ophthalmol Strabismus 19(4):47, 1982.

1079. Weisenthal R and others: Follicular thyroid cancer metastatic to the iris, Arch Ophthalmol 107:494, 1989.

1080. Whitcup S and others: Intraocular lymphoma, Ophthalmology 100:1399, 1993.

1081. Wilson DJ and others: Intraocular lymphoma, Arch Ophthalmol 110:1455, 1992.

1082. Williams AT and others: Osseous choristoma of the choroid simulating a choroidal melanoma. Association with a positive 32$_p$ test, Arch Ophthalmol 96:1874, 1978.

1083. Wyzinski P, Rootman J, and Wood W: Simultaneous bilateral iris metastases from renal cell carcinoma, Ophthalmology 92:206, 1981.

1084. Yanoff M: In discussion of Robb RM, Ervin L, and Sallan SE: A pathological study of the eye involvement in acute leukemia of childhood, Trans Am Ophthalmol Soc 76:100, 1978.

1085. Yeo JH and others: Metastatic carcinoma masquerading as scleritis, Ophthalmology 90:183, 1983.

1086. Zakka KA and others: Leukemic iris infiltration, Am J Ophthalmol 89:204, 1980.

Neuroepithelial tumors of the ciliary body

1087. Andersen S: Medulloepithelioma of the retina, Int Ophthalmol Clin 2:483, 1962.

1088. Apt L and others: Dictyoma (embryonal medulloepithelioma): recent review and case report, J Pediatr Ophthalmol 10:30, 1973.

1089. Badal J and Lagrange F: Carcinome primitif des procès et du corps ciliare, Arch Ophthalmol 12:143, 1892.

1090. Bateman JB, Foos RY: Coronal adenomas, Arch Ophthalmol 97:2379, 1979.

1091. Broughton WL and Zimmerman LE: A clinicopathologic study of 56 cases of intraocular medulloepitheliomas, Am J Ophthalmol 85:407, 1978.

1092. Brown HH, Glasgow BJ, and Foos RY: Ultrastructural and immunohistochemical features of coronal adenomas, Am J Ophthalmol 112:34, 1991.

1093. Brownstein S and others: Nonteratoid medulloepithelioma of the ciliary body, Ophthalmology 91:1118, 1984.

1094. Campochiaro PA and others: Ciliary body adenoma in a 10-year-old girl who had a rhabdomyosarcoma, Arch Ophthalmol 110:681, 1992.

1095. Canning CR, McCartney ACE, and Hungerford J: Medulloepithelioma (diktyoma), Br J Ophthalmol 72:764, 1988.

1096. Capo H, Palmer E, and Nicholson DH: Congenital cysts of the iris stroma, Am J Ophthalmol 116:228, 1993.

1097. Carrillo R and Streeten BW: Malignant teratoid medulloepithelioma in an adult, Arch Ophthalmol 97:695, 1979.

1098. Chang M, Shields JA, and Wachtel DL: Adenoma of the pigment epithelium of the ciliary body simulating a malignant melanoma, Am J Ophthalmol 88:40, 1979.

1099. Coden DH and Hornblass A: Photoreceptor cell differentiation in intraocular medulloepithelioma: an immunohistopathologic study, Arch Ophthalmol 108:481, 1990.

1100. Cogan D and Kuwabara T: Tumors of the ciliary body, Int Ophthalmol Clin 11:27, 1971.

1101. Conway VH, Brownstein S, and Chisholm IA: Lacrimal gland choristoma of the ciliary body, Ophthalmology 92:449, 1985.

1102. de Buen S and Gonzalez-Angelo A: Diktyoma (embryonal medulloepithelioma): review of the literature and report of a case, Am J Ophthalmol 49:606, 1960.

1103. Doro S and others: Fetal adenoma of the pigmented ciliary epithelium associated with persistent hyperplastic primary vitreous, Ophthalmology 93:1343, 1986.

1104. Dryja TP, Albert DM, and Horns D: Adenocarcinoma arising from the epithelium of the ciliary body, Ophthalmology 88:1290, 1981.

1105. Dugmore WN: 11-year follow-up of a case of iris leiomyosarcoma, Br J Ophthalmol 56:366, 1972.

1106. Eagle RC: Iris pigmentation and pigmented lesions: an ultrastructural study, Trans Am Ophthalmol Soc 86:581, 1988.

1107. Elsas FJ and others: Clinicopathologic report: Primary rhabdomyosarcoma of the iris, Arch Ophthalmol 109:982, 1991.

1108. Fan JT, Robertson DM, and Campbell RJ: Clinicopathologic correlation of a case of adenocarcinoma of the retinal pigment epithelium, Am J Ophthalmol 91:469, 1981.

1109. Ferry AP and others: Pathologic examination of ciliary body melanoma treated with proton beam irradiation, Arch Ophthalmol 103:1849, 1985.

1110. Floyd BB, Minckler DS, and Valentin L: Intraocular medulloepithelioma in a 79-year-old man, Ophthalmology 89:1088, 1982.

1111. Foos AJE and others: Are most intraocular "leiomyomas" really melanocytic lesions? Ophthalmology 101:919, 1994.

1112. Fralick F and Wilder H: Intraocular diktyoma and glioneuroma, Trans Am Ophthalmol Soc 47:317, 1949.

1113. Fuchs" E: Wucherungen und Geschwülste des Ziliarepithels, Graefes Arch Ophthalmol 68:534, 1908.

1114. Gifford H: A cystic diktyoma, Surv Ophthalmol 11:557, 1966.

1115. Green W, Hill W, and Trotter R: Malignant teratoid medulloepithelioma of the optic nerve, Arch Ophthalmol 91:451, 1974.

1116. Grossnilaus HE, Zimmerman LE, and Kachmer ML: Pleomorphic adenocarcinoma of the ciliary body, Ophthalmology 97:763, 1990.

1117. Hamburg A: Medulloepithelioma arising from the posterior pole, Ophthalmologica 181(3-4):152, 1980.

1118. Harry J and Morgan G: Pathology of a unique type of teratoid medulloepithelioma, Br J Ophthalmol 63:132, 1979.

1119. Hillemann J and Naumann G: Beitrag zum benignen Epithliom (Fuchs") des Ziliarkörpers, Ophthalmologica 164:321, 1972.

1120. Holbach I, Volcker HE, and Naumann GOH: Malignes teratoides Medulloepitheliom des Ziliarkorpers und saures Gliafaserprotein. Klinishe, histochemische und immunhistochemische Berfunde, Klin Monatsbl Augenbeilkd 187:282, 1985.

1121. Horie A and others: Electron microscopic study on the so-called malignant medullo-epithelioma (ciliary epithelial carcinoma), Virchows Arch (A) 355:284, 1972.

1122. Hunt LM and others: Congenital hypertrophy of the retinal pigment epithelium and mandibular osteomata as markers in familial colorectal cancer, Br J Cancer 70:173, 1994.

1123. Ide CH: Dictyoma, Br J Ophthalmol 55:553, 1971.

1124. Iwamoto T, Witmer R, and Landolt E: Diktyoma, a clinical histological and electron-microscopical observation, Graefes Arch Clin Exp Ophthalmol 172:293, 1967.

1125. Jakobiec FA and others: Electron microscopic diagnosis of medulloepithelioma, Am J Ophthalmol 79:321, 1975.

1126. Jakobiec FA, Witschel H, Zimmerman LE: Choroidal leiomyoma of vascular origin, Am J Ophthalmol 82:205, 1976.

1127. Jakobiec FA and others: Metastatic colloid carcinoma versus primary carcinoma of the ciliary epithelium, Ophthalmology 94:1469, 1987.

1128. Jampel HD and others: Retinal pigment epithelial hyperplasia assuming tumor-like proportions. Report of two cases, Retina 6:105, 1986.

1129. Johnson MW and others: Malignant melanoma of the iris in xeroderma pigmentosum, Arch Ophthalmol 107:402, 1989.

1130. Kahn D, Goldberg MF, and Jednock N: Combined retinal-retina pigment epithelial hamartoma presenting as a vitreous hemorrhage, Retina 4:40, 1984.

1131. Kivela T and Tarkkanen A: Recurrent medulloepithelioma of the ciliary body: immunohistochemical characteristics, Ophthalmology 95:1565, 1988.

1132. Kivela T and others: Glioneuroma associated with colobomatous dysplasia of the anterior uvea and retina. A case simulating medulloepithelioma, Ophthalmology 96:1799, 1989.

1133. Kivela and others: Congenital intraocular teratoma, Ophthalmology 100:782, 1993.

1134. Klien B: Diktyoma retinae, Arch Ophthalmol 22:432, 1939.

1135. Knowles DM II and others: Ophthalmic striated muscle neoplasms, Surv Ophthalmol 21:219, 1976.

1136. Kuhlenbeck H and Haymaker W: Neuroectodermal tumors containing neoplastic neuronal elements—ganglioneuroma, spongioncuroblastoma and glioneuroma—with a clinicopathologic report of eleven cases, and a discussion of their origin and classification, Milit Surg 99:273, 1946.

1137. Lang GK and others: Ocular reticulum cell sarcoma. Clinicopathologic correlation of a case with multifocal lesions, Retina 5:79, 1985.

1138. Li Z-Y, Tso MOM, and Sugar J: Leiomyoepithelioma of iris pigment epithelium, Arch Ophthalmol 105:819, 1987.
1139. Lieb WE and others: Cystic adenoma of the pigmented ciliary epithelium. Clinical, pathologic, and immunohistopathologic findings, Ophthalmology 97:1489, 1990.
1140. Litricin O and Latkovic Z: Malignant teratoid medulloepithelioma in an adult, Ophthalmologica 191(1):17, 1985.
1141. Llopis MD and Menezo JL: Congenital hypertrophy of the retinal pigment epithelium and familial polyposis of the colon, Am J Ophthalmol 103:235, 1987.
1142. Lloyd WC and others: Congenital hypertrophy of the retinal pigment epithelium, Ophthalmology 97:1052, 1990.
1143. Malone R: Diktyoma, Br J Ophthalmol 39:429, 1955.
1144. Manz H and others: Neuroectodermal tumor of anterior lip of the optic cup: glioneuroma transitional to teratoid medulloepithelioma, Arch Ophthalmol 89:382, 1973.
1145. Meyer SL and others: Leiomyoma of the ciliary body. Electron microscopic verification, Am J Ophthalmol 66:1061, 1968.
1146. Minckler D and Allen AW: Adenocarcinoma of the retinal pigment epithelium, Arch Ophthalmol 96:2252, 1978.
1147. Morris AT and Garner A: Medulloepithelioma involving the iris, Br J Ophthalmol 59:276, 1975.
1148. Mullaney D: Primary malignant medulloepithelioma of the retinal stalk, Am J Ophthalmol 77:499, 1974.
1149. Munden PM and others: Ocular findings in Turcot syndrome (glioma-polyposis), Ophthalmology 98:111, 1991.
1150. Naumann GOH and others: Primary rhabdomyosarcoma of the iris, Am J Ophthalmol 74:110, 1972.
1151. Nordman J: Les tumeurs de la retine ciliare, Ophthalmologica 102:257, 1941.
1152. Offret H and Saraux H: Adenoma of the iris pigment epithelium, Arch Ophthalmol 98:875, 1980.
1153. Orellana J and others: Medulloepithelioma diagnosed by ultrasound and vitreous aspirate: electron microscopic observations, Ophthalmology 90:1531, 1983.
1154. Panda A, Dayal Y, and Mohan M: Medulloepithelioma of the ciliary body, Indian J Ophthalmol 33(3):183, 1985.
1155. Papale JJ and others: Adenocarcinoma of the ciliary body pigment epithelium in a child, Arch Ophthalmol 102:100, 1984.
1156. Patrinely JR and others: Hamartomatous adenoma of the nonpigmented ciliary epithelium arising in iris-ciliary body coloboma, Ophthalmology 90:1540, 1983.
1157. Pe'er J and Hidayat AA: Malignant teratoid medulloepithelioma manifesting as a black epibulbar mass with expulsive hemorrhage, Arch Ophthalmol 102:1523, 1984.
1158. Pollak A and Friede RL: Fine structure of medulloepithelioma, J Neuropathol Exp Neurol 36:712, 1977.
1159. Rodrigues M, Hidayat A, and Karesh J: Pleomorphic adenocarcinoma of ciliary epithelium simulating an epibulbar tumor, Am J Ophthalmol 106:595, 1988.
1160. Ryan SJ Jr and others: Bilateral inflammatory pseudotumors of the ciliary body, Am J Ophthalmol 72:586, 1971.
1161. Shields CL and others: Transscleral leiomyoma, Ophthalmology 98:84, 1991.
1162. Shields CL and others: Differentiation of adenoma of the iris pigment epithelium from iris cyst and melanoma, Am J Ophthalmol 100:678, 1985.
1163. Shields JA and others: Observations on seven cases of intraocular leiomyoma, Arch Ophthalmol 112:521, 1994.
1164. Shields JA and others: Mesectodermal leiomyoma of the ciliary body managed by partial lamellar iridocyclochoroidectomy, Ophthalmology 96:1369, 1989.
1165. Shields JA and others: Adenoma of the iris-pigment epithelium, Ophthalmology 90:735, 1983.
1166. Shields JA, Shields CL, and Schwartz RL: Malignant teratoid medulloepithelioma of the ciliary body simulating persistent hyperplastic primary vitreous, Am J Ophthalmol 107:296, 1989.
1167. Shivde AV, Kher A, and Junnarkar RV: Diktyoma, Br J Ophthalmol 53:352, 1969.
1168. Sirsat MV, Shrikhande SS, and Sampat MB: Medullo-epithelioma (diktyoma) of the eye, Br J Ophthalmol 56:362, 1972.
1169. Spencer W and Jesberg D: Glioneuroma (choristomatous malformation of the optic cup margin): a report of two cases, Arch Ophthalmol 89:387, 1973.
1170. Streeten B and McGraw J: Tumor of the ciliary pigment epithelium, Am J Ophthalmol 74:420, 1972.
1171. Takagi T and others: Mesectodermal leiomyoma of the ciliary body. An ultrastructural study, Arch Ophthalmol 103:1711, 1985.
1172. Verhoeff F, Fralick F, and Wilder H: Intraocular diktyoma and glioneuroma, Trans Am Ophthalmol Soc 47:317, 1949.
1173. Verhoeff FH: A rare tumor arising from the pars ciliaris retinae (teratoneuroma), of a nature hitherto unrecognized, and its relation to the so-called glioma retinae, Trans Am Ophthalmol Soc 10:351, 1904.
1174. Virji MA: Medulloepithelioma (diktyoma) presenting as a perforated, infected eye, Br J Ophthalmol 61:229, 1977.
1175. Wadsworth J: Epithelial tumors of the ciliary body, Am J Ophthalmol 32:1487, 1919.
1176. Wilensky J and Holland M: A pigmented tumor of the ciliary body, Arch Ophthalmol 92:219, 1974.
1177. Woyke S and Chwirot R: Rhabdomysarcoma of the iris. Report of the first recorded case, Br J Ophthalmol 56:60, 1972.
1178. Wilson ME, McClatchey SK, and Zimmerman LE: Rhabdomyosarcoma of the ciliary body, Ophthalmology 97:1484, 1990.
1179. Yanko L and Behar A: Teratoid intraocular medulloepithelioma, Am J Ophthalmol 85:350, 1978.
1180. Zaidman GW and others: Fuchs'" adenoma affecting the peripheral iris, Arch Ophthalmol 101:771, 1983.
1181. Zimmerman LE: Verhoeff's "terato-neuroma": a critical reappraisal in light of new observations and current concepts of embryonic tumors, Am J Ophthalmol 72:1039, 1971.
1182. Zimmerman LE, Font RL, and Anderson S: Rhabdomyosarcomatous differentiation in malignant intraocular medulloepitheliomas, Cancer 30:817, 1972.

CHAPTER 8
FUNDUS

Embryology and anatomy[1-117]

FUNCTIONAL ANATOMY

Light is received by the sensory retina (Figs. 8-1–8-13) and transformed photochemically into an electric impulse for transmission through the optic nerve to the primary and secondary visual centers of the brain. The other components of the eye exist to support this photoreceptive function, serving primarily as refractive media (cornea and lens), for nourishment (uvea), or for protection (cornea and sclera).

The retina (tunica nervosa)[28] is the innermost of the three tunics of the eyeball (Fig. 1-1). In contrast to the invertebrate retina, in which the photoreceptors are anatomically oriented so that their apices face directly toward the incoming light, rods and cones are located in the outermost posterior layers of the retina, directly adjacent to the pigment epithelium (Figs. 8-2 to 8-6). The photoreceptive apices of the rods and cones in the human retina are, therefore, not directed toward incoming light; they are "inverted" or actually separated from incoming light by the other elements of the retina. This arrangement, however, makes possible an active metabolic exchange between the photoreceptors and the adjacent pigment epithelium and choriocapillaris, apparently compensating for the disadvantage that the light waves must first pass through the entire thickness of the retina to reach the photoreceptors.

The inverted retinal configuration also dictates that the nerve fibers must be located anterior to the photoreceptors. They must, therefore, converge and penetrate the sensory retina at some point, the optic nerve head, to leave the eye. This blind spot is typical of the inverted retina. In a noninverted retina the nerve fibers are posterior to the photoreceptors; therefore, this site of penetration is not required.

The fact that light must first pass through the retinal vascular layers before reaching the photoreceptors provides the basis for the clinically useful entoptic phenomenon, in which a patient's visual function can be tested despite opaque media. When appropriately tested, patients with intact retinal function can see the "shadows" of their own retinal vessels, which are cast on their sensory retina (and hence on their visual field) by the overlying retinal vessels.

The retina extends from the optic nerve head to its "sawtooth" edged peripheral margin, the ora serrata (Figs. 8-10 and 8-11). It is firmly attached to the underlying pigment epithelium at these two sites; at all other loci the attachment is relatively tenuous. For this reason, separation of the sensory retina from the pigment epithelium frequently occurs, not only in vivo in a retinal detachment (Figs. 8-71 and 8-74–8-76; Color Plates 8-36) but also as a very common artifact of fixation and tissue preparation (Fig. 8-77). The latter occurrence results from a relatively greater shrinkage (Figs. 8-1 and 8-2) of the sensory retina

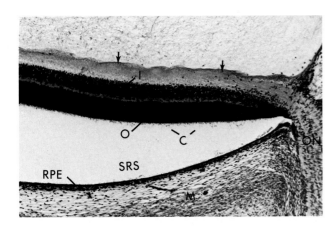

Fig. 8-1. Embryonic sensory retina. *Small arrows,* Vitreoretinal interface; vitreous fibrils *(above); I,* inner nuclear layer; *O,* outer nuclear layer; *C,* cilia of embryonic photoreceptors; *SRS,* subretinal space opened because of processing artifact; *RPE,* retinal pigment epithelium; *M,* mesenchyme forming choroidal and scleral tunics; *ON,* optic nerve. (H & E stain; ×90.) (From Naumann GOH and Apple DJ: In Doerr W, Seifert G, and Uehlinger E, editors: Handbuch der speziellen pathologischen Anatomie, Band Auge, Berlin, 1980, Springer-Verlag.)

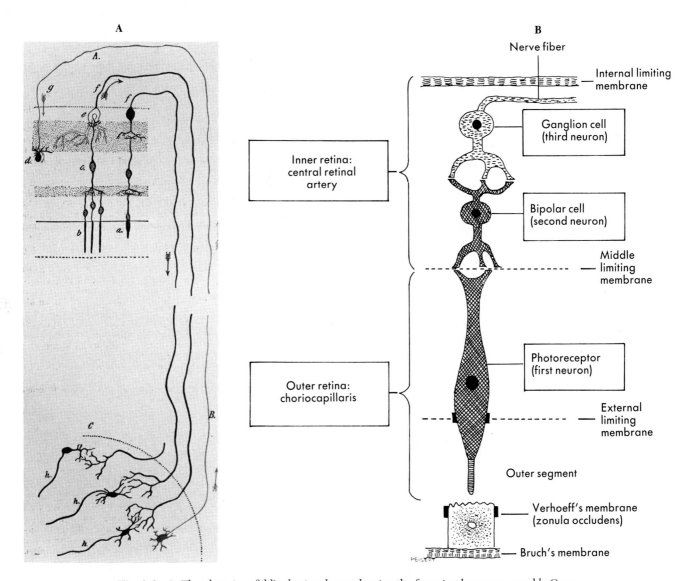

Fig. 8-2. A, Theodore Axenfeld's classic scheme showing the four visual neurons. *a* and *b,* Cones and rods; *c,* bipolar cells; *e,* ganglion cells forming *f,* nerve fiber layer that synapses with cells and fibers *(h)* in lateral geniculate body *(below).* **B,** Vascular supply and functional neuronal division of the sensory retina. (**A** from Axenfeld T: Lehrbuch und Atlas der Augenheilkunde, Jena, 1912, Gustav Fischer.)

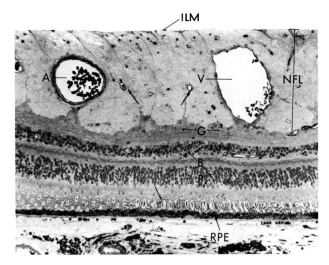

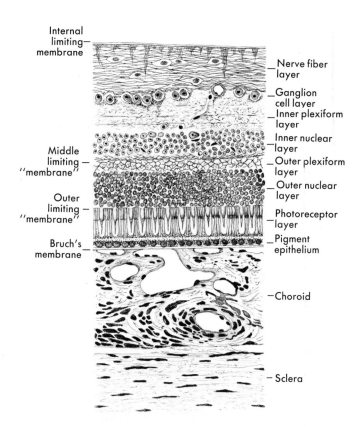

Fig. 8-3. Sensory retina in peripapillary region, where nerve fiber layer *(NFL)* is very prominent. A relatively thick-walled retinal arteriole *(A)* derived from the central retinal artery, a thin-walled venule *(V)*, and numerous capillaries *(large arrows)* represent the primary vascular supply to the inner half of the retina. *ILM*, Internal limiting membrane; *G*, plane of ganglion cell layer (cell body of nerve fiber layer axons); *B*, intermediate bipolar cell layer or inner nuclear layer; *P*, photoreceptor cell nuclei or outer nuclear layer; *small arrow*, processes of rods and cones; *RPE*, retinal pigment epithelium overlying the choroid *(below)*. (Mallory blue stain; ×180.) (From Apple DJ, Goldberg MF, and Wyhinny G: Am J Ophthalmol 75:595, 1973.)

Fig. 8-4. Diagram of retinal layers and limiting "membranes." (Modified from Salzmann M: The anatomy and histology of the human eyeball in the normal state: its development and senescence, Chicago, 1931, University of Chicago Press [Translated by EVL Brown].)

in most fixatives compared to that of the adjacent pigment epithelium, choroid, and sclera.

The retina is extremely thin and exhibits a cellophanelike transparency. Its thickness at the posterior pole in the peripapillary region is approximately 0.6 mm; at the equator, 0.2 to 0.3 mm; and at the ora serrata, approximately 0.1 to 0.2 mm. Gross examination of the macular region (Fig. 8-7) reveals a circular focus of orange-yellow discoloration, which encircles the fovea centralis. This yellow color (from which the term *macula lutea* is derived) is best seen in postmortem retinas in which slight opacification following enucleation has occurred. In freshly enucleated eyes in which postmortem autolysis is not yet advanced, the yellow coloration of the xanthophyll is more difficult to perceive.

EMBRYOLOGY

Only the posterior portion of the original embryonic optic cup, the pars optica retinae, is capable of an optical function (Figs. 1-9–1-11). The segment of the cup anterior to the future ora serrata (pars caeca retinae; Latin, *caecum,* blind) forms the epithelia of the ciliary body and iris.

In the early stages of development, during the original invagination of the primary optic vesicle (Fig. 1-7, *A*), the distal, or anterior, wall of the vesicle (the primordia of the sensory retina) begins to thicken, and the nuclei within the cells are arranged so that a nucleus-containing zone and a nucleus-free zone are formed (Fig. 1-10). The latter zone forms a syncytium, and the fibrils therein form the anlage of the Müller supportive fibers. The entire outer wall of the optic vesicle is lined by a basement membrane. The distal or anterior aspect of the membrane, corresponding

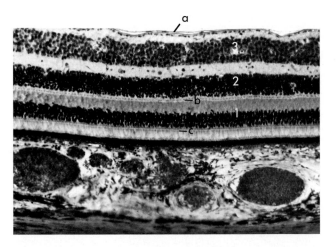

Fig. 8-5. Sensory retina showing the first three neurons of the visual system *(1, 2,* and *3)* and the three limiting "membranes." *a,* Internal limiting membrane; *b,* middle limiting membrane; *c,* external limiting membrane. (From Naumann GOH and Apple DJ: In Doerr W, Seifert G, and Uehlinger E, editors: Handbuch der speziellen pathologischen Anatomie, Band Auge, Berlin, 1980, Springer-Verlag.)

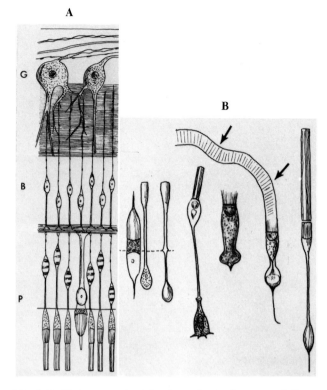

Fig. 8-6. Early anatomists' drawings of retinal neurons. **A,** Interconnections of photoreceptors *(P)* with bipolar cells *(B)* and ganglion cells *(G).* **B,** Various types of photoreceptors in different species. Lamellar plates in photoreceptor outer segments *(arrows)* were recognized long before the advent of the electron microscope. (Redrawn by Dr. Steven Vermillion, University of Iowa, from von Graefe A and Saemisch T: Handbuch der gesammten Augenheilkunde, Leipzig, 1874, Wilhelm Engelman.)

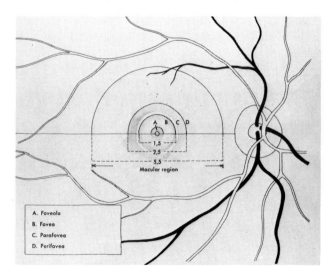

Fig. 8-7. Boundaries of the macular region. (From Spitznas M: Dtsch Ophthalmol Gesellschaft 73:26, 1973.)

to the location of the future sensory retina, forms the retinal internal limiting membrane. The proximal, or posterior, epithelium of the vesicle is the rudimentary retinal pigment epithelium, and its basement membrane contributes to Bruch's membrane.

As the optic cup develops from the vesicle during its first 6 weeks, extensive mitotic activity occurs within the cells of the future sensory retina (Figs. 1-8 and 1-9). The original monolayered epithelium becomes multilayered, and the retina greatly increases in thickness. During this period the newly formed retinal cells or retinoblasts remain relatively undifferentiated. At the time of closure of the embryonic fissure (about 6 weeks) they begin to divide into two layers, the inner and outer neuroblastic layers. These layers are separated by the transient layer of Chievitz (Figs. 1-11 and 8-1) Although this area forms a plexiform layer between the two neuroblastic layers, it is not a true predecessor of the future definitive inner or outer plexiform layers of the retina. Its existence is only temporary, and it disappears after more complex migration of retinoblasts within the sensory retina.

The first retinal cells to differentiate are those of the inner neuroblastic layer. The ganglion cells and their processes, the future nerve fiber layer of the retina, begin to develop first, but maturation of the ganglion cells is very slow and approaches completion only in the eighth fetal month. Ganglion cell maturity is signaled by the appearance of Nissl granules composed of rough endoplasmic reticulum within the cytoplasm. The growing axons of the ganglion cells forming the nerve fiber layer course parallel to the retinal surface and exit from the globe through the embryonic fissure, reaching the brain through the optic stalk.

In addition to forming ganglion cells, the inner neuroblastic layer contributes to the cell bodies of the amacrine cells and Müller cells. The cells of the outer neuroblastic layer differentiate into photoreceptors, bipolar cells, and horizontal cells. The transient layer of Chievitz is retained until the time of birth but eventually disappears because cells continuously migrate across this layer until the nuclear layers have reached their adult configuration (Fig. 8-1). The final development of the rods and cones is accomplished only after birth. The fovea is not functional until a few months following birth.

HISTOLOGY

As with other portions of the brain, one can classify the projections of the nerve fibers of the retina into two types: vertical and horizontal.

The vertical fibers (Figs. 8-2–8-6) provide a direct connection between the photoreceptors and the visual centers through a series of four neurons (Fig. 8-2, *A*). The first three are in the retina itself (Fig. 8-2, *B*): (1) the photoreceptors, (2) the bipolar cells, and (3) the ganglion cells. The fourth neuron of the visual system is situated within the lateral geniculate body of the thalamus (Fig. 8-3).

The horizontal interconnections within the retina, which provide neurosensory informational integration between overlapping fields of the ocular fundus, are mediated by the amacrine and horizontal cells.

The first neuron of the retina (photoreceptors or sensory epithelium) subserves the function of light reception. This layer contains no blood vessels and is fully dependent on the choriocapillaris for nutritive support (Figs. 8-2, *B*, and 8-13).

The nucleus of the second neuron, the bipolar cell, is situated within the inner nuclear layer. This cell is intermediary between the photoreceptors and the third retinal neuron, the ganglion cell. The dendritic processes of the ganglion cell receive the sensory impulse from the bipolar cells. The visual impulse then proceeds through the axis cylinder of the ganglion cell forming the nerve fiber layer. This axon courses successively through the retinal nerve fiber layer, the optic nerve, optic chiasm, and optic tract to the lateral geniculate body. The optic radiations into the visual cortex are derived from the fourth neuron within the lateral geniculate body.

Microscopic examination of the sensory retina (Figs. 8-2–8-6) reveals nine layers. These are closely associated with the pigment epithelium and Bruch's membrane. The layers (Fig. 8-4) listed from inward (vitreal) toward the outside (sclera) are

1. Internal limiting membrane
2. Nerve fiber layer
3. Ganglion cell layer
4. Inner plexiform layer
5. Inner nuclear layer
    a. Bipolar cells
    b. Amacrine and horizontal cells
    c. Müller cells
6. Outer plexiform layer
    a. Middle limiting membrane
    b. Henle's fiber layer (in macular region)
7. Outer nuclear layer
8. External (outer) limiting membrane
9. Rod and cone layer (photoreceptors)
    a. Inner segment
    b. Outer segment
10. Pigment epithelium
11. Bruch's membrane

Internal limiting membrane

The internal limiting membrane, which is derived from Müller cells, forms the interface between retina and vitreous. The fibrils of the vitreous merge with its inner lamallae, and the basal foot processes of the Müller cells insert directly into the undersurface of this periodic acid-Schiff (PAS)-positive basement membrane (Fig. 8-4). These processes are occasionally visible clinically as small yellow-white spots (Gunn's dots). At the ora serrata the internal limiting membrane is continuous with the inner bordering membrane of the nonpigmented epithelium of the ciliary body.

Nerve fiber layer

The unmyelinated axons of the ganglion cells form the nerve fiber layer of the retina. The nerve fibers converge at the optic nerve head, pass through the lamina cribrosa and, following ensheathment by myelin posterior to the lamina, course toward the lateral geniculate body. The nerve fiber layer contains not only sensory fibers extending from the retina toward the brain but also occasionally fibers running in the reverse direction (Fig. 8-5). The origin and function of these efferent fibers is unclear.

In contrast to the remaining sensory retina fibers, which course vertically, or perpendicular to the surface of the retina, the fibers within the nerve fiber layer course parallel to the surface. Nasally the fibers converge toward the disc radially, or in a "spoke-wheel pattern." The temporal fibers run in an arcuate manner when viewed frontally because the temporal fibers coursing toward the optic nerve must pass around the fovea. They arch above and below the fovea forming a horizontal raphe in the meridian of the fovea. Arcuate scotomas, characteristic field defects that occur in glaucoma and other diseases, can be explained by this anatomic pattern.

The arrangement of fibers of the nerve fiber layer is also responsible for ophthalmoscopically visible flame-shaped hemorrhages that result from pathologic deposits of blood within this layer (Figs. 8-45, 8-46, *A*, and 8-49; Color Plates 8-12 and 8-13). The extravasated blood is deposited parallel to the adjacent nerve fibers. The resultant flame-shaped lesions are oriented radially to the optic nerve. Hemorrhagic deposits in the deeper layers of the retina are usually more nonspecific in appearance, as in dot or blot hemorrhages, because the extravasated (Fig. 8-6) blood between the fibers does not have such a specific orientation.

Sagittal sections through the nerve fiber layer reveal that the fibers derived from the most peripheral ganglion cells are situated deeply, and the more central or posterior fibers (e.g., from the macular or peripapillary ganglion cells) lie more superficially within the layer. The thickness of the nerve fiber layer decreases significantly toward the periphery and within a few millimeters of the ora serrata consists merely of occasional fibers.

In addition to the nerve fibers themselves and the basal processes of the Müller cells, the nerve fiber layer contains occasional glial cells, primarily astrocytes. These may proliferate in pathologic states such as massive retinal gliosis (Fig. 10-37) or rare astrocytic tumors, such as the astrocytic hamartoma seen in tuberous sclerosis (Fig. 10-40; Color Plates 10-14 and 10-15).

Ganglion cell layer

The ganglion cell layer forms the cell body (nucleus and perikaryon) of the retinal nerve fiber. The ganglion cell nucleus is chromatin-poor. The cytoplasm contains abundant Nissl substance. These hematoxylin-positive, basophilic granules correspond to endoplasmic reticulum.

Throughout most of the retina the ganglion cell layer is composed of a single row of cells (Fig. 8-4). In the peripapillary region the cells are close together, but more peripherally the cells become more scattered, and at the region of the ora serrata they are seen only occasionally. In the macular region the ganglion cell layer becomes multilayered, increasing to six to eight layers of cells (Figs. 7-5, 8-5, and 8-8).

Inner plexiform layer

The inner plexiform layer contains the synaptic processes between the bipolar cell (the second neuron) and the ganglion cells (the third neuron of the visual pathway). Synaptic connections from the amacrine cells are also present. In addition to these neuronal synaptic processes, fibers from the Müller cells course vertically through this layer.

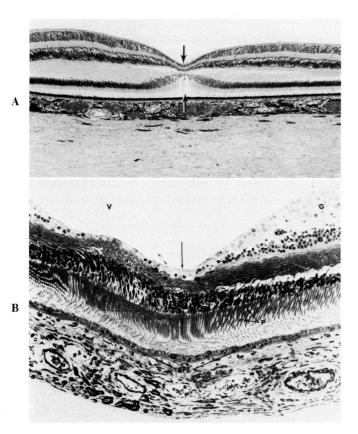

Fig. 8-8. Fovea centralis. **A,** Paraffin section showing outlines of fovea interna *(upper arrow)* and fovea externa *(lower arrow).* (H & E stain; ×80.) (Same case as Fig. 7-4.) **B,** Epon section of foveal region demonstrating characteristic decrease in retinal thickness *(arrow).* V, Vitreous cavity overlying internal limiting membrane; *G,* ganglion cell layer, which is several cell layers thick in macular region but is thinned out in center of fovea; *B,* bipolar cell layer; *H,* Henle's fiber layer, or outer plexiform layer; *P,* photoreceptor layer of cones, which are composed of nuclei and outer elongated processes; *small arrows,* outer limiting membrane; *RPE,* retinal pigment epithelium. External light stimuli are first received by the photoreceptor cells. The generated electrical impulse is then transmitted to the bipolar layer through Henle's fiber layer. The final pathways to the occipital cortex consist of the ganglion cell, the retinal nerve fiber layer, and the central projections of the optic nerve. (Mallory blue stain; ×200.) (**A** from Naumann GOH and Apple DJ: In Doerr W, Seifert G, and Uehlinger E, editors: Handbuch der speziellen pathologischen Anatomie, Band Auge, Berlin, 1980, Springer-Verlag.)

Inner nuclear layer

The cell bodies of four cell types can be distinguished in the inner nuclear layer.

Bipolar cells

The most numerous cells within the inner nuclear layer are the bipolar cells. Their cell processes synapse outwardly with the photoreceptors forming the middle limiting "membrane" and inwardly with the dendrites of the ganglion cells.

Amacrine and horizontal cells

The amacrine cells are situated at the inner surface of the inner nuclear layer. The horizontal cells are located at the outer aspect of this layer. The amacrine and horizontal cells provide numerous "horizontal" associative and neuronal interconnections between groups or fields of retinal sensory neurons. The amacrine cells and the horizontally spread terminals of the ganglion cell dendrites synapse within the inner plexiform layer. The horizontal cells terminate at the basal processes of the rods and cones within the outer plexiform layer.

Müller cells

The extra neuronal space of the retina is filled almost entirely by the cell bodies and elongated cytoplasmic processes, or "fibers," of the Müller glial cells. The nucleus and perikaryon of the Müller cells are located within the inner nuclear layer. In contrast to most other elements of the retina, which possess either a photoreceptive or neurotransmission function, the Müller cell provides structural support and contributes to the metabolism of the sensory retina.

In sagittal sections the Müller fibers course vertically through the retina (Figs. 8-67 and 8-68; Color Plate 8-31) between the neural elements and terminate internally at the internal limiting membrane by formation of basal foot processes. They form vertical columns between the nerve fiber bundles and within the two reticular layers. Outwardly the apical aspects of the Müller cells terminate in the region of the external limiting membrane of the retina. These apical processes are characterized by abundant microvilli, which project toward the underlying retinal pigment epithelium. The extracellular space between the apical processes, the outer segments of the photoreceptors, and the underlying pigment epithelium contains abundant mucopolysaccharides.

Because the Müller cells are situated between neural elements, it is possible that they provide an insulatory function between photoreceptors, perhaps producing a relative isolation between cells needed for neural transmission. At the level of the external limiting membrane no contact occurs between adjacent photoreceptors; a Müller cell process is always sandwiched between them. The photoreceptors and Müller cells at this level are connected by intercellular bridges of the zonula adherens type, forming the external limiting "membrane."

Besides Müller cells the retina contains other glial cells, particularly astrocytes (Fig. 10-41; Color Plates 10-14 and 10-15), which are primarily situated around blood vessels. The astrocyte ensheathe the vessels by broad foot process. These probably contribute to the blood-retina barrier. Oligodendroglia—glial cells that elaborate myelin—are found in the retina only in cases of myelinated (medullated) retinal nerve fibers.

Outer plexiform layer

The outer plexiform layer contains the synapses between the rods and cones and the dendritic processes of the bipolar cells. The synapses frequently can be clearly seen in histologic sections as a row of delicate punctate foci of increased staining. This area is often termed the *middle limiting membrane* (Figs. 8-4 and 8-5), although it is not a true membrane in the sense of the inner limiting membrane. Thus the outer plexiform layer can be divided into two subdivisions on either side of the "membrane": an inner, which consists of the dendrites of the bipolar cells and the horizontally coursing processes of the horizontal cells, and an outer, which consists of the basal aspects of the photoreceptors.

Awareness of the middle limiting "membrane" is useful in that it divides the sensory retina into two halves, that is, forms a border between the inner (vitreal) aspect and the outer portion of the retina. The retina internal to the middle limiting membrane contains the second and third neurons of the projective neuronal system; the outer portion corresponds to the entire length of the photoreceptor cell. This "membrane" also forms the approximate border between the vascular inner retina and the avascular outer portion. The central retinal artery supplies the retina internally from the middle limiting membrane to the internal limiting membrane. The outer layers of the retina from the middle limiting membrane to the pigment epithelium contain no vessels; they are supplied by the choriocapillaris, which is derived from the ciliary vascular system. Distinguishing these two nonanastomotic vascular systems is necessary to understand the various vascular diseases affecting these two systems (p. 370).

In the macular region the outer plexiform layer is slightly modified and is designated Henle's fiber layer (p. 362).

Outer nuclear layer

The outer nuclear layer contains the nuclei of the photoreceptor cells. Except for the cone-dominated macular region, rod nuclei form the bulk of the multilayered outer nuclear layer. Most cone nuclei lie in a single layer immediately internal to the external limiting membrane. They are somewhat larger than the rod nuclei and can also be distinguished from the latter by their chromatin pattern. Occasionally, cone nuclei may be seen deeper in the outer nuclear layer or, rarely, may actually lie external to the outer limiting membrane. The significance of these ectopic cone nuclei is uncertain, but this probably represents a harmless histologic variation.

External (outer) limiting membrane

The external limiting membrane is not a continuous basement membrane but rather a series of encircling or girdling modifications of the plasma membranes of the photoreceptor and Müller cells. In sagittal sections at low magnification this row of densities appears continuous, thus the designation "membrane." At higher magnification it is fenestrated, composed of intercellular bridges situated just external to the photoreceptor nuclei near the base of the photoreceptor inner segment. These cell junctions interconnect the photoreceptor cells to Müller cells. The cell junctions are of the zonula adherens type. By definition this type of junction does not create a physiologic barrier to fluid flow between cells.

In simplified terms intercellular junctions within the eye are of three important types.

1. Zonula occludens (tight junctions) are situated between pigment epithelial cells and between endothelial cells of the retinal capillaries. They form a physiologic barrier to the intercellular passage of fluids or exudates or fluorescein dye. By fluorescein angiography a normal retinal capillary does not show leakage, and the dye does not diffuse through a normal retinal pigment epithelium.

2. Zonula adherens (e.g., external limiting membrane) differ from the tight junctions in that a functional "space" remains between the epithelial cells at the site of the junction. It, therefore, does not form a barrier to the intercellular passage of fluids. Both types of cell junctions often occur in the same cell, forming a junctional complex.

3. Macula adherens (desmosome) is physiologically similar to the zonula adherens; that is, fluid may pass freely between cells, but the intercellular bridges forming the desmosomes are much thicker and more easily viewed by light microscopy. These large membrane densities, and the tonofibrils that anchor them into their respective cells, are particularly visible in the malpighian layer or stratum spinosum of skin epithelium, forming typical intercellular bridges between squamous cells (Fig. 11-4). Their identification is sometimes useful in the diagnosis of squamous cell carcinoma.

Rod and cone layer (photoreceptors)

The photoreceptors (neurosensory epithelium, rods and cones) are the light-sensitive elements of the retina. They depend heavily on the pigment epithelium and choroid for support.

Each photoreceptor (Figs. 8-6 and 10-11) consists of (1) the nucleus and cell body within the outer nuclear layer, (2) a basal region that extends into the outer plexiform layer as far as the middle limiting membrane, and (3) the apical aspect of the cell that is external to the nucleus and is subdivided into inner and outer segments. The long axis of the photoreceptor is oriented perpendicular to the retinal surface.

The rods primarily subserve peripheral vision and vision in low illumination (scotopic vision). The cones, which in histologic sections are distinguished by their broader, flask-shaped profiles in contrast to the thinner cylindric shape of the rods, are primarily responsible for photopic vision and for highly discriminatory central vision and color vision. In the foveal region, rods are lacking or extremely rare. The retinal periphery contains a marked decrease in numbers of both types of photoreceptors.

The rods contain visual purple (rhodopsin) within their outer segments. Visual purple accumulates in darkness and bleaches after exposure to light to initiate the visual impulse. The apical outer segments of the photoreceptor are directly apposed to and enmeshed within the apical microvilli of the pigment epithelium.[41]

The outer segments of the rods and cones are composed of lipoprotein membranes, or discs, which form the actual light-receptive portion of the cell. Although best seen by ultrastructural examination, these discs have been recognized for more than a century, and their functional significance was known long before the advent of the electron microscope (Fig. 8-6). The inner segment is connected to the outer segment by an apical 9 + 0 type of cilium, that is, a cilium containing nine circumferentially arranged neurotubules with no microtubules central to this ring. All motile cilia of the body (kinetocilia), such as respiratory of fallopian tube cilia, differ from the cilia of photoreceptors by the presence of nine circumferential and two central microtubules within the cilium (9 + 2 configuration). The inner segments contain abundant mitochondria. These are enzyme-rich cell organelles that reflect a very active metabolism within the photoreceptors during the visual process.

Pigment epithelium and Bruch's membrane

The pigment epithelium and the inner portion of Bruch's membrane are derived from the outer layer of the optic cup and are continuous anteriorly with the pigmented ciliary epithelium (Fig. 1-11).[117] This layer remains throughout life as a single-layered cuboidal or low columnar epithelium (Figs. 8-3, 8-4, 8-8, and 8-13). Pigmentation begins very early in development, and the pigment granules develop in situ within the optic cup. This differs from the pigmentation of the uveal stroma, in which the pigment cells and granules migrate into the tissue from the neural crest.

Pigment epithelium

The characteristics color and granular appearance of the fundus is largely dependent on the pigment epithelium. In the foveal region it is slightly more densely pigmented. Throughout the entire fundus there is usually a slight variation in pigmentation so that the general pattern is not homogeneous.[31]

In flat preparations the pigment epithelial cells are hexagonal. The pigment granules, which are either elliptic or spheric, are primarily situated within the inner aspect of the cell, particularly extending into the apical microvilli. The outer half of the cell contains the nucleus, numerous mitochondria, and other cell organelles that mediate the active metabolic, fluid exchange, and phagocytotic functions of these cells. The pigment epithelium mediates metabolic processes between the choriocapillaris and the rods and cones. It also plays a decisive role in the biochemical processes of vision. The pigment epithelium is rich in enzymes and has phagocytic capabilities. Discarded outer segments of photoreceptors, which undergo a continuous physiologic cyclic degradation, are phagocytosed by intracellular lysosomes within the pigment epithelium.[115]

The epithelial cells are bound together by junctional complexes (footnote, p. 00).[82] Exchange of fluid between pigment epithelial cells is hindered by the zonula occludens type of cell junction, which is a major component of the junctional complex.[42] Fluid exchange is forced to occur under active metabolic control from within and through the cell, rather than intercellularly between the cells.

Because the retina-pigment epithelium attachment is firm only at the ora serrata (Figs. 8-10 and 8-11) and optic nerve (Figs. 10-1–10-3), the retina is susceptible to pathologic separation from the underlying pigment epithelium.[31] A retinal detachment or separation represents a reopening of the embryonic lumen of the optic vesicle or optic cup. The protruding microvilli of the pigment epithelial cells that surround the tips of the photoreceptors, the presumably viscous acid mucopolysaccharides that bathe the photoreceptors and pigment epithelial cells, and the intraocular pressure exerted on the retina from within the cavity of the eye are probably the three main factors that prevent retinal detachments.

Bruch's membrane

Bruch's membrane, particularly its inner aspect, is closely connected and associated with the pigment epithelium.

By light microscopy two main layers are seen: it consists of two visible layers: (1) the basal membrane of the retinal pigment epithelium (lamina basalis) and (2) the lamina elastica, which consists of fibroelastic connective tissue of the choroid and the endothelial basement membrane of adjacent choriocapillaris capillaries. Thus, in simplified terms, Bruch's membrane is a structure consisting of connective-elastic tissue sandwiched between two basement membranes. It *does not* form a barrier for the free flow of fluid between choriocapillaris and adjacent pigment epithelium and photoreceptors (Fig. 8-7).

Ultrastructurally Bruch's membrane has five distinct layers. Subjacent to the pigment epithelium is the basement membrane of this cell. Directly external to this is a layer of collagen, followed by a core of elastic tissue. The fourth layer consists of a second thin layer of collagen. The fifth and outermost layer is a basement membrane elaborated by the endothelial cells of the choriocapillaris.

Hyaline excrescences, or drusen (Figs. 8-89 and 8-90), and elastic degeneration and calcification of Bruch's membrane are common aging processes. These changes may be physiologic and clinically harmless; however, they may represent a pathologic degeneration. Increased numbers of drusen may occur in patients with disciform macular degeneration (p. 442). Pathologic degeneration with calcification and breaks in Bruch's membrane is seen in angioid streaks (p. 429, Figs 8-95 and 8-97).

MACULAR REGION

The macula lutea is a differentiated region of retina that lies 2 disc diameters temporal to the optic nerve head (Figs. 8-7–8-9).[5] Spitznas[98] describes the macular region as approximately 5.5 mm in diameter, the nasal margin being

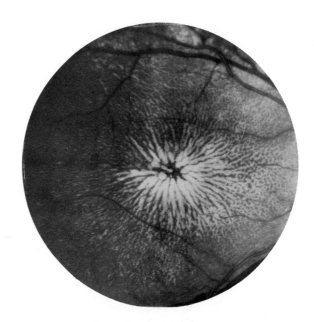

Fig. 8-9. Macular star figure in a case of von Hippel–Lindau disease. The fluid and lipid deposits conform to the lines of Henle's fiber layer as the fibers course radially away from the central foveal region. (From Watzke R, Weingeist T, and Constantine J: In Peyman GA, Apple DJ, and Sanders DR, editors: Intraocular tumors, New York, 1977, Appleton-Century-Crofts.)

at the temporal border of the optic nerve (Fig. 8-7). A yellow substance, xanthochrome, is deposited within the retina in this region. This lipid-soluble pigment is responsible for the name macula lutea (Latin, *lutea,* yellow). In addition to the yellow coloration, the macula often appears more deeply pigmented than the remaining fundus because the underlying pigment epithelium is more heavily pigmented.

The macula is subdivided into four zones: foveola, fovea, parafovea, and perifovea. The central depression of 1.5 mm in diameter contains the foveola and the fovea centralis, the site subserving central vision and color vision. The central foveola covers an area of 0.2 mm. Here the retina is maximally thinned, and its entire thickness consists entirely of photoreceptors and their nuclei. The internal limiting membrane follows the contour of the surface of the retina, and the depression at the center is obvious in histologic sections (fovea interna) (Fig. 8-8). In addition, the external limiting membrane of the sensory retina bows slightly forward in the central region and, therefore, forms the so-called fovea externa, which is probably a fixation artifact (Fig 8-8, *A*).

The fovea immediately surrounds the foveola and is 1.5 mm in diameter. The central border of the fovea is defined as the site where the nuclei of the inner nuclear layer and ganglion cell layers reappear. The retina approaches its greatest thickness at the peripheral edge of the fovea, where the ganglion cells become stratified into six to eight layers (Figs. 7-5, 8-5, and 8-8). The parafovea and perifovea surround the central foveola fovea depression.

Rods are absent or rare in the region corresponding to the foveola and fovea. The cones within these regions are more elongated and slender than the cones of the extra macular region (Fig. 8-9).

The lack of rods centrally may be important for a reason other than the obvious functional considerations. Rods possess a special relationship to the pigment epithelium because their apical outer segments are rather closely enmeshed within the apical villous processes of the retinal pigment epithelium. This probably enhances the adherence between the neural retina and pigment epithelium. In contrast, cone outer segments are shorter than those of rods and have much less contact with the pigment epithelial villous processes. The adherence of retina to pigment epithelium in the rod-free central retina might, therefore, be expected to be less firm. This may partially explain why even small transudates or exudates that originate in the foveal region may spread quickly to produce a localized detachment of the neuroepithelium, for example, central serous chorioretinopathy (p. 434).[98]

The thinning of the retina at the foveal depression is not caused by an actual reduction in number of cells, but rather the second and third neurons of the retina are displaced circumferentially from the central depression, leaving only photoreceptors centrally. The synaptic interconnection of photoreceptor cells with bipolar cells occurs in Henle's fiber layer. The axons of the outer plexiform layer that form Henle's layer must course obliquely for a relatively great distance to reach the site of synapse with the dendritic processes of the cells in the inner nuclear layer (Fig. 8-8).

Retinal capillaries derived from the central retinal artery normally supply the inner half of the retina, terminating externally in the region of the outer border of the inner nuclear layer. Because this inner half of the retina is obviously absent at the foveola-fovea depression, this vascular network does not exist and a capillary-free zone of approximately 0.4 to 0.5 mm in diameter exists centrally. Occasionally, fluorescein angiography demonstrates small capillaries coursing through this otherwise capillary-free zone; these channels perhaps represent remnants of embryonic vessels. The capillary-free zone corresponds anatomically to the rod-free zone. It is possible that the absence of vascular channels centrally is partly responsible for increased foveal visual acuity: the slight but significant hindrance that these vessels would impose on light as it passes through the retina toward the photoreceptors is negated (p. 365).

The neuronal arrangement of the central retina is such that every cone is interconnected with a single bipolar cell, which in turn synapses with a single ganglion cell and its corresponding nerve fiber. This provides a direct one-to-one relationship between the first three visual neurons. This differs from the arrangement in the extra macular retina in which many sensory cells have input into a single ganglion cell. The importance of the macular region for visual function is emphasized by the fact that a third of all fibers entering the optic nerve originate in this region. The macular fibers (papillomacular bundle) enter the optic nerve at its temporal edge but immediately penetrate the central or axial region of the nerve as they course toward the brain.

In summary, there are several ways to histologically identify the macular region and its substructures.

1. Sagittal sections through the foveola-fovea (Fig. 8-8) clearly reveals the thinning of the retina, because most of the cells of the inner half of the retina are shoved or displaced to the edge of the foveal depression. The center of the foveola is the thinnest portion of the retina.

2. In contrast to the central thinning, the retina immediately surrounding the border of the fovea, including the peripapillary area, is the thickest portion of the retina. It is characterized by a ganglion cell layer that is stratified (six to eight layers thick) (Fig. 7-5) in contrast to the single-cell layer thickness in all other regions of the fundus. This fact is of direct importance in explaining the characteristics of the cherry-red spots seen in storage diseases such as the sphingolipidoses (Fig. 8-82). The lipid deposits occur in the ganglion cells and are, therefore, most visible where the ganglion cell layer is thickest, leaving the central ganglion cell-free zone a relatively red color.

3. The photoreceptor elements of the macular region are mostly cones; however, these are modified in appearance in that they are long and slender and the microscopist must avoid confusing them with rods.

4. The retinal pigment epithelial cells are slightly more columnar and more richly pigmented in the central retina than in the extra macular regions.

5. The outer plexiform layer in the macular region has a unique appearance forming Henle's fiber layer (Fig. 8-8). The fibers of this layer course obliquely and actually run almost parallel to the retinal surface in contrast to the vertical orientation (perpendicular to the retinal surface) in the extra macular retina. This oblique course of the fibers results from the fact that the foveal cones and their processes are extremely closely grouped and every cone has

a 1:1 relationship with its corresponding bipolar cell and ganglion cell. This requires the presence of an extremely large number of interconnecting fibers. Because of space limitations, the bipolar (Fig. 8-9) cells and ganglion cells are dislocated relatively distantly from the photoreceptors. The fibers of Henle's layer must, therefore, diverge and course obliquely to reach them. Because the fibers in Henle's fiber layer are delicate and loosely arranged, this layer is susceptible to deposition of transudates, exudates, blood, and other products. Cystoid edema is common (Figs. 8-84 and 8-86), the Müller fibers forming the walls of the cyst cavities in a manner similar to that seen in peripheral microcystoid degeneration (Figs. 8-67 and 8-68; Color Plate 8-31). Exudates within Henle's fiber layer typically form a macular star figure, corresponding to the radial arrangement of the fibers as they diverge from the fovea (Fig. 8-9).

6. The vascular-free zone of the foveola-fovea can be readily contrasted, particularly in flat preparations by the trypsin digest technique, from the rich intraretinal capillary network that characterizes the parafoveal and perifoveal zones. The central fovea is totally devoid of vessels, but the peripheral macular region is richly vascularized by three arcades of capillaries within the inner half of the retina.

7. The inferior oblique muscle overlies the macular region, inserting directly into the sclera without an intervening tendon (Figs. 1-2 and 1-3). When a microscopic section shows skeletal muscle fibers inserting directly into the posterior sclera, in the absence of a tendon, one can be sure that the macular region lies near this insertion.

RETINAL PERIPHERY[28–31]

At the ora serrata the embryonic pars optica retinae continues anteriorly as the pars caeca retinae. Only the former has potential for vision (Fig. 1-11).

The ora serrata is the "tooth-like" junction between the peripheral retina and the pars plana (Figs. 4-4 and 8-10).[28–31] It is composed of alternating forward extensions of retina known as dentate processes and intervening backward extensions of ciliary epithelium, or oral bays. The dentate processes and oral bays are much more prominent nasally. Because the pars plana epithelium anterior to the ora serrata is firmly attached to its adjacent pigment epithelium by cell junctions, detachment of the sensory retina usually does not extend anteriorly past the ora serrata into the ciliary epithelium.

With the exception of the foveola-fovea depression, the retina is much thinner peripherally than at the posterior pole (Fig. 8-11) because of a loss of neuronal elements and a partial fusing together of the rows of nuclei. The number of rods and cones decreases measurably, and vascularization is sparse. Most holes and tears (Figs. 8-10, 8-72, 8-73, and 8-74; Color Plates 8-27, 8-29, and 8-31) develop in this area. At the juncture of retina and ciliary body at the ora, the retina is often reduced to a single-layered columnar epithelium.

Characteristic foci of cystoid degeneration occur in the retinal periphery of almost all adults (Figs. 8-10, 8-67, and 8-68; Color Plate 8-31) and are termed *Blessig-Iwanoff cysts* (senile microcystoid degeneration). These occur occasionally in children, but significant cyst formation generally begins in the second and third decades and its extent in-

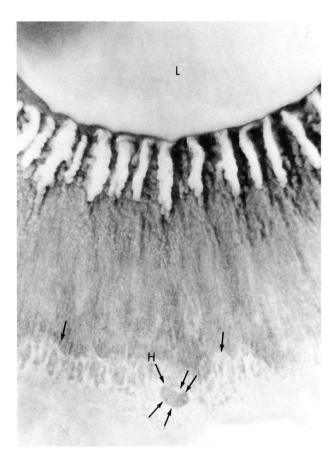

Fig. 8-10. Peripheral retina and ciliary body. Gross photograph of peripheral retina *(bottom)*, ora serrata *(arrows)*, ciliary body, and lens *(L)*. A retinal hole *(H)* is present in the area of peripheral microcystoid degeneration. (From Daicker B: Anatomie und Pathologie der menschlichen retino-ziliaren Fundusperipherie, Basel, 1972, S Karger, AG.)

creases throughout life. The temporal quadrants are more commonly and severely involved. Clinical fundus examination or viewing of flat preparations of the cysts reveals a dendrite-like, or branched, configuration forming a network of intertwining channels. Initially the cysts form in the outer plexiform and inner nuclear layers but may enlarge to involve almost the entire thickness of the retina. The lateral walls are composed of vertically coursing Müller fibers. The spaces may become confluent after breakdown of the Müller cells, leading to a flat retinoschisis (p. 410).

A second type of peripheral retinal cystoid degeneration is termed *reticular cystoid degeneration* (p. 411). Reticular degeneration reveals a different pattern of branching of the cystoid spaces in which the intertwining cystoid channels are smaller and form a more delicate "reticular" pattern than that of the Blessig-Iwanoff type. Reticular cystoid degeneration also differs from the latter type in that the cavity formation primarily occurs in the nerve fiber layer rather than in the outer plexiform layer.

BLOOD SUPPLY OF THE RETINA AND PIGMENT EPITHELIUM

The primary arterial supply to the eye is the ophthalmic artery, which is the first branch of the internal carotid

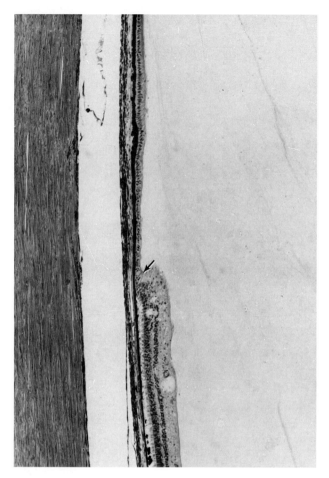

Fig. 8-11. Ora serrata *(arrow)*, junction of thin peripheral retina *(below)*, and cuboidal pars plana epithelium. Delicate fibrils, which comprise a portion of the vitreous base *(right)*, straddle the ora. (H & E stain; ×40.)

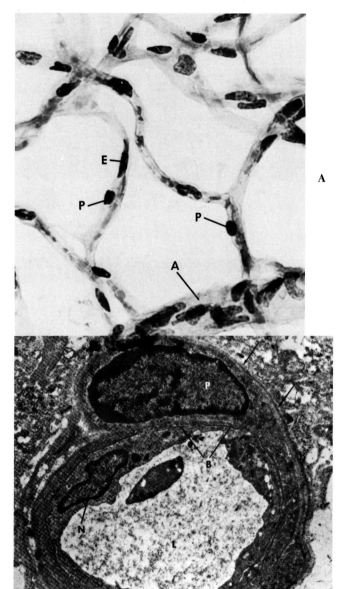

Fig. 8-12. A, Trypsin digest flat preparation of a retinal arteriole *(A)* and capillaries. The neural retinal elements are digested by the enzyme, leaving the easily visible vascular channels. The capillary is composed of two cells: (1) the intramural pericyte *(P)*, which is situated on the external aspect of the capillary wall and is spheric to oval in appearance, and (2) the endothelial cell *(E)*, which lines the lumen of the capillary and is much more elongated or spindle shaped than the pericyte. (Flat preparation, PAS stain; ×625.) **B,** Electron micrograph of a normal retinal capillary. The lumen *(L)* is lined by the endothelial cell *(N,* endothelial cell nucleus), which possesses a basement membrane *(B)*. The mural cell (pericyte, *P)* also is rimmed by an outer membrane *(arrows)*. (Uranyl acetate and lead citrate stain; ×3040.) (**A** courtesy Dr. Samuel J Vainisi; **B** from Apple DJ, Goldberg MF, and Wyhinny G: Am J Ophthalmol 75:595, 1973.)

artery.° The ophthalmic artery enters the orbit with the optic nerve through the optic canal and then divides into two major subdivisions (Figs. 7-1, 7-5, 7-6, 8-2, *B*, 8-12, 8-13, 10-8, and 10-9).

1. The retinal system, in particular the central retinal artery, which supplies the inner half of the retina (Fig. 8-2, *B*).
2. The ciliary system, which supplies the uvea, the outer half of the sensory retina (Fig. 8-2, *B*), and the optic nerve (p. 531) (Fig. 8-11).

Retinal system

The central retinal artery enters the optic nerve parenchyma (Fig. 10-8) posterior to the globe by passing through the meningeal spaces and enters the globe itself at the optic nerve head, forming the clinically visible central retinal artery. At this point the vessel is a true artery rather than an arteriole; therefore, it is susceptible to atherosclerotic occlusive disease (Fig. 8-4). The secondary and tertiary branches of the central retinal artery, branching from the optic nerve head, form the primary blood supply to the

---

° References 51, 60, 92, 93, 112, 114.

four quadrants of the fundus (Fig. 8-7). Structurally these vessels more closely resemble arterioles (Fig. 8-3). Diseases affecting them are, therefore, similar to those of other arterioles of the body, for example, the renal arterioles. Occlusive disease of the fundus vessels leading to such clinical signs as copper or (Fig. 8-12) silver wiring is best described as an arteriolosclerosis rather than atherosclerosis. These arterioles and corresponding venules supply the inner half of the retina, which includes the second and third neurons and all other tissues internal to the middle limiting membrane.[32]

The four primary fundus arterioles lie superficially in the nerve fiber layer. The arterioles can easily be distinguished from the venules not only clinically by their smaller diameter and color and reflex differences but also histologically by evaluation of the vessel wall thickness (Fig. 8-3). At arteriovenous crossings, the arterioles are generally situated above (internal to) the venules, and both vessels are enclosed within a common adventitial sheath. Arteriovenous crossing phenomena (e.g., arteriosclerotic retinopathy) are discussed on page 372.

The terminal fundus arterioles bend sharply and dip almost vertically into the retina, forming a rich capillary network (Fig. 8-12). The capillaries extend as deeply as the outer aspect of the inner nuclear layer, sometimes just into the outer plexiform layer to the dividing line formed by the middle limiting "membrane."

In the posterior pole the temporal pair of retinal vessels course in an arcuate manner toward the macula. The macula is sometimes supplied by a cilioretinal artery from the ciliary circulation that appears at the temporal optic disc (p. 387; Figs. 8-41 and 8-42). In 15% of patients this artery supplies the primary nourishment for the macular region.

The capillary network in the perifoveal zone is especially well developed and contains three layers of capillaries. As they approach the central foveola, the capillaries gradually decrease in number until the fovea and foveola are free of vessels.

In the peripapillary retina, an additional layer of capillaries is also present. These four layers nourish the extremely thick nerve fiber layer characteristic of this region (Figs. 7-34, *B*, 8-3, 10-2, and 10-3). Most of the extra macular and extra papillary fundus is supported by two layers of capillaries; peripherally this is reduced to a scanty single layer as the ora serrata is approached.

The retinal capillaries consist of two distinct cell types: the endothelial cell and the pericyte, or mural cell (Fig. 8-12).[60,85] The endothelial cell encircles the lumen of the capillary and is in turn encircled by its basement membrane. The endothelial cells of a normal retinal capillary are closely bound about the lumen by intercellular junctions of the zonula occludens type (tight junctions). These intercellular bridges normally prohibit a free flow of fluids from the vascular lumen into the retinal interstitium outside the capillary. Normal capillary permeability is, therefore, minimal and typically does not leak fluorescein dye.* These junctions, in association with the astrocyte and Müller cell foot processes that encircle the retinal capillaries, probably

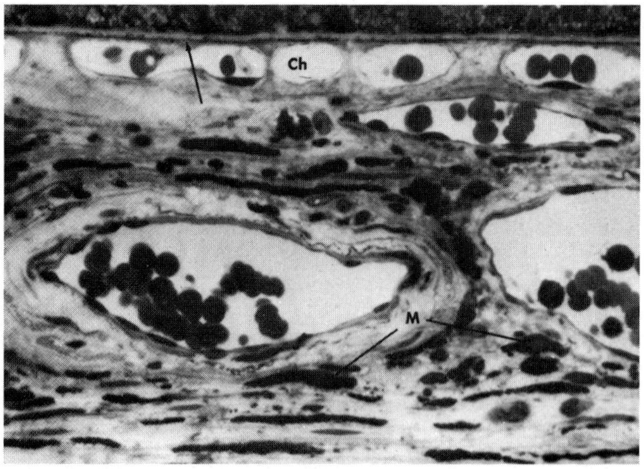

Fig. 8-13. Normal choroid showing the large vessels (Haller's layer), the deeper medium-sized vessels (Sattler's layer), and the choriocapillaris *(Ch)*, adjacent to Bruch's membrane *(arrow)*. Elongated, deeply staining melanocytes *(M)* are within the choroid. The cells are analogous embryologically and morphologically to those in the iris (Fig. 7-2) and are further discussed in Chapter 7. (Mallory blue stain; ×275.) (From Apple DJ, Goldberg MF, and Wyhinny G: Am J Ophthalmol 75:595, 1973.)

contribute to the blood-retina barrier. Newly formed vessels (e.g., neovascularization in diabetic retinopathy or Coats' syndrome) characteristically leak fluorescein dye after fluorescein angiography, perhaps because of qualitatively and/or quantitatively deficient intercellular tight junctions.[6]

The pericytes form a "cap" around the outer aspects of the endothelial cell basement membrane. The pericyte itself also elaborates a basement membrane around the outer circumference of a capillary. Normally the endothelial cells and pericytes are present in a one-to-one ratio in young persons; however, as an aging process there is a gradual decrease in the number of endothelial cells. On the other hand, various diseases cause a relative decrease in the number of pericytes. The most important of these diseases is diabetic retinopathy (p. 375).

Ciliary system

By way of the posterior ciliary arteries, the ciliary system provides the source for the choroidal vessels that nourish the outer half of the retina (Figs. 7-1, 7-5, 7-6, and 10-9). Blood flows freely from the outer layer of large vessels (Haller's layer) into the layer of medium-sized vessels (Sattler's layer) directly into the single-layered row of large capillary-like channels, the choriocapillaris (Fig. 8-13). This free flow between the various layers causes a rapid fall in the rate of flow and in the perfusion pressure. Vessels in the macular region form a rich plexus because of the heavy responsibility for adequate nourishment to the photoreceptors in this critical area.

In contrast to the retinal capillaries the walls of the choriocapillaris channels are porous and fluids move in a relatively unhindered manner between choroid, Bruch's membrane, and adjacent pigment epithelium. The most important barrier to free flow between choroidal vessels

---

* References 3, 4, 9, 26, 42, 43, 54.

and the sensory elements of the retina is found within the pigment epithelium, where the adjacent cuboidal cells of the pigment epithelium are tightly bound by junctional complexes, including intact zonulae occludens. Because the fluid exchange through the intercellular spaces of the pigment epithelium is hindered, the normal flow of fluid from choroid to sensory retina is regulated by active metabolic processes within organelles in the cell, and the fluid exchange is, therefore, an *intra*cellular process.

The choriocapillaris is not, as previously presumed, a freely anastomotic plexus of vessels that perfuses the entire fundus without regard to segmental distribution. Studies have shown that discrete areas of the choroid are actually divided into lobules according to their primary vascular supply.[51,108] Although some overlap of flow occurs, the choroidal vascular supply actually resembles that of the liver, in which discrete lobules are supplied by primary efferent vessels. This may have practical consequences during photocoagulation, for example, for subpigment epithelial neovascularization when ciliary or choroidal vessels are destroyed by the treatment.[7] One cannot always assume that a freely anastomotic system can compensate for the destroyed vasculature and thus prevent choroidal infarction.

Because the outer half of the retina is supplied by the ciliary vascular system through the choriocapillaris, it follows that ciliary-choroidal vascular diseases would affect the corresponding outer portion of the sensory retina. Just as diseases of the central retinal artery characteristically damaged the *inner* retina, diseases of choroidal vasculature characteristically first affect the *outer* retina (Fig. 8-13).

VITREOUS (HYALOID)

During the first month of fetal life the space between the lens and the retina contains the primary vitreous hyaloid (Figs. 1-9, 2-23, 2-24, and 8-14). It consists of two parts:

1. mesodermally derived tissue, including the hyaloid vessel and its branches[6,12]
2. a fibrillar meshwork, or scaffolding, of uncertain origin°

These delicate supporting fibers, which form a network between the hyaloid vessels, are possibly derived from the cells of the inner layer of the optic cup, and many authors consider them to be neuroectodermal in origin. However, it is also possible that the lens, especially in the earlier stages of its development, takes part in formation of fibers within the primary vitreous, thus suggesting a component derived from the surface ectoderm. Following development of the lens capsule, however, it is probable that the lens plays no further role in the development of the vitreous. The ground substance, or gel component, of the primary as well as the secondary (adult) vitreous consists of hyaluronic acid.

In the second month of embryonic development the adult, or secondary, vitreous begins to develop in the form of an active secretion of collagen fibrils and hyaluronic acid, which begin to replace the vascular elements that predominate in the primary vitreous (Fig. 8-14). By the fifth to sixth month of development the cavity of the eye is filled with the secondary vitreous. The primary vitreous is thus reduced to a small **S**-shaped, central space—Cloquet's canal (Fig. 8-14)—which courses between the optic nerve head and the posterior surface of the lens. In sagittal sections the canal is funnel shaped, with the broad opening of the funnel bordering the posterior lens surface and with the stem of the funnel curved in an **S**. By the end of embryonic development no vascular channels remain within the secondary vitreous.

The tertiary vitreous forms the zonules of Zinn (suspensory ligament of the lens). It forms in the fourth month of gestation with an elaboration of fibrils between the lens and ciliary body.

The secondary or definitive adult vitreous occupies almost the entire space between the lens and retina and represents about two thirds of the volume of the eye. Ninety-nine percent of the vitreous humor is water bound with collagen and hyaluronic acid. This forms a hydrogel of high viscosity. Hyaluronic acid actually received its name when first isolated in the hyaloid body. The vitreous substance, in conjunction with aqueous humor, which maintains the intraocular pressure, is responsible for maintenance of the spheric form of the globe. The pressure of the vitreous humor on the retinal surface provides protection against retinal detachment.

The fibrillar network is denser in the periphery, forming the vitreous base. It straddles the ora serrata and extends about 1.5 mm anterior and an equal distance posterior to the ora. The vitreous base is one of two sites where the vitreous is firmly attached to the adjacent retina. It is also firmly attached to the retina at the outer circumference of the optic nerve head, the ring of Martegiani. The attachment of vitreous to retina in all other sites between the ring of Martegiani and the vitreous base is much less firm; posterior detachment of the vitreous is a common clinical finding (Fig. 8-73).

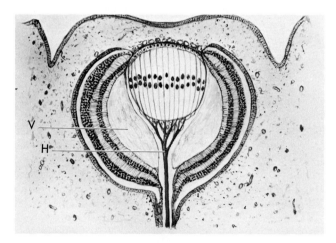

Fig. 8-14. Drawing of embryonic optic cup showing hyaloid artery *(H)* within Cloquet's canal and the developing adult (secondary) vitreous, V, filling the remainder of the cavity. (From Apple DJ, Hamming NA, and Gieser DK: In Peyman GA, Apple DJ, and Sanders DR, editors: Intraocular tumors, New York, 1977, Appleton-Century-Crofts.)

° Abnormalities related to persistence of elements of the embryonic vitreous and hyaloid vasculature are discussed in Chapter 2.

The anterior border of the vitreous at the posterior surface of the lens forms a flattened spheric surface, the patellar fossa. Here the anterior vitreous face shows a membrane-like condensation of fibrils known as Wieger's ligament or the ligamentum hyaloideo-capsulario. The space between the lens and this posteriorly arching vitreous face is the retrolenticular space or Berger's space and is normally very narrow—hardly more than a potential space. In pathologic circumstances this area can be greatly enlarged, for example, through engorgement by blood or exudates. An anterior condensation of vitreous fibrils lateral to the lens equator forms the remainder of the anterior hyaloid face, extending laterally and posteriorly to the vitreous base. The lining of Cloquet's canal, that is, the border between what was previously the primary and secondary vitreous, also consists of a linear condensation of vitreous fibrils rather than a true basement membrane.

The vitreous presses firmly against the retinal surface and holds it against the pigment epithelium. Normally, the posterior fibers of the vitreous merge into the internal limiting membrane of the retina; therefore, the term *posterior vitreous face* does not apply to the normal vitreous but only to a vitreous that has undergone a degenerative or pathologic change and has detached posteriorly with condensation of the fibrils forming a new "face" (Fig. 8-73).

The cortex of the vitreous contains scattered cells, termed *hyalocytes*, of uncertain origin. They may originate in situ in the vitreous or may migrate from the bloodstream. Otherwise the vitreous contains mostly extracellular elements and in itself has a meager metabolism. For this reason the vitreous often reforms poorly after disease or injury and has a tendency to liquefy with age. The fibrillar network often has a tendency to thicken, forming fine opacities that may cause an optical inhomogeneity and opacities.

Asteroid hyalosis (Fig. 8-15 and Color Plate 8-1) consists of compounds that are visible clinically as punctate white intravitreal opacities and that may be annoying to the affected person because of the "floaters" in the visual field.° The iridescent particles consists of complex lipids embedded in an amorphous matrix containing calcium and phosphorous attached to the vitreous framework. This condition is sometimes seen with diabetes mellitus and ocular vascular diseases.

Histologically the particles consist of amorphous PAS and acid-mucopolysaccharide-positive bodies that show birefringence when viewed with polarized light. They are composed of complex lipids and phospholipids.

Asteroid hyalosis should be distinguished from synchesis scintillans, which also is clinically characterized by a unilateral accumulation of "golden" particles. These bodies are composed of cholesterol and represent blood breakdown products following intravitreal hemorrhage. Age-related degeneration and liquefaction of the vitreous may be considered normal aging processes usually occurring unilaterally in elderly individuals.

The basement membrane of the Müller cells forms the principal part of the internal limiting membrane of the retina, and the remaining inner portion is formed by vitreous fibrils and mucopolysaccharide. Several pathologic processes may occur at the vitreoretinal interface that may affect vision. Sub, intra-, or epiretinal membranes may occur as a result of idiopathic gliosis or fibrosis, or may occur secondary to other conditions such as retinal detachment, chronic glaucoma, diabetes, proliferative retinopathy, and vitreous hemorrhage and following intraocular surgery or photocoagulation. Epiretinal macular membranes that often occur without known cause (idiopathic) or that occur following retinal surgery or other conditions are designated as macular puckers or cellophane maculopathy. Extensive gliosis of the inner or of the outer surfaces of the retina may cause fixed folds, especially after retinal detachment. When the membranous proliferation is extensive and associated with retinal detachment it is termed a *proliferative vitreoretinopathy* (p. 420).[49,68]

Histologically, in both the idiopathic and the secondary varieties of epiretinal membranes, a variety of cells, including retinal pigment epithelial (RPE) cells, fibrocytes, and myofibroblasts (see Table 1-2). The immune system is activated during the proliferative process. Depending on the composition of the membrane, immunohistochemical staining may be positive for cytokeratin, glial fibrillary acidic protein, vimentin, actin, and fibronectin (see Table 1-2).

Trauma

TRAUMATIC CHORIORETINOPATHIES

Ocular trauma is a serious public health problem.[118–239] Detailed reports of traumatic chorioretinopathies begin to appear by the midnineteenth century. In 1854 von Graefe[230] described the crescent-shaped choroidal ruptures that are typically associated with blunt trauma (p. 447). Almost 20 years later Berlin[126] described a postcontusion injury—a milky-white opacification of the posterior pole of the eye. When it involves the macular region it is often referred to as "Berlin's edema." Golzieher[156] in 1901 reported the clinical findings of chorioretinitis sclopetaria in the eyes of patients with bullet injuries to the orbit. Purtscher[204,205] in 1912 described the soft exudates concentrated in the posterior pole of the eye following injury to the head and chest. These four entities remain the predominant types of traumatic chorioretinopathy. In late stages of most forms of this entity an infiltration of pigment epithelial pigment into the retina may occur, producing a clinical picture of pseudoretinitis pigmentosa (p. 406, Fig. 8-63).

Commotio retinae (Berlins' edema)

Berlin[126] in 1873 invoked the Latin term for retinal contusion, *commotio retinae,* to describe a transient whitening of the retina resulting from blunt ocular trauma.° It may occur peripherally or within the posterior pole region. In the latter case it is referred to as "Berlin's edema." Extensive posterior pole involvement may give rise to a cherry-red spot. Although Berlin considered edema to be responsible for the appearance of commotio retinae, there has been no evidence of intraretinal or subretinal dye accumulation in uncomplicated cases.

Experimental, clinical, and histologic evidence have confirmed that the lesion is not an edema, but rather consists

---

° References 65, 66, 87, 100, 107, 262.

° References 120, 123, 124, 127, 139, 148, 152, 154, 161, 189, 203, 210, 216.

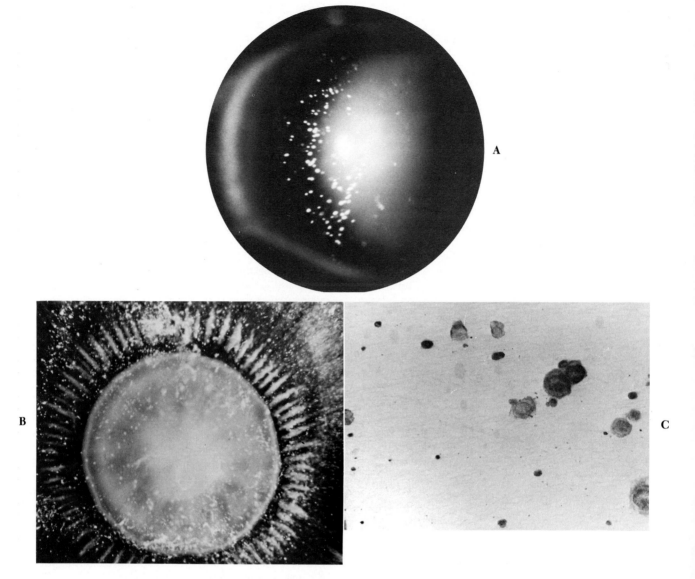

Fig. 8-15. Asteroid hyalosis. **A,** Clinical photograph. **B,** Gross photograph of vitreous and retro-lental area viewed from behind showing asteroid hyalosis (*multiple white dots*) in the vitreous. **C,** Photomicrograph. Round, amorphous opacities are suspended among vitreous fibrils. (H & E stain; ×430.) (**B** from Daicker B: Anatomie und Pathologie der menschlichen retino-ziliaren Fundusperipherie, Basel, 1972, S Karger, AG.)

of changes at the junction of photoreceptor outer segments and retinal pigment epithelium in the macular region.[189,216] Photoreceptor vacuolization and disruption and damage to the retinal pigment epithelium occurs. The retinal pigment epithelium then phagocytizes outer segment materials, undergoes hyperplasia, and may migrate into the neural retina. Although the process may resolve without sequelae or the damage to photoreceptors, vision loss may occur as a sequelae to microcystoid degeneration of the fovea, macrocyst formation, lamellar hole formation, or through-and-through neural retinal hole formation.

Chorioretinal rupture, retinitis, and sclopetaria

Goldzieher[156] in 1901 introduced the term *chorioretinitis plastica sclopetaria* to describe the appearance of direct choroidal and retinal rupture in the peripheral retina fol-lowing trauma from a bullet wound in the orbital area. The term now connotes a specific type of traumatic chorioretinopathy that results indirectly from blunt injury produced by a missile entering the orbit and ricocheting off the sclera.[192,200,208] Fundus examination shows an exuberant fibroglial scar with sharp serrated borders and pigment proliferation. The projectile does not penetrate the globe but passes in close proximity to it, inducing a rupture of the retina and choroid. The visual prognosis depends on the extent and location of intraocular injury. Choroidal rupture, a lesion that may progress toward disciform macular degeneration, is described on page 447.[119,217,238]

Purtscher's retinopathy

In 1910 Purtscher[202,204,205] described a syndrome of sudden blindness in five severely traumatized patients. Several areas of superficial retinal whitening were located primarily in the posterior pole of both eyes. This lesion that bears his name generally follows chest compression and is characterized by superficial white exudates, cotton-wool spots, and hemorrhages in the retina.[128,133] The clinical picture probably is caused by damage to retinal vessels secondary to sudden changes in intraluminal pressure, which are related directly or indirectly to the compression of the chest. Microemboli as a cause, however, cannot be ruled out. Several mechanisms have been proposed for the pathogenesis of Purtscher's retinopathy. These include:

1. fat embolization, occurring as a result of long-bone fractures or after acute pancreatitis with enzymatic digestion of omental fat[164]
2. air embolization from compressive chest injuries
3. venous reflux with endothelial cell swelling and capillary engorgement of the upper body
4. severe angiospastic response following a sudden increase in venous pressure
5. complement-induced granulocyte aggregation. Leukocyte aggregation by activated complement factor 5 (C5A) has been shown to occur in such diverse conditions as trauma, acute pancreatitis, and connective tissue disease.

Retinal hemorrhages and Terson's syndrome

Retinal hemorrhages after trauma may assume virtually all configurations ranging from flame-shaped to globular. Terson's syndrome consists of hemorrhages in the vitreous compartment associated with intracranial subarachnoid or subdural hemorrhage.[137,150,229] Vitreous hemorrhage frequently obscures visualization of the fundus.* Organization of vitreoretinal hemorrhages may result in formation of membranes on the internal surface of the retina, leading to epiretinal membranes (see Fig. 8-79), cellophane retinopathy, proliferative vitreoretinopathy, pigmentary macular changes, perimacular neural retinal folds, and fixed retinal folds. Many of the delicate epiretinal and preretinal membranes, especially those of the macular region, result from proliferation of glial cells normally present in the nerve fiber and ganglion cell layers and retinal pigment epithelial cells, fibrocytes, and myofibroblasts.

Shaken baby syndrome

The presenting signs of child abuse include eye trauma in 4% to 6% of cases (Fig. 8-16; Color Plates 8-2 and 8-3).† Diagnosis requires a high index of suspicion and knowledge of the manifestations of child abuse. The most common ocular manifestation includes retinal hemorrhages followed by periorbital ecchymosis and vitreoretinal damage. Retinal hemorrhages occur in 11% to 23% of all physically abused children and in 50% to 80% of shaken babies. The term *whiplash shaken baby syndrome* was coined by Caffey to describe the occurrence in infants of retinal, subdural, or subarachnoid hemorrhages, with minimal or absent signs of external trauma. While the term *shaken baby syndrome* has become well entrenched in the

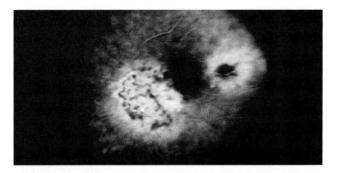

Fig. 8-16. Fluorescein angiogram of a patient with retinal toxicity due to light from a surgical microscope (same patient as Color Plate 8-2), showing the two discrete burns. The small lesion on the right being from the original cataract surgery and (see also Color Plate 8-4) the larger region on the left being from the later vitrectomy procedure.

literature of child abuse, it is characteristic that a history of shaking is usually absent. Shaking is often assumed. The diagnosis is usually based on finding a triad of skeletal injuries (metaphyseal avulsions, rib fractures, and stripping of periosteum), with computed tomographic (CT) findings of intracranial bleeding and retinal hemorrhages. The baby's head constitutes 10% of the total volume and weight of the infant, and infants have poor neural control of the muscles of the neck. During shaking the head experiences severe accelerations and decelerations with resultant shear and tensile strains in the infant's soft, poorly myelinated brain. When external signs of trauma are lacking, the ophthalmologist is often called upon to establish the diagnosis. The syndrome carries a 15% mortality rate and a 50% morbidity rate.

Splinter and flame-shaped hemorrhages may also be seen in some otherwise normal newborns.[125] These are probably caused by a mechanical rise in pressure inside the skull during labor, increased blood viscosity, and obstetric instrumentation during delivery. The presence of such hemorrhages, however, must always lead one to be aware of and rule out this syndrome.

PHOTIC RETINAL INJURY

Light can damage the retina by photochemical, thermal, or mechanical effects or some combination of the three.* Although solar retinopathy was once believed to be caused by retinal photocoagulation, it was shown in 1971 that solar-induced retinal temperature increases are generally too low for thermal damage.[149] Most forms of solar retinopathy probably represent photochemical retinal damage, perhaps enhanced by thermal changes. The clinical entity of solar retinopathy typically presents as a small yellow-white foveolar lesion. Over a period of 1 or 2 weeks, the lesion fades, often replaced by a foveolar depression or lamellar hole.

Ultraviolet radiation has long been implicated as a cause of both age-related macular degeneration (AMD) and cataracts. The evidence linking environmental light exposure

* References 146, 147, 180, 215, 223, 231, 232.
† References 125, 132, 134, 135, 142, 151, 159, 166, 179, 193, 209, 233.

* References 118, 121, 122, 138, 143, 158–160, 167, 173, 174, 176, 178, 183–188, 190, 191, 195–198, 201, 211, 219, 220, 224–227, 234–236, 239.

to these conditions remains circumstantial; however, recent studies continue to demonstrate increasingly this cause and effect. Macular light damage caused by illumination from various ophthalmic instruments and the surgical operating microscope is now well established. Although there had been warnings of potential light injury as early as the 1970s, it was not until the 1980s that reports of operating microscope injury following various operations such as cataract surgery with and without an intraocular lens (IOL), vitrectomy, corneal transplant, and keratorefractive surgery appeared.[136] The most common potential cause of photic injury occurs following insertion of an IOL in which the light from the operating microscope focuses onto the retina. Retinal damage has also been demonstrated with intraocular fiberoptic illuminators used in vitreous surgery.

Operating microscope injuries are typically round to oval retinal lesions, one-half to two disk areas in extent, located in the inferior macula or adjacent to it. The lesions are ophthalmoscopically (Color Plate 8-4), angiographically (Fig. 8-16), and histologically distinct from cystoid macular edema (CME). They show characteristics of both photochemical and thermal retinal damage. The lesions are located at the level of the pigment epithelium and occasionally have an overlying serious retinal detachment. Their initial yellow-white fundus appearance gradually fades, leaving behind pigment.

Retinal vascular diseases

As noted in the previous section, the inner aspect of the sensory retina receives its vascular supply from the central retinal arterial system. Intraretinal arterioles, venules, and capillaries constituting this system are illustrated in Figs. 8-2, *B* and 8-3.

The outer half of the retina, bordering the inner portion at the middle limiting membrane and devoid of vessels, is composed almost entirely of the photoreceptor cells and their processes. Diffusion of nutrients from the underlying choriocapillaris, which is derived from the ciliary vessels, sustains the outer retina (Fig. 8-13).

This subdivision of the retina into inner and outer portions is of practical value because certain categories of retinal disease primarily affect one portion or the other in a selective manner.[240–579]

A. Initial damage to the inner retina
   1. Retinal vascular diseases
      a. Hypertensive and arteriosclerotic retinopathy
      b. Proliferative retinopathies, for example, diabetes mellitus (microangiopathy and proliferative retinopathy)
      c. Central artery obstruction (ischemic infarction of inner retina)
      d. Central vein obstruction (venous stasis retinopathy and hemorrhagic infarction of inner retina)
   2. Glaucoma (ganglion cells, nerve fiber layer)
   3. Optic nerve and nerve fiber layer degeneration (optic nerve hypoplasia, optic neuritis, papilledema, optic atrophy, and damage from intracranial lesions)
B. Initial damage to the outer retina
   1. Primary photoreceptor and/or pigment epithelial dystrophies, including several forms of macular dystrophy or the retinitis pigmentosa syndromes. The perivascular pigmentation and retinal vascular attenuation in the latter are secondary phenomena

   2. Retinal detachment
   3. Lesions of pigment epithelium and Bruch's membrane
   4. Choroidal diseases, including subpigment epithelial neovascularization, choroidal vascular insufficiency, inflammations, degenerations, and dystrophies

Histopathologic localization of the site of retinal injury helps determine the pathogenesis of the disease. For example, glaucoma and lesions of the optic nerve, both of which are often characterized by eventual destruction of axons in the nerve fiber layer and retinal ganglion cells, and diseases of the intraretinal vasculature necessarily manifest first in the inner retina. In contrast, selective degeneration of the outer retina signifies a different category of pathogenesis. Outer retinal degeneration should provoke the pathologist to search for conditions such as primary disease of the photoreceptors, pigment epithelial disease, and choroidal vascular insufficiency. For example, simple retinal detachment initially creates outer retinal (photoreceptor) degeneration caused by separation of the retina from the underlying choroidal vascular supply. In the early stages of retinal detachment, the inner layers of the retina remain relatively intact because of retention of an uncompromised vascular supply from the retinal circulation.

These principles are valuable in obtaining information concerning the basic pathogenesis of a disease process when the tissue is examined microscopically in relatively early stages of the disease. During later stages of retinal disease there is usually a more diffuse involvement of all retinal layers, and the distinction between inner and outer retinal layer damage is not so apparent. When the damage, which initially involves only selected layers, becomes more widespread with degeneration of previously uninvolved layers, the degenerative process is sometimes described as spreading transsynaptically. In early glaucoma, for example, retinal degeneration may be confined to the ganglion cell layer. In later stages, subsequent damage and attenuation of the inner nuclear layer, which is separated from the ganglion cell layer by the row of synapses in the inner plexiform layer, often occur.

HYPERTENSIVE AND ARTERIOSCLEROTIC RETINOPATHY

Hypertensive retinopathy (Figs. 8-17 and 8-18) is commonly classified according to changes that provide prognostic clues to the course of the disease. Although any division of hypertensive retinopathy into stages is necessarily arbitrary and oversimplified, it provides a useful basis for understanding the primary changes and evaluating prognosis. Because arteriosclerotic changes often occur in close association with hypertensive retinopathy, both conditions are considered together.[240–274] The Scheie[260] and the Keith-Wagener[251,266] classifications, which assign stages to these diseases, are useful not only to ophthalmologists but particularly to internists concerned about the general course of these diseases.

Hypertension-related vascular effects primarily involve diminution in diameter of the retinal vessels. They may manifest as acute focal spasms (as in acute toxemia of pregnancy or malignant hypertension) or, more commonly, as a more diffuse, slowly progressive narrowing, such as that of ordinary essential hypertension.[242,249,268]

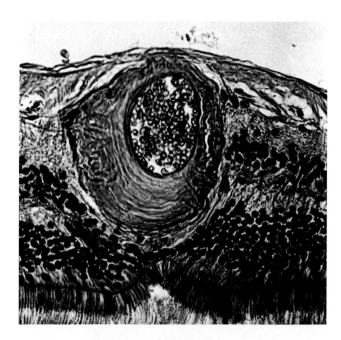

Fig. 8-17. Arteriosclerosis. Cross-section through the retina shows a great thickening of the media. (H & E stain; ×380.) (From Blodi FC and Allen L: Stereoscopic manual of the ocular fundus in local and systemic disease, vol I, St. Louis, 1964, The CV Mosby Co.)

A

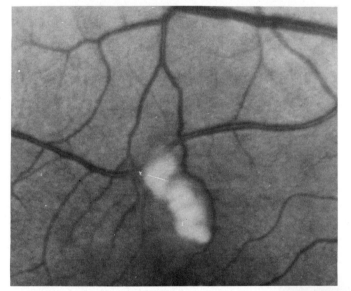

Fig. 8-18. A, Gross photograph of a cotton-wool exudate (cytoid body). This white lesion is not a true exudate but clusters of swollen nerve fiber layer axons. Degeneration with subsequent focal bulbous swelling of each affected fiber often occurs in diseases that lead to retinal ischemia. In histopathologic sections the swollen terminus of the fiber superficially resembles a round or fusiform cell, hence the term *cytoid body.* In contrast to this lesion the hard, yellow waxy exudate frequently seen in diabetic retinopathy does represent an exudative process resulting from passage of fluid, lipid, and other materials out of the affected vessel. **B,** Early drawing of retinal cytoid bodies. (It has long been appreciated that cytoid bodies are clusters of bulbous swelling of ischemic nerve fiber layer axons.) **C,** Photomicrograph of cytoid bodies in nerve fiber layer. Note continuity with nerve axons *(arrows).* (H & E stain; ×450.) (**B** from Schieck F: In Henke F and Lubarsch O: Handbuch der speziellen pathologischen Anatomie und Histologie, Berlin, 1928, Julius Springer; **C** from Naumann GOH and Apple DJ: In Doerr W, Seifert G, and Uehlinger E, editors: Handbuch der speziellen pathologischen Anatomie, Band Auge, Berlin, 1980, Springer-Verlag.)

B

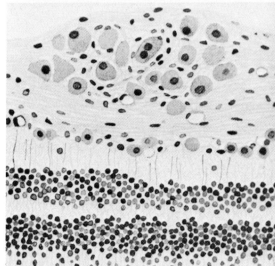

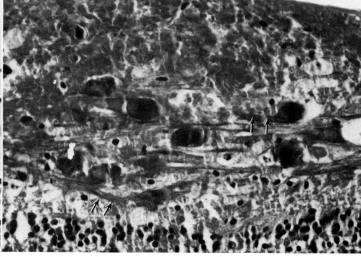

C

Sclerotic changes of the arteriolar wall invariably occur in long-standing cases. The intraocular arteriolar change represents an arteriolosclerosis analogous to the process of nephrosclerosis, which often occurs concurrently. Histopathologically a hyaline or "onionskin" thickening of the vessel wall occurs with marked diminution of lumen diameter (Fig. 8-17). These arteriolar lesions differ from the process of atherosclerosis, which affects larger-caliber arteries (Figs. 7-17, 8-16, 8-43, and 10-19).

The various arteriolovenous crossing changes ("AV nicking"), which may or may not be associated with hypertension, are the clinical manifestations of arteriolosclerosis.[73] There is mural thickening of the arteriole as it nears and crosses the retinal venule. At the site of crossing, the vessels are in a common adventitial sheath. Arteriovenous crossing phenomena are probably caused for the most part by a partial obscuration of the venous blood column by the optical effect of the thickened overlying arteriolar walls.[73]

Copper-wire and silver-wire changes that occur with more advanced sclerotic change are also caused simply by a diminution in the reflection of the red blood column back to the eye of the examiner. This diminution results from sclerosis and relative opacity of the overlying arteriolar wall. When the wall is sufficiently opaque to reflect only a portion or none of the red color of the intravascular blood into the eye of the examining ophthalmoscopist, the vessel assumes first a copper-wire pattern and ultimately a silver-wire pattern.

The flame-shaped hemorrhage seen in hypertensive retinopathy and in many other retinal vascular diseases, such as central vein occlusions (Figs. 8-45, 8-46, *A*, and 8-49), assumes this typical shape because the extravasated erythrocytes are deposited in the retinal nerve fiber layer. The blood deposits are, therefore, confined within spaces between the nerve fibers, which are nearly parallel with one another. The nerve fibers are grouped in an arcuate pattern temporally and in a radial (spoke-wheel pattern) nasally. Accumulation of blood between the fibers causes the flame-shaped appearance on fundus examination.*

The cotton-wool "exudate" (cytoid body, soft exudate), often seen in hypertensive retinopathy, lupus erythematosus retinopathy, preproliferative and proliferative diabetic retinopathy, and many other forms of retinal disease, is actually not an exudate (Fig. 8-18).[258] It is composed of clusters of ganglion cell axons in the nerve fiber layer, which have undergone a bulbous dilatation at a site of ischemic damage or infarction. When scores of fibers are affected, the multitude of swollen terminals becomes clinically visible. These aggregates resemble a tuft of cotton or wool when viewed during ophthalmoscopic examination (Fig. 8-18, *A*). Histopathologically the segment of the fiber that undergoes such bulbous thickening assumes a shape reminiscent of a cell, hence the term *cytoid* (cell-like) *bodies* (Fig. 8-18, *B* and *C*). Cytoid body refers by definition to the histopathologic rather than the clinical appearance of such lesions; however, use of this term in the clinical sense is not altogether undesirable because it continually reminds the clinician of the histopathologic basis of this frequently encountered lesion.

Direct vascular changes, including a decrease in arterio-

---

* References 241, 243, 256, 257, 271, 272.

lar caliber and changes indicative or arteriolosclerotic disease comprise grades I and II of the Keith Wagener scheme.[251,266] Grade III indicates formation of cotton-wool spots, hard exudates, including the macular star figure (Fig. 8-9), hemorrhages, and arteriolar attenuation. In grade IV, the superimposition of papilledema (Figs. 10-13, 10-15, and 10-16; Color Plate 10-4) on these earlier changes often signals initiation of the malignant phase of hypertension and a more ominous prognosis.[240,267]

PROLIFERATIVE RETINOPATHY

Proliferative retinopathy occurs in several different pathologic conditions, which have in common a proliferation of fibrovascular tissue that may form membranes and

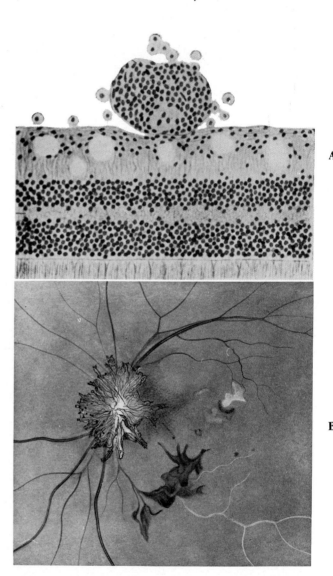

A

B

Fig. 8-19. A, Early schematic drawing illustrating an early stage of preretinal neovascularization. This solid glomeruloid bud of endothelial cells has broken through the internal limiting membrane. **B,** Early fundus drawing showing florid neovascularization of the optic disc. (**A** from Schieck F: In Henke F and Lubarsch O, editors: Handbuch der speziellen pathologischen Anatomie und Histologie, vol I, Berlin, 1928, Julius Springer; **B** from the collection of Professor Wolfgang Stock, University of Tübingen, Tübingen, Germany.)

traction bands in the retina and vitreous cavity (Figs. 8-19, 8-20, and 8-24–8-26; Color Plates 8-5 and 8-6).[275–478]

The two basic types, with some overlap in certain cases, are (1) that which follows organization of intraocular hemorrhages, exudates, or inflammatory infiltrates and (2) that occurring as a sequela of hypoxia-induced retinal neovascularization.

1. Posthemorrhagic, posttraumatic, or postinflammatory with organization of blood or exudate remnants
2. Ischemic or hypoxia-induced
   a. Diabetes mellitus
   b. Central retinal vein occlusion (venous stasis and hemorrhagic retinopathy) and branch retinal vein occlusion; association with central artery occlusion is less common[486,524]
   c. Eales' disease
   d. Hemoglobinopathies, for example, sickle retinopathy
   e. Sarcoidosis
   f. Hypertensive retinopathy
   g. Carotid and ciliary arterial insufficiency, anterior ischemic optic neuropathy[543]
   h. Collagen diseases[310,311,420]
   i. Uveitis, Behçet's disease
   j. Coats' syndrome and Leber's miliary aneurysms
   k. Persistent hyperplastic primary vitreous (PHPV)
   l. Retinopathy of prematurity

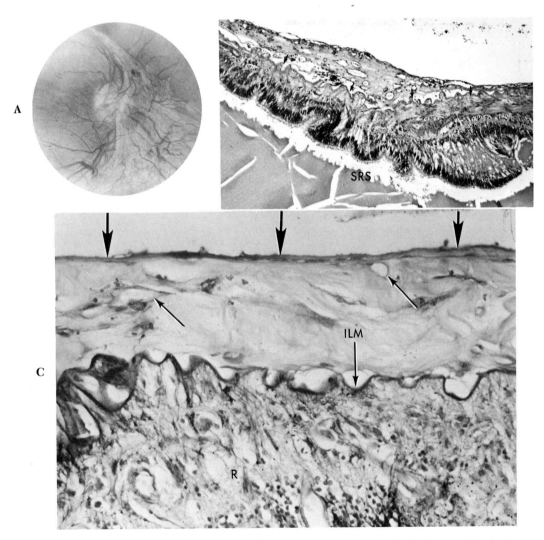

Fig. 8-20. A, Proliferative diabetic retinopathy with preretinal neovascularization and formation of fibrovascular tufts on the retinal surface extending into the vitreous. **B,** Diabetic retinopathy, preretinal neovascularization, and fibrosis. *Arrows,* Wrinkling of the vitreoretinal interface. Retinal detachment is indicated by presence of fluid in the subretinal space *(SRS)*. (H & E stain; ×100.) **C,** Vitreoretinal interface from a patient with proliferative diabetic retinopathy. The inner aspect of the retina *(R)* shows loss of normal neural architecture. The internal limiting membrane *(ILM)* is wrinkled because of traction exerted by a preretinal fibrovascular membrane *(large arrows)* containing newly formed vessels *(small arrows)*. Neovascular tissue originates in the inner retina and grows along the anterior surface of the retina. Rupture and penetration of the internal limiting membrane frequently occurs, with subsequent ingrowth of the neovascular fronds into the vitreous. Such new vessels characteristically leak fluorescein. (PAS stain; ×325.)

m. Norrie's disease
n. Incontinentia pigmenti
o. Prolonged hypoxic cyanosis
p. Dysproteinemias, for example, macroglobulinemia

In all of the diseases in which neovascularization is prominent (group 2 in the preceding list), the common mechanism is a localized or generalized retinal ischemia or hypoxia. Apparently the presence of living tissue is essential for neovascularization: new vessels seldom invade a necrotic area. Vasoproliferation is only rarely seen in diseases involving total anoxia, for example, central retinal artery occlusion. Regardless of the disease producing the retinal ischemia, it is probable that the hypoxic retina elaborates a vasoformative substance that stimulates the growth of new vessels on the retina and the optic disc.[306,320,433] Most neovascular tufts occur in or adjacent to areas of retinal ischemia or capillary dropout and grow into the ischemic zone.

Important variants of intraocular neovascularization are rubeosis iridis and subpigment epithelial neovascularization.[275,407,430,447] Both of these also represent a proliferative response to ischemia and differ from retinal and preretinal neovascularization mainly in location. Rubeosis iridis can occur in almost all of the diseases listed, causing a proliferative retinopathy. It may occur as a result of a space-occupying intraocular mass, including any intraocular tumor or in association with long-standing retinal detachment. It causes the dread complication of neovascular glaucoma.

In the normally developing retina the vascular network is formed by a process of budding from embryonic mesoderm. In the fetus the new vessels ordinarily develop from an advanced matrix of vasoformative mesenchyme, which forms solid cords of endothelial cells that bud out from the parent vessels. The same basic origin is found in neovascularization in the retina (Fig. 8-19). Initially the proliferating buds are within the retina and may be invisible ophthalmoscopically, particularly without the benefit of fluorescein angiography.

The initial anastomoses are intraretinal, but preretinal vascularization occurs when the new vessels break through the internal limiting membrane onto the inner surface of the retina (Fig. 8-20, *B* and *C*). As the new vessels grow into the vitreous, the delicate vessels form a rich plexus of capillaries, or rete mirabile (Fig. 8-19, *B*), for example, the "sea fan" of sickle retinopathy (Fig. 8-34) or the neovascular tufts seen in retinopathy of prematurity (p. 496; Figs. 9-28 and 9-29; Color Plates 9-11 and 9-12). The newly formed channels are extremely delicate and friable, and some histologic evidence indicates that the tight junctions (intercellular bridges of the zonula occludens type) between endothelial cells are absent, thus explaining the fluorescein leakage of new vessels.

Diabetic retinopathy

Diabetes mellitus, which affects about 5% of the population, is the most common cause of proliferative retinopathy.* Because of advances in therapy, the life span of diabetic persons is significantly improved.[25] Relatively mild ocular symptoms, usually related to refractive changes, may occur early in the disease.[305] However, because the occurrence and severity of diabetic retinopathy often relates to duration of the disease, the prevalence of the retinal disease has greatly increased. About 60% of diabetic patients develop retinopathy 15 to 20 years after the initial diagnosis. Women are more commonly affected. Diabetic retinopathy now ranks with glaucoma, macular disease, and cataract as a major cause of blindness in the United States and Europe.

Diabetic retinopathy may be classified into three subgroups: (1) background, or nonproliferative, retinopathy, (2) preproliferative retinopathy, and (3) proliferative retinopathy.*

A. Background retinopathy
  1. Capillary microangiopathy
    a. Microvascular obstructions and permeability changes; nonperfusion of capillaries
    b. Retinal capillary microaneurysms
    c. Basement membrane thickening
    d. Loss of pericytes
    e. Intraretinal microvascular abnormalities (IRMA)
  2. Venous abnormalities: dilatation, duplications, beadings, and central or branch vein obstruction
  3. Intraretinal hemorrhages
  4. Exudates
    a. Hard (yellow, waxy) exudates
    b. Soft "exudates" (cytoid bodies)
  5. Macular changes
    a. Macular edema; progression to macular retinoschisis (cyst) or macular hole
    b. Macular ischemia caused by retinal vascular occlusions
B. Preproliferative retinopathy (any or all of the changes of background diabetic retinopathy plus the following)
  1. Significant venous beading
  2. Cotton-wool exudates
  3. Extensive formation of IRMA
  4. Extensive retinal ischemia
C. Proliferative retinopathy
  1. Neovascularization and fibrous tissue proliferation
    a. Intraretinal
    b. On retinal surface
    c. On surface of optic disc
    d. Elevation of disc or retinal new vessels into vitreous
  2. Vitreous alterations and hemorrhage
  3. Macular disease
  4. Retinal detachment

Background retinopathy. The changes in the nonproliferative, or simple, phase of the disease are intraretinal, while the proliferative, or malignant, phase is largely characterized by preretinal and vitreous involvement. The background changes are the first to occur. They may or may not be followed by preproliferative or proliferative changes.

Capillary microangiopathy. The initial lesion of diabetic retinopathy is a microangiopathy, which by definition primarily affects capillaries, small arterioles, and ven-

---

* References 318, 319, 332, 335, 350, 374, 376–378, 382, 383, 386–388, 390, 391, 398, 400, 403–405, 408, 409, 412, 419, 421, 427, 431, 435, 439, 442, 444, 446, 451, 453, 454, 458, 459, 468, 469.

* References 281, 302, 304, 306, 312, 314, 320, 339, 354, 379, 393, 396, 464, 476.

ules (Fig. 8-21).° Five histopathologically documented changes in small vessels cause major secondary effects.

Microvascular obstructions and permeability changes; nonperfusion of capillaries. The earliest changes are retinal capillary bed obstructions and capillary dropout. The nonperfusion, which is visible by fluorescein angiography (Fig. 8-21, *B*), provides a basis for the hypoxia that later can lead to proliferative changes. Larger areas of ischemia may follow occlusion of a precapillary arteriole; this explains the presence of ophthalmoscopically visible cotton-wool spots (p. 372).

The small-vessel occlusion is often preceded by angiographic evidence of narrowing of the lumen of the arteriole at its origin. This obstruction is caused by mural deposition of PAS-positive plasma derivatives passing through a defective endothelium (plasmatic vasculosis). The abnormal permeability can also be seen angiographically as a staining of the wall of the vessel, or aneurysm, or as frank leakage of fluorescein into the surrounding retina.

Retinal capillary microaneurysms. Microaneurysms often develop adjacent to or surrounding areas of capillary nonperfusion (Fig. 8-21). Patent microaneurysms show positive fluorescence by fluorescein angiography. These can be contrasted with dot hemorrhages or small lipid exudates, which typically do not fluoresce. However, a microaneurysm may hyalinize and become occluded because of deposition of PAS-positive material. It then appears as a yellow or white spot that does not show fluorescence.

Basement membrane thickening. Basement membrane thickening occurs not only in vascular structures (e.g., renal glomeruli and retinal and skeletal muscle capillaries) but also in nonvascular structures (renal tubules and ciliary body epithelium; Figs. 8-31 and 8-32).[474] Progressive basement membrane thickening associated with plasmatic vasculosis probably contributes to the gradual closure of small retinal arterioles described previously (Fig. 8-21) and to nonperfusion of the capillaries that they supply.

Loss of pericytes. The ratio of pericytes to endothelial cells in retinal capillaries of a normal young person is approximately 1:1 (Fig. 8-12). As a normal aging process, a relative decrease of capillary endothelial cells occurs; however, this is reversed in diabetic retinopathy, in which retinal capillary pericytes, or mural cells are gradually lost. Pericytes are normally wrapped about the outer circumference of the vascular channel. They have a contractible function, regulate microvascular blood flow, react to vasoactive substances, and function to provide structural integrity to the vessel.[308,325,475] The loss of pericytes may diminish the carrying out of these functions and may create a weakness in the vessel wall that could provide a partial explanation for the predisposition to formation of aneurysms.

Intraretinal microvascular abnormalities (IRMA). Formation of intraretinal vascular shunts may occur in foci of ischemic retina. Nonleaking or very slowly leaking intraretinal vascular channels—IRMA—indicate a progression toward the preproliferative phase and can be demonstrated by fluorescein angiography.[463] These form as a compensatory response to the hypoxic stimulant.

° References 285–292, 297, 303, 307, 308, 314, 339, 341, 357, 462.

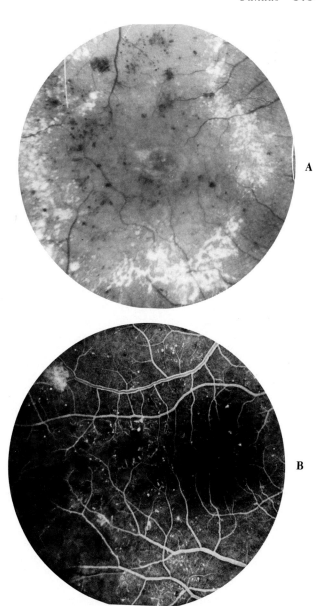

Fig. 8-21. Background diabetic retinopathy. **A,** Severe case with multiple microaneurysms, dot hemorrhages, yellow exudates in a circinate pattern, neurosensory detachment, and macular edema and degeneration. **B,** Fluorescein angiogram from another case, showing distinct, multiple microaneurysms.

Venous abnormalities: dilatation, duplications, beading, and central or branch vein obstruction. Generalized dilatation of the retinal veins is a feature of diabetic retinopathy.[355,1530,1778] Beading and formation of venous loops can occur as a response to local ischemia. This finding is among those that signify a progression toward the preproliferative state. Obstruction of the central vein (p. 390) or of a retinal branch vein (p. 391) may be superimposed on the clinical picture of a diabetic retinopathy or may occur in a diabetic person with little other evidence of retinopathy.

Intraretinal hemorrhages. The initial microvascular changes partially provide a structural basis to explain the more advanced stages of background diabetic retinopathy and proliferative retinopathy. Various types of hemorrhages are important complications (Figs. 8-21 and 8-26; Color Plates 8-5 and 8-6).[423] Flame-shaped hemorrhages assume their characteristic appearance because the blood is deposited in the superficial retina between the nearly parallel coursing fibers of the nerve fiber layer.

The bleeding may break through the inner limiting membrane and form layered preretinal or intravitreal hemorrhages.[329,330] Dot and blot hemorrhages represent focal deposits of blood deposited primarily in the deeper inner nuclear and outer plexiform layers of the retina. As the blood permeates the middle layers, often breaking through the confines of the Müller cell processes, the hemorrhages enlarge and multiple hemorrhages may become confluent.

Exudates. The two kinds of exudate are hard and soft.

Hard (yellow, waxy) exudates. Common sequelae of the microvascular changes in background retinopathy described previously are exudates of the hard, yellow, waxy type, sometimes deposited within Henle's fiber layer in a circinate fashion about the macula, forming a macular star figure (Figs. 8-21, *A*, and 8-22). They consist of proteinaceous and lipid material. They may be derived from exudation of serum components of leaking vessels or from an accumulation of lipid products from degenerating neural elements within the retina. Absorption of hard exudates, primarily mediated by a macrophagic (microglial) resorption (Fig. 8-22, *B*), is sometimes a slow process, often requiring months. This is because they are generally deposited in the outer plexiform layer within the avascular zone of the retina, thereby making drainage of lipid more difficult.

Soft "exudates" (cytoid bodies). Because cotton-wool "exudates" often accompany retinal ischemic processes, it is not surprising that they occur in diabetic retinopathy in or near zones of microvascular occlusion and nonperfusion, particularly in the preproliferative form. The nature and pathogenesis of cytoid bodies is described on page 372.

Macular changes. The pathologic changes in diabetic maculopathy may be divided on an anatomic basis into two broad categories: (1) intraretinal changes, including macular edema and hard exudates (which result from increased retinal vascular permeability) and macular ischemia (Fig. 8-21, *A*) and (2) preretinal and vitreoretinal changes, which are described in the section on proliferative retinopathy.[299,410,443,452,457]

Macular edema; progression to macular retinoschisis (cyst) or macular hole. Microcystoid macular edema, which may significantly worsen the visual prognosis, is best viewed by contact lens examination and fluorescein angiography (Fig. 8-84).* It is caused by severe capillary and neovascular leakage, primarily into the outer plexiform layer (Henle's fiber layer). It may progress to macular retinoschisis and even partial or complete macular hole formation (Figs. 8-87 and 8-88). Edema residues or hard yellow exudates around the macula may lead to the formation of a macular star figure (Fig. 8-9) or circinate retinopathy. Sometimes a marked diffuse edema of the posterior pole

occurs. This is termed *florid diabetic retinopathy* and is usually seen in young juvenile-onset diabetic patients.[350]

Macular ischemia caused by retinal vascular occlusions. An inadequate blood supply leading to macular ischemia may in itself be a cause of decreased vision or may compound the visual problem in an eye with macular edema. The presence of ischemia is confirmed if ophthalmoscopy shows cotton-wool spots or white, attenuated arterioles in or around the macula. Fluorescein angiography is the most accurate method of evaluating the blood supply. A focal capillary dropout or an enlargement of the foveal avascular zone caused by occlusion of perifoveal capillaries or occlusion of larger precapillary arterioles can cause macular ischemia with severe visual loss.

Preproliferative retinopathy. This form of diabetic retinopathy is intermediate between the background and the proliferative forms.* The four major features that characterize preproliferative retinopathy are listed below and illustrated in Fig. 8-23. The characteristics of proliferative retinopathy (Figs. 8-19, 8-20, and 8-24–8-26; Color Plates 8-5 and 8-6) are usually changes superimposed on the changes of background retinopathy described previously. However, the proliferation may occur in the absence of clinically visible background retinopathy.

Proliferative retinopathy.

Neovascularization and fibrous tissue proliferation. The proliferative phase is characterized by the growth of fibrovascular and glial tissue in response to underlying retinal hypoxia and probable release of an angiogenesis factor.†

Associated with these proliferative changes are alterations of the vitreous, which may include retinal wrinkling and macular heterotropia, contraction of the vitreous body, detachment of the posterior hyaloid surface, and thickening of the posterior hyaloid membrane.[300,301] The ultimate disastrous sequelae that may occur are based primarily on two processes: (1) opacification of the vitreous caused by hemorrhage from new vessels (Figs. 8-22–8-24) and dense fibrous or glial tissue formation and (2) detachment of the retina because of traction from the contracting vitreous body.

Neovascularization is almost always found posterior to the equator in diabetic retinopathy, ordinarily on the optic disc and along the course of the major retinal vessels, usually within three disc diameters from the disc (Figs. 8-13, 8-20, and 8-24–8-26; Color Plates 8-5–8-7).

In addition to being a site of predilection for neovascularization, which often grows into Cloquet's canal, retrobulbar neuritis, papillitis, optic disc edema, and optic atrophy may occasionally occur. These are ischemic manifestations of diabetic microangiopathy within the optic nerve head when collateral circulation is inadequate. Transient bilateral optic disc edema and minimal impairment of function may develop in juvenile onset diabetics.

The proliferation begins with the formation of new vessels with very little fibrous tissue component. They arise from primitive mesenchymal elements that differentiate into vascular endothelial cells (Fig. 8-19). The newly

---

* References 351, 384, 426, 443, 459, 530, 1778.

* References 277, 295, 296, 362, 368, 428, 473.

† References 278, 279, 306, 320, 326, 340, 353, 372, 401, 416, 433, 448.

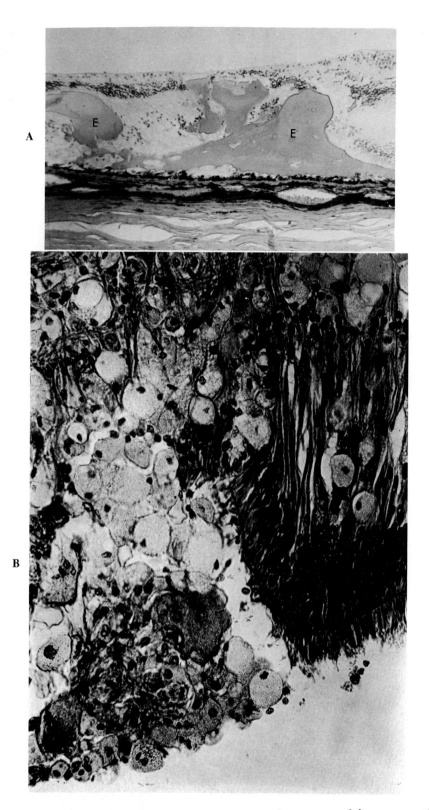

Fig. 8-22. Background diabetic retinopathy. **A,** Extensive degeneration of the sensory retina. *E,* Deposition of exudates within the sensory retina and subretinal space. (H & E stain; ×150.) **B,** Later stage of a deep waxy exudate in diabetic retinopathy than that shown in **A.** In this case the fatty material has been engulfed and is phagocytized by numerous foam cells, forming lipid-laden macrophages. (H & E stain; ×400.) (From Blodi FC and Allen L: Stereoscopic manual of the outer fundus in local and systemic disease, vol I, St. Louis, 1964, The CV Mosby Co.)

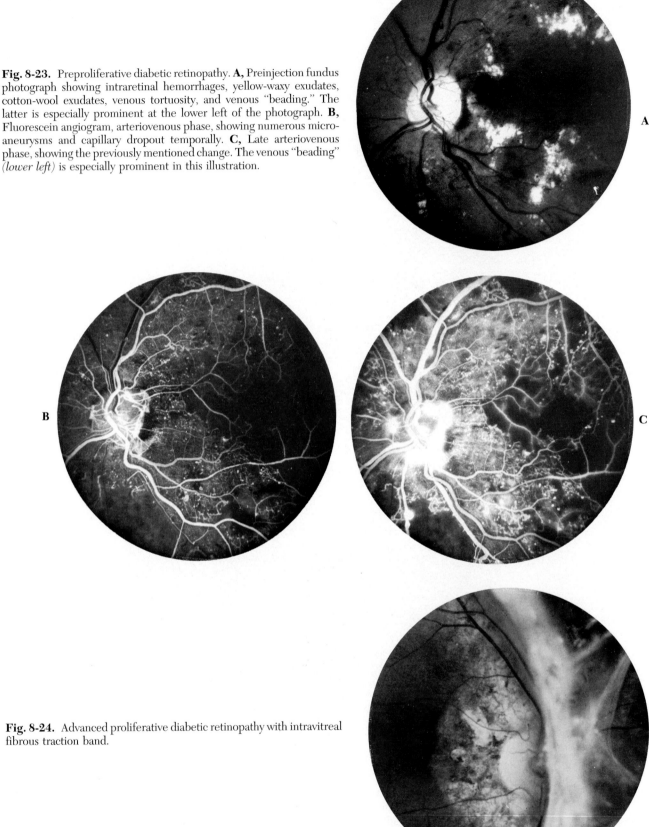

Fig. 8-23. Preproliferative diabetic retinopathy. **A,** Preinjection fundus photograph showing intraretinal hemorrhages, yellow-waxy exudates, cotton-wool exudates, venous tortuosity, and venous "beading." The latter is especially prominent at the lower left of the photograph. **B,** Fluorescein angiogram, arteriovenous phase, showing numerous microaneurysms and capillary dropout temporally. **C,** Late arteriovenous phase, showing the previously mentioned change. The venous "beading" (*lower left*) is especially prominent in this illustration.

Fig. 8-24. Advanced proliferative diabetic retinopathy with intravitreal fibrous traction band.

formed vascular channels, often termed a *rete mirabile* (Fig. 8-19, *B*), then undergo fibrous metaplasia; that is, the angioblastic buds are transformed into fibrous tissue.

The new vessels do not share the permeability characteristics of normal retinal vessels.[463] Thus they leak fluorescein, sometimes so profusely as to rapidly obscure retinal detail during angiography. The new vessels and fibrous tis-

sue break through the internal limiting membrane and arborize at the interface between the internal limiting membrane and the posterior hyaloid membrane (Fig. 8-20, *B* and *C*).

The fibrovascular tissue may form preretinal membranes that create dense adhesions with the posterior hyaloid membrane. The membranes are composed of blood vessels, fibroblasts, glial cells, scattered B and T lymphocytes, and monocytes, along with immunoglobulin, complement deposits, and class II major histocompability complex antigens. These adhesions are extremely important because they are responsible for transmitting the forces of vitreous traction to the retina during the later stage of vitreous shrinkage.

Vitreous alterations and hemorrhage. Before the development of vitreous changes and formation of fibrovascular traction bands, the new vessels remain flat, usually do not bleed, and may produce no symptoms despite extensive fundus disease.[327,328,479] Contraction of the vitreous and detachment of the posterior hyaloid produce elevation of the newly formed fibrovascular tissue caused by the adhesions between these structures (Fig. 8-24). Progressive traction on the fibrovascular tissue may eventually lead to a localized area of retinal detachment. Vitreous traction on the neovascular membranes or on retinal vessels frequently causes avulsion of the vessels, which in turn may lead to vitreous hemorrhage. If the hemorrhage is subhyaloid, it may assume a boat shape with a rounded bottom and a horizontal fluid level (Fig. 8-26). Blood breakdown products may present as hemosiderin-laden macrophages (positive with Prussian Blue stain) (Table 1-1) or cause synchesis scintillans (p. 367). Organization of hemorrhage and gliosis may cause secondary complications such as epiretinal membrane and proliferative vitreoretinopathy (pp. 420 and 421).

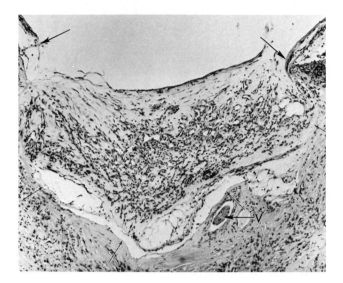

Fig. 8-25. Extensive vascularization of the optic nerve head in a patient with diabetes mellitus. The optic nerve head is deeply cupped as a result of secondary glaucoma. *Small arrows,* Base of the cup, which is filled with numerous capillarylike vascular channels. *V,* Central retina vein containing an artifactitious field of endothelium prolapsed into its lumen. The inner retinal layers are greatly attenuated as they course around the margin of the glaucomatous disc *(large arrows).* (H & E stain; ×175.)

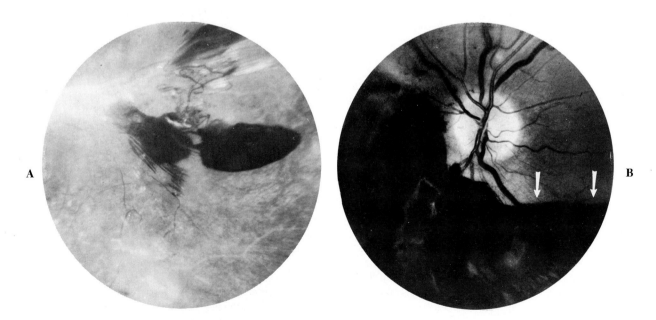

Fig. 8-26. Proliferative diabetic retinopathy. **A,** Focal preretinal hemorrhages from a neovascular membrane. **B,** Massive intravitreal hemorrhage with formation of horizontal fluid level *(arrows)* due to gravity.

Macular disease. In addition to macular edema (Fig. 8-21, *A*), several proliferative changes may compromise macular function[443,452,457]:

1. Progressive thickening of the posterior vitreous can occur on the surface of a slowly resorbing preretinal hemorrhage. If the preretinal hemorrhage covers the macula, the result may be a dense posterior hyaloid membrane that obscures the macula and causes significant visual impairment, even after the blood clears. Persistence of blood in front of the macula may be an indication for vitrectomy to release the trapped blood and to remove the preretinal fibrous tissue.
2. Preretinal membranes may form that may wrinkle the inner retinal surface and cause macular heterotropia ("cellophane" or "surface wrinkling" retinopathy).[300,301] These can be removed by vitrectomy (Fig. 8-20, *B* and *C*).
3. Direct or indirect traction on the macula may lead to detachment of the macula.

Retinal detachment. Retinal detachment at the macula, or peripherally, is a major complication of proliferative retinopathy with or without vitreous hemorrhage. Most retinal detachments resulting from proliferative diabetic retinopathy begin as tractional detachments without holes, but they may become rhegmatogenous by the formation of retinal holes at some later point in the disease. The tractional detachments are caused by abnormal vitreoretinal adhesions with subsequent shrinkage of the fibrous bands and elevation of the retina.

Prognosis and treatment. The course followed by eyes with proliferative diabetic retinopathy is extremely varied and unpredictable.[347,352,369,373,385] Some eyes run a protracted course over many years, developing small areas of neovascularization, repeated small vitreous hemorrhages, and localized areas of traction. Others run a severe course with rapid deterioration of vision resulting from massive proliferative changes, extensive tractional detachment of the retina, and/or large vitreous hemorrhages. A relatively small group may show a spontaneous regression in which the new vessels dry up and the hemorrhagic activity ceases. Optic atrophy and retinal arteriolar attenuation may accompany the regression.

Clinical and experimental evidence suggests that good control of the metabolic aspects of diabetes delays the onset of retinopathy and decreases its severity. Medical agents, for example, clofibrate, may be of some limited use in causing resorption and clearing of edema residues and hard exudates from the retina. Photocoagulation therapy can also induce the resorption of exudate; therefore, a combination of photocoagulation and clofibrate therapy may be more effective than either modality alone. Pituitary ablation may be helpful in maintaining visual acuity in proliferative diabetic retinopathy, but the positive results are relatively short-term and the side effects too severe.

The treatment most widely used today for diabetic retinopathy is panretinal photocoagulation with the argon laser, krypton laser (p. 447). A federally funded study has clearly shown that photocoagulation is beneficial in slowing the course of the disease in many instances.°

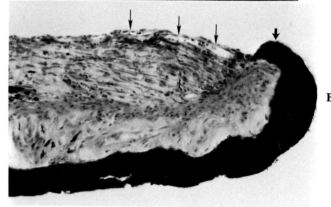

Fig. 8-27. A, Clinical photograph of multiple new vessels on iris surface. **B,** Rubeosis iridis and ectropion uveae in severe diabetic retinopathy. This photomicrograph of the pupillary margin of the iris reveals a proliferation of small, delicate, newly formed vessels on the anterior iris surface *(arrows)*. Rubeosis not only is associated with the various diseases characterized by widespread retinal neovascularization but also is frequently seen in uveitis or in association with intraocular tumors. The fibrovascular membrane eventually contracts and exerts traction on the posterior iris pigment epithelium at the pupillary margin. The shrunken membrane draws the epithelium around the pupillary margin onto the anterior iris surface *(short arrow)*. Ectropion is visible clinically as a black rim encircling pupillary margin. *I,* Iris stroma. (H & E stain; ×245.)

Effects of diabetes mellitus on other eye tissues. [283,356]Conjunctival microaneurysms may occur, but these are not pathognomonic. Lipid imbibition into the walls of conjunctival capillaries can be seen by biomicroscopy. Rubeosis iridis, or iris neovascularization, is not only frequently associated with proliferative diabetic retinopathy (Figs. 8-28) but also occurs in several diverse conditions.° It has many causes.

1. Diabetes mellitus and other forms of proliferative retinopathy
2. Central retinal vein occlusion
   a. Central retinal artery occlusion (rare)
   b. Temporal arteritis
   c. Carotid artery disease
   d. Ocular ischemic syndrome

° References 281, 316, 392, 477, 478.

° References 283, 306, 320, 340, 354, 371, 395, 417, 422, 430, 434, 447, 465.

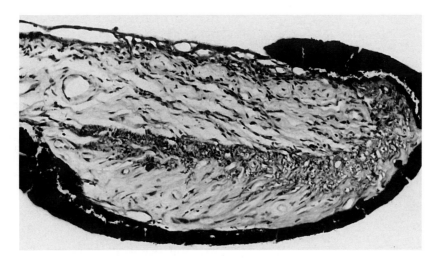

Fig. 8-28. High power photomicrograph showing advanced rubeosis iridis (*small channels on surface*), with migration of pigment onto the anterior surface ectropion uveae (*large arrows*). (H & E stain; ×100.)

3. Neoplastic
   a. Uveal malignant melanoma
   b. Retinoblastoma
   c. Metastatic carcinoma (uveal)
   d. Embryonal medulloepthelioma
   e. Metastatic tumors
4. Chronic uveitis, Fuchs' heterochromic iridocyclitis
   a. Fungal endophthalmitis
5. Chronic glaucoma
6. Posttrauma (surgical or nonsurgical)
   a. Postretinal detachment surgery
   b. Postradiation therapy
7. Childhood diseases
   a. Coats' disease
   b. Persistent hyperplastic primary vitreous
   c. Leber's military microaneurysms
   d. Norrie's disease
8. Chronic retinal detachment

The stimulus for new vessel formation is probably caused by an angiogenic factor released by the retina.[276,277] The fibrovascular membrane is situated on the anterior surface of the iris stroma. Ectropion uveae (Fig. 8-27 and Figs. 8-29–8-32) commonly results from contraction or shrinkage of the fibrovascular membrane. The shrunken membrane exerts traction on the iris pigment epithelium, which in turn contracts and pulls the epithelium around the pupillary margin.[370] Rubeosis occurring within the angle itself can cause secondary closed-angle glaucoma (neovascular glaucoma).[461] This is a result of anterior synechiae formation and hemorrhage into the angle from the delicate newly formed iris vessels. Diabetic persons have an increased incidence of chronic simple glaucoma.

Lacy vacuolation of the iris pigment epithelium is a relatively unusual but highly characteristic finding (Figs. 8-29 and 8-30).[311,323,414,456] It usually occurs in association with high blood sugar levels, that is, it correlates directly with an elevation of serum glucose. The intraepithelial vacuoles contain glycogen. Irritation of these vacuoles during ante-

rior chamber surgery results in a release of iris epithelial pigment into the posterior chamber (so-called Schwarzwasser or black water); the pigment may be seen flowing as a stream through the pupil into the anterior chamber.

The basement membrane of the ciliary pigmented epithelium often shows a diffuse thickening (Fig. 8-31).[324,474] This finding is not surprising, because capillary basement membrane thickening is also a major finding in retinal microangiopathy. A similar thickening of capillary basement membrane sometimes occurs within skeletal muscles. In equivocal cases, a tissue diagnosis of diabetes mellitus may be obtained by gastrocnemius muscle biopsy.

The thickening of the ciliary epithelial basement membrane should not be confused with the process of hyalinization of the entire stroma of the ciliary processes that occurs as a nonspecific aging process or as a degenerative change following chronic diseases such as glaucoma (Fig. 6-27).[411]

Corneal epithelium and its basement membrane may be abnormal, epithelial lesions are common, corneal sensation and tear production may be reduced, and the stroma may be thickened. Decreased penetration of "anchoring" fibrils from the corneal epithelial basement membrane into the corneal stroma may be responsible for the loose adhesion between the corneal epithelium and the stroma.[*]

Refractive changes in the lens from osmotic causes are well documented and usually consist of a transient myopia during periods of hyperglycemia.[305] In juvenile patients the snowflake cataract consists of subcapsular opacities with vacuoles and chalky white cortical deposits, or flakes.[399] The incidence and progression of adult age-related cataracts are increased in diabetic patients.[†] Aldose reductase may play a role in diabetic cataracts. The histopathologic findings are similar to those of the age-related cataract discussed in Chapter 4 (Fig. 8-30).

Kidney and systemic vascular changes. The histopathologic correlation is high between the microan-

---

[*] References 291, 358, 359, 375, 445, 449, 460.
[†] References 317, 360, 361, 380, 381, 455, 466.

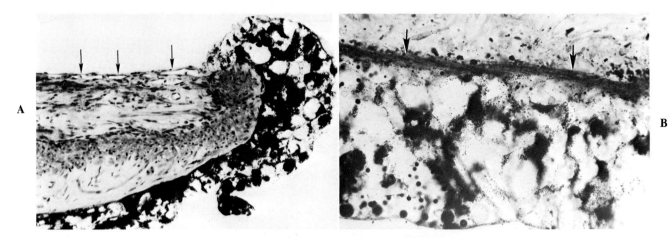

Fig. 8-29. A, Photomicrograph of the iris in a patient with long-standing diabetes mellitus and diabetic retinopathy. Three noteworthy findings are evident: (1) "lacy" vacuolation of the posterior pigment epithelial layers caused by infiltration by glycogen; (2) rubeosis iridis (note the formation of delicate, thin-walled vessels on the anterior iris surface, *arrows*); and (3) ectropion uveae caused by pulling on the iris pigment epithelium at the pupillary margin by the contracting fibrovascular membrane. The marginal pigment epithelium is drawn around the pupillary margin onto the anterior iris surface. (H & E stain; ×200.) **B,** Higher power photomicrograph of "lacy" vacuolation showing glycogen droplets within the posterior iris epithelium. *Arrows,* Dilator muscle. (PAS stain; ×350.)

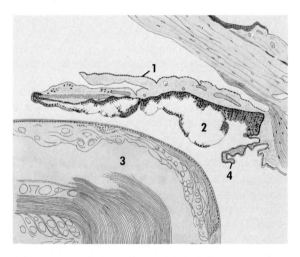

Fig. 8-30. One of the earliest published illustrations showing many of the important anterior segment complications of diabetes. *1,* Rubeosis iridis; *2,* "lacy" vacuolation of iris pigment epithelium; *3,* diabetic cortical cataract; *4,* thickening of the ciliary body epithelial basement membrane. (Redrawn by Dr. Steven Vermillion, University of Iowa, from Kamocki, 1887. Cited by Ginsburg S: In Henke F and Lubarsch O, editors: Handbuch der speziellen pathologischen Anatomie und Histologie, Berlin, 1928, Julius Springer.)

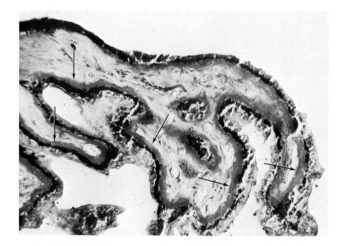

Fig. 8-31. The ciliary processes (pars plicata or corona ciliaris) of the eye of a 37-year-old patient with juvenile diabetes. The marked thickening of the basement membrane *(arrows)* of the ciliary pigment epithelium is highly characteristic of this disease. Normally this basement membrane is extremely thin and would be only faintly visible at this magnification. (PAS stain; ×175.)

giopathic changes observed in diabetic retinopathy and microvascular changes observed in diabetic nephropathy (Kimmelstiel-Wilson disease, or nodular glomerulosclerosis; Fig. 8-32).[334] Clinically visible retinal microangiographic changes usually connote the simultaneous occurrence of small vessel disease of the kidneys that may induce either subclinical or clinically manifest renal insufficiency.

The onset of generalized arteriosclerosis occurs at a younger age in diabetic persons than in the general population, with a sharp increase in incidence beyond age 50.

Retinal arterial macroaneurysms. Because retinal arterial macroaneurysms are considered in the differential diagram of background diabetic retinopathy with microaneurysms, they are described here.[389,391,432]

Aneurysms of the retinal vasculature occur in many systemic and ocular disease states, most commonly diabetes and the retinal telangiectasias, which include the diseases of Coats and Leber (pp. 493 and 496).[437] Aneurysmal changes are also seen with von Hippel angiomatosis, retinal

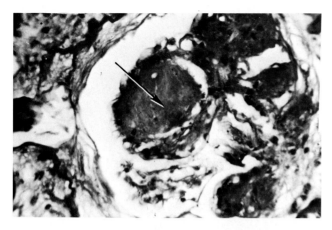

Fig. 8-32. Nodular glomerulosclerosis (Kimmelstiel-Wilson disease) of the kidney in a patient with diabetes mellitus. The PAS-positive nodules of basement membrane-like material *(arrow)* within the glomerulus are highly characteristic of diabetic nephropathy. (PAS stain; ×400.)

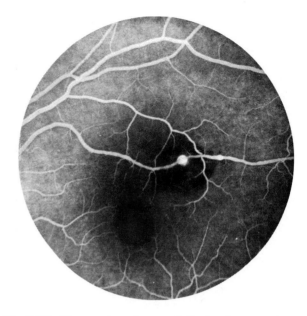

Fig. 8-33. Fluorescein angiogram of a fundus demonstrating two macroaneurysms involving the superior temporal artery.

vein occlusion, retinal arteritis, Eales' disease, cytomegalovirus retinitis, radiation retinopathy, sickle cell retinopathy, Takayasu's disease, and the hyperviscosity and aortic arch syndromes.

The first published report of an isolated retinal artery aneurysm was by Loring in 1880, in which he described a "peculiar bulging" within the first bifurcation of a retinal artery in an otherwise healthy 26-year-old man with normal vision and no other ocular abnormalities.[437]

Retinal arterial macroaneurysms represent a distinct clinical entity. Macroaneurysms are most commonly seen in the elderly with a marked female predominance and a strong association with hypertension and arteriosclerotic vascular changes. Most cases are unilateral.

Although acute loss of vision is the most common presenting symptom, patients with retinal arterial macroaneurysms may be visually asymptomatic, with the abnormality found only on routine funduscopic examination. If there is macular involvement with exudation, edema, or hemorrhage or if vitreous hemorrhage is present, patients may complain of insidious or sudden onset of decreased vision. Patients may also describe central shadows, scotomas, or floating spots.

Ophthalmoscopic examination typically reveals round or fusiform, sometimes pulsatile, dilations of the arterial wall (Fig. 8-33; Color Plates 8-8–8-10); however, they may be enlarged up to several times the size of the artery. Multiple macroaneurysms, either along the same or a different artery, are present in up to 20% of cases. Macroaneurysms are most commonly located along the temporal arcade arteries.

Approximately 50% of patients have an associated retinal hemorrhage surrounding the macroaneurysm. Subretinal, preretinal, or vitreous hemorrhages are usually seen in association with intraretinal hemorrhage. Subretinal hemorrhage may mimic a disciform process, a choroidal melanoma, and unusual cystic retinal lesions, vitreous hemorrhages, secondary to arterial macroaneurysmal rupture, have been reported in approximately 10% of cases.

Generalized arteriolar narrowing and irregularity and mild-to-marked arteriovenous crossing changes are frequently observed with macroaneurysms. The presence of a circinate ring should prompt a search for a leaking lesion in the center. Infrequently, macular edema without a lipid response is also observed. Neurosensory retinal detachment can frequently be seen surrounding a macroaneurysm, usually in association with edema, hemorrhage, or exudate. If the macroaneurysm is close enough to the fovea, the retinal detachment may be a cause of decreased vision.

An exudative retinopathy, consisting of intraretinal yellow or white ("hard") lipid deposits, is a common finding (Color Plate 8-9). Frequently, these deposits adopt a circinate pattern surrounding the macroaneurysm but may also appear as a dense accumulation of lipid exudate in the macular region, irrespective of the location of the macroaneurysm.

Retinal arterial macroaneurysms may remain stationary over long periods. Eventually, the majority follow a course of thrombosis, fibrosis, and spontaneous involution with a return to, or preservation of, prior visual function.[437] However, extensive hemorrhagic activity may be present because of a ruptured lesion or blood oozing from a small dehiscence in the wall of the aneurysm (Color Plate 8-10). The ultimate prognosis often depends on the location of the hemorrhage and exudate or the severity and duration of macular involvement.

Intraretinal hemorrhages generally resolve completely, with little or no effect on vision. Similarly, vitreous hemorrhages gradually resorb over 6 to 10 weeks, with visual function returning to normal or near normal in the vast majority of cases. Vitreous floaters may persist because of incomplete resorption of vitreous hemorrhage, recurrent hemorrhage, or chronic structural changes induced by blood in the vitreous. Hemorrhages in the preretinal space generally resolve, and prior visual acuity is resumed; however, epiretinal membrane formation can result in incomplete visual recovery and metamorphopsia.

Hemorrhages in the subretinal space may produce secondary morphologic changes within the macula, causing permanent architectural damage to the retinal pigment epithelium and photoreceptors, usually resulting in permanent central visual loss.

The macular exudative response may resolve with involution of the macroaneurysm, but most often such a response results in permanent structural damage. Late complications resulting from chronic macular edema include epiretinal membrane, cystoid macular edema, and macular hole formation. Chronic macular edema and structural damage from macular exudate are the most common causes of poor visual outcome in patients with retinal arterial macroaneurysms.

Histopathologically, aneurysmal sites typically show thickening of the vessel wall secondary to a fibrinlaminated clot with accompanying hypertrophy of the muscularis. Hyaline deposits, hemorrhage, and occasional foamy macrophages may be seen in the vessel wall. Commonly a fresh or organized thrombus partially fills the aneurysm. Cholesterol crystals are frequently seen, suggesting the possibility of embolization. Thickened hyaline walls are common in the arterioles adjacent to the macroaneurysm. The surrounding retina may show dilation of the capillary bed, edema, fatty exudate, hemorrhage, and secondary photoreceptor degeneration.

Trypsin digest studies have demonstrated four types of aneurysmal changes (Color Plate 8-11): (1) round ones at sites of large-vessel branching, (2) small "cuff-type" aneurysms on smaller arteries or arterioles (Color Plate 8-8), (3) large, single, "blowout" aneurysms, ranging from 70 to 75 mm, and (4) loops formed by fusion of adjacent blowout aneurysms. Blowout aneurysms appear as linear splits along the vessel wall through which the aneurysmal sac protrudes.

Histopathologic findings support the pathogenetic hypothesis that focal arterial wall damage produced by embolic or occlusive disease may predispose hypertensive patients to formation of arterial aneurysms.

Macroaneurysms have been termed a *masquerade syndrome*. They can mimic other ocular diseases and have been frequently misdiagnosed. The differential diagnosis includes diabetic retinopathy, retinal telangiectasia, venous macroaneurysms or retinal vein occlusion, angiomatosis retinae, retinal cavernous hemangioma, age-related macular degeneration with macular disciform scar, idiopathic vitreous hemorrhage, idiopathic preretinal gliosis, and malignant melanoma.

The natural history is usually one of gradual and spontaneous involution with good visual prognosis in the majority of cases; however, complications of retinal or vitreous hemorrhage and macular edema, with resultant loss of vision, can occur.

Treatment is recommended when there is visual loss as a result of macular edema, macular exudate, serous neurosensory retinal detachment, or recurrent vitreous hemorrhage. It remains unclear whether indirect treatment is superior to direct treatment and whether dye of yellow

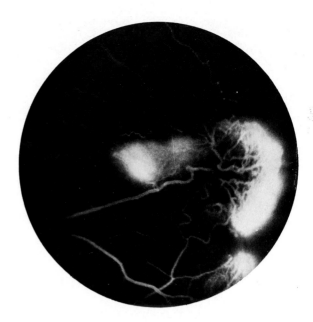

Fig. 8-34. Sickle retinopathy. This fluorescein pattern of the "sea fan" occurs particularly in SC and S-thal hemoglobinopathy. The peripheral focus of neovascularization arises in response to retinal arteriolar occlusions (microthrombi), which produce ischemia in the immediate area. The ischemia process apparently stimulates formation of arteriovenous anastomoses and new vessels. (Courtesy Dr. Morton F. Goldberg.)

wave length is preferable to argon green or blue-green wave lengths.[*]

Sickle retinopathy

Goldberg[344–346] has emphasized that sickle cell disease is a significant cause of retinopathy (Figs. 8-34–8-36; Color Plate 8-11).[†] This finding does not reflect the fact that the disease has become more common; rather it signifies increased awareness by ophthalmologists and internists that ocular involvement may occur in this disease. Although perifoveal capillary-arteriolar occlusion may occasionally lead to impairment of central visual acuity (Fig. 8-36), with rare exceptions sickle retinopathy is more commonly characterized by midperipheral or peripheral retinal lesions, including arteriolar occlusions, neovascularization, proliferative retinopathy, and preretinal hemorrhage.[‡] This condition has certain similarities to Eales' disease (discussed later), in which the majority of tissue changes primarily occur in the peripheral fundus. Many cases diagnosed in the past as Eales' disease in black persons were probably sickle retinopathy.

Sickle cell disease affecting the eye may occur in sickle cell disease, sickle cell thalassemia (S-thal), and is often particularly severe in sickle cell–hemoglobin C (SC) disease (Figs. 8-35 and 8-36). The classification proposed by Goldberg[344] defines five stages that concisely indicate the

---

[*] References 298, 309, 315, 336, 337, 343–346, 349, 362, 363, 402, 406, 424, 425, 429, 437, 438, 441.
[†] References 298, 309, 315, 336–338, 343, 348, 349, 362–365, 402, 406, 413, 424, 425, 429, 436, 438, 441.
[‡] References 331, 336, 362, 414, 424, 429.

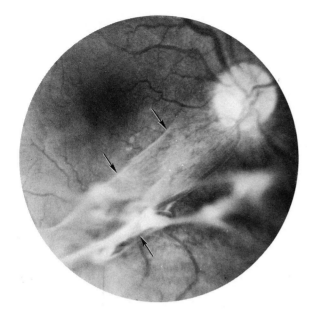

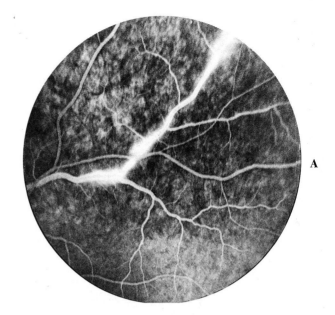

Fig. 8-35. Proliferative retinopathy *(arrows)* from a patient with SC hemoglobinopathy. Involvement of the posterior pole as illustrated here is less common than involvement of the midperiphery.

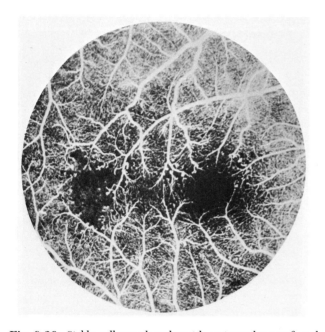

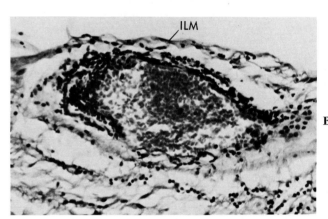

Fig. 8-37. Eales' disease. **A,** Fluorescein angiogram showing leakage of an affected venule. **B,** Photomicrograph of a retinal venule. Infiltration of deeply staining round cells (primarily lymphocytes) has occurred within and around the vessel wall. The lumen of the vessel is greatly congested, and degeneration of the affected sensory retina about the vessel is advanced. *ILM,* Internal limiting membrane. (H & E stain; ×200.)

Fig. 8-36. Sickle cell maculopathy with an irregular parafoveal avascular zone, venular hairpin loops, and capillary telangiectasia. Vascular occlusion of terminal arterioles may lead to impairment of central visual acuity.

important changes occurring during the pathogenesis of sickle retinopathy (Fig. 8-37):

Stage I	Arteriolar occlusions
Stage II	Arteriolovenous anastomoses
Stage III	Neovascularization
Stage IV	Vitreous hemorrhage
Stage V	Retinal detachment

Stage I consists of peripheral arteriolar occlusions with formation of ghost vessels (silver wiring). The peripheral small arterioles are presumably obstructed by microthrombi and/or lodgment of clusters of erythrocytes within the vessel. Because of an increase in viscosity of the blood and resultant stagnation of blood flow, the formed elements tend to adhere to one another. The resultant zones of ischemic, avascular retina are first seen in the peripheral (equatorial) retina, but the process spreads in a centripetal manner, so that the area of involvement tends to move toward the posterior pole.

Stages II (peripheral arteriolovenous anastomoses) and III (neovascular and fibrous proliferation; Figs. 8-34 and 8-35) are probably compensatory phenomena in which the retinal vasculature attempts to compensate for the relative ischemia induced by the peripheral arteriolar occlusions. These newly formed channels arise in patches of ischemic retina, presumably in response to hypoxic stimuli. The "sea fan" (Fig. 8-34) is a highly characteristic clinical sign, which reveals a striking fluorescein angiographic pattern. The neovascular tufts that form on the inner surface of the retina and invade the vitreous cavity are similar in pathogenesis and morphology to those of diabetic and other proliferative retinopathies. However, the peripheral localization of the proliferative process usually seen in sickle retinopathy differs from the more posteriorly located neovascular processes that involve the paramacular region and optic disc in most cases of diabetic retinopathy. The "sea fan" is most commonly associated with SC and S-thal hemoglobinopathy.

Stage IV (vitreous hemorrhage) and stage V (retinal detachment) are natural sequelae of the proliferative phase of the disease. These sequelae are similar to those in advanced cases of diabetic retinopathy.

Two distinctive fundus lesions, salmon patches and black sunbursts, are highly characteristic, if not pathognomonic, of sickle retinopathy. They appear to be caused by subretinal, intraretinal, or preretinal hemorrhage.

The salmon patch (Color Plate 8-11), a well-circumscribed, slightly elevated, red-orange retinal lesion, is most commonly found in the midperiphery of the fundus. This lesion is usually caused by hemorrhage within the superficial (inner) layers of the retina immediately beneath the internal limiting membrane. The color is due to extravasated blood deposited immediately below the inner limiting membrane. As the salmon patch resorbs, a schisis cavity forms between the internal limiting membrane and the remaining retina. Iridescent spots, which may be striking by ophthalmoscopy, are created by reflection of light from hemosiderin-laden macrophages, which collect in the inner retina after degradation of the blood.

The black sunburst sign consists of a round, sharply circumscribed, hyperpigmented chorioretinal scar in the peripheral fundus, which probably reflects hemorrhage into deeper layers of the retina than is seen with the salmon patch. The deep pigmentation of the lesion results from the combined presence of hemosiderin-laden macrophages and, more important, increased density of the pigment epithelial melanin. The deep permeation of extravasated blood probably stimulates a reactive hyperplasia of the pigment epithelium. When melanin pigment migrates into the sensory retina, it may collect around vessels producing a focal bone spicule pattern similar to that seen in some of the inherited pigmentary retinopathies.

An eye with proliferative sickle retinopathy rarely shows spontaneous regression of neovascular lesions. The natural course of this condition thus reflects a progressive chain of events, in many cases leading ultimately to retinal detachment (stage V). Intervention by xenon arc or argon laser photocoagulation can retard or postpone the progression of the disease.

Eales' disease

Eales' disease generally affects young men and is usually diagnosed in the second or third decade of life.[321,471] It is relatively uncommon in the United States, but for unexplained reasons it is extremely common, almost endemic, in India. Generally Eales' disease is not associated with systemic disease and, although tuberculosis has been implicated, a consistent factor responsible for the pathogenesis of the condition has not been determined.

The eye involvement is usually unilateral, and the patient suffers from intermittent episodes of decreased vision. This decrease is sometimes a result of haziness in the vitreous caused by hemorrhage from newly formed retinal vessels. The retinal vascular involvement, a periphlebitis (Fig. 8-37), is especially severe in the periphery of the fundus. Common complications of Eales' disease include peripheral retinal neovascularization and recurrent peripheral intravitreous hemorrhage. The distribution of peripheral retinal neovascularization is similar to that of sickle retinopathy.

RETINAL VASCULAR OCCLUSIONS

Hayreh[515–519,521,571] has proposed the following terminology for central retinal vascular occlusions.[479–579]

1. Ischemic retinopathy, caused by a temporary or prolonged stoppage of circulation in the central retinal artery (commonly referred to as a central retinal artery occlusion)
2. Venous stasis retinopathy, caused by occlusion of the central retinal vein alone, unaccompanied by total or incomplete occlusion of the central retinal artery (sometimes termed incipient or impending central retinal vein occlusion)
3. Hemorrhagic retinopathy, caused by occlusion of the central retinal vein associated with partial or total central retinal arterial involvement and retinal ischemia (commonly called central retinal vein occlusion)

Ischemic retinopathy

Ischemic retinopathy, or occlusion of the central retinal artery (Figs. 8-38 and 8-39; Color Plates 8-12 and 8-13), is typically associated with a sudden onset of unilateral amaurosis.* The retinal circulation may reestablish itself within a few hours or days, and in some cases the retinal ischemia may be transitory or partial because the artery is only partially occluded.

Sudden occlusion of the central retinal artery produces a predictable clinical picture (Figs. 8-38 and 8-39; Color Plates 8-12 and 8-13). Ischemic necrosis of the retina is caused by direct obstruction of its nutritive blood supply. The decreased retinal blood flow leads to cloudy swelling, edema, and necrosis, all of which cause a diminution of the red reflex. Hayreh and Weingeist[522,523] have shown in monkeys that irreversible retinal damage occurs within 90 minutes of total arterial occlusion (Figs. 8-38–8-41).

In a total central artery occlusion the whitish discoloration affects the entire fundus, with the exception of a foveal cherry-red spot (Figs. 8-38 and 8-42; Color Plates 8-12 and 8-13). This red circular area can be easily explained, because the foveal retina is normally thinned and avascular and the underlying choriocapillaris channels that normally nourish the fovea are intact. The foveal retina, which is not dependent on the central retinal artery and is, therefore, not infarcted, remains transparent and transmits the red reflex from the choroid. This contrasts with the remainder of the infarcted eyegrounds where the gray discoloration of the retina partially obscures the normal red reflex of the pigment epithelium and choriocapillaris.

---

* References 367, 480, 482, 488, 489, 499, 501, 531, 532, 535, 538, 547, 556, 563, 566, 577, 578.

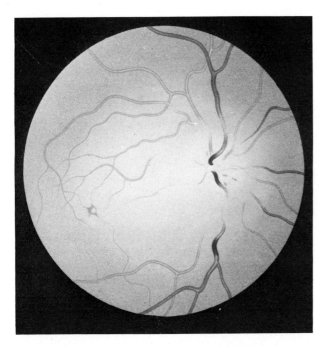

Fig. 8-38. Early fundus drawing of artist's conception of an embolic central retinal artery occlusion showing the attenuation of arterioles and retinal pallor. (From Oeller J: Atlas seltener ophthalmoskopischer Befunde, Wiesbaden, 1903, JF Bergmann.)

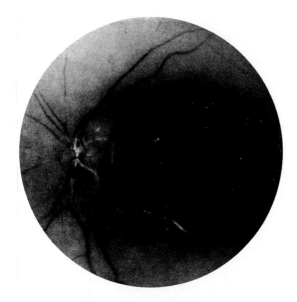

Fig. 8-39. Central retinal artery occlusion. Fluorescein angiogram, 49 seconds after injection, showing only minimal perfusion of some of the arterioles. (From Blodi FC, Allen L, and Frazier O: Stereoscopic manual of the ocular fundus in local and systemic disease, vol II, St. Louis, 1970, The CV Mosby Co.)

The cherry-red spot in arterial occlusion should be differentiated from the cherry-red spot of the lipid storage diseases, or gangliosidoses (p. 423; Fig. 8-82). In the latter group of diseases, lipid accumulates within the ganglion cells occurring throughout the retina. The lipid deposits produce a gray-white discoloration of the fundus, particu-

larly around the borders of the fovea where the ganglion cell layer is stratified. However, because the foveola is devoid of ganglion cells, lipid deposits at this site are necessarily absent and the normal red reflex is retained.

An occlusion of a branch arteriole supplying a quadrant or quadrants of the fundus (Fig. 8-40) may cause similar fundus changes corresponding to the sector supplied by the vessel. Figure 8-40 shows an occlusion in the inferior temporal quadrant of the left eye in which the "cloudy swelling" is confined to that region. Color Plate 8-14 illustrates an ischemic necrosis affecting the entire inferior aspect of the fundus and caused by arterial occlusion supplying this region.

As noted on p. 365, the macula is sometimes supplied by a cilioretinal artery that appears at the temporal optic disc.[487] In 15% of patients, the supply from this artery is the primary nourishment to the macular region. The presence of this vessel may be a blessing or a curse. In cases of central retinal artery occlusion in which a cilioretinal artery is present, the macular region may be spared, with reasonable retention of visual acuity (Fig. 8-41). In instances of occlusion of the cilioretinal artery itself (Color Plate 8-15), the ischemic and necrotic process may be totally confined to the macular region, leading to devastating visual loss in the presence of an otherwise normal retina (Fig. 8-42).

Most central retinal artery occlusions occur just before emergence of the artery from the nerve head into the retina. At this point the artery retains the structure of a true artery and is, therefore, susceptible to atherosclerosis. The atherosclerotic changes here differ very little from similar changes seen in other major arteries of the body, such as the aorta, the coronary arteries, or the cerebral arteries, but they do differ from the arteriolar narrowing observed in the fundus vessels in hypertensive and arteriolosclerotic retinopathy (Fig. 8-17). After branching of the central retinal artery into the four major fundus vessels, the channels diminish in diameter, lose a large portion of their muscular coat and internal elastic lamina, and are, therefore, categorized as arterioles. Embolization from a distant source is a very important cause of central, branch, and cilioretinal arterial occlusion.*

Examination of the occluded artery in the optic nerve may show evidence of atherosclerosis (Fig. 8-43). This is histologically manifest by such features as proliferation of the vascular endothelium and deposition of foamy lipid-laden histiocytes within the vessel lumen. Older, longstanding lesions show organization of the intraluminal contents, with formation of calcareous fibrous plaques (Fig. 10-19) or cholesterol clefts, which represent the residua of the intraluminal lipid deposits.

The acute visual loss typical of ischemic retinopathy follows the formation of a platelet-fibrin thrombus within the already compromised lumen of the atherosclerotic vessel. Stagnation and increased turbulence of flow are largely responsible for superimposition of the thrombus on the atherosclerotic plaque (Fig. 8-43). This is essentially the same mechanism that follows acute blockage of atherosclerotic coronary and cerebral vessels. The superimposition of

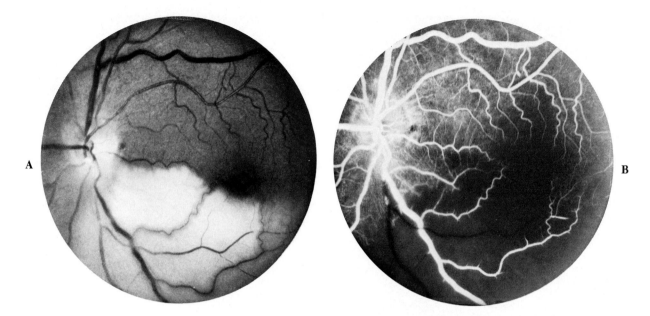

Fig. 8-40. A, Occlusion of the inferior temporal branch arteriole leading to retinal necrosis and "cloudy swelling" to the quadrant supplied by that vessel. **B,** Fluorescein angiogram of the same case during the venous phase showing the occluded inferior temporal arteriole and its branches and lack of blood flow to this region.

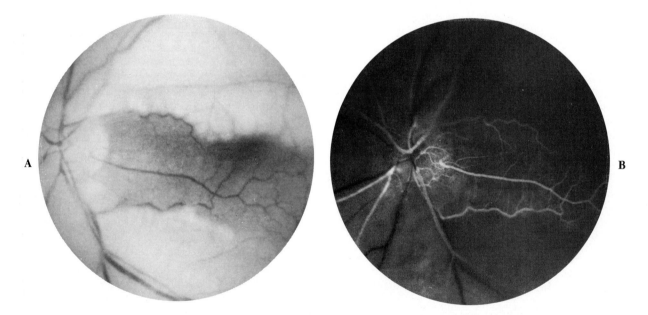

Fig. 8-41. A, Fundus photograph of an occlusion of the central retinal artery in the presence of a patent cilioretinal artery that supplies the macula and, in this case, has led to sparing of the macular region. Note the retention of the red reflex at the posterior pole as opposed to dense cloudy swelling throughout the outer quadrants of the fundus. **B,** Fluorescein angiogram from the same case, very early arterial phase, showing beginning filling of the retinal arterioles but complete filling of the cilioretinal artery supplying the macular region. The latter vessel fills early during the choroidal phase because it is derived from the choroidal (ciliary) circulation.

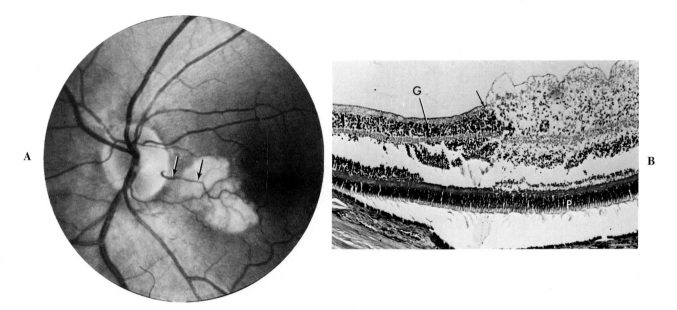

Fig. 8-42. A, Occlusion of the cilioretinal artery *(arrows)*, which has recanalized at this stage. Cloudy swelling and necrosis of the involved area has occurred. **B,** Presumed occlusion of the cilioretinal artery. *Arrow,* Junction of the normal macula *(left)* with the necrotic retina *(right)*. The edema and necrosis primarily involve the inner retina, with relative sparing of photoreceptors *(P)*. G, Thickened ganglion cell layer, indicative of the macular region. (**A** courtesy Dr. Victor Zion; **B** courtesy Dr. Jerry Kobrin, University of Iowa.)

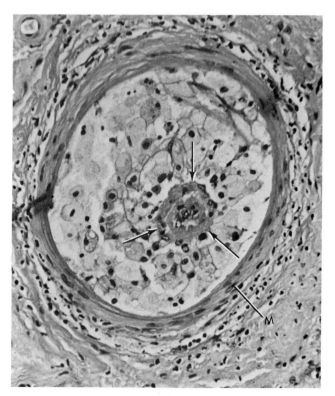

Fig. 8-43. Photomicrograph of the occluded central retinal artery in the optic nerve. The artery is identified by the presence of the thick, muscular coat *(M)*. The lumen contains round-to-oval pale cells, which exhibit a clear cytoplasm and distinct, deeply staining, round nuclei. These cells are proliferating, lipid-laden endothelial cells and macrophages. These elements signify a primary atherosclerotic process. *Arrows,* A central area of dense-staining material representing a focus of acute thrombosis with deposition of fibrin and platelets. This acute insult, which totally occludes the already compromised lumen, is responsible for the acute clinical course characteristic of most central retinal artery occlusions. The thrombus is induced by stagnation of flow and increased turbulence of flow through the constricted lumen. (H & E stain; ×275.)

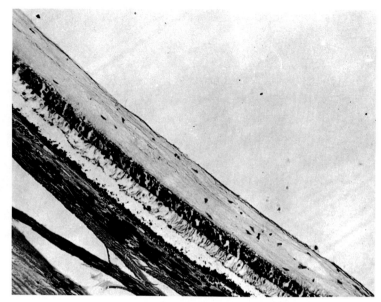

Fig. 8-44. Anemic infarct of the retina caused by occlusion of the central retinal artery. The inner layers of the retina are atrophic and devoid of viable cells and fibers. The outer layers (rods and cones), which derive their blood supply by diffusion from the choriocapillaris, are not affected. (H & E stain; ×120.) (From Blodi FC and Allen L: Stereoscopic manual of the ocular fundus in local and systemic disease, vol I, St. Louis, 1964, The CV Mosby Co.)

a thrombus with sudden occlusion of the vessel is similarly responsible for the acute nature of a myocardial infarction or a cerebrovascular accident.

Treatment with means such as aqueous paracentesis, massage, ocular hypotensive agents, anticoagulants, and vasodilators has been largely unsuccessful in the majority of cases.

The retinal ischemia and necrosis first affects the inner retinal layers (Figs. 8-42 and 8-44).* This is predictable because these inner layers were formerly supplied by the now-occluded vessel (p. 364; Fig. 8-2, *B*). The cellular elements are rapidly destroyed and resorbed. Normal and necrotic portions of the retina are easily compared in Fig. 8-42, *B*. The sharp demarcation between normal and affected retina in the macular region conforms to the borders of a region supplied by an occluded cilioretinal artery (on the right) and one of the major retinal arterial branches (on the left).[487]

Usually an infarction of the nerve fiber layer and ganglion cells occurs, and the inner nuclear layer and adjacent plexiform layers undergo varying degrees of destruction.[499] The photoreceptor cells remain intact in early stages because of retention of choriocapillaris nourishment; however, late in the course of the disease even the outer portions of the retina atrophy. Replacement gliosis is minimal in most cases of central retinal artery occlusion; therefore, as the necrotic tissue is resorbed, extensive thinning of the retina typically occurs. Neovascularization is a rare complication, particularly if carotid arterial insufficiency is concomitant.[488,574]

Venous stasis and hemorrhagic retinopathies

Experimental and clinical studies by Hayreh[515–518] have shown that central retinal vein occlusion consists of two distinct entities—venous stasis retinopathy and hemor-

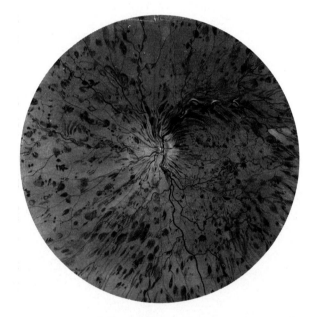

Fig. 8-45. Turn-of-the-century artist's drawing of a central vein occlusion (hemorrhagic retinopathy). (From the collection of Professor Wolfgang Stock, University of Tübingen, Tübingen, Germany.)

rhagic retinopathy—which differ in their clinical picture, prognosis, and management (Figs. 8-45–8-49; Color Plate 8-16).* Most cases are actually venous stasis retinopathy; hemorrhagic retinopathy is a comparatively (Figs. 8-45–8-47) uncommon disease. Diagnosis of each is made by evaluating a combination of symptoms, visual acuity, visual fields, ophthalmoscopic picture, and fluorescein angiographic appearance (Table 8-1). The findings in some patients fall into the gray zone between these two types.

---

* References 511, 555 (for an unusual syndrome of outer retinal ischemic infarction), 483, 494, 500, 502, 510, 512, 513, 515–518, 539–542, 545, 546, 553, 563, 570, 572.

* References 483, 494, 500, 502, 504, 507, 510, 512, 513, 515–518, 525, 539, 542, 545, 553, 554, 559, 562–565, 567, 568, 570, 572, 573.

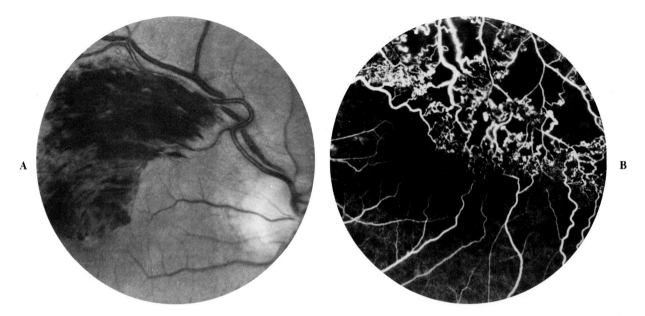

Fig. 8-46. A, Branch vein occlusion, right eye, superior temporal vein. **B,** Superior temporal vein occlusion, left eye, from another case: arteriovenous phase fluorescein angiogram. The obstructed retinal vein fills later than the other nonobstructed veins. Note the hypofluorescence in the region of the branch vein and the dilated tortuous capillary bed.

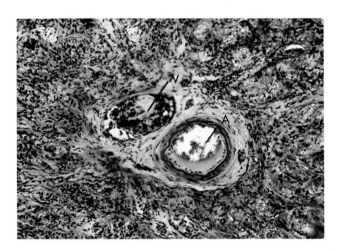

Fig. 8-47. Central retinal vein *(V)* containing a thrombus. The adjacent artery *(A)* shares a common adventitial sheath with the vein. (H & E stain; ×200.)

Venous stasis retinopathy is thought to result from complete occlusion of the central retinal vein alone without any significant retinal hypoxia.[515–518,521] These cases have often been diagnosed as "partial," "incipient," or "impending" central vein occlusion. Venous stasis retinopathy can be divided into two subgroups: (1) that seen in young persons (probably inflammatory in origin, from phlebitis of the central retinal vein, which produces venous thrombosis) and (2) that seen in older persons with arteriosclerosis (arteriosclerosis of the neighboring central retinal artery probably plays an important role in the venous occlusion).

The site of occlusion may be in the lamina cribrosa or more likely at some place posterior to the laminar region

(Fig. 8-47). Following occlusion, branches of the central vein anterior to the site of occlusion show compensatory enlargement. These branches develop into collateral vessels that help drain the blood from the occluded segment to the adjacent venous territories. Therefore, in all probability, the severity of the clinical picture depends on the site of venous occlusion within the optic nerve—the farther back the occlusion, the greater the availability of the collaterals and the less severe the retinopathy.

Available clinical and experimental evidence indicates that hemorrhagic retinopathy is caused by occlusion of the central retinal vein associated with retinal ischemia or significant hypoxia. This condition often leads to rubeosis iridis and neovascular glaucoma. The sequence of events in the pathogenesis of hemorrhagic retinopathy is thought by Hayreh to be as follows: central retinal arterial occlusion (partial or complete, transitory or prolonged) leads to stasis of the retinal circulation, which in turn produces venous stasis. Venous stasis precipitates thrombosis and completes occlusion in a central retinal vein already unhealthy and stenosed because of endothelial proliferation, the presence of partial thrombosis, or arteriosclerosis of the adjacent central retinal artery. Some retinal arterial circulation is almost always restored within a few hours or days. Because of the blocked central retinal vein, the blood cannot leave the retinal vascular bed. The rise of intraluminal pressure in retinal capillaries produced by the perfusing blood, therefore, causes the retinal capillaries to rupture, resulting in hemorrhagic retinopathy.

Branch vein occlusion

Most retinal branch vein occlusions seem to result from obstruction of venous flow at arteriovenous crossings, where the arteriole and venule share a common adventitial

Table 8-1. Comparisons of clinical features of venous stasis retinopathy and hemorrhagic retinopathy

Clinical feature	Venous stasis retinopathy	Hemorrhagic retinopathy
Age	Young adults and past middle age	More common in those past middle age
Symptoms	May have nonblurred or vaguely blurred vision	Always marked deterioration of vision
Visual acuity	May be normal or only mildly to moderately defective, rarely marked defective	Markedly defective
Visual fields	Peripheral—normal; central—normal or with relative/absolute central scotoma	Peripheral—usually markedly abnormal; central—almost always abnormal with central scotoma
Ophthalmoscopy		
EARLY CASES		
Retinal	Markedly engorged, turgid, and tortuous	Greatly engorged, turgid, and tortuous
Retinal hemorrhage	Vary from few flame-shaped and punctate hemorrhages to large number in central part and punctate in peripheral regions	Central part covered with gross hemorrhages; progressive during initial stages, less in periphery
Cotton-wool spots	Rare	Very common
Optic disc	Hyperemic and may be edematous	Swollen and usually covered with hemorrhages
Macula	Normal or may show edema	Gross hemorrhages and edema
Retinal arterioles	Normal or arteriosclerotic	Usually arteriosclerotic and narrow
LATE CASES (6–9 MONTHS OR LONGER)		
Retinal veins	Mildly to moderately engorged; sometimes sheathed	Mildly to moderately engorged; frequently sheathed
Retinal hemorrhages	May be none or usually a few; mainly in periphery	Maybe none or only a few
Retina	Normal	Frequently microaneurysms, dilated capillaries, and neovascularization; may have preretinal or vitreous hemorrhages
Optic disc	Normal or slightly hyperemic with retinociliary veins	May be pale disc, usually with retinociliary veins
Macula	Normal or may show cystoid degeneration	Macular degeneration and pigmentary disturbances: sometimes preretinal fibrosis
Fluorescein fundus angiography		
Early cases	Retinal venous stasis, engorged capillaries, some microaneurysms; fluorescein staining of retina maximum along main veins; fluorescence of macula when macular edema is present	Retina venous stasis, engorged capillaries and microaneurysms, masked by gross hemorrhages; may have delayed retinal arterial filling; late fluorescein staining of retina and main veins
Late cases	Mild-to-moderate retinal venous stasis, retinociliary veins on optic disc and possible microaneurysms; no neovascularization or obliterations of retinal capillaries	Mild-to-moderate, retinal venous stasis, retinociliary veins on optic disc, areas of retinal capillary obliteration, arteriovenous shunts, neovascularization, and microaneurysms; late staining of retina and veins
Prognosis	Good (40% recover normal function without therapy)	Poor
Course	Self-limited; does not progress to hemorrhagic retinopathy	Progressive
Complications	Macular edema, cystoid macular degeneration, central scotoma	Macular degeneration, preretinal or vitreous hemorrhages, retinitis proliferans, rubeosis iridis, neovascular glaucoma
Pathology	Central retinal vein occlusion with stasis	Red infarct due to central retinal vein occlusion with arterial ischemia
Treatment	If macular edema develops, systemic corticosteroids usually effective; otherwise no treatment required	Usually no treatment seems effective; photocoagulation of neovascularization (experimental)

Modified from Hayreh SS: Ophthalmologica 172:1, 1976.

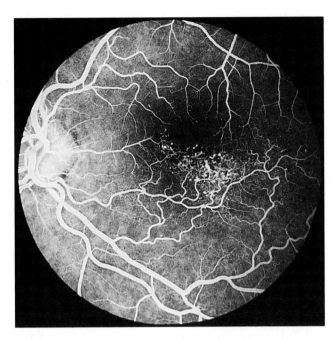

Fig. 8-48. Macular branch vein occlusion. Fluorescein angiogram, early venous phase. There is dilation of the capillary bed as is evidenced by multiple areas of hyperfluorescence.

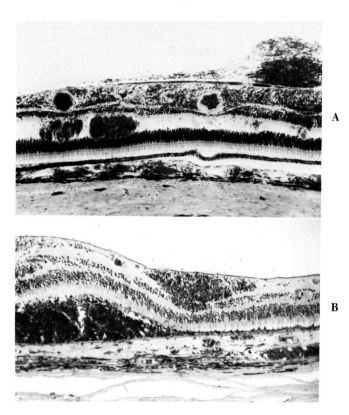

Fig. 8-49. Retinal hemorrhages in venous stasis retinopathy. **A,** Preretinal (*upper right*) nerve fiber layer and outer plexiform layer hemorrhage. (H & E stain; ×110.) **B,** Nerve fiber layer and subretinal hemorrhage. (H & E stain; ×90.)

sheath.* The clinicopathologic features are similar to those of central vein obstruction, except the changes are localized to a single quadrant (Figs. 8-46 and 8-48; Color Plate 8-17). The superior temporal vein seems to be most often affected; this may be because the macular region is affected and the patient seeks medical assistance earlier.[534] Hemicentral vein occlusion also may occur (Fig. 8-49).[520]

Unlike with the optic nerve, no short-circuiting vessels are normally available in the retina; that is, the chance of developing collateral channels to help drain the blocked area is decreased.[557] Fluorescein angiography reveals that the obstructed retinal vein fills much later than normal (Fig. 8-46, *B*) and the affected tertiary vessels become dilated and tortuous. Furthermore, a branch vein occlusion produces secondary arterial ischemia with a pattern of hypofluorescence (Fig. 8-46, *B*). It drains this segment of the retina by converting the segment into a closed circulation. Occlusion of the retinal branch vein alone, therefore, can result in sectoral hemorrhagic retinopathy with severe, although more localized, sequelae of the latter (Table 8-1).

Pathologic findings

Gross examination of a globe enucleated after venous stasis retinopathy or hemorrhagic retinopathy shows findings similar to the ophthalmoscopic observations listed in Table 8-1. They differ primarily in degree of retinal destruction. Predictably, because of a relatively good prognosis, eyes with venous stasis retinopathy are rarely enucleated, and the pathologic findings described here apply more directly in cases of hemorrhagic retinopathy.

In contrast to a central arterial occlusion, which produces an ischemic infarct of the retina, hemorrhagic retinopathy represents a hemorrhagic infarct of the retina.[481] The hemorrhage extends throughout all quadrants of the globe (Fig. 8-45; Color Plate 8-16) or in branch vein occlusions involves only the affected quadrant of the fundus (Table 8-1) (Fig. 8-46; Color Plate 8-17). In addition to intraretinal hemorrhage, breakthrough into the vitreous may be a complication (Fig. 8-49). The pattern of hemorrhage is usually more diffuse and widespread than that seen in other hemorrhagic diseases (such as hypertensive retinopathy or leukemic infiltrates). The hemorrhages are usually flame-shaped because of involvement of the nerve fiber layer, but they may be the "dot" or "blot" types when they involve deeper layers of the retina.

Macular edema (Fig. 8-86, *A*), a subsequent neovascularization, and hemorrhagic glaucoma are common sequelae of acute hemorrhagic retinopathy.

In contrast to central arterial occlusion in which the retina usually, but not always, becomes thinned and atrophic, with minimal gliosis, hemorrhagic retinopathy often causes thickening of the retina by organization of neovascular tissue and blood products, with subsequent reactive gliosis.[487,496] Hemosiderin derived from extravasated blood is deposited in old lesions. This iron-containing substance is most apparent in retinal sections stained by the Prussian blue technique for iron (Table 1-1).

In globes enucleated months or years after central vein occlusion, the histopathologic diagnosis is often difficult to confirm by examination of the retina alone. However,

---

* References 481, 484, 495, 498, 506, 508, 514, 526–528, 551, 558, 579.

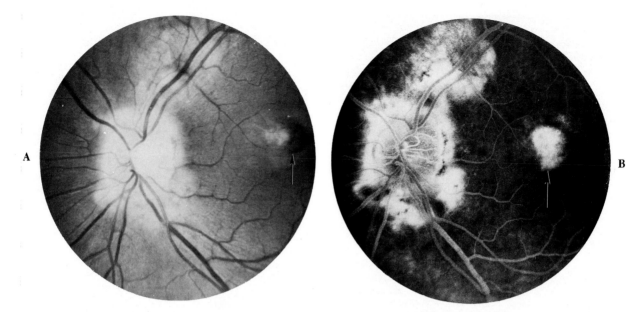

Fig. 8-50. Presumed histoplasmic chorioretinitis. **A,** Hemorrhagic disciform detachment of the macula, peripapillary atrophy, and peripheral chorioretinal scars are the clinical hallmarks of this syndrome. Leakage of serous fluid, blood, or both into the subretinal and subpigment epithelial spaces characteristically occurs at the macula *(arrow).* Subpigment epithelial neovascularization of the macular region may frequently be demonstrated by fluorescein angiography. **B,** Fluorescein angiogram from the same case as in **A.** Note the intense fluorescein staining in the peripapillary retina and leakage of dye from subpigment epithelial neovascular tissue at the macula *(arrow).*

remnants of the intravenous thrombus, which initially was composed of fibrin and platelets, may persist (Fig. 8-47). The thrombus is transformed into a permanent, fibrous mass. In more favorable cases in which the acute process resolves, the thrombus may recanalize or be partially or completely resorbed.

Chorioretinal inflammation

HISTOPLASMOSIS

Peripapillary inflammation and atrophy with pigment proliferation, peripheral scars, and (less often) disciform detachment of the macula are the clinical hallmarks of presumed histoplasmic chorioretinitis (Fig. 8-50; Color Plate 8-18).[580–950] This condition is called presumed histoplasmosis syndrome because the organism has rarely been demonstrated in affected eyes. In many cases the triad of ocular findings occurs without historical, clinical, or histopathologic evidence of exposure to the organism.* The fundus lesions, particularly the macular lesions, are less frequent in blacks. In affected patients the onset of symptoms usually occurs after the third decade of life. The presumed responsible organism, *Histoplasma capsulatum,* is a fungus that propagates well in soil enriched with foul excrement.[584,604] The organism is inhaled and occasionally spreads systemically to the lung, liver, spleen, and eye. The region of the United States in which histoplasmosis is endemic is a triangular area with its apices near Omaha, Ne-

braska, Columbus, Ohio, and Natchez, Mississippi. It includes most of the Ohio and Mississippi River valleys. In a large portion of this histobelt, 60% or more of the young adult, lifelong residents react positively to histoplasmin skin testing.[26,609]

In contrast to the *Toxoplasma* organism, which at least in its initial stages demonstrates an affinity for retinal tissue and vitreous, the initial destructive lesion of *Histoplasmosis* invasion occurs in the choroid. The peripapillary changes, which in most cases occur bilaterally, are usually confined to the choroid or, secondarily, to the outer retinal layers.[595] Therefore, they do not cause nerve fiber bundle defects as one would expect from a primary retinitis, for example, toxoplasmic retinochoroiditis.

Foci of nodular granulomatous choroiditis, perhaps caused by an allergic reaction to the organism, also appear in the periphery. The resultant peripheral atrophic lesions are probably residual of such granulomas. In distinct contrast to toxoplasmosis, inflammatory cells are not noted within the vitreous.[602,603,613,615,617]

The inflammatory focus in the macula causes damage to Bruch's membrane, with resultant invasion of neovascular tissue and leakage of serum and blood into the subpigment epithelial and subretinal spaces.[588,599] The neovascular tissue and extravasated fluid from these channels can be appreciated by fluorescein angiography (Fig. 8-50, *B*). The hemorrhagic macular lesion tends to organize, forming a disciform scar similar to that of the Junius-Kuhnt type (pp. 442–447). Photocoagulation may be useful in destroying the neovascular tissue before severe hemorrhage ensues.[580,594,611,614]

---

* References 583, 585, 587, 589, 591, 593, 596–598, 600, 605, 607, 608, 610, 613.

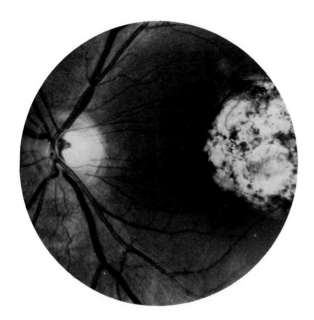

Fig. 8-51. Healed toxoplasmosis of the macula.

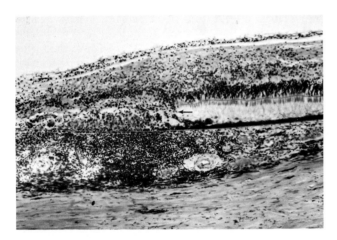

Fig. 8-52. Toxoplasmic granulomatous retinochoroiditis. *Arrow,* Junction of a relatively intact portion of retina *(right)* with a focus of necrotic, inflamed retina and choroid *(left)*. (H & E stain; ×120.)

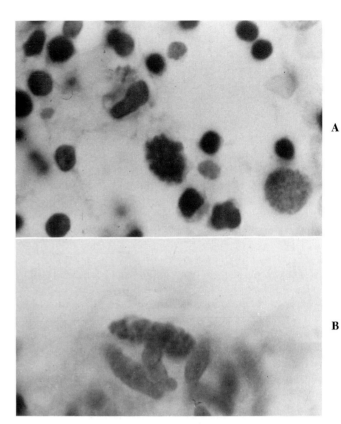

Fig. 8-53. *Toxoplasma gondii* organisms (faint punctate dots) within chorioretinal exudate. (**A,** H & E stain; ×430; **B,** H & E stain; ×470.) (From the collection of Professor Wolfgang Stock, University of Tübingen, Tübingen, Germany, and from Naumann GOH and Apple DJ: In Doerr W, Seifert G, and Uehlinger E, editors: Handbuch der speziellen pathologischen Anatomie, Band Auge, Berlin, 1980, Springer-Verlag.)

TOXOPLASMOSIS

Toxoplasmic retinochoroiditis, caused by an intracellular protozoan parasite of approximately 4 μm to 7 μm, may be either congenital or acquired (Figs. 8-51–53 Color Plates 8-19 and 8-26).[618–643]

The congenital form may be manifest only in the eye or may be associated with jaundice, hepatosplenomegaly, encephalitis, hydrocephalus, and intracranial calcification. Congenital toxoplasmosis is sometimes confused with infantile rubella, cytomegalic inclusion disease, and herpes simplex. This differential diagnosis is sometimes designated the "TORCH" syndrome. Children with congenital toxoplasmosis usually have bilateral ocular involvement. The bilateral and symmetric nature of the lesions has prompted some authors to consider *Toxoplasma gondii* a causative factor in the pathogenesis of at least some types of congenital macular colobomas (Fig. 2-22; Color Plate 2-13; p. 28).[619]

The macular lesions usually progress to a chronic stage with scar formation and pigmentation. Later recurrences of congenital lesions often appear as satellite lesions near preexisting scars, and peripheral atrophic scars may also develop. Chorioretinal atrophy occurs, and proliferated retinal pigment epithelium often borders the lesion (Fig. 8-51; Color Plates 8-19 and 8-20).

The acute, acquired lesion, which, like the congenital form has no sex predilection, consists of a necrotizing granulomatous retinitis with heavy exudation into the vitreous.[628,629,636,643,935] The granulomatous process extends secondarily to the choroid and adjacent sclera (Fig. 8-52).[639] Histoplasmic choroiditis typically does not show a vitritis.

Toxoplasmosis is probably one of the most common causes of so-called Jensen's juxtapapillary retinochoroiditis. The peripapillary lesions of toxoplasmosis differ from histoplasmosis in that the retina and nerve fiber layer are destroyed, creating arcuate scotomas radiating from the blind spot. This finding is absent in histoplasmosis choroiditis. Acquired toxoplasmosis is usually diagnosed in patients between the ages of 10 and 40 and, unlike the congenital form, is rarely associated with central nervous system involvement. In addition to the fundus abnormalities, sometimes a proteinaceous and cellular reaction occurs within the anterior chamber, with formation of keratic precipitates on the corneal endothelium.

The acute, active granulomatous lesion usually resolves into a chronic quiescent form or undergoes gliosis and/or fibrosis with proliferation of retinal pigment epithelium similar to that seen in the congenital form. Choroidal neovascularization and retinochoroidal vascular anastomoses may occur as late complications.[620,631] In the chronic state, so-called pseudocysts may form. These contain many organisms enclosed by a fibrous membrane (Fig. 8-53). They have a tendency to rupture later, causing reexacerbations of the retinitis. The complement fixation, hemagglutination, and methylene blue dye tests detect antibodies to the toxoplasmic antigen.[616,624]

The classic treatment regimen for ocular toxoplasmosis consists of pyrimethamine, sulfadiazine, and corticosteroids and is often known as "triple drug therapy." Steroids are added to the antibiotics to minimize the damage to other ocular structures caused by the inflammatory response. Similarly, topical corticosteroids and cycloplegics are used to treat any associated anterior uveitis.

ACQUIRED IMMUNE DEFICIENCY SYNDROME AND CYTOMEGALIC INCLUSION DISEASE

The acquired immune deficiency syndrome (AIDS)[658,860] was first recognized as a clinical syndrome in the summer of 1981 when the Centers for Disease Control (CDC) reported five cases of *Pneumocystis carinii* pneumonia in young homosexual males.[658,680] It rapidly became clear that this syndrome, commonly associated with a wide variety of opportunistic infectious agents and malignancies, was associated with an underlying cellular immunodeficiency that usually occurred in a person who had otherwise no discernible cause of such a deficiency. It has been determined that *P. carinii* pneumonia is the most common secondary infection seen in AIDS patients. Almost two thirds of AIDS patients have *P. carinii* pneumonia at some point in their disease.[668,709,860] Kaposi's sarcoma is the most common malignancy associated with this disease. Until the recent development of regimens such as "cocktails" composed of various agents such as protease inhibitors and reverse transcriptase inhibitors, which have provided some hope of improvement in at least some cases, there has been little effective treatment.

Between 1982 and 1988 the number of reported AIDS cases increased from fewer than 500 to more than 72,000.[847,860] From 1 to 1.5 million people in the United States are infected with the human immunodeficiency virus (HIV)[103] As of 1993, there have been approximately 300,000 deaths from AIDS in the United States.

More than 75% of patients diagnosed with AIDS before 1985 have died, the highest incidence of the disease in the United States being in San Francisco, Los Angeles, and New York.[658,739] At least six groups have been found to be at risk for developing AIDS, the largest group being homosexual/bisexual male nonintravenous (non-IV) drug abusers (65%). Of the remaining cases, IV drug abusers constitute 17%, homosexual/bisexual male IV drug abusers 8%, heterosexual contacts 1%, hemophiliacs and transfu-

sion recipients 3%, and others with no identifiable risk 6%.[*]

In the United States over 60% of the AIDS patients are white, the majority being males ranging in age from 20 to 49 years.[646,728,860] In addition, workers in the health professions are also at risk of acquiring the HIV infection.[717,721,892,894] In a study performed by the CDC, four out of 870 health care workers who had puncture wounds from contaminated needles developed the infection.[658] A survey from San Francisco showed that of 184 men who were known HIV seroconverters, 48% of those developed AIDS within 10 years.[658]

A condition has been described that most commonly occurs among homosexual males, a constellation of symptoms that includes fever, night sweats, loss of weight, lymphadenopathy, and malaise. This has been described as AIDS-related complex (ARC). Individuals with ARC are at increased risk of developing full-blown AIDS. Twenty-nine percent of these patients go on to develop AIDS within 54 months after the onset of ARC.[728,809,860]

The AIDS virus was initially known as the human T-lymphotrophic virus type III (HTLV-III) in the United States and the lymphadenopathy-associated virus (LAV) in France. Once it was determined that these viruses were one and the same, the term *human immunodeficiency virus (HIV)* has been adopted by most researchers.[647,660] The virus has been isolated from many tissues and fluids, including blood, semen, urine, saliva, breast milk, pulmonary secretions, lymph node secretions, cerebrospinal fluid, cervical and vaginal secretions, tears, and the eyes.[†] It does not appear that the virus can be spread by casual contact such as holding hands, kissing, or sharing of utensils.

The most common test in use today to detect the presence of viral antibody to HIV is the enzyme-linked immunosorbent assay (ELISA) test.[647,685,740] Because this test has a number of false-positive results, especially in a population with a low prevalence of HIV, seropositive specimens must be reexamined using a more specific test, the Western Blot test.

Immunology

The HIV is a member of the retrovirus family, which uses the enzyme reverse transcriptase to produce DNA on an RNA template.[647,685] The virus directly infects lymphocytes and causes an increased general susceptibility to infection. The most severely affected component of the human immune system is the T-cell–mediated response, a response that is directly responsible systemically for limiting all types of microbial infections.[779,784,789]

Laboratory studies reveal that although the B- to T-cell ratio is normal, an absolute leukopenia occurs with a reduction in number of both B and T cells.[647,723,779] Within the T-cell subsets there is a decrease in the number of T-helper cells and a normal-to-increased number of T-suppressor cells.[647] This leads to a decreased helper-to-suppressor cell ratio. As a result, the affected patient shows a poor-to-absent response to antigens and/or mitogens and cutaneous anergy.[647,685,779] In addition, there is a decreased cytotoxic

---

[*] References 646, 701, 702, 728, 739, 750, 809, 834, 847.
[†] References 646, 670, 687, 701, 716, 717, 728, 834, 854, 860.

response with decreased numbers of natural killer (NK) cells available for destruction of invading organisms.[647,860] In addition to defective cell-mediated immunity, immunoglobulin levels may be normal or increased.° Increased levels of both IgG and IgA are found in adults; increased levels of IgM have been found in children.[647,685,860] Increased numbers of circulating immune complex have also been found in AIDS patients.[733]

Ocular involvement

The HIV was first isolated from the tears of a patient with AIDS in 1985.[717] The virus has been isolated from conjunctival epithelium, corneal epithelium, the iris, the aqueous humor, and the vitreous humor.† To date, there has been no reported transmission of the virus by direct contact with ocular tissues or fluids of infected patients.[863] Although the corneal epithelium may be infected by the virus, there has been no report of HIV transmission by penetrating keratoplasty.[711] Nevertheless, all corneal donors are screened for antibodies to the HIV.[793,831]

Nonepidemic Kaposi's sarcoma is the most common malignancy involving the eye and adnexa (see Chapter 11, p. 581). Before the AIDS epidemic, the "classic" form of Kaposi's sarcoma was well recognized as a usually slow growing tumor, most commonly seen in males of Mediterranean descent; it continues to be a significant tumor affecting equatorial African blacks.[853] The classic nonepidemic form common in Central Africa does not appear to be associated with AIDS.[853,860] This classic Kaposi's sarcoma had a relatively low (10%) incidence of multiple organ involvement. In sharp contrast, Kaposi's sarcoma seen in almost one fourth of patients with AIDS has greater than a two-thirds incidence of visceral involvement.[691,742,860] As opposed to the classic Kaposi's sarcoma, the sarcoma seen in AIDS patients may involve multiple tissues and organs such as the skin, lymph nodes, lungs, bone, and gastrointestinal (GI) tract.[714,727,805]

Ocular adnexal involvement by Kaposi's sarcoma in AIDS patients may occur.‡ The tumor may be confused with hemangiomas, chalazia, or hordeola. The lesions are typically vascular and reddish-purple. Adnexal Kaposi's sarcoma may be the first clinical presentation in AIDS.[864]

Burkitt's lymphoma, now seen increasingly in individuals infected with AIDS, is a tumor that was originally confined to areas of Central Africa.[661,727] Like Kaposi's sarcoma, Burkitt's lymphoma may involve the orbit and/or eyelid, often with symptoms similar to those of Kaposi's sarcoma.[661,813]

Although the majority of severe intraocular complications of AIDS involve the retina and choroid (Color Plates 8-18 and 8-19), significant involvement of the cornea, anterior segment, and orbit may occur.§ Common infectious organisms include herpes simplex and herpes zoster viruses,[855] cytomegalovirus (CMV), *Candida* species and other fungi, and several species of mycobacteria and toxoplasmosis.‖

The most common fundus lesions (Color Plates 8-21–8-23) seen in AIDS are cotton-wool spots.° These occur in over half of AIDS patients and differ from spots seen in hypertensive or diabetic individuals in that they are not associated with either atherosclerotic changes or the hemorrhages and exudates typical of diabetic retinopathy.[753,791,817] The spots typically are white and reveal feathered edges. They are usually present at the posterior pole in the superficial nerve fiber layer of the retina.[706,751,782] These lesions usually resolve after a period of about 6 weeks with new lesions developing as old ones disappear.[817,860] The spots are frequently confused with the lesions of CMV infection.[827] However, the lesions of CMV retinitis, in contrast to cotton-wool spots, quickly increase in size and intensity.

It is believed that elevated levels of circulating immune complexes in AIDS patients may be partially responsible for the pathogenesis of both cotton-wool spots and other forms of AIDS vasculitis.[710,733,771,814] The vascular endothelial cells themselves may be infected with HIV.[817,841] This vasculitis may lead to extensive retinal ischemia and necrosis. AIDS patients with CMV retinitis have a higher incidence of perivasculitis.[817,827,862] The HIV may directly infect the retina and, when the virus invades the capillary endothelium, the infection probably contributes to the cause of the cotton-wool spots.†

Cytomegalic inclusion disease‡ is described here because it is frequently associated with AIDS. It is caused by a DNA virus of the same name. Other viruses documented as causing a necrotic retinitis or chorioretinitis include herpes simplex, herpes zoster, and measles (rubeola) viruses.§ Fungi such as *Cryptococcus* have also been implicated. Newborn or infant cytomegalic inclusion disease usually results in gross malformation or death. A CMV infection occurs in approximately 1% of all live births worldwide, making it a major cause of intrauterine infection in man.[786,736] The virus can gain access to the developing fetus via the transplacental circulation or via cervical secretions during passage through the birth canal.[815] Approximately 5% to 10% of congenitally infected neonates have clinically significant disease that involves the reticuloendothelial and central nervous systems. Ocular manifestations of CMV include chorioretinitis, optic atrophy, and cataract formation.[669] Ninety percent of infected infants have subclinical or minimal disease; many remain undiagnosed or have subtle deficits such as sensorineural hearing loss or psychomotor disturbance. Intracranial involvement with calcification, involvement of the salivary glands, acute hemorrhagic phenomena reflecting a thrombocytopenia, hepatosplenomegaly, pneumonitis, mental retardation, and motor disability are in important component of the systemic form. This systemic form of the infantile disease is much less common than the localized form of the disease, in which the virus is limited to the salivary glands.

As AIDS has increased in incidence in recent years, the adult form of cytomegalic inclusion retinitis has been re-

---

° References 648, 685, 723, 784, 785, 789.
† References 651, 670, 716, 793, 816, 854, 860, 866.
‡ References 661, 714, 727, 759, 813, 864, 874, 882, 887, 890, 891.
§ References 657, 672, 684, 698, 777, 781, 823, 835–838, 842, 875, 880.
‖ References 663, 677, 678, 680, 696, 790, 828, 830, 842, 855, 856, 863, 869, 871.

° References 712, 752, 760, 772, 804, 812, 817, 835, 837.
† References 670, 733, 791, 841, 910, 916, 918, 935, 940, 943, 947, 950.
‡ References 659, 673, 729, 730, 747, 811, 877, 931, 947, 950.
§ References 906, 921, 923, 931, 934, 946.

ported with increasing frequency. It also occurs in patients treated with immunosuppressive drugs and in patients debilitated with terminal diseases such as leukemia.

Pathologic lesions characteristic of CMV infection were first described by Ribbert in 1904.[843] He observed "protozoan-like" cells in the kidney and salivary glands of stillborn babies. In 1921 Goodpasture and Talbot postulated a viral cause for what was then termed *salivary gland inclusion disease* in infants.[725]

In 1959 Foerster reported a case of chorioretinitis in a 59-year-old white female with a 2-year history of unilateral uveitis.[703] Histopathologic sections of the eye showed focal retinal necrosis and granulomatous inflammation. Foerster demonstrated retinal cells with intranuclear inclusions similar to those found in other CMV-infected tissue and proposed CMV as the causative agent.[667] Smith[867] reported the first histopathologic study of CMV retinitis in 1964, and Wyhinny and associates in 1973 reported a detailed electron microscopic examination of retinal tissue.[895] The patient was a 61-year-old black female who died of Hodgkin's disease after treatment with chemotherapy and irradiation.

Active CMV infection accounts for significant morbidity and mortality in immunocompromised patients, including those with AIDS, recipients of bone marrow and solid organ transplants who are on immunosuppressive agents, and neonates.* Cytomegalovirus is a double-stranded DNA herpes virus that infects many organs, including the eyes, lungs, kidneys, GI tract, and reticuloendothelial system.

Only three cases of CMV retinitis were reported in the literature before the 1970s.[838] During the past two decades, an increase in the incidence of CMV retinitis has occurred in conjunction with the rapid rise in the number of AIDS cases and with the wider clinical use of a variety of new immunosuppressive medications.[656] CMV retinitis is the most common ophthalmic infection in AIDS patients and occurs in 15% to 40% of patients.[1666] It may be the initial manifestation of AIDS. As many as one in three patients with AIDS may develop CMV retinitis at some point.†

Transmission of CMV infection occurs by several modes. The virus has been isolated from many body fluids, including cervical secretions, breast milk, amniotic fluid, blood, semen, urine, saliva, tears, and a variety of solid tissues.[741,889] Cytomegalovirus nucleic acid has also been detected in peripheral blood lymphocytes.[702,844] The mechanisms of immunity, intracellular viral latency, and reactivation are not well understood but are presumably regulated by cell-mediated immune response.[644,783]

In adults, the seroprevalence of antibodies to CMV varies with respect to differences in geographic location, age, and immune status.[893] Seroprevalence ranges from 50% to 70% in industrial nations and approaches 100% in less developed countries.[695,773] Seropositivity increases with age, reaching the highest incidence in individuals older than 50 years of age.[783] Most immunocompetent individuals with a positive serology have an asymptomatic infection. In these individuals, primary infection or reactivation results in a subclinical or mild disease. A mild disease may present as a mononucleosis-like syndrome with fever, malaise, atypical lymphocytosis, and liver function test abnormalities.

Active CMV infection accounts for significant morbidity and mortality in immunocompromised patients.[665,762,796,857] Active CMV infection occurs in 50% to 100% of bone marrow and organ transplant patients and is the result of either reactivation while on immunosuppressive medication or transmission from seropositive tissue and blood to a seronegative recipient.[671,702,768] Active CMV infection in immunocompromised individuals may take many forms: retinitis, pneumonitis, hepatitis, colitis, sialoadenitis, and nephritis.[841]

Diagnostic modalities for CMV infection currently used in the clinical virology laboratory include isolation of the virus in culture with detection of viral cytopathic effect.* Viral isolation in culture is considered to be the "standard" for CMV diagnosis but is slow and often takes weeks to yield positive results.[845,868] The presence of antibody to early viral nuclear antigen is considered a marker of active infection. Active CMV retinitis may or may not be accompanied by positive viral isolation in cultures of subretinal and aqueous fluid.[694,801] In addition, other body fluids such as tears, urine, blood leukocytes, and nasopharyngeal secretions may be cultured. One must be cautious in interpreting positive culture results because prolonged viral shedding may persist for up to 1 year after primary infection or reactivation.[783]

Serologic studies have limited usefulness in the diagnosis of systemic CMV infection. Infection by CMV can produce symptomatic, asymptomatic, primary, latent, or reactivated infection with variable elevations in antibody titer. Different methods of serodiagnosis include enzyme-linked immunoassay, indirect hemagglutination, radioimmunoassay, and complement fixation. The presence of IgM instead of IgG antibody may signify either an early primary infection or a recent reactivation of disease.

Recent advances in molecular biology have provided cloned DNA sequences for diagnosis of viral infection by DNA hybridization.[797] In situ DNA hybridization allows the specific histologic localization of CMV DNA. Hybridization occurs between labeled DNA probes and complimentary viral DNA sequences present in tissue sections or cultured cell samples. Use of biotinylated DNA probes with affinity histochemical detection avoids the potentially hazardous and time-consuming procedures that use radioactively labeled probes. DNA hybridization is more useful as a research tool because it requires fresh or specially fixed tissue specimens.[737]

Patients with CMV retinitis may be asymptomatic or may have a variety of visual complaints that correlate closely with the area of retinal involvement (Color Plates 8-21 and 8-23).[1791] In the asymptomatic patient, early lesions of the peripheral retina may cause mild visual impairment or may go undetected if indirect ophthalmoscopy is not performed. In light of this and the fact that CMV retinitis is the major cause of visual loss in AIDS patients, it is very important to perform frequent fundoscopic examinations

---

* References 699, 713, 757, 783, 829, 888.
† References 681, 707, 753, 773, 820, 829, 862.

* References 683, 690, 726, 738, 801, 825.

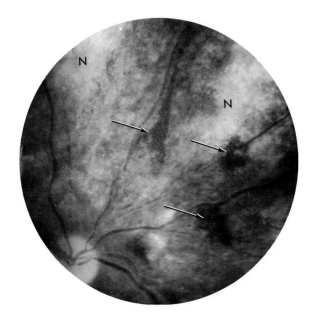

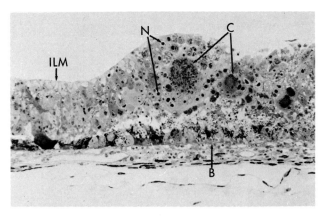

Fig. 8-55. Total loss of the normal parallel architecture of the retinal neurons. The sensory retina is fused with the markedly degenerate pigment epithelium, which shows extensive pigment dispersion. *N*, Dense intranuclear inclusions; *C*, more diffuse, granular, cytoplasmic inclusions. The choroid is uninvolved, apparently because of the barrier created by Bruch's membrane *(B)*. *ILM*, Internal limiting membrane. (Mallory blue stain; ×150.)

Fig. 8-54. Cytomegalic inclusion retinitis in an adult following immunosuppression after renal transplantation. The ophthalmoscopic appearance of this relatively uncommon condition is characteristic in fully developed cases. The broad areas of yellow discoloration are not exudates but areas of marked retinal necrosis *(N)* resulting from direct invasion of the vein. *Arrows,* Patchy distribution of irregular intraretinal hemorrhages.

in patients with impaired immunity.[746,820] With vitreous involvement, the patient may complain of blurred vision and floaters. If the disease process involves the macula, patient complaints may include a rapid decrease in visual acuity, metamorphopsia, and micropsia.

The fundoscopic appearance of CMV retinitis is distinct. (Fig. 8-54)[652,885] The disease may be unilateral or bilateral and often begins as focal discrete lesions that progress to diffuse retinal involvement.[676] The initial findings include retinal edema, yellow-white granular dots, which are localized areas of RPE involvement, and vascular sheathing and attenuation (Fig. 8-54).[713,765,788,810] The characteristic fundus appearance has been described by some as resembling "pizza pie."[720] Vascular sheathing occurs and is caused by a perivascular mononuclear cell infiltrate.[771] Fluorescein angiography may demonstrate focal retinal vascular occlusions with increased vascular permeability.[814] Cotton-wool spots, intraretinal hemorrhage, exudates, vascular aneurysms, and areas of retinal necrosis and atrophy may develop. Retinal hemorrhages first occur in the superficial layers of the retina, and the flame-shaped lesions may resemble those of branch retinal vein occlusion. In addition, white-centered hemorrhages (Roth spots) may be seen, resembling those found in leukemic retinitis and other retinal infectious processes.[913] The white core is thought to be a collection of white cells and fibrin sequestered as the clot forms. This is analogous to the buffy coat, which forms after centrifugation of blood.

Retinitis of CMV often progresses as a "brush fire–like" extension from each discrete lesion. The optic disc is usually spared.[796] Necrotizing may cause a marked thinning and atrophy of the retina, which may progress to both exu-

dative and rhegmatogenous retinal detachment.* Few conditions cause such widespread and massive destruction of the retina.

Clinical diagnosis of CMV retinitis is usually established by characteristic ophthalmoscopic findings. Chorioretinal tissue biopsy is usually considered an unsafe procedure but may be indicated in certain situations. One such indication would be the biopsy of a blind eye of a patient in which the differential diagnosis includes leukemic infiltration, sarcoidosis, or opportunistic infection.[769] The choice of treatment in these conditions differs greatly in efficacy and potential side effects. Viral isolation, detection of viral DNA, and serodiagnosis are not sufficient to diagnose CMV retinitis, but may be helpful as corroborative studies in the diagnosis of CMV infection.

Histopathologically the retina typically reveals a hemorrhagic necrotizing retinitis that involves all layers and the RPE (Fig. 8-55).[683,686,765,867,895] There is often total loss of the normal parallel architecture of the retinal neurons. The sensory retina frequently fuses with the RPE. In the chronic phase of the disease, sensory retinal and RPE atrophy occur and dense fibrouslike tissue forms.[720] Initially the underlying choroid is not primarily involved or inflamed. However, a secondary diffuse granulomatous choroiditis frequently develops with progression of the disease.

The histologic hallmark of CMV infection is the "owl's eye" nuclear inclusion (Fig. 8-56).[683,686,765,867,895] This consists of an enlarged oval or reniform host cell that contains the characteristic intranuclear viral inclusion that is eosinophilic in hematoxylin and eosin-stained or periodic acid–Schiff-stained tissue. In addition, eosinophilic and/or basophilic cytoplasmic inclusions may be found. Infected cells with viral inclusions are located in the RPE and vascular endothelium. Electron microscopy has shown that these inclusions contain viral particles that measure approximately 150 nm in diameter.[690,825,895] The characteristic

---

* References 655, 662, 688, 708, 719, 787, 802, 813, 835, 850, 907.

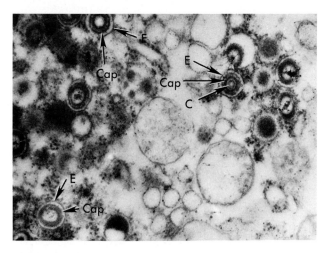

Fig. 8-56. Electron micrograph of the retina. The characteristic three-layered substructure of the cytomegalovirus, which is similar to that of several virus classes, is visible: (1) the central nucleic acid core *(C)*, (2) the intermediate capsid *(Cap)*, and (3) the outer envelope *(E)*, which probably functions as a determinant for antigenic properties. Note the swollen, degenerate mitochondria and other cytoplasmic organelles injured during the inflammatory process. (×28,940.) (From Wyhinny GJ and others: Am J Ophthalmol 76:773, 1973.)

three-layered substructure of the cytomegalovirus is composed of the central nucleic acid core, the intermediate capsid, and the outer envelope (Fig. 8-56). The latter probably functions as an important determinant of antigenic properties.[655,868]

In the past, attempts at treating CMV retinitis with broad spectrum antibiotics, steroids, α-interferon, and antiviral agents such as vidarabine and acyclovir have been variable.[645,693,753,798,883] The use of trisodium phosphonoformate hexahydrate (Foscarnet) has met with only limited success because of poor penetration of the blood-ocular barrier.[883] Ganciclovir, 10-[2-hydroxy-1-(hydroxymethyl) ethoxymethyl]guanine, or 10-(1,3-dihydroxy-2-propoxymethyl)guanine has been found to have in vitro activity against CMV.* The drug is an acyclic nucleoside analogue of guanine. Though structurally related to acyclovir, differing only in the acrylic side chain, ganciclovir has markedly more in vitro activity against CMV.[788,792] The drug is taken up by both CMV-infected and noninfected cells where it is phosphorylated to a triphosphate form by the host cell enzymes. The triphosphate form specifically inhibits CMV deoxyribonucleic acid polymerase and viral DNA synthesis. Although such side effects as bone marrow suppression occur, maintenance therapy is necessary to prevent disease reactivation and progression of retinopathy.[666,754] Recent trials with this agent show that it is effective in the control of the proliferative phase of the virus, but the drug does not eradicate the infection. Reactivation of retinitis may occur after cessation of therapy.[650,754,758,848] Response rates as high as 87% to 92% have been reported in several different studies.[653,705,754,799,821] Response to treatment has been demonstrated by the resolution of retinal hemor-

rhage, exudates, and perivascular lesions with reduction in retinal opacification.[683]

Toxoplasmic retinitis (see p. 395) may be seen in AIDS patients, frequently developing as a newly acquired primary infection.* It is probably the second most common cause of retinochoroiditis after CMV.[680,755] Toxoplasmosis may be the cause of initial signs and symptoms of AIDS. Patients initially complain of such symptoms as blurred vision, photophobia, and floaters.[886] These symptoms are usually secondary to granulomatous iridocyclitis and vitritis.[827,843] Retinal lesions include focal areas of coagulative necrotizing retinitis and are frequently bilateral and multifocal.[744,859] As opposed to congenital reactivation, these lesions are not located next to preexisting scars but may be found anywhere within the retina. Resolution often leaves an irregular pigmented scar. In addition, secondary rhegmatogenous retinal detachments may occur. If the lesions involve the macula or optic nerve head, there may be significant visual loss.

It is important to note that, compared to infections seen in immunocompetent individuals, toxoplasmic retinitis seldom spontaneously resolves in AIDS patients.[680] It is, therefore, important that antiprotozoan therapy be begun promptly. Most patients must be continued on maintenance drug therapy because of multiple recurrences. The two most commonly used treatment modalities include either pyrimethamine or clindamycin.[680]

Although rarely associated with AIDS, both *Candida* and *Cryptococcus* may produce a retinochoroiditis.[689,941] *Candida* retinitis is especially common in AIDS patients who are also IV drug abusers.[860] The retinal lesions vary in size from one to several disc diameters and are fluffy, yellow-white retinal infiltrates with irregular borders.[675] The vitreous may be secondarily involved, and retinal detachments have also been associated with *Candida* retinitis.[743]

Many AIDS patients may have an associated syphillis.[766,794] The syphillis seen in AIDS patients is especially difficult to treat and is often chronic.[824,873] A unilateral focal area of coagulative necrotizing syphilitic retinitis with mild-to-severe secondary vitritis often occurs, causing the patient to complain of blurred vision and floaters.[680,873] Syphilitic retinitis is often associated with neurosyphillis.[680,766]

Retinal involvement with herpes simplex or herpes zoster virus may be seen in AIDS patients in the form of the acute retinal necrosis syndrome.† There is sometimes an associated involvement of skin by the virus.[664] Examination usually reveals a granulomatous anterior uveitis with an associated mild-to-moderate vitritis, and the retina is usually involved peripherally with a necrotizing reaction, thus sparing the macula and posterior pole.[681,552] Presently, the most common mode of treatment involves the use of intravenous acyclovir.[678]

ACUTE RETINAL NECROSIS

In 1971, Urayama and coworkers[946] first reported six cases of what appeared to be a new syndrome characterized

---

* References 649, 700, 735, 749, 778, 788, 800, 803, 832, 846, 858, 881.

* References 718, 731, 732, 744, 755, 806, 822, 833, 869, 886.
† References 612, 674, 680, 682, 780, 795, 829, 830, 911, 915, 919, 926, 927.

by acute necrotizing retinitis, vitritis, retinal arteritis, choroiditis, and late-onset rhegmatogenous retinal detachment. The acute retinal necrosis (ARN) syndrome is characterized by the initial onset of episcleritis or scleritis, periorbital pain, and anterior uveitis, which may be granulomatous or stellate in appearance.* This is followed by decreased vision resulting from vitreous opacification, necrotizing retinitis and, in some cases, optic neuritis or neuropathy. The retinitis appears as deep, multifocal yellow-white patches, typically beginning in the peripheral fundus and then becoming concentrically confluent and spreading toward the posterior pole; the macula is frequently spared. An active vasculitis is present, with perivascular hemorrhages, sheathing, and terminal obliteration of arterioles by thrombi. The phase of active retinitis usually lasts 4 to 6 weeks, during which time an exudative retinal detachment may occur.

About 50% of cases are bilateral. The condition is typically caused by both the varicella-zoster and herpes simplex viruses. It may result from activation of latent, previously acquired infection, usually herpes zoster dermatitis (shingles) or may develop during the course of primary varicella-zoster (chickenpox) infection.[901] Viral antibodies have been found in intrathecally produced cerebrospinal fluid from patients who have ARN, suggesting CNS involvement.[896]

Histologically, by light microscopy, Cowdry type A intranuclear inclusions and, by electron microscopy, intranuclear aggregates of viral particles can be seen in the areas of disorganized necrotic retina.[917,928]

Whereas ARN represents a distinct syndrome, its differential diagnosis includes CMV retinopathy, syphilitic retinitis, toxoplasmosis (particularly in immunocompromised hosts), large-cell lymphoma, and acute multifocal hemorrhagic retinal vasculitis. A more extensive differential diagnosis includes toxocariasis, fungal or bacterial retinitis, pars planitis, Behçet's disease, sarcoidosis, commotio retinae, central retinal artery or ophthalmic artery occlusion, the ischemic ocular syndrome, collagenvascular disease, and retinoblastoma.

Retinal dysplasia

A dysplasia is a failure of tissue to develop normally during embryonic life. The tissue never achieves maturity. The noxious influence responsible for growth retardation, for example, a chromosome abnormality, usually causes a deviation in the growth pattern so that the final structure of the tissue is distinctly abnormal. Embryonic tissues are relatively pluripotential in their capacity to develop along several lines, and dysplastic growth often reflects this state when bizarre tissue differentiation occurs.

During normal retinal embryogenesis, retinal development probably reaches a point at which noxious influences are less likely to create growth deviations characteristic of retinal dysplasia. This postulated point or time interval has not been documented experimentally or clinically; however, it follows that noxious insults very early in gestation are more likely to create abnormal growth of the pluripo-

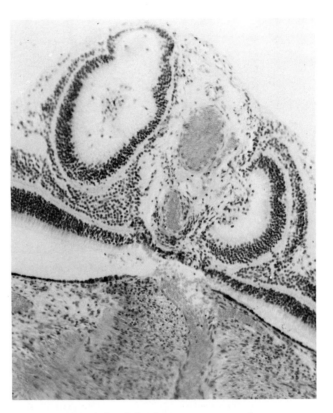

Fig. 8-57. Two isolated dysplastic rosettes near the optic nerve head, seen in the absence of other congenital intraocular defects. (H & E stain; ×275.)

tential neuroepithelium of the optic cup than are later insults.

Retinal dysplasia is considered a lesion with specific morphologic characteristics rather than a disease or syndrome in itself (Figs. 2-56–2-58, 8-57, 8-58, 9-10, and 9-35).[951–955] It may occur in otherwise normal individuals as an isolated, unilateral lesion (Fig. 8-57), or it may be observed as a component of several syndromes with intraocular involvement. Examples of the latter are trisomy 13 (p. 41; Figs. 2-56–2-58 and 8-58) and Norrie's disease (p. 501; Fig. 9-35).[6]

The primary histopathologic feature of retinal dysplasia is the formation of rosettes. A rosette represents an attempt to form embryonic retinal tissue, primary rods and cones (Fig. 9-10). The nuclei lining the rosette are analogous to the nuclei in the outer nuclear layer of the retina. The apparent membrane that often lines the outer margin of the lumen of the rosette is analogous to the external limiting membrane. The benign rosettes of retinal dysplasia, which show no anaplasia, should be clearly distinguished from the malignant Flexner-Wintersteiner rosettes formed in retinoblastoma (p. 485). The latter rosettes possess the same propensity toward formation of rods and cones, but unlike dysplastic rosettes, they exhibit neoplastic differentiation with malignant behavior.

In addition to formation of rosettes, retinal dysplasia occasionally shows an attempt by the faulty neuroepithelium to form simple cuboidal epithelium resembling that of embryonic retina or ciliary body (Fig. 9-35, *B*).

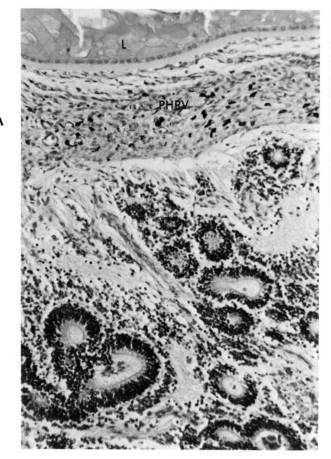

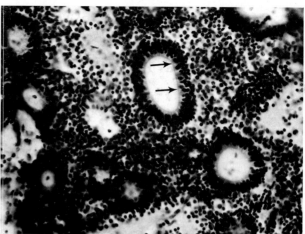

Fig. 8-58. Retinal dysplasia in trisomy 13. **A,** Numerous rosettes are within a mass of dysplastic retina behind a retrolental fibrous membrane (PHPV). *L,* Cataractous lens. (H & E stain; ×225.) **B,** Higher power micrograph of dysplastic rosettes. The "membrane" lining the lumens *(arrows)* is characteristic (see Figs. 9-10 and 9-11). (H & E stain; ×250.)

Retinal dysplasia should be distinguished from retinal dystrophy and retinal degeneration. While a dysplasia signifies an embryonic aberration in which the tissue fails to mature, a dystrophy is the process by which a mature tissue undergoes atrophy or regression. This is sometimes termed an *abiotrophy*. By definition, the term *dystrophy* usually applies to diseases related to genetic influences. The retinitis pigmentosa syndromes are examples of retinal dystrophies. Degeneration in the strictest sense connotes a deterioration or atrophy of tissue caused by an acquired influence such as trauma, toxicity, vascular disease, or inflammatory insults.

Peripheral retinal and choroidal dystrophies and degenerations

RETINITIS PIGMENTOSA SYNDROMES

The retinitis pigmentosa syndromes are retinal dystrophies.[956–1090] The primary retinal dystrophies should be clearly distinguished from secondary or pseudoretinitis pigmentosa conditions (p. 406). The term *retinal pigmentary degeneration*, although often used interchangeably with the term *dystrophy* (as in the syndromes with a retinitis pigmentosa-like pigmentary degeneration, p. 404), is perhaps less accurate because, in the strictest sense, it connotes a deterioration or atrophy of retinal tissue resulting from acquired influences as opposed to developmental or genetic influences.

Most forms of inherited retinal dystrophy share the common feature of a deterioration of selected retinal elements that have previously matured but undergo regression or abiotrophy at a later date.[777] The human retinitis pigmentosa syndromes are sometimes called *tapetoretinal degenerations*. This term was coined by early anatomists, who designated the retinal pigment epithelium the tapetum nigrum, or black carpet; it underscores the point that the pigment epithelium and sensory retina are intimately involved in this condition from pathogenetic and morphologic standpoints.

Two pathogenetic theories are presently debated: one theory postulates a primary, genetically induced degeneration of photoreceptors; the other points toward a primary aberration in function of the retinal pigment epithelium. It has been postulated that pathogenesis may involve defective interaction between pigment epithelium and photoreceptors, including an inadequate capacity of the pigment epithelium to phagocytose outer segment discs shed normally from photoreceptor cells, which may be responsible.

Isolated retinitis pigmentosa

Retinitis pigmentosa (retinopathia pigmentosa, pigmentary retinopathy, pigmentary retinal dystrophy, peripheral tapetoretinal degeneration, and peripheral tapetoretinal dystrophy) may occur as an isolated ocular defect without associated systemic changes.[952,995,1016,1021,1045] It is not an inflammatory disease, and the suffix *-itis*, although entrenched in clinical usage, is inaccurate.

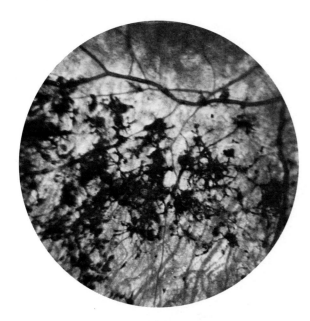

Fig. 8-59. Fundus photograph of retinitis pigmentosa with "bone spicules," causing baring background choroidal vessels and attenuation of retinal arterioles.

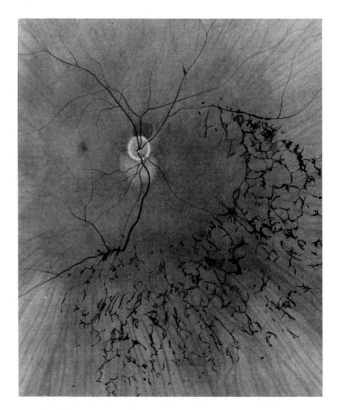

Fig. 8-60. Artist's drawing of sector retinitis pigmentosa.

Isolated retinitis pigmentosa is usually transmitted as an autosomal-recessive trait, but it may also be inherited in an autosomal-dominant and, rarely, in an **X**-linked recessive manner. Because of this multimodal pattern of inheritance, genetic counseling is possible only after definite determination of the genetic pattern by family studies. Ocular involvement is usually bilateral and symmetric.[1077]

Although usually hereditary, the visual signs and symptoms often first appear in early adult life. The important clinical symptoms of classic retinitis pigmentosa include night blindness and a progressive limitation of the visual field that begins as an equatorial, or ring, scotoma and contracts from the periphery, leading to tubular vision and eventually to total blindness. Progression of the disease and contraction of the field are associated with changes in the dark-adaptation curve and an abnormal or extinguished electroretinogram (ERG) and electrooculogram. Fishman and colleagues have reported macular lesions associated with retinitis pigmentosa.[990,991,994] These may include atrophic hypopigmentation of the retinal pigment epithelium or cystoid macular lesions.

Because the visual field loss begins in the midperiphery and far periphery and leaves only central vision as the disease progresses, it is unfortunate that an associated component of this disease in some cases is a posterior polar cataract (cataracta complicata).[989] Such a cataract causes an exaggerated loss of vision because of its central location in the already compromised visual field.

In addition to cataract, retinitis pigmentosa is sometimes associated with keratoconus, marginal corneal dystrophy, macular cystoid degeneration, Coats's syndrome, optic disc drusen (Fig. 8-61), astrocytic hematomas of the optic nerve head, and myopia.[982,1015,1055]

The primary funduscopic changes (Figs. 8-59–8-61; Color Plates 8-25–8-27) include deposition of the typical bone spicules or bone corpuscles in the retinal periphery, associated attenuation of the retinal vessels, and a pale, "waxy" discoloration of the disc with eventual optic atrophy.[1029] The choroidal vessels become increasingly visible as the epithelial pigment is dispersed or destroyed.[1031]

The earliest histopathologic changes in the sensory retina occur in the outer half of the retina. This region corresponds to the entire span of the photoreceptor cell (see diagram on p. 355). The rods are primarily affected, but cone degeneration also occurs. Eventually all layers of the retina are attenuated, and thinning, gliosis, and atrophy of the entire retina occur in long-standing cases.[1016,1020,1037,1069]

Melanin pigment, derived from retinal pigment epithelium, migrates into the sensory retina and is deposited in and around the walls of the retinal vessels (Fig. 8-62). The perivascular deposition of pigment in the vessel walls and within the glial network around the vessels is responsible for the bone spicule pattern observed clinically. The pigment follows the contour of the branching retinal vessels. Attenuation of the retinal vasculature is a secondary phenomenon. Formation of a glial membrane on the optic disc may partially explain the peculiar yellow waxy discoloration of this structure.

"Atypical" forms of retinitis pigmentosa

In addition to the isolated typical or classic form of retinitis pigmentosa, atypical forms include the following:

1. Retinitis pigmentosa without pigment (sine pigmento) is similar to the typical form except for an absence of pigmented bone spicules in clinical examination.
2. When the changes are confined to a single sector of the fundus, it is known as a sector retinitis pigmentosa (Fig. 8-60).[1019,1061]

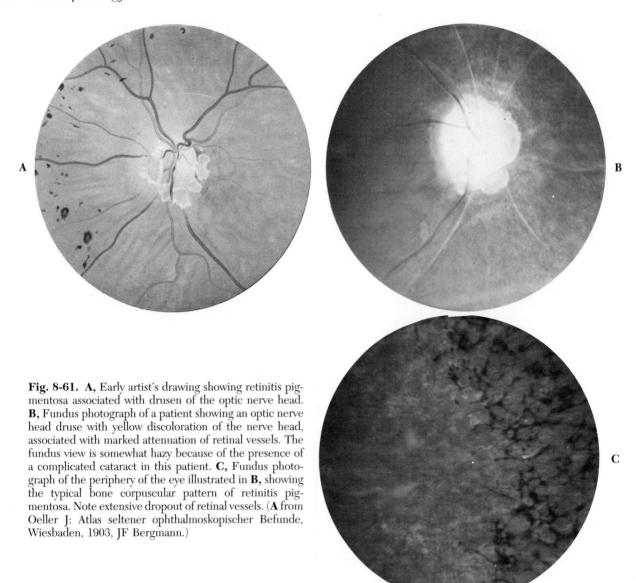

Fig. 8-61. A, Early artist's drawing showing retinitis pigmentosa associated with drusen of the optic nerve head. **B,** Fundus photograph of a patient showing an optic nerve head druse with yellow discoloration of the nerve head, associated with marked attenuation of retinal vessels. The fundus view is somewhat hazy because of the presence of a complicated cataract in this patient. **C,** Fundus photograph of the periphery of the eye illustrated in **B,** showing the typical bone corpuscular pattern of retinitis pigmentosa. Note extensive dropout of retinal vessels. (**A** from Oeller J: Atlas seltener ophthalmoskopischer Befunde, Wiesbaden, 1903, JF Bergmann.)

3. Central retinitis pigmentosa occurs when the changes are confined to the macular region (p. 429).[1062]
4. Leber's congenital amaurosis might be considered as a congenital form of retinitis pigmentosa.[1023,1040,1046] Affected children are born blind or with severe visual handicap. The ERG is extinct, even when done at an early age. The fundus is initially normal or may show abnormal tapetal reflexes or pigmentary changes at the macula, or it may reveal a picture of retinitis punctata albescens. Later in life, the fundus becomes more and more pigmented until the typical bone corpuscles and attenuated vessels appear. It is also frequently associated with keratoconus and/or cataract.
5. Retinitis punctata albescens (progressive albipunctate dystrophy) involves functional abnormalities of the retina similar to those of retinitis pigmentosa, but the ophthalmoscopic findings are different.[988] The fundus shows multiple, diffusely scattered white dots together with abnormal fundal reflexes. The disease is slowly progressive. No histopathologic study has been made.
6. Some syndromes have a retinitis pigmentosa-like pigmentary degeneration. Pigmentary retinopathy is sometimes associ-

ated with systemic disorders.[*] Most are inherited in an autosomal-recessive pattern, and many reflect defects in enzyme synthesis and metabolism. This is in keeping with a general rule that genetic diseases associated with enzyme imbalance are often inherited as recessive traits. Genetic diseases associated with a structural protein abnormality are more often inherited in a dominant mode.[992]

The following is an outline of various syndromes with a retinitis pigmentosa-like pigmentary deficit[†]:

A. The mucopolysaccharidoses
   1. Scheie's syndrome (mucopolysaccharidosis, type I-S)
      a. Autosomal recessive
      b. Normal intelligence
      c. Thickening of joints with limitation of motion
      d. Clawing of hands

---

[*] References 962, 966, 978–980, 1022, 1042, 1067, 1081, 1087.
[†] Courtesy Dr. Gerald Fishman, University of Illinois, Chicago.

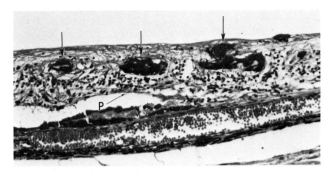

Fig. 8-62. Retinitis pigmentosa, late stage. Perivascular distribution of intraretinal pigment *(arrows)* causes the bone spicule appearance seen clinically. Pigment derived from the adjacent pigment epithelium follows the contours of the walls of the network of intraretinal vessels and their glial sheaths. The total destruction of the photoreceptor cell layer *(P)* and degeneration of the retinal pigment epithelium are considered early changes. In later stages, such as that illustrated here, subsequent diffuse degeneration of the entire thickness of retina affects all layers. The vessels (lined by pigment) show marked attenuation of their lumens. (H & E stain; ×80.)

    e. Broad facies but not gargoylism

    f. Increase in urine dermatan sulfate levels

    g. Corneal clouding

    h. Some cases: atypical retinitis pigmentosa with abnormal ERG; others: normal fundi and normal ERG

  2. Hunter's syndrome (mucopolysaccharidosis, type II)

    a. X-linked recessive

    b. Gargoylelike facies

    c. Hepatosplenomegaly

    d. Dwarfism

    e. Dementia

    f. Deafness

    g. Stiff joints

    h. Onset in early childhood, with death from cardiac failure between 20 and 40 years of age

    i. Deficiency of β-galactosidase activity

    j. Increase in urine dermatan sulfate levels

    k. Increase in urine heparitin sulfate levels

    l. Metachromatic granules in lymphocytes

    m. Clear cornea

    n. Atypical retinitis pigmentosa with degeneration of retinal pigment epithelium and loss of rods and cones; subnormal ERG

    o. Pseudopapilledema

  3. Sanfilippo's syndrome (mucopolysaccharidosis, type III)

    a. Autosomal recessive

    b. Severe mental retardation

    c. Stiff joints

    d. Hernias

    e. Hirsutism

    f. Onset in early childhood, with death in early adolescence

    g. Increase in urine heparitin sulfate levels

    h. Metachromatic granules in lymphocytes

    i. Absence of corneal clouding

    j. Atypical retinitis pigmentosa

 B. Batten-Mayou syndrome

  1. Autosomal recessive[1004,1072]

  2. Onset between 5 and 8 years of age; Vogt-Spielmeyer disease onset between 2 and 4 years of age in Jewish families

  3. Mental retardation

  4. Upper and lower motor neuron palsies

  5. Ataxia, starting in lower limbs

  6. Convulsions

  7. Inclusion in cytoplasm of lymphocytes in blood and conjunctival fluid

  8. Retinal pigmentary degeneration with loss of rods and cones

 C. Laurence-Moon-Bardet-Biedl syndrome°

  1. Autosomal recessive

  2. Obesity

  3. Hypogenitalism

  4. Mental retardation (85%)

  5. Polydactyly (80%)

  6. Nerve deafness (4%)

  7. Wide fluctuations in body temperature

  8. Shortening of metacarpals and metatarsals

  9. Congenital heart disease

  10. Keratoconus[1001]

  11. Retinitis pigmentosa–like pigmentary degenerations (15%)

 D. Bassen-Kornzweig syndrome[977]

  1. Autosomal recessive; onset in infancy

  2. Acanthocytosis (thorn-shaped erythrocytes)

  3. Celiac disease with inability to absorb lipids

  4. High frequency in persons of Jewish extraction

  5. Abetalipoproteinemia with inability to transport lipids

  6. Low serum cholesterol and phospholipid levels

  7. Steatorrhea in childhood

  8. Mental retardation in early childhood

  9. Gait disturbance, ataxia, dysdiadochokinesia, absent tendon reflexes

  10. Glycosuria, low sedimentation rate, nonspecific aminoaciduria

  11. Elevated cerebrospinal fluid protein levels

  12. Atypical pigmentary tapetoretinal degeneration beginning around age 10 to 14 with progression

 E. Refsum's syndrome[967,1081]

  1. Autosomal recessive

  2. Chronic and progressive symmetric paresis of distal limb parts

  3. Cerebellar ataxia

  4. Onset in childhood

  5. Progressive deafness

  6. Failure to oxidize phytanic acid, with resulting accumulation of phytanic acid in serum, urine, and tissues

  7. Increased cerebrospinal fluid protein levels without cells

  8. Increased serum copper, ceruloplasmin, and *N*-acetylneuraminic acid levels

  9. Cataracts

  10. Night blindness, with an atypical retinitis pigmentosa infrequent, starting in the macula, often sine pigmento

 F. Sjögren-Larsson syndrome

  1. Autosomal recessive

  2. Ichthyosis

  3. Spastic diplegia

° References 973, 976, 1001, 1008, 1022, 1204.

4. Oligophrenia with cortical central nervous system atrophy of neurons and secondary gliosis throughout the gray matter
5. Hyperreflexia
6. Life expectancy half normal
7. Atypical retinitis pigmentosa with macular and perimacular pigment degeneration in 20% to 30% of affected persons; however, normal ERG

G. Hallgren's syndrome
1. Autosomal recessive
2. Congenital deafness
3. Vestibulocerebellar ataxia (90%)
4. Mental deficiency (25%)
5. Retinitis pigmentosa–like pigmentary degeneration, with night blindness present at preschool age

H. Alström's syndrome
1. Autosomal recessive
2. Severe nerve deafness
3. Obesity, generally truncal
4. Absence of mental retardation
5. Acanthosis nigricans
6. In males, hypogonadism associated with normal secondary sex characteristics
7. Hyperuricemia
8. Hypertriglyceridemia with elevated pre-β-lipoprotein levels
9. Baldness
10. Hyperostosis frontalis interna
11. Chronic nephropathy occurring in adulthood with aminoaciduria, nephrogenic diabetes insipidus, and uremia
12. Generalized cell membrane thickening and hyalinization of connective tissues
13. No polydactyly, syndactyly, or brachydactyly
14. Resistance to insulin, causing diabetes mellitus in adulthood
15. Resistance to vasopressin and gonadotropins
16. Cataracts
17. Nystagmus
18. Retinal pigmentary degeneration with profound blindness between 1 and 2 years of age

I. Usher's syndrome[964,975,993]
1. Autosomal dominant
2. Deaf-mutism, beginning in early childhood
3. Ataxia
4. Mental deficiency
5. Hypophosphatemic glycosuric rickets
6. Muscle wasting
7. Retinal pigmentary degeneration

J. Amalric-Dialinos syndrome
1. Deaf-mutism
2. Atypical retinitis pigmentosa with small, scattered, fine, pigmented deposits in the macular region accompanied by small white and yellow spots; larger choroidal vessels prominent; changes not associated with night blindness or abnormalities of ERG

K. Cockayne's syndrome[1026]
1. Autosomal recessive
2. Onset generally within second year of life
3. Mental retardation
4. Dwarfish appearance
5. Disproportionately long limbs, with large hands and feet
6. Progressive infantile deafness

7. Progeria (precocious senile appearance)
8. Hepatosplenomegaly
9. Intracranial calcifications
10. Sensitivity to sunlight, with skin pigmentation and scarring
11. Cataracts
12. Enophthalmos
13. Poor pupillary response to mydriatics
14. Retinitis pigmentosa–like retinal degeneration

L. Hallervorden-Spatz syndrome[1030,1069]
1. Autosomal recessive
2. Basal ganglia symptoms
3. Dementia
4. Early death
5. Retinitis pigmentosa–like fundus changes

M. Pelizaeus-Merzbacher syndrome
1. X-linked recessive
2. Dementia and cerebellar ataxia
3. Retinitis pigmentosa–like fundus changes

N. Alport's syndrome
1. Autosomal dominant
2. Hereditary familial hemorrhagic nephritis
3. Early death in males; normal lifespan in females
4. Hearing loss
5. Juvenile arcus
6. Thinning of lens capsule, anterior lenticonus, subcapsular cataracts
7. Fundus albipunctatus (rare)

O. Kearns-Sayre syndrome[959,986,987]
1. Autosomal
2. Chronic external ophthalmoplegia
3. Cardiac abnormalities
4. Retinal pigmentary degeneration

P. Zellweger's syndrome[1002]
1. Cerebral degeneration
2. Hepatic degeneration
3. Pigmentary retinopathy

Pseudoretinitis pigmentosa

Some nonhereditary, acquired diseases may produce a unilateral or bilateral pigmentary retinopathy with fundus changes resembling retinitis pigmentosa.[976,981,1073]

1. Trauma (retinitis sclopedaria or late stage of commotio retinae)
2. Inflammation or infection
   a. Syphilis
   b. Toxoplasmosis
   c. Measles
   d. Rubella
   e. Herpes
   f. Cytomegalic inclusion disease
3. Toxic (drug-induced)
   a. Chloroquine
   b. Chlorpromazine
   c. Thioridazine[1039]
4. After retinal or choroidal arterial occlusion
5. Senile degeneration in an otherwise normal eye

Trauma

Posttraumatic migration of retinal pigment epithelium into the sensory retina may occasionally occur, often as a se-

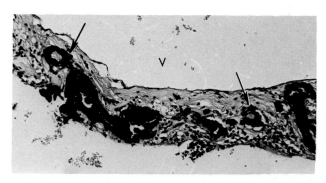

Fig. 8-63. Posttraumatic pseudoretinitis pigmentosa. The patient suffered blunt trauma several years before. Examination of the globe after enucleation for other causes revealed melanin pigment distributed around retinal vessels *(arrows)*. This perivascular deposition of melanin is responsible for the bone corpuscle pattern observed clinically. Traumatic pseudoretinitis pigmentosa must be differentiated from other causes of pigmentary degeneration of the retina, such as true retinitis pigmentosa, toxic pigmentary degeneration, and infectious (syphilitic) pigmentary degeneration. Note the massive destruction of all retinal layers occurring in late stages of the disease. V, Vitreous. (H & E stain; ×100.) (From Crouch E and Apple DJ: Am J Ophthalmol 78:251, 1974.)

quela to commotio retinae or Berlin's edema.[960,961,981,1073] Berlin's edema was formerly thought to be a true transudation of edema fluid into the sensory retina. The edematous appearance is actually probably due to primary structural or mechanical damage to photoreceptors and pigment epithelium, which causes a partial loss of the normal red fundus reflex. The clinical and histopathologic picture of posttraumatic pseudoretinitis pigmentosa is similar to the pattern observed in true retinitis pigmentosa, particularly in its later stages (Fig. 8-63; Color Plate 8-24). In the late stages of both true and pseudoretinitis pigmentosa, perivascular deposition of melanin pigment occurs and creates the familiar spicular pattern, attenuation of vessels, and destruction of all layers of the sensory retina, particularly the photoreceptors.

Inflammation

Syphilis is an important example of a postinfectious pseudoretinitis pigmentosa. The microscopic appearance of the retina in postsyphilitic pigmentary retinopathy resembles or duplicates that of true retinitis pigmentosa.

Pigmentary retinopathy may occur in patients after intrauterine exposure to rubella virus (maternal rubella syndrome), but true migration of pigment epithelium into the perivascular spaces of sensory retina is rare. Most cases of rubella "salt-and-pepper" fundus result from simple alternating hypoplasia and hyperplasia of the pigment epithelium, without important clinical sequelae or electroretinographic exchanges (p. 132; Fig. 4-36).

Toxins

Chloroquine produces a toxic retinopathy, which initially creates a central macular lesion and shows peripheral pigmentary changes in later stages (Fig. 8-98).[1060] At first a diffuse mottling of the affected macular area occurs. Then a pale ring composed of degenerate or atrophic retinal pig-

ment epithelium forms and surrounds the central focus, which remains more pigmented. This bull's-eye appearance is highly characteristic of this condition. Ultimately an attenuation of retinal vessels and constriction of the visual fields follows the initial macular lesion, and a pigmentary retinopathy and optic atrophy not unlike that seen in retinitis pigmentosa eventually develop.

CHOROIDAL DEGENERATIONS AND DYSTROPHIES

Although not primarily retinal in origin, three choroidal diseases affect the peripheral fundus in areas corresponding to that seen in retinitis pigmentosa and are, therefore, briefly described here.[968,1017,1018,1078,1085]

Primary diffuse choroidal sclerosis

Primary choroidal sclerosis is a degenerative vascular condition, which often occurs in families.[1070,1074,1080] The macular form, geographic atrophy of the pigment epithelium and choriocapillaris, formerly termed *central areolar choroidal dystrophy*, is described on page 429. Both the macular form and the diffuse form are characterized by a disappearance of the pigment epithelium and the choriocapillaris, which permits the vessels of the choroid to be seen, causing a tigroid background throughout the fundus. Optic atrophy, constriction of the visual fields, and blindness are the usual sequelae.

Choroideremia

Choroideremia and gyrate atrophy of the choroid are classified as tapetochoroidal degenerations.* Choroideremia is a sex chromosome–transmitted, X-linked condition, which affects males and is carried, usually without symptoms, by females. This progressive condition is characterized by defective scotopic vision, and, in later stages of the disease, by a severely constructed visual field. Dark-adaptation curves show severe impairment, and blindness eventually ensues.

The fundus of the affected male shows scattered flecks of pigment; the pigment particles are confined to the choroid and do not invade the retina as in retinitis pigmentosa (Color Plate 8-28). In advanced cases the choroidal vessels are almost entirely destroyed and the white sclera is bared. The pigment epithelium and retina are markedly atrophic (Fig. 8-64). The optic nerve remains normal in appearance, and the retinal vessels show few changes. Although asymptomatic, female carriers of the disease show minor fundus changes, including minimal pigmentary changes. Vision is normal in carriers, or there may be a slight enlargement of the blind spot or a slight defect in dark adaptation.

Gyrate atrophy

Gyrate atrophy, choroideremia, and retinitis pigmentosa have been noted in the same pedigree, suggesting that they are in some cases possibly forms of the same disease, although the pathogenesis is entirely unclear.[1089] Gyrate atrophy has been associated with hyperornithinemia.[1014,1035,1079] This hereditary disease is characterized by patchy and progressive atrophy of the choroid in the equatorial region, forming a girdle or ring-shaped area of

---

* References 958, 972, 1010, 1033, 1054, 1059, 1071, 1083.

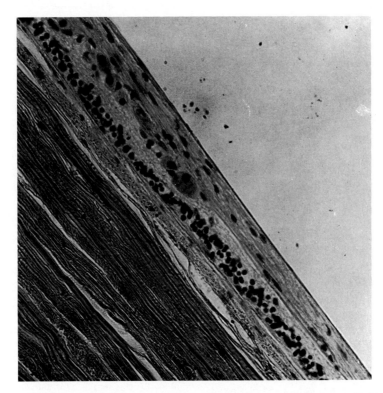

Fig. 8-64. Histologic section through an eye with choroideremia. The retina is highly atrophic and thin. Neither pigment epithelium nor intact choroid is present. (H & E stain; ×140.) (From Blodi F and Allen L: Stereoscopic manual of the ocular fundus in local and systemic disease, vol I, St. Louis, 1964, The CV Mosby Co.)

atrophy, sparing initially the central area and the far periphery of the fundus.[1035,1079] The patches of atrophy are characterized by disappearance of the choriocapillaris and later the large vessels, leaving the sclera exposed. Admixed with the wide areas of atrophy are areas of pigment clumping. The visual field shows peripheral constriction with a scotoma subtending the belt-shaped area of atrophy. A central scotoma and envelopment of central vision does not occur until late stages of the disease. No histologic reports are available.

Retinal degenerations, retinal breaks, and retinal detachment[1091–1252]

RETINAL DEGENERATIONS

The term *retinal degeneration* connotes a deterioration or atrophy of retinal tissue resulting from aging, vascular disease, exudative or inflammatory insults, mechanical forces, trauma, or toxicity. Certain degenerative lesions of the peripheral retina and vitreous, particularly those which lead to retinal breaks, play a significant role in the pathogenesis of retinal detachment. Other lesions may reveal a specific clinical picture but have little or no correlation with retinal detachment.[1065]

The unique anatomy and histology of the peripheral retina and vitreous, the two structures most intimately involved in the pathogenesis of retinal breaks and detachment, are discussed on pages 363 and 366.

The following outline (modified from a classification of Dr. Michael Goldbaum, Department of Ophthalmology, University of California, San Diego) categorizes the most common type of peripheral cilioretinal degenerations. The entities in group A are generally clinically innocuous and rarely lead to retinal detachment. Those in group B are more likely to result in retinal detachment.

A. Peripheral congenital or degenerative cilioretinal lesions that rarely produce retinal breaks
   1. Pars plana and pars plicata
      a. Cysts and cystic excavations
   2. Ora serrata[1226]
      a. Enclosed oral bays
      b. Pearls
      c. Meridional folds
   3. Sensory retina
      a. Microcystoid degeneration
      b. Degenerative ("senile") retinoschisis
   4. Retinal pigment epithelium
      a. Drusen
      b. Congenital hypertrophy of the retinal pigment epithelium
      c. Bear tracks
      d. Senile reticular hyperpigmentation
   5. Choroid retina
      a. Cobblestone degeneration
      b. Senile peripheral tapetochoroidal degeneration
   6. Retinovitreal interface
      a. White with or without pressure
      b. Retinal pits
B. Lesions causing retinal breaks
   1. Retinovitreal interface
      a. Lattice degeneration and snail track degeneration

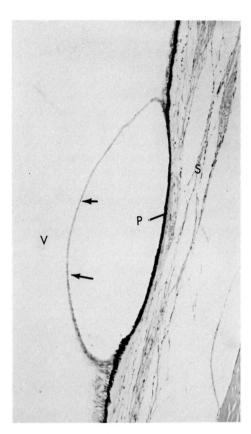

Fig. 8-65. Typical cyst of the pars plana. The inner nonpigmented epithelium *(arrows)* is separated from the outer pigmented layer *(P). S,* Stroma of the pars plana; *V,* vitreous cavity. (H & E stain; ×80.)

b. Granular tags
c. Zonuloretinal traction tufts
d. Pigmented chorioretinal scars with vitreous traction
e. Angioids (remnants of embryonic retinovitreal vessels of the vasa hyaloidea propria)
f. Round atrophic holes (rare cause)

In this section the most common entities that have a distinct histopathologic appearance are considered. These are cysts and cystic excavations of the pars plana and pars plicata, microcystoid degeneration and retinoschisis, peripheral drusen, cobblestone degeneration, and lattice degeneration.

Cysts of the pars plana and pars plicata

Typical cysts of the pars plana and pars plicata are acquired, translucent, or transparent teardrop-shaped or round cysts that are present in up to 20% of individuals.[1143,1152,1171,1194] They increase in frequency with age. Unless very large, the pars plana cysts are seen only when the ora and pars plana are examined during depression ophthalmoscopy. These discrete cystic structures are usually easily differentiated from tumors and do not cause retinal holes or detachment (Fig. 4-27, *A*).

They may arise as a simple separation of the two ciliary epithelial layers (Fig. 8-65). They contain hyaluronic acid, a fact that is not surprising when the embryology of the retinal layers is considered.[1249] Both layers of the original optic cup normally possess the capability to secrete muco-

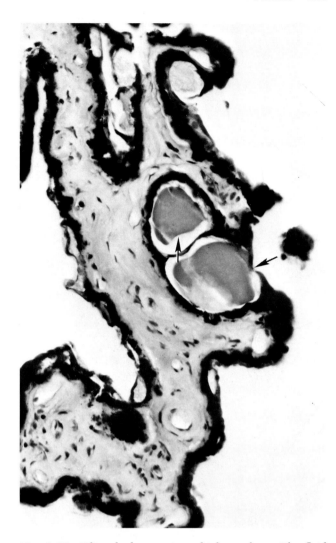

Fig. 8-66. Ciliary body cysts in multiple myeloma. The fluid *(arrows)* contains myeloma protein. (H & E stain; ×220.)

polysaccharides, including hyaluronic acid. The matrix of the vitreous human, which is predominantly hyaluronic acid, and the acid mucopolysaccharides that normally engulf the photoreceptor cells represent a physiologic formation of this substance. In addition to pars plana cysts, other diseases in which mucopolysaccharides form from the ocular neuroepithelium include peripheral senile cystoid retinal degeneration, senile retinoschisis, and neuroepithelial tumors of the ciliary body (p. 329). In the latter condition, hyaluronic acid is a secretory product of neoplastic neuroepithelial cells.

Senile retinoschisis with inner and outer holes and holes at the base of meridional folds, particularly when located temporally, are rare causes of retinal breaks.

So-called microcysts of the pars plana, sometimes known as cystic excavations of the pars plana, are smaller than the typical cysts. These are multiple cysts within the nonpigmented inner layer of the ciliary epithelium produced by proliferation and separation of the individual epithelial cells.

Pars plana cysts may be prominent in patients with multiple myeloma (Fig. 8-66; Color Plate

Table 8-2. Classification of peripheral microcystoid degeneration and retinoschisis

Microcystoid degeneration	Retinoschisis
Outer plexiform layer	
Typical type (Blessig-Iwanoff)	Degenerative "senile" retinoschisis
No specific precursor	Secondary retinoschisis (tumors, trauma, exudative)
Nerve fiber layer	
Reticular type	Reticular retinoschisis
No specific precursor	Juvenile (**X**-linked) retinoschisis

8-29).[1093,1121,1159,1160] However, in contrast to simple cysts, they turn white after fixation. This is a result of denaturation and fixation of the myeloma immunoglobulins that fill the cystic cavities.

Peripheral retinal microcystoid degeneration and retinoschisis

Retinal microcystoid degenerative lesions and retinoschisis may affect the central or peripheral retina and are divided into two categories according to the layer of retina primarily involved: those initially occurring in the outer plexiform layer and those initially affecting the nerve fiber layer (Table 8-2).[1137,1150,1155,1195,1232] Diseases causing microcystoid edema of the outer plexiform layer at the macula are listed on page 424.

Microcystoid changes in the nerve fiber layer are relatively uncommon. Three conditions known to primarily involve this layer are reticular cystoid degeneration with or without retinoschisis; **X**-linked, or juvenile, retinoschisis (p. 422); and the schisis cavity associated with the "salmon patch" that forms in sickle retinopathy as a sequela of intraretinal hemorrhage (p. 384).

Peripheral "senile" microcystoid degeneration of the retina

Peripheral microcystoid (The term *cystoid* is used to distinguish this process from the formation of true "cysts." In the latter, a fluid accumulates progressively in a cavity that possesses its own epithelial lining, as in epithelial cysts.) degeneration is a process in which cavities are formed within the retinal tissue (Figs. 8-10, 8-67, and 8-68; Color Plates 8-30 and 8-31). It usually is an innocuous lesion that does not require treatment. It is bilaterally symmetric and is usually more significant temporally. It occurs in almost all persons after the first decade of life but increases in severity with age and is extensive in myopia. The cystoid cavities are sometimes designated "Blessig-Iwanoff cysts" after the investigators who described them (Blessig's cysts, Iwanoff's edema).

Peripheral cystoid degeneration is best seen clinically by depression ophthalmoscopy or mirror lens slitlamp examination. Oblique viewing of the retina reveals myriad small interconnecting channels or lacunae. The degeneration usually begins at the ora serrata and extends posteriorly, and the temporal retina usually shows the most involvement.

The cystoid spaces arise by rarefaction of the nervous elements of the retina and may be associated with degenerative or sclerotic changes in the underlying choriocapillaris, choroidal tumors, choroidal inflammation, trauma, retinal detachment, myopia, or retinal dystrophies.

The outer plexiform layer is primarily affected. At an early stage the cystoid spaces form rows of small hyaluronic acid–containing vesicles or lacunae in the outer plexiform layer, but as they enlarge they involve the nuclear layers on either side, and they coalesce to form columns or tunnels, which are separated by Müller fibers (Figs. 8-67 and 8-68). With further progression they extend from the outer to inner limiting membranes and, after breakdown of the Müller fiber columns, a retinoschisis develops (Fig. 8-68). Even at an early stage the inner wall of a cyst may give way, resulting in the formation of an inner layer lamellar

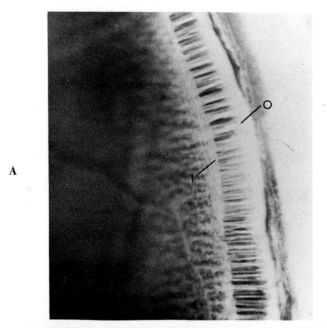

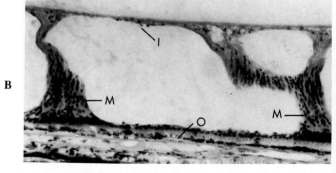

Fig. 8-67. Peripheral microcystoid degeneration. **A,** Gross photograph showing Müller cell columns lining the cystoid spaces. *O,* Outer retinal layer; *I,* inner retinal layer. (See Color Plates 8-30 and 8-31.) **B,** Photomicrograph of peripheral retinal microcystoid degeneration. The cavities (Blessig's space) are lined by Müller cell columns (*M*). the inner retina (*I*), and the outer retina (*O*), which is composed of residual photoreceptors. The process begins in the outer plexiform layer but in this case has broken through several layers. (H & E stain; ×280.) (**A** from Daicker B: Anatomie und Pathologie der menschlichen retino-ziliaren Fundusperipherie, Basel, 1972, S Karger, AG.)

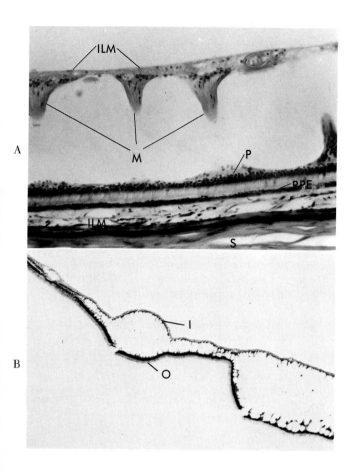

Fig. 8-68. Peripheral senile retinoschisis arising in an area of microcystoid degeneration. **A,** In advanced cases of peripheral cystoid retinal degeneration, the walls of the individual cavities may break down, leading to confluence of the cystoid spaces and to retinoschisis. The inner wall of this schisis cavity is composed primarily of the internal limiting membrane *(ILM)* and the inner portion of the Müller cells *(M)*. The outer wall of the schisis cavity is lined by nuclei of the photoreceptor cells *(P)*. RPE, Retinal pigment epithelium; *S,* sclera. (H & E stain; ×250.) **B,** Low-power photomicrograph of another case of peripheral flat retinoschisis showing rupture of Müller columns and confluence of the intraretinal cavities. *I,* Inner layer; *O,* outer layer. (H & E stain; ×35.)

hole. These never lead to retinal detachment in the absence of an outer layer hole.

Degenerative retinoschisis

Retinoschisis is defined as a cleavage or splitting of the retina into two layers.* There are two varieties of senile retinoschisis: flat, degenerative ("senile") retinoschisis and reticular retinoschisis.[1173] Although degenerative retinoschisis occasionally may produce retinal holes and detachment if an outer layer hole forms, it is described here because it is the consequence of a coalescence of the cavities of typical microcystoid degeneration.

Degenerative retinoschisis is a relatively common condition in elderly patients, is usually bilateral, and most com-

monly involves the lower temporal quadrant. It is usually limited to the preequatorial retina and tends to progress slowly with few complications. It is rarely seen before the third decade of life, is usually asymptomatic, and is commonly discovered incidentally during indirect ophthalmoscopy. The nearly transparent inner layer may appear tense, does not have folds, and may reveal a characteristic "beaten metal" appearance. White spots in a finely stippled pattern may be seen near the edge. These white spots ("glistening dots" or "snowflakes") are remnants of Müller cells that have recently split and that cling to the internal limiting membrane (Color Plate 8-31).[1064] Commensurate with the fact that the schisis arises from microcystic cavities, foci of microcystic degeneration surround and merge with the schisis cavity.

The splitting of the retina in the area of retinoschisis produces an absolute scotoma subtending the involved area. This may differentiate it from a flat retinal detachment that usually does not produce an early absolute visual field defect. Degenerative retinoschisis may also be clinically significant when it extends posteriorly to the fovea, but this is rare. Holes may form in either layer. Outer layer holes are often obvious and may have rolled edges. When there are holes in both the inner and outer layers of the schisis, a full-thickness retinal break exists and rhegmatogenous detachment is possible.[1115,1229]

Treatment is considered when posterior extension threatens the macula, an extremely rare state, or when there is risk of retinal detachment. A barrier of photocoagulation just outside the schisis may be used when the schisis threatens the macula. Cryopexy may be placed around retinal holes, and if it is desired to collapse the retinoschisis, cryopexy or photocoagulation can be scattered throughout the area of involvement at the risk of creating more holes in either layer.

Degenerative retinoschisis merely represents an advanced stage of the Blessig-Iwanoff type of peripheral retinal degeneration. Confluence of the cystoid spaces eventually results primarily from breakdown of the Müller fibers, which form the lateral walls of each space. The lamellar splitting begins in the outer plexiform layer, but the adjacent layers internal and external to this layer are eventually destroyed. The separation of the two walls may be so extreme that a macrocyst forms. (Fig. 8-69)[1116,1182]

The inner wall in advanced retinoschisis is thinner than the outer and is usually made up of the internal limiting membrane, the inner portions of Müller cells, remnants of the nerve fiber layer, and blood vessels. The outer wall consists mainly of degenerate outer plexiform layer, the outer nuclear layer, and the photoreceptors.

Reticular cystoid degeneration

Foos and Feman[1137] describe a second form of peripheral cystoid degeneration, which they term *reticular cystoid degeneration* (Color Plate 8-32). It often exists concurrently with typical "senile" cystoid degeneration but exhibits distinctive clinical and histopathologic features that warrant its being classified separately.

It is characterized by a fine, delicately stippled surface and an arborizing superficial vascular pattern. This pattern contrasts with the relatively large cystoid spaces seen in cysts of the Blessig-Iwanoff type. The reticular lesions usu-

---

* References 1109, 1176, 1210, 1225, 1250, 1251.

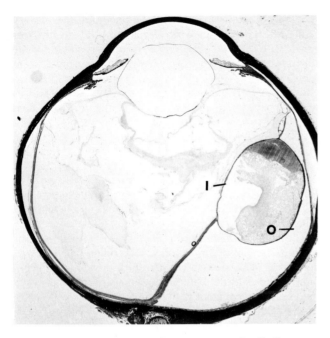

Fig. 8-69. Retinal macrocyst forming as a result of bullous retinoschisis. *I,* Inner layer of schisis; *O,* outer layer of schisis. (H & E stain; ×2.) (From the collection of Professor Wolfgang Stock, University of Tübingen, Tübingen, Germany, and from Naumann GOH and Apple DJ: In Doerr W, Seifert G, and Uehlinger E, editors: Handbuch der speziellen pathologischen Anatomie, Band Auge, Berlin, 1980, Springer-Verlag.)

ally occur immediately posterior to a band of typical cystoid degeneration. The borders of the lesion tend to be angular, linear, and often limited by larger vessels. There is a definite predilection for the temporal quadrants.

Histopathologically reticular cystoid degeneration differs from typical microcystoid degeneration in that the early splitting occurs in the nerve fiber layer (Table 8-2). Although initially located completely within the nerve fiber layer, the cavities may later extend from the internal limiting membrane toward the inner plexiform layer.

Drusen

Drusen (German, *druse,* crystal-like nodule) are deposits of hyaline material on Bruch's membrane (Figs. 8-89 and 8-90). They may occur as a senile process without clinically obvious antecedent disease or may arise as degenerative sequelae to many types of intraocular conditions, including overlying choroidal nevi or tumors, inflammatory diseases, vascular insufficiency, trauma or retinal detachment, and phthisic eyes. They are more common in the posterior pole rather than in the retinal periphery and are frequently associated with disciform degeneration of the macula (p. 442). Familial (dominant) drusen are considered on page 426.

Cobblestone degeneration

Cobblestone, or paving-stone, degeneration is a chorioretinal atrophic process that is primarily an aging change produced by relative ischemia of the peripheral retina.[1196] The yellow-white patches usually have scalloped, sharply demarcated and often pigmented borders.

The lesions are mostly round or oval, may occur singly or in groups, or may be confluent. They occur in 25% of autopsy eyes and occur most frequently inferior temporally. They are usually separated from the ora serrata by a zone of normal retina. Prominent choroidal vessels frequently may be seen at the base of the lesions. They are of little clinical significance because they do not cause retinal breaks.

Microscopic sections of a focus of cobblestone degeneration reveal a nonspecific thinning of the entire retina, particularly the outer layers. This predilection to outer retinal layer atrophy, which occurs concurrently with atrophy of the pigment epithelium and choriocapillaris, suggests that choroidal vascular insufficiency is probably responsible for the characteristic changes. While the pigment epithelium within the focus of cobblestone degeneration shows atrophy, the pigment epithelium rimming the lesion may actually undergo a hyperplasia, thus causing an ophthalmoscopically visible hyperpigmentation at the outer borders.

The atrophic sensory retina becomes adherent to Bruch's membrane; therefore, not only does cobblestone degeneration not result in retinal detachment, it may actually be protective because of the chorioretinal adhesion.

Lattice degeneration and snail-track degeneration

Lattice, or palisade, degeneration represents a specific type of peripheral retinal degeneration and thinning with associated vitreous traction (Fig. 8-70; Color Plate 8-33).* It is significant because it can lead to retinal breaks and retinal detachment.

Snail-track degeneration is characterized by lesions that are the same size and shape as those of lattice degeneration. White dots are often present, creating a frost-like appearance ophthalmoscopically. Although some authors make a distinction between snail-track and lattice degeneration, the clinical course and potential for retinal detachment are the same in both types. Some authors consider snail-track degeneration a form of early lattice degeneration.

No sex predilection is involved, and lattice lesions can appear relatively early in life, sometimes by age 20. Lattice degeneration is usually bilateral and is most often encountered in the upper temporal quadrant. The lesions are sharply circumscribed, cigar-shaped patches that usually involve the retina circumferentially (parallel to the limbus) between the equator and the ora serrata. They range from 0.5 to 2 mm in width and from 1.5 mm to more than a quadrant in length.

Early lesions reveal a retinal thinning visible only when the retina is viewed almost on end during depression ophthalmoscopy. As the lesions age, sclerosis of retinal vessels within the lesion gives rise to the characteristic crisscross pattern or latticework (Color Plate 8-33).[1207] The retinal pigment epithelium may clump in the midst of the intertwining white lines, creating patches of alternating hyperpigmentation and hypopigmentation. The retinal thinning may lead to atrophic holes, and, when vitreous traction is present, horseshoe tears may develop.

Lattice degeneration affects 7% of the population. Al-

---

* References 997, 1103, 1108, 1110, 1111, 1114, 1141, 1217, 1227, 1228, 1235.

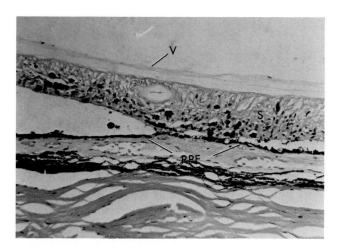

Fig. 8-70. Photomicrograph of lattice degeneration. The sensory retina *(S)* is greatly thinned and shows atrophy and degeneration of all layers. The pigmented clinical appearance of this lesion is caused by migration of pigment epithelium into the sensory retina. The intraretinal vessels show marked hyalinization of the wall with almost complete obliteration of the lumens. This vascular sclerosis represents the histopathologic counterpart of the lattice line. The underlying choroid is thinned, the retinal pigment epithelium *(RPE)* is atrophied, and the overlying vitreous *(V)* is condensed. (H & E stain; ×140.)

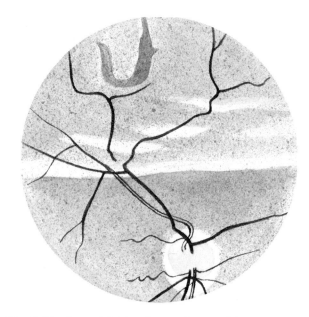

Fig. 8-71. Original fundus drawing by Greef showing superior retinal detachment associated with a horseshoe tear. (From Greef R: In Orth J, editor: Lehrbuch der speziellen pathologischen Anatomie, Berlin, 1902, Hirschwald.)

though lattice degeneration is found in a significant percentage of eyes with rhegmatogenous retinal detachment and, therefore, clearly contributes to the pathogenesis of detachment, most cases of lattice degeneration do not progress to detachment.

Fewer than 0.5% of patients with lattice degeneration progress toward detachment; those most likely to do so have a past history of detachment in the other eye, recently acquired retinal breaks, or a family history of retinal detachment. Prophylactic treatment methods designed to increase the retinal–pigment epithelial adhesion around the lesion include transconjunctival cryopexy and peripheral photocoagulation.

Histopathologic findings

The white lines of lattice degeneration correlate histopathologically with small retinal vessels that show thickening and "hyalinization" of the vessel wall (Fig. 8-70). Fluorescein angiography shows nonperfusion of these channels. The circumscribed, "punched-out" thinning of the retina affects the inner layers initially, and the inner limiting membrane may be destroyed. The inner retinal degeneration is possibly related to ischemia produced by impaired blood perfusion through the "sclerotic" vessels. However, because retinal degeneration of this type may occur in the absence of lattice lines, and because lattice degeneration often occurs in young individuals who otherwise show no signs of vascular "sclerosis," other causes of degeneration must be considered.

Alternating condensation and liquefaction of the overlying vitreous occur (Fig. 8-70). The condensed vitreous remains adherent to the edges of the lattice lines and may exert traction on the retina, causing tears and detachment.

The retinal pigment epithelium shows alternating clumping and rarefaction of pigment granules and migration of pigment into the sensory retina, thus accounting for the hyperpigmentation characteristic of most lattice lesions.

RETINAL BREAKS

The previous section emphasized that most peripheral retinal degenerations do not lead to retinal breaks or perforations (see p. 408). Although rhegmatogenous retinal detachments (p. 415) are caused by retinal breaks, the majority of retinal holes do not necessarily lead to retinal detachment; nevertheless, careful clinical follow-up and/or prophylactic treatment is indicated in patients with various types of retinal breaks.[1113,1123]

A retinal break is a through-and-through opening in the neurosensory retina, which forms a communication between the vitreous cavity and the subretinal space (Figs. 8-10 and 8-70–8-72; Color Plates 8-34–8-36).* Breaks are of several types and are classified by their pathogenesis (senile, degenerative, arteriosclerotic, inflammatory, myopic, traumatic) or by their appearance. The morphologic appearance often provides a clue to the pathogenesis of the break. The following paragraphs discuss some commonly accepted terms.

A *hole* is an opening, often round, occurring singly or in groups with or without an attached flap of retina (operculum).[1140,1231] An *atrophic hole* is a primary focal atrophic disintegration of retinal tissue in an otherwise relatively normal-appearing area. Retinal holes without opercula generally do not produce symptoms.

Many holes are caused by traction. A piece of retina is pulled away from the rest of the retina by vitreous strands

---

* References 1097, 1118, 1125, 1138, 1193, 1203, 1206, 1232.

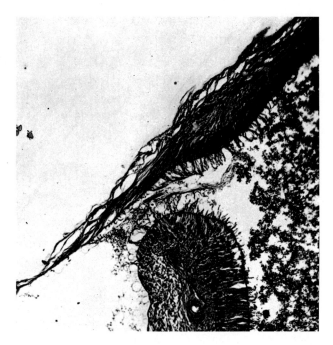

Fig. 8-72. Cross-section through a retinal tear. The posterior lip of the tear, which is in the lower part of the photomicrograph, has a characteristic rounded edge. The anterior lip (*above*) tapers off into a strand of vitreous that is adherent to this area. The vitreous lies on the left side of the picture, whereas the subretinal fluid is visible on the right side. (H & E stain; ×100.) (From Blodi FC and Allen L: Stereoscopic manual of the ocular fundus in local and systemic disease, vol I, St. Louis, 1964, The CV Mosby Co.)

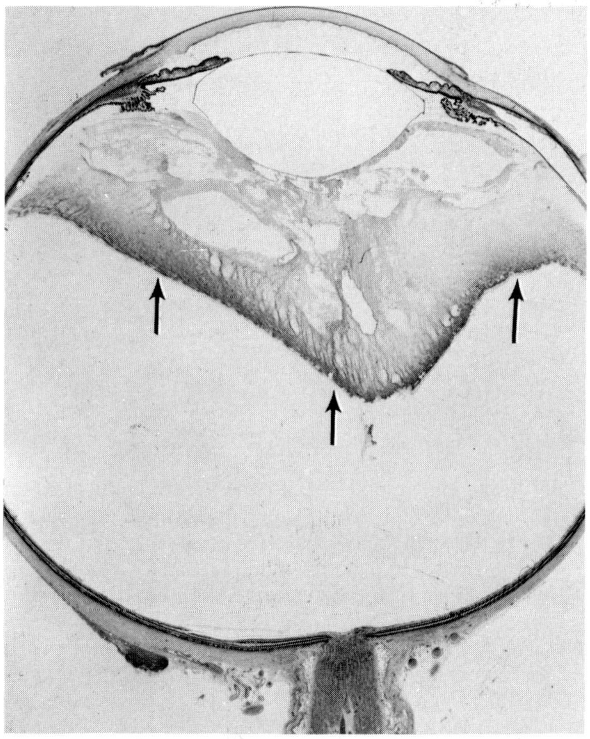

Fig. 8-73. Photomicrograph of condensed posterior detached vitreous. *Arrows,* Posterior vitreous face. (H & E stain; ×4.) (From the collection of Professor Wolfgang Stock, University of Tübingen, Tübingen, Germany, and from Naumann GOH and Apple DJ: In Doerr W, Seifert G, and Uehlinger E, editors: Handbuch der speziellen pathologischen Anatomie, Band Auge, Berlin, 1980, Springer-Verlag.)

or a detached vitreous (Fig. 8-73).* When the piece of retina attached to the detached vitreous face floats internal (anterior) to the hole, the piece of retina is called an operculum, and the hole is an operculated hole.

A hole may occur in either layer of retinoschisis. A simple inner layer hole is usually innocuous. A full-thickness hole in retinoschisis may lead to retinal detachment.

The margins of most retinal holes are smooth and rounded. Areas of cystoid degeneration of the retina often surround the defect (Figs. 8-72 and 8-88). Some vitreous remains attached to the margins. An operculum, when present, floats free in the vitreous, attached to the condensed face of the detached vitreous. Macular holes are considered on page 424 and in Figs. 8-87 and 8-88.

A *retinal tear*[1136] is a break ripped open by traction, most often by the vitreous[1218] and rarely from a zonule (zonuloretinal traction tuft).[1134,1136,1218] This often produces irritating symptoms such as flashing lights. Showers of black dots can be seen when a retinal vessel is torn and a small hemorrhage occurs. Often the tear is shaped like a horseshoe, with the two ends pointing anteriorly and the closed convexity usually pointing toward the posterior pole. The horse "walks" toward the posterior pole (Figs. 8-71 and 8-74, *A*; Color Plates 8-34–8-36). The tongue of retina inside the horseshoe is a flap. Condensed vitreous is often attached to the flap. A retinal break caused by traction

where traction still persists (e.g., a horseshoe tear) has a significant chance of progression to retinal detachment.

Distortion of the globe from blunt trauma may stretch the retina to the point where it tears.[1120,1124] A retinal tear induced by blunt injury often overlies a tear in Bruch's membrane and can lead to retinal detachment. A giant tear is a limbus parallel tear; it is often greater than 90 degrees, or 3 clock hours, in length. Such tears may even extend 360 degrees.[1214]

A *retinal dialysis* (Color Plate 8-36), a linear break at the ora serrata, also is often caused by blunt trauma.[1164,1218,1220, 1252] It is bordered anteriorly by ciliary epithelium and posteriorly by retina. Often the vitreous base remains attached to the retina posterior in this type of tear but is detached from the ciliary epithelium anterior to the tear. Most peripheral dialyses occur in young persons with emmetropia and affect the lower temporal quadrant. Almost all cases are traumatic.

The presence of subretinal fluid extending more than two disc diameters from the edge of a break increases the risk of clinical or symptomatic detachment, whether the break is traction induced or atrophic. A sound vitreous helps prevent a retinal break from leading to retinal detachment. Diseases with vitreous degeneration (e.g., myopia or Wagner-Stickler disease) are more likely to progress to retinal detachment from a retinal break. Aphakia greatly

---

* References 1120, 1135, 1156, 1157, 1166, 1230.

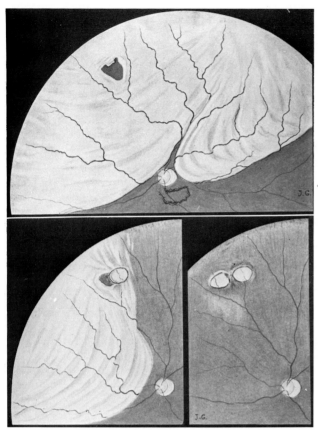

Fig. 8-74. Fundus drawings by Professor J Gonin (see also Color Plate 8-29), showing how he developed the principle that retinal detachments can be treated by closing a retinal hole. **A,** Large superior retinal detachment with a horseshoe tear in a patient with high myopia. **B,** *Left,* Treatment over the hole by a single spot of thermal cautery showing marked regression of the detachment. *Right,* After application of a second treatment, the detachment is entirely resolved and the retina is flat. (From Gonin J: Le décollement de la rétine, Lausanne, 1934, Librairie Payot & Cie.)

increases the risk of a break progressing to detachment.[1101,1103,1133,1186,1198]

Prophylactic photocoagulation and transconjunctival cryopexy increase the adhesion between the retina and choroid and are, therefore, often used to prevent retinal detachment.

RETINAL DETACHMENT

In strict terms, a retinal detachment actually connotes a separation rather than a "detachment" between the neurosensory retina and the retinal pigment epithelium.* The potential space between the retina and pigment epithelium, the subretinal space, is the vestige of the original cavity of the embryonic optic vesicle (Figs. 1-7, *A,* 1-9, and 8-1). Normally, the retina is firmly attached to the pigment epithelium only at the optic disc and the ora serrata. Throughout the remaining fundus areas, the retina is less

---

* References 1098, 1112, 1120, 1126, 1142, 1144, 1145, 1154, 1168, 1186, 1189, 1190, 1200, 1215, 1241.

firmly attached, and many pathologic alterations of the retina-vitreous may create a reopening of this cavity.

Retinal detachments are one of two types:

1. Rhegmatogenous (Greek, *rhegma,* break or rupture, and *gen,* source), in which a retinal break is present. Fluid from the vitreous passes through the break (a hole or tear) and accumulates in the subretinal space.
2. Nonrhegmatogenous, in which fluid or other abnormal tissue accumulates under an intact sensory retina. These are either exudative or tractional. Distinguishing clinical features of each type are listed in Table 8-3.

Rhegmatogenous detachments

The occurrence of holes and tears in the retina (described on p. 413) and their high incidence in cases of retinal detachment had been noted in the nineteenth century (Fig. 8-71).[40] However, Jules Gonin (Color Plate 8-36) was the first to stress that the primary factor in the pathogenesis of many "idiopathic" detachments of vitreous through a break into the subretinal space. He showed that the retina can be reattached by localization and obliteration or occlusion of the hole (Fig. 8-74).[1098–1100]

The incidence of retinal holes in the population is much higher than the incidence of retinal detachment.[1210] About one third of all nontraumatic retinal detachment occur in myopes. About 1% to 2% of patients with high myopia develop a detachment. Aphakic retinal detachments were much more prevalent before the era of extracapsular cataract common extraction and lens implantation. About 20% of all detachments occurred in aphakes, and about 2% to 5% of all aphakes developed a neural retinal detachment. With extracapsular cataract extraction, retinal detachment occurs in much less than 1 percent of cases. Every rhegmatogenous retinal detachment begins with a retinal break, but by no means does every retinal break lead to a retinal detachment, proving that factors other than the simple presence of a hole are important. The most important factor is degeneration or detachment of the overlying vitreous and traction exerted by the vitreous on the retinal tissue adjacent to the break.[1091,1157,1180,1230]

Nonrhegmatogenous detachments

Exudative detachments. Exudative detachments (Color Plate 8-37) signify an accumulation of fluid exudate or tumor below the sensory retina in the absence of a retinal break.[1105,1146] The following outline, modified from that of Dr. Michael Goldbaum, University of California, San Diego, lists the conditions that may cause exudative retinal detachment:

A. Inflammatory disorders[1127]
  1. Harada's disease
  2. Posterior and peripheral uveitis (peripheral exudative detachment), pars planitis
  3. Choroidal effusion[1103]
  4. Viral retinitis (cytomegalic inclusion retinitis)
  5. Sympathetic ophthalmia
  6. Excessive cryopexy
  7. Scleritis
  8. Extensive photocoagulation

Table 8-3. Distinguishing features of retinal detachment

Feature	Rhegmatogenous	Nonrhegmatogenous exudative	Nonrhegmatogenous tractiona
Retinal break	Always	No	No
Surface	Convex; may be bullous	Convex: may not reach ora unless caused by peripheral uveitis	Dentate or scalloped; rarely if ever reaches ora unless caused by peripheral uveitis
Fluid	Rarely shifts	Shifting is common: fluid is often dependent	No shifting; subretinal fluid appears "sucked" into space under pulled-up retina
Height	Bullous from superior hole; shallow from inferior hold; never touches lens	Often high; only type that may touch lens	Generally not high
Flourescein	No leak or pooling; window defect if long-standing	Leaking and pooling of flourescein in subretinal fluid	No leak or pooling; window defect possible
Natural history	Progresses or remains detached usually does not spontaneously resolve	Waxes and wanes according to cause; may spontaneously resolve	Generally progresses; may develop hole and become rhegmatogenous
Treatment	Surgical	Medical—treat underlying cause; for example, apply photocoagulation to leaking vascular channels	Observation; may buckle or band; vitrectomy

Modified from Dr. Michael Goldbaum, University of California, San Diego.

B. Systemic disorders[1172]
  1. Renal failure, Goodpasture's syndrome
  2. Hypertension
  3. Toxemia of pregnancy (Color Plate 8-37)
  4. Dysproteinemias and macroglobulinemias
C. Retinal pigment epithelial defect
  1. Pigment epithelial detachment
  2. Central serous choroidopathy
D. Subretinal neovascularization
  1. Senile disciform macular degeneration
  2. Presumed ocular histoplasmosis syndrome
  3. Angioid streaks, choroidal rupture, or myopia
E. Tumors
  1. Malignant[1170]
    a. Malignant melanoma
    b. Retinoblastoma
    c. Metastases
  2. Benign
    a. Hemangioma of the choroid
    b. Angiomatosis retinae
    c. Coats's disease

Tractional detachment. Traction exerted from the vitreous may lead to detachment in the absence of a retinal break.[1166,1185,1222] Organization of vitreous hemorrhages or inflammatory exudates, posttraumatic vitreous condensation and fibrosis, surgical or nonsurgical vitreous loss, and any cause of proliferative retinopathy (p. 376) may produce tractional detachment.* Following are diseases with increased incidence of retinal detachment as a result of traction or vitreous degeneration (modified from Dr. Michael Goldbaum, University of California, San Diego):

1. Traction
  a. Trauma (with or without foreign body) with vitreous traction bands to retina
  b. Vitreous loss due to cataract extraction

  c. Diabetic retinopathy
  d. Central and branch vein occlusion
  e. Retinopathy of prematurity
  f. Persistent hyperplastic primary vitreous (PHPV)
  g. Sickle retinopathy
  h. Eales' disease and other peripheral retinal vasoproliferative diseases
  i. Congenital toxoplasmosis
  j. Intravitreal parasite
2. Vitreous degeneration
  a. Goldmann-Favre disease
  b. Wagner-Stickler hereditary vitreoretinal degeneration[1101,1184]
  c. Marfan's syndrome
  d. Homocystinuria
  e. Ehlers-Danlos syndrome

Neovascularization from the retina leads to the formation of vascular strands extending into the vitreous from the nerve head or elsewhere in the fundus. Contraction of these strands causes partial or complete retinal detachment.

Recently developed techniques of vitrectomy have been major advances in the treatment of these conditions.

Signs and symptoms

Depending on the predisposing cause, the early symptoms of retinal detachment are often minimal. As the posterior vitreous face pulls away from the retina during syneresis, the retina may be stimulated to produce flashing lights. If contraction of the vitreous causes an operculated hole or horseshoe tear in the retina, bright flashes are observed that are indistinguishable from those produced by syneresis without retinal break. The sparks and flashes result from irritation of rods and cones in the involved area. In addition, the small vessels torn by the retinal break may bleed a small amount into the vitreous, producing floaters, which appear to the patient as spiderwebs or a shower of black dots (muscae volitantes).[1213]

*References 1122, 1147, 1154, 1177, 1181, 1240.

When an actual detachment occurs and spreads, the patient may become aware of a shadow, curtain, or dark area in the quadrants opposite the site of the detachment. The visual field shows a relative scotoma corresponding to the detached retina, and the borders of the field defect slope gradually, indicating a wide separation of the isopters of the visual field. In contrast, in retinoschisis the scotoma is absolute and the borders are steep. Eventually, as the detachment approaches or passes through the macula, metamorphopsia and blurring of vision may occur.[1107]

The fundus shows a gray discoloration in the area of the detachment that contrasts with the normal red reflex (Figs. 8-71 and 8-74; Color Plate 8-36). The higher the retinal elevation, the grayer the involved area seems. Superior holes that cause rapid detachment (hours to days) lead to large, bullous detachments. A very shallow detachment or a shallow region in a retinal detachment has nearly normal color and choroidal pattern and may be extremely difficult to distinguish from attached retina. A chronic detachment several months old causes atrophy of the detached retina. "Cysts," really a splitting or schisis of the detached retina, connote a retinal detachment of several months' duration.

Corrugation of the outer surface of the retina produces a fine ripple effect where it exists. Retinal folds may show a pattern of "hills and valleys" and may shift from day to day or, in long-standing cases, may be fixed or "star-shaped" folds that do not move with movements of the eye.

The intraocular pressure is usually decreased in retinal detachment. Nonneoplastic detachments usually can be distinguished from choroidal tumors by the methods discussed in Chapter 7.

Histopathologic findings

The microscopic appearance of the peripheral retinal degenerations that lead to retinal breaks and the morphology of the breaks have been described earlier.

Because the retina has a high rate of metabolism, which is supported by the central retinal artery and choriocapillaris, a detachment separates the outer layers from the choriocapillaris and thus from their immediate source of nourishment. The inner retinal layers retain their blood supply from the central retinal artery.

The subretinal fluid, which, depending on the origin of the detachment, is composed of serous fluid, protein or lipid-rich exudates, inflammatory exudates, blood, or tumor, contains some nutrients. As time passes, however, the diffusion of nutrients through the vitreous to the retina becomes inadequate and the outer retina suffers. The macula undergoes cystic changes and degeneration of the rods and cones if it is separated from the choroid for more than 4 to 6 weeks. The retina elsewhere also tends to become edematous and atrophic, particularly in the outer layers, after 2 to 3 months' detachment.

Microscopically the earliest change is degeneration of rods and cones (Figs. 8-75 and 8-76). Cystoid degeneration occurs in the outer plexiform layer, followed by coalescence of the cystoid spaces to form larger and larger cysts. These cysts produce the orange-peel effect seen clinically in a long-standing detachment. Glial and connective tissue proliferation also occurs in detached retinas (proliferative vitreoretinopathy).[1147,1174,1178,1239,1242] This proliferation

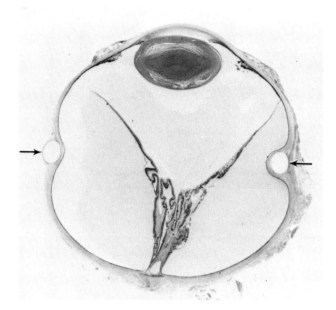

Fig. 8-75. Retinal detachment. Total detachment with retinal folds and degeneration. *Arrows,* Encircling bands placed at scleral buckling operation. (H & E stain; ×2.) (Courtesy Dr. Morton Smith.)

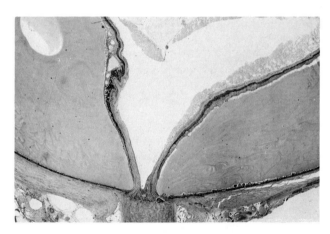

Fig. 8-76. Total retinal detachment with especially protein-rich, densely staining subretinal transudate. Retinal folds and degeneration are on the left and degenerative drusen on the pigment epithelium at the lower right. (H & E stain; ×15.) (From Naumann GOH and Apple DJ: In Doerr W, Seifert G, Uehlinger E, editors: Handbuch der speziellen pathologischen Anatomie, Band Auge, Berlin, 1980, Springer-Verlag.)

can result in shortening of the retina so that it becomes more flattened and tightly stretched between the ora serrata and disc. Fibroglial membranes on the internal or external surface of the retina may cause macula pucker (cellophane maculopathy) and may shrink and cause fixed retinal and epiretinal folds.[846]

Outer segments can continue to regenerate only to a limited degree.[1247] When the retina has been detached for some time, the neuronal elements are eliminated and the retina is reduced to a glial membrane. Shortening and folding may produce so-called star folds and progress to a complete end-stage, funnel-shaped detachment (Fig. 8-75).

An artifactitious retinal detachment frequently occurs after fixation (Figs. 1-1 and 8-7). Three features help differentiate this from a true detachment.

1. The presence of a subretinal fluid proves the existence of a true detachment; it is never present in a postmortem detachment. The fluid underlying a true detachment, however, may occasionally disappear during tissue processing, so this criterion alone is not sufficient to differentiate a true or artifactitious detachment.
2. A true detachment causes varying degrees of destruction of the photoreceptors. This degeneration of rods and cones does not occur with artifactious detachment.
3. In a true detachment, a "clean break" occurs between photoreceptors and the underlying pigment epithelium. In an artifactitious detachment, the rods and cones are "wrenched away" from the apices of the pigment cell, and pigment granules cling to the outer portion of the photoreceptors (Fig. 8-77).

Proliferative and degenerative changes also occur in the pigment epithelium, Bruch's membrane, and choroid.[1179,1234] Bruch's membrane thickens, drusen form, and the choriocapillaris undergoes "hyalinization" (Fig. 8-76). The proliferating pigment epithelium lays down basement membrane and undergoes fibrous metaplasia, forming clinically visible demarcations at the margin of the detachment.[1161] A similar but not extensive pigment epithelial proliferation at the ora is known as ringschwiele (Fig. 8-78).

A major cause of failure of retinal reattachment surgery is proliferative vitreoretinopathy (PVR).° This disorder is characterized by the formation of cellular membranes on both surfaces of the retina and within the vitreous cavity.† These cellular membrane contract and, thereby, cause traction retinal detachments.

The contractile cellular membranes found within the vitreous cavity and along both surfaces of the retina are composed of retinal pigment epithelial (RPE) cells, glial cells, fibrocytes, and macrophages.‡

Diseases of the macular region

Maumenee and Emery[1596] have classified macular diseases according to the anatomic location of the lesion in the retina, pigment epithelium, or choroid.[1253–1808] Maumenee[1595] has modified this classification by combining aspects of the clinical appearance of macular lesions and their pathogenesis with the original purely anatomic scheme.[1596] Because we emphasize the anatomic-pathologic changes in this book, we retain the original classification for descriptive purposes.

I. Vitreoretinal surface
    A. Preretinal hemorrhage and subinternal limiting membrane hemorrhage
    B. Vitreous traction on the macula and contraction of the inner surface of the retina

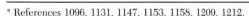

° References 1096, 1131, 1147, 1153, 1158, 1209, 1212.
† References 1095, 1117, 1175, 1205, 1243, 1246.
‡ References 7, 12, 14, 20, 23, 24, 26, 28–32, 35, 40, 42, 44, 47, 52, 64, 65.

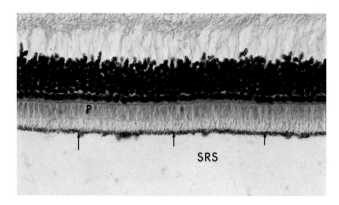

Fig. 8-77. Artifactitious separation of the sensory retina from the pigment epithelium (see also Fig. 1-1). The photoreceptor inner and outer segments *(P)* are intact and fragments of pigment remain attached to their tips *(arrows). SRS,* Subretinal space, which contains no fluid. The pigment epithelium lies below, out of this photograph. (H & E stain; ×150.)

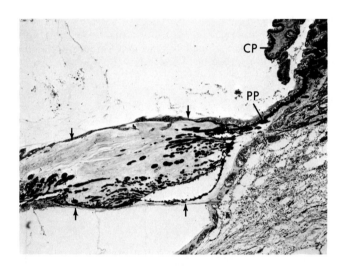

Fig. 8-78. Ringschwiele (German, *Schwiele,* callous or stripe) associated with chronic retinal detachment. This is plaque *(arrows)* formed by hyperplasia and fibrous metaplasia of the peripheral retina and pars plana of the ciliary epithelium at the ora serrata. It is seen as a degenerative phenomenon in long-standing detachments. *CP,* Ciliary process; *PP,* pars plana epithelium. Note the edematous choroidal stroma, signifying hypotony, at lower right. (H & E stain; ×45.)

    C. Idiopathic epiretinal membranes, massive preretinal proliferation (MPP)
    D. Vitreoretinal dystrophies
        1. Macular degeneration in juvenile sex-linked retinoschisis
        2. Goldmann-Favre recessive vitreoretinal dystrophy
II. Nerve fiber–ganglion cell layers
    A. Hereditary cerebromacular degenerations
        1. Sphingolipidoses
            a. Tay-Sachs (GM_2 gangliosidosis, type I)
            b. Sandhoff's disease (GM_2 gangliosidosis, type II)
            c. Niemann-Pick disease

d. Lactosyl ceramidosis

e. Metachromatic leukodystrophyand Kraffe's disease[1314,1349,1381]

f. Gaucher's disease[1346]

2. Mucolipidosis

a. Farber's lipogranulomatosis

b. Sea-blue histiocyte syndrome (chronic Niemann-Pick disease)

c. Generalized gangliosidosis (GM_1 gangliosidosis, type I)

d. Mucolipidosis I (lipomucopolysaccharidosis)

3. Goldberg's disease (unclassified syndrome with features of mucopolysaccharidoses, sphingolipidoses, and mucolipidoses)

4. Other

a. Jansky-Bielschowsky disease (late infantile)

b. Batten-Mayou, Vogt-Spielmeyer-Stock disease (juvenile)

III. Nerve fiber, ganglion cell, inner plexiform, inner nuclear, and outer plexiform layers

A. Ischemia secondary to inadequate perfusion of central and branch arterioles and venules

B. Senile macular degeneration (inner type)

IV. Outer plexiform layer

A. Cystoid macular edema and degeneration

1. With retinal vascular leakage

a. Postoperative (Irvine-Gass)

b. Acute nongranulomatous iridocyclitis

c. Acute cyclitis

d. Peripheral posterior segment inflammation (pars planitis)

e. Vascular anomalies

f. Hypertension

g. Diabetes

h. Low-grade venous obstruction

i. Radiation retinopathy

2. Without obvious retinal vascular leakage

a. Vitreous traction of the macula

b. Serous detachment of sensory epithelium

c. Serous detachment of pigment epithelium

d. Hemorrhagic detachment of macula

e. Choroidal tumors

f. Senile?

B. Lipid deposits in macula secondary to vascular disease in retina

1. Stellate retinopathy

a. Hypertensive retinopathy

b. Diabetic retinopathy

c. Coats's disease

d. Trauma

e. Retinal arterial or venous occlusion

f. Retinal periphlebitis

g. Juxtapapillary choroiditis

h. Papilledema

i. Angiomatosis retinae

j. Idiopathic

2. Circinate retinopathy

a. Senile vascular disease

b. Venous obstruction

c. Diabetic retinopathy

d. Coats's disease

e. Retinal detachment

f. Anemia

g. Leukemia

h. Idiopathic (primary)

3. Diabetic retinopathy

V. Outer nuclear rod and cone layers (neuroepithelium, sensory epithelium)

A. Congenital hereditary color vision defects

1. Trichromatism (anomalous)

2. Dichromatism

3. Monochromatism

B. Hereditary macular dystrophies

1. Stargardt's disease (atrophic macular dystrophy with fundus flavimaculatus)

2. Dominant progressive foveal dystrophy (dominant Stargardt's disease)

3. Progressive cone dystrophy

4. Central retinopathy pigmentosa (inverse pigmentary dystrophy)

C. Olivopontocerebellar degeneration[1745,1748]

D. Solar burn (idiopathic foveomaculopathy)[1259,1465]

VI. Pigment epithelium

A. Hereditary macular dystrophies

1. Vitelliform dystrophy (Best's)

2. Fundus flavimaculatus

3. Dominant drusen (Doyne's honeycomb degeneration, Hutchinson-Tay)

4. Reticular dystrophy (Sjögren)

5. Butterfly-shaped pigment dystrophy (Deutman)

6. Albipunctate dystrophy

7. Sjögren-Larsson syndrome

B. Inflammatory lesions

1. Rubella[1647]

2. Acute posterior multifocal placoid pigment epitheliopathy

C. Toxic lesions

1. Chloroquine[1356,1693,1768]

2. Phenothiazine

3. Sparsomycin

4. Ethambutol

5. Indomethacin

6. Griseofulvin

D. Drusen (senile degenerative)

E. Refsum's disease

VII. Bruch's membrane

A. Angioid streaks associated with

1. Pseudoxanthoma elasticum (Gronblad-Stranberg)

2. Senile elastosis of skin

3. Osteitis deformans (Paget's disease)

4. Fibrodysplasia hyperelastica (Ehlers-Danlos)

5. Sickle cell disease

6. Acromegaly

B. Senile fracture of Bruch's membrane (a type of angioid streaks?)

VIII. Pigment epithelium, Bruch's membrane; choriocapillaris

A. Serous detachment of neuroepithelium or pigment epithelium associated with

1. Idiopathic leak from choriocapillaris

2. Hemangioma of choroid

3. Malignant melanoma

4. Pitting of optic disc

5. Hypotony

6. Leukemic infiltrates of choroid

7. Terminal illness
8. Trauma
9. Uveitis
10. Optic neuritis
11. Papilledema
12. Acute hypertension
13. Vitreous traction
14. Angioid streaks
15. Harada's disease
16. Toxocara canis
17. Myopic choroidal degeneration
18. Metastatic carcinoma
19. Choroidal nevus
20. Collagen vascular disease
21. Hemorrhagic or organized disciform detachment

B. Degenerative lesions
1. Disciform macular degeneration (senile, juvenile)
2. Pseudoinflammatory macular dystrophy of Sorsby[1322,1373,1480]
3. Senile macular degeneration (outer type)
4. Adult hereditary cerebromacular degeneration (Kufs)
5. Congenital cystic macular degeneration

C. Lipoid proteinosis (Urbach-Wiethe)

IX. Choroid[1552]
A. Degenerative lesions[1562]
1. Central areolar choroidal atrophy
2. Myopic choroidal atrophy[1360,1470,1545]
3. Helicoid peripapillary chorioretinal atrophy?

B. Inflammatory lesions
1. Histoplasmosis[1281,1694,1742]

C. Vascular occlusive lesions

X. Miscellaneous
A. Retinal inflammations (multilayer alterations that may involve the macula)
1. Toxoplasma gondii
2. Toxocara canis
3. Septic emboli
a. Candida
b. Bacteria

B. Congenital anomalies of the macula
1. Aplasia
2. Hypoplasia
3. Heterotopia
4. Colobomas
5. Aberrant macular vessels

Some aspects of the Maumenee-Emery classification must be considered tentative and possibly subject to future modification (e.g., it is unknown whether some dystrophies primarily affect photoreceptors, pigment epithelium, or both). This classification, however, is one of the most accurate to date and is excellent for descriptive purposes. Other important detailed references on diseases of the macula have been published by Deutman,[1367] Gass,[1425] The German Ophthalmological Society,[1371] Krill,[1558] and Rabb.[1663]

Unfortunately, the histopathologic appearance of many macular diseases remains undocumented, and clinicopathologic correlation often rests on speculation from indirect evidence, such as the fluorescein angiographic appearance, as to the localization of the various lesions within the af-

fected retina.* Although a detailed discussion of each disease is beyond the scope of this chapter and pathologic examples of each condition are often unavailable, brief discussions of selected macular lesions are included, based primarily on the anatomic scheme of Maumenee and Emery[1596] and in part on Deutman's classification[1367] of hereditary macular diseases.

VITREORETINAL INTERFACE

Various types of cells may gain access to the inner surface of the retina and affect the macular region.† After retinal hole/detachment formation, such cells may also migrate both under and above the surface of the retina (periretinal proliferation). These cells may proliferate and engage in secretory activities that result in fibrocellular tissue formation. These various proliferations are often broadly lumped together and are termed *epiretinal membranes* (ERMs) (Fig. 8-79, *A–D*; Color Plates 8-38 and 8-39). Membranes occurring unassociated with other known ocular problems and are called idiopathic ERMs. The ERMs that occur with or after ocular inflammatory disease and chronic diseases are called secondary ERMs.

The terminology of periretinal proliferation has been extensive, with overlapping and duplications; many clinical variations have emerged. In an effort to bring uniformity to the terminology, the Retina Society Terminology committee provided a classification of periretinal proliferation based on intensity or involvement under the general category of proliferative vitreoretinopathy.

An excellent review of pathogenesis and pathologic features of epiretinal and vitreous membranes has been provided by Kampik and coworkers.[1524] They observed that membranes growing on the inner retinal surface (ERM) occur in a number of conditions, for example:

1. In proliferative retinopathies
2. In ocular inflammatory conditions
3. In nonproliferative retinal vascular disorders
4. After blunt or penetrating injuries
5. After vitreous hemorrhage
6. Associated with rhegmatogenous retinal detachment or after otherwise successful retinal reattachment surgery
7. After retinal photocoagulation or cryotherapy
8. As an idiopathic process in otherwise normal eyes

In some of these conditions, abnormal membranes may also be present within the vitreous gel. Epiretinal membranes in eyes with proliferative retinopathies are usually vascularized, while in the other conditions listed the epiretinal tissue usually is avascular. These membranes often exert traction on the underlying retina, and visual acuity may be reduced if the epiretinal tissue covers, distorts, or causes traction detachment of the macula.[1524]

---

* References 1642, 1674, 1681, 1778, 1786, 1787, 1805.
† References 270, 273, 274, 1165, 1167, 1219, 1221, 1248, 1257, 1261–1264, 1268, 1271, 1272, 1278, 1282–1285, 1299, 1300, 1305, 1319, 1333, 1335, 1341, 1363, 1394, 1398, 1406, 1407, 1418, 1442, 1443, 1456, 1463, 1467, 1473, 1482, 1483, 1517, 1523–1525, 1527, 1533, 1537, 1544, 1547, 1556, 1567, 1568, 1576, 1581, 1598, 1599, 1602, 1605, 1608–1611, 1613, 1617, 1623, 1632, 1643, 1669, 1672, 1673, 1677, 1679, 1685, 1703, 1707, 1710, 1714–1717, 1724, 1725, 1727–1729, 1734, 1739, 1740, 1760–1763, 1773, 1778, 1783, 1792, 1804.

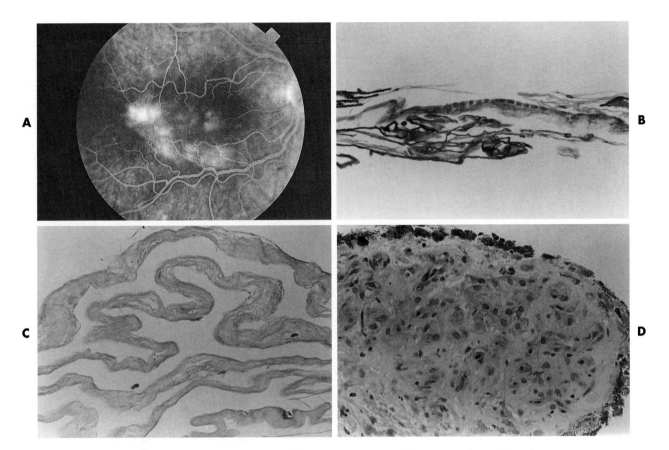

Fig. 8-79. Epiretinal membranes. **A,** Fluorescein angiogram of an epiretinal membrane showing marked hyperfluorescence due to leakage of dye with the lesion. **B,** Photomicrograph of a membrane consisting mostly of cortical basement membrane material and a row of cuboidal epithelium dermoid from RPE. (PAS stain; ×250.) **C,** Photomicrograph of a membrane composed almost entirely of fibroglial tissue without discernable cellular elements. (H & E stain; ×275.) **D,** Photomicrograph of a membrane, which in sharp contrast to **B** is highly cellular. Note row of RPE cells around the periphery. (H & E stain; ×150.)

The stimuli causing epiretinal and intravitreal cellular proliferation and secondary membrane formation are not well defined as are the pathogenetic mechanisms accounting for the variations in morphologic features of these membranes. In an ultrastructural study of 56 cases of epiretinal and vitreous membranes obtained surgically from eyes with various ocular diseases, Kampik and coworkers[1183] concluded that the cells of origin of various forms of macular and extramacular membranes were of five morphologic types:

1. RPE cells that were evident only in association with retinal detachment
2. Fibrous astrocytes that were characteristic of all disease groups
3. Macrophages
4. Fibrocytes
5. Myofibroblast-like cells that had primarily the characteristics of fibrocytes and, occasionally, those of RPE cells or fibrous astrocytes

Other cells such as hyalocytes, inflammatory cells, vascular endothelium, and perithelial cells may contribute to epiretinal and intravitreal membranes.[1524] The combination of cell types varied in different types of membranes, but the formation of collagen and the development of cells with myofibroblast-like properties were common features, their genesis apparently being within the capacity of several cell types. These two features seem to be the basis for the contractile properties of epiretinal and vitreous membranes.

Of the cell types that have been documented to account for the formation of ERMs, certain types may dominate in various clinical conditions. Fibrous astrocytes have been implicated most frequently; these have been observed in eyes with (1) idiopathic membranes without other serious disorders, (2) pars planitis, (3) nonproliferative retinal vascular conditions and vitreous hemorrhage, and (4) rhegmatogenous retinal detachment or macular pucker after retinal reattachment surgery. Cells derived from the RPE are believed to be the major cell type contributing to epiretinal and intravitreal membranes in eyes with rhegmatogenous retinal detachment complicated by massive periretinal proliferation (MPP), which is also known as proliferative vitreoretinopathy (PVR).

Retinal glial cells gain access to the inner retinal surface at a number of sites where the retinal internal limiting membrane (ILM) is normally thin or discontinuous, such as at the optic nerve head, the fovea, along major blood vessels, and at retinal tufts. Acquired sites of discontinuity of the ILM include retinal tags, pits (lamellar holes), holes and tears, avulsed retinal vessels, areas of regenerative remodeling, lattice degeneration, and random sites of vitreous traction. The RPE gains access to the vitreous cavity and inner surface of the retina, principally at point of retinal holes, tears, and dialyses. Other sites include the ora serrata and posterior aspect of the pars plana within the vitreous base and in areas of lattice degeneration. It is apparent, however, that RPE may also extend through an intact retina in some instances, such as some cases of idiopathic macular pucker.

Vitreoretinal dystrophies

Macular degeneration in juvenile sex-linked retinoschisis, Goldmann-Favré recessive vitreoretinal dystrophy, and Wagner-Stickler dominant vitreoretinal dystrophy have in common the formation of a schisis cavity at the level of the nerve fiber layer and ganglion cell layers, accompanied by vitreous anomalies. Only the first two dystrophies listed affect the macula.

Sex-linked juvenile retinoschisis (congenital vascular veils in the vitreous) is a condition in which ophthalmologic evidence of the disease is usually present at birth (Fig. 8-80).[*] It typically affects boys and is often associated with hypermetropia. The expression of the gene is low so that the multiple signs characteristic of the disease are seen in only a small percentage of cases.

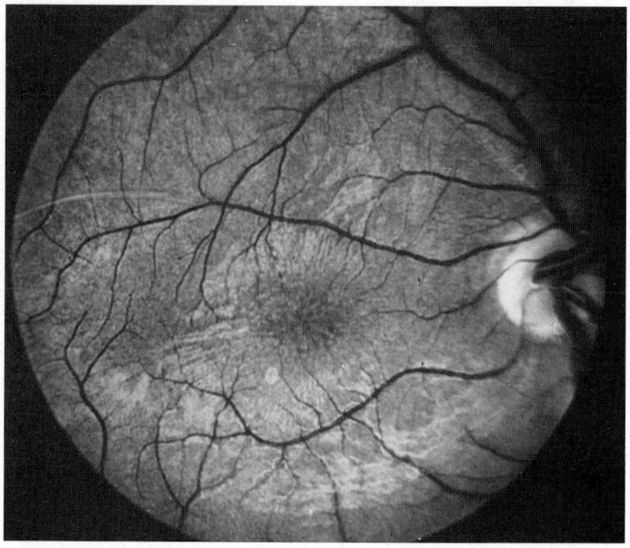

Because the fovea is almost always involved, this disease is a potential source of significant visual loss. Extensive macular cystoid degeneration and/or a marked pigmentary degeneration are common. This is sometimes accompanied by choroidal sclerosis. The presence of foveal retinoschisis, which is typically bilateral and symmetric, is pathognomonic. Ophthalmoscopically foveal retinoschisis consists of an optically empty zone from which radial, spokelike folds may emanate (Fig. 8-81). Actual vitreous veils appear in fewer than 30% of cases. The veils are translucent, often perforated by lacunae, and sometimes do not contain vessels.

A common complication of this disease is hemorrhage into the vitreous from ruptured retinal vessels (usually venules) in the areas of retinoschisis; however, true retinal detachment is rarely a complication. Visual acuity can remain normal for a long period, but vision gradually diminishes with increasing age. Complete blindness, however, is rare.

The plane of cleavage in the retina is at the level of the nerve fiber layer. Therefore, the inner stratum of the schisis cavity, that is, the "vitreous veil," is composed of the internal limiting membrane and immediately adjacent fragments of neuroglial tissue. This plane of cleavage resembles that seen in reticular cystoid degeneration and reticular retinoschisis (p. 411) but differs from that observed in simple peripheral cystoid degeneration of the Blessig-Iwanoff type and from that seen in senile retinoschisis (p. 410). In these conditions, splitting and/or cavitation occurs in the outer plexiform layer.

---

[*] References 1292, 1317, 1336, 1452, 1588, 1704, 1796.

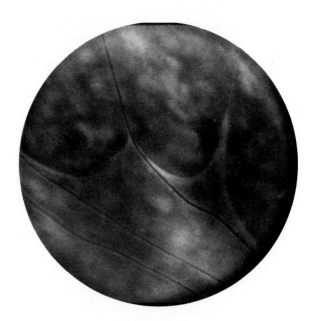

Fig. 8-80. Juvenile (X-linked) retinal schisis. Note typical macular pattern associated with the cystic lesions in the nerve fiber layer. The schisis cleft is in the nerve fiber layer. Note also the preretinal vitreous veil seen superior temporally to the macula (*arrows*).

Fig. 8-81. X-linked juvenile retinoschisis. The inner schisis wall is displaced in a vitreal direction, forming so-called vascular veils within the vitreous. The plane of cleavage is at the level of the nerve fiber layer.

The recessive vitreoretinal dystrophy of Goldmann-Favré is characterized by bilateral central and peripheral retinoschisis occurring in young people of either sex and is transmitted in an autosomal-recessive manner. It involves chorioretinal atrophy, a degeneration of the vitreous with the formation of peripheral condensations and preretinal membranes, night blindness, abolition of the ERG, complicated cataract, and slow but progressive loss of vision.

Table 8-4. Differential diagnosis of sphingolipidoses and mucolipidoses causing a cherry-red spot (all autosomal recessive)

Disorders	Enzyme deficiency
Sphingolipidoses	
GM$_2$ ganggliosidosis, type I (Tay-Sachs disease)	Hexosaminidase A
GM$_2$ ganggliosidosis, type II (Sandhoff's disease)	Total hexosaminidase (A and B)
Essential lipid histiocytosis (infantile Neimann-Pick disease)	Sphingomylinase
Infantile mentachromatic leukodystrophy (sulfatide lipidosis)	Lysosomal sulfate enzymes (arylsulfatase-A)
Primary splenomegaly (Gaucher's disease)	β-Glucosidase
Mucolipidoses	
Lipogranulomatosis (Farber's disease)	Ceramidase
Sea-blue histiocyte syndrome (chronic Neimann-Pick disease)	Unknown
GM$_2$ ganggliosidosis, type I (generalized ganggliosidosis; Norman-Landing disease)	β-Galactosidase A, B, and C
Syndrome of cherry-red spot and corneal clouding (Goldberg's disease)	Sialidase, α-N-acetylneuraminidase; β-galactosidase

Table 8-5. Hereditary cerebromacular degeneration (neuronal ceroid-lipofuscinosis) with macular degeneration but usually without a cherry spot

Disorder	Enzyme deficiency
Jansky-Bielschowsky disease (late infantile)	Peroxidase
Batten-Mayou or Vogt-Spielmeyer-Stock disease (juvenile)	Peroxidase

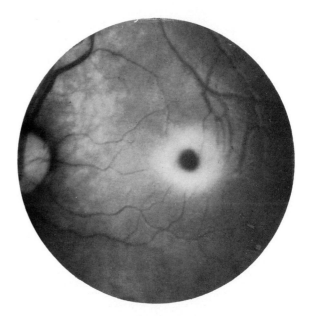

Fig. 8-82. Cherry-red spot of Tay-Sachs disease. Accumulation of lipid in retinal ganglion cells characterizes lipid storage diseases. These deposits impart a white discoloration to the involved fundus. The perifoveal region is even more involved (white, cloudy appearance) because the affected ganglion cell layer is several layers thick (p. 358). This contrasts with all other areas of the fundus, in which the ganglion cell stratum is only one cell layer thick. The central foveal region is normally devoid of ganglion cells; therefore the normal red color of the underlying choriocapillaris is ophthalmoscopically visible and prominent, forming the cherry-red spot. (Courtesy Dr. Edward Cotlier.)

NERVE FIBER LAYER AND GANGLION CELL LAYERS

Hereditary cerebromacular degenerations

The hereditary cerebromacular degenerations with and without cherry-red spots are classified in Tables 8-4 and 8-5.* These cerebromacular degenerations should be differentiated from the group of heredomacular dystrophies. The former are characterized by bilateral degenerative changes in the retina and central nervous system, usually with lipid deposits in retinal ganglion cells and in neurons of the brain. Diseases in the latter group might be classified as macular tapetoretinal dystrophies or abiotrophies usually affecting the eye only, without brain involvement. They are sometimes named according to the age of onset: (1) infantile type of Best, (2) juvenile type of Stargardt, and (3) adult type of Behr.

Tay-Sachs disease. Tay-Sachs disease (infantile cerebromacular degeneration) is the prototype lipid storage disease.[1345,1347,1352,1353,1522] It usually affects Jewish children and is transmitted as an autosomal recessive trait. There is early visual deterioration with formation of a macular cherry-red spot (Fig. 8-82; Color Plate 8-40), mental retardation, progressive muscular weakness, and death.

The histopathologic hallmark of all lipidoses and mucolipidoses is stored lipid within retinal ganglion cells and brain cells. The lipid material induces swelling and eventual degeneration of the ganglion cells. There is associated atrophy of the nerve fiber layer and optic nerve in late phases.

The pale color of the fundus is caused by the deposition of lipid within the retinal ganglion cells (Fig. 8-83). This pallor is accentuated in the perifoveal region because the ganglion cell layer is thicker than elsewhere (Figs. 7-5, 8-5, 8-8, and 8-82). The cherry-red spot is present at the foveola because the central foveal region is normally devoid of ganglion cells; therefore, it remains unaffected by the lipid deposits, allowing the normal choriocapillaris color to be retained.

A disease consisting of a cherry-red spot associated with corneal clouding has been described by Goldberg and coworkers.[1449] This syndrome combines the features of two storage diseases: the sphingolipidoses (cherry-red spot) and the mucopolysaccharidoses (corneal clouding). In short, this disease (a mucolipidosis) represents a combination of a typical Tay-Sachs-like condition as a result of abnormal lipid storage and Hurler's disease because of abnormal mucopolysaccharide storage.

---

* References 1302, 1315, 1337, 1339, 1345, 1352, 1353, 1361, 1380, 1384, 1411, 1419, 1446, 1449, 1499, 1503, 1592, 1593, 1618, 1629, 1630, 1648, 1670, 1671, 1722–1724, 1733, 1747, 1749, 1756, 1771, 1803.

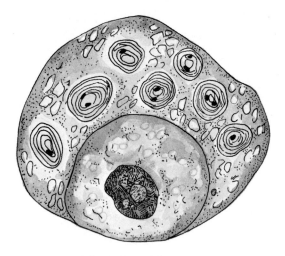

Fig. 8-83. One of the earliest known microscopic illustrations of a retinal ganglion cell in Tay-Sachs disease. Even in the preelectron microscope era, the laminated cytoplasmic sphingomyelin lipid inclusions were observed. (Compare with the appearance of normal myelin, Fig. 10-5, *B.*) (Redrawn by Dr. Steven Vermillion, University of Iowa, from Schieck F: In Henke F and Lubarsch O, editors: Handbuch der speziellen pathologischen Anatomie und Histologie, Berlin, 1928, Julius Springer.)

Table 8-6. Causes of cystoid macular edema

General factors	Specific factors
Ophthalmologic surgery	Cataract extraction (Irvine-Gass syndrome with or without intraocular lens insertion), retinal reattachment, penetrating keratoplasty, filtering procedures, vitrectomy, photocoagulation, cryotherapy
Retinal vascular diseases	Diabetic retinopathy, hypertensive retinopathy, central retinal vein occlusion, branch vein occlusion, papillophlebitis, retinal telangiectasis, subretinal neovascularization, retinopathy, syphilitic retinitis
Inflammation	Pars planitis, posterior uveitis, vitritis, choriorentinitis, papillitis
Drugs	Epinephrine, nicotinic acid, grisofulvin
Radiation Dystrophies	Retinitis pigmentosa, dominant cystoid macular edema
Ocular tumors	Melanoma, hemangioma, metastic tumor, nevus
Others	Vitreoretinal traction, preretinal gliosis, hypotony

Modified from Vine AK: Int Ophthalmol Clin 21(3):157, 1981.

Late infantile and juvenile cerebromacular degenerations. The syndromes of neuronal ceroid-lipofuscinosis,° including the late infantile (Jansky-Bielschowsky) type and the juvenile (Batten-Mayou, Vogt-Spielmeyer-Stock) variant, are also hereditary cerebromacular degen-

° References 1004, 1072, 1298, 1311, 1372, 1447, 1448, 1493, 1528, 1701.

erations. They differ, however, from the other forms because the lipid infiltration and degeneration of ganglion cells progress more slowly. A cherry-red spot, therefore, is usually not seen.

Jansky-Bielschowsky disease appears between 2 and 4 years of age and has a more prolonged clinical course than Tay-Sachs disease; however, it has the same neurologic symptoms as Tay-Sachs disease and, like it, ends in blindness and death.

The juvenile (Batten-Mayou, Vogt-Spielmeyer-Stock) form of amaurotic family idiocy differs from the infantile form in its later onset (between the fifth and eighth years) and its longer duration.[1324,1325,1723] The primary degeneration occurs both in the outer retinal layers and in the ganglion cells. The pathologic picture in the retina thus resembles a combination of the features of typical amaurotic family idiocy and pigmentary retinopathy. On the one hand, the ganglion cells undergo lipid degeneration, and, on the other, the outer retinal layers disappear and are replaced by neuroglial proliferation and a migration of retinal pigment epithelium. Lafora's disease is a disorder of carbohydrate metabolism in which polyglucosans are deposited in retinal ganglion cells and inner retinal layer.[1288,1702,1795] These PAS-positive deposits are termed *Lafora bodies.* This is a progressive disease that is universally fatal in childhood. It is characterized by Unverricht's syndrome (myoclonia, grand mal seizures, amaurosis, ataxia, dysenthia and dyshenesia, and dementia).

OUTER PLEXIFORM LAYER

Cystoid macular edema and degeneration

Cystoid degeneration of the retina shows a predilection for the two places where the retina is thinnest and least vascularized: the periphery and the macular region.° The tissues within the outer plexiform layer are less tightly packed than elsewhere in the retina and any intraretinal transudate or exudate tends to migrate into this region. This layer, therefore, is highly susceptible to cystoid changes caused by the numerous diseases listed on page 419 (section IV, A of the outline) and in Table 8-6.

Clinically a cystoid macular edema produces a honeycomb appearance corresponding to the walls of the lacunar cavities. By fluorescein angiography a flower petal pattern is characteristic (Fig. 8-84). As degenerative changes proceed, the small spaces in the outer plexiform layer (Figs. 8-85 and 8-86) may rupture and in so doing produce a macular retinoschisis or a lamellar hole (Figs. 8-87 and 8-88). The hole may be confined to the inner layer of the retina or eventually may produce a complete macular hole.† The cystoid spaces and a resultant hole cause a permanent defect in central vision, regardless of cause.

Stellate and circinate retinopathy. When an intraretinal transudation or outpouring of lipid is significant and affects a wide area, the fluid in the outer plexiform layer

° References 1254, 1299, 1301, 1313, 1358, 1382, 1399, 1424, 1426, 1429, 1430, 1484, 1490, 1506, 1508, 1509, 1514, 1530, 1582, 1607, 1618, 1631, 1682, 1751–1753, 1757, 1778, 1779, 1789, 1797.
† References 1253, 1254, 1262, 1277, 1312, 1318, 1342, 1412, 1417, 1436, 1437, 1439, 1475, 1486, 1492, 1519, 1572, 1584, 1585, 1666, 1706, 1744, 1750, 1799, 1802.

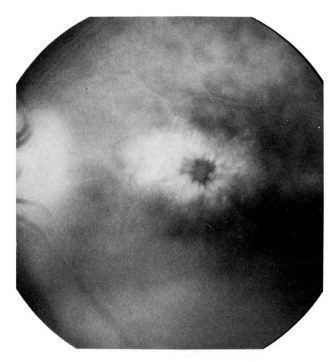

Fig. 8-84. Cystoid macular edema following cataract extraction (Irvine-Gass syndrome). This fluorescein angiogram demonstrates the characteristic flower petal appearance of the fluid accumulating within the retinal cystoid spaces in the outer plexiform layer.

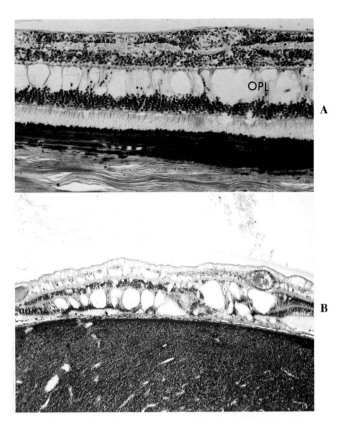

Fig. 8-86. Cystoid macular edema. **A,** The retina in venous stasis retinopathy (central vein occlusion). Extravasated erythrocytes have engorged the inner layers of the retina. Blood deposited in the nerve fiber layer is responsible for the flame-shaped hemorrhage observed clinically. Extensive cystoid degeneration involves the outer plexiform layer *(OPL)*. (H & E stain; ×175.) **B,** Retina overlying choroidal malignant melanoma with cystoid spaces in the outer plexiform layer. (H & E stain; ×120.)

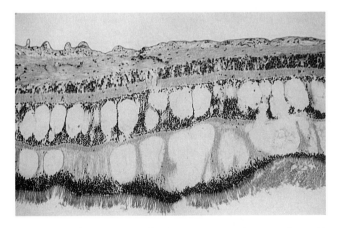

Fig. 8-85. Photomicrograph of sensory retina showing advanced microcystoid degeneration affecting both inner and outer plexiform layers. The inner retinal layers, including the ganglion cell layer, are intact (H & E stain; ×50.)

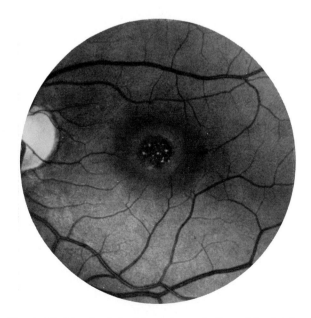

Fig. 8-87. Macular hole. Macrophages (yellow-white dots) are present in the depths of the hole. These cells probably phagocytose degenerate photoreceptor outer segments.

may be distributed in an arrangement determined by the radiating architecture of the fibers of Henle (p. 362). This produces a macular star figure, or stellate retinopathy (Fig. 8-9).[1332,1786,1787]

Circinate retinopathy is not a single clinical entity but is a pathologic process occurring as a local response to retinal vascular leakage caused by a wide variety of diseases. A partial or complete ring of lipids is deposited within the outer plexiform layers, often but not invariably, in the macular region (Fig. 8-108).

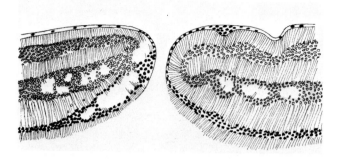

Fig. 8-88. Artist's drawing of macular hole. The edges are smooth and rounded. (Redrawn by Dr. Steven Vermillion, University of Iowa, from Fuchs E: Reproduced by Schieck F: In Henke F and Lubarsch O, editors: Handbuch der speziellen pathologischen Anatomie und Histologie, vol I, Berlin, 1928, Julius Springer.)

PHOTORECEPTORS, PIGMENT EPITHELIUM, BRUCH'S MEMBRANE, AND CHOROID

Because of the close relationship and interactions between the retinal photoreceptors, pigment epithelium, Bruch's membrane, and choroid, and because the exact site of the primary lesion is unclear in several of these entities, hereditary diseases arising primarily in one or more of these structures are described together.* The congenital hereditary color vision defects are primarily functional biochemical defects and histopathologic reports are rare; therefore, the lesions are not considered here. Deutman's classification of the hereditary dystrophies of the posterior pole of the eye follows[1367]:

1. Sex-linked juvenile retinoschisis primarily affects the inner retina and has been discussed on page 422.† The hereditary dystrophies of the posterior pole of the eye primarily affect the inner retina and have been discussed on page 423.
2. Stargardt's disease
3. Dominant progressive foveal atrophy
4. Progressive cone dystrophy
5. Central retinitis pigmentosa
6. Vitelliform dystrophy of the fovea
7. Fundus flavimaculatus
8. Reticular dystrophy of the retinal pigment epithelium (Sjögren's syndrome)
9. Butterfly-shaped pigment dystrophy of the fovea
10. Grouped pigmentations of the foveal area
11. Dominant drusen of Bruch's membrane
12. Pseudoinflammatory dystrophy (Sorsby)
13. Geographic atrophy of the pigment epithelium and choriocapillaris (formerly known as central areolar choroidal dystrophy)

Although a detailed discussion of each disease is beyond the scope of this chapter and pathologic examples of each condition are generally unavailable, brief discussions of five diseases within this category are presented: (1) dominant (familial) drusen, (2) fundus flavimaculatus and Stargardt's disease, (3) Best's vitelliform dystrophy of the fovea, (4) geographic atrophy of the pigment epithelium and chorio-

capillaris (areolar choroidal dystrophy), and (5) central (inverse) retinitis pigmentosa.

Drusen

The term *drusen* is derived from the German *druse* (singular), *drusen* (pleural) signifying a crystallike nodule (Figs. 8-89 and 8-90). These lesions are seen in both dominant drusen (familial drusen, Tay's central guttate choroiditis, Doyne's honeycomb choroiditis) and acquired age-related drusen. Drusen are multiple colloid bodies or excrescences on Bruch's membrane, which are localized predominantly in the posterior pole.* The familial disease is inherited as an autosomal-dominant trait, and the bilateral retinal lesions generally become manifest in early adulthood or middle age. Deutman[1368] believes that the pathogenesis of inherited drusen is an inborn error of metabolism localized in the cells of the pigment epithelium; however, no enzymatic defect has yet been demonstrated to account for the deposits on Bruch's membrane. The visual acuity may remain normal for many years, but in late middle age the vision becomes progressively affected due to macular degeneration.

Familial and age-related drusen. These are at least two fundamental types of age-related drusen. Nodular hard discrete drusen consist of focal thickenings of the basement membrane of the retinal pigment epithelium. These are congenital or acquired early in life and have a relatively good prognosis. The presence of nodular drusen probably does not represent a high-risk factor for the development of exudative (wet) age-related macular degeneration. It is unclear whether or not it represents a high-risk factor for the development of dry (nonexudative) macular degeneration.

The second form is a limited (or focal) separation of the relatively normal basement membrane of the RPE from its attachment to Bruch's membrane at the inner collagenous zone. The sub pigment epithelial space is filled in by a wide variety of materials differing in their consistency. These include lesions with a clinical appearance that is often designated as soft exudative of fluffy drusen. These usually are acquired at 50 years of age or beyond and represent the earliest sign of age-related macular degeneration.

Both inherited and degenerative drusen show hyperfluorescence when studied angiographically. This hyperfluorescence is probably the result of two factors: (1) a window defect is created by depigmentation of the overlying pigment epithelium (Fig. 8-90, *B*), thereby permitting observation of background choroidal fluorescence, and (2) some dye is probably taken up by the drusen themselves. This direct staining of these lesions is particularly evident in late sequences of the fluorescein angiogram.

Dominantly inherited drusen and age-related senile drusen are fundamentally identical in histopathological appearance.[1388] The lesion consists of an eosinophilic, PAS-positive, hyaline deposit forming a bulbous thickening or excrescence on Bruch's membrane (Fig. 8-90). This material represents an accumulation of secretory and breakdown products derived from the pigment epithelium.

The pigment epithelium normally secretes the inner

---

* References 1256, 1260, 1289, 1326, 1367, 1425, 1549, 1558, 1596, 1601.
† References 1270, 1349, 1362, 1513, 1536, 1620.

* References 1237, 1344, 1386, 1387, 1510, 1566, 1571, 1691, 1785.

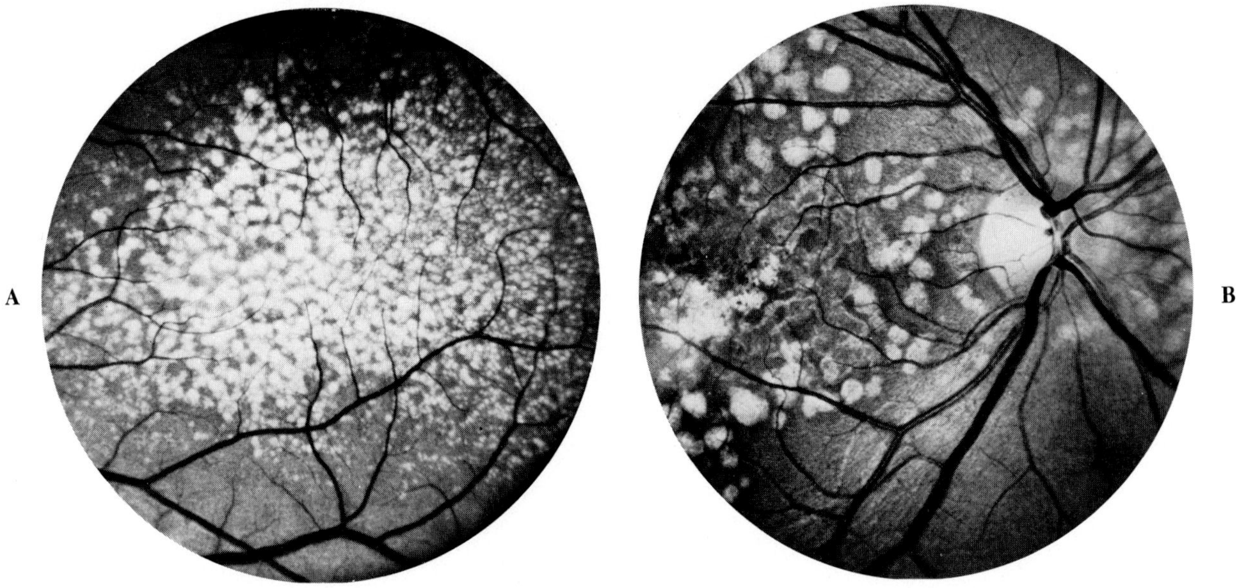

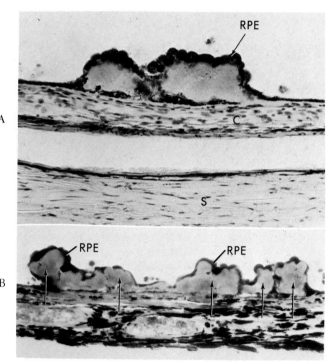

Fig. 8-89. A, Multiple drusen in the left eye, with no family history of dominant inheritance. **B,** Multiple drusen in the right eye of a different patient. In general, the individual lesions are larger than those seen in **A.**

Fig. 8-90. "Senile" drusen. **A,** The drusen represents a focal excrescence or thickening of Bruch's membrane composed primarily of mucopolysaccharides, which are secretory, and degeneration products of the adjacent retinal pigment epithelium (*RPE*). The overlying sensory retina is artifactitiously removed in this section. *C.* Choroid; *S*, sclera. (H & E stain; ×120.) **B,** Multiple confluent drusen. *Arrows*, hyaline mucopolysaccharide deposits between Bruch's membrane and retinal pigment epithelium (*RPE*). (H & E stain; ×130.)

"cuticular" or PAS-positive basement membrane portion of Bruch's membrane, somewhat analogous to the secretion of Descemet's membrane by corneal epithelium.[1391,1392] Indeed, drusen on Bruch's membrane are structurally analogous to the Hassall-Henle bodies of Descemet's membrane in that they are focal excrescences composed of basement membrane–like material. In early stages a druse shows a finely granular appearance, and the overlying pigment epithelium appears normal. At a later stage the druse shows a more homogenous appearance, and the pigment epithelium may become flattened or atrophic. These mucopolysaccharide-rich excrescences are accompanied by destruction, depigmentation, and migration of the involved pigment epithelium and overlying retina. In later stages, particularly (but not exclusively) in phthisic eyes, a druse may show a concentric lamination and calcification. Ossification of drusen is common in phthisis bulbi (p. 304).

Fundus flavimaculatus and Stargardt's disease

Franceschetti[1080,1081] coined the term *fundus flavimaculatus*, describing a bilateral, symmetric, slowly progressive fundus condition with yellow or yellowish white, round and linear disciform flecks that vary not only in size and shape but also in apparent density.° The borders of the lesions are fuzzy, with a tendency toward confluence (Fig. 8-91). They are usually limited to the posterior pole but occasionally extend to the equator. The disease is usually transmitted in an autosomal-recessive manner, and the patient is either asymptomatic or, more frequently, has a decrease in visual acuity from invasion of the fovea by the flecks or from an associated Stargardt's atrophic macular dystrophy.

° References 1255, 1294, 1350, 1376, 1401, 1408, 1409, 1477, 1507, 1543, 1553, 1559, 1577, 1600, 1624, 1628, 1637, 1726.

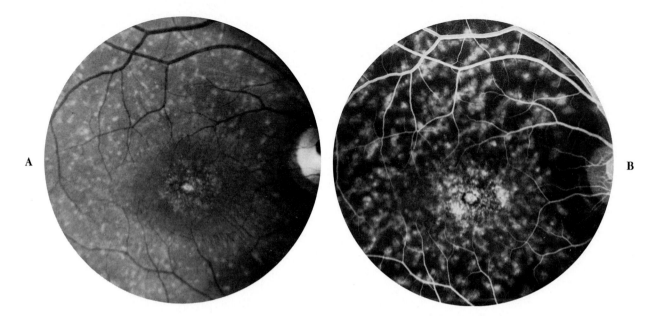

Fig. 8-91. Fundus flavimaculatus. **A,** Typical flecks and atrophic (Stargardt's type) macular lesion. These lesions are often less discrete than drusen and exhibit a tendency toward confluence. The lesions probably represent an accumulation of mucopolysaccharide material within the pigment epithelial cells. **B,** Fluorescein angiogram, same case as in **A.** As with drusen, each lesion has a hyperfluorescent pattern.

In 1967 Klien and Krill[1554] performed a histopathologic study of fundus flavimaculatus. They determined that the primary changes were in the retinal pigment epithelium, a finding that correlates with electrooculogram changes in this disease. These included displacement of the nucleus from the base of the cell to the center or inner surface, variation in size and shape in the pigment epithelial cells, and accumulation of mucopolysaccharide substance, largely within the inner half of the cell. They considered these findings to be slightly different from those in inherited or nospecific drusen, in which mucopolysaccharide material is deposited within the outer aspect of the pigment epithelial cell and in Bruch's membrane.

Stargardt's disease is a slowly progressive dystrophy affecting the posterior pole.° It can occur alone or, in 50% of patients, with fundus flavimaculatus. It is usually transmitted recessively, rarely in an autosomal-dominant manner (dominant progressive foveal dystrophy). The lesions are bilateral and symmetric. There is an initial loss of the foveal reflex, the retinal reflexes become grayish or metallic, mottled pigmentary spots accumulate at the macula, and a slow loss of central vision occurs. (Color Plate 8-41)

Histopathologically photoreceptors and pigment epithelium are completely lost, and the overlying retina exhibits cystoid degeneration.

Best's vitelliform dystrophy

Best's vitelliform dystrophy of the fovea (exudative central detachment of the macula) is transmitted as an autosomal-dominant trait with a highly variable expres-

sion.° Deutman[1367] described the evolution of this bilateral condition in detail and classified the evolutional process as follows. In early stages the fovea appears normal, but the electrooculogram is abnormal. This previtelliform stage is followed by the vitelliform ("egg-yolk") stage (Fig. 8-92, *A;* Color Plate 8-42), the "scrambled egg" stage, the cyst stage, the pseudohypopyon stage, and an end-stage of pigmented chorioretinal atrophy. Eventually a central scotoma develops. The peripheral fields, the dark-adaptation curve, and the ERG remain normal. Because of the high variation in expressivity, each stage can be skipped and various transitional forms exist.

Clinicopathologic correlation is rare because no histopathologic studies of the early stages of Best's disease are available. Microscopic sections from a case in the stage of multifocal pigmented chorioretinal atrophy revealed that a homogenous substance is deposited at the level of the retinal pigment epithelium and Bruch's membrane, probably a product of abnormally proliferating pigment epithelial cells (Fig. 8-92).

Cone-rod dystrophy

Cone-rod dystrophy is a heterogeneous group of disorders frequently characterized by a significant and progressive decrease of visual acuity, abnormal color vision, and abnormal photopic and, to a lesser extent, scotopic ERG responses. Both autosomal-dominant and autosomal-recessive patterns have been reported.

Patients with autosomal-recessive cone-rod dystrophy

° References 1338, 1403, 1440, 1445, 1477, 1507, 1731, 1772, 1806.

° References 1265, 1569, 1279, 1287, 1291, 1328, 1352, 1383, 1402, 1410, 1413, 1428, 1495, 1538, 1557, 1560, 1587, 1615, 1616, 1621, 1634, 1639, 1640, 1645, 1650, 1684, 1769.

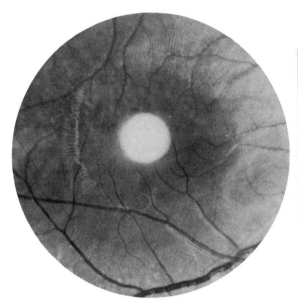
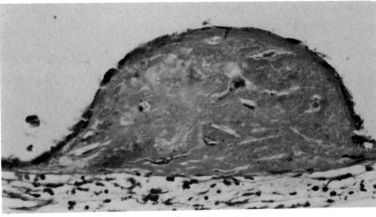

Fig. 8-92. Best's vitelliform macular dystrophy. **A,** "Egg-yolk" appearance. **B,** Later stage. A material of unknown nature is deposited between the retinal pigment epithelium and Bruch's membrane. (H & E stain; ×160.) (Case of Drs. Jerry Kobrin, David Apple, Robert Watzke, and Thomas Weingeist, University of Iowa.)

usually have a decrease in visual acuity during the first two decades of life and may have a characteristic bull's-eye macular lesion. Some patients also demonstrate a diffuse spotty clumping of pigment in the macula and elsewhere in the posterior pole as well as characteristic electrophysiologic findings in this disorder. Patients with cone-rod dystrophy usually exhibit color vision abnormalities.

Clinical, histopathologic, and electron microscopic tests were performed on two postmortem eyes from a 29-year-old black man and the clinical and electrophysiologic findings of his 33-year-old sister, both of whom had bilateral atrophic macular lesions with cone-rod dystrophy (Fig. 8-93, *A–C*).[1665,1736] Light microscopy revealed a loss of photoreceptor cells primarily in the peripheral retina and macula, with relative preservation of both rod and cone cells in the equatorial area. Electron microscopy showed abundant lipofuscin-like granules aggregated in the basal portion of the retinal pigment epithelial cells. In the macular area, many retinal pigment epithelial cells were atrophic. The phagocytic capacity of the retinal pigment epithelium appeared to remain intact. The accumulation of lipofuscin-like granules in the retinal pigment epithelium was considered to be one of the significant pathologic changes of this dystrophy.

Geographic atrophy of the pigment epithelium and choriocapillaris

The condition, also known as central areolar choroidal dystrophy or atrophy, is a bilateral condition of unknown pathogenesis affecting elderly persons.° The most striking clinical finding is a local, circumscribed area of "sclerosis"

of the choroidal vessels at the macular region (Fig. 8-94). The inheritance pattern may be either autosomal-dominant or recessive. A simple pigment mottling occurs in early stages. Ultimately, however, pigment epithelial atrophy leads to exposure of the larger choroidal vessels, which are visible as white streaks. The large choroidal vessels are striking by fluorescein angiography (Fig. 8-94, *B*). Eventually a central scotoma develops. The lesion should not be compared with the condition of geographic serpinginous chroiditis, which is believed to be an inflammatory disease (Color Plate 8-43).

Histopathologically there is total degeneration and virtual absence of choriocapillaris channels in late stages. Bruch's membrane remains intact, but a corresponding atrophy of the overlying pigment epithelium and retina occurs.

Central (inverse) retinitis pigmentosa

Central (inverse) pigmentary dystrophy, in which the pigment deposits are confined to the macular region, is rare. Although central vision is severely affected, dark adaptation and the ERG are only slightly altered. The histopathologic changes in the affected macula are identical to the more peripheral retinal changes of classic retinitis pigmentosa (Fig. 8-62).

RETINAL PIGMENT EPITHELIUM AND BRUCH'S MEMBRANE

Angioid streaks

Angioid streaks are a network of streaks radiating from the peripapillary region irregularly toward the equator (Figs. 8-95 and 8-96; Color Plate 8-44).° They are usually

° References 1275, 1295, 1323, 1395, 1396, 1516, 1532, 1636, 1690, 1720, 1781.

° References 1257, 1258, 1276, 1296, 1340, 1374, 1390, 1429, 1441, 1453, 1478, 1496, 1497, 1548, 1604, 1625, 1649, 1662, 1756, 1784.

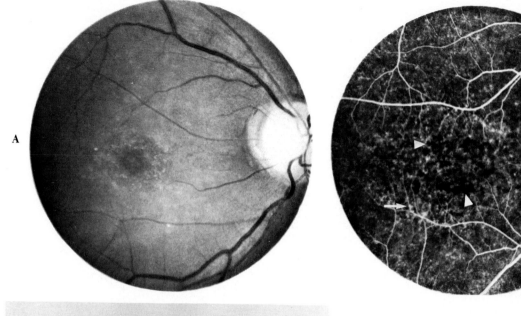

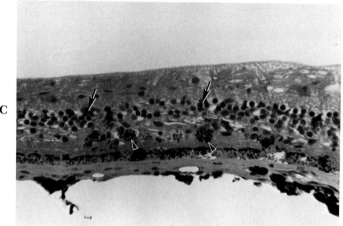

Fig. 8-93. A, Fundus photograph of an eye with cone-rod dystrophy showing pigment mottling in the macular area. **B,** Fluorescein angiogram of another case of cone-rod dystrophy in the midvenous phase showing large areas of hyperfluorescent spots in the macular and perimacular regions. **C,** Posterior retina of a patient with cone-rod dystrophy. Occasional ganglion cells are present. The internuclear layer *(arrows)* is thin. The outer nuclear layer has largely disappeared. Pigment-laden macrophages *(arrowheads)* are noted in the subretinal space. The retinal pigment epithelium appears irregularly pigmented. (H & E stain; ×80.) (From Rabb MF, Tso MOM, and Fishman GA: Ophthalmology 93: 1443, 1986.)

bilateral and are often associated with drusen, subpigment, epithelial neovascularization, and disciform hemorrhagic macular lesions (p. 422). The macular lesions are the most important visual complications of angioid streaks.[1427] In addition to hemorrhage, the pigment epithelium undergoes abnormal pigmentation and atrophy.

Pigmentary deposits (peau d'orange) throughout the peripheral fundus, patches of choroidal atrophy, and drusen may occur. The electrooculographic response of patients with angioid streaks is decreased. This decrease probably occurs because the electrical barrier normally present at the level of the pigment epithelium and Bruch's membrane is disrupted in the involved areas, thus contributing to an abnormal electrooculographic response.

Because elastic tissue is primarily affected, systemic diseases producing elastic tissue degeneration such as pseudoxanthoma elasticum and the other conditions listed in section VII of the outline not infrequently have associated angioid streaks (Fig. 8-97).

Pseudoxanthoma elasticum (Gronblad-Stanberg syndrome) inherited mostly as an autosomal recessive but also as an autosomal dominant, involves mainly the skin, the eyes, and the cardiovascular system. The skin of the face and neck becomes thickened and grooved with the areas

between the grooves diamond shaped, rectangular, polygonal, elecated, and yellowish (resembling chicken skin). The skin in the involved areas becomes lax, redundant, and relatively inelastic. The eyes show angioid streaks often with subretinal neovascularization. Examination of the fundus may show a background pattern, called peau d'orange. These are caused by multiple breaks in Bruch's membrane.

The primary defect lies at the level of Bruch's membrane and involves degeneration of the elastic tissue components. Imbibition of calcium into the damaged focus occurs after degeneration of the elastic tissue. Subsequent fragmentation and breakage of the membrane, with associated defects in the overlying pigment epithelium, create the clinically visible streaks and an opportunity for choroidal vessels to grow and/or bleed beneath the retina, causing a disciform degeneration.

Acute posterior multifocal placoid pigment epitheliopathy

Gass[1421] first described acute posterior multifocal placoid pigment epitheliopathy (APMPPE) in 1968.* The affected patient characteristically has a rapid loss of central

---

* References 1266, 1370, 1404, 1508, 1512, 1683, 1788.

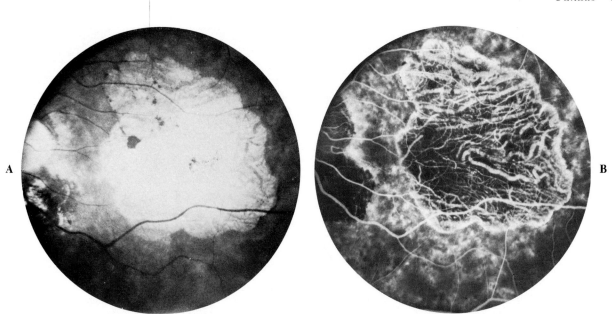

Fig. 8-94. Geographic atrophy of the pigment epithelium and choriocapillaris (central areolar choroidal atrophy). **A,** Fundus photograph showing white discoloration in the region of retinochoroidal degeneration. **B,** Fluorescein angiogram of the same case, showing that the involvement is confined to the macular region. The choriocapillaris vessels have atrophied, the overlying pigment epithelium and sensory retina have undergone degeneration. The larger choroidal vessels are visible as a network of white lines. Several drusen are also present around the central lesion.

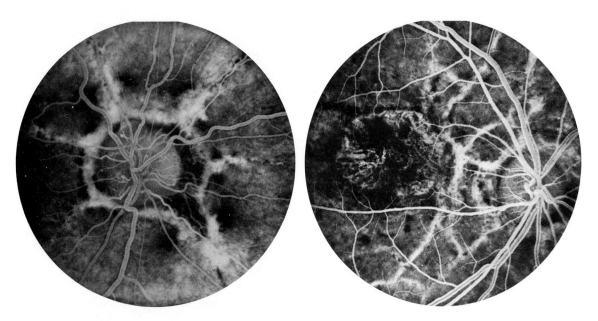

Fig. 8-95. Fluorescein angiograms from two cases of angioid streaks showing hyperfluorescence at the sites of rupture of Bruch's membrane. The choriocapillaris circulation is bared at the site of the defects in Bruch's membrane and the overlying pigment epithelium. These streaks cross under branches of both arterioles and venules, whereas true retinal vessels never cross both types of channels.

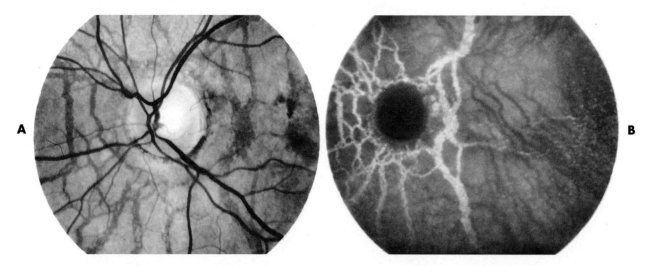

Fig. 8-96. Angioid streaks, defects in elastic tissue components at the level of Bruch's membrane. **A,** Red-free photograph showing classic angoid streaks. **B,** Indocyanine green, showing discrete hyperfluorescence of angioid streaks. In this particular case the indocyanine green angiography demonstrated the streaks much better than standard fluorescein angiography.

Fig. 8-97. Pseudoxanthoma elasticum. **A,** Characteristic skin lesions affecting the neck. **B,** Photomicrograph of the deep dermis from the skin of another patient with pseudoxanthoma elasticum and angioid streaks of the fundus (calcium stain). Intradermal elastic tissue is swollen *(arrows)*, irregularly clumped, fragmented, and calcified *(dense staining)*, a process essentially the same as that occurring in Bruch's membrane, which is also rich in elastic tissue. In normal skin the broad, deeply staining clumps of elastic tissue, as seen in this section, would not occur; the normal delicate elastic fibrils would be only faintly visible. (von Kossa stain; × 200.)

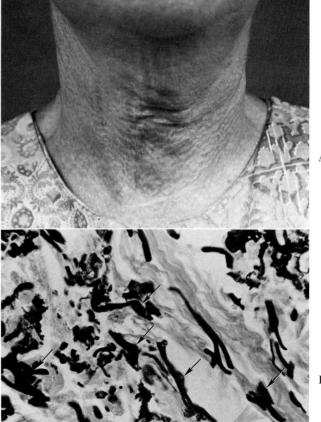

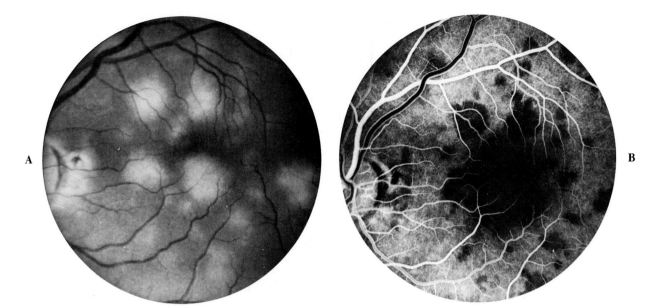

Fig. 8-98. Acute posterior multifocal placoid pigment epitheliopathy. **A,** Patchy and confluent yellowish white placoid retinal lesions. The retinal vessels are characteristically normal. Visual acuity in such cases is greatly decreased because of direct macular involvement. In most cases the acute lesions resolve, leaving a residual chorioretinal scar. Vision generally returns to normal. **B,** Fluorescein angiogram of the same case as in **A.** Although the acute lesions characteristically obscure the background choroidal fluorescence in the early stages of the angiogram as seen here, these areas fluoresce brightly in the late phase.

acuity caused by yellow-white placoid lesions at the level of the pigment epithelium and choroid (Fig. 8-98). Generally the acute lesions are rapidly resolved, and vision often returns to normal or near normal; however, residual alterations frequently occur in the pigment epithelium, including areas of atrophy and clumping. Retinal vasculitis, papillitis, serous retinal detachment, and anterior uveitis have also been reported in some cases.

Because no involved tissue has been analyzed histopathologically, the primary site of involvement is uncertain. Ophthalmoscopic and fluorescein angiography indicates that the pigment epithelium and the smaller choroidal vessels are most affected. The fluorescein angiogram is characteristic in the acute stages. In the early arterial phase, yellow-white lesions obscure the underlying fluorescence from choroidal vessels (Fig. 8-98, *B*); later stages show localized hyperfluorescence within these areas. Although no abnormal systemic factors have been observed consistently in these patients, several cases have followed an influenza-like illness, and APMPPE has been seen in patients with erythema nodosum.

Toxic maculopathy

Numerous toxic, infectious, metabolic, and degenerative conditions may lead to pigmentary degeneration of the retina (p. 402).

Chloroquine, frequently used in the treatment of rheumatoid arthritis and dermatologic disorders, is the prototype of a toxic retinopathy that creates a central macular lesion (Fig. 8-99).[1667] The lesion first shows a diffuse mottling of the affected central area. Then a pale ring, corresponding to a ring of degenerate or atrophic retinal pig-

ment epithelium, forms and surrounds the central focus, which remains more pigmented. The bull's-eye appearance is highly characteristic of this condition. Ultimate attenuation of retinal vessels, loss of ganglion cells, and constriction of the visual fields follow the initial macular lesion. These are caused by a peripheral pigmentary retinopathy and optic atrophy not unlike that seen in retinitis pigmentosa.

A bull's-eye macula can be seen in several conditions (Fig. 8-100), as indicated in the following list for differential diagnosis:*

1. Chloroquine retinopathy
2. Progressive cone dystrophy
3. Macular bull's-eye dystrophy without cone dysfunction
4. Vogt-Spielmeyer-Stock disease
5. Benign, dominant bull's-eye macular dystrophy

Many conditions (see the following list) that affect the pigment epithelium, Bruch's membrane, and choroid may lead to temporary or permanent visual loss by producing serous exudation or hemorrhage beneath the sensory retina and pigment epithelium.†

1. Idiopathic central serous chorioretinopathy or choroidopathy
2. Choroidal hemangioma
3. Malignant melanoma
4. Optic pit
5. Hypotony
6. Leukemic choroidal infiltrates
7. Terminal illness

---

* References 1303, 1355, 1371, 1466, 1619, 1770.
† References 1267, 1275, 1286, 1304, 1320, 1421, 1425, 1549–1552, 1594.

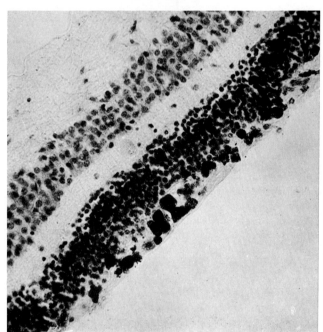

Fig. 8-99. Chloroquine retinopathy. **A,** Characteristic bull's-eye lesion. The "normal" central red region is surrounded by atrophic retinal pigment epithelium. **B,** In the early arteriovenous phase the bull's-eye appearance of the macula is conspicuous. The hyperpigmented center blocks the background fluorescence. **C,** Histologic section showing the pigmentary retinopathy. The ganglion cells are rarefied. A dark, black pigmentation is visible in the outer-most layers of the retina. (H & E stain; × 150.) (**A** and **B** from Blodi FC, Allen L, and Frazier O: Stereoscopic manual of the ocular fundus in local and systemic disease, vol II, St. Louis, 1970, The CV Mosby Co. **C** from Blodi FC and Allen L: Stereoscopic manual of the ocular fundus in local and systemic disease, vol I, St. Louis, 1964, The CV Mosby Co.)

8. Trauma
9. Uveitis
10. Optic neuritis
11. Papilledema
12. Acute hypertension
13. Vitreous traction
14. Angioid streaks
15. Harada's disease
16. Toxocara canis
17. Myopic chorioretinal degeneration
18. Metastatic carcinoma
19. Choroidal nevus
20. Collagen vascular disease

Many of these conditions are described elsewhere in this text. In contrast to the idiopathic choroidopathy, which rarely progresses, most of these factors lead to severe visual impairment with cystoid macular degeneration, reti-

noschisis, or macular hole if the underlying primary cause is not corrected.

In this section we consider (1) idiopathic central serous chorioretinopathy, in which visual loss is usually transient and permanent sequelae are rare; (2) serous detachment of the retinal pigment epithelium; and (3) the various forms of senile macular degeneration, including hemorrhagic disciform degeneration, in which severe and permanent loss of visual function often occurs.

Idiopathic central serous chorioretinopathy (central serous retinopathy)

Idiopathic central serous chorioretinopathy or choroidopathy affects healthy young adults, usually men.* In most

---

* References 1416, 1425, 1487, 1490, 1565, 1596, 1699, 1706, 1774–1776.

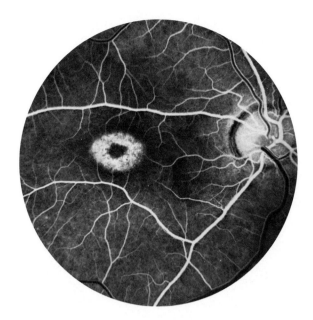

Fig. 8-100. Early arteriovenous phase fluorescein angiogram showing a prominent bull's-eye lesion of the macula.

cases the effect is unilateral; if bilateral, it is usual for the onset in the second eye to be delayed for a few weeks.

Initially there may be a history of premonitory transient attacks of blurred vision, but when the lesion develops, a positive scotoma results. The visual acuity is usually only moderately decreased, and the induced hyperopia caused by elevation of the retina can often be corrected with plus lenses. Micropsia and metamorphopsia often occur because of separation of the cones by the fluid and changes in retinal contour. Color perception is sometimes decreased, dark adaption may be prolonged, and stereopsis may be impaired.

In most cases the lesion persists from 2 to 3 months and then gradually subsides, leaving minimal residual macular pigmentation but normal vision. In a minority of cases it may recur one or more times. In rare instances, usually those characterized by multiple recurrences in which the serous detachment has persisted for a long period (6–8 months) or in which an associated pigment epithelial detachment is large, irreversible changes may occur. Subretinal neovascularization or hemorrhagic detachment is rare.[1743]

Uncomplicated central serous chorioretinopathy consists of a circular raised area in the macular region (Fig. 8-101) that is caused by serous detachment of the sensory retina from the underlying retinal pigment epithelium. The early phases of fluorescein angiography often reveal a focal spot of hyperfluorescence that indicates the retinal pigment epithelial defect (Fig. 8-101, *B*). As the dye passes through the defect it may assume an appearance that at times resembles a smokestack (Fig. 8-101, *C*). In the mid-arteriovenous and late phases the hyperfluorescence increases in area but increases only minimally to moderately in intensity. (Fig. 8-101, *D*).

The subretinal proteinaceous fluid is easily recognized in microscopic sections by the pink-staining serous fluid in the space between the elevated sensory retina and the underlying pigment epithelium (Fig. 8-102; Color Plate 8-

45). Histopathologic localization of the much smaller pigment defect often requires serial sectioning. Except in prolonged cases, the retinal photoreceptors are normal, and the retina rarely shows advanced cystoid changes or degeneration. Figure 8-103 illustrates how the serous detachment of the retina may coexist with a simultaneous detachment of the underlying pigment epithelium. The latter may even precede the sensory detachment.

Serous detachment of the retinal pigment epithelium

As the name implies, this disease connotes a condition characterized by a detachment of retinal pigment epithelium, which may occur with or without associated detachment of the overlying sensory retina (Figs. 8-103 and 8-104).*

Patients with RPE detachment are usually older than 30 and younger than 55 years of age and, in the idiopathic variety, have no underlying systemic disease. When an RPE detachment occurs in older patients, one should be alert to an underlying disease process.

Initial symptoms vary and depend largely on whether the fovea is involved. Persons with detachments involving the fovea are more likely to have visual disturbance, such as metamorphopsia or a mild positive scotoma. Occasionally, the detachment is totally asymptomatic and is an incidental finding during examination.

Pigment epithelial detachments vary widely in number, location, size, and evolution. They may be solitary and focal, involving only the pigment epithelium (Figs. 8-104, *A* and 8-105); multiple (Fig. 8-106); or accompanied by a detachment of the sensory retina (Figs. 8-101, 8-102, *B*, and 8-107).

Multiple detachments are more common than solitary detachments and are usually bilateral. The small multiple pigment epithelial detachments that are located away from the macula tend not to be associated with serious detachments of the sensory retina.

In general, RPE detachments in younger patients are smaller, are multiple, and have underlying clear fluid, in contrast to the larger lesions with turbid fluid seen in older persons. The detachments are often dome shaped and well circumscribed with distinct boundaries. Sensory detachments of the retina are less well circumscribed, often with poorly defined boundaries, and are shallow and less dome shaped. Both RPE and sensory retinal detachments show anterior bowing of the slit beam during biomicroscopic examination with the slit-lamp and contact lens; however, the beam is split whenever there is an associated sensory retinal detachment (Figs. 8-75, 8-103, and 8-104, *B*) but not with a pure pigment epithelial detachment (Figs. 8-105 and 8-106).

At times linear pigment bands are visible on the dome of the pigment epithelial detachment similar to those on a "hot cross bun" (Fig. 8-105). The bands are usually present in more long-standing detachments and are caused by pigment proliferations and deposition.

Drusen may occur in association with RPE detachments (Fig. 8-108). Differentiation of the two conditions is sometimes difficult.

When an RPE detachment is caused by subretinal neo-

---

* References 1385, 1431–1433, 1515, 1580, 1586, 1664, 1698, 1758, 1794.

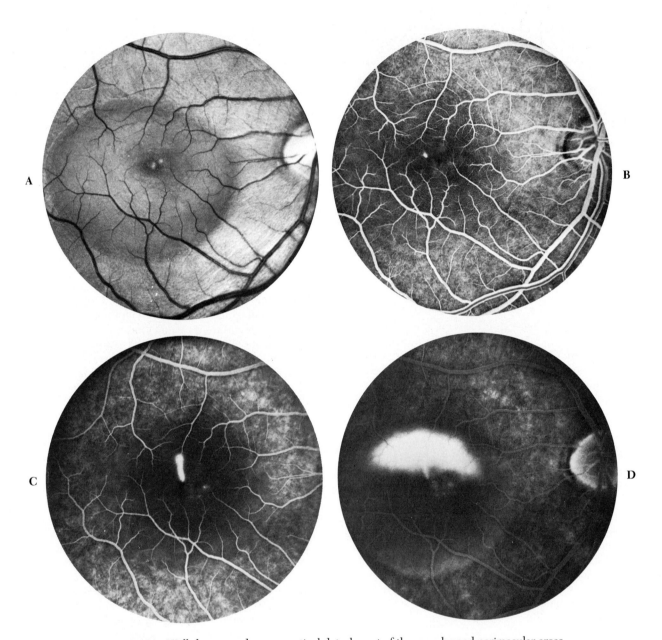

Fig. 8-101. Well-demarcated sensory retinal detachment of the macular and perimacular areas. **A,** Red-free photograph showing distinct borders and a few retinal pigment epithelial changes in the foveal region. **B,** Early arteriovenous phase angiogram showing a hyperfluorescent spot at the level of the retinal pigment epithelium. **C,** Later arteriovenous phase angiogram showing an area of hyperfluorescence extending upward, beginning to assume a "smokestack" appearance. **D,** In the late phase of the angiogram, the upward and lateral spread of the fluorescein has created an increase in intensity and size; fluorescence is present around the margins of the sensory retinal detachment. (From Rabb MF and Morgan BS: Perspect Ophthalmol 3:81, 1979.)

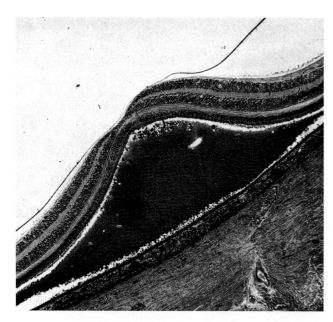

Fig. 8-102. A central serous chorioretinopathy is usually characterized by a circumscribed retinal detachment in the macular area. The macular area can be recognized by a thickening of the ganglion cell layer. Outside of the macula this layer consists of only one row of nuclei. (H & E stain; × 100.) (From Blodi FC and Allen L: Stereoscopic manual of the ocular fundus in local and systemic disease, vol I, St. Louis, 1964, The CV Mosby Co.)

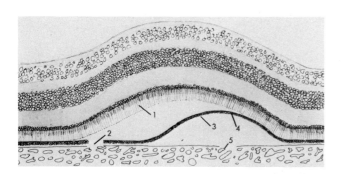

Fig. 8-103. Schematic drawing showing various possible mechanisms of neurosensory detachment: *(1)* detachment of the sensory retina, *(2)* a defect in Bruch's membrane and pigment epithelium without pigment epithelial detachment, *(3)* detachment of the retinal pigment epithelium, and *(4)* a break in the detached retinal pigment epithelium overlying *(5)* another break in Bruch's membrane. (Drawn by Dr. Steven Vermillion, University of Iowa.)

vascularization, other telltale findings are usually present. These may include the "dirty-gray" neovascular membrane itself, widespread RPE atrophic and/or drusen-like changes, surrounding lipid rings or exudate, and subretinal hemorrhage. The fluorescein angiogram in these cases shows early lacy hyperfluorescence, a "hot spot" corresponding to the site of the pigment epithelial detachment, and late hyperfluorescence with fuzzy irregular borders.

Small multiple pigment epithelial detachments (Fig. 8-106) in younger persons tend to have a good prognosis and little evidence of progression to the type of pigment epithelial detachments associated with subretinal neovas-

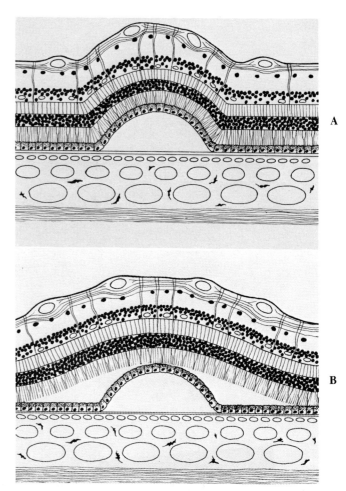

Fig. 8-104. Pigment epithelial detachment. **A,** The pigment epithelium is separated from Bruch's membrane. The sensory retina is attached to the pigment epithelium. **B,** The pigment epithelium is separated from Bruch's membrane. The overlying sensory retina is also detached from the pigment epithelium; however, the retina lies flat on the dome of the pigment epithelial detachment. (From Schatz H and others, editors: Interpretation of fundus fluorescein angiography: a comprehensive text and atlas, St. Louis, 1978, The CV Mosby Co.)

cularization. The detachments may increase in size while good central visual acuity is maintained and may disappear as mysteriously as they originally appeared, in some instances after many years. However, in older patients the detachments, whether single or multiple, tend not to regress spontaneously and are often associated with subretinal neovascularization.[1541]

Once subretinal neovascularization occurs, the visual prognosis is poor. Nevertheless, if RPE detachments are unassociated with serous detachment of the sensory retina, exudate, or hemorrhage, they tend to have a better prognosis. The longer the large pigment epithelial detachments remain in an area, particularly near the macula, the greater the chance of focal pigment epithelial degeneration, which further lessens the visual prognosis.

Because the prognosis of uncomplicated RPE detachment in the younger age group is good, any therapeutic modality for this group must be scrutinized regarding value

Text continues on p. 442.

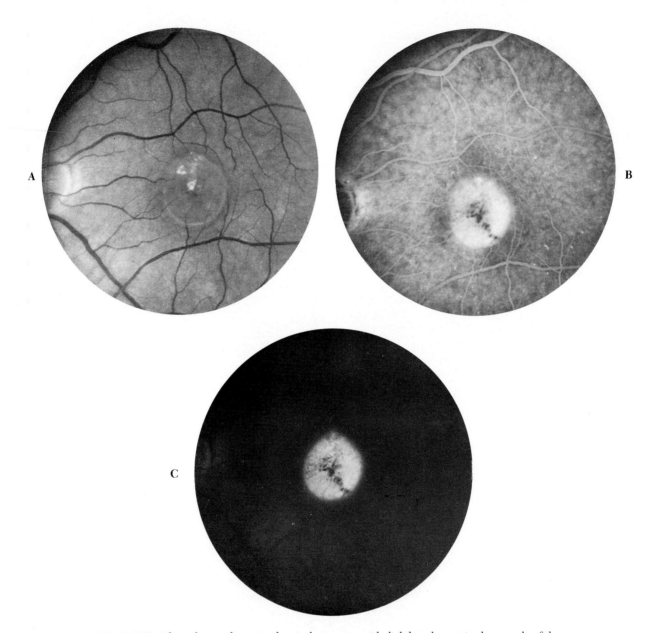

Fig. 8-105. Idiopathic medium-sized retinal pigment epithelial detachment in the macula of the left eye. **A,** Monochromatic red-free photograph. **B** and **C,** Early and midarteriovenous phase angiograms showing a homogeneous filling of the subepithelial space. Irregular bands of hypofluorescence occur on the dome of the detachment ("hot cross bun"). (From Rabb MF and Morgan BS: Perspect Ophthalmol 3:81, 1979.)

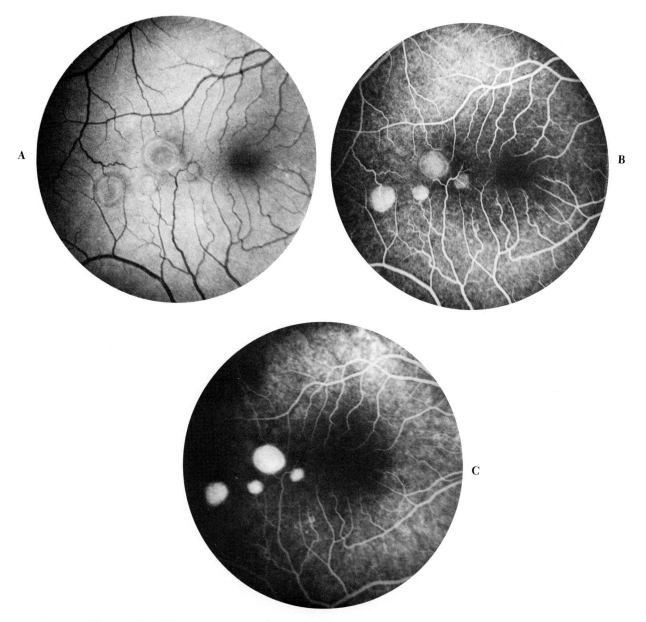

Fig. 8-106. Multiple retinal pigment epithelial detachments temporal to the right macula. **A,** Monochromatic red-free photograph. **B,** Midvenous phase angiogram showing four discrete detachments. **C,** Late venous phase angiogram again demonstrating a discrete hyperfluorescence of each lesion. An increase in intensity has occurred without an increase in size. (From Rabb MF and Morgan BS: Perspect Ophthalmol 3:81, 1979.)

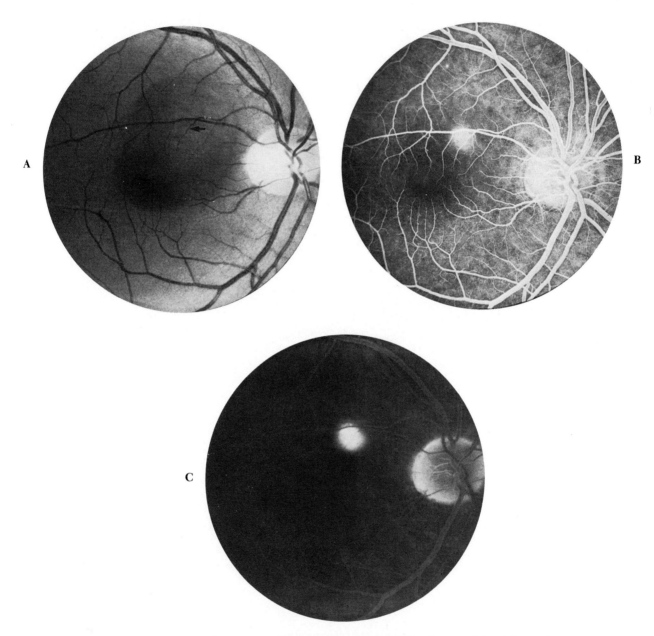

Fig. 8-107. Combined sensory retinal and pigment epithelial detachment of the right eye (see also Figs. 8-103 and 8-104, *B*). **A,** Red-free photograph demonstrating the entire area of the serous detachment of the sensory retina. The underlying retinal pigment epithelial detachment *(arrow)* is barely visible. **B,** Arteriovenous phase angiogram revealing a fuzzy hyperfluorescent spot at the site of the pigment epithelial detachment. **C,** Late venous phase angiogram clearly showing the entire extent of the pigment epithelial detachment. (From Rabb MF and Morgan BS: Perspect Ophthalmol 3:81, 1979.)

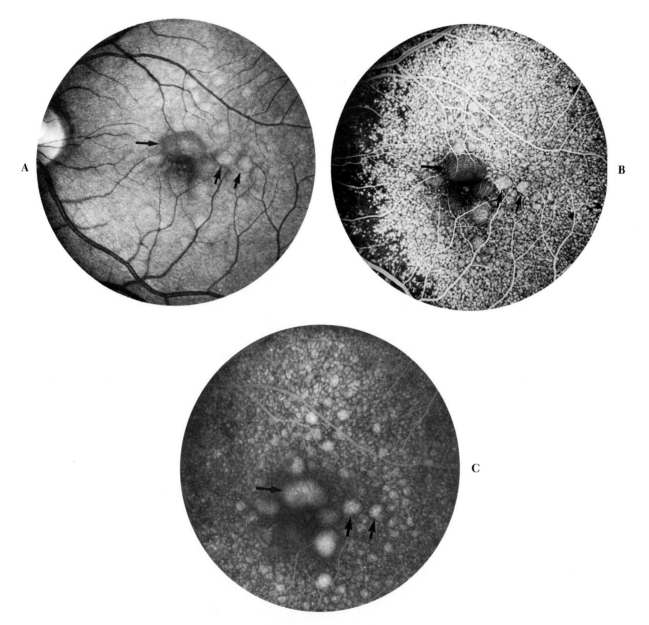

Fig. 8-108. Multiple drusen with multiple retinal pigment epithelial detachments. **A,** Red-free photograph showing multiple drusen in the posterior pole with associated elevated multiple retinal pigment epithelial detachments *(arrows).* **B,** Arteriovenous phase angiogram vividly demonstrating fine, discrete drusen throughout the posterior pole. The retinal pigment epithelial detachments in the macular area have less intense hyperfluorescence *(arrows).* **C,** Late venous phase angiogram. The retinal pigment epithelial detachments *(arrows)* stain more intensely, facilitating differentiation from the drusen. (From Rabb MF and Morgan BS: Perspect Ophthalmol 3:81, 1979.)

versus risks being initiated.[1541,1606,1664] To date, no randomized prospective study involving strictly defined patients has been carried out; however, the use of photocoagulation to seal a leaking pigment epithelial detachment is efficacious both in simple RPE detachment and in those combined with sensory retinal detachment. In the latter group of patients, photocoagulation of the area of leakage shortens the period of visual morbidity from approximately 5 months to 5 weeks, without influencing the final visual acuity in comparison with that of untreated persons.

When pigment epithelial detachments are unassociated with sensory retinal detachment and present for less than 6 months, a conservative approach may be followed. For pigment epithelial detachment combined with sensory retinal detachment, the risks of photocoagulation should be weighed against the patient's age, visual acuity, severity and duration of symptoms, initial versus recurrent attacks, severity of pigmentary changes, and presence or absence of underlying neovascularization.

We recommend photocoagulation for patients with a visual acuity of 20/80 or worse, visual disability symptoms for 3 months or longer, recurrence, and extensive pigmentary disturbance without any fluorescein angiographic evidence of subretinal neovascularization.

When subretinal neovascularization complicates the retinal pigment epithelial detachment, a high-quality angiogram showing the foveal avascular zone is of utmost importance in deciding whether photocoagulation should be performed. Only lesions that are situated at least ¼ disc diameter or 375 μm from the center of the foveal avascular zone should be considered for treatment. The pigment epithelial detachment and subretinal neovascularization are treated with overlapping intense burns, as is thick subretinal neovascular membrane. Careful follow-up examinations are necessary to detect any recurrent or inadequately treated neovascular net.

Age-related macular degeneration (nondisciform and disciform)

Age-related macular degeneration is the most prevalent cause of legal blindness in the United States; a similar frequency of blindness is seen in the dry and the exudative disciform forms (Figs. 8-109–8-112); (Color Plates 8-16 to 8-48).

Age-related macular degeneration consists of a gradual, often bilateral decrease of vision that occurs without hereditary influence. It is probably caused by aging and vascular disease in the choriocapillaris or the afferent retinal vessels. There are basically two morphologic types: nondisciform (or predisciform) and disciform.

Nondisciform (dry, atrophic) macular degeneration occurs in elderly patients, causing a slow visual loss in both eyes.[1414,1531] It is caused by partial or total obliteration of the underlying choriocapillaris. Two main features are apparent ophthalmoscopically:

1. Degeneration and hypopigmentation of the retinal pigment epithelium. In long-standing cases, a secondary cystoid degeneration, schisis, or hole formation in the overlying sensory retina may occur.
2. Subpigment epithelial deposition of yellow, often calcified material, which probably represents degenerative products derived from the pigment epithelium and Bruch's membrane. They vary in size from small focal drusen to large plaques caused by diffuse thickening of Bruch's membrane.[1334,1651–1653,1705]

In most cases of nondisciform macular degeneration, the secondary retinal changes evolve slowly and the loss of vis-

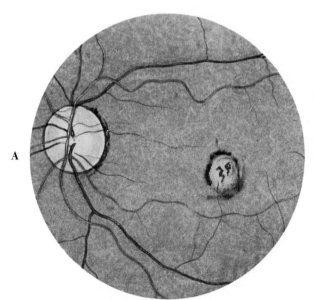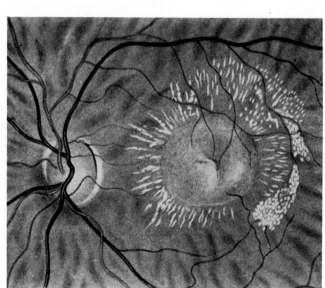

Fig. 8-109. Disciform macular degeneration: fundus drawings. **A,** Subretinal pigment epithelial neovascular membrane, early stage. **B,** Exudative neurosensory detachment with circinate deposition of lipids within the retina surrounding the elevated lesion. (From Junius P and Kuhnt H: Die scheibenförmige Entartung der Netzhautmitte; Degeneratio maculae luteae disciformis, Berlin, 1926, S Karger.)

ual acuity is gradual; however, in a small percentage of cases a severe loss of vision results. Exposure to sunlight and soft and hard drusen have been implicated as risk factors, but proof is lacking. The atrophy of the retinal pigment epithelial tends to spread and form well-demarcated borders, called geographic atrophy of macular degeneration. The atrophic areas often are bilateral and relatively symmetrical and are multifocal in about 40% of eyes. They tend to follow the disappearance of flattening of soft drusen. The underlying choriocapillaris is atrophic. Histologi-

cally the choriocapillaris may be partially or completely obliterated. Bruch's membrane may be thickened and may show basophilic changes. The pigment epithelium is atrophic with depigmentation, hypertrophy, or even hyperplasia. In advanced cases the overlying retina may show microcystoid changes or retinoschisis. Hole formation may occur in the inner wall of the macrocyst. A disciform degeneration with subsequent serous and hemorrhagic detachment of the pigment epithelium and retina may evolve in a small percentage of cases.

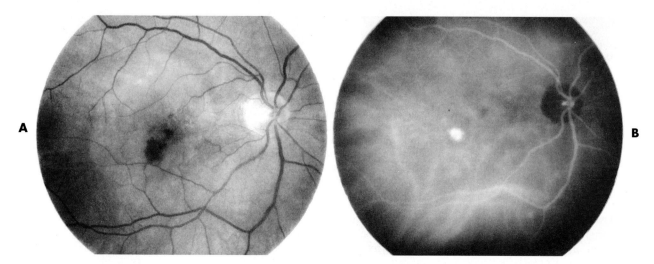

Fig. 8-110. Age-related macular degeneration. These photographs demonstrate the value of indocyan green angioscopy in delineating a focus of neovascularization. **A,** Red-free photograph showing a detachment of the sensory retina with underlying subretinal blood. **B,** Indocyanine green angiography clearly delineates a central focus of hyperfluorescence ("hot spot"), demonstrating the area of neovascularization.

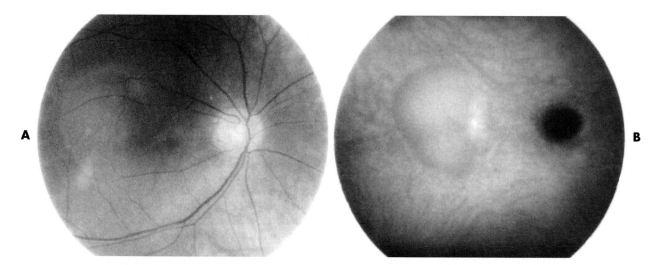

Fig. 8-111. Age-related macular degeneration with a focus of hyperfluorescence demonstrated only by indocyan green angiography. **A,** Fundus photograph showing an obvious retinal pigment epithelial detachment with an overlying sensory detachment. A distinct focus is not seen. **B,** Indocyanine green angiography from the same patient clearly showing a focus of hyperfluorescence (neovascularization) *(arrow)* at the nasal edge of the retinal pigment epithelial detachment. These foci are termed "hot spots," and sometimes are amenable to laser therapy if outside the fovea, such as in this case.

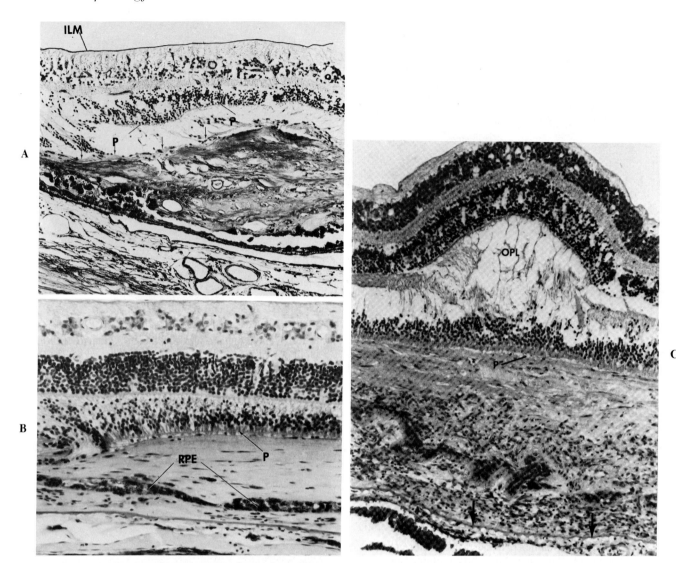

Fig. 8-116. Three photomicrographs of advanced hemorrhagic disciform detachment of the sensory retina and pigment epithelium (Kuhnt-Junius disease) of the macula. **A,** Previous serous and hemorrhagic detachment of the sensory retina and pigment epithelium, with subsequent organization of the hemorrhage, has formed a pigmented, fibrous plaque *(arrows)* below the retina. There is destruction of the overlying photoreceptor layer *(P)*. The pigment epithelial melanin is continuous with the fibrovascular plaque. Some of the fibrous tissue forms because of fibrous metaplasia of the pigment epithelium. Because of staining by the PAS technique, the internal limiting membrane *(ILM)* is exceptionally prominent. In addition to the major degeneration seen in the outer photoreceptor cell layer, extensive secondary damage to all other retinal layers has occurred. (PAS stain; ×115.) **B,** Evidence of a previous hemorrhagic detachment of the retinal pigment epithelium. The fibrous plaque between the retinal pigment epithelium *(RPE)*, the retinal photoreceptors above *(P)*, and the underlying Bruch's membrane below *(B)* consists of fibrous tissue derived from organized hemorrhage and metaplastic pigment epithelium. Both subretinal and subpigment epithelial involvement are evident. Because such lesions contain hemosiderin and dispersed pigment epithelial melanin, they are occasionally mistaken for malignant melanoma. The thickened ganglion cell layer (top layer of cells) is characteristic of the macular region. (H & E stain; ×180.) **C,** A dense, slightly pigmented plaque separates photoreceptors from Bruch's membrane *(arrows)*. There is marked cystoid macular edema in the outer plexiform layer *(OPL)*. (H & E stain; ×80.)

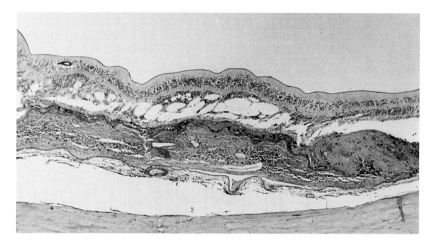

Fig. 8-117. Photomicrograph showing age-related macular degeneration, disciform type. Note the large disciform-shaped fibrosplak situated between the sensory retina, which shows the vast degeneration of retinal outer layers and choroid. (H & E stain; ×25.)

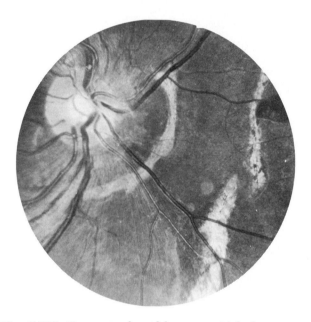

Fig. 8-118. Traumatic choroidal rupture. Multiple crescent-shaped choroidal defects have caused baring of the underlying sclera.

from nevi, malignant melanoma, or pigment epithelial tumors is sometimes difficult.

A disciform lesion may develop after trauma. The lesion may follow a direct hemorrhage under the subretinal space or may develop later after bleeding and exudation from a choroidal neovascular membrane, which may form at the site of the old choroidal rupture (Fig. 8-115).

Nonperforating and perforating wounds may cause intrachoroidal hemorrhage because of choroidal rupture.[1416,1529,1718] In most cases the clinical picture of a choroidal rupture includes a crescent-shaped tear or tears (Fig. 8-118; Color Plate 8-50). The shape is caused by the nature and direction of the lines of force applied to the choroid at injury. Hemorrhage into the choroid, subretinal space, and even into the vitreous can occur. In some cases a retinal

whitening (commotio retinae, or Berlin's edema) accompanies the injury. As the hemorrhage is resorbed, the choroidal and pigment epithelial ruptures become visible as crescent-shaped, yellow-white lines that are usually concentric with the optic nerve. The white color results from baring of the sclera.

Histopathologic changes induced by photocoagulation

The therapeutic application of light coagulation, introduced by Meyer-Schwickerath[1835] in the late 1940s and early 1950s, represented a major breakthrough in the treatment of numerous ocular diseases, particularly many of the fundus diseases described in this chapter. Prominent examples initiate the treatment of diabetic retinal disease and macular lesions.

The major instrument used today, the blue-green light of the argon laser, produces a specific tissue reaction on the retina and choroid, which make it highly amendable to treatment of diseases affecting these tissues. Selected references regarding the development of photocoagulation, its clinical application, and the histopathology of laser lesions, topics beyond the scope of this text, are listed in the references sections.[1809–1864] A more extensive clinicopathologic discussion and list of references are available (Apple DJ: Histopathology of xenon arc and argon laser photocoagulation. In L'Esperance FA Jr, editor: Current diagnosis and management of chorioretinal diseases, St. Louis, 1977, The CV Mosby Co).

References

General references

1. Abramov I and others: The retina of the newborn infant, Science 217:265, 1982.
2. Albert DM: Jaeger's atlas of diseases of the ocular fundus, Philadelphia, 1972, WB Saunders Co.
3. Anders B, Törnquist P, and Alm A: Permeability of the intraocular blood vessels, Trans Ophthalmol Soc UK 100:332, 1980.
4. Apple DJ: Histopathology of xenon-arc and argon laser photocoagulation. In L'Esperance FA Jr, editor: Current diagnosis and management of chorioretinal diseases, St Louis, 1977, The CV Mosby Co.

5. Apple DJ: Anatomy and histopathology of the macular region, Int Ophthalmol Clin 21(3):1, 1981.

6. Apple DJ, Hamming N, and Gieser D: Differential diagnosis of leukocoria. In Peyman GA, Apple DJ, and Sanders DR, editors: Intraocular tumors, New York, 1977, Appleton-Century-Crofts.

7. Archer DB and Gardiner TA: Experimental subretinal neovascularization, Trans Ophthalmol Soc UK 100:363, 1980.

8. Arroyo JG and Irvine AR: Retinal distortion and cotton-wool spots associated with epiretinal membrane contraction, Ophthalmology 102:662, 1995.

9. Ashton N: Oxygen and the retinal blood vessels, Trans Ophthalmol Soc UK 100:359, 1980.

10. Axenfeld T: Lehrbuch und Atlas der Augenheilkunde, Jena, 1912, Gustav Fischer.

11. Ballantyne AJ and Michaelson IC: Textbook of the fundus of the eye, ed 2, Baltimore, 1970, The Williams & Wilkins Co.

12. Bellhorn RW: Control of blood vessel development, Trans Ophthalmol Soc UK 100:328, 1980.

13. Bergren RL, Brown GC, and Duker JS: Prevalence and association of asteroid hyalosis with systemic disease, Am J Ophthalmol 111:289, 1991.

14. Blach RK: Clinical understanding in the management of retinal vascular disease, Trans Ophthalmol Soc UK 96:211, 1976.

15. Blodi FC and Allen L: Stereoscopic manual of the ocular fundus in local and systemic disease, vol I, St Louis, 1964, The CV Mosby Co.

16. Blodi FC, Allen L, and Frazier O: Stereoscopic manual of the ocular fundus in local and systemic disease, vol II, St Louis, 1970, The CV Mosby Co.

17. Braley AE: The retina, Int Ophthalmol Clin 3:3, 1962.

18. Brazitikos PD and others: Erbium: YAG laser surgery of the vitreous and retina, Ophthalmology 102:278, 1995.

19. Brockhurst RJ, Albert DM, and Zakov ZN: Pathologic findings in familiar exudative vitreoretinopathy, Arch Ophthalmol 99:2143, 1981.

20. Buettner H and Machemer R: Histopathologic findings in human eyes after pars plana vitrectomy and lensectomy, Arch Ophthalmol 95:2029, 1977.

21. Byer NE: Lattice degeneration of the retina, Surv Ophthalmol 23:213, 1978.

22. Cant J: The ocular circulation in health and disease, St Louis, 1969, The CV Mosby Co.

23. Chase J: The evolution of retinal vascularization in mammals: a comparison of vascular and avascular retinae, Ophthalmology 89:1518, 1982.

24. Chester EM: The ocular fundus in systemic disease: a clinical pathological correlation, Chicago, 1973, Year Book Medical Publishers, Inc.

25. Cibis GW, Watzke RC, and Chau J: Retinal hemorrhages in posterior vitreous detachment, Am J Ophthalmol 80:1043, 1975.

26. Cunha-Vaz JG: Blood-retinal barriers in health and disease, Trans Ophthalmol Soc UK 100:337, 1980.

27. Daicker B and Guggenheim R: Studies on fibrous and fibro-glial surface wrinkling retinopathy by scanning electron microscopy (German), Albrect von Graefes Archiv fur Klinische und Experimentelle Ophthalmologie 207:229, 1978 (author's translation).

28. Davson H: The Bowman lecture, 1979: the little brain, Trans Ophthalmol Soc UK 99:21, 1979.

29. Diabetic Retinopathy Study Research Group: Photocoagulation treatment of proliferative diabetic retinopathy: the second report of diabetic retinopathy study findings, Ophthalmology 85:82, 1978.

30. Duke-Elder S: System of ophthalmology, vol X, Diseases of the retina, St Louis, 1967, The CV Mosby Co.

31. Eisner G: Biomicroscopy of the peripheral fundus, New York, 1973, Springer Publishing Co, Inc.

32. Ernest JT: Blood flow in normal and abnormal retinal vessels, Trans Ophthalmol Soc UK 100:343, 1980.

33. Federman JL and others: Retina and vitreous. In Podos SM, Yanoff M, Textbook of ophthalmology, vol 9, London, 1994, The CV Mosby Co.

34. Feeney-Burns L, Berman ER, and Rothman H: Lipofuscin of human retinal pigment epithelium, Am J Ophthalmol 90:783, 1980.

35. Fine BS: Retinal structure: light- and electron-microscopic observations. In McPherson A, editor: New and controversial aspects of retinal detachment, New York, 1968, Harper & Row, Publishers.

36. Folkman J and Haudenschild C: Angiogenesis by capillary endothelial cells in culture, Trans Ophthalmol Soc UK 100:346, 1980.

37. Foos RY and Kopelow SM: Development of retinal vasculature in paranatal infants, Surv Ophthalmol 18:117, 1973.

38. Foos RY and Roth AM: Surface structure of the optic nerve head. 2. Vitreopapillary attachments and posterior vitreous detachment, Am J Ophthalmol 76:662, 1973.

39. Foos RY: Ultrastructural features of posterior vitreous detachment, Albrecht von Graefes Arch Klin Ophthalmol 196:103, 1975.

40. Foos RY and Wheeler NC: Vitreoretinal juncture: synchysis senilis and posterior vitreous detachment, Ophthalmology 89:1502, 1982.

41. Foulds WS: The retinal-pigment epithelial interface, Br J Ophthalmol 63:71, 1979.

42. Foulds WS and others: Vitreal, retinal and pigment epithelial contributions to the posterior blood-ocular barrier, Trans Ophthalmol Soc UK 100:341, 1980.

43. Frost W: The fundus oculi, New York, 1896, Macmillan & Co.

44. Fuchs E: Lehrbuch der Augenheilkunde, Vienna, 1889, Franz Deuticke.

45. Gariano RF, Kalina RE, and Hendrickson AE: Normal and pathological mechanisms in retinal vascular development, Surv Ophthalmol 40:481, 1996 (review).

46. Garner A: Ocular angiogenesis, Int Rev Exp Pathol 28:249, 1986.

47. von Graefe A and Saemisch T: Handbuch der gesammten Augenheilkunde, Leipzig, 1874, Wilhelm Engelmann.

48. Greef R: Die pathologische Anatomie des Auges. In Orth J editor: Lehrbuch der speziellen pathologischen Anatomie, Berlin, 1902, Hirschwald.

49. Gross JG and others: Experimental endoretinal biopsy, Am J Ophthalmol 110:619, 1990.

50. Grossniklaus HE and others: Hemoglobin spherulosis in the vitreous cavity, Arch Ophthalmol 106:961, 1988.

51. Hayreh SS: The choriocapillaris, Graefes Arch Clin Exp Ophthalmol 182:165, 1974.

52. Hendrickson AE and Yuodelis C: The morphological development of the human fovea, Ophthalmology 91:603, 1984.

53. Henke F and Lebarsch O, editors: Handbuch der speziellen pathologischen Anatomie und Histologie, Berlin, 1928, Julius Springer.

54. Henkind P: Some observations about retinal vascular-neuronal interrelationships, Br J Ophthalmol 62:361, 1978.

55. Katz B, Hoyt WF: Intrapapillary and peripapillary hemorrhage in young patients with incomplete posterior vitreous detachment. Signs of vitreopapillary traction, Ophthalmology 102:349, 1995.

56. Kimura S and Caygill W, editors: Retinal diseases, Philadelphia, 1966, Lea & Febiger.

57. Klein BR and others: Fundus photographic and fluorescein angiographic characteristics of pseudoholes of the macula in eyes with epiretinal membranes, Ophthalmology 102:768, 1995.

58. Korte GE and D'Aversa G: The elastic tissue of Bruch's membrane. Connections to choroidal elastic tissue and the ciliary epithelium of the rabbit and human eyes, Arch Ophthalmol 107:1654, 1989.

59. Krill AE: Hereditary retinal and choroidal diseases, vol 1, Evaluation, New York, 1972, Harper & Row, Publishers.

60. Kuwabara T and Cogan DG: Studies of retinal vascular patterns: normal architecture, Arch Ophthalmol 64:904, 1960.

61. Laatikainen L, Immonen I, and Summanen P: Peripheral retinal angioma-like lesion and macular pucker, Am J Ophthalmol 108:563, 1989.

62. Lanum J: The damaging effects of light on the retina: empirical findings, theoretical and practical implications, Surv Ophthalmol 22:221, 1978.

63. Larsen HW: The ocular fundus: a color atlas, Philadelphia, 1976, WB Saunders Co.

64. L'Esperance FA Jr, editor: Current diagnosis and management of chorioretinal diseases, St Louis, 1977, The CV Mosby Co.

65. Luxenberg M and Sime D: Relationship of asteroid hyalosis to diabetes mellitus and plasma lipid levels, Am J Ophthalmol 67:406, 1969.

66. March W, Shoch D, and O'Grady R: Composition of asteroid bodies, Invest Ophthalmol 13:701, 1974.

67. Marchesani O and Sautter H: Atlas of the ocular fundus, New York, 1959, Hafner Publishing Co (Translated by A Philipp).

68. McLaren MJ: Kinetics of rod outer segment phagocytosis by cultured retinal pigment epithelial cells. Relationship to cell morphology, Invest Ophthalmol Vis Sci 37:1213, 1996.

69. Michaelson IC, editor: Textbook of the fundus of the eye, ed 3, New York, 1981, Churchill Livingstone, Inc.

70. Miller H and others: Asteroid bodies—an ultrastructural study, Invest Ophthalmol Vis Sci 24:133, 1983.

71. Morse PH: Vitreoretinal disease: a manual for diagnosis and treatment, Chicago, 1979, Year Book Medical Publishers, Inc.

72. Murakami K and others: Vitreous floaters, Ophthalmology 90:1271, 1983.

73. New Orleans Academy of Ophthalmology: Symposium on retina and retinal surgery: transactions of the New Orleans Academy of Ophthalmology, St Louis, 1969, The CV Mosby Co.

74. New Orleans Academy of Ophthalmology: Symposium on retinal diseases: transactions of the New Orleans Academy of Ophthalmology, St Louis, 1977, The CV Mosby Co.

75. Nover A: The ocular fundus, Philadelphia, 1974, Lea & Febiger (Translated by FC Blodi).

76. Oeller J: Atlas seltener ophthalmoskopischer Befunde, Wiesbaden, 1903, JF Bergmann.

77. Panda-Jonas S, Jonas JB, and JakobczykZmija M: Retinal pigment epithelial cell count, distribution, and correlations in normal human eyes, Am J Ophthalmol 121:181, 1996.

78. Pandolfi M: Hemorrhages in ophthalmology, Stuttgart, 1979, Georg Thieme Verlag.

79. Pauleikhoff D and others: Aging changes in Bruch's membrane. A histochemical and morphologic study, Ophthalmology 97:171, 1990.

80. Pauleikhoff D and others: Correlation between biochemical composition and fluorescein binding of deposits in Bruch's membrane, Ophthalmology 99:1548, 1992.

81. Peyman GA and Sanders DR: Advances in uveal surgery, vitreous surgery and the treatment of endophthalmitis, New York, 1975, Appleton-Century-Crofts.

82. Peyman GA, Spitznas M, and Straatsma BR: Peroxidase diffusion in the normal and photocoagulated retina, Invest Ophthalmol 10:181, 1971.

83. Pruett RC and Regal CDJ, editors: Retina Congress, New York, 1974, Appleton-Century-Crofts.

84. Radius RL and Anderson DR: The histology of retinal nerve fiber layer bundles and bundle defects, Arch Ophthalmol 97:948, 1979.

85. Rahi A and Ashton N: Contractile proteins in retinal endothelium and other non-muscle tissues of the eye, Br J Ophthalmol 62:627, 1978.

86. Ramrattan RS and others: Morphometric analysis of Bruch's membrane, the choriocapillaris, and the choroid in aging, Invest Ophthalmol Vis Sci 35:2857, 1994.

87. Rodman HI, Johnson FB, and Zimmerman LF: New histopathological and histochemical observations concerning asteroid hyalitis, Arch Ophthalmol 66:552, 1961.

88. Roizenblatt J, Grant S, and Foos RY: Vitreous cylinders, Arch Ophthalmol 98:739, 1980.

89. Roy F: Ocular differential diagnosis, ed 2, Philadelphia, 1975, Lea & Febiger.

90. Salzmann M: The anatomy and histology of the human eyeball in the normal state: its development and senescence, Chicago, 1931, University of Chicago Press (Translated by EVL Brown).

91. Sautter H, Straub W, and Rossmann H: Atlas of the ocular fundus, Philadelphia, 1977, JB Lippincott Co.

92. Schatz H and others, editors: Fundus fluorescein angiography: a comprehensive text and atlas, St Louis, 1978, The CV Mosby Co.

93. Seitz R: The retinal vessels, St Louis, 1964, The CV Mosby Co (Translated by FC Blodi).

94. Shimizu K: Fluorescein microangiography of the ocular fundus, Baltimore, 1973, The Williams & Wilkins Co.

95. Sivalingam A and others: Visual prognosis correlated with the presence of internal-limiting membrane in histopathologic specimens obtained from epiretinal membrane surgery, Ophthalmology 97:1549, 1990.

96. Sorsby A: Diseases of the fundus oculi, London, 1975, Butterworth & Co (Publishers), Ltd.

97. Spencer LM, Foos RY: Paravascular vitreoretinal attachments, Arch Ophthalmol 84:557, 1970.

98. Spitznas M: Der normale ephthalmoskopische und histologische Befund der Maculazone und seine Varianten, Dtsch Ophthalmol Gesellschaft 73:26, 1973.

99. Straatsma B and others: The retina, UCLA Forum in Medical Sciences, No 8, Berkeley, 1969, University of California Press.

100. Streeten BW: Vitreous asteroid bodies: ultrastructural characteristics and composition, Arch Ophthalmol 100:969, 1982.

101. Streeten BW: The nature of the ocular zonule, Trans Am Ophthalmol Soc 80:823, 1982.

102. Svarc ED and Werner D: Isolated retinal hemorrhages associated with oral contraceptives, Am J Ophthalmol 84:50, 1977.

103. Tasman W: Retinal diseases in children, New York, 1971, Harper & Row, Publishers.

104. Tasman W: Retina and optic nerve, Arch Ophthalmol 94:1201, 1976.

105. Tasman W and Shields JA: Disorders of the peripheral fundus, New York, 1980, Harper & Row, Publishers.

106. Tolentino FI, Schepens CL, and Freeman HM: Vitreoretinal disorders: diagnosis and management, Philadelphia, 1976, WB Saunders Co.

107. Topilow HW and others: Asteroid hyalosis, Arch Ophthalmol 100:964, 1982.

108. Torczynski E and Tso MOM: The architecture of the choriocapillaris at the posterior pole, Am J Ophthalmol 81:428, 1976.

109. von Graefe A and Saemisch T: Handbuch der gesammten Augenheilkunde, Leipzig, 1874, Wilhelm Engelmann.

110. Watzke R, Weingeist T, and Constantine J: Diagnosis and management of von Hippel-Lindau disease. In Peyman GA, Apple DJ, and Sanders DR, editors: Intraocular tumors, New York, 1977, Appleton-Century-Crofts.

111. Weinberg RS, Peyman GA, and Apple DJ: Histopathology after vitrectomy with the vitreophage, Graefes Arch Clin Exp Ophthalmol 196:133, 1975.

112. Wessing A: Fluorescein angiography of the retina: textbook and atlas, St Louis, 1969, The CV Mosby Co (Translated by GK von Noorden).

113. Wilmer W: Atlas fundus oculi, New York, 1934, The Macmillan Co.

114. Wise GN, Dollery CT, and Henkind P: The retinal circulation, New York, 1971, Harper & Row, Publishers.

115. Young RW: The Bowman Lecture, 1982: biological renewal—applications to the eye, Trans Ophthalmol Soc UK 102:42, 1982.

116. Zhao DS: An ultrastructural histopathological study of the membrane formation in retinal detachment (Chinese). Yen Ko Hsueh Pao (Eye Science) 2:53, 1986.

117. Zinn KM and Marmor MF: The retinal pigment epithelium, Cambridge, Mass, 1979, Harvard University Press.

Trauma

118. Abramov I and Hainline L: Light and the developing visual system. In Marshall J, editor-The susceptible visual apparatus, vision and visual dysfunction, vol 16, London, 1991, Macmillan Press.

119. Aguilar JP and Green WR: Choroidal rupture: a histopathologic study of 47 eyes, Retina 4:269, 1984.

120. Archer DB and Canavan YM: Contusional eye injuries: retinal and choroidal lesions, Aust J Ophthalmol 11:251, 1983.

121. Azzolini C and others: Updating on intraoperative light-induced retinal injury, International Ophthalmology 18:269, 1994 (review).

122. Azzolini C, Docchio F, and Brancato R: Refractive hazards of intraoperative retinal photocoagulation, Ophthalmic Surgery 24:16, 1993.

123. Benson WE: The effects of blunt trauma on the posterior segment of the eye, Trans Penn Acad Ophthalmol 2:26, 1982.

124. Benson WE, Shakin J, and Sarin LK: Blunt trauma. In Tasman W and Jaeger EA, editors: Clinical ophthalmology, vol 3, Philadelphia, 1988, JB Lippincott Co.

125. Bergen R and Margolis S: Retinal hemorrhages in the newborn, Ann Ophthalmol 8:53, 1976.

126. Berlin R: Zur sogenannten Commotio retinae, Klin Monatbl Augenheilka 11:42, 1873.

127. Blight R and Hard JCD: Structural changes in the outer retinal layers following blunt mechanical non-perforating trauma to the globe: an experimental study, Br J Ophthalmol 61:573, 1977.

128. Blodi B and others: Purtscher's-like retiopathy after childbirth, Ophthalmology 97:1654, 1990.

129. Boldery EE, Ho BT, and Griffith RD: Retinal burns occurring at cataract extraction, Ophthalmology 91:1297, 1984.

130. Brod RD and others: Phototoxic retinal damage during refractive surgery, Am J Ophthalmol 102:121, 1986.

131. Brod RD and others: The site of operating microscope induced light injury on the human retina, Am J Ophthalmol 107:390, 1989.

132. Budenz DL and others: Ocular and optic nerve hemorrhages in abused infants with intracranial injuries, Ophthalmol 107:390, 1989.

133. Burton TC: Unilateral Purtscher's retinopathy, Ophthalmology 87:1096, 1980.

134. Buys UM and others: Retinal findings after head trauma in infants and young children, Ophthalmology 99:1718, 1992.

135. Caffey J: The whiplash shaken infant syndrome: manual shaking by the extremities with whiplash-induced intracranial and intraocular bleedings, linked with residual permanent brain damage and mental retardation, Pediatrics 54:396, 1974.

136. Calkins JL and Hochhiemer BF: Retinal light exposure from operation microscopes, Arch Ophthalmol 97:2363, 1979.

137. Clarkson JG, Glynn HW Jr, and Daily MJ: Vitrectomy in Terson's syndrome, Am J Ophthalmol 90:549, 1980.

138. Cordes FC: A type foveomacular retinitis observed in the U.S. Navy, Am J Ophthalmol 27:308, 1944.

139. Delori F, Pomerantzeff O, and Cox MS: Deformation of the globe under high speed impact: its relation to contusion injuries, Invest Ophthalmol Vis Sci 8:290, 1969.

140. Delori FC, Pomerantz O, and Mainster MA: Light level in ophthalmic diagnostic instruments, Proc Soc Photo Optical Instrum Engl 229:154, 1980.

141. Dobson V: Editorial: phototherapy and retinal damage, Invest Ophthalmol Vis Sci 15:595, 1976.

142. Elner SC and others: Ocular and associated systemic findings in suspected child abuse: a necropsy study, Arch Ophthalmol 108:1094, 1990.

143. Ewald RA and Richey CL: Sun gazing as the cause of Foveomacular retinitis, Am J. Ophthalmol 70:491, 1970.

144. Feist RM and Farber MD: Ocular trauma epidemiology, Arch Ophthalmol 107:503, 1989.

145. Fishman GA: Light-induced maculopathy from surgical microscopes during cataract surgery. In Ernest JT, editor: The 1985 Year Book of Ophthalmology, St. Louis, 1985, Mosby-Year Book, Inc.

146. Forrester JV, Lee WR, and Williamson J: The pathology of vitreous hemorrhagem, I. Gross and histological appearances, Arch Ophthalmol 96:703, 1978.

147. Forrester JV, Brierson I, and Lee WR: The pathology of vitreous hemorrhage, II. Ultrastructure, Arch Ophthalmol 97:2368, 1979.

148. Fuchs E: Zur Vernderung der Macula lutea nach Contusion, Z Augenheilkd 6:181, 1901.

149. Fuller D, Machemer R, and Knighton RW: Retinal damage produced by intraocular fiber optic light Am J Ophthalmol 85:519, 1978.

150. Garcia Arumi J and others: Epiretinal membranes in Terson's syndrome, Retina 14:351, 1994.

151. Gaynon MW and others: Retinal folds in the shaken baby syndrome, Am J Ophthalmol 106:423, 1988.

152. Giovinazzo VJ and others: The ocular complications of boxing, Ophthalmol 94:587, 1987.

153. Gladstone GJ and Tasman W: Solar retinitis after minimal exposure, Arch Ophthalmol 96:1368, 1978.

154. Goldberg MF: Chorioretinal vascular anastomoses after blunt trauma to the eye, Am J Ophthalmol 82:892, 1976.

155. Goldberg MF: Chorioretinal vascular anastomeses after perforating trauma to the eye, Am J Ophthalmol 85:171, 1978.

156. Goldzieher W: Beitrag zur Pathologie der orbitalen Schussverletzungen, Z Augenheilkd 6:277, 1901.

157. Gomolin JE and Koenekoop RK: Presumed photic retinopathy after cataract surgery: an angiographic study, Can J Ophthalmol 28:221, 1993.

158. Green WR and Robertson D: Pathologic findings of photic retinopathy in the human eye, Am J Ophthalmol 112:520, 1991.

159. Greenwald MJ and others: Traumatic retinoschisis in battered babies, Ophthalmology 93:618, 1986.

160. Grey RHB: Foveo-macular retinitis, solar retinopathy, and trauma, Br J Ophthalmol 62:543, 1978.

161. Hart JCD and Frank HJ: Retinal opacification after blunt nonperforating concussional injuries to the globe: a clinical and retinal fluorescein angiographic study, Trans Ophthalmol Soc UK 95:94, 1975.

162. Henry MM, Henry LM, and Henry LM: A possible cause of chronic cystic maculopathy, Ann Ophthalmol 9:455, 1977.

163. Herschler J: Trabecular damage due to blunt anterior segment injury and its relationship to traumatic glaucoma, Trans am Acad Ophthalmol Otolaryngol 83:239, 1977.

164. Inkeles DM, Walsh JB, and Matz R: purtscher's retinopathy in acute pancreatitis, Am J Med Sci 272:335, 1976.

165. Irvine Ar, Wood I, and Morris BW: Retinal damage from the illumination of the operating microscope. An experimental study in pseudophakic monkeys, Arch Ophthalmol 102:1358, 1984.

166. Jensen AD, Smith RE, and Olson MI: Ocular clue to child abuse, J Pediatr Ophthalmol 8:270, 1971.

167. Kerr LM and Little HL: Foveomacular retinitis, Arch Ophthalmol 76:498, 1966.

168. Khwarg SG, Geoghegan M, and Hanscom TA: Ligh-induced maculopathy from the operating microscope, Am J Ophthalmol 98:628, 1984.

169. Khwarg SG and others: Incidence, risk factors and morphology in operating microscope light retinopathy, Am J Ophthalmol 103:255, 1987.

170. Klopfer J and others: Ocular trauma in the United States: eye injuries resulting in hospitalization, Arch Ophthalmol 110:838, 1992.

171. Kraff Mc and others: Effect of ultraviolet-filtering intraocular lens on cystoid macular edema, Ophthalmol 92:366, 1985.

172. Kuhn F, Morris R, and Massey M: Photic retinal injury from endoillumination during vitrectomy, Am J Ophthalmol 111:42, 1991.

173. Kuming BS: Foveomacular retinitis, Br J Ophthalmol 70:816, 1986.

174. Lanum J: The damaging effects of light on the retina. Empirical findings, theoretical and practical implications, Surv Ophthalmol 22:221, 1978.

175. LaRoche GR, Mc Intyre L, and Scherter RM: Epidemiology of severe eye injuries in childhood, Ophthalmology 95:1603, 1988.

176. Lawwill T: Three major pathologic processes caused by light in the primate retina: a search for mechanisms, Trans Am Ophthalmol Soc 80:517, 1982.

177. Leonardy NJ, Dabbs CN, and Sternberg PS: Subretinal neovascularization after operating microscope burn, Am J Ophthalmol 109:224, 1982.

178. Lerman S: Ocular phototoxicity. In Davidson SI and Fraunfelder FT, editors: Recent advances in ophthalmology, London, 1985, Churchill Livingstone, Inc.

179. Levin AV: Ocular manifestations of child abuse, Ophthalmology Clin North Am 3:249, 1990.

180. Lewis H and others: Tissue plasminogen activator treatment of experimental subretinjal hemorrhage, Am J Ophthalmol 111:197, 1991.

181. Liggett PE and others: Ocular trauma in an urban population: review of 1132 cases, Ophthalmology 97:581, 1990.

182. Macy JI and Baerveldt G: Pseudophakic serous maculopathy, Arch Ophthalmol 101:228, 1983.

183. Mainster MA: Solar retinitis, photic maculopathy and the pseudophakic eye, Am Intra Ocular implant Soc J 4:84, 1978.

184. Mainster MA: Ham WT Jr, and Delori FC: Potential retinal hazards. Instrument and environmental ligh sources, Ophthalmol 90:927, 1983.

185. Mainster MA: The spectra, classification, and rationale of ultraviolet-protected intraocular lenses, Am J Ophthalmol 102:727, 1986.

186. Mainster MA: Light and macular degeneration: a biophysical and clinical perspective, Eye 1:304, 1987.

187. Mainster MA: Photic retinal injury. In Ryan SJ, editor: Retina, vol 1, St. Louis, 1989, Mosby-Year Book, Inc.

188. Mainster MA: Photic retinal injury. In Ryan SJ, editor: Retina, ed 2, vol 3, St. Louis, 1994, Mosby-Year Book, Inc.

189. Mansour AM, Green WR, and Hogge C: Histopathology of commotio retinae, Retina 12:24, 1992.

190. Marlor RL and others: Foveomacular retinitis, an important problem in military medicine: epidemiology, Invest Ophthalmol Vis Sci 12:5, 1973.

191. Marshall J: Radiation of the aging eye, Ophthalmol Physiol Opt 5:241, 1985.

192. Martin DF and others: Treatment and pathogenesis of traumatic

chorioretinal rupture (sclopetaria), Am J Ophthalmol 117:190, 1994.

193. Massicotte SJ and others: Vitreoretinal traction and perimacular folds in the eyes of deliberately traumatized children, Ophthalmol 98:1124, 1991.

194. McDonald Hr, Irvine Ar: Light induced maculopathy from the operating microscope in extracapsular cataract extraction and intraocular lens implantation, Ophthalmology 90:945, 1983.

195. Messner Kh, Maisels MJ, and Leure-DuPree AE: Phototoxicity to the newborn primate retina, Invest Ophthalmol Vis Sci 17:178, 1978.

196. Michels RL: Light toxicity, Surv Ophthalmol 34:237, 1990 (review).

197. Noell WK: Possible mechanisms of photoreceptors damage by light in mammalian eyes, Vision Res 20:1163, 1980.

198. Organisciak DT and others: Retinal light exposure in rats exposed to intermittent light. Comparison with continuous ligh exposure, Invest Ophthalmol Vis Sci 30:795, 1989.

199. Parver LM, Auker Cr, and Fine BS. Observations on monkey eyes exposed to light from an operating microscope, Ophthalmology 90: 964, 1983.

200. Perry HD and Rahn EK: Chorioretinitis sclopetaria, Arch Ophthalmol 95:328, 1977.

201. Pollak VA and Romanchuk KG: The risk of retina damage from high intensity ligh sources, J Am Indust Hygiene Assoc 41:322, 1980.

202. Pratt MV and De Venecia G: Purtscher's retinopathy: a clinicopathological correlation, Surv Ophthalmol 14:417, 1970.

203. Pulido JR and Blair NP: The blood-retinal barrier in Berlin's edema. Retina 7:233, 1987.

204. Purtscher O: Noch unbekannte Befunde nach Schaedeltrauma, Berl Dtsch Ophthal Ges 36:294, 1910.

205. Purtscher O: Angiopathia retinae traumatica: Lymphorrhagien des Augengrundes, Graefes Arch Klin Exp Ophthalmol 82:347, 1912.

206. Rapoport I and others: Eye injuries in children in Israel: a nationwide collaborative study, Arch Ophthalmol 108:376, 1990.

207. Ravin JG and Meyer RF: Fluoreschein angiographic findings in a case of traumatic asphyxia, Am J Ophthalmol 75:643, 1973.

208. Richards RD, West CE, and Meisels AA: Chorioretinitis sclopetaria, Am J Ophthalmol 66:852, 1968.

209. Riffenburg RS and Sathyavagiswaran L: Ocular findings at autopsy of child abuse victims, Ophthalmology 98:1519, 1991.

210. Rimmer S and Schuler JD: Severe ocular trauma from a driver's-side air bag, Arch Ophthalmol 109:774, 1991.

211. Robertson DM and Erickson GJ: The effect of prolonged indirect ophthalmoscopy on the human eye, Am J Ophthalmol 87:652, 1979.

212. Robertson DM and Feldman RB: Photic retinopathy from the operating room microscope, Am J Ophthalmol 101:561, 1986.

213. Robertson DM and McLaren JW: Photic retinopathy from the operating room microscope. Study with filter, Arch Ophthalmol 107:373, 1989.

214. Schein Od and others: The spectrum and burden of ocular injury, Ophthalmology 95:300, 1988.

215. Shaw HE Jr, Landers MB III, and Sydnor CF: The significance of intraocular hemorrhages due to subarachnoid hemorrhage, Ann Ophthalmol 9:1403, 1977.

216. Sipperley JO, Quigley HA, and Gass JDM: Traumatic retinopathy in primate; the explanation of commotio retinae, Arch Ophthalmol 96:2267, 1978.

217. Smith RE, Kelley JS, and Harbin TS: Late macular complication of horiodal ruptures, Am J Ophthalmol 77:650, 1974.

218. Sternberg P and Aaberg TM: The persistent challenge of ocular trauma, Am J Ophthalmol 4:421, 1989.

219. Taylor HR and others: The long-term effect of visible light on the eye, Arch Ophthalmol 110:99, 1992.

220. Taylor HR and others: Effect of ultraviolet radiation on cataract formation, New Engl J Med 319:1429, 1988.

221. Tielsch JM and Parver LM: Determinants of hospital charges and length of stay for ocular trauma, Ophthalmology 97:231, 1990.

222. Tielsch JM, Parver L, and Shankar B: Time trends in the incidence of hospitalized ocular trauma, Arch Ophthalmol 107:519, 1989.

223. Toth CA and others: Fibrin directs early retinal damage after experimental subretinal hemorrhage, Arch Ophthalmol 109:723, 1991.

224. Tso MO, Fine BS, and Zimmerman LE: Photic maculopathy produced by the indirect ophthalmoscope, I. Clinical and histopathologic study, Am J Ophthalmol 73:686, 1972.

225. Tso MO and La Piana FG: The human fovea after sungazing, Trans Am Acad Ophthalmol Otolaryngol 79:OP-788, 1975.

226. Tso MO and Woodford BJ: Effect of photic injury on the retinal tissues, Ophthalmol 90:952, 1983.

227. Tso MO: Retinal photic injury in normal scorbutic monkeys, Trans Am Ophthalmol Soc 85:498, 1987.

228. Van der Hoeve J: Eye lesions produced by ligh rich in ultraviolet rays: senile cataract, senile degeneration of the macula, Am J Ophthalmol 3:178, 1920.

229. Velikay M and others: Retinal detachment with severe proliferative vitreoretinopathy in Terson's syndrome, Ophthalmology 101:35, 1994.

230. Von Grafe A: Zwei Faelle von Ruptur der Choriordea, Graefes Arvh Ophthalmol Klin Exp Ophthalmol 1:402, 1854.

231. Walsh FB and Hedges TR: Optic nerve sheath hemorrhage, Am J Ophthalmol 34:509, 1951.

232. Weingeist TA and others: Terson's syndrome. Clinicopatholic correlations, Ophthalmol 93:1435, 1986.

233. Weissbold DJ and others: Ruptured vascular malformation masquerading as battered/shaken baby syndrom: a nearly tragic mistake, Surv Ophthalmol 39:509, 1995.

234. Wergerland FL Jr and Brenner EH: Solar retinopathy and foveomacular retinitis, Ann Ophthalmol 7:495, 1975.

235. West SK and others: Exposure to sunlight and other risk factors for age related macular degeneration, Arch Ophthalmol 107:875, 1989.

236. White TJ and others: Chorioretinal temperature increases from solar observation, Bull Math Biophys 33:1, 1971.

237. Wolter JR: Coup-contrecoup mechanism of ocular injuries, Am J Ophthalmol 56:785, 1963.

238. Wyzynski Re, Grossnicklaus HE, and Frank KE: Indirect choroidal rupture, secondary to blunt ocular trauma: a review of eight eyes, Retina 8:237, 1988.

239. Yannuzzi LA and others: Solar retinopathy: A photobiological and geophysical analysis, Trans Am Ophthalmol Soc 85:120, 1987.

Retinal vascular diseases

Hypertensive and arteriosclerotic retinopathy

240. Ashton N: The eye in malignant hypertension Trans Am Acad Ophthalmol Otolaryngol 76:17, 1972.

241. Ashton N and Harry J: The pathology of cotton-wool spots and cytoid bodies in hypertensive retinopathy and other diseases, Trans Ophthalmol Soc UK 83:91, 1963.

242. Capoor S and others: White-centered retinal hemorrhages as an early sign of preeclampsia, Am J Ophthalmol 119:804, 1995.

243. Christensen L: The nature of the cytoid body, Trans Am Ophthalmol Soc 56:451, 1958.

244. de Venecia G and others: The eye in accelerated hypertension. I. Elschnig's spots in nonhuman primates, Arch Ophthalmol 98:913, 1980.

245. Friedman and others: Choroidal vascular patterns in hypertension, Arch Ophthalmol 71:842, 1964.

246. Garner and others: Pathogenesis of hypertensive retinopathy. Br J Ophthalmol 59:3, 1975.

247. Gass JDM: A fluorescein angiographic study of macular dysfunction secondary to retinal vascular disease. III. Hypertensive retinopathy, Arch Ophthalmol 80:569, 1968.

248. Gass JDM: A fluorescein angiographic study of macular dysfunction secondary to retinal vascular disease. I. Embolic retinal artery obstruction. II. Retinal vein occlusion. III. Hypertensive retinopathy. IV. Diabetic retinal angiography. V. Retinal telangiectasis. VI. X-ray irradiation, carotid artery occlusion, collagen vascular disease, and vitritis, Arch Ophthalmol 80:535, 550, 569, 583, 592, 606, 1968.

249. Hayreh SS, Servais GE, and Virdi PS: Fundus lesions in malignant hypertension. IV. Focal intraretinal periarteriolar transudates, Ophthalmology 92:60, 1985.

250. Irinoda K, editor: Color atlas and criteria of fundus changes in hypertension, Philadelphia, 1970, JB Lippincott Co.

251. Keith N, Wagener H, and Barker N: Some different types of essential hypertension: their courses and prognosis, Am J Med Sci 197: 332, 1939.

252. Kennedy J and Wise G: Clinicopathological correlation of retinal lesions, Arch Ophthalmol 74:658, 1965.

253. Kishi S, Tso MOM, and Hayreh SS: Fundus lesions in malignant

hypertension. I. A pathologic study of experimental hypertensive choroidopathy, Arch Ophthalmol 103:1189, 1985.

254. Kishi S, Tso MOM, and Hayreh SS: Fundus lesions in malignant hypertension. II. A pathologic study of experimental hypertensive optic neuropathy, Arch Ophthalmol 103:1198, 1985.

255. Klein R and others: Hypertension and retinopathy, anteriolar narrowing, and arteriovenous nicking in a population, Arch Ophthalmol 112:92, 1994.

256. Klien B: Comments on the cotton-wool lesions of the retina, Am J Ophthalmol 59:17, 1965.

257. McLeod D and others: The role of axoplasmic transport in the pathogenesis of retinal cotton-wool spots, Br J Ophthalmol 61:177, 1977.

258. McLeod D and Kohner EM: Cotton-wool spots and giant cell arteritis, Ophthalmology 103:701, 1996 (letter).

259. Morse, P: Elschnig's spots and hypertensive choroidopathy, Am J Ophthalmol 66:844, 1968.

260. Scheie H: Evaluation of ophthalmoscopic changes of hypertension and arteriolar sclerosis, Arch Ophthalmol 49:117, 1953.

261. Schwartz B, editor: Perspective on ocular hypertension, Surv Ophthalmol 25:123, 1980 (special issue).

262. Topilow HW and others: Asteroid hyalosis. Biomicroscopy, ultrastructure, and composition, Arch Ophthalmol 100:964, 1982.

263. Tso MOM and Jampol LM: Pathophysiology of hypertensive retinopathy, Ophthalmology 89:1132, 1982.

264. Tso MOM and Woodford BJ: Effect of photic injury on the retinal tissues, Ophthalmology 90:952, 1983.

265. Velikay M and others: Retinal detachment with severe proliferative vitreoretinopathy in Terson's syndrome, Ophthalmology 101:35, 1994.

266. Wagener H and Keith N: Diffuse arteriolar disease with hypertension and the associated retinal lesions, Medicine 18:317, 1939.

267. Walsh FB, Hedges TR, Optic nerve sheath hemorrhage, Am J Ophthalmol 34:509, 1951.

268. Wallow IHL and others: Systemic hypertension produces pericyte changes in retinal capillaries, Invest Ophthalmol Vis Sci 34:420, 1993.

269. Weingeist TA and others: Terson's syndrome. Clinicopathologic correlation.

270. Wilkes SR, Mansour AM, and Green WR: Proliferative vitreoretinopatholy. Histopathology of retroretinal membranes, Retina 7:94, 1987.

271. Wolter J: Pathology of a cotton-wool spot, Am J Ophthalmol 48:473, 1959.

272. Wolter J and Liss L: The evolution of hyaline corpuscles (cytoid bodies) in the human optic nerve, Am J Ophthalmol 43:885, 1957.

273. Yamashita H and others: Glial cells in culture of preretinal membrane of proliferative vitreoretinopathy, Jpn J Ophthalmol 29:42, 1985.

274. Zarbin MA, Michels RG, and Green WR: Epiretinal membrane co-intracture associated with macular prolapse, Am J Ophthalmol 110:610, 1990.

Proliferative retinopathy (diabetic retinopathy, retinal arterial macroaneurysms, sickle retinopathy, Eales' disease)

275. Anderson D, Morin D, and Hunter W: Rubeosis iridis, Can J Ophthalmol 6:138, 1971.

276. Adamis AP and others: Inhibition of vascular endothelial growth factor prevents retinal ischemia-associated iris neovascularization in a nonhuman primate, Arch Ophthalmol 114:66, 1996.

277. Adamis AP and others: Increased vascular endothelial growth factor levels in the vitreous of eyes with proliferative diabetic retinopathy, Am J Ophthalmol 118:445, 1994.

278. Aiello LM, Wand M, and Liang G: Neovascular glaucoma and vitreous hemorrhage following cataract surgery inpatients with diabetes mellitus, Ophthalmology 90:814, 1983.

279. Alzaid AA and others: The role of growth hormone in the development of diabetic retinopathy, Diabetes Care 17:531, 1994.

280. Appen RE and others: Diabetic papillopathy, Am J Ophthalmol 90:203, 1980.

281. Apple DJ: Pathology. In L'Esperance FA Jr and James WA Jr, editors: Diabetic retinopathy: clinical evaluation and management, St Louis, 1981, The CV Mosby Co.

282. Archer DB: Intraretinal, preretinal, and subretinal new vessels, Trans Ophthalmol Soc UK 97:449, 1977.

283. Armaly M and Balogion P: Diabetes mellitus and the eye. I. Changes in the anterior segment, Arch Ophthalmol 77:485, 1967.

284. Asdourian G and others: Evolution of the retinal black sunburst in sickling haemoglobinopathies, Br J Ophthalmol 59:710, 1975.

285. Ashton N: Vascular changes in diabetes with particular reference to retinal vessels, Br J Ophthalmol 33:407, 1949.

286. Ashton N: Arteriolar involvement in diabetic retinopathy, Br J Ophthalmol 37:282, 1953.

287. Ashton N: Diabetic micro-angiopathy, Adv Ophthalmol 8:1, 1958.

288. Ashton N: Diabetic retinopathy: a new approach, Lancet 2:625, 1959.

289. Ashton N: Studies of retinal capillaries in relation to diabetic and other retinopathies, Br J Ophthalmol 47:521, 1963.

290. Ashton N: Vascular basement membrane changes in diabetic retinopathy, Br J Ophthalmol 58:344, 1974.

291. Azar DT and others: Decreased penetration of anchoring fibrils into the diabetic stroma, Arch Ophthalmol 107:1520, 1989.

292. Ballantyne A and Loewenstein A: The pathology of diabetic retinopathy, Trans Ophthalmol Soc UK 63:95, 1943.

293. Ballantyne A and Loewenstein A: Retinal microaneurysms and punctate haemorrhages, Br J Ophthalmol 28:593, 1944.

294. Barr CC, Glaser JS, and Blankenship G: Acute disc swelling in juvenile diabetes. Clinical profile and natural history of 12 cases, Arch Ophthalmol 98:2185, 1980.

295. Baudouin C and others: Immunohistopathologic findings in proliferative diabetic retinopathy, Am J Ophthalmol 105:383, 1988.

296. Baudouin C and others: Class II antigen expression in diabetic preretinal membranes, Am J Ophthalmol 109:70, 1990.

297. Bloodworth J Jr: Diabetic microangiopathy, Diabetes 12:99, 1963.

298. Boase DL: Sickle cell retinopathy: is there a case for treatment? Trans Ophthalmol Soc UK 96:220, 1976.

299. Bresnick GH: Diabetic macular edema: a review, Ophthalmology 93:989, 1986.

300. Bresnick GH, Haight B, and de Venecia G: Retinal wrinkling and macular heterotopia in diabetic retinopathy, Arch Ophthalmol 97:1890, 1979.

301. Bresnick GH, Smith V, and Pokorny J: Visual function abnormalities in macular heterotopia caused by proliferative diabetic retinopathy, Am J Ophthalmol 92:83, 1981.

302. Bresnick GH and others: Clinicopathologic correlations in diabetic retinopathy, Arch Ophthalmol 95:1215, 1977.

303. Brooks PC, Clark RAF, and Cheresh DA: Requirement of vascular integrin for angiogenesis, Science 264:569, 1994.

304. Brotherman DP: Diabetic retinopathy: a perspective, Surv Ophthalmol 16:359, 1972.

305. Brown C and Burman D: Transient cataracts in a diabetic child with hyperosmolar coma, Br J Ophthalmol 57:429, 1973.

306. Brown GC, MaGargal LE, and Federman JL: Ischaemia and neovascularization, Trans Ophthalmol Soc UK 100:377, 1980.

307. Caird F, Pirie M, and Ramsell T: Diabetes and the eye, Oxford, England, 1969, Blackwell Scientific Publications, Ltd.

308. Cogan D, Toussaint D, and Kuwabara T: Retinal vascular patterns. IV. Diabetic retinopathy, Arch Ophthalmol 66:366, 1961.

309. Condon PI, Hayes RJ, and Serjeant GR: Retinal and choroidal neovascularization in sickle cell disease, Trans Ophthalmol Soc UK 100:434, 1980.

310. Coppeto J and Lessell S: Retinopathy in systemic lupus erythematosus, Arch Ophthalmol 95:794, 1977.

311. Cotter PB Jr and Weiter JJ: Retinopathy in a patient with systemic lupus erythematosus, Ann Ophthalmol 14:470, 1982.

312. Cunha-Vaz JG: Pathophysiology of diabetic retinopathy, Br J Ophthalmol 62:351, 1978.

313. Cunliffe IA and others: Extracapsular cataract surgery with lens implantation in diabetics with and without proliferative retinopathy, Br J Ophthalmol 75:9, 1991.

314. de Venecia G, Davis M, and Engerman R: Clinicopathologic correlations in diabetic retinopathy, Arch Ophthalmol 94:1766, 1976.

315. Dizon RV and others: Choroidal occlusive disease in sickle cell hemoglobinopathies, Surv Ophthalmol 23:297, 1979.

316. Ederer F and Hiller R: Clinical trials, diabetic retinopathy and photocoagulation: a reanalysis of five studies, Surv Ophthalmol 19:267, 1975.

317. Ederer F, Hiller R, and Taylor HR: Senile lens changes and diabetes in two population studies, Am J Ophthalmol 91:381, 1981.

318. Engerman RL: Pathogenesis of diabetic retinopathy, Diabetes 38: 1203, 1989.

319. English FP and Harrison M: Diabetic retinopathy following lipid disease of the capillary endothelium, Arch Ophthalmol 114:106, 1996 (letter).

320. Federman JL and others: Experimental ocular angiogenesis, Am J Ophthalmol 89:231, 1980.

321. Ffytche TJ: Retinal vasculitis: a review of the clinical signs, Trans Ophthalmol Soc UK 97:457, 1977.

322. Fichte C, Streeten BW, and Friedman AH: A histopathologic study of retinal arterial aneurysms, Am J Ophthalmol 85:509, 1978.

323. Fine B, Berkow J, and Helfgott J: Diabetic lacy vacuolation of iris pigment epithelium, Am J Ophthalmol 69:197, 1970.

324. Fisher RF: Factors which influence the thickness of basement membrane in diabetes: evidence of humoral control, Trans Ophthalmol Soc UK 99:10, 1979.

325. Fisher RF: Comparison of the size of pericytes of the retinal capillaries in the normal and diabetic state, Trans Ophthalmol Soc UK 100:90, 1980.

326. Flaxel CJ and others: Partial laser ablation of massive peripapillary subretinal neovascularization, Ophthalmology 103:1250, 1996.

327. Foos RY and others: Posterior vitreous detachment in diabetic subjects, Ophthalmology 87:122, 1980.

328. Foos RY, Kreiger AE, and Nofsinger K: Pathologic study following vitrectomy for proliferative diabetic retinopathy, Retina 5:101, 1985.

329. Forrester JV, Grierson I, and Lee WR: The pathology of vitreous hemorrhage. II. Ultrastructure, Arch Ophthalmol 97:2368, 1979.

330. Forrester JV, Lee WR, and Williamson J: The pathology of vitreous hemorrhage. I. Gross and histological appearances, Arch Ophthalmol 96:703, 1978.

331. Frank RN and Cronin MA: Posterior pole neovascularization in a patient with hemoglobin SC disease, Am J Ophthalmol 88:680, 1979.

332. Frank RN: On the pathogenesis of diabetic retinopathy. A 1990 update, Ophthalmology 98:586, 1991.

333. Frieberg TR and others: The effect of long-term near normal glycemic control on mild diabetic retinopathy, Ophthalmology 92: 1051, 1985.

334. Friedman EA and L'Esperance FA Jr: Diabetic renal-retinal syndrome, New York, 1980, Grune & Stratton, Inc.

335. Fryczkowski AW, Sato SE, and Hodes BL: Changes in the diabetic choroidal vasculature: scanning electron microscopy findings, Ann Ophthalmol 20:299, 1988.

336. Galinos SO and others: Spontaneous remodeling of the peripheral retinal vasculature in sickling disorders, Am J Ophthalmol 79:853, 1975.

337. Galinos SO and others: Multifocal Best's disease and sickle cell trait, Ann Ophthalmol 13:1181, 1981.

338. Gagliano DA and Goldberg MF: The evolution of salmon-patch hemorrhages in sickle cell retinopathy, Arch Ophthalmol 107:1814, 1989.

339. Garner A: Pathology of diabetic retinopathy, Br Med Bull 26:137, 1970.

340. Gartner S and Henkind P: Neovascularization of the iris (rubeosis iridis), Surv Ophthalmol 22:291, 1978.

341. Gass JDM: A fluorescein angiographic study of macular dysfunction secondary to retinal vascular disease. IV. Diabetic retinal angiopathy, Arch Ophthalmol 80:583, 1968.

342. Gass JD and Braunstein R: Sessile and exophytic capillary angiomas of the juxtapapillary retina and optic nerve head, Arch Ophthalmol 98:1790, 1980.

343. Goldbaum M and others: Proliferative sickle retinopathy. In L'Esperance FA Jr, editor: Current diagnosis and management of chorioretinal diseases, St Louis, 1977, The CV Mosby Co.

344. Goldberg M: Classification and pathogenesis of proliferative sickle retinopathy, Am J Ophthalmol 71:649, 1971.

345. Goldberg M: Natural history of untreated proliferative sickle retinopathy, Arch Ophthalmol 85:428, 1971.

346. Goldberg M and Acacio I: Argon laser photocoagulation of proliferative sickle retinopathy, Arch Ophthalmol 90:35, 1973.

347. Goldberg M and Fine S: Symposium on the treatment of diabetic retinopathy, Airlie, 1968, US Public Health Service Pub No 1890. Washington DC, 1969, US Government Printing Office.

348. Goldberg MF, Charache S, and Acacio I: Ophthalmologic manifestations of sickle cell thalassemia, Arch Intern Med 128:33, 1971.

349. Goldberg MF and Tso MOM: Rubeosis iridis and glaucoma associated with sickle cell retinopathy: a light and electron microscopic study, Ophthalmology 85:1028, 1978.

350. Goldstein DE and others: Glycemic control and development of retinopathy in youth-onset insulin-dependent diabetes mellitus, Ophthalmology 100:1125, 1993.

351. Guyer DR, D'Amico DJ, and Smith CW: Subretinal fibrosis after laser photocoagulation for diabetic macular edema, Am J Ophthalmol 113:652, 1992.

352. Han DP and others: Vitrectomy for proliferative diabetic retinopathy with severe equatorial fibrovascular proliferation, Am J Ophthalmol 119(5):563, 1995.

353. Hanneken A and others: Altered distribution of basic fibroblast growth factor in diabetic retinopathy, Arch Ophthalmol 109:1005, 1991.

354. Henkind P: Ocular neovascularization, Am J Ophthalmol 85:287, 1978.

355. Hersh PS, Green WR, and Thomas JV: Tractional venous loops in diabetic retinopathy, Am J Ophthalmol 92:661, 1981.

356. Hidayatt AA and Fine BS: Diabetic choroidopathy. Light and electron microscopic observations of seven cases, Ophthalmology 92: 512, 1985.

357. Hutton W and others: Retinal microangiopathy without associated glucose intolerance, Trans Am Acad Ophthalmol Otolaryngol 76: 968, 1972.

358. Hyndiuk RA and others: Neurotrophic corneal ulcers in diabetes lipemia retinalis, Arch Ophthalmol 89:120, 1973.

359. Ishida NR and others: Corneal nerve alterations in diabetes mellitus, Arch Ophthalmol 102:1380, 1984.

360. Jaffe GJ and Burton TC: Progression of nonproliferative diabetic retinopathy following cataract extraction, Arch Ophthalmol 106: 745, 1988.

361. Jaffe GJ and others: Progression of nonproliferative diabetic retinopathy and visual outcome after extracapsular cataract extraction and intraocular lens implantation, Am J Ophthalmol 114:448, 1992.

362. Jampol LM and Goldbaum MH: Peripheral proliferative retinopathies, Surv Ophthalmol 25:1, 1980.

363. Jampol LM and others: A randomized clinical trial of feeder vessel coagulation of proliferative sickle cell retinopathy. I. Preliminary results, Ophthalmology 90:540, 1983.

364. Jampol LM and others: Calcification of Bruch's membrane in angioid streaks with homozygous sickle cell disease, Arch Ophthalmol 105:93, 1987.

365. Jampol LM and others: Salmon-patch hemorrhages after central retinal artery occlusion in sickle cell disease, Arch Ophthalmol 99: 237, 1981.

366. Jampol LM, Ebroon DA, and Goldbaum MH: Peripheral proliferative retinopathies: an update on angiogenesis, etiologies and management, Surv Ophthalmol 38:519, 1994 (review).

367. Jampol LM, Wong AS, and Albert DM: Atrial myxoma and central retinal artery occlusion, Am J Ophthalmol 75:242, 1973.

368. Jerdan JA, Michels RG, and Glaser BM: Diabetic preretinal membranes. An immunohistochemical study, Arch Ophthalmol 104: 286, 1986.

369. Jerneld B and Algvere P: Relationship of duration and onset of diabetes to prevalence of diabetic retinopathy, Am J Ophthalmol 102:431, 1986.

370. John T, Sassani JW, and Eagle RC Jr: The myofibroblastic component of rubeosis iridis, Ophthalmology 90:721, 1983.

371. John T, Sassani JW, and Eagle RC: Scanning electron microscopy of rubeosis iridis, Trans Pa Acad Ophthalmol Otolaryngol 35:119, 1982.

372. Joondeph BC, Joondeph HC, and Flood TP: Foveal neovascularization in diabetic retinopathy, Arch Ophthalmol 105:1672, 1987.

373. Kador PF and others: Prevention of retinal vessel changes associated with diabetic retinopathy in galactose-fed dogs by aldose reductase inhibitors, Arch Ophthalmol 108:1301, 1990.

374. Kahn H and Hiller R: Blindness caused by diabetic retinopathy, Am J Ophthalmol 78:58, 1974.

375. Keoleian GM and others: Structural and functional studies of the corneal ulcers in diabetes mellitus, Arch Ophthalmol 95:2193, 1977.

376. Kern TS and Engerman RL: A mouse model of diabetic retinopathy, Arch Ophthalmol 114:986, 1996.

377. Kimmel AS and others: Diabetic retinopathy under age 20. A review of 71 cases, Ophthalmology 92:1047, 1985.

378. Kincaid MC and others: An ocular clinicopathologic correlative study of six patients from the diabetic retinopathy study, Retina 3: 218, 1983.

379. Kingsley and others: Severe diabetic retinopathy in adolescents, Br J Ophthalmol 67:73, 1983.

380. Kinoshita JH: Aldose reductase in the diabetic eye, 43rd Edward Jackson Memorial Lecture, Am J Ophthalmol 102:685, 1986.

381. Klein BEK, Klein R, and Moss SE: Prevalence of cataract in a population-based study of persons with diabetes mellitus, Ophthalmology 91:1101, 1985.

382. Klein R, Klein BEK, and Moss SE: Visual impairment in diabetes, Ophthalmology 91:1, 1984.

383. Klein R, Klein BEK, and Moss SE: The Wisconsin epidemiologic study of diabetic retinopathy. III. Prevalence and risk of diabetic retinopathy when age at diagnosis is 30 or more years, Arch Ophthalmol 102:527, 1984.

384. Klein R and others: The Wisconsin epidemiologic study of diabetic retinopathy. IV. Diabetic macular edema, Ophthalmology 91:1464, 1984.

386. Klein R and others: Glycosylated hemoglobin predicts the incidence and progression of diabetic retinopathy, JAMA 260:2864, 1988.

386. Klein R and others: The Wisconsin epidemiologic study of diabetic retinopathy. IX. Four-year incidence and progression of diabetic retinopathy when age at diagnosis is less than 30 years, Arch Ophthalmol 107:237, 1989.

387. Klein R and others: Wisconsin epidemiologic study of diabetic retinopathy. XII. Relationship of C-peptide and diabetic retinopathy, Diabetes 39:1145, 1990.

388. Klein R and others: The Wisconsin epidemiologic study of diabetic retinopathy. XIV. Ten-year incidence and progression of diabetic retinopathy, Arch Ophthalmol 112:1217, 1994.

389. Klein R and others: Retinal microaneurysm counts and 10-year progression of diabetic retinopathy, Arch Ophthalmol 113:1386, 1995.

390. Klein R and others: Incidence of retinopathy and associated risk factors from time of diagnosis of insulin-dependent diabetes, Arch Ophthalmol 115:391, 1994.

391. Klein R and others: The relationship of retinal microaneurysm counts to the 4-year progression of diabetic retinopathy, Arch Ophthalmol 107:1780, 1989.

392. Koerner F, Schlegel D, and Koerner U: Diabetic retinopathy study: preliminary results from 215 patients treated uniocularly with photocoagulation, Graefes Arch Clin Exp Ophthalmol 200:99, 1976.

393. Kohner EM and Porta M: Vascular abnormalities in diabetes and their treatment, Trans Ophthalmol Soc UK 100:440, 1980.

394. Kushner MS, Jampol LM, and Haller JA: Cavernous hemangioma of the optic nerve, Retina 14:359, 1994.

395. Laatikainen L: Development and classification of rubeosis iridis in diabetic eye disease, Br J Ophthalmol 63:150, 1979.

396. Larsen H: Diabetic retinopathy, Acta Ophthalmol 38:(suppl 60), 1960.

397. Lass JH and others: A morphologic and fluorophotometric analysis of the corneal endothelium in type I diabetes mellitus and cystic fibrosis, Am J Ophthalmol 100:783, 1985.

398. Lee VS and others: The diagnosis of diabetic retinopathy, Ophthalmology 100:1504, 1993.

399. Leginger TG, Goldmana KN, and Saenger P: Bilateral cataracts as the initial sign of insulin-dependent diabetes mellitus in a child, Am J Dis Child 137:602, 1983.

400. Lewis H, Abrams GW, and Foos RY: Clinicopathologic findings in anterior hyaloidal fibrovascular proliferation after diabetic vitrectomy, Am J Ophthalmol 104:614, 1987.

401. Leys AM and Bonnet S: Case report: Associated retinal neovascularization and choroidal hemangioma, Retina 13:22, 1993.

402. Liang JC and Jampol LM: Spontaneous peripheral chorioretinal neovascularization in association with sickle cell anemia, Br J Ophthalmol 67:107, 1983.

403. Lincoff H and others: Tractional elevations of the retina in-patients with diabetes, Am J Ophthalmol 113:235, 1992.

404. Lister J: The clinical syndrome of diabetes mellitus, London, 1959, HK Lewis & Co, Ltd.

405. Luxenberg M and Sime D: Relationship of asteroid hyalosis to diabetes mellitus and plasma lipid levels, Am J Ophthalmol 67: 406, 1969.

406. Madigan J Jr and others: Peripheral retinal neovascularization in sarcoidosis and sickle cell anemia Am J Ophthalmol 83:387, 1977.

407. Madsen P: Rubeosis of the iris and hemorrhagic glaucoma inpatients with proliferative diabetic retinopathy, Br J Ophthalmol 55: 368, 1971.

408. Madson CE Jr and Chester EM: The pathogenesis of the cotton-wool spot in diabetic retinopathy, Doc Ophthalmol 37:217, 1974.

409. Malinowski SM, Pulido JS, and Flickinger RR: The protective effect of the tilted disc syndrome in diabetic retinopathy, Arch Ophthalmol 114:230, 1996.

410. Mansour AM and others: Foveal avascular zone in diabetes mellitus, Retina 13:125, 1993.

411. Mapstone R and Clark CV: Prevalence of diabetes in glaucoma, Br Med J 291:93, 1985.

412. Marshall G and others: Factors influencing the onset and progression of diabetic retinopathy in subjects with insulin-dependent diabetes mellitus, Ophthalmology 100:1133, 1993.

413. McLeod DS, Goldberg MF, and Lutty GA: Dual-perspective analysis of vascular formation in sickle cell retinopathy, Arch Ophthalmol 111:1234, 1993.

414. Merritt JC, Risco JM, and Pantell JP: Bilateral macular infarction in S S disease, J Pediatr Ophthalmol Strabismus 19:275, 1982.

415. Messmer E and others: Nine cases of cavernous hemangioma of the retina, Am J Ophthalmol 95:383, 1983.

416. Miller H and others: Diabetic neovascularization: permeability and ultrastructural, Invest Ophthalmol Vis Sci 25:1338, 1984.

417. Miller JW and others: Phthalocyanine photodynamic therapy of experimental iris neovascularization, Ophthalmology 98:1711, 1991.

418. Miller JW, Stinson WG, and Folkman J: Regression of experimental iris neovascularization with systemic alpha-interferon, Ophthalmology 100:9, 1993.

419. Miyamoto K and others: Evaluation of retinal microcirculatory alterations in the goto-kakizaki rat. A spontaneous model of non-insulin-dependent diabetes, Invest Ophthalmol Vis Sci 37:898, 1996.

420. Moloney JBM and Drury MI: The effect of pregnancy on the natural course of diabetic retinopathy, Am J Ophthalmol 93:745, 1982.

421. Moss SE, Klein R, and Klein BEK: Ten-year incidence of visual loss in a diabetic population, Ophthalmology 101:1061, 1994.

422. Moss SE and others: The association of iris color with eye disease in diabetes, Ophthalmology 94:1226, 1987.

423. Muraoka K and Shimizu K: Intraretinal neovascularization in diabetic retinopathy, Ophthalmology 91:1440, 1984.

424. Nagpal KC, Goldberg MF, and Rabb MF: Ocular manifestations of sickle hemoglobinopathies, Surv Ophthalmol 21:391, 1977.

425. Nagpal KC and others: Angioid streaks and sickle hemoglobinopathies, Br J Ophthalmol 60:31, 1976.

426. Nasrallah FP and others: The role of the vitreous in diabetic macular edema, Ophthalmology 95:1335, 1988.

427. Niki T, Muraoka K, and Shimizu K: Distribution of capillary nonperfusion in early-stage diabetic retinopathy, Ophthalmology 91: 1431, 1984.

428. Nork TM and others: Mueller's cell involvement in proliferative diabetic retinopathy, Arch Ophthalmol 105:1424, 1987.

429. Ober RR and Michels RG: Optic disk neovascularization in hemoglobin SC disease, Am J Ophthalmol 85:711, 1978.

430. Ohrt V: The frequency of rubeosis iridis in diabetic patients, Acta Ophthalmol 49:301, 1971.

431. Okun E, Johnston G, and Boniuk I: Management of diabetic retinopathy: a stereoscopic presentation, St Louis, 1971, The CV Mosby Co.

432. Palestine AG, Robertson DM, and Goldstein BG: Macroaneurysms of the retinal arteries, Am J Ophthalmol 93:164, 1982.

433. Patz A: Clinical and experimental studies on retinal neovascularization: 39th Edward Jackson Memorial Lecture, Am J Ophthalmol 94:715, 1982.

434. Pavan and others: Diabetic rubeosis and panretinal photocoagulation: a prospective controlled, masked trial using iris fluorescein angiography, Arch Ophthalmol 101:882, 1983.

435. Pavan PR and others: Optic disc edema in juvenile-onset diabetes, Arch Ophthalmol 98:2193, 1980.

436. Peachey NMS, Gagliano DA, and Jacobson MS: Correlation of electroretinographic findings and peripheral retinal nonperfusion inpatients with sickle cell retinopathy, Arch Ophthalmol 108:110, 1990.

437. Rabb MF, Gagliano DA, and Teske MP: Retinal arterial macroaneurysms, Surv Ophthalmol 33:73, 1988.

438. Raichand M and others: Evolution of neovascularization in sickle cell retinopathy, Arch Ophthalmol 95:1543, 1977.

439. Regillo CD and others: Diabetic papillopathy. Patient characteristics and fundus findings, Arch Ophthalmol 113:889, 1995.

440. Rodrigues MM and Currier CA: Histopathology of argon laser photocoagulation in juvenile diabetic retinopathy, Ophthalmology 90: 1023, 1983.

441. Romayananda N, Goldberg MF, and Green WR: Histopathology of sickle cell retinopathy, Trans Am Acad Ophthalmol Otolaryngol 77:652, 1973.

442. Rothova A and others: Uveitis and diabetes mellitus, Am J Ophthalmol 106:17, 1988.

443. Schatz H and Patz A: Cystoid maculopathy in diabetics, Arch Ophthalmol 94:761, 1976.

444. Schröder S, Palinski W, and Schmid-Schönbein GW: Activated monocytes and granulocytes, capillary nonperfusion, and neovascularization in diabetic retinopathy, Am J Pathol 139:81, 1991.

445. Schultz RO and others: Diabetic keratopathy, Trans Am Ophthalmol Soc 74:180, 1981.

446. Schultz RO and others: Corneal endothelial changes in type I and type II diabetes mellitus, Am J Ophthalmol 98:401, 1984.

447. Schulze R: Rubeosis iridis, Am J Ophthalmol 63:487, 1967.

448. Sebag J and McMeel JW: Diabetic retinopathy: pathogenesis and the role of retina-derived growth factor in angiogenesis, Surv Ophthalmol 30:377, 1986.

449. Shetlar DJ, Bourne WM, and Campbell RJ: Morphologic evaluation of Descemet's membrane and corneal endothelium in diabetes mellitus, Ophthalmology 96:247, 1989.

450. Shields CL and others: Vasoproliferative tumors of the ocular fundus. Classification and clinical manifestations in 103 patients, Arch Ophthalmol 113:615, 1995.

451. Shorb SR: Anemia and diabetic retinopathy, Am J Ophthalmol 100: 434, 1985.

452. Sigelman J: Diabetic macular edema in juvenile and adult-onset diabetes, Am J Ophthalmol 90:287, 1980.

453. Sinclair SH: Macular retinal capillary hemodynamics in diabetic patients, Ophthalmology 98:1580, 1991.

454. Sinclair SH and others: Macular edema and pregnancy in insulin-dependent diabetes, Am J Ophthalmol 97:154, 1984.

455. Skalka HW and Prchal JT: The effect of diabetes mellitus and diabetic therapy on cataract formation, Ophthalmology 88:117, 1981.

456. Smith M and Glickman P: Diabetic vacuolation of the iris pigment epithelium, Am J Ophthalmol 79:875, 1975.

457. Stevens TS: Diabetic maculopathies, Int Ophthalmol Clin 21(3): 11, 1981.

458. Sussman EJ, Tsiaras WG, and Soper KA: Diagnosis of diabetic eye disease, JAMA 247:3231, 1982.

459. Tachi N and Ogino N: Vitrectomy for diffuse macular edema in cases of diabetic retinopathy, Am J Ophthalmol 122:258, 1996.

460. Taylor HR and Kimsey RA: Corneal epithelial basement membrane changes in diabetes, Invest Ophthalmol 20:548, 1981.

461. Tolentino MJ and others: Vascular endothelial growth factor is sufficient to produce iris neovascularization and neovascular glaucoma in a nonhuman primate, Arch Ophthalmol 114:964, 1996.

462. Toussaint D and Dustin P: Electron microscopy of normal and diabetic retinal capillaries, Arch Ophthalmol 70:96, 1963.

463. Tso MOM and others: Clinicopathologic study of blood retinal barrier in experimental diabetes mellitus, Arch Ophthalmol 98: 2032, 1980.

464. Urrets-Zavalia A: Diabetic retinopathy, Paris, 1977, Masson & Cie, Editeurs.

465. Vander JF, Brown GC, and Benson WE: Iris neovascularization after central retinal artery obstruction despite previous panretinal photocoagulation for diabetic retinopathy, Am J Ophthalmol 109: 464, 1990.

466. Vinding T and Nielsen NV: Two cases of acutely developed cataract in diabetes mellitus, Acta Ophthalmol 62:373, 1984.

467. Vine AK: Severe periphlebitis, peripheral retinal ischemia, and preretinal neovascularization in-patients with multiple sclerosis, Am J Ophthalmol 113:28, 1992.

468. Vinores SA and others: Immunohistochemic localization of blood-retinal barrier breaking down in human diabetes, Am J Pathol 134: 231, 1989.

469. Wallow I and others: Chorioretinal and choriovitreal neovascularization after photocoagulation for proliferative diabetic retinopathy: a clinicopathologic correlation, Ophthalmology 92:523, 1985.

470. Wautier JO and others: Increased adhesion of erythrocytes to cells in diabetes mellitus and its relation to vascular complication, N Engl J Med 305:237, 1981.

471. Wessing A and Meyer-Schwickerath G: Fluorescein studies in Eales' disease and related lesions of the retina. In Proceedings of the International Symposium on Fluorescein Angiography, Albi, 1971, Basel, 1971, S Karger, AC.

472. West RH and Barnett AJ: Ocular involvement in scleroderma Br J Ophthalmol 63:845, 1979.

473. Williams JM Sr, de Juan E Jr, and Machemer R: Ultrastructural characteristics of new vessels in proliferative diabetic retinopathy, Am J Ophthalmol 105:491, 1988.

474. Yamashita T and Becker B: The basement membrane in the human diabetic eye, Diabetes 10:167, 1961.

475. Yanoff M: Diabetic retinopathy. N Engl J Med 174:1344, 1966.

476. Yanoff M: Ocular pathology of diabetes, Am J Ophthalmol 67:21, 1969.

477. Yassur Y and others: Optic disc neovascularization in diabetic retinopathy. I. A system for grading proliferation at the optic nerve head in patients with proliferative diabetic retinopathy. Br J Ophthalmol 61:69, 1980.

478. Yassur Y and others: Optic disc neovascularization in diabetic retinopathy. II, Natural history and results of photocoagulation treatment, Br J Ophthalmol 64:77, 1980.

Retinal vascular occlusions

479. Anderson B Jr: Activity and diabetic vitreous hemorrhages, Ophthalmology 87:173, 1980.

480. Appen R, Wray S, and Cogan D: Central retinal artery occlusion, Am J Ophthalmol 79:374, 1975.

481. Archer D, Ernest J, and Newell F: Classification of branch retinal vein obstruction, Trans Am Acad Ophthalmol Otolaryngol 78:148, 1974.

482. Arruga J and Sanders MD: Ophthalmologic findings in 70 patients with evidence of retinal embolism, Ophthalmology 89:1336, 1982.

483. Behrman S: Retinal vein obstruction, Br J Ophthalmol 46:336, 1962.

484. Bowers DK and others: Branch retinal vein occlusion. A clinicopathologic case report, Retina 7:252, 1987.

485. Brazitikos PD and others: Erbium: YAG laser surgery of the vitreous and retina, Ophthalmology 102:278, 1995.

486. Brown GC: Isolated central retinal artery obstruction in association with ocular neovascularization, Am J Ophthalmol 96:110, 1983.

487. Brown GC, Shields JA: Cilioretinal arteries and retinal arterial occlusion, Arch Ophthalmol 97:84, 1979.

488. Brown GC and others: Preretinal arterial loops and retinal arterial occlusion, Am J Ophthalmol 87:6, 1979.

489. Brown GC and others: Arterial obstruction and ocular neovascularization, Ophthalmology 89:139, 1982.

490. Brownstein S, Font RL, and Alper MG: Atheromatous plaques of the retinal blood vessels, Arch Ophthalmol 90:49, 1973.

491. Caltrider ND and others: Retinal emboli inpatients with mitral valve prolapse, Am J Ophthalmol 90:534, 1980.

492. Carr JM, McKinney M, and McDonagh J: Diagnosis of disseminated intravascular coagulation, Am J Clin Pathol 91:280, 1989.

493. Castanon C and others: Ocular vaso-occlusive disease in primary antiphospholipid syndrome, Ophthalmology 102:256, 1995.

494. Chan C and Little HL: Infrequency of retinal neovascularization following central retinal vein occlusion, Ophthalmology 86:256, 1979.

495. Clemett R, Kohmer E, and Hamilton A: The visual prognosis in retinal branch vein occlusion, Trans Ophthalmol Soc UK 93:523, 1973.

496. Cogan D and Wray S: Vascular occlusions in the eye from cardiac myxomas, Am J Ophthalmol 80:396, 1975.

497. Cohen SM, Davis JL, and Gass JDM: Branch retinal arterial occlusions in multifocal retinitis with optic nerve edema, Arch Ophthalmol 113:1271, 1995.

498. Cousins SW, Flynn HW, and Clarkson JG: Macroaneurysms associated with retinal branch vein occlusion, Am J Ophthalmol 109:567, 1990.

499. Dahrling B: Histopathology of early central retinal artery occlusion, Arch Ophthalmol 73:506, 1965.

500. Dodson PM and others: β-thromboglobulin and platelet factor 4 levels in retinal vein occlusion, Br J Ophthalmol 67:143, 1983.

501. Dougal MA and others: Central retinal artery occlusion in systemic lupus erythematosus, Ann Ophthalmol 15:38, 1983.

502. Dryden R: Central retinal vein occlusion and chronic simple glaucoma, Arch Ophthalmol 73:659, 1965.

503. Duane TD, Osher RH, and Green WR: White-centered hemorrhages: their significance, Ophthalmology 87:66, 1980.

504. Duker JS, Magargat LE, and Stubbs GW: Quadrantic venous-stasis retinopathy secondary to an embolic branch retinal artery obstruction, Ophthalmology 97:167, 1990.

505. Ernest JT: Blood flow in normal and abnormal retinal vessels, Trans Ophthalmol Soc UK 100:3, 1980.

506. Finkelstein D and others: Branch vein occlusion: retinal neovascularization outside the involved segment, Ophthalmology 89:1357, 1982.

507. Fong ACO and Schatz H: Central retinal vein occlusion in young adults, Surv Ophthalmol 37:393, 1993.

508. Frangieh GT and others: Histopathologic study of nine branch vein occlusions, Arch Ophthalmol 100:1132, 1982.

509. Gass JDM: A fluorescein angiographic study of macular dysfunction secondary to retinal vascular disease. I. Embolic retinal artery obstruction, Arch Ophthalmol 80:535, 1968.

510. Gass JDM: A fluorescein angiographic study of macular dysfunction secondary to retinal vascular disease. II. Retinal vein obstruction, Arch Ophthalmol 80:550, 1968.

511. Gass JDM and Parrish R: Outer retinal ischemic infarction—a newly recognized complication of cataract extraction and closed vitrectomy. I. A case report, Ophthalmology 89:1467, 1982.

512. Green WR and others: Central retinal vein occlusion: a prospective histopathologic study of 29 eyes in 28 cases, Retina 1:27, 1981.

513. Gutman FA: Evaluation of a patient with central retinal vein occlusion, Ophthalmology 90:481, 1983.

514. Gutman FA and Zegarra II: The natural course of temporal-retinal branch occlusion, Trans Am Acad Ophthalmol Otolaryngol 78:178, 1974.

515. Hayreh SS: Occlusion of the central retinal vessels, Br J Ophthalmol 49:626, 1965.

516. Hayreh SS: Pathogenesis of occlusion of the central retinal vessels, Am J Ophthalmol 72:998, 1971.

517. Hayreh SS: So-called "central retinal vein occlusion." I. Pathogenesis, terminology, clinical features, Ophthalmologica 172:1, 1976.

518. Hayreh SS: So-called "central retinal vein occlusion." II. Venous stasis retinopathy, Ophthalmologica 172:14, 1976.

519. Hayreh SS: Classification of central retinal vein occlusion, Ophthalmology 90:458, 1983.

520. Hayreh SS and Hayreh MS: Hemi-central retinal vein occlusion: pathogenesis, clinical features, and natural history, Arch Ophthalmol 98:1600, 1980.

521. Hayreh SS, Van Heuven WAJ, and Hayreh MS: Experimental retinal vascular occlusion. I. Pathogenesis of central retinal vein occlusion, Arch Ophthalmol 96:311, 1978.

522. Hayreh SS and Weingeist TA: Experimental occlusion of the central artery of the retina. I. Ophthalmoscopic and fluorescein fundus angiographic studies, Br J Ophthalmol 64:896, 1980.

523. Hayreh SS and Weingeist TA: Experimental occlusion of the central artery of the retina. IV. Retinal tolerance time to acute ischaemia, Br J Ophthalmol 64:818, 1980.

524. Hayreh SS and others: Ocular neovascularization with retinal vascular occlusion. III. Incidence of ocular neovascularization with retinal vein occlusion, Ophthalmology 90:488, 1983.

525. Hayreh SS, Zimmerman MB, and Podhajsky P: Incidence of various types of retinal vein occlusion and their recurrence and demographic characteristics, Am J Ophthalmol 117:429, 1994.

526. Hockley DJ, Tripathi RC, and Ashton N: Experimental retinal branch vein occlusion in the monkey: histopathological and ultrastructural studies, Trans Ophthalmol Soc UK 96:202, 1976.

527. Hockley DJ, Tripathi RC, and Ashton N: Experimental retinal branch vein occlusion in rhesus monkeys. III. Histopathological and electron microscopical studies, Br J Ophthalmol 63:393, 1979.

528. Irazazabal FJ, Suarez LC, and Domingo EO: Hemispheric retinal branch vein occlusion, Ophthalmologica 193:14, 1986.

529. Irvine AR, Shorb SR, and Morris BW: Optociliary veins. Trans AM Acad Ophthalmol Otolaryngol 83:541, 1977.

530. Jacobson DM: Systemic cholesterol microembolization syndrome masquerading as giant cell arteritis, Surv Ophthalmol 35:23, 1991.

531. Jampol LM: Arteriolar occlusive diseases of the macula, Ophthalmology 90:534, 1983.

532. Jampol LM and Rabb MF: Vasocclusive diseases of the posterior pole, Int Ophthalmol Clin 21(3):201, 1981.

533. Jampol LM, Wong A, and Albert D: Atrial myxoma and central retinal artery occlusion, Am J Ophthalmol 75:242, 1973.

534. Joffe, L and others: Macular branch vein occlusion, Ophthalmology 87:91, 1980.

535. Käfter O: Die Macula lutea beim Zentralarterienverschluss. Klin, Monatsbl Augenheilkd 164:773, 1974.

536. Kahn M and others: Ocular features of carotid occlusive disease, Retina 6:239, 1986.

537. Kahn M, Knox DL, and Green WR: Clinicopathologic studies of a case of aortic arch syndrome, Retina 6:228, 1986.

538. Kearns TP, Younge BR, and Piepgras DG: Resolution of venous stasis retinopathy after carotid artery bypass surgery, Mayo Clin Proc 55:342, 1980.

539. Kearns TP: Differential diagnosis of central retinal vein obstruction, Ophthalmology 90:475, 1983.

540. Khawly JA and Pollock SC: Litten's sign (Roth's spots) in bacterial endocarditis, Arch Ophthalmol 112:683, 1994.

541. Kohner, EM: pathophysiology of retinal vein occlusion, Tran Ophthalmol Soc UK 96:189, 1976.

542. Kohner EM, Laatikainen L, and Oughton J: The management of central retinal vein occlusion, Ophthalmology 90:484, 1983.

543. Knox DL: Ocular aspects of cervical vascular disease, Surv Ophthalmol 13:245, 1969.

544. Kushner MS, Jampol LM, and Haller JA: Cavernous hemangioma of the optic nerve, Retina 14:359, 1994.

545. Laatikainen L: Vascular changes after central retinal vein occlusion, Trans Ophthalmol 96:190, 1976.

546. Laatikainen L and Blach RK: Behavior of the iris vasculature in central retinal vein occlusion: a fluorescein augiographic study of the vascular response of the retina and the iris, Br J Ophthalmol 61:272, 1977.

547. Lang GE and Lang GK: Ocular manifestations of carotid artery disease, Current Opinion in Ophthalmology 1:167, 1990.

548. Mansour AM and others: Foveal avascular zone in diabetes mellitus, Retina 13:125, 1993.

549. McCluskey PJ, Wakefield D: Ocular involvement in the acquired immunodeficiency syndrome (aids), Aust J Ophthalmol 13:293, 1985.

550. McLeod D and others: The roll of axoplasmic transport in the pathogenesis of retinal cotton-wool spots, Br J Ophthalmol 61:177, 1977.

551. Michels R and Gass JDM: The natural history of retinal branch vein obstruction, Trans Am Acad Ophthalmol Otolaryngol 78:166, 1974.

552. Om A, Ellahham S, and Disciascio G: Cholesterol embolism. An underdiagnosed clinical entity. Am Heart J 124(5):1321, 1992.

553. Orth DH, and Patz A: Retinal branch vein occlusion, Surv Ophthalmol 22:357, 1978.

554. Ortiz JM and others: Disseminated intravascular coagulation in infancy and in the neonate. Ocular findings, Arch Ophthalmol 100:1413, 1982.

555. Parrish R, Gass JDM, and Anderson DR: Outer retina ischemic infarction—a newly recognized complication of cataract extraction and closed vitrectomy. 2. An animal model, Ophthalmology 89:1472, 1982.

556. Perraut, L and Zimmerman LE: The occurrence of glaucoma following occlusion of the central retinal artery, Arch Ophthalmol 61:845, 1959.

557. Pieris SJP and Hill DW: Collateral vessels in branch vein occlusion, Trans Ophthalmol Soc UK 102:178, 1982.

558. Priluck IA, Robertson DM, and Hollenhorst RW: Long-term follow-up of occlusion of the central retinal vein in young adults, Am J Ophthalmol 90:190, 1980.

559. Quinlan PM and others: The natural course of central retinal vein occlusion, Am J Ophthalmol 110:118, 1990.

560. Rabb MF and others: Retinal periphlebitis in-patients with acquired immunodeficiency syndrome with cytomegalovirus retinitis mimics acute frosted retinal periphlebitis, Arch Ophthalmol 110: 1257, 1992.

561. Radius RL, Anderson DR: The histology of retinal nerve fiber layer bundles and bundle defects, Arch Ophthalmol 97:943, 1979.

562. Rath EZ and others: Risk factors for retinal vein occlusions, Ophthalmology 99:509, 1992.

563. Rothstein T: Bilateral central retinal vein closure as the initial manifestation of polycythemia, Am J Ophthalmol 74:256, 1972.

564. Schatz H and others: Central retinal vein occlusion associated with retinal arteriovenous malformation, Ophthalmology 100:24, 1993.

565. Schwartz AC and others: Cavernous hemangioma of the retina, cutaneous angiomas, and intracranial vascular lesion by computed tomography and nuclear magnetic resonance imaging, Am J Ophthalmol 98:483, 1984.

566. Sher NA and others: Central retinal artery occlusion complicating Fabry's disease, Arch Ophthalmol 96:815, 1978.

567. Sinclair S II and Gragoudas ES: Prognosis for rubeosis iridis following central retinal vein occlusion, Br J Ophthalmol 63:735, 1979.

568. Smith P and others: Central retinal vein occlusion in Reye's syndrome, Arch Ophthalmol 98:1256, 1980.

569. Soushi S and others: Demonstration of varicella-zoster virus antigens in the vitreous aspirates of patients with acute retinal necrosis syndrome, Ophthalmology 95:1394, 1988.

570. Trope GE and others: Abnormal blood viscosity and haemostasis in long-standing retinal vein occlusion, Br J Ophthalmol 67:137, 1983.

571. Van Heuven WAJ, Hayreh MS, and Hayreh SS: Experimental central retinal vascular occlusion: blood-retinal barrier alterations and retinal lesions, Trans Ophthalmol Soc UK 97:588, 1977.

572. Verhoeff F: Obstruction of the central retinal vein, Arch Ophthalmol 36:1, 1907.

573. Weinberg D and others: Exudative retinal detachment following central and hemicentral retinal vein occlusions, Arch Ophthalmol 108:271, 1990.

574. Willerson D and Aaberg TM: Acute central retinal artery occlusion and optic disc neovascularization: occurrence in a patient with carotid artery disease, Arch Ophthalmol 96:451, 1978.

575. Wilson RS and Ruiz RS: Bilateral central retinal artery occlusion in homocystinuria. A case report, Arch Ophthalmol 82:267, 1969.

576. Wolter JR and Hansen KD: Intimo-intimal intussusception of the central retinal artery, Am J Ophthalmol 92:486, 1981.

577. Zamora RL and others: Branch retinal artery occlusion caused by a mitral valve papillary fibroelastoma, Am J Ophthalmol 119(3): 325, 1994.

578. Zamora RL and others: Branch retinal artery occlusion caused by a mitral valve papillary fibroelastoma-correlation, Am J Ophthalmol 120:126, 1995 (letter).

579. Zegarra H and others: Partial occlusion of the central retinal vein, Am J Ophthalmol 96:330, 1983.

Chorioretinal inflammation

Histoplasmosis

580. Anonymous: Five-year follow-up of fellow eyes of individuals with ocular histoplasmosis and unilateral extrafoveal or juxtafoveal choroidal neovascularization, Macular Photocoagulation Study Group, Arch Ophthalmol 114:677, 1996.

581. Baskin MA: Macular lesions in blacks with the presumed ocular histoplasmosis syndrome, Am J Ophthalmol 89:77, 1980.

582. Cantrill Ill and Burgess D: Peripapillary neovascular membranes in presumed ocular histoplasmosis, Am J Ophthalmol 89:192, 1980.

583. Casady J and others: The etiology of retinochoroiditis and uveitis, Arch Ophthalmol 54:28, 1955.

584. Craig E and Suie T: Histoplasma capsulatum in human ocular tissue, Arch Ophthalmol 92:285, 1974.

585. Damato BE, Trope GA, and Dudgeon J: Presumed ocular histoplasmosis, Trans Ophthalmol Soc UK 101:403, 1981.

586. Feman SS, Podgorski SF, and Penn MK: Blindness from presumed ocular histoplasmosis in Tennessee, Ophthalmology 89:1295, 1982.

587. Gass JDM and Wilkinson C: Follow-up study of presumed ocular histoplasmosis, Trans Am Acad Ophthalmol Otolaryngol 76:562, 1972.

588. Jester JV and Smith RE: Subretinal neovascularization after experimental ocular histoplasmosis in a subhuman primate, Am J Ophthalmol 100:252, 1985.

589. Khalil MK: Histopathology of presumed histoplasmosis, Am J Ophthalmol 94:369, 1982.

590. Klein ML and others: Follow-up study in eyes with choroidal neovascularization caused by presumed ocular histoplasmosis, Am J Ophthalmol 83:830, 1977.

591. Klintworth G and others: Granulomatous choroiditis in a case of disseminated histoplasmosis, Arch Ophthalmol 90:45, 1973.

592. Krause H, and Hopkins W: Ocular manifestations of histoplasmosis, Am J Ophthalmol 34:564, 1951.

593. Krill AE and Archer D: Choroidal neovascularization in multifocal (presumed histoplasmin) choroiditis, Arch Ophthalmol 84:595, 1970.

594. Macular Photocoagulation Study Group: Persistent and recurrent neovascularization after krypton laser photocoagulation for neovascular lesions of ocular histoplasmosis, Arch Ophthalmol 107:344, 1989.

595. Meredith TA and Aaberg TM: Hemorrhagic peripapillary lesions in presumed ocular histoplasmosis, Am J Ophthalmol 84:160, 1977.

596. Meredith TA and others: Ocular histoplasmosis: clinicopathologic correlation of 3 cases, Surv Ophthalmol 22:189, 1977.

597. Ronday MHJ and others: Presumed acquired ocular toxoplasmosis, Arch Ophthalmol 113:1524, 1995.

598. Roth AM: Histoplasma capsulatum in the presumed ocular histoplasmosis syndrome, Am J Ophthalmol 84:293, 1977.

599. Ryan SJ Jr: De novo subretinal neovascularization in the histoplasmosis syndrome, Arch Ophthalmol 94:321, 1976.

600. Schlaegel TF Jr: Ocular histoplasmosis, New York, 1977, Grune & Stratton, Inc.

601. Schlaegel TF Jr, editor: Update on ocular histoplasmosis, Int Ophthalmol Clin 23(2), 1983.

602. Schlaegel TF Jr and Weber J: Follow-up study of presumed histoplasmic choroiditis, Am J Ophthalmol 71:1192, 1971.

603. Schlaegel TJ Jr and others: Presumed histoplasmic choroiditis, Am J Ophthalmol 63:919, 1967.

604. Scholz R and others: Histoplasma capsulatum in the eye, Ophthalmology 91:1100, 1984.

605. Sheffer A and others: Presumed ocular histoplasmosis syndrome: a clinicopathologic correlation of a treated case, Arch Ophthalmol 98:335, 1980.

606. Shields JA and others: Adenocarcinoma of retinal pigment epithelium arising from a juxtapapillary histoplasmosis scar, Arch Ophthalmol 112:650, 1994.

607. Smith RE: Studies of the presumed ocular histoplasmosis syndrome, Trans Ophthalmol Soc UK 101:328, 1981.

608. Smith RE: Natural history and reactivation studies of experimental ocular histoplasmosis in a primate model, Trans Am Ophthalmol Soc 80:695, 1982.

609. Smith RE and Ganley JP: Presumed ocular histoplasmosis. I. Histoplasmin skin test sensitivity in cases identified during a community survey, Arch Ophthalmol 87:245, 1972.

610. Spaeth G: Absence of so-called histoplasma uveitis in 34 cases of proven histoplasmosis, Arch Ophthalmol 77:41, 1967.

611. Thomas MA and Ibanez HE: Subretinal endophotocoagulation in the treatment of choroidal neovascularization, Am J Ophthalmol 116:279, 1993.

612. Thompson WS and others: Acute retinal necrosis caused by reactivation of herpes simplex virus type 2, Am J Ophthalmol 118:205, 1994.

613. Van Metre T Jr and Maumenee AE: Specific ocular uveal lesions in patients with evidence of histoplasmosis, Arch Ophthalmol 71: 314, 1964.

614. Watzke RC and Claussen RW: The long-term course of multifocal choroiditis (presumed ocular histoplasmosis). Am J Ophthalmol 91: 750, 1981.

615. Watzke R and Leaverton P: Light coagulation in presumed histoplasmic choroiditis: a controlled clinical study, Arch Ophthalmol 86:127, 1971.

616. Weiss MJ, Velazquez N, and Hofeldt AJ: Serologic tests in the

diagnosis of presumed toxoplasmic retinochoroiditis, Am J Ophthalmol 109:407, 1990.

617. Woods, AC and Wahlen HE: The probable role of benign histoplasmosis in the etiology of granulomatous uveitis, Am J Ophthalmol 49:205, 1960.

Toxoplasmic retinochoroiditis

618. Akstein RB, Wilson LA, and Teutsch SM: Acquired toxoplasmosis, Ophthalmology 89:1299, 1982.
619. Dobbie J: Toxoplasma retinochoroiditis: successful isolation of Toxoplasma gondii from subretinal fluid of the living human eye, Ann Ophthalmol 2:509, 1970.
620. Fine SL and others: Choroidal neovascularization as a late complication of ocular toxoplasmosis, Am J Ophthalmol 91:318, 1981.
621. Frenkel J and Jacobs I: Ocular toxoplasmosis: pathology, diagnosis and treatment, Arch Ophthalmol 59:260, 1958.
622. Hogan M: Ocular toxoplasmosis, AM J Ophthalmol 46:467, 1958.
623. Hogan M, Kumura S, and O'Connor G: Ocular toxoplasmosis, Arch Ophthalmol 72:592, 1961.
624. Kaufman H: Uveitis accompanied by a positive toxoplasma dye test, Arch Ophthalmol 63:767, 1960.
625. Kazacos KR and others: The raccoon ascarid: a probable cause of human ocular larva migrans, Ophthalmology 92:1735, 1985.
626. Matthews JD and Weiter JJ: Outer retinal toxoplasmosis, Ophthalmology 95:941, 1988.
627. Maumenee AE: Toxoplasmosis: Symposium by the Council for Research on Glaucoma and Allied Diseases, Nov 20–22, 1960, Surv Ophthalmol 6:699, 1961.
628. Michelson JB and others: Retinitis secondary to acquired systemic toxoplasmosis with isolation of the parasite, Am J Ophthalmol 86:548, 1978.
629. Nicholson DII and Wolchok E: Ocular toxoplasmosis in an adult receiving long-term corticosteroid therapy, Arch Ophthalmol 94:248, 1976.
630. O'Connor G: Ocular toxoplasmosis, Jpn J Ophthalmol 19:1, 1975.
631. Owens PL, Goldberg MF, and Busse BJ: Prospective observation of vascular anastomoses between the retina and choroid in recurrent toxoplasmosis, AM J ophthalmol 88:402, 1979.
632. Perkins E: Ocular toxoplasmosis, Br J Ophthalmol 57:1, 1973.
633. Rao NA and Font RL: Toxoplasmic retinochoroiditis, Arch Ophthalmol 95:273, 1977.
634. Remington J, Jacobs L, and Kaufman D: Studies on chronic toxoplasmosis: the relation of infective dose to residual infection and to the possibility of congenital transmission, Am J Ophthalmol 46:261, 1958.
635. Ronday MHJ and others: Presumed acquired ocular toxoplasmosis, Arch Ophthalmol 113:1524, 1995.
636. Saari M and others: Acquired toxoplasmic chorioretinitis, Arch Ophthalmol 94:1485, 1976.
637. Sabates R, Pruett RC, and Brockhurst RJ: Fulminant ocular toxoplasmosis, Am J Ophthalmol 92:497, 1981.
638. Schlaegel TF Jr: Ocular toxoplasmosis and pars planitis, New York, 1978, Grune & Stratton, Inc.
639. Schuman JS and others: Toxoplasmic scleritis, Ophthalmology 95:1399, 1988.
640. Scott EH: New concepts in toxoplasmosis, Surv Ophthalmol 18:255, 1974.
641. Tessler HH: Ocular toxoplasmosis, Int Ophthalmol Clin 21(3):185, 1981.
642. Walsh FB, Hogan MJ, and Sabin AB: Symposium: toxoplasmosis, Am Acad Ophthalmol Otolaryngol 54:177, 1950.
643. Wilder II: Toxoplasma chorioretinitis in adults, Arch Ophthalmol 48:127, 1952.

Acquired immune deficiency syndrome, CMIR, and ARN

644. Aaberg TM, Cesarz TJ, and Rytel MW: Correlation of virology and clinical course of cytomegalovirus retinitis, Am J Ophthalmol 74:407, 1972.
645. Acheson JF and others: Treatment of CMV retinitis in an AIDS patient, Br J Ophthalmol 71:810, 1987.
646. Allen JR: Heterosexual transmission of human immunodeficiency virus (HIV) in the United States, Bull NY Acad Med 64:464, 1988.
647. Ammann AJ: The immunology of AIDS, Int Ophthalmol Clin 29(2):77, 1988.

648. Ammann AJ and others: B-cell immunodeficiency in acquired immune deficiency syndrome, JAMA 251:1447, 1984.
649. Anand R and others: Pathology of cytomegalovirus retinitis treated with sustained release intravitreal ganciclovir, Ophthalmology 100:1032, 1993.
650. Anonymous: Combination foscarnet and ganciclovir therapy vs monotherapy for the treatment of relapsed cytomegalovirus retinitis in patients with aids. The cytomegalovirus retreatment trial. The studies of ocular complications of AIDS research group in collaboration with the AIDS clinical trials group, Arch Ophthalmol 114:23, 1996.
651. Anonymous: Special issue: AIDS and the eye, Arch Ophthalmol 114:791, 1996.
652. Anonymous: Assessment of cytomegalovirus retinitis. Clinical evaluation vs centralized-grading of fundus photographs. Studies of ocular complications of AIDS research group, AIDS clinical trials group, Arch Ophthalmol 114:791, 1996.
653. Anonymous: Clinical vs photographic assessment of treatment cytomegalovirus retinitis. Foscarnet-ganciclovir cytomegalovirus retinitis trial report 8. Studies of ocular complications of AIDS research group, AIDS clinical trials group, Arch Ophthalmol 114:848, 1996.
654. Arevalo JF and others: Correlation between intraocular pressure and cd4 + t-lymphocyte counts in patients with human immunodeficiency virus with and without cytomegalovirus retinitis, Am J Ophthalmol 122:91, 1996.
655. Augsburger JJ and Henry RY: Retinal aneurysms in adult cytomegalovirus retinitis, Am J Ophthalmol 86:794, 1978.
656. Bachman DM and others: Culture-proven cytomegalovirus retinitis in a homosexual man with the acquired immunodeficiency syndrome, Ophthalmology 89:797, 1982.
657. Benson WH, Linberg JV, and Weinstein GW: Orbital pseudotumor in a patient with AIDS, Am J Ophthalmol 105:697, 1988.
658. Bolan RK: AIDS—The struggle to survive: a clinician's perspective, Int Ophthalmol Clin 29(2):70, 1988.
659. Boniuk I: The ctyomegaloviruses and the eye, Int Ophthalmol Clin 12:169, 1972.
660. Broder S and Gallo RC: A pathogenic retrovirus (HTLV-III) linked to AIDS, N Engl J Med 311:1292, 1984.
661. Brooks HL Jr and others: Orbital Burkitt's lymphoma in a homosexual man with acquired immune deficiency, Arch Ophthalmol 102:1533, 1984.
662. Broughton WL, Cupples HP, and Parver LM: Bilateral retinal detachment following cytomegalovirus retinitis, Arch Ophthalmol 96:618, 1978.
663. Brown HH and others: Cytomegalovirus infection of the conjunctiva in AIDS, Am J Ophthalmol 106:102, 1988.
664. Browning DJ and others: Association of varicella zoster dermatitis with acute retinal necrosis syndrome, Ophthalmology 94:602, 1987.
665. Buechi ER and others: Can AZT treatment in AIDS patients aggravate pre-existing CMV retinitis? Br J Ophthalmol 72:239, 1988 (letter to the editor).
666. Burd EM and others: Maintenance of replicative intermediates in ganciclovir-treated human cytomegalovirus-infected retinal glia, Arch Ophthalmol 114:856, 1996.
667. Burd EM and others: Replication of human cytomegalovirus in human retinal glial cells, Invest Ophthalmol Vis Sci 37:1957, 1996.
668. Burkes RL and others: Simultaneous occurrence of *Pneumocystis carinii* pneumonia, cytomegalovirus infection, Kaposi's sarcoma, and β-immunoblastic sarcoma in a homosexual man, JAMA 253:3425, 1985.
669. Burns R: Cytomegalic inlusion disease uveitis, Arch Ophthalmol 61:376, 1959.
670. Cantrill HL and others: Recovery of human immunodeficiency virus from ocular tissues in patients with acquired immune deficiency syndrome, Ophthalmology 95:1458, 1988.
671. Carson S and Chatterjee SN: Cytomegalovirus retinitis: two cases occurring after renal transplantation, Ann Ophthalmol 10:275, 1978.
672. Chang M and others: Clinicopathologic correlation of ocular and neurologic findings in AIDS: case report, Ann Ophthalmol 18:105, 1986.
673. Chawla HB and others: Ocular involvement in cytomegalovirus infection in a previously healthy adult, Br Med J 2:281, 1976.
674. Chess J and others: Candida retinitis in bare lymphocyte syndrome, Ophthalmology 93:696, 1986.

675. Chess J and Marcus DM: Zoster-related bilateral acute retinal necrosis syndrome as presenting sign in AIDS, Ann Ophthalmol 20: 421, 1988.

676. Chumbley LC and others: Adult cytomegalovirus inclusion retinouveitis, Am J Ophthalmol 80:807, 1975.

677. Cohen DB and Glasgow BJ: Bilateral optic nerve cryptococcosis in sudden blindness in-patients with acquired immune deficiency syndrome, Ophthalmology 100:1689, 1993.

678. Cole EL and others: Herpes zoster ophthalmicus and acquired immune deficiency syndrome, Arch Ophthalmol 102:1027, 1984.

679. Cooper HM and Beer PM: Spontaneous regression and successful laser prophylaxis in progressive outer retinal necrosis syndrome, Am J Ophthalmol 121:723, 1996.

680. Culbertson WW: Infections of the retina in AIDS, Int Ophthalmol Clin 29(2):108, 1989.

681. Culbertson WW and others: Varicella zoster virus is a cause of the acute retinal necrosis syndrome, Ophthalmology 93:559, 1986.

682. Cunningham ET and others: Acquired immunodeficiency syndrome-associated herpes simplex virus retinitis. Clinical description and use of a polymerase chain reaction-based assay as a diagnostic tool, Arch Ophthalmol 114:834, 1996.

683. D'Amico DJ and others: Ophthalmoscopic and histologic findings in cytomegalovirus retinitis treated with BW-B759U, Arch Ophthalmol 104:1788, 1986.

684. Davis JL and others: Endogenous bacterial retinitis in AIDS, Am J Ophthalmol 107:613, 1989.

685. de Martini RM and Parker JW: Immunologic alterations in human immunodeficiency virus infection: review, J Clin Lab Anal 3(1):56, 1989.

686. de Venecia G and others: Cytomegalic inclusion retinitis: a clinical, histopathologic, and ultrastructural study, Arch Ophthalmol 86:44, 1971.

687. Dennehy PJ and others: Ocular manifestations in pediatric patients with acquired immunodeficiency syndrome, Arch Ophthalmol 107:978, 1989.

688. Dodds EM and others: Serous retinal detachments in a patients with clinically resistant cytomegalovirus retinitis, Arch Ophthalmol 114:896, 1996.

689. Doft BH and Curtin VT: Combined ocular infection with cytomegalovirus and cryptococcosis, Arch Ophthalmol 100:1800, 1982.

690. Donnellan WL, Chantra-Umporn S, and Kidd JM: The cytomegalic inclusion cell: an electron microscopic study, Arch Pathol 82:336, 1966.

691. Drew WL and others: Cytomegalovirus and Kaposi's sarcoma in young homosexual men, Lancet II:125, 1982.

692. Dugel PU and others: Ocular adnexal Kaposi's sarcoma in acquired immunodeficiency syndrome, Am J Ophthalmol 110:500, 1990.

693. Duker JS and others: Long-term, successful maintenance of bilateral cytomegalovirus retinitis using exclusively local therapy, Arch Ophthalmol 114:881m, 1996 (letter).

694. Egbert PR and others: Cytomegalovirus retinitis in immunosuppressed hosts. II. Ocular manifestations, Ann Intern Med 93:664, 1980.

695. England AC III, Miller SA, and Maki DG: Ocular findings of acute cytomegalovirus infection in an immunologically competent adult, N Engl J Med 307:94, 1982.

696. Engstrom RE and Holland GN: Chronic herpes zoster virus keratitis associated with the acquired immunodeficiency syndrome, Am J Ophthalmol 105:556, 1988.

697. Engstrom RE Jr and others: Hemorheologic abnormalities in patients with human immunodeficiency virus infection and ophthalmic microvasculopathy, Am J Ophthalmol 109:153, 1990.

698. Fay MT and others: Atypical retinitis in patients with the acquired immunodeficiency syndrome, Am J Ophthalmol 105:483, 1988.

699. Fekrat S and others: Cytomegalovirus retinitis in HIV-infected patients with elevated Cd4 + counts, Arch Ophthalmol 113:18, 1995 (letter).

700. Felsenstein D and others: Treatment of cytomegalovirus retinitis with 9-[2-hydroxy-1-(hydroxymethyl)ethoxymethyl]guanine, Ann Intern Med 103:377, 1985.

701. Feorino PM and others: Transfusion-associated acquired immunodeficiency syndrome: evidence for persistent infection in blood donors, N Engl J Med 312:1293, 1985.

702. Fiala M and others: Epidemiology of cytomegalovirus infection after transplantation and immunosuppression, J Infect Dis 132: 421, 1975.

703. Foerster HW: Pathology of granulomatous uveitis, Surv Ophthalmol 4:283, 1959.

704. Foster DJ and others: Rapidly progressive outer retinal necrosis in the acquired immunodeficiency syndrome, Am J Ophthalmol 110:341, 1990.

705. Freeman WR: New developments in the treatment of CMV retinitis, Ophthalmology 103:999, 1996 (editorial, comment).

706. Freeman WR and O'Connor GR: Acquired immune deficiency syndrome retinopathy, pneumocystis, and cotton-wool spots, Am J Ophthalmol 98:235, 1984.

707. Freeman WR and others: A prospective study of the ophthalmologic findings in the acquired immune deficiency syndrome, Am J Ophthalmol 97:133, 1984.

708. Freeman WR and others: Prevalence, pathophysiology, and treatment of rhegmatogenous retinal detachment in treated cytomegalovirus retinitis, Am J Ophthalmol 103:527, 1987.

709. Freeman WR and others: Pneumocystis carinii choroidopathy: a new clinical entity, Arch Ophthalmol 107:863, 1989.

710. Freeman WR and others: Prevalence and significance of acquired immunodeficiency syndrome-related retinal microvasculopathy, Am J Ophthalmol 107:229, 1989.

711. Friedberg DN and others: Microsporidial keratoconjunctivitis in acquired immunodeficiency syndrome, Arch Ophthalmol 108:504, 1990.

712. Friedman AH: The retinal lesions of the acquired immune deficiency syndrome. Trans Am Ophthalmol Soc 82:447, 1984.

713. Friedman AH and others: Cytomegalovirus retinitis: a manifestation of the acquired immune deficiency syndrome (AIDS), Br J Ophthalmol 67:372, 1983.

714. Friedman-Kien AE, and others: Disseminated Kaposi's sarcoma in homosexual men, Ann Intern Med 96(6): Part 1:693, 1982.

715. Friedman SM and Margo CE: Bilateral central retinal vein occlusions in a patient with acquired immunodeficiency syndrome—clinicopathologic correlation, Arch Ophthalmol 113:1184, 1995.

716. Fujikawa LS and others: Human T-cell leukemia/lymphotropic virus type III in the conjunctival epithelium of a patient with AIDS, Am J Ophthalmol 100:507, 1985.

717. Fujikawa LS and others: HTLV-III in the tears of AIDS patients, Ophthalmology 93:1479, 1986.

718. Gagliuso DJ and others: Ocular toxoplamosis in AIDS patients, Trans Am Ophthalmol Soc 88:63, 1990.

719. Gal A, Pollack A, and Oliver M: Ocular findings in the acquired immunodeficiency syndrome, Br J Ophthalmol 68:238, 1984.

720. Gass JDM: Stereoscopic atlas of macular diseases: diagnosis and treatment, ed 3, St Louis, 1987, The CV Mosby Co.

721. Gerberding JL: Occupational health issues for providers of care to patients with HIV infection, Infect Dis Clin North Am 2(2):321, 1988.

722. Glasgow BJ and Weisberger AK: A quantitative and cartographic study of retinal microvasculopathy in acquired immunodeficiency syndrome, Am J Ophthalmol 118:46, 1994.

723. Goedert JJ and others: Determinants of retrovirus (HTLV-III) antibody and immunodeficiency conditions in homosexual men, Lancet II:711, 1984.

724. Gomez-Ulla F and others: Chroidal vascular abnormality in Purtscher's retinopathy shown by indocyaninee green angiography, Am J Ophthalmol 122:261, 1996.

725. Goodpasture EW and Talbot FB: Concerning the nature of "protozoan-like" cells in certain lesions of infancy, Am J Dis Child 21: 415, 1921.

726. Griffiths PD and others: Rapid diagnosis of cytomegalovirus infection in immunocompromised patients by detection of early antigen fluorescent foci, Lancet II:1242, 1984.

727. Groopman JE: Kaposi's sarcoma and other neoplasms. In Gottlieb MS, moderator: The acquired immunodeficiency syndrome, Ann Intern Med 99(2):208, 1983.

728. Groopman JE and others: Seroepidemiology of human T-lymphotropic virus type III among homosexual men with the acquired immunodeficiency syndrome or generalized lymphadenopathy and among asymptomatic controls in Boston, Ann Intern Med 102:334, 1985.

729. Gross JG and others: Longitudinal study of cytomegalovirus retini-

tis in acquired immune deficiency syndrome, Ophthalmology 97: 681, 1990.

730. Grossniklaus HE, Frank KE, and Tomsak RL: Cytomegalovirus retinitis and optic neuritis in acquired immune deficiency syndrome: report of a case, Ophthalmology 94:1601, 1987.

731. Grossniklaus HE and others: Toxoplasma gondii retinochoroiditis and optic neuritis in acquired immunodeficiency syndrome. Report of a case, Ophthalmology 97:1342, 1990.

732. Grossniklaus HE and others: Toxoplasma gondii retinochoroiditis and optic neuritis in acquired immune deficiency syndrome. Report of a case, Ophthalmology 97:1342, 1990.

733. Gupta S and Licorish K: Circulating immune complexes in AIDS, N Engl J Med 310:1530, 1984 (letter to the editor).

734. Guarda LA and others: Acquired immunodeficiency syndrome: postmortem findings, Am J Clinicopathologic Pathol 81:549, 1984.

735. Guyer DR and others: Regression of cytomegalovirus retinitis with zidovudine: a clinicopathologic correlation, Arch Ophthalmol 107: 868, 1989.

736. Guyton TB and others: New observations in generalized cytomegalic inclusion disease of the new born, N Engl J Med 257:803, 1957.

737. Haase AT: Analysis of viral infections by in situ hybridization, J Histochem Cytochem 34:27, 1986.

738. Hackman RC and others: Rapid diagnosis of cytomegaloviral pneumonia by tissue immunofluorescence with a murine monoclonal antibody, J Infect Dis 151:325, 1985.

739. Hahn RA: Prevalence of HIV infection among intravenous drug users in the United States, JAMA 261:2677, 1989.

740. Handsfield HH: Screening for HTLV-III antibody, N Engl J Med 313:888, 1985 (letter to the editor).

741. Hanshaw JB and others: Acquired cytomegalovirus infection: association with hepatomegaly and abnormal liver-function tests, N Engl J Med 272:602, 1965.

742. Haverkos HW, Drotman DP, and Morgan M: Prevalence of Kaposi's sarcoma among patients with AIDS, N Engl J Med 312: 1518, 1985 (letter to the editor).

743. Heinemann MH, Bloom AF, and Horowitz J: Candida albicans endophthalmitis in a patient with AIDS, Arch Ophthalmol 105: 1172, 1987.

744. Heinemann MH, Gold JM, and Maisel J: Bilateral toxoplasma retinochoroiditis in a patient with acquired immune deficiency syndrome, Retina 6(4):224, 1986.

745. Helm CJ, Holland GN: Ocular tuberculosis, Surv Ophthalmol 38: 229, 1993.

746. Henderly DE and others: Cytomegalovirus retinitis and response to therapy with ganciclovir, Ophthalmology 94:425, 1987.

747. Henderly DE and others: Cytomegalovirus retinitis as the initial manifestation of the acquired immune deficiency syndrome, Am J Ophthalmol 103:316, 1987.

748. Hennis HL, Scott AA, and Apple DJ: Clinical pathological review, Surv Ophthalmol 4(3):193, 1989.

749. Henry K and others: Use of intravitreal ganciclovir (dihydroxy propoxymethyl guanine) for cytomegalovirus retinitis in a patient with AIDS, Am J Ophthalmol 103:17, 1987.

750. Ho DD, Pomerantz RJ, and Kaplan JC: Pathogenesis of infection with human immunodeficiency virus, N Engl J Med 317:278, 1987.

751. Holland GN, Gottlieb, MS, and Foos, RY: Retinal cotton-wool patches in acquired immunodeficiency syndrome, N Engl J Med 307:1704, 1982 (letter to the editor).

752. Holland GN and others: Ocular disorders associated with a new severe acquired cellular immunodeficiency syndrome, Am J Ophthalmol 93:393, 1982.

753. Holland GN and others: Acquired immune deficiency syndrome: ocular manifestations, Ophthalmology 90:859, 1983.

754. Holland GN and others: Treatment of cytomegalovirus retinopathy with ganciclovir, Ophthalmology 94:815, 1987.

755. Holland GN and others: Ocular toxoplasmosis in patients with the acquired immunodeficiency syndrome, Am J Ophthalmol 106:653, 1988.

756. Holland GN, MacArthur LJ, and Foos RY: Choroidal pneumocystosis, Arch Ophthalmol 109:1454, 1991.

757. Hoover DR and others: Occurrence of cytomegalovirus retinitis after human immunodeficiency virus immunosuppression, Arch Ophthalmol 114:821, 1996.

758. Hooymans JMM, Sprenger HG, and Weits J: Treatment of cyto-

megalovirus retinitis with DHPG in a patient with AIDS, Doc Ophthalmol 67:5, 1987.

759. Howard GM, Jakobiec FA, and DeVoe AG: Kaposi's sarcoma of the conjunctiva, Am J Ophthalmol 79:420, 1975.

760. Humphry RC, Parkin JM, and Marsh RJ: The ophthalmological features of AIDS and AIDS related disorders, Trans Ophthalmol Soc UK 105:505, 1986.

761. Jabs DA: Acquired immunodeficiency syndrome and the eye—1996, Arch Ophthalmol 114:863, 1996 (editorial, review).

762. Jabs DA, Enger C, and Bartlett JG: Cytomegalovirus retinitis and acquired immunodeficiency syndrome, Arch Ophthalmol 107:75, 1989.

763. Jabs DA and others: Treatment of cytomegalovirus retinitis with ganciclovir, Ophthalmology 94:824, 1987.

764. Jabs DA and others: Ocular manifestations of acquired immune deficiency syndrome, Ophthalmology 96:1092, 1989.

765. Jensen OA and others: Cytomegalovirus retinitis in the acquired immunodeficiency syndrome (AIDS): light-microscopical, ultrastructural and immunohistochemical examination of a case, Acta Ophthalmol 62:1, 1984.

766. Johns DR, Tierney M, and Felsenstein D: Alteration in the natural history of neurosyphilis by concurrent infection with the human immunodeficiency virus, N Engl J Med 316:1569, 1987.

767. Johnston WH and others: Recurrence of presumed varicella-zoster virus retinopathy in-patients with acquired immunodeficiency syndrome, Am J Ophthalmol 116:42, 1993.

768. Kanich RE, and Craighead JE: Cytomegalovirus infection and cytomegalic inclusion disease in renal homotransplant recipients, Am J Med, 40:874, 1966.

769. Karma A: Ophthalmic changes in sarcoidosis, Acta Ophthalmol Suppl 141, 1979.

770. Keefe KS and others: Atypical healing of cytomegalovirus retinitis, significance of persistent border opacification, Ophthalmology 99: 1377, 1992.

771. Kestelyn P, Lepage P, and Van de Perre P: Perivasculitis of the retinal vessels as an important sign in children with AIDS-related complex, Am J Ophthalmol 100:614, 1985 (letter to the editor).

772. Kestelyn P and others: A prospective study of the ophthalmologic findings in the acquired immune deficiency syndrome in Africa, Am J Ophthalmol 100:230, 1985.

773. Khadem M and others: Ophthalmologic findings in acquired immune deficiency syndrome (AIDS), Arch Ophthalmol 102:201, 1984.

774. Kirsch LS and others: Intravitreal cidofovir (HPMPC) treatment of cytomegalovirus retinitis in-patients with acquired immune deficiency syndrome, Ophthalmology 102:533, 1995.

775. Kirsch LS and others: Phase I/II study of intravitreal cidofovir for the treatment of cytomegalovirus retinitis in-patients with the acquired immunodeficiency syndrome, Am J Ophthalmology 119: 466, 1995.

776. Klein S, Roschlau G, and Ryssel D: Augenveränderungen bei Zytomegalie, Ophthalmologica 160:209, 1970.

777. Kohn SR: Molluscum contagiosum in patients with acquired immunodeficiency syndrome, Arch Ophthalmol 105:458, 1987 (letter to the editor).

778. Koretz SH and others in Collaborative DHPG Treatment Study Group: treatment of serious cytomegalovirus infections with 9-(1,3-dihydroxy-2-propoxymethyl) guanine in patients with AIDS and other immunodeficiencies, N Engl J Med 314:802, 1986.

779. Krowka JF, Moody DJ, and Stites DP: Immunological effects of HIV infection. In Levy JA, editor: AIDS pathogenesis and treatment, New York, 1988, Marcel Dekker.

780. Kupperman BD and others: Clinical and histopathologic study of varicella zoster virus retinitis in patients with the acquired immunodeficiency syndrome, Am J Ophthalmol 118:589, 1994.

781. Kurosawa A and others: Sporothrix schenckii endophthalmitis in a patient with human immunodeficiency virus infection, Arch Ophthalmol 106:376, 1988.

782. Kwok S, O'Donnell JJ, and Wood IS: Retinal cotton-wool spots in a patient with Pneumocystis carinii infection, N Engl J Med 307: 184, 1982 (letter to the editor).

783. Lamberson HV: Cytomegalovirus (CMV): the agent, its pathogenesis, and its epidemiology. In Infection, immunity and blood transfusion, New York, 1985, Alan R Liss, Inc.

784. Lane HC and others: Qualitative analysis of immune function in

patients with the acquired immunodeficiency syndrome: evidence for a selective defect in soluble antigen recognition, N Engl J Med 313:79, 1985.

785. Lerner CW: B-cell abnormalities in AIDS, N Engl J Med 310:258, 1984 (letter to the editor).

786. Lonn LI: Neonatal cytomegalic inclusion disease chorioretinitis, Arch Ophthalmol 88:434, 1972.

787. Lurain NS, Thompson KD, and Farrand SK: Rapid detection of cytomegalovirus in clinical specimens by using biotinylated DNA probes and analysis of cross-reactivity with herpes simplex virus, J Clin Microbiol 24:724, 1986.

788. Macdonald EA: Treatment of cytomegalovirus retinitis in a patient with AIDS with 9-(1,3-dihydroxy-2-propoxymethyl) guanine, Can J Ophthalmol 22:48, 1987.

789. Macher AM: Infection in the acquired immunodeficiency syndrome. In Fauci AS, moderator: Acquired immunodeficiency syndrome: epidemiologic, clinical, immunologic and therapeutic considerations, Ann Intern Med 100:92, 1984.

790. Macher A and others: Disseminated bilateral choriorentinitis due to histoplasma capsulatum in a patient with the acquired immunodeficiency syndrome, Ophthalmology 91:1159, 1985.

791. Mansour AM and others: Cotton-wool spots in acquired immunodeficiency syndrome compared with diabetes mellitus, systemic hypertension, and central retinal vein occlusion, Arch Ophthalmol 106:1074, 1988.

792. Mar E-C, Cheng Y-C, and Huang E-S: Effect of 9-(1,3-dihydroxy-2-propoxymethyl)guanine on human cytomegalovirus replication in vitro, Antimicrob Agents Chemother 24:518, 1983.

793. Margo CE: Should corneal transplant donors be screened for human T-cell lymphotropic virus type III antibody? Arch Ophthalmol 103:1643, 1985.

794. Margo CE and Harmed LM: Ocular syphilis, Surv Ophthalmol 37(3):203, 1992.

795. Margolis TP and others: Varicella-zoster virus retinitis in-patients with the acquired immunodeficiency syndrome, Am J Ophthalmol 112:119, 1991.

796. Marmor and others: Optic nerve head involvement with cytomegalovirus in an adult with lymphoma, Arch Ophthalmol 96:1252, 1978.

797. Martin DC and others: Cytomegalovirus viremia detected by molecular hybridization and electron microscopy, Ann Intern Med 100:222, 1984.

798. Marx JL and others: Use of the ganciclovir implant in the treatment of recurrent cytomegalovirus retinitis, Arch Ophthalmol 114:815, 1996.

799. Masur H and others: Effect of 9-(1,3-dihydroxy-2-propoxymethyl)-guanine on serious cytomegalovirus disease in eight immunosupressed homosexual men, Ann Intern Med 104:41, 1986.

800. Maurice DM: Use of intravitreal ganciclovir (dihydroxy propoxymethyl guanine) for cytomegalovirus retinitis in a patient with AIDS, Am J Ophthalmol 103:842, 1987.

801. McGavran MH and Smith MG: Ultrastructural, cytochemical, and microchemical observations on cytomegalovirus (salivary gland virus) infection of human cells in tissue culture, Exp Mol Pathol 4:1, 1965.

802. Meredith TA, Aaberg TM, and Reeser FH: Rhegmatogenous retinal detachment complicating cytomegalovirus retinitis, Am J Ophthalmol 87:793, 1979.

803. Mills J and others: Treatment of cytomegalovirus retinitis in patients with AIDS, Rev Infect Dis 10(suppl 3):S522, 1988.

804. Mines JA and Kaplan HJ: Acquired immunodeficiency syndrome (AIDS): the disease and its ocular manifestations, Int Ophthalmol Clin 26(2):73, 1986.

805. Mitsuyasu RT: AIDS-related Kaposi's sarcoma: a review of its pathogenesis and treatment, Blood Rev 2(4):222, 1988.

806. Moorthy RS, Smith RE, and Rao NA: Progressive ocular toxoplasmosis in-patients with acquired immunodeficiency syndrome, Am J Ophthalmol 115:742, 1993.

807. Morinelli EN and others: Infectious multifocal choroiditis in-patients with acquired immune deficiency syndrome, Ophthalmology 100:1014, 1993.

808. Morley MG, Duker JS, and Zacks C: Successful treatment of rapidly progressive outer retinal necrosis in the acquired immunodeficiency syndrome, Am J Ophthalmol 264, 1994.

809. Moss AR and others: Seropositivity for HIV and the development of AIDS or AIDS related condition: three year follow up of the San Francisco General Hospital cohort, Br Med J 296:745, 1988.

810. Murray HW and others: Cytomegalovirus retinitis in adults: a manifestation of disseminated viral infection, Am J Med 63:574, 1977.

811. Neuwith J and others: Cytomegalovirus retinitis in a young homosexual man with acquire immunodeficiency, Ophthalmology 89:805, 1982.

812. Newman NM and others: Clinical and histologic findings in opportunistic ocular infections: part of a new syndrome of acquired immunodeficiency, Arch Ophthalmol 101:396, 1983.

813. Newsome DA: Noninfectious ocular complications of AIDS, Int Ophthalmol Clin 29(2):95, 1989.

814. Newsome and others: Microvascular aspects of acquired immune deficiency syndrome retinopathy, Am J Ophthalmol 98:590, 1984.

815. Numazaki and others: Primary infection with cytomegalovirus: virus isolation from healthy infants and pregnant women, Am J Epidemiol 91:410, 1970.

816. O'Day DM: The risk posed by HTLV-III-infected corneal donor tissue, Am J Ophthalmol 101:246, 1986 (editorial).

817. O'Donnell JJ and Jacobson MA: Cotton-wool spots and cytomegalovirus retinitis in AIDS, Int Ophthalmol Clin 29(2):105, 1989.

818. Ormerod LDd and others: Ophthalmologic manifestations of acquired immune deficiency syndrome-associated progressive multifocal leukoencephalopathy, Ophthalmology 103:899, 1996.

819. Pakola SJ and Nichols CW: Cd8 + t-lymphocytes and cytomegalovirus retinitis in patients with the acquired immunodeficiency syndrome, Am J Ophthalmol 121:455, 1996 (letter; comment).

820. Palestine AG and others: Ophthalmic involvement in acquired immunodeficiency syndrome, Ophthalmology 91:1092, 1984.

821. Palestine AG and others: Treatment of cytomegalovirus retinitis with dihydroxy propoxymethyl guanine, Am J Ophthalmol 101:95, 1986.

822. Parke DW II and Font RL: Diffuse toxoplasmic retinochoroiditis in a patient with AIDS, Arch Ophthalmol 104:571, 1986.

823. Parrish CM, O'Day DM, and Hoyle TC: Spontaneous fungal corneal ulcer as an ocular manifestation of AIDS, Am J Ophthalmol 104:302, 1987.

824. Passo MS and Rosenbaum JT: Ocular syphilis in patients with human immunodeficiency virus infection, Am J Ophthalmol 106:1, 1988.

825. Patrizi G and others: Human cytomegalovirus: electron microscopy of a primary viral isolate, J Lab Clin Med 65:825, 1966.

826. Pepose JS: Infectious retinitis: diagnostic modalities, Ophthalmology 93:570, 1986.

827. Pepose JS and others: An analysis of retinal cotton-wool spots and cytomegalovirus retinitis in the acquired immunodeficiency syndrome, Am J Ophthalmol 95:118, 1983.

828. Pepose JS and others: Concurrent herpes simplex and cytomegalovirus retinitis and encephalitis in the acquired immune deficiency syndrome (AIDS), Ophthalmology 91:1669, 1984.

829. Pepose JS and others: Acquired immune deficiency syndrome: pathogenic mechanisms of ocular disease, Ophthalmology 92:472, 1985.

830. Pepose JS and others: Immunocytologic locations of herpes simplex type I viral antigens in herpetic retinitis and encephalitis in an adult, Ophthalmology 92:160, 1985.

831. Pepose JS and others: The impact of the AIDS epidemic on corneal transplantation, Am J Ophthalmol 100:610, 1985 (editorial).

832. Pepose JS and others: Pathologic features of cytomegalovirus retinopathy after treatment with the antiviral agent ganciclovir, Ophthalmology 94:414, 1987.

833. Perkins ES: Ocular toxoplasmosis, Br J Ophthalmol 57:1, 1973.

834. Peterman TA and others: Transfusion-associated acquired immunodeficiency syndrome in the United States, JAMA 254:2913, 1985.

835. Pezzi and others: Retinal cotton-wool-like spots: a marker for AIDS? Ann Ophthalmol 21:31, 1989.

836. Pflugfelder SC, Saulson R, and Ullman S: Peripheral corneal ulceration in a patient with AIDS-related complex, Am J Ophthalmol 104:542, 1987.

837. Pollard RB and others: Cytomegalovirus retinitis in immunosuppressed hosts. I. Natural history and effects of treatment with adenine arabinoside, Ann Intern Med 93:655, 1980.

838. Pomerantz RJ and others: Infection of the retina by human immunodeficiency virus type I, N Engl J Med 317:1643, 1987.

839. Rabb MF and others: Retinal periphlebitis in-patients with acquired immunodeficiency syndrome with cytomegalovirus retinitis mimics acute frosted retinal periphlebitis, Arch Ophthalmol 110:1257, 1992.

840. Rahhal FM and others: Intravitreal cidofovir for the maintenance treatment of cytomegalovirus retinitis (see comments), Ophthalmology 103:1078, 1996.

841. Rao NA and others: A clinical, histopathologic, and electron microscopic study of Pneumocystis carinii choroiditis, Am J Ophthalmol 107:218, 1989.

842. Rehder JR and others: Acute unilateral toxoplasmic iridocyclitis in an AIDS patient, Am J Ophthalmol 106:740, 1988 (letter to the editor).

843. Ribbert H: Ueber protozoenartige Zellen in der Niere eines syphilitischen Neugeborenen und in der Parotis von Kidern, Centralbl f allg Path, u path Anat, Jena XV:945, 1904.

844. Rice GPA, Schrier RD, and Oldstone MBA: Cytomegalovirus infects human lymphocytes and monocytes: virus expression is restricted to immediate-early gene products, Proc Natl Acad Sci USA 81:6134, 1984.

845. Richman DD and others: Rapid viral diagnosis, J Infect Dis 149:298, 1984.

846. Robinson MR and others: Treatment of cytomegalovirus optic neuritis with dihydroxy propoxymethyl guanine, Am J Ophthalmol 102:533, 1986 (letter to the editor).

847. Ronald AR and others: A review of HIV-1 in Africa, Bull NY Acad Med 64:480, 1988.

848. Rosecan LR and others: Antiviral therapy for cytomegalovirus retinitis in AIDS with dihydroxy propoxymethyl guanine, Am J Ophthalmol 101:405, 1986.

849. Rosecan LR and others: Antiviral therapy with ganciclovir for cytomegalovirus retinitis and bilateral exudative retinal detachments in an immunocompromised child, Ophthalmology 93:1401, 1986.

850. Rosenberg PR and others: Acquired immunodeficiency syndrome: ophthalmic manifestations in ambulatory patients, Ophthalmology 90:874, 1983.

851. Rummelt V and others: Triple retinal infection with human immunodeficiency virus Type I, Cytomegalovirus, and herpes simplex virus Type 1. Light and electron microscopy, immunohistochemistry, and in situ hybridization, Ophthalmology 101:270, 1994.

852. Rungger-Braendle E, Roux L, and Leuenberger PM: Bilateral acute retinal necrosis (BARN): identification of the presumed infectious agent, Ophthalmology 91:1648, 1984.

853. Safai B and Good RA: Kaposi's sarcoma: a review and recent developments, Cancer 31:2, 1981.

854. Salahuddin SZ and others: Isolation of the human T-cell leukemia/lymphotropic virus type III from the cornea, Am J Ophthalmol 101:149, 1986.

855. Sandor EV and others: Herpes zoster ophthalmicus in patients at risk for the acquired immune deficiency syndrome (AIDS), Am J Ophthalmol 101:153, 1986.

856. Santos C and others: Bilateral fungal corneal ulcers in a patient with AIDS-related complex, Am J Ophthalmol, 102:118, 1986 (letter to the editor).

857. Sarkies NJC and Blach RK: Ocular disease in immunosuppressed patients, Trans Ophthalmol Soc UK 104:243, 1985.

858. Schulman J and others: Intraocular 9[2-hydroxy-1-(hydroxy methyl)] ethoxymethylguanine levels after intravitreal and subconjunctival administration, Ophthalmic Surg 17:429, 1986.

859. Schuman JS and Friedman AH: Retinal manifestations of the acquired immune deficiency syndrome (AIDS): cytomegalovirus, Candida albicans, cryptococcus, toxoplasmosis and Pneumocystis carinii, Trans Ophthalmol Soc UK 103:177, 1983.

860. Schuman JS and others: Acquired immunodeficiency syndrome (AIDS), Surv Ophthalmol 31:384, 1987.

861. A and others: Pathologic features and immunofluorescent antibody demonstration of ocular microsporidiosis (encephalitozoon hellem) in seven patients with acquired immunodeficiency syndrome, Am J Ophthalmol 115:285, 1993.

862. Severin M and Hartmann C: Endothelial alterations in AIDS with cytomegalovirus infection, Ophthalmologica 196:7, 1988.

863. Shuler JD, Engstrom RE Jr, and Holland GN: External ocular disease and anterior segment disorders associated with AIDS, Int Ophthalmol Clin 29:98, 1989.

864. Shuler JD and others: Kaposi sarcoma of the conjunctiva and eyelids associated with the acquired immunodeficiency syndrome, Arch Ophthalmol 107:858, 1989.

865. Sidikaro Y and others: Rhegmatogenous retinal detachments in-patients with AIDS and necrotizing retinal infections, Ophthalmology 98:129, 1991.

866. Skolnik PR and others: Dual infection of retina with human immunodeficiency virus type 1 and cytomegalovirus, Am J Ophthalmol 107:361, 1989.

867. Smith ME: Retinal involvement in adult cytomegalic inclusion disease, Arch Ophthalmol 72:44, 1964.

868. Smith MG: Propagation in tissue cultures of a cytopathogenic virus from human salivary gland virus (SVG) disease, Proc Soc Exp Biol Med 92:424, 1956.

869. Smith RE: toxoplasmic retinochoroiditis as an emerging problem in AIDS patients, Am J Ophthalmol 106:738, 1988 (editorial).

870. Spaide RF and others: Frosted branch angiitis associated with cytomegalovirus retinitis, Am J Ophthalmol 113:522, 1992.

871. Specht CS and others: Ocular histoplasmosis with retinitis in a patient with acquired immune deficiency syndrome, Ophthalmology 98:1356, 1991.

872. Stanton CA and others: Acquired immunodeficiency syndrome—related primary intraocular lymphoma, Arch Ophthalmology 110:1614, 1992.

873. Stoumbos VD and Klein ML: Syphilitic retinitis in a patient with acquired immunodeficiency syndrome-related complex, Am J Ophthalmol 103:103, 1987.

874. Teich SA: Conjunctival vascular changes in AIDS and AIDS-related complex, Am J Ophthalmol 103:332, 1987.

875. Teich SA and others: Viral particles in the conjunctiva of a patient with the acquired immune deficiency syndrome, Am J Med 82:151, 1987.

876. Tenhula WN and others: Morphometric comparisons of optic nerve axon loss in acquired immunodeficiency syndrome, Am J Ophthalmol 113:14, 1992.

877. Theobald GD: Cytomegalic inclusion disease: report of a case, Am J Ophthalmol 47:52, 1959.

878. Thierfelder S, Linnert D, and Grehn F: Increased prevalence of HIV-related retinal microangiopathy syndrome in patients with hepatitis C, Arch Ophthalmol 114:899, 1996 (letter).

879. Tufail A, Weisz JM, and Holland GN: Endogenous bacterial endophthalmitis as a complication of intravenous therapy for cytomegalovirus retinopathy, Arch Ophthalmol 114:879, 1996 (letter).

880. Ullman S, Wilson RP, and Schwartz L: Bilateral angle-closure glaucoma in association with the acquired immune deficiency syndrome, Am J Ophthalmol 101:419, 1986.

881. Ussery FM III and others: Intravitreal ganciclovir in the treatment of AIDS-associated cytomegalovirus retinitis, Ophthalmology 95:640, 1988.

882. Visser OHE and Bos PJM: Kaposi's sarcoma of the conjunctiva and CMV-retinitis in AIDS, Doc Ophthalmol 64:77, 1986.

883. Walmsley SL, Crew E, and Read SE: Treatment of cytomegalovirus retinitis with trisodium phosphonoformate hexahydrate (Foscarnet), J Infect Dis 157:569, 1988.

884. Walter KA and others: Corneal endothelial deposits in patients with cytomegalovirus retinitis, Am J Ophthalmol 121:391, 1996.

885. Weinberg RS and Zaidman GW: Acquired syphilitic uveitis in homosexuals. In Saari KM, editor: Uveitis update, Amsterdam, 1984, Elsevier Science Publishers, BV.

886. Weiss A and others: Toxoplasmic retinochoroiditis as an initial manifestation of the acquired immune deficiency syndrome, Am J Ophthalmol, 101:248, 1986 (letter to the editor).

887. Weiter JJ, Jakobiec FA, and Iwamoto T: The clinical and morphologic characteristics of Kaposi's sarcoma of the conjunctiva, Am J Ophthalmol 89:546, 1980.

888. Weller TH: The cytomegaloviruses: ubiquitous agents with protean clinical manifestations (first of two parts), N Engl J Med 285:203, 1971.

889. Winston DJ and others: Cytomegalovirus infections associated with leukocyte transfusions, Ann Intern Med 93:671, 1980.

890. Winward KE and Curtin VT: Conjunctival squamous cell carcinoma in a patient with human immunodeficiency virus infection, Am J Ophthalmol 107:554, 1989.

891. Winward KE, Hamed LM, and Glaser JS: The spectrum of optic nerve disease in human immunodeficiency virus infection, Am J Ophthalmol 107:373, 1989.

892. Wofsy CB: Prevention of HIV transmission, Infect Dis Clin North Am 2(2):307, 1988.

893. Wong T-W and Warner NE: Cytomegalic inclusion disease in adults: report of 14 cases with review of literature, Arch Pathol 74(11):403, 1962.

894. Wormser GP and others: Human immunodeficiency virus infections: considerations for health care workers, Bull NY Acad Med 64:203, 1988.

895. Wyhinny J and others: Adult cytomegalic inclusion retinitis, Am J Ophthalmol 76:773, 1973.

Acute retinal necrosis syndromes

896. el Azazi M and others: Intrathecal antibody production against viruses of the herpes virus family in acute retinal necrosis syndrome, Am J Ophthalmol 112:76, 1991.

897. Avila MP and others: Manifestations of Whipple's disease in the posterior segment of the eye, Arch Ophthalmol 102:384, 1984.

898. Besen G and others: Long-term therapy for herpes retinitis in an animal model with high-concentrated liposome-encapsulated HPMPC, Arch Ophthalmol 113:661, 1995.

899. Blumenkranz MS and others: Acute multifocal hemorrhagic retinal vasculitis, Ophthalmology 95:1663, 1988.

900. de Boer JH and others: Detection of intraocular antibody production to herpes viruses in acute retinal necrosis syndrome, Am J Ophthalmol 117:201, 1994.

901. Browning DJ and others: Association of varicella zoster dermatitis with acute retinal necrosis syndrome, Ophthalmology 94:602, 1987.

902. Carney MD and others: Acute retinal necrosis, Retina 6:85, 1996.

903. Char and others: Primary intraocular lymphoma (ocular reticulum cell sarcoma): diagnosis and management, Ophthalmology 95:625, 1988.

904. Charles NC, Bennett TW, and Margolis S: Ocular pathology of the congenital varicella syndrome, Arch Ophthalmol 95:2034, 1977.

905. Chess J and others: Candida retinitis in bare lymphocyte syndrome, Ophthalmology 93:696, 1986.

906. Cibis GW, Flynn JT, and Davis EB: Herpes simplex retinitis, Arch Ophthalmol 96:299, 1978.

907. Clarkson JG and others: Retinal detachment following the acute retinal necrosis syndrome, Ophthalmology 91:1665, 1984.

908. Cochereau I and others: Ocular involvement in Epstein-Barr virus associated T-cell lymphoma, Am J Ophthalmol 121:322, 1996.

909. Culbertson WW and others: Chickenpox-associated acute retinal necrosis syndrome, Ophthalmology 98:1641, 1991.

910. Culbertson WW and others: The acute retinal necrosis syndrome. 2. Histopathology and etiology. Ophthalmology 89:1317, 1982.

911. Culbertson WW and others: Varicella zoster virus is a cause of the acute retinal necrosis syndrome, Ophthalmology 93:559, 1986.

912. Davis JL and others: Silicone oil repair of retinal detachments caused by necrotizing retinitis in HIV, Am J Ophthalmol 113:1401, 1995.

913. Duane TD, Osher RH, and Green WR: White centered hemorrhages: their significance, Ophthalmology 87:66, 1980.

914. Duker JS and Blumenkranz MS: Diagnosis and management of the acute retinal necrosis (ARN) syndrome, Surv Ophthalmol 35: 327, 1991.

915. Duker JS and others: Rapidly progressive acute retinal necrosis secondary to herpes simplex virus, type 1, Ophthalmology 97:1638, 1990.

916. Fisher JP and others: The acute retinal necrosis syndrome. 1. Clinical manifestations, Ophthalmology 89:1309, 1982.

917. Freeman WR and others: Demonstration of herpes group virus in acute retinal necrosis syndrome, J Ophthalmol 102:701, 1986.

918. Gass JDM and others: Diffuse unilateral subacute neuroretinitis, Ophthalmology 85:521, 1978.

919. Grevin CM and others: Progressive outer retinal necrosis syndrome secondary to caricella zoster virus in acquired immunodeficiency syndrome, Retina 15:14, 1995.

920. Grossnicklaus HE and others: Retinal necrosis in X-linked lymphoproliferative disease, Ophthalmology 101:705, 1994.

921. Haltia M and others: Measles retinopathy during immuno-suppression, Br J Ophthalmol 62:356, 1978.

922. Hedges TR III and Albert DM: The progression of the ocular abnormalities of herpes zoster. Histopathologic observations of nine cases, Ophthalmology 89:165, 1982.

923. Johnson BL and Wisotzkey HM: Neuroretinitis associated with

924. Karbassi, Raizman MB, and Schuman JS: Herpes zoster ophthalmicus, Surv Ophthalmol 36, 395, 1992 (major review).

925. Karma A and others: Diagnosis and clinical characteristics of ocular lyme borreliosis (see comments), Am J Ophthalmol 119:127, 1995.

926. Lewis ML and others: Herpes simplex virus type 1: a cause of the acute retinal necrosis syndrome, Ophthalmology 96:875, 1989.

927. Ludwig IH, Zegarra H, and Zakov ZN: The acute retinal necrosis syndrome: possible herpes simplex retinitis, Ophthalmology 91: 1659, 1984.

928. Matsuo T and others: Immune complex containing herpes virus antigen in a patient with acute retinal necrosis, Am J Ophthalmol 101:368, 1986.

929. Matsuo T and others: A proposed type of acute retinal necrosis syndrome, Am J Ophthalmol 105:579, 1988.

930. Nanda M and others: Ocular histopathologic findings in a case of human herpes b virus infection, Arch Ophthalmol 108:713, 1990.

931. Naumann G, Gass JDM, and Font RL: Histopathology of herpes zoster ophthalmicus, Am J Ophthalmol 65:533, 1968.

932. Naumann GOH and Apple DJ: Pathology of the eye, New York, 1985, Springer-Verlag, Inc (Translation, modification, and update by DJ Apple).

933. Newsom RW, Martin TJ, and Wasilauskas B: Cat-scratch disease diagnosed serologically using an enzyme immunoassay in a patient with neuroretinitis, Arch Ophthalmol 114:493, 1996.

934. Partamian LG, Morse PH, and Klein HZ: Herpes simplex type I retinitis in an adult with herpes zoster, Am J Ophthalmol 92:215, 1981.

935. Price FW and Schlaegel TF Jr: Bilateral acute retinal necrosis, Am J Ophthalmol 89:419, 1980.

936. Reynolds JD and others: Congenital herpes simples retinitis, Am J Ophthalmol 102:33, 1986.

937. Rummelt V and others: Detection of varicella zoster virus DNA and viral antigen in the late stage of bilateral acute retinal necrosis syndrome, Arch Ophthalmol 110:1132, 1992.

938. Rungger-Braendle E, Roux L, and Leuenberger PM: Bilateral acute retinal necrosis (BARN): identification of the presumed infectious agent, Ophthalmology 91:1648, 1984.

939. Rutzen AR and others: Clinicopathologic study of retinal and choroidal biopsies in intraocular inflammation, Am J Ophthalmol 119: 597, 1995.

940. Saari KM and others: Bilateral acute retinal necrosis, Am J Ophthalmol 93:103, 1982.

941. Shields JA and others: Cryptococcal chorioretinitis, Am J Ophthalmol 89:210, 1980.

942. Soushi S and others: Demonstration of varicella-zoster virus antigens in the vitreous aspirates of patients with acute retinal necrosis syndrome, Ophthalmology 95:1394, 1988.

943. Sternberg P Jr and others: Acute retinal necrosis syndrome, Retina 2:145, 1982.

944. Ulrich GG and others: Cat scratch disease associated with neuroretinitis in a 6 year old girl, Ophthalmology 99:246, 1992.

945. Uninsky E and others: Disseminated herpes simplex infection with retinitis in a renal allograft recipient, Ophthalmology 90:175, 1983.

946. Urayama A and others: Unilateral acute uveitis with retinal periarteritis and detachment, Jpn J Clin Ophthalmol 25:607, 1971.

947. Willerson D, Aaberg TM, and Reeser FH: Necrotizing vasoocclusive retinitis, Am J Ophthalmol 84:209, 1977.

948. Yanoff M, Allman MI, and Fine BS: Congenital herpes simplex virus, type 2 bilateral endophthalmitis, Trans Am Ophthalmol Soc 75:325, 1977.

949. Yoser SL, Forster DJ, and Rao NA: Systemic viral infections and their retinal and choroidal manifestations, Surv Ophthalmol 37: 313, 1993 (major review).

950. Young NJA and Bird AC: Bilateral acute retinal necrosis, Br J Ophthalmol 62:581, 1978.

Retinal dysplasia

951. Fulton AB and others: Human retinal dysplasia, Am J Ophthalmol 85:690, 1978.

952. Hunter WS and Zimmerman LE: Unilateral retinal dysplasia, Arch Ophthalmol 74:23, 1965.

953. Lahav M, Albert DM, and Wyand S: Clinical and histopathologic classification of retinal dysplasia, Am J Ophthalmol 75:648, 1973.

954. Reese AB and Blodi FC: Retinal dysplasia, Am J Ophthalmol 33: 23, 1950.

955. Reese AB and Straatsma BR: Retinal dysplasia, Am J Ophthalmol 45:199, 1958.

Peripheral retinal and choroidal dystrophies and degenerations

956. Adler R: Mechanisms of photoreceptor death in retinal degenerations. From the cell biology of the 1990s to the ophthalmology of the 21st century? Arch Ophthalmol 114:79, 1996 (review).

957. Albert DM, Pruett RC, and Craft JL: Transmission electron microscopic observation of vitreous abnormalities in retinitis pigmentosa, Am J Ophthalmol 101:665, 1986.

958. Ayazi A: Choroideremia, obesity and congenital deafness, Am J Ophthalmol 92:63, 1981.

959. Bachynski BN and others: Hyperglycemic acidotic coma and death in Kearns-Sayre syndrome, Ophthalmology 93:391, 1986.

960. Bastek JV, Foos RY, and Heckenlively J: Traumatic pigmentary retinopathy, Am J Ophthalmol 92:621, 1981.

961. Bastek JV, Foos RY, and Heckenlively J: Traumatic pigmentary retinopathy, Am J Ophthalmol 92:624, 1981.

962. Bateman JB and others: Heterogeneity of retinal degeneration and hearing impairment syndromes, Am J Ophthalmol 90:755, 1980.

963. Berson EL: Retinitis pigmentosa, Invest Ophthalmol Vis Sci 34: 671, 1993.

964. Berson EL and Adamian M: Ultrastructural findings in an autopsy eye from a patient with Usher's syndrome type II, Am J Ophthalmol 114:748, 1992.

965. Berson EL and others: Natural course of retinitis pigmentosa over a three-year interval, Am J Ophthalmol 99:240, 1985.

966. Betten MG, Bilchik RC, and Smith ME: Pigmentary retinopathy of myotonic dystrophy, Am J Ophthalmol 72:720, 1971.

967. Billimoria JD and others: Metabolism of phytanic acid in Refsum's disease, Lancet 1:194, 1982.

968. Bloome MA and Garcia CA: Manual of retinal and choroidal dystrophies, New York, 1982, Appleton-Century-Crofts.

969. Brosnahan DM and others: Pathology of hereditary retinal degeneration associated with hypobetalipoproteinemia, Ophthalmology 101:38, 1994.

970. Brown GC and others: Radiation retinopathy, Ophthalmology 89: 1494, 1982.

971. Buchanan TAS, Gardiner TA, and Archer DB: an ultrastructural study of retinal photoreceptor degeneration associated with bronchial carcinoma, Am J Ophthalmol 97:277, 1984.

972. Cameron JD, Fine BS, and Shapiro I: Histopathologic observations in choroideremia with emphasis on vascular changes of the uveal tract, Ophthalmology 94:187, 1987.

973. Campo RV and Aaberg TM: Ocular and systemic manifestations of the Bardet-Biedl syndrome, Am J Ophthalmol 91:750, 1982.

974. Chen JC, Fitzke FW, and Bird AC: Long-term effect of acetazolamide in a patient with retinitis pigmentos, Invest Ophthalmol Vis Sci 31:1914, 1990.

975. Cherry PM: Usher's syndrome, Ann Ophthalmol 5:743, 1973.

976. Cogan DG: Pseudorentinitis pigmentosa, Arch Ophthalmol 81:45, 1969.

977. Cogan DG and others: Ocular abnormalities in abetalipoproteinemia: a clincopathologic correlation, Ophthalmology 91:991, 1984.

978. Corwin JM and Weiter JJ: Immunology of chorioretinal disorders, Surv Ophthalmol 25:287, 1984.

979. Cotlier E, Maumenee IH, and Berman ER, editors: Genetic eye diseases—retinitis pigmentosa and other inherited eye disorders: proceedings of the International Symposium on Genetics and Ophthalmology, Sept 1981, Jerusalem, NY, 1982, Alan R Liss, Inc.

980. Cross HE: Genetic counseling, Trans Am Acad Ophthalmol Otolaryngol 76:1203, 1972.

981. Crouch, ER Jr and Apple DJ: Posttraumatic migration of retinal pigment epithelial melanin, Am J Ophthalmol 78:251, 1974.

982. DeBustros S and others: Bilateral astrocytic hamartomas of the optic nerve heads in retinitis pigmentosa, Retina 3:21, 1983.

983. De Jong TVM and Delleman JW: Pigment epithelial pattern dystrophy. Four different manifestations in a family, Arch Ophthalmol 100:1416, 1982.

984. Detrick B and others: Expression of HLA-DR antigen on retinal pigment epithelial cells in retinitis pigmentosa, Am J Ophthalmol 101:584, 1986.

985. Dryja TP and others: A point mutation of the rhodopsin gene in one form of retinitis pigmentosa, Nature 343, 1990.

986. Eagle RC Jr, Hedges TR, and Yanoff M: The Kearns-Sayre syndrome: a light and electron microscopic study, Trans Am Ophthalmol Soc 80:218, 1982.

987. Eagle RC Jr, Hedges TR, and Yanoff M: The atypical pigmentary retinopathy of Kearns-Sayer syndrome. A light and electron microscopic study, Ophthalmology 89:1433, 1982.

988. Ellis DS and Heckenlively JR: Retinitis punctata albescens: fundus appearance and functional abnormalities, Retina 3:27, 1983.

989. Eshaghian J, Rafferty NS, and Gossens W: Ultrastructure of human cataract in retinitis pigmentosa, Arch Ophthalmol 98:2227, 1980.

990. Fishman GA, Fishman M, and Maggiano J: Macular lesions associated with retinitis pigmentosa, Arch Ophthalmol 95:798, 1977.

991. Fishman GA, Maggiano JM, and Fishman M: Foveal lesions seen in retinitis pigmentosa, Arch Ophthalmol 95:1993, 1977.

992. Fishman GA, Alexander KR, and Anderson RJ: Autosomal dominant retinitis pigmentosa. A method of classification, Arch Ophthalmol 103:366, 1985.

993. Fishman GA and others: Usher's syndrome. Ophthalmic and neuro-otologic findings suggesting genetic heterogeneity, Arch Ophthalmol 101:1367, 1983.

994. Fishman GA, Lam BL, and Anderson RJ: Racial differences in the prevalence of atrophic-appearing macular lesions between black and white patients with retinitis pigmentosa, Am J Ophthalmol 118:33, 1994.

995. Flannery JG and others: Degenerative changes in a retina affected with autosomal dominant retinitis pigmentosa, Invest Ophthalmol Vis Sci 30:191, 1989.

996. Fogle JA, Welch RB, and Green WB: Retinitis pigmentosa and exudative vasculopathy, Arch Ophthalmol 96:696, 1978.

997. Foos RY and Simons KB: Vitreous in lattice degeneration of retina, Ophthalmology 91:452, 1984.

998. Franceschetti A, Francois J, and Babel J: Chorioretinal heredodegenerations, Springfield, Ill, 1974, Charcles C Thomas, Publisher.

999. Francois J: The differential diagnosis of tapetoretinal degenerations, Arch Ophthalmol 59:88, 1958.

1000. Francois J: Metabolic tapetoretinal degenerations, Surv Ophthalmol 26:293, 1982.

1001. Francois J and Neetens A: Bardet-Biedl syndrome and keratoconus, Ophthalmic Paediatr Genet 2:199, 1983.

1002. Garner A and others: Tapetoretinal degeneration in the cerebro-hepato-renal (Zellweger's) syndrome, Br J Ophthalmol 66:422, 1982.

1003. Gartner S and Henkind P: Pathology of retinitis pigmentosa, Ophthalmology 89:1425, 1982.

1004. Goebel HH, Zeman W, and Damaske E: An ultrastructural study of the retina in the Jansky-Bielschowsky type of neuronal ceroid-lipofuscinosis, Am J Ophthalmol 83:70, 1977.

1005. Goldberg MF and others: Histopathologic study of autosomal dominant vitreoretinochoroidopathy. Peripheral annular pigmentary dystrophy of the retina, Ophthalmology 96:1736, 1989.

1006. Gorin MB and others: A peripherin/retinal degeneration slow mutation (Pro-210-Arg) associated with macular and peripheral retinal degeneration, Ophthalmology 102:246, 1995.

1007. Green JL and Rabb MF: Degeneration of Bruch's membrane and retinal pigment epithelium, Int Ophthalmol Clin 23(3)27, 1981.

1008. Green JS and others: The cardinal manifestation of Bardet-Biedl syndrome, a form of Laurence-Moon-Biedl syndrome, N Engl J Med 321:1002, 1989.

1009. Grizzard WS, Deutman AF, and Pinckers AJLG: Retinal dystrophies associated with peripheral retinal vasculopathy, Br J Ophthalmol 62:188, 1978.

1010. Grützer P and Vogel M: Klinischer Verlauf und histologischer Befund bei progressive tapetochoriodealer Degeneration (Choroideremie), Klin Monatsbl Augenheilkd 162:206, 1973.

1011. Hansen RI and others: The association of retinitis pigmentosa with preretinal macular gliosis, Br J Ophthalmol 61:597, 1977.

1012. Hsich RC, Fine BS, and Lyons JS: Patterned dystrophies of the retinal pigment epithelium, Arch Ophthalmol 95:429, 1977.

1013. Kaiser-Kupfer MI and others: Clinical biochemical correlations in Bietti's crystalline dystrophy, Am J Ophthalmol 118:569, 1994.

1014. Kennaway NG, Weleber RG, and Buist NRM: Gyrate atrophy of the choroid and retina with hyperornithinemia. Biochemical and histologic studies and response to vitamin B6, Am J Hum Genet 32:529, 1980.

1015. Khan JA, Ide CH, and Strickland MP: Coats-type retinitis pigmentosa, Surv Ophthalmol 32:317, 1988.

1016. Kolb H and Gouras P: Electron microscopic observations of human retinitis pigmentosa, dominantly inherited, Invest Ophthalmol 13:487, 1974.

1017. Krill AE: Hereditary retinal and choroidal diseases, vol I, Evaluation, 1972; vol II, Clinical consideration, 1977, New York, Harper & Row, Publishers.

1018. Krill AE and Archer D: Classification of the choroidal atrophies, Am J Ophthalmol 72:562, 1971.

1019. Krill AE, Archer D, and Martin D: Sector retinitis pigmentosa, Am J Ophthalmol 69:977, 1970.

1020. Lahav M and others: Advanced pigmentary retinal degeneration: an ultrastructural study. Retina 2:65, 1982.

1021. Landers MB III, editors: Retinitis pigmentosa: clinical implications of current research, New York, 1977, Plenum Publishing Corp.

1022. Laurence JZ and Moon RC: Four cases of retinitis pigmentosa occuring the same family and accompanied by general imperfections of development, Ophthalmol Rev 2:32, 1866.

1023. Leber T: Ueber Retinitis pigmentosa und angeborene Amaurose, Graefes Arch Ophthalmol 15:1, 1869.

1024. L'Esperence FA Jr, editor: Current diagnosis and management of chorioretinal diseases, St Louis, 1977, The CV Mosby Co.

1025. Leveille AS, Morse PH, and Kiernan JP: Autosomal dominant central pigment epithelial and choroidal degeneration, Ophthalmol 89:1407, 1982.

1026. Levin PS and others: Histopathology of the eye in Cocayne's syndrome, Arch Ophthalmol 101:1093, 1983.

1027. Lewis H and others: Reticular degeneration of the pigment epithelium, Ophthalmology 92:1485, 1985.

1028. Little CW and others: Transplantation of human fetal retinal pigment epithelium rescues photoreceptor cells from degeneration in the royal college of surgeons rat retina, Invest Ophthalmol Vis Sci 37:204, 1996.

1029. Li ZY, Possin DE, and Milam AH: Histopathology of bone spicule pigmentation in retinitis pigmentosa, Ophthalmology 102:805, 1995.

1030. Luckenbach MW and others: Ocular clinicopathologic correlation of Hallervorden-Spatz syndrome with acanthocystosis and pigmentary retinopathy, Am J Ophthalmol 95:369, 1983.

1031. Marmor MF and Byers B: Pattern dystrophy of the pigment epithelium, Am J Ophthalmol 84:32, 1977.

1032. Marmor MF and others: Retinitis pigmentosa: a symposium on terminology and methods of examination, Ophthalmology 90:126, 1983.

1033. McCulloch JC: The pathologic findings in two cases of choroideremia, Trans Am Acad Ophthalmol Otolaryngol 54:565, 1950.

1034. McCulloch, JC and others: Hyperornithinemia and gyrate atrophy of the choroid and retina, Ophthalmology 85:918, 1978.

1035. Merin S and Auerbach A: Retinitis pigmentosa, Surv Ophthalmol 20:303, 1976.

1036. Meyer KT: Dominant retinitis pigmentosa: a clinicopathologic correlation, Ophthalmology 89:1414, 1982.

1037. Michaelson IC, editor: Textbook of the fundus of the eye, ed 3, New York, 1981, Churchill Livingstone, Inc.

1038. Milam AH and others: Clinicopathologic effects of the q64ter rhodopsin mutation in retinitis pigmentosa, Invest Ophthalmol Vis Sci 37:753, 1996.

1039. Miller FS III, Bunt-Milam AH, and Kalina RE: Clinical ultrastructural study of thioridazine retinopathy, Ophthalmology 89:1478, 1982.

1040. Mizuno K and others: Leber's congenital amaurosis, Am J Ophthalmol 83:32, 1977.

1041. Nakazawa M and others: Variable expressivity in a Japanese family with autosomal dominant retinitis pigmentosa closely linked to chromosome 19q, Arch Ophthalmol Surv Ophthalmol 34:237, 1990.

1042. Newsome DA and others: Clinical and serum lipid findings in a large family with autosomal dominant retinitis pigmentosa, Ophthalmology 95:1691, 1988.

1043. Newsome DA and Michaels RG: Detection of lymphocytes in the vitreous gel of patients with retinitis pigmentosa, Am J Ophthalmol 105:596, 1988.

1044. Newsome DA and others: Cellular immune status in retinitis pigmentosa, Ophthalmology 95:1696, 1988.

1045. Nishida S and Mizuno K: Electron microscopy of pigmentary degeneration of the human retina, Acta Soc Ophthalmol Jpn 75:1779, 1971.

1046. Noble KG and Carr RE: Leber's congenital amaurosis: A retrospective study of 33 cases and a histopathological study of one case, Arch Ophthalmol 96:818, 1978.

1047. Noble KG and Carr RE: Peripapillary pigmentary retinal degeneration, Am J Ophthalmol 86:65, 1978.

1048. Noble KG, Care RE, and Siegel, IM: Pigment epithelial dystrophy, Am J Ophthalmol 83:751, 1977.

1049. Noble KG: Peripapillary (pericentral) pigmentary retinal degeneration, Am J Ophthalmol 108:686, 1989.

1050. Noble KG: Hereditary pigmented paravenous chorioretinal atrophy, Am J Ophthalmol 108:365, 1989.

1051. Noble KG and Carr RE: Pigmented paravenous chorioretinal atrophy, Am J Ophthalmol 96:338, 1983.

1052. Novack RL and Foos RY: Drusen of the optic disk in retinitis pigmentosa, Am J Ophthalmol 103:44, 1987.

1053. Pagon RA: Retinitis pigmentosa, Surv Ophthalmol 33:137, 1988.

1054. Pameyer J, Waardenberg P, and Henkes H: Choroideremia, Br J Ophthalmol 44:724, 1960.

1055. Pillai S, Limaye SR, and Saimovici L-B: Optic disc hamartoma associated with retinitis pigmentosa, Retina 3:24, 1983.

1056. Porta A and others: Preserved para-arteriolar retinal pigment epithelium retinitis pigmentosa, Am J Ophthalmol 113:161, 1992.

1057. Pruett RC: Retinitis pigmentosa: clinical observations and correlations, Trans Am Ophthalmol Soc 81:693, 1983.

1058. Puck A, Tso, MOM, and Fishman GA: Drusen of the optic nerve associated with retinitis pigmentosa, Arch Ophthalmol 103:231, 1985.

1059. Rafuse EV, and McCulloch, JC: Choroideremia: a pathologic report, Can J Ophthalmol 3:347, 1968.

1060. Ramsey MS and Fine BS: Chloroquine toxicity in the human eye: histopathologic observations by electron microscopy, Am J Ophthalmol 73:229, 1972.

1061. Rayborn, ME, Moorhead, LC, and Hollyfield JG: A dominantly inherited chorioretinal degeneration resembling sectoral retinitis pigmentosa, Ophthalmology 89:1441, 1982.

1062. Reinstein NM and Chalfin AE: Inverse retinitis pigmentosa, deafness and hypogenitalism, Am J Ophthalmol 72:332, 1971.

1063. Richards SC and Creel DJ: Pattern dystrophy and retinitis pigmentosa caused by a pareipherin/RDS mutation, Retina 15:68, 1995.

1064. Robertson DM, Link FP, and Rostvold JA: Snowflake degeneration of the retina, Ophthalmology 89:1513, 1982.

1065. Rodger RC: Further study of the relation of vitamin A to retinal degeneration, Trans Ophthalmol Soc UK 98:128, 1978.

1066. Rodrigues MM and others: Retinitis pigmentosa with segmental massive retinal gliosis. An immunohistochemical, biochemical, and ultrastructural study, Ophthalmology 94:180, 1987.

1067. Roth, AM and others: Pigmentary retinal dystrophy in Hallervorden-Spatz disease: clinicopathologic report of a case, Surv Ophthalmol 16:24, 1971.

1068. Runge P and others: Histopathology of mitochondrial cytopathy and the Laurence-Moon-Biedl syndrome, Br J Ophthalmol 70:782, 1986.

1069. Santos-Anderson RM, Tso MOM, and Fishman GA: A histopathologic study of retinitis pigmentosa, Ophthalmol Paediatr Genet 1:151, 1982.

1070. Sarks S II: Senile choroidal sclerosis, Br J Ophthalmol 57:98, 1973.

1071. Schmoger E, Busch I, and Lukassek B: Histologischer Beitrag zur Choroideremie, Ophthalmologica 166:144, 1973.

1072. Schochet SS, Font RL, and Morris HH III: Jansky-Bielschowsky form of neuronal ceroid-lipofuscinosis: ocular pathology of the Batten-Vogt syndrome, Arch Ophthalmol 98:1083, 1980.

1073. Shields JA, Green WR, and McDonald PR: Uveal psuedomelanoma due to post-traumatic pigmentary migration, Arch Ophthalmol 89:519, 1973.

1074. Sorsby A: Choroidal angiosclerosis, Br J Ophthalmol 22:443, 1939.

1075. Straatsma BR and others: Fluorescein angiography in reticular degeneration of the pigment epithelium, Am J Ophthalmol 100:202, 1985.

1076. Szamier RB: Ultrastructure of the preretinal membrane in retinitis pigmentosa, Invest Ophthalmol Vis Sci 21:227, 1981.

1077. Szamier RB and Berson EL: Retinal histopathology of a carrier of X-chromosome-linked retinitis pigmentosa, Ophthalmology 92: 271, 1985.

1078. Takki K: Differential diagnosis between the primary total choroidal vascular atrophies, Br J Ophthalmol 58:24, 1974.

1079. Takki K: Gyrate atrophy of the choroid and retina associated with hyperornithinaemia, Br J Ophthalmol 58:3, 1974.

1080. Tolentino F, Schopens C, and Freeman H: Vitreoretinal disorders, Philadelphia, 1976, WB Saunders Co.

1081. Toussaint D and Danis P: An ocular pathologic study of Refsum's syndrome, Am J Ophthalmol 72:342, 1971.

1082. Traboulsi E, O'Neill JF, and Maumenee I: Autosomal recessive pericentral pigmentary retinopathy, Arch Ophthalmol 106:5321, 1988.

1083. Vainisi SJ, Beck BB, and Apple DJ: Retinal degeneration in a baboon, Am J Ophthalmol 78:279, 1974.

1084. Watzke RC, Folk JC, and Lang RM: Pattern dystrophy of the retinal pigment epithelium, Ophthalmology 89:1400, 1982.

1085. Weiter J and Fine BS: A histologic study of regional choroidal dystrophy, Am J Ophthalmol 83:741, 1977.

1086. Weleber RG and others: Phenotypic variation including retinitis pigmentosa, pattern dystrophy, and fundus flavimaculatus in a single family with a deletion of codon 153 or 154 of the peripheral RDS gene, Arch Ophthalmol 111:1531, 1993.

1087. Wilson DJ and Green WR: Systemic diseases with retinitis pigmentosa-like changes, Md Med J 35:1011, 1986.

1088. Wilson DJ and others: Bietti's crystalline dystrophy, Arch Ophthalmol 107:213, 1989.

1089. Wilson DJ, Weleber RG, and Green WR: Ocular clinicopathologic study of gyrate atrophy, Am J Ophthalmol 111:24, 1991.

1090. Wong F: Photoreceptor apoptosis in animal models; implications for retinitis pigmentosa research, Arch Ophthalmol 113:1245,

Retinal degenerations, retinal breaks, and retinal detachments

1091. Anonymous: The repair of rhegmatogenous retinal detachments, American Academy of Ophthalmology, Ophthalmology 103:1313, 1996.

1092. Arroyo JG and Irvine AR: Retinal distortion and cotton-wool spots associated with epiretinal membrane contraction, Ophthalmology 102:662, 1995.

1093. Baker T and Spencer W: Ocular findings in multiple myeloma, Arch Ophthalmol 91:110, 1974.

1094. Bastek JV and others: Chorioretinal juncture. Pigmentary patterns of the peripheral fundus, Ophthalmology 89:1455, 1982.

1095. Baudouin C and others: Immunohistologic study of epiretinal membranes in proliferative vitreoretinopathy, Am J Ophthalmol 108:387, 1989.

1096. Baudouin C and others: Immunohistologic study of proliferative vitreoretinopathy, Am J Ophthalmol 110:593, 1990.

1097. Bedord M and Chegnell A: U-shaped retinal tear associated with presumed malignant melanoma of the choroid, Br J Ophthalmol 54:200, 1970.

1098. Benson WE: Retinal detachment: diagnosis and management, New York, 1980, Harper & Row, Publishers.

1099. Benson WE, Nantawan P, and Morse PH: Characteristics and prognosis of retinal detachments with demarcation lines, Am J Ophthalmol 84:641, 1977.

1100. Binder S and Riss B: Advances in intraocular techniques in the treatment of retinal detachments arising from holes in the posterior pole, Br J Ophthalmol 67:147, 1983.

1101. Blair NP and others: Hereditary progressive arthro-ophthalmopathy of Stickler, Am J Ophthalmol 88:876, 1979.

1102. Blight R and Hart JCD: Histological changes in the internal retinal layers produced by concussive injuries to the globe: an experimental study, Trans Ophthalmol Soc UK 98:270, 1978.

1103. Boehringer HR: Statistisches zur Häufigkeit und Risiko der Netzhautablösung, Ophthalmologica 131:331, 1956.

1104. Boldrey EE and others: The histopathology of familial exudative vitreoretinopathy: a report of two cases, Arch Ophthalmol 103:238, 1985.

1105. Brockhurst R and Schepens C: Uveal effusion, Arch Ophthalmol 70:101, 1963.

1106. Brubaker RJ and Pederson JE: Ciliochoroidal detachment, Surv Ophthalmol 27:281, 1983.

1107. Burton TC: Recovery of visual acuity after retinal detachment involving the macula, Trans Am Ophthalmol Soc 80:175, 1982.

1108. Burton TC: The influence of the refractive error and lattice degeneration on the incidence of retinal detachment, Trans Am Ophthalmol Soc 87:143, 1989.

1109. Byer NE: Clinical study of senile retinoschisis, Arch Ophthalmol 79:36, 1968.

1110. Byer NE: Changes in and prognosis of lattice degeneration of the retina, Trans Am Acad Ophthalmol Otolaryngol 78:114, 1974.

1111. Byer NE: Lattice degeneration of the retina, Surv Ophthalmol 23: 213, 1979.

1112. Byer NE: Cystic retinal tufts and their relationship to retinal detachment, Arch Ophthalmol 99:1788, 1981.

1113. Byer NE: The natural history of asymptomatic retinal breaks, 89: 1033, 1982.

1114. Byer NE: Long-term natural history of lattice degeneration of the retina, Ophthalmology 96:1396, 1989.

1115. Byer NE: Long-term natural history study of senile retinoschisis with implication for management, Ophthalmology 93:1127, 1986.

1116. Campo RV, Reeser FH, and Flindall RJ: Vascular leakage, neovascularization and vitreous hemorrhage in senile bullous retinoschisis, Am J Ophthalmol 95:826, 1983.

1117. Charteris DG and others: Proliferative vitreoretinopathy. Lymphocytes in epiretinal membranes, Ophthalmology 99:1364, 1992.

1118. Christmas NJ and others: Treatment of retinal breaks with autologous serum in an experimental model, Ophthalmology 102:263, 1995.

1119. Cibis GW, Watzke RC, and Chau J: Retinal hemorrhages in posterior vitreous detachment, Am J Ophthalmol 80:1043, 1975.

1120. Cibis P: Vitreoretinal pathology and surgery in retinal detachment, St Louis, 1965, The CV Mosby Co.

1121. Clark E: Ophthalmological complications of multiple myelomatosis, Br J Ophthalmol 39:233, 1955.

1122. Cleary PE, Minckler DS, and Ryan SJ: Ultrastructure of traction retinal detachment in rhesus monkey eyes after a posterior penetrating ocular injury, Am J Ophthalmol 90:829, 1980.

1123. Combs JL and Welch RB: Retinal breaks without detachment: natural history, management and long-term follow-up, Trans Am Ophthalmol Soc 80:64, 1982.

1124. Cox M, Schepens C, and Freeman H: Retinal detachment due to ocular contusion, Arch Ophthalmol 76:678, 1966.

1125. Davis M: The natural history of retinal breaks without detachment, Trans Am Ophthalmol Soc 71:343, 1973.

1126. Delaney WV Jr, Oates RP: Retinal detachment in the second eye, Arch Ophthalmol 96:629, 1978.

1127. DeLuise VP and others: Syphilitic retinal detachment and uveal effusion, Am J Ophthalmol 94:757, 1982.

1128. Eagle RC Jr, Yanoff M, and Morse P: Anterior segment necrosis following scleral buckling in hemoglobin SC disease, Am J Ophthalmol 75:426, 1973.

1129. Eisner G: Biomicroscopy of the peripheral fundus, Surv Ophthalmol 17:1, 1972.

1130. El Baba F and others: Clinicopathologic correlation of lipidization and detachment of the retinal pigment epithelium, Am J Ophthalmol 101:576, 1986.

1131. Elner SG and others: Anterior proliferative vitreoretinopathy: clinicopathologic, light microscopic, and ultrastructural findings, Ophthalmology 95:1349, 1988.

1132. Feman SS and Lam KW: An enzyme histochemical analysis of human subretinal fluid, Arch Ophthalmol 96:129, 1978.

1133. Folk JC and Burton TC: Bilateral aphakic retinal detachment, Retina 3:1, 1983.

1134. Foos, RY: Zonular traction tufts of the peripheral retina in cadaver eyes, Arch Ophthalmol 82:620, 1969.

1135. Foos, RY: Posterior vitreous detachment, Trans Am Acad Ophthalmol Otolaryngol 76:480, 1972.

1136. Foos, RY and Allen R: Retinal tears and lesser lesions of the peripheral retina in autopsy eyes, Am J Ophthalmol 64:643, 1967.

1137. Foos RY and Feman S: Reticular cystoid degeneration of the peripheral retina, Am J Ophthalmol 69:392, 1970.

1138. Foos RY, Spencer L, and Straatsma, BR: Trophic degeneration of the peripheral retina. In New Orleans Academy of Ophthalmology: Symposium on retina and retinal surgery: transaction of the New

Orleans Academy of Ophthalmology, St Louis, 1969, The CV Mosby Co.

1139. Foos RY: Ultrastructural features of posterior vitreous detachment, Albrecht von Graefes Arch Klin Ophthalmol 196:103, 1975.

1140. Foos RY: Retinal holes, Am J Ophthalmol 86:354, 1978.

1141. Foos RY and Simons KB: Vitreous in lattice degeneration of retina, Ophthalmology 91:452, 1984.

1142. Fuhshuku N and Ohba N: Congential retinal non-attachment associated with the Dandy-Walker syndrome, Ophthalmol Paediatr Genet 2:21, 1983.

1143. Gärtner J: Fine structure of pars plana cysts, Am J Ophthalmol 73:971, 1972.

1144. Gass JDM: Retinal detachment and narrow-angle glaucoma, Am J Ophthalmol 64:612, 1967.

1145. Gass JDM: Bullous retinal detachment: an unusual manifestation of idiopathic central serous choroidopathy, Am J Ophthalmol 75:810, 1973.

1146. Gass JDM and Little H: Bilateral bullous exudative retinal detachment complicating idiopathic central serous chorioretinopathy during systeming corticosteroid therapy, Ophthalmology 102:737, 1995.

1147. Glaser BM, Cardin A, and Biscoe B: Proliferative vitreoretinopathy. The mechanism of development of vitreoretinal traction, Ophthalmology 94:327, 1987.

1148. Glazer LC and others: Improved surgical treatment of familial exudative vitreoretinopathy in children, Am J Ophthalmol 120, 471, 1995.

1149. Gonin J: Le décollement de la rétine, Lausanne, 1934, Librairie Payot & Cie.

1150. Göttiner W: Senile retionoschisis: morphological relationship of the formation of spaces within the peripheral retina to senile retinoschisis and to schisis detachment, Stuttgart, 1978, Georg Thieme Verlag.

1151. Green WR and Wilson DJ: Choroidal neovascularization, Ophthalmology 93:1169, 1986.

1152. Grignolo A, Schepens C, and Health P: Cysts of the pars plana ciliaris, Arch Ophthalmol 58:530, 1957.

1153. Hardwick C and others: Pathologic human vitreous promotes contraction by fibroblasts; implication for proliferative vitreoretinopathy, Arch Ophthalmol 113:1545, 1995.

1154. Hilton G and others: The classification of retinal detachment with proliferative vitreoretinopathy, Ophthalmology 90:121, 1983.

1155. Inomata H: Electron microscopic observations on cystoid degeneration in the peripheral retina, Jpn J Ophthalmol 10:26, 1966.

1156. Jaffe NS: Vitreous traction at the posterior pole of the fundus due to alterations in the posterior vitreous, Trans Am Acad Ophthalmol Otolaryngol 71:642, 1967.

1157. Jaffe NS: The vitreous in clinical ophthalmology, St Louis, 1969, The CV Mosby Co.

1158. Jerdan JA and others: Proliferative vitreoretinopathy membranes. An immunohistochemical study, Ophthalmology 96:801, 1989.

1159. Johnson B: Proteinaceous cysts of the ciliary epithelium. II. Their occurrence in nonmyelomatous hypergammaglobulinemic conditions, Arch Ophthalmol 84:171, 1970.

1160. Johnson B and Storey J: Proteinaceous cysts of the ciliary epithelium. I. Their clear nature and immuno-electrophoretic analysis in a case of multiple myeloma, Arch Ophthalmol 84:166, 1970.

1161. Johnson NF and Foulds WS: Observations on the retinal pigment epithelium and retinal macrophanges in experimental retinal detachment, Br J Ophthalmol 61:564, 1977.

1162. Kaplan HJ and Aaberg TM: Birdshot retinochoroidopathy, Am J Ophthalmol, 90:773, 1980.

1163. Katz B and Hoyt WF: Intrapapillary and peripapillary hemorrhage in young patients with incomplete posterior vitreous detachment. Signs of vitreopapillary traction, Ophthalmology 102:349, 1995.

1164. Kinyoun JL and Knobloch WH: Idiopathic retinal dialysis, Retina 4:9, 1984.

1165. Klein BR and others: Fundus photographic and fluorescein angiographic characteristics of pseudoholes of the macula in eyes with epiretinal membranes, Ophthalmology 102:768, 1995.

1166. Kloess G: Ueber Strangbildungen im Glaskörper, Klin Monatsbl Augenheilkd 88:161, 1932.

1167. Kono T, Kohno T, and Inomata H: Epiretinal membrane formation. Light and electron microscopic study in an experimental rabbit model, Arch Ophthalmol 113:359, 1995.

1168. Knorr HL and Jonas JB: Retinal detachments by squash ball accidents, Am J Ophthalmol 122:260, 1996.

1169. Krill AE: Hereditary retinal and choroidal diseases, vol 1, Evaluation, New York, 1972, Harper & Row, Publishers.

1170. Knapp AJ, Gartner S, and Henkind P: Multiple myeloma and its ocular manifestations, Surv Ophthalmol 31:343, 1987.

1171. Kozart D and Scheie H: Spontaneous cysts of ciliary epithelium, Trans Am Acad Ophthalmol Otolaryngol 74:534, 1970.

1172. Lambert SR and others: Serous retinal detachments in thrombotic thrombocytopenic purpura, Arch Ophthalmol 103:1172, 1985.

1173. Landers MB III and Robinson CH: Photocoagulation in the diagnosis of senile retinoschisis, Am J Ophthalmol 84:18, 1977.

1174. Laqua H and Machemer R: Glial cell proliferation in retinal detachment (massive periretinal proliferation), Am J Ophthalmol 80:602, 1975.

1175. Lewis H and others: Subretinal membranes in proliferative vitreoretinopathy, Ophthalmology 96:1403, 1989.

1176. Lincoff H and others: Retinoschisis associated with optic nerve pits, Arch Ophthalmol 106:61, 1988.

1177. Lopez PF and others: Pathogenetic mechanisms in anterior proliferative vitreoretinopathy, Am J Ophthalmol 114:257, 1992.

1178. Machemer R: Pathogenesis and classification of massive periretinal proliferation, Br J Ophthalmol 62:737, 1978.

1179. Machemer R, Van Horn D, and Aaberg, TM: Pigment epithelial proliferation in human retinal detachment with massive periretinal proliferation, Am J Ophthalmol 85:181, 1978.

1180. Machemer R: The importance of fluid absorption, traction, intraocular currents, and chorioretinal scars in the therapy of rhegmatogenous retinal detachments, Am J Ophthalmol 98:681, 1984.

1181. Machemer R and others: An updated classification of retinal detachment with proliferative vitreoretinopathy, Am J Ophthalmol 112:159, 1991.

1182. Marcus DF and Aaberg TM: Intraretinal macrocysts in retinal detachment, Arch Ophthalmol 97:1273, 1979.

1183. Matsuo N and others: Photoreceptor outer segments in the aqueous humor in rhegmatogenous retinal detachment, Am J Ophthalmol 101:673, 1986.

1184. Maumenee IH, Stoll HU, and Mets MB: The Wagner syndrome versus hereditary arthoophthalmopathy. Tran Am Ophthalmol Soc 80:349, 1982.

1185. McDonald HR, Johnson RN, and Schatz H: Surgical results in the vitreomacular traction syndrome, Ophthalmology 101:1397, 1994.

1186. McPherson A: New and controversial aspects of retinal detachment, New York, 1968, Harper & Row, Publishers.

1187. Meyer E and Kurz GH: Retinal pits: a study of pathologic findings in two cases, Arch Ophthalmol 70:102, 1963.

1188. New Orleans Academy of Ophthalmology: Symposium on retina and retinal surgery: transaction of the New Orleans Academy of Ophthalmology, St Louis, 1969, The CV Mosby Co.

1189. Nork TM and others: Selective loss of blue cones and rods in human retinal detachment, Arch Ophthalmol 113:1066, 1995.

1190. O'Connor P, editor: Retinal detachment, Int Ophthalmol Clin 16, 1976.

1191. Okun E: Gross and microscopic pathology in autopsy eye. I. Introduction and long posterior ciliary nerves, Am J Ophthalmol 50:424, 1960.

1192. Okun E: Gross and microscopic pathology in autopsy eyes. II. Peripheral chorioretinal atrophy, Am J Ophthalmol 50:574, 1960.

1193. Okun E: Gross and microscopic pathology in autopsy eyes. III. Retinal breaks without detachment, Am J Ophthalmol 51:369, 1961.

1194. Okun E: Gross and microscopic pathology in autopsy eyes. IV. Pars plana cysts, Am J Ophthalmol 51:1221, 1961.

1195. O'Malley P and Allen RA: Peripheral cystoid degeneration of the retina: incidence and distribution of 1,000 autopsy eyes, Arch Ophthalmol 77:769, 1965.

1196. O'Malley P and others: Paving stone degeneration of the retina, Arch Ophthalmol 73:169, 1965.

1197. Palestine AG and others: Progressive subretinal fibrosis and uveitis, Br J Ophthalmol 68:667, 1984.

1198. Percival SPB, Anand V, and Das SK: Prevalence of aphakic retinal detachment, Br J Ophthalmol 67:43, 1983.

1199. Peyman GA and Sanders DR: Advances in uveal surgery, vitreous surgery, and the treatment of endophthalmitis, West Nyack, NJ, 1975, Prentice-Hall, Inc.

1200. Phelps C and Burton T: Glaucoma and retinal detachment, Arch Ophthalmol 95:418, 1977.

1201. Pruett R and Regan C, editors: Retina Congress: 25th Anniversary Meeting of the Retina Service, Massachusetts Eye and Ear Infirmary, New York, 1972, Appleton-Century-Crofts.

1202. Pruett R and Schepens C: Posterior hyperplastic primary vitreous, Am J Ophthalmol 69:535, 1970.

1203. Regenbogen L and others: Retinal breaks secondary to vascular accidents, Am J Ophthalmol 84:187, 1977.

1204. Rizzo JF III, Berson EL, and Lessell S: Retinal and neurologic findings in the Laurence-Moon-Bardet-Biedl phenotype, Ophthalmology 93:1452, 1986.

1205. Robbins SG and others: Immunolocalization of integrins in proliferative retinal membranes, Invest Ophthalmol 35:3475, 1994.

1206. Robertson D and Curtin V: Rhegmatogenous retinal detachment and choroidal melanoma, Am J Ophthalmol 72:351, 1971.

1207. Robinson MR and Streeten BW: The surface morphology of retinal breaks and lattice retinal degeneration: a scanning electron microscopic study, Ophthalmology 93:237, 1986.

1208. Roth AM and Foos RY: Surface wrinkling retinopathy in eyes enucleated at autopsy, Trans Am Acad Ophthalmol Otolaryngol 75:1047, 1971.

1209. Rubsamen PE and others: Prevention of experimental proliferative vitreoretinopathy with a biodegradable intravitreal implant for the sustained release of fluorouracil, Arch Ophthalmol 112:407, 1994.

1210. Ruiz R: Traumatic retinal detachment, Br J Ophthalmol 53:59, 1969.

1211. Ryan S and Goldberg MF: Anterior segment ischemia following scleral buckling in sickle cell hemoglobinopathy, Am J Ophthalmol 72:35, 1971.

1212. Schepens C, editor: Importance of the vitreous body in retina surgery, St Louis, 1960, The CV Mosby Co.

1213. Schepens C and Marsden B: Data on the natural history of retinal detachment, Am J Ophthalmol 61:213, 1966.

1214. Scott JD: Equatorial giant tears affected by massive vitreous retraction, Trans Ophthalmol Soc UK 96:309, 1976.

1215. Scott JD: Lens epithelial proliferation in retinal detachment, Trans Ophthalmol Soc UK 102:385, 1982.

1216. Shea M, Schepens C, and von Pirquet S: Retinoschisis. I. Senile type: a clinical report on one hundred seven cases, Arch Ophthalmol 63:1, 1960.

1217. Shukla M and Ahuja OP: A possible relationship between lattice and snail track degenerations of the retina, Am J Ophthalmol 92:482, 1981.

1218. Sigelman J: Vitreous base classification of retinal tears: clinical application, Surv Ophthalmol 25:59, 1980.

1219. Sivalingam A and others: Visual prognosis correlated with the presence of internal-limiting membrane in histopathologic specimens obtained from epiretinal membrane surgery, Ophthalmology 97:1549, 1990.

1220. Smiddy WE and Green WR: Retinal dialysis: pathology and pathogenesis, Retina 2:94, 1982.

1221. Smiddy WE and others: Idiopathic epiretinal membranes. Ultrastructural characteristics and clinicopathologic correlation, Ophthalmology 96:811, 1989.

1222. Smiddy WE and others: Ultrastructural studies of vitreomacular traction syndrome, Am J Ophthalmol 107:177, 1989.

1223. Spencer L and Foos RY: Paravascular vitreoretinal attachments, Arch Ophthalmol 84:557, 1970.

1224. Sramek SJ and others: Immunostaining of preretinal membranes for actin, fibronectin, and glial fibrillary acidic protein, Ophthalmology 96:935, 1989.

1225. Straatsma BR and Foos RY: Typical and reticular degenerative retinoschisis, Am J Ophthalmol 75:551, 1973.

1226. Straatsma BR, Landers M, and Kreiger A: The ora serrata in the adult human eye, Arch Ophthalmol 80:3, 1968.

1227. Straatsma BR and others: Lattice degeneration of the retina, Am J Ophthalmol 77:619, 1974.

1228. Streeten B and Bert M: The retinal surface in lattice degeneration of the retina, Am J Ophthalmol 74:1201, 1972.

1229. Sulonen JM and others: Degenerative retinoschisis with giant outer layer breaks with retinal detachment, Am J Ophthalmol 99:114, 1985.

1230. Teng C and Chi H: Vitreous changes and the mechanisms of retinal detachment, Am J Ophthalmol 44:335, 1957.

1231. Teng C and Katzin H: An anatomic study of the periphery of the retina. I. Nonpigmented epithelial cell proliferation and hole formation, Am J Ophthalmol 34:1237, 1951.

1232. Teng C and Katzin H: An anatomical study of the peripheral retina. II. Peripheral cystoid degeneration of the retina: formation of cysts and holes, Am J Ophthalmol 36:29, 1953.

1233. Teng C and Katzin H: An anatomic study of the peripheral retina. III. Congenital retinal rosettes, Am J Ophthalmol 36:69, 1953.

1234. Theodossiadis GP and Kokolakis SN: Macular pigment deposits in rhegmatogenous retinal detachment, Br J Ophthalmol 63:498, 1979.

1235. Tillery WV and Lucier AC: Round atrophic holes in lattice degeneration—an important cause of phakic retinal detachment, Trans Am Acad Ophthalmol Otolaryngol 84:509, 1976.

1236. Tolentino F, Schepens C, and Freeman H: Vitreoretinal disorders: diagnosis and management, Philadelphia, 1976, WB Saunders Co.

1237. Topilow HW and Ackerman AL: Massive exudative retinal and choroidal detachments following scleral buckling surgery, Ophthalmology 90:143, 1983.

1238. Urrets-Zavalia A Jr: Acute scleral necrosis; a hitherto unrecognized complication of retinal detachment surgery, Trans Am Acad Ophthalmol Otolaryngol 75:1035, 1971.

1239. Van Horn DL and others: Glial cell proliferation in human retinal detachment with massive periretinal proliferation, Am J Ophthalmol 84:383, 1977.

1240. Velikay M and others: Retinal detachment with severe proliferative vitreoretinopathy in Terson's syndrome, Ophthalmology 101:35, 1994.

1241. Verdaguer TJ: Juvenile retinal detachment, Am J Ophthalmol 93:145, 1982.

1242. Wallow IHL and Miller SA: Preretinal membrane by retinal pigment epithelium, Arch Ophthalmol 96:4643, 1978.

1243. Wilkes SR, Mansour AM, and Green WR: Proliferative vitreoretinopathy. Histopathology of retroretinal membranes, Retina 7:94, 1987.

1244. Willshaw HE and Rubinstein K: Azelaic acid in the treatment of ocular and adnexal malignant melanoma, Br J Ophthalmol 67:54, 1983.

1245. Wilson DJ and Green WR: histopathologic study of the effect of retinal detachment surgery on 49 eyes obtained post mortem, Am J Ophthalmol 103:167, 1987.

1246. Yamashita H and others: Glial cells in culture of preretinal membrane of proliferative vitreoretinopathy, Jpn J Ophthalmol 29:42, 1985.

1247. Young RW: The Bowman lecture, 1982, biological renewal—applications to the eyes, Trans Ophthalmol Soc UK 102:42, 1982.

1248. Zarbin MA, Michels RG, and Green WR: Epiretinal membrane co-intracture associated with macular prolapse, Am J Ophthalmol 110:610, 1990.

1249. Zimmerman, LE and Fine BS: production of hyaluronic acid by cysts and tumors of the ciliary body, Arch Ophthalmol 72:365, 1964.

1250. Zimmerman LE and Naumann GOH: Pathology of retinoschisis. In McPherson A, editor: New and controversial aspects of retinal detachment, St Louis, 1968, The CV Mosby Co.

1251. Zimmerman LE and Spencer W: The pathologic anatomy of retinoschisis, with a report of two cases diagnosed clinically as malignant melanoma, Arch Ophthalmol 63:10, 1960.

1252. Zion VM and Burton TC: Retinal dialysis, Arch Ophthalmol 98:1971, 1980.

Retinal and choroidal dystrophies: degenerations affecting the macular region

1253. Aaberg, TM: Macular holes: a review, Surv Ophthalmol 15:139, 1970.

1254. Aaberg TM, Blain C, and Gass JDM: Macular holes, Am J Ophthalmol 69:555, 1970.

1255. Aaberg TM: Stargardt's disease and fundus flavimaculatus: evaluation of morphologic progression and intrafamilial co-existence, Trans Am Ophthalmol Soc 84:453, 1986.

1256. Adler R: Mechanisms of photoreceptor death in retinal degenerations—from the cell biology of the 1990s to the ophthalmology of the 21st century, Arch Ophthalmol 114:79, 1996.

1257. Aessopos A and others: Angioid streaks in sickle-thalassemia, Am J Ophthalmol 117:589, 1994.

1258. Aessopos A and others: Angioid streaks in homozygous thalassemia, Am J Ophthalmol 108:356, 1989.

1259. Aiello LP and others: Solar retinopathy associated with hypoglycemic insulin reaction, Arch Ophthalmol 112:982, 1994.

1260. Aish SFS and Dajani B: Benign familial fleck retina, Br J Ophthalmol 64:652, 1980.

1261. Akiba J, Quiroz MA, and Trempe CL: Role of posterior vitreous detachment in idiopathic macular holes, Ophthalmology 97:1610, 1990.

1262. Akiba J, Yoshida A, and Trempe CL: Risk of developing a macular hole, Arch Ophthalmol 108:1088, 1990.

1263. Alexander LJ: Pre-retinal membrane formation, J Am Optometric Assoc 51:567, 1980.

1264. Allen AW and Gass JDM: Contraction of a perifoveal epiretinal membrane simulating a macular hole, Am J Ophthalmol 82:684, 1976.

1265. Anderson S: Ocular pathology in hereditary (vitelliform) macular degeneration, European Ophthalmic Pathology Society, Ghent, May 28, 1970. Cited By Francois J: Vitelliform macular degeneration, Ophthalmologica 163:12, 1971.

1266. Annesley W, Tomer T, and Shields JA: Multifocal placoid pigment epitheliopathy, Am J Ophthalmol 76:511, 1973.

1267. Annesley WH Jr: Peripheral exudative hemorrhagic chorioretinopathy, Trans Am Ophthalmol Soc 78:321, 1980.

1268. Appaiah A, Hirose T: Secondary cause of premacular fibrosis, Ophthalmology 96:389, 1989.

1269. Apple DJ: Anatomy and histopathology of the macular region, Int Ophthalmol Clin 21(3):1, 1981.

1270. Arden GB, Gorin MB, and Polinghorne PJ: Detection of the carrier state of X-linked retinoschisis, Am J Ophthalmol 105:590, 1988.

1271. Arkefeld DF and Brockhurst RJ: Vascularized vitreous membranes in congenital retinoschisis, Retina 7:20, 1987.

1272. Arroyo JG and Irvine AR: Retinal distortion and cotton-wool spots associated with epiretinal membrane contraction, Ophthalmology 102:662, 1995.

1273. Asdourian GK, Goldberg MF, and Busse B: Optic disc neovascularization of uveal (choroidal or posterior ciliary) origin, Arch Ophthalmol 95:998, 1977.

1274. Asdourina GK and others: Retinal macroaneurysms, Arch Ophthalmol 95:624, 1977.

1275. Ashton N: Central areolar choroidal sclerosis: a histopathological study, Br J Ophthalmol 37:140, 1953.

1276. Awan KJ: Ocular melanocytosis and angioid streaks, J Pediatr Ophthalmol Strabismus 17:300, 1980.

1277. Azar P and others: Acute posterior multifocal placoid pigment epitheliopathy associated with an adenovirus type 5 infection, Am J Ophthalmol 80:1003, 1975.

1278. Barr CC, Michels RG: Idiopathic nonvascularized epiretinal membranes in young patients: report of 6 cases, Annals of Ophthalmol 14:335, 1982.

1279. Barricks ME: Vitelliform lesions developing in normal fundi, Am J Ophthalmol 83:324, 1977.

1280. Bartel PR and others: Visual function and long-term chloroquine treatment, S Afr Med J 84:32, 1994.

1281. Baskin MA and others: Macular lesions in blacks with the presumed ocular histoplasmosis syndrome, Am J Ophthalmol 89:77, 1980.

1282. Bastek JV and others: choriorentinal juncture: pigmentary patterns of the peripheral fundus, Ophthalmology 89:1455, 1982.

1283. Baudouin C and others: Immunohistologic study of epiretinal membranes in proliferative vitreoretinopathy, Am J Ophthalmol 110:593, 1990.

1284. Baudouin C and others: Immunohistologic study of epiretinal membranes in proliferative vitreoretinopathy, Am J Ophthalmol 110:593, 1990.

1285. Bellhorn MB and others: ultrastructure and clinicopathologic correlation of idiopathic preretinal macular fibrosis, Am J Ophthalmol 79:366, 1975.

1286. Benner JD and others: Fibrinolytic-assisted removal of experimental subretinal hemorrhage within seven days reduces outer retinal degeneration, Ophthalmology 101:672, 1994.

1287. Benson W and others: Best's vitelliform macular dystropyhy, Am J Ophthalmol 79:59, 1975.

1288. Berard-Badier M and others: The retina in Lafora disease: light and electron microscopy, Graefes Arch Klin Exp Ophthalmol 212:285, 1980.

1289. Bergsma D, Bron A, and Cotlier E: The eye and inborn errors of metabolism, New York, 1976, Alan R Liss Inc.

1290. Berkow J and Font R: Disciform macular degeneration with subpigment epithelial hematoma, Arch Ophthalmol 82:51, 1969.

1291. Best F: Ueber eine hereditäre Maculaaffektion: Beitra;uge zur Vererbungslehre, Z Augenheilkd 13:199, 1905.

1292. Bird A and Blach R: X-linked recessive fundus dystrophies and their carrier states, Trans Ophthalmol Soc UK 40:127, 1970.

1293. Bird A and Teeters V: The evolution of subpigment epithelial neovascularization in senile disciform macular degeneration, Trans Ophthalmol Soc UK 92:413, 1972.

1294. Birnbach CD and others: Histopathology and immunocytochemistry of the neurosensory retina in fundus flavimaculatus, Ophthalmology 101:1211, 1994.

1295. Blumenkranz MS, Gass JDM, and Clarkson JG: Atypical serpiginous choroiditis, Arch Ophthalmol 100:1773, 1982.

1296. Böck, J: Zur Klinik und Anatomic der gefassähnlichen Streifen im Augenhintergrund, Z Augenheilkd 95:1, 1983.

1297. Boldrey EE: Foveal ablation for subfoveal choroidal neovascularization, Ophthalmology 96:1430, 1989.

1298. Bolmers D and others: Some patients with cerebro-macular degeneration in the cadre of Batten's disease, Ophthalmologica 169:241, 1974.

1299. Bonnet M: Bull's-eye maculopathy, Klin Monatsbl Augenheilkd 168:297, 1976.

1300. Bonnet M: Clinical factors predisposing to massive proliferative vitreoretinopathy in rhegmatogenous retinal detachment, Ophthalmologica 188:148, 1984.

1301. Boozalis GT, Schachat AP, and Green WR: Subretinal neovascularization from the retina in radiation retinopathy, Retina 7:156, 1987.

1302. Borit A, Sugarman GI, and Spencer WH: Ocular involvement in I-cell disease (mucolipidosis II) light and electron microscopic findings, Albrecht von Graefes Arch Klin Ophthalmol 198:25, 1976.

1303. Bornfield N, Laqua H, and El-Hifnawi E: Ultrastrukturelle Befunde an epiretinalen Membranen bei spontanem "macular pucker," Fortschr Ophthalmol 80:326, 1983.

1304. Braunstein RA and Gass JDM: Serous detachment of the retinal pigment epithelium in patients with senile macular disease, Am J Ophthalmol 88:652, 1979.

1305. Brazitikos PD and others: Erbium: YAG laser surgery of the vitreous and retina, Ophthalmology 102:278, 1995.

1306. Bressler NM, Bressler SB, and Fine SL: Age-related macular degeneration, Surv Ophthalmol 32:375, 1988.

1307. Bressler NM and others: Clinicopathologic correlation of drusen and retinal pigment epithelial abnormalities in age-related macular degeneration, Retina 14:130, 1994.

1308. Bressler SB and others: Relationship of drusen and abnormalities of the retinal pigment epithelium to the prognosis of neovascular macular degeneration, Arch Ophthalmol 108:1442, 1990.

1309. Bressler NM and Bressler SB: Preventive ophthalmology age-related macular degeneration, Ophthalmology 102:1206, 1995.

1310. Bressler SB and others: Clinicopathologic correlation occult choroidal neovascularization in age-related macular degeneration, Arch Ophthalmol 110:827, 1992.

1311. Brod RD, Packer AJ, and Van Dyk JL: Diagnosis of neuronal ceroid lipofuscinosis by ultrastructural examination of peripheral blood lymphocytes, Arch Ophthalmol 105:1388, 1987.

1312. Bronstein MA, Trempe CL, and Freeman HM: Fellow eyes of eyes with macular holes, Am J Ophthalmol 92:757, 1981.

1313. Brown GC and others: Radiation retinopathy, Ophthalmology 89:1494, 1982.

1314. Brownstein S and others: Optic nerve in globoid leukodystrophy (Krabbe's disease), Arch Ophthalmol 96:864, 1978.

1315. Brownstein S and others: Sandhoff's disease (GM2 gangliosidosis type 2): histopathology and ultrastructure of the eye, Arch Ophthalmol 98:1089, 1980.

1316. Buchanan TAS and others: Retinal ultrastructural findings in cone degenerations, Am J Ophthalmol 106:405, 1988.

1317. Burns R, Lovrien E, and Cibis A: Juvenile sex-linked retinoschisis: clinical and genetic studies, Trans Am Acad Ophthalmol Otolaryngol 75:1011, 1971.

1318. de Bustros S: Early stages of macular holes, Arch Ophthalmol 108:1085, 1990.

1319. Bynoe LA and others: Histopathologic examination of vascular patterns in subfoveal neovascular membranes, Ophthalmology 101: 1112, 1994.

1320. Campbell RJ and others: Pathologic findings in the retinal pigment epitheliopathy associated with the amyotrophic lateral sclerosis/parkinsonism-dementia complex of guam, Ophthalmology 100:37, 1993.

1321. Campochiaro PA and others: Spontaneous involution of subfoveal neovascularization, Am J Ophthalmol 109:688, 1990.

1322. Capon RC, Marshall J, and Krafft JI: Sorby's fundus dystrophy. A light and electron microscopic study, Ophthalmology 96:1769, 1989.

1323. Carr RE and Nobel KG: Geographic (serpiginous) choroidopathy, Ophthalmology 87:1065, 1980.

1324. Carr RE, Nobel KG: Juvenile macular degeneration, Ophthalmology 87:83, 1980.

1325. Carr RE and Noble KG: Disorders of the fundus. I. Juvenile macular degeneration, Ophthalmology 87:83, 1980.

1326. Carr RE, Noble KG, and Nasaduke I: Hereditary hemorrhagic macular dystrophy, Am J Ophthalmol 85:318, 1978.

1327. Castro-Correi J, Coutinho MF, and Moreira R: Drusen of Bruch's membrane, Acta Oftalmologica 3:7, 1992.

1328. Cavender JC: Best's macular dystrophy, Arch Ophthalmol 100: 1067, 1982 (editorial).

1329. Chandra S and others: Natural history of disciform degeneration of the macula, Am J Ophthalmol 78:579, 1974.

1330. Chang B and others: Choroidal neovascularization in second eyes of patients with unilateral exudative age-related macular degeneration, Ophthalmology 102:1380, 1995.

1331. Chang TS and others: Clinicopathologic correlation of choroidal neovascularization demonstrated by indocyaninee green angiography in a patient with retention of good vision for almost four years, Retina 14:114, 1994.

1332. Change B and others: Retinal degeneration in motor neuron degeneration: a mouse model of ceroid lipofuscinosis, Invest Ophthalmol Vis Sci 35:1071, 1994.

1333. Charteris DG and others: Proliferative vitreoretinopathy. Lymphocytes in epiretinal membranes, Ophthalmology 99:1364, 1992.

1334. Chen JC and others: Functional loss in age-related Bruch's membrane change with choroidal perfusion defect, Invest Ophthalmol Vis Sci 33:334, 1992.

1335. Cherfan GM and others: Clinicopathologic correlation of pigmented epiretinal membranes, Am J Ophthalmol 106:536, 1988.

1336. Chew E and Pinckers A: Bilateral retinal detachments in X-linked juvenile retinoschisis, Ophthalmic Paediatr Genet 2:89, 1983.

1337. Chu FC and others: Ocular manifestations of familial highdensity lipoprotein deficiency (Tangier disease), Arch Ophthalmol 97: 1926, 1979.

1338. Cibis GW, Morey M, and Harris DJ: Dominantly inherited macular dystrophy with flecks (Stargardt), Arch Ophthalmol 98:1785, 1980.

1339. Cibis GW and others: Mucolipidosis I, Arch Ophthalmol 101:933, 1983.

1340. Clarkson JG and Altman RD: Angioid streaks, Surv Ophthalmol 26:235, 1982.

1341. Clarkson JG, Green WR, and Massof D: A histopathologic review of 168 cases of preretinal membrane, Am J Ophthalmol 84:1, 1977.

1342. Cleary PE and Leaver PK: Macular abnormalities in the reattached retina, Br J Ophthalmol 62:595, 1978.

1343. Cohen SY and others: Etiology of choroidal neovascularization in young patients, Ophthalmology 103:1241, 1996.

1344. Coffey AJH and Brownstein S: The prevalence of macular drusen in postmortem eyes, Am J Ophthalmol 102:164, 1986.

1345. Cogan DG and Kuwabara T: The sphingolipidoses and the eye, Arch Ophthalmol 79:437, 1968.

1346. Cogan DG and others: Fundal abnormalities of Gaucher's disease, Arch Ophthalmol 98:2202, 1980.

1347. Cogan DG and others: Gangliosidoses and the fetal retina, Ophthalmology 91:508, 1984.

1348. Cogan DG, Kuwabara T, and Moser H: Metachromatic leukodystrophy, Ophthalmologica 160:2, 1970.

1349. Condon GP and others: Congenital hereditary (juvenile X-linked) retinoschisis: histopathologic and ultrastructural findings in three eyes, Arch Ophthalmol 104:576, 1986.

1350. Cortin P and others: A patterned macular dystrophy with yellow plaques and atrophic changes, Br J Ophthalmol 64:127, 1980.

1351. Coskuncan NM and others: The eye in bone marrow transplantation, Arch Ophthalmol 112:372, 1994.

1352. Cotlier E: Tay-Sachs' retina: deficiency of acetyl hexosaminidase A, Arch Ophthalmol 86:352, 1971.

1353. Cotlier E: Biochemical detection of inborn errors of metabolism affecting the eye, Trans Am Acad Ophthalmol Otolaryngol 76:1165, 1972.

1354. Cox TA and others: A retinopathy on guam with high prevalence in lytico-bodig, Ophthalmology 96:1731, 1989.

1355. Craythorn JM, Swartz M, and Creel DJ: Clofazimine-induced bull's-eye retinopathy, Retina 6:50, 1986.

1356. Cruess AF and others: Chloroquine retinopathy. Is fluorescein angiography necessary? Ophthalmology 92:1127, 1985.

1357. Cruickshanks KJ, Klein R, and Klein BEK: Sunlight and age-related macular degeneration, Arch Ophthalmol 111:514, 1993.

1358. Cunha-Vaz JG and Travassos A: Breakdown of the blood-retinal barriers and cystoid macular edema, Surv Ophthalmol 28(suppl): 485, 1984.

1359. Curcio CA, Medeiros NE, and Millican CL: Photoreceptor loss in age-related macular degeneration, Invest Ophthalmol Vis Sci 37: 1236, 1996.

1360. Curtin BJ, Iwamoto T, and Renaldo DP: Normal and staphylomatous sclera of high myopia. An electron microscopic study, Arch Ophthalmol 97:912, 1979.

1361. Dabbs ME, Bremer DL, and Rogers GL: Treatment of corneal opacification in mucolipidosis IV with conjunctival transplantation, Am J Ophthalmol 74:579, 1990.

1362. Dahl N and Peterson U: Use of linked DNA probes for carrier detection and diagnosis of x-linked juvenile retinoschisis, Arch Ophthalmol 106:1414, 1988.

1363. Daicker B: Anatomie und Pathologie der menschlichen retinoziliaren funduseperiphierie, Basel, 1972, S Karger AG.

1364. Das A and others: Ultrastructural immunocytochemistry of subretinal neovascular membranes in age-related macular degeneration, Ophthalmology 99:1368, 1992.

1365. Dastgheib K and Green R: Granulomatous reaction to Bruch's membrane in age-related macular degeneration, Arch Ophthalmol 112:813, 1994.

1366. Destro M and Puliafito CA: Indocyanineine green video angiography of choroidal neovascularization, Ophthalmology 96:846, 1989.

1367. Deutman AF: The hereditary dystrophies of the posterior pole of the eye, Springfield, III, 1971, Charles C Thomas, Publisher.

1368. Deutman AF and Jansen L: Dominantly inherited drusen of Bruch's membrane, Br J Ophthalmol 54:373, 1970.

1369. Deutman AF and Lion F: Choriocapillaris nonperfusion in acute multifocal placoid pigment epitheliopathy, Am J Ophthalmol 84: 652, 1977.

1370. Deutman AF and others: Acute posterior multifocal placoid pigment itheliopathy: pigment epitheliopathy or choriocapillaritis, Br J Ophthalmol 56:863, 1972.

1371. Deutsche Ophthalmologische Gesellschaft (1973 Proceedings): Erkrankungen der Macula, Munich, 1975, JF Bergmann.

1372. de Venecia G and Shapiro M: Neuronal ceroid lipofuscinosis: a retinal trypsin digest study, Ophthalmology 91:1406, 1984.

1373. Dreyer RF and Hidayat AA: Pseudoinflammatory macular dystrophy, Am J Ophthalmol 106:154, 1988.

1374. Duker JS, Belmont J, and Bosley TM: Angioid streaks associated with abetalipoproteinemia, Arch Ophthalmol Arch Ophthalmol 105:1173, 1987.

1375. Eagle RC Jr: Mechanisms of maculopathy, Ophthalmology 91:613, 1984.

1376. Eagle RC Jr and others: Retinal pigment epithelial abnormalities in fundus flavimaculatus, Ophthalmology 87:1189, 1980.

1377. El Baba and others: Massive hemorrhage complicating age-related macular degeneration: clinicopathologic correlation and role of anticoagulants, Ophthalmology 93:1581, 1986.

1378. Eisner A and others: Visual function and the subsequent development of exudative age-related macular degeneration, Invest Ophthalmol Vis Sci 33:3091, 1992.

1379. Elman MJ and others: The natural history of serous retinal pigment epithelium detachment in patients with age-related macular degeneration, Ophthalmology 93:224, 1986.

1380. Emery J and others: Niemann-Pick disease (type C): histopathology and ultrastructure, Am J Ophthalmol 74:1144, 1972.

1381. Emery JM, Green WR, and Huff DS: Krabbe's disease. Histopathology and ultrastructure of the eye, Am J Ophthalmol 74:400, 1972.

1382. Epstein D: Cystoid macular edema occurring 13 years after cataract extraction, Am J Ophthalmol 83:501, 1977.

1383. Epstein GA and Rabb MF: Adult vitelliform macular degeneration: diagnosis and natural history, Br J Ophthalmol 64:733, 1980.

1384. Falls H: A classification and clinical description of hereditary macular lesions, Trans Am Acad Ophthalmol Otolaryngol 70:1034, 1966.

1385. Farkas TG: Drusen of the retinal pigment epithelium, Surv Ophthalmol 16:75, 1972.

1386. Farkas TG, Sylvester VM, and Archer D: The histochemistry of drusen, Am J Ophthalmol 71:1206, 1971.

1387. Farkas TG, Sylvester VM, and Archer D: The ultrastructure of drusen, Am J Ophthalmol 71:1196, 1971.

1388. Farkas TG and others: Familial and secondary drusen: histologic and functional correlations, Trans Am Acad Ophthalmol Otolaryngol 75:333, 1971.

1389. Farmer SG and others: Fleck retina in Kjellin's syndrome, Am J Ophthalmol 99:45, 1985.

1390. Federman J, Shields J, and Tomer T: Angioid streaks. II. Fluorescein angiographic features, Arch Ophthalmol 93:951, 1975.

1391. Feeney-Burns L and Ellersieck MR: Age-related changes in the ultrastructure of Bruch's membrane, Am J Ophthalmol 100:686, 1985.

1392. Feeney-Burns L, Burns RP, and Gao CL: Age-related macular changes in humans over 90 years old, Am J Ophthalmol 109:265, 1990.

1393. Feeney-Burns L, Berman ER, and Rothman H: Lipofuscin of human retinal pigment epithelium, Am J Ophthalmol 90:783, 1980.

1394. Fekrat S and others: Clinicopathologic correlation of an epiretinal membrane associated with a recurrent macular hole, Retina 15:53, 1995.

1395. Ferry A, Llovera I, and Shafer D: Central arcolar choroidal dystrophy, Arch Ophthalmol 88:39, 1972.

1396. Fetkenhour CL and others: Central areolar pigment epithelial dystrophy, Am J Ophthalmol 81:745, 1976.

1397. Fielder AR, Garner A, and Chambers TL: Ophthalmic manifestations of primary oxalosis, Br J Ophthalmol 64:782, 1980.

1398. Fine BS: Limiting membranes of the sensory retina and pigment epilthelium:an electron microscope study, Arch Ophthalmology 66:847, 19961.

1399. Fine BS and Brucker AJ: Macular edema and cystoid macular edema, Am J Ophthalmol 92:466, 1981.

1400. Fish G and others: The dark choroid in posterior retinal dystrophies, Br J Ophthalmol 65:359, 1981.

1401. Fishman GA: Fundus flavimaculatus: a clinical classification, Arch Ophthalmol 94:2061, 1976.

1402. Fishman GA and others: Pseudovitelliform macular degeneration, Arch Ophthalmol 95:73, 1977.

1403. Fishman GA and others: Visual acuity loss in patients with Stargardt's macular dystrophy, Ophthalmology 94:809, 1987.

1404. Fitzpatrick P and Robertson D: Acute posterior multifocal placoid pigment epitheliopathy, Arch Ophthalmol 89:373, 1973.

1405. Folk JC and others: Early retinal adhesion from laser photocoagulation, Ophthalmology 96:1523, 1989.

1406. Foos RY: Vitreoretinal juncture; epiretinal membranes and vitreous, Invest Ophthalmology Vis Sci 16:416, 1977.

1407. Foos RY: Vitreoretinal juncture; healing of experimental wounds, Albrecht von Graefes Archiv fur Klinische und Experimentelle Ophthalmologie 196:213, 1975.

1408. Franceschetti A: A special form of tapetoretinal degeneration: fundus flavimaculatus, Trans Am Acad Ophthalmol Otolaryngol 69:1048, 1965.

1409. Franceschetti A and François J: Fundus flavimaculatus, Arch Ophthalmol 25:505, 1965.

1410. François J: Vitelliform macular degeneration, Ophthalmologica 163:312, 1971.

1411. François J: Ocular manifestations of inborn errors of carbohydrate and lipid metabolism, Basel, 1975, S Karger, AG.

1412. Frangieh GT, Green WR, and Engel HM: A histopathologic study of macular cysts and holes, Retina 1:311, 1981.

1413. Frangieh GT, Green WR, and Fine SL: A histopathologic study of Best's macular dystrophy, Arch Ophthalmol 100:1115, 1982.

1414. Frank R, Green W, and Pollack I: Senile macular degeneration:

1415. Frayer W: Elevated lesions of the macular area; a histopathologic study emphasizing lesions similar to disciform degeneration of the macula, Arch Ophthalmol 53:82, 1955.

1416. Fuller B and Gitter K: Traumatic choroidal rupture with late serous detachment of macula, Arch Ophthalmol 89:354, 1973.

1417. Funata M and others: Clinicopathologic study of bilateral macular holes treated with parts plana vitrectomy and gas tamponade, Retina 12:289, 1992.

1418. Garcia-Arumi J and others: Epiretinal membranes in Terson's syndrome, Retina 14:351, 1994.

1419. Garner A: Ocular pathology of GM2 gangliosidosis type 2 (Sandhoff's disease), Br J Ophthalmol 57:514, 1973.

1420. Gass JDM: Pathogenesis of disciform detachment of the neuropithelium. I. General concepts and classification, Am J Ophthalmol 63:573, 1967.

1421. Gass JDM: Acute posterior placoid pigment epitheliopathy, Arch Ophthalmol 80:177, 1968.

1422. Gass JDM: Drusen and disciform macular detachment and degeneration, Arch Ophthalmol 90:206, 1973.

1423. Gass JDM: Symposium: the value of fluorescein angiography in the study of choroidal and pigment epithelial disease. Choroidal neovascular membranes—their visualization and treatment, Trans Am Acad Ophthalmol Otolaryngol 77:310, 1973.

1424. Gass JDM: Lamellar macular hole: a complication of cystoid macular edema after cataract extraction: a clinicopathologic case report, Trans Am Ophthalmol Soc 73:321, 1975.

1425. Gass JDM: Stereoscopic atlas of macular diseases: diagnosis and treatment, ed 2, St Louis, 1977, The CV Mosby Co.

1426. Gass JDM, Anderson DR, and Davis EB: A clinical, fluorescein angiographic, and electron microscopic correlation of cystoid macular edema, Am J Ophthalmol 100:82, 1985.

1427. Gass JDM and Clarkson J: Angioid streaks and disciform detachment in Paget's disease (osteitis deformans), Am J Ophthalmol 75:576, 1973.

1428. Gass JDM, Jallow S, and Davis B: Adult vitelliform macular detachment occuring in patients with basal laminar drusen. Am J Ophthalmol 99, 45.

1429. Gass JDM and Norton EWD: Cystoid macular edema and papilledema following cataract extraction, Arch Ophthalmol 76:646, 1966.

1430. Gass JDM and Norton EWD: Follow-up study of cystoid macular edema following cataract extraction, Trans Am Acad Ophthalmol Otolaryngol 73:665, 1969.

1431. Gass JDM, Norton EWD, and Justice J Jr: Serous detachment of the retinal pigment epithelium, Trans Am Acad Ophthalmol Otolaryngol 70:990, 1966.

1432. Gass JDM: Pathogenesis of disciform detachment of the neuroepithelium. I. General concepts and classification. II. Idiopathic central serous choroidopathy. III. Senile disciform macular degeneration. V. Disciform macular degeneration secondary to heredodegenerative, neoplastic and traumatic lesions of the choroid, Am J Ophthalmol 63:573, 587, 617, 661, 689, 1967.

1433. Gass JDM: Serous retinal pigment epithelial detachment with a notch. A sign of occult choroidal neovascularization, Retina 4:205, 1984.

1434. Gass JDM: Biomicroscopic and histopathologic considerations regarding the feasibility of surgical excision of subfoveal neovascular membranes, Am J Ophthalmol 118:285, 1994.

1435. Gass JDM: A fluorescein angiographic study of macular dysfunction secondary to retinal vascular disease. I. Embolic retinal artery obstruction. II. Retinal vein occlusion. III. Hypertensive retinopathy. IV. Diabetic retinal angiography. V. Retinal telangiectasis. VI. X-ray irradiation, carotid artery occlusion, collagen vascular disease, and vitritis, Arch Ophthalmol 80:535, 550, 569, 583, 592, 606, 1968.

1436. Gass JDM and Joondeph BC: Observations concerning patients with suspected impending macular holes, Am J Ophthalmol 109:638, 1990.

1437. Gass JDM: Reappraisal of biomicroscopic classification of stages of development of a macular hole, Am J Ophthalmol 119:752, 1995.

1438. Gass JD and Taney BS: Flecked retina associated with café au lait spots, microcephaly, epilepsy, short stature, and right 17 chromosome, Arch Ophthalmol 112:738, 1994.

1439. Gass JDM: Clinicopathologic correlation of surgically removed macular hole opercula, Am J Ophthalmol 121:453, 1996 (letter; comment).

1440. Gerber S and others: Stargardt's disease is not alleic to the genes for neuronal ceroid lipofuscinoses, J Med Genet 31:222, 1994.

1441. Gibson JM, Chaudhuri PR, and Rosenthal AR: Angioid streaks in a case of beta thalassemia major, Br J Ophthalmol 67:29, 1983.

1442. Gilbert C and others: Inflammation and the formation of epiretinal membranes, Eye 2 (suppl):S140, 1988 (review).

1443. Glaser BM, Cardin A, and Biscoe B: Proliferative vitreoretinopathy. The mechanism of development of vitreoretinal traction, Ophthalmology 94:327, 1987.

1444. Glatt HH and Machemer R: Experimental subretinal hemorrhage in rabbits, Am J Ophthalmol 94:762, 1982.

1445. Glenn AM and others: Effect of vitamin A treatment on the prolongation of dark adaptation in Stargardt's dystrophy, Retina 14:27, 1994.

1446. Goebel HH, Fix JD, and Zeman W: Retinal pathology in GM1 gangloisidosis, type II, Am J Ophthalmol 75:434, 1973.

1447. Goebel HH, Fix JD, and Zeman W: The fine structure of the retina in neuronal ceroid-lipofuscinosis, Am J Ophthalmol 77:25, 1974.

1448. Goebel HH, Zeman W, and Damaske E: An ultrastructural study of the retina in the Jansky-Bielschowsky type of neuronal ceroid-lipofuscinosis, Am J Ophthalmol 83:70, 1977.

1449. Goldberg MF and others: Macular cherry-red spot, corneal clouding, and beta-galactosidase deficiency: clinical, biochemical, and electron microscopic study of a new autosomal recessive storage disease, Arch Intern Med 128:387, 1971.

1450. Gorin MB and others: A peripherin/retinal degeneration slow mutation (Pro-210-Arg) associated with macular and peripheral retinal degeneration, Ophthalmology 102:246, 1995.

1451. Grand MG, Isserman MJ, and Miller CW: Angioid streaks associated with pseudoxanthoma elasticum in a 13-year-old patient, Ophthalmology 94:197, 1987.

1452. Green JL Jr and Jampol LM: Vascular opacification and leakage in X-linked (juvenile) retinoschisis, Br J Ophthalmol 63:368, 1979.

1453. Green W, Friedman-Kien A, and Banfield W: Angioid streaks in Ehlers-Danlos syndrome, Arch Ophthalmol 76:197, 1966.

1454. Green W and Gass JDM: Senile disciform degeneration of the macula: retinal arterialization of the fibrous plaque demonstrated clinically and histopathologically, Arch Ophthalmol 86:487, 1971.

1455. Green WR, McDonnell PJ, and Yeo JH: Pathologic features of senile macular degeneration, Ophthalmology 92:615, 1985.

1456. Green WR and others: Ultrastructure of epiretinal membranes causing macular pucker after retinal re-attachment surgery, Trans Ophthalmol Soc UK 99:65, 1979.

1457. Green WR and others: Parafoveal retinal telangiectasis: light and electron microscopy studies, Trans Ophthalmol Soc UK 100:162, 1980.

1458. Green WR: Clinicopathologic studies of treated choroidal neovascular membranes, Retina 11:328, 1991.

1459. Green WR and Enger C: Age-related macular degeneration histopathologic studies. The 1992 Lorenz E. Zimmerman Lecture, Ophthalmology 100:1519, 1993.

1460. Green WR and Robertson DM: Pathologic findings of photic retinopathy in the human eye, Am J Ophthalmol 112:520, 1991.

1461. Green WR and Wilson DJ: Choroidal neovascularization, Ophthalmology 93:1169, 1986.

1462. Gregor Z, Bird AC, and Chisholm IH: Senile disciform macular degeneration in the second eye, Br J Ophthalmol 61:141, 1977.

1463. Greven CM, Slusher MM, and Weaver RG: Epiretinal membrane release and posterior vitreous detachment, Ophthalmology 95:902, 1988.

1464. Greven CM, Moreno RJ, and Tasman W: Unusual manifestations of Bardet-Biedl syndrome, a form of Laurence-Moon-Biedl syndrome, N Engl J Med 321:1002, 1989.

1465. Grey RHB: Foveo-macular retinitis, solar retinopathy, and trauma, Br J Ophthalmol 62:543, 1978.

1466. Grey RHB, Blach RK, and Barnard WM: Bull's eye maculopathy with early cone degeneration, Br J Ophthalmol 61:702, 1977.

1467. Grierson I and Forrester JV: Vitreous haemorrhage and vitreal membranes, Trans Ophthalmol Soc UK 100:140, 1977.

1468. Gross JG and others: Subfoveal neovascular membrane removal in patients with traumatic choroidal rupture, Ophthalmology 103:579, 1996.

1469. Gross JG and others: Experimental endoretinal biopsy, Am J Ophthalmol 110:619, 1990.

1470. Grossniklaus HE and Green WR: Pathologic findings in pathologic myopia, Retina 12:127, 1992.

1471. Grossniklaus HE and others: Clinicopathologic features of surgically excised choroidal neovascular membranes, Ophthalmology 101:1099, 1994.

1472. Grossniklaus HE and others: Immunohistochemical and histochemical properties of surgically excised subretinal neovascular membranes in age-related macular degeneration, Am J Ophthalmol 114:464, 1992.

1473. Guerin CJ and others: Immunocytochemical identification of Müller's glia as a component of human epiretinal membranes, Invest Ophthalmol Vis Sci 31:1483, 1990.

1474. Guidry C: Isolation and characterization of porcine muller cells. Myofibroblastic dedifferentiation in culture, Invest Ophthalmol Vis Sci 37:740, 1996.

1475. Guyer DR and others: Histopathologic features of idiopathic macular holes and cysts, Ophthalmology 97:1045, 1990.

1476. Guyer DR and others: Indocyanineine green-guided laser photocoagulation of focal spots at the edge of plaques of choroidal neovascularization (see comments), Arch Ophthalmol 82:527, 1976.

1477. Hadden O and Gass JDM: Fundus flavimaculatus and Stargardt's disease, Am J Ophthalmol 82:527, 1976.

1478. Hagedoorn A: Angioid streaks, Arch Ophthalmol 21:746, 1939.

1479. Halperin LS: Choroidal neovascular membrane and other chorioretinal complications of acquired syphilis, Am J Ophthalmol 108:554, 1989.

1480. Hamilton WK and others: Sorby's fundus dystrophy, Ophthalmology 96:1755, 1989.

1481. Hampton GR, Kohen D, and Bird AC: Visual prognosis of disciform degeneration in myopia, Ophthalmology 90:923, 1983.

1482. Hardwick C and others: Pathologic human vitreous promotes contraction by fibroblasts; implication for proliferative vitreoretinopathy, Arch Ophthalmol 113:1545, 1995.

1483. Haut J and others. Surgery of idiopathic epiretinal macular membranes. A retrospective statistical study of the functional result. Apropos of 42 treated cases (French), J Francais d Ophthalmologie 12:81, 1989.

1484. Hayreh SS: Postradiation retinopathy: flourescence fundus angiographic study, Br J Ophthalmol 54:705, 1970.

1485. Hayreh SS: Submacular choroidal vascular pattern, Graefes Arch Clin Exp Ophthalmol 192:181, 1974.

1486. Hee MR and others: Optical coherence tomography of macular holes, Ophthalmology 102:748, 1995.

1487. Hee MR and others: Optical coherence tomography of central serous chorioretinopathy, Am J Ophthalmol 120:65, 1995.

1488. Heher KL and Johns DR: A maculopathy associated with the 15257 mitochondrial DNA mutation, Arch Ophthalmol 111:1495, 1993.

1489. Henkind P: Ocular neovascularization (Krill Memorial Lecture), Am J Ophthalmol 85:287, 1978.

1490. Henkind P, editor: The first international cystoid macular edema symposium, Surv Ophthalmol 28(suppl):431, 1984.

1491. Heriot WJ and others: Choroidal neuvascularization can digest Bruch's membrane: a prior break is not essential, Ophthalmology 91:1603, 1984.

1492. Hikichi T, Akiba J, and Trempe CL: Effect of the vitreous on the prognosis of full-thickness idiopathic macular hole, Am J Ophthalmol 116:273, 1993.

1493. Hittner H and Zeller R: Ceroid-lipofuscinosis (Batten disease), Arch Ophthalmol 93:178, 1975.

1494. Ho AC and others: The natural history of idiopathic subfoveal choroidal neovascularization, Ophthalmology 102:782, 1995.

1495. Hodes BL, Feiner LA, and Sherman SH: Progression of pseudovitelliform macular dystrophy, Arch Ophthalmol 111:1495, 1993.

1496. Hogan MJ: Bruch's membrane and disease of the macula, Trans Ophthalmol Soc UK 87:111, 1967.

1497. Hogan MJ and Alvarado J: Studies on the human macula. IV. Aging changes in Bruch's membrane, Arch Ophthalmol 77:410, 1967.

1498. Holz FG and others: Autosomal dominant macular dystrophy simulating North Carolina macular dystrophy, Arch Ophthalmol 113:178, 1995.

1499. Holz FG and others: Analysis of lipid deposits extracted from human macular and peripheral Bruch's membrane, Arch Ophthalmol 112:402, 1994.

1500. Holz FG and others: Bilateral macular drusen in age-related macular degeneration. Prognosis and risk factors, Ophthalmology 101: 1522, 1994.

1501. Hotchkiss ML and Fine SL: Pathologic myopia and choroidal neovascularization, Am J Ophthalmol 91:177, 1981.

1502. Howe LJ and others: Choroidal hypoperfusion in acute posterior multifocal placoid pigment epitheliopathy, an idocyanine green angiography study, Ophthalmology 102:790, 1995.

1503. Howes E and others: Ocular pathology of infantile Niemann-Pick disease: study of fetus of 23 weeks' gestation, Arch Ophthalmol 93:494, 1975.

1504. Hsu JK and others: Clinicopathologic studies of an eye after submacular membranectomy for choroidal neovascularization, Retina 15: 43, 1995.

1505. Hutton WL and others: Focal parafoveal retinal telangiectasis, Arch Ophthalmol 96:1362, 1978.

1506. Irvine AR: Cystoid maculopathy, Surv Ophthalmol 21:1, 1976.

1507. Irvine AR and Wergeland FL Jr: Stargardt's hereditary progressive macular degeneration, Br J Ophthalmol 56:817, 1972.

1508. Irvine AR and others: Macular edema after cataract extraction, Ann Ophthalmol 3:1234, 1971.

1509. Irvine SR: A newly defined vitreous syndrome following cataract extraction: interpreted according to recent concepts of the structure of the vitreous (Seventh Francis I. Proctor Lecture), Am J Ophthalmol 36:599, 1953.

1510. Ishibashi T and others: Formation of drusen in the human eye, Am J Ophthalmol 101:342, 1986.

1511. Ishibashi T and others: Pericytes of newly formed vessels in experimental subretinal neovascularization, Arch Ophthalmol 113:227, 1995.

1512. Jacklin HN: Acute posterior multifocal placoid pigment epitheliopathy and thyroiditis, Arch Ophthalmol 95:995, 1977.

1513. Jacobson DM, Thompson S, and Bartley JA: X-linked progressive cone dystrophy, Ophthalmology 96:885, 1989.

1514. Jacobson D and Dellaporta A: Natural history of cystoid macular edema after cataract extraction, Am J Ophthalmol 77:445, 1974.

1515. Jaffe GJ and Schatz H: Histopathologic features of adult-onset foveomacular pigment epithelial dystrophy, Arch Ophthalmol 106: 958, 1988.

1516. Jampol LM and others: Subretinal neovascularization with geographic (serpiginous) choroiditis, Am J Ophthalmol 88:683, 1979.

1517. Jerdan JA and others: Proliferative vitreoretinopathy membranes. An immunohistochemical study, Ophthalmology 96:801, 1989.

1518. Johnson MW, Hassan TS, and Elner VM: Laser photocoagulation of the choroid through experimental subretinal hemorrhage, Arch Ophthalmol 113:364, 1995.

1519. Johnson RNK and Gass JDM: Idiopathic macular holes. Observations, stages of formation, and implications for surgical intervention, Ophthalmology 95:917, 1988.

1520. Junius P: Erscheinungsformen und Ablauf der juvenilen Retinitis exsudativa macularis, Z Augenheilkd 70:129, 1930.

1521. Junuis P and Kuhnt H: Die scheibenförmige Entartung der Netzhautmitte (Degeneratio maculae luteae disciformis), Berlin, 1926, S Karger.

1522. Kaback M and others: Tay-Sachs disease-carrier screening, prenatal diagnosis, and the molecular era, JAMA 270:2307, 1993.

1523. Kampik A and others: Ultrastructural features of progressive idiopathic epiretinal membrane removed by vitreous surgery, Am J Ophthalmol 99:797, 1980.

1524. Kampik A and others: Epiretinal and vitreous membranes: comparative study of 56 cases, Arch Ophthalmol 99:1445, 1981.

1525. Kampik A: Proliferative vitreoretinal reaction (German), Fortschritte der Medizin 102:75, 1984.

1526. Kandori F and others: Fleck retinal, Arch Ophthalmol 73:673, 1972.

1527. Katz B and Hoyt WF: Intrapapillary and peripapillary hemorrhage in young patients with incomplete posterior vitreous detachment, Ophthalmology 102:349, 1995.

1528. Katz ML and Rodrigues M: Juvenile ceroid lipofuscinosis. Evidence for methylated lysine in neural storage body protein, Am J Ophthalmol 138:323, 1991.

1529. Kauffer G and Zimmerman LE: Direct rupture of choroid, Arch Ophthalmol 75:384, 1966.

1530. Kearns M, Hamilton AM, and Kohner EM: Excessive permeability in diabetic maculopathy, Br J Ophthalmol 63:489, 1979.

1531. Keeney A and Jain M: Macular disease of involutional type: classification and therapeutic approaches, Trans Am Ophthalmol Soc 56: 247, 1958.

1532. Keithahn MAZ and others: The variable expressivity of a family with central areolar pigment epithelial dystrophy, Ophthalmology 103:406, 1996.

1533. Kenyon KR and Michels RG: Ultrastructure of epiretinal membrane removed by pars plana vitreoretinal surgery, Am J Ophthalmol 83:815, 1977.

1534. Kenyon KR and others: Diffuse drusen and associated complications, Am J Ophthalmol 100:119, 1985.

1535. Kenyon KR and others: Mucolipidosis IV. Histopathology of conjunctiva, cornea and skin, Arch Ophthalmol 97:1106, 1979.

1536. Khouri G and others: X-linked congenital stationary nightblindness. Review and report of a family with hyperopia, Arch Ophthalmol 106:1417, 1988.

1537. Kimmel AS and others: Idiopathic premacular gliosis in children and adolescents, Am J Ophthalmol 108:578, 1989.

1538. Kingham JD and Lochen GP: Vitelliform macular degeneration, Am J Ophthalmol 84:526, 1977.

1539. Kivela T and others: Clinically successful contact transscleral krypton laser cyclophotocoagulation, long-term histopathologic and immune histochemical autopsy findings, Arch Ophthalmol 113:1447, 1995.

1540. Khwarg SG and others: Incidence, risk factors and morphology in operating microscope light retinopathy, Am J Ophthalmol 103:255, 1987.

1541. Klein ML and others: Follow-up study of detachment of the retinal pigment epithelium, Br J Ophthalmol 64:412, 1980.

1542. Klein ML, Mauldin WM, and Stoumbous VD: Heredity and age-related macular degeneration. Observations in monozygomatic twins, Arch Ophthalmol 112:932, 1994.

1543. Klein R and others: Subretinal neovascularization associated with fundus flavimaculatus, Arch Ophthalmol 96:2054, 1978.

1544. Klein R and others: The epidemiology of epiretinal membranes, Trans Am Ophthalmol Soc 92:403, 1994.

1545. Klein RM and Green S: The development of lacquer cracks in pathologic myopia, Am J Ophthalmol 106:282, 1988.

1546. Klein RM and others: The relationship of age-related maculopathy, cataract, and glaucoma to visual acuity, Invest Ophthalmol Vis Sci 36:182, 1995.

1547. Klein BR and others: Fundus photographic and fluorescein angiographic characteristics of pseudoholes of the macula in eyes with epiretinal membranes, Ophthalmology 102:768, 1995.

1548. Klien BA: Clinical and histopathologic aspects of angioid streaks, Am J Ophthalmol 32:1134, 1949.

1549. Klien BA: The heredodegenerations of the macula lutea, Am J Ophthalmol 33:371, 1950.

1550. Klien BA: Macular lesions of vascular origin, Am J Ophthalmol 34: 1279, 1951.

1551. Klien BA: Macular lesions of various origin. II. Functional vascular conditions leading to damage of the macula lutea, Am J Ophthalmol 36:1, 1953.

1552. Klien BA: Retinal lesions associated with uveal disease. I. Am J Ophthalmol 42:831, 1956.

1553. Klien BA: Diseases of the macula, Arch Ophthalmol 60:175, 1958.

1554. Klien BA and Krill AE: Fundus flavimaculatus: clinical functional, and histopathologic observations, Am J Ophthalmol 64:3, 1967.

1555. Kliffen M and others: Identification of glycosaminoglycans in age-related macular deposits, Arch Ophthalmol 114:1009, 1996.

1556. Kono T, Kohno T, and Inomata H: Epiretinal membrane formation. Light and electron microscopic study in an experimental rabbit model, Arch Ophthalmol 113:359, 1995.

1557. Kobrin JL, Apple DJ, and Hart WB: Vitelliform dystrophy, Int Ophthalmol Clin 21(3):167, 1981.

1558. Krill AE: Hereditary retinal and choroidal diseases, vol I, Evaluation, New York, 1972, Harper & Row, Publishers.

1559. Krill AE and Klien BA: Flecked retina syndrome, Arch Ophthalmol 74:496, 1965.

1560. Krill AE and others: Hereditary vitelliruptive macular degeneration, Am J Ophthalmol 61:1405, 1966.

1561. Krill AE and Deutman AE: Dominant macular degeneration, Am J Ophthalmol 73:352, 1972.

1562. Krill AE and Archer D: Classification of the choroid atrophies, Am J Ophthalmol 75:562, 1971.

1563. Kvanta A and others: Subfoveal fibrovascular membranes in age-related macular degeneration express vascular endothelial growth factor, Invest Ophthalmol Vis Sci 37:1929, 1996.

1564. Laatikainen L, Immonen I, and Summanen P: Peripheral retinal angiomalike lesion and macular pucker, Am J Ophthalmol 108:563, 1989.

1565. Levine R, Brucker AJ, and Robinson F: Long-term follow-up of idiopathic central serous chorioretinopathy by fluorescein angiography, Ophthalmology 96:854, 1989.

1566. Lewis H, Straatsma BR, and Foos RY: Chorioretinal juncture: multiple extramacular drusen, Ophthalmology 93:1098, 1986.

1567. Lewis H and others: Subretinal membranes in proliferative vitreoretinopathy, Ophthalmology 96:1403, 1989.

1568. Lewis H and Verdaguer JI: Surgical treatment for chronic hypotony and anterior proliferative vitreoretinopathy, Am J Ophthalmol 122:228, 1996.

1569. Lewis H and others: Tissue plasminogen activator treatment of experimental subretinal hemorrhage, Am J Ophthalmol 111:197, 1991.

1570. Lewis RA and others: Familial foveal retinoschisis, Arch Ophthalmol 95:1190, 1977.

1571. Liem ATA, Keunen JEE, and van Norren D: Foveal densitometry in adult-onset diffuse drusen, Am J Ophthalmol 114:149, 1992.

1572. Liggett PE and others: Human autologous serum for the treatment of full-thickness macular holes. A preliminary study, Ophthalmology 102:1071, 1995.

1573. Lindsey PS and others: Ultrastructure of epiretinal membrane causing retinal starfold, Ophthalmology 90:578, 1983.

1574. Lopez PF and others: Bone marrow transplant retinopathy, Am J Ophthalmol 112:635, 1991.

1575. Lopez and others: Pathogenetic mechanisms in anterior proliferative vitreoretinopathy, Am J Ophthalmol 114:257, 1992.

1576. Lopez PF and others: Pathologic features of surgically excised subretinal neovascular membranes in age-related macular degeneration, Am J Ophthalmol 112:647, 1995.

1577. Lopez PF and others: Autosomal-dominant fundus flavimaculatus. Clinicopathologic correlation, Ophthalmology 97:798, 1990.

1578. Lopez PF and others: Retinal pigment epithelial wound healing in vivo, Arch Ophthalmol 113:1437, 1995.

1579. Lopez PF and others: Transdifferentiated retinal pigment epithelial cells are immunoreactive for vascular endothelial growth factor in surgically excised age-related macular degeneration-related choroidal neovascular membranes, Invest Ophthalmol Vis Sci 37:855, 1996.

1580. MacCumber MW and others: Clinicopathologic correlation of the multiple recurrent serosanguineous retinal pigment epithelial detachments syndrome, Retina 14:143, 1994.

1581. Machemer R and others: An updated classification of retinal detachment with proliferative vitreoretinopathy, Am J Ophthalmol 112:159, 1991.

1582. Mackool RJ and others: Epinephrine-induced cystoid macular edema in aphakic eyes, Arch Ophthalmol 95:791, 1977.

1583. Madigan MC and others: Intermediate filament expression in human retinal macroglia, Retina 14:65, 1994.

1584. Madreperla SA and others: Clinicopathologic correlation of a macular hole treated by cortical vitreous peeling and gas tamponade, Ophthalmology 101:682, 1994.

1585. Madreperla SA and others: Clinicopathologic correlation of surgically removed macular hole opercula, Am J Ophthalmol 120:197, 1995.

1586. Maguire JI, Benson WE, and Brown GC: Treatment of foveal pigment epithelial detachments with contiguous extrafoveal choroidal neovascular membranes, Am J Ophthalmol 109:523, 1990.

1587. Maloney WF, Robertson DM, and Duboff SM: Hereditary vitelliform macular degeneration: variable fundus findings within a single pedigree, Arch Ophthalmol 95:979, 1977.

1588. Manschot W: Pathology of hereditary juvenile retinoschisis, Arch Ophthalmol 88:131, 1972.

1589. Marchesani O and Sautter H: Atlas of the ocular fundus, New York, 1959, Hafner Publishing Co (Translated by A Philipp).

1590. Marmor MF and others: Diagnostic clinical findings of a new syndrome with night blindness, maculopathy, and enhanced s cone sensitivity, Am J Ophthalmol 110:124, 1996.

1591. Marmor MF: Long-term follow-up of the physiologic abnormalities and fundus changes in fundus albipunctatus, Ophthalmology 97:380, 1990.

1592. Martin NF, Green WR, and Martin LW: Retinal phlebitis in the Irvine-Gass syndrome, Am J Ophthalmol 83:377, 1977.

1593. Matthews JD, Weiter JJ, and Kolodny EH: Macular halos associated with Niemann-Pick type B disease, Ophthalmology 93:933, 1986.

1594. Maumenee AE: Serous and hemorrhagic disciform detachment of the macula, Trans Pac Coast Otoophthalmol Soc 40:139, 1959.

1595. Maumenee AE: Symposium: macular diseases—pathogenesis, Trans Am Acad Ophthalmol Otolaryngol 69:691, 1965.

1596. Maumenee AE and Emery J: An anatomic classification of diseases of the macula, Am J Ophthalmol 74:594, 1972.

1597. McDonald HR and Irvine AR: Light induced maculopathy from the operating microscope in extracapsular cataract extraction and intraocular lens implantation, Ophthalmology 90:945, 1983.

1598. McDonald HR, Johnson RN, and Schatz H: Surgical results in the vitreomacular traction syndrome, Ophthalmology 101:1397, 1994.

1599. McDonald HR and others: Clinicopathologic results of vitreous surgery for epiretinal membranes in patients with combined retinal and retinal pigment epithelial hamartomas, Am J Ophthalmol 100:806, 1985.

1600. McDonnell PJ: Fundus flavimaculatus without maculopathy: a clinicopathologic study, Ophthalmology 93:116, 1986.

1601. McFarland C: Heredodegeneration of the macula lutea: study of the clinical and pathologic aspects, Arch Ophthalmol 53:224, 1955.

1602. McGuinness R: Epiretinal membrane formation associated with spontaneous massive periretinal proliferation, Br J Ophthalmol 64:102, 1980.

1603. McKusick V: Heritable disorders of connective tissue, ed 4, St Louis, 1972, The CV Mosby Co.

1604. McLane NJ and others: Angioid streaks associated with hereditary spherocytosis, Am J Ophthalmol 97:444, 1984.

1605. McLeod D, Marshall J, and Grierson I: Epimacular membrane peeling, Trans Ophthalmol Soc UK 101:170, 1981.

1606. Meredith TA, Bradley RE, and Aaberg TM: Natural history of serous detachments of the retinal pigment epithelium, Am J Ophthalmol 88:643, 1979.

1607. Michael JC and de Venecia G: Retinal trypsin digest study of cystoid macular edema associated with choroidal melanoma, Am J Ophthalmol 119:152, 1995.

1608. Michel J: Über Geschwülste des Uvealtractus, Graefes Arch Ophthalmol 24:131, 1878.

1609. Michel J: Lehrbuch der Augenheilkunde, Wiesbaden, 1890, JF Bergmann.

1610. Michels RG: Surgical management of epiretinal membranes, Trans Ophthalmol Soc UK 99:54, 1979.

1611. Michels RG: A clinical and histopathologic study of epiretinal membranes affecting the macula and removed by vitreous surgery, Trans Am Ophthalmol Soc 80:580, 1982.

1612. Michelson JB, Michelson PE, and Chisari FV: Subretinal neovascular membrane and disciform scar in Behçet's disease, Am J Ophthalmol 90:182, 1980.

1613. Miller B, Miller H, and Ryan SJ: Experimental epiretinal proliferation induced by intravitreal red blood cells, Am J Ophthalmol 103:2, 188, 1986.

1614. Miller H, Miller B, and Ryan SJ: Newly formed subretinal vessels. Fine structure and fluorescein leakage, Invest Ophthalmol Vis Sci 27:204, 1986.

1615. Miller SA: Multifocal Best's vitelliform dystrophy, Arch Ophthalmol 95:984, 1977.

1616. Miller SA: Fluorescence in Best's vitelliform dystrophy, lipofuscin, and fundus flavimaculatus, Br J Ophthalmol 62:256, 1978.

1617. Mills PV: Preretinal macular fibrosis, Trans Ophthalmol Soc UK 99:50, 1979.

1618. Miyake K, Sakamura S, and Miura H: Long-term follow-up study on prevention of aphakic cystoid macular edema by topical indomethacin, Br J Ophthalmol 64:324, 1980.

1619. Miyake Y and others: Bull's eye maculopathy and negative electroretinogram, Retina 9:210, 1989.

1620. Miyake Y and others: Focal macular electroretinogram in x-linked congenital retinoschisis, Invest Ophthalmol Vis Sci 34:512, 1993.

1621. Mohler CW and Fine SL: Long-term evaluation of patients with Best's vitelliform dystrophy, Ophthalmology 88:688, 1981.

1622. Moorfields Macular Study Group: Treatment of senile disciform macular degeneration: a single-blind randomised trial by argon photocoagulation, Br J Ophthalmol 66:745, 1982.

1623. Morino I and others: Variation in epiretinal membrane components with clinical duration of the proliferative tissue (see comments), Br J Ophthalmol 74:393, 1990.

1624. Morse PH and others: Fundus flavimaculatus with cystoid macular changes and abnormal Stiles-Crawford effect, Am J Ophthalmol 91:190, 1981.

1625. Nagpal KC and others: Angioid streaks and sickle haemoglobinopathies, Br J Ophthalmol 60:31, 1976.

1626. Nasr YG and others: Goldmann-Favre maculopathy, Retina 10: 178, 1990.

1627. Neetens A and Burvenich H: Presumed inflammatory maculopathies, Trans Ophthalmol Soc UK 98:160, 1978.

1628. Newell F, Krill AE, and Farkas TG: Drusen and fundus flavimaculatus: clinical, functional and histologic characteristics, Trans Am Acad Ophthalmol Otolaryngol 76:88, 1972.

1629. Newell F, Matalon R, and Meyer S: A new mucolipidosis with psychomotor retardation, corneal clouding, and retinal degeneration, Am J Ophthalmol 80:440, 1975.

1630. Newman NJ and others: Corneal surface irregularities and episodic pain in a patient with mucolipidosis IV, Arch Ophthalmol 108:251, 1990.

1631. Newsom WA and others: Cystoid macular edema: histopathologic and angiographic correlations; a clinicopathologic case report, Trans Am Acad Ophthalmol Otolaryngol 76:1005, 1972.

1632. Newsome DA, Rodrigues MM, and Machemer R: Human massive periretinal proliferation: in vitro characteristics of cellular components, Arch Ophthalmol 99:873, 1981.

1633. Newsome DA and others: Oral zinc in macular degeneration, Arch Ophthalmol 106:192, 1988.

1634. Nichols BE and others: Refining the locus for Best vitelliform macular dystrophy and mutation analysis of the candidate gene ROM1, Am J Hum Genet 54:95, 1994.

1635. Nielsen CE: Stickler's syndrome, Acta Ophthalmol 59:286, 1981.

1636. Noble KG: Central areolar choroidal dystrophy, Am J Ophthalmol 84:310, 1977.

1637. Noble KG and Carr RE: Stargardt's disease and fundus flavimaculatus, Arch Ophthalmol 97:1281, 1979.

1638. Noble KG and Carr RE: Acquired macular degeneration. I. Nonexudative (dry) macular degeneration, Ophthalmology 92:591, 1985.

1639. Noble KG, Scher BM, and Carr RE: Polymorphous presentations in vitelliform macular dystrophy: subretinal neovascularization and central choroidal atrophy, Br J Ophthalmol 62:561, 1978.

1640. Noble KG and Chang S: Adult vitelliform macular degeneration progressing to full-thickness macular hole. Case report, Arch Ophthalmol 109:325, 1991.

1641. Noble KG and Sherman J: Central pigmentary sheen dystrophy, Am J Ophthalmol 108:255, 1989.

1642. Norton EWD and others: Symposium: macular diseases: diagnosis; fluorescein in the study of macular diseases, Trans Am Acad Ophthalmol Otolaryngol 69:631, 1965.

1643. Ober RR and others: Autosomal dominant exudative vitreoretinopathy, Br J Ophthalmol 64:112, 1980.

1644. O'Donnell FE and Welch RB: Fenestrated Sheen macular dystrophy: a new autosomal dominant maculopathy, Arch Ophthalmol 97:1292, 1979.

1645. O'Gorman S and others: Histopathologic findings in Best's vitelliform macular dystrophy, Arch Ophthalmol 106:1261, 1988.

1646. Ormerod LD, Puklin JE, and Frank RN: Long-term outcomes after the surgical removal of advanced subfoveal neovascular membranes in age-related macular degeneration, Ophthalmology 101: 1201, 1994.

1647. Orth DH and others: Rubella maculopathy, Br J Ophthalmol 64: 201, 1980.

1648. Palmer M and others: Niemann-Pick disease—type C: ocular histopathologic and electron microscopic study, Arch Ophthalmol 103: 817, 1985.

1649. Paton D: The relation of angioid streaks to systemic disease, Springfield, Ill, 1972, Charles C Thomas, Publisher.

1650. Patrinely JR, Lewis RA, and Font RL: Foveomacular vitelliform dystrophy, adult type: a clinicopathologic study including electron microscopic observations, Ophthalmology 92:1712, 1985.

1651. Pauleikhoff D and others: Aging changes in Bruch's membrane.

A histochemical and morphologic study, Ophthalmology 97:171, 1990.

1652. Pauleikhoff D and others: Correlation between biochemical composition and fluorescein binding of deposits in Bruch's membrane, Ophthalmology 99:1548, 1992.

1653. Pauleikhoff D and others: Choroidal perfusion abnormality with age-related Bruch's membrane change, Am J Ophthalmol 109:211, 1990.

1654. Pauleikhoff D and others: Drusen as risk factors in age-related macular disease, Am J Ophthalmol 109:38, 1990.

1655. Pavan PR and Margo CE: Submacular neovascular membrane and focal granulomatous inflammation, Ophthalmology 103:586, 1996.

1656. Peachey NS and others: A form of congenital stationary night blindness with apparent defect of rod phototransduction, Invest Ophthalmol Vis Sci 31:237, 1990.

1657. Perry HD, Zimmerman LE, and Benson WE: Hemorrhage from isolated aneurysm of a retinal artery, Arch Ophthalmol 95:281, 1977.

1658. Pitta CG and others: Small unilateral foveal hemorrhages in young adults, Am J Ophthalmol 89:96, 1980.

1659. Poliner LS and others: Natural history of retinal pigment epithelial detachments in age-related macular degeneration, Ophthalmology 93:543, 1986.

1660. Prensky JG and Bresnick GH: Butterfly-shaped macular dystrophy in four generations, Arch Ophthalmol 101:1198, 1983.

1661. Pruett RC, Carvalho ACA, and Trempe CL: Microhemorrhagic maculopathy, Arch Ophthalmol 99:425, 1981.

1662. Quaranta M and others: Indocyanineine green videoangiography of angioid streaks, Am J Ophthalmol 119:136, 1995.

1663. Rabb MF, editor: Macular disease, Int Ophthalmol Clin 21(3), 1981.

1664. Rabb MF and Morgan BS: Serous detachment of the retinal pigment epithelium, Perspect Ophthalmol 3:81, 1979.

1665. Rabb MF, Tso MOM, and Fishman GA: Cone-rod dystrophy: a clinical and histopathologic report, Ophthalmology 93:1443, 1986.

1666. Raichand M and others: Macular holes associated with proliferative sickle cell retinopathy, Arch Ophthalmol 96:1592, 1978.

1667. Ramsey M and Fine B: Chloroquine toxicity in the human eye: histopathologic observations by electron microscopy, Am J Ophthalmol 73:229, 1972.

1668. Reddy BM, Zamora RL, and Kaplan HJ: Distribution of growth factors in subfoveal neovascular membranes in age-related macular degeneration and presumed ocular histoplasmosis syndrome, Am J Ophthalmol 120:291, 1995.

1669. Rentsch FJ: The ultrastructure of preretinal macular fibrosis, Graefes Arch Clin Exp Ophthalmol 203:321, 1977.

1670. Riedel KG and others: Ocular abnormalities in mucolipidosis IV, Am J Ophthalmol 99:125, 1985.

1671. Robb RM and Kuwabara T: The ocular pathology of type A Niemann-Pick disease: a light and electron microscopic study, Invest Ophthalmol 12:366, 1973.

1672. Robbins SG and others: Immunolocalization of integrins in proliferative retinal membranes, Invest Ophthalmol Vis Sci 35:3475, 1994.

1673. Robertson DM and Buettner H: Pigmented preretinal membranes, Am J Ophthalmol 83:824, 1977.

1674. Rodger FC: Some practical conclusions following a longitudinal study of common macular lesions, Trans Ophthalmol Soc UK 102: 187, 1982.

1675. Rodrigues MM and others: Choroideremia: a clinical, electron microscopic, and biochemical report, Ophthalmology 91:873, 1984.

1676. Rosa RH, Thomas MA, and Green WR: Clinicopathologic correlation of submacular membranectomy with retention of good vision in a patient with age-related macular degeneration, Arch Ophthalmol 114:480, 1996.

1677. Roth A and Foos R: Surface wrinkling retinopathy in eyes enucleated at autopsy, Trans Am Acad Ophthalmol Otolaryngol 75:1047, 1971.

1678. Roy M and Kaiser-Kupfer M: Second eye involvement in age-related macular degeneration. A four-year prospective study, Eye 4:813, 1990.

1679. Rubsamen PE and others: Prevention of experimental proliferative vitreoretinopathy with a biodegradable intravitreal implant for the sustained release of fluorouracil, Arch Ophthalmol 112:407, 1994.

1680. Rumelt S, Kraus E, and Rehany U: Retinal neovascularization and cystoid macular edema in punctata albescens retinopathy, Am J Ophthalmol 114:507, 1992.

1681. Rush JA: Acute macular neuroretinopathy, Am J Ophthalmol 83: 490, 1977.

1682. Ryan S: Cystoid maculopathy in phakic retinal detachment procedures, Am J Ophthalmol 76:519, 1973.

1683. Ryan S and Maumenee A: Acute posterior multifocal placoid pigment epitheliopathy, Am J Ophthalmol 74:1066, 1972.

1684. Sabates R, Pruett RC, and Hirose T: Pseudovitelliform macular degeneration, Retina 2:197, 1982.

1685. Sakamoto T and others: Inhibition of experimental proliferative vitreoretinopathy by retroviral vector mediated transfer of suicide gene. Can proliferative vitreoretinopathy be a target of gene therapy? Ophthalmology 102:1417, 1995.

1686. Sandberg MA and others: Iris pigmentation and extent of disease in patients with neovascular age-related macular degeneration, Invest Ophthalmol Vis Sci 35:2734, 1994.

1687. Sandberg MA and others: Hyperopia and neovascularization in age-related macular degenearation, Ophthalmology 100:1009, 1993.

1688. Sarks S: New vessel formation beneath the retinal pigment epithelium in senile eyes, Br J Ophthalmol 57:951, 1973.

1689. Sarks SH and others: Softening of drusen and subretinal neovascularization, Trans Ophthalmol Soc UK 100:414, 1980.

1690. Sarks SH: Drusen patterns predisposing to geographic atrophy of the retinal pigment epithelium, Aust J Ophthalmol 10:91, 1982.

1691. Sarks SH: Drusen and their relationship to senile macular degeneration, Aust J Ophthalmol 8:117, 1980.

1692. Sarks SH: Ageing and degeneration in the macular region. A clinicopathological study, Br J Ophthalmol 60:324, 1976.

1693. Sassani JW and others: Progressive chloroquine retinopathy, Ann Ophthalmol 15:19, 1983.

1694. Saxe SJ and others: Ultrastructural features of surgically excised subretinal neovascular membranes in the ocular histoplasmosis syndrome, Arch Ophthalmol 111:88, 1993.

1695. van der Schaft TL and others: Histologic features of the early stages of age-related macular degeneration, Ophthalmology 99:278, 1992.

1696. van der Schaft TL, de Bruijn WC, and Mooy CM: Is basal laminar deposit unique for age-related macular degeneration? Arch Ophthalmol 109:420, 1991.

1697. Schatz H and others, editors: Interpretation of fundus fluorescein angiography: a comprehensive text and atlas, St Louis, 1978, The CV Mosby Co.

1698. Schatz H, McDonald R, and Johnson RN: Retinal pigment epithelial folds associated with retinal pigment epithelial detachment in macular degeneration, Ophthalmology 97:658, 1990.

1699. Schatz H and others: Subretinal fibrosis in central serous chorioretinopathy, Ophthalmology 102:1077, 1995.l

1700. Schatz H and McDonald HR: Atrophic macular degeneration, Ophthalmology 96:1541, 1989.

1701. Schochet SS Jr, Font RI, and Morris HH III: Jansky-Bielschowsky form of neuronal ceroid-lipofuscinosis. Ocular pathology of the Batten-Vogt syndrome, Arch Ophthalmol 98:1083, 1980.

1702. Schwarz GA and Yanoff M: Lafora bodies, corpora amylacea and Lewey bodies—a morphologic and histochemical study, Arch Neurobiol (Madr) 28:801, 1965.

1703. Schwartz D and others: Proliferative vitreoretinopathy. Ultrastructural study of 20 retroretinal membranes removed by bitreous surgery, Retina 8:275, 1988.

1704. Sheehan B: Congenital vascular veils in the vitreous, Trans Ophthalmol Soc UK 72:623, 1952.

1705. Sheraidah G and others: Correlation between lipids extracted from Bruch's membrane and age, Ophthalmology 100:47, 1993.

1706. Sheta SM and others: Cyanoacrylate tissue adhesive in the management of recurrent retinal detachment caused by macular hole, Am J Ophthalmol 109:28, 1990.

1707. Shirakawa H and Ogino N: Idiopathic epiretinal membranes with spontaneous posterior vitreous separation, Ophthalmologica 194: 90, 1987.

1708. Sigurdsson R and Begg IS: Organized macular plaques in exudative diabetic maculopathy, Br J Ophthalmol 64:392, 1980.

1709. Singerman LJ, Berkow JW, and Patz A: Dominant slowly progressive macular dystrophy, Am J Ophthalmol 83:680, 1977.

1710. Sivalingam A and others: Visual prognosis correlated with the presence of internal limiting membrane in histopathologic specimens obtained from epiretinal membrane surgery, Ophthalmology 97: 1549, 1990.

1711. Slusher MM and Tyler ME: Choroidoretinal vascular anastomoses, Am J Ophthalmol 90:217, 1980.

1712. Small KW and Gehrs K: Clinical study of a large family with autosomal dominant progressive cone degeneration, Am J Ophthalmol 121:1, 1996.

1713. Small M and others: Senile macular degeneration: a clinicopathologic correlation of two cases with neovascularization beneath the retinal pigment epithelium, Arch Ophthalmol 94:599, 1976.

1714. Smiddy WE and others: Idiopathic epiretinal membranes. Ultrastructural characteristics and clinicopathologic correlation, Ophthalmology 96:811, 1989.

1715. Smiddy WE and others: Ultrastructural studies of vitreomacular traction syndrome, Am J Ophthalmol 107:177, 1989.

1716. Smiddy WE and others: Histopathology of tissue removed during vitrectomy for impending idiopathic macular holes, Am J Ophthalmol 108:360, 1989.

1717. Smiddy WE and others: Morphology, pathology, and surgery of idiopathic vitreoretinal macular disorders. A review, Retina 10:288, 1990.

1718. Smith R, Kelley J, and Harbin T: Late macular complications of choroidal ruptures, Am J Ophthalmol 77:650, 1974.

1719. Sneed SR and Sieving PA: Fenestrated sheen macular degeneration, Am J Ophthalmol 112:1, 1991.

1720. Sorsby A and Crick R: Central areolar choroidal sclerosis, Br J Ophthalmol 37:129, 1953.

1721. Soubrane G and others: Occult subretinal new vessels in age-related macular degeneration. Natural history and early laser treatment, Ophthalmology 97:649, 1990.

1722. Spaeth G: Ocular manifestations of the lipidoses. In Tasman W, editor: Retinal diseases in children, New York, 1971, Harper & Row, Publishers.

1723. Spalton DJ, Taylor DSI, and Sanders MD: Juvenile Batten's disease: an ophthalmological assessment of 26 patients, Br J Ophthalmol 64:726, 1980.

1724. Spitznas M and Leuenberger R: Die primäre epiretinale Gliöse, Klin Monatsbl Augenheilkd 171:410, 1977.

1725. Sramek SJ and others: Immunostaining of preretinal membranes for actin, fibronectin, and glial fibrillary acidic protein, Ophthalmology 96:835, 1989.

1726. Steinmetz RL and others: Histopathology of incipient fundus flavimaculatus, Ophthalmology 98:953, 1991.

1727. Stern WH and others: Epiretinal membrane formation after vitrectomy, Am J Ophthalmol 93:757, 1982.

1728. Stern WH and others: Fluorouracil therapy for proliferative vitreoretinopathy after vitrectomy, Am J Ophthalmol 96:33, 1983.

1729. Sternberg P Jr and Machemer R: Subretinal proliferation, Am J Ophthalmol 98, 456, 1984.

1730. Sternberg P and others: Occult choroidal neovascularization. Influence on visual outcome in patients with age-related molecular degeneration, Arch Ophthalmol 114:400, 1996.

1731. Stone EM and others: Clinical features of a Stargardt-like dominant progressive macular dystrophy with genetic linkage to chromosome 6q, Arch Ophthalmol 112:765, 1994.

1732. Straatsma B and others: The retina, UCLA Forum in Medical Sciences, no 8, Berkeley, 1969, University of California Press.

1733. Sugita M, Dulaney J, and Moser H: Ceramidase deficiency in Farber's disease (lipogranulomatosis). Science 178:1100, 1972.

1734. Sumner KD and others: Spontaneous separation of epiretinal membranes, Arch Ophthalmol 98:318, 1980.

1735. Sunness JS, Bressler NM, and Maguire MG: Scanning laser ophthalmoscopic analysis of the pattern of visual loss in age-related geographic atrophy of the macula, Am J Ophthalmol 119:143, 1994.

1736. Szlyk JP and others: Clinical subtypes of cone-rod dystrophy, Arch Ophthalmol 111:781, 1994.

1737. Tach AB and others: Accidental Nd:YAG laser injuries to the macula, Am J Ophthalmol 119:143, 1995.

1738. Talbot JF and Bird AC: Krypton laser in the management of disciform macular degeneration, Trans Ophthalmol Soc UK 100:423, 1980.

1739. Tang SB and Scheiffarth OF: Expression of HLA-DR antigen in epiretinal and vitreous membranes, Yen Ko Hsueh Pa (Eye Science) 5:28, 1989.

1740. Tani PM, Buettner H, and Robertson DM: Massive vitreous hemorrhage and senile macular choroidal degeneration, Am J Ophthalmol 90:525, 1980.

1741. Teeters V and Bird A: The development of neovascularization of senile disciform macular degeneration, Am J Ophthalmol 76:1, 1973.

1742. Thomas MA and Kaplan HJ: Surgical removal of subfoveal neovascularization in the presumed ocular histoplasmosis syndrome, Am J Ophthalmol 111:1, 1991.

1743. Thomas JW and others: Ultrastructural features of surgically excised idiopathic subfoveal neovascular membranes, Retina 13:93, 1993.

1744. Thompson JT and others: Fluorescein angiographic characteristics of macular holes before and after vitrectomy with transforming growth factor Beta-2, Am J Ophthalmol 117:291, 1994.

1745. To KW and others: Olivopontocerebellar atrophy with retinal degeneration. An electroretinographic and histopathologic investigation, Ophthalmology 100:15, 1993.

1746. Toth CA, Pasquale AC III, and Graichen DF: Clinicopathologic correlation of spontaneous retinal pigment epithelial tears with choroidal neovascular membranes in age-related macular degeneration, Ophthalmology 102:272, 1995.

1747. Traboulsi EI and Maumenee IH: Ophthalmologic findings in mucolipidosis III (pseudo-Hurler polydystrophy), Am J Ophthalmol 102:592, 1986.

1748. Traboulsi EI and others: Olivopontocerebellar atrophy with retinal degeneration. A clinical and ocular histopathologic study, Arch Ophthalmol 106:801, 1988.

1749. Tremblay M and Szots F: GM2 type 2–gangliosidosis (Sandhoff's disease): ocular and pathological manifestations, Can J Ophthalmol 9:338, 1974.

1750. Trempe CL, Weiter JJ, and Furukawa H: Fellow eyes in cases of macular hole. Biomicroscopic study of the vitreous, Arch Ophthalmol 104:93, 1986.

1751. Trese MT and Foos RY: Infantile cystoid maculopathy, Br J Ophthalmol 64:206, 1980.

1752. Tso MOM: Pathological study of cystoid macular oedema, Trans Ophthalmol Soc UK 100:408, 1980.

1753. Tso MOM: Pathology of cystoid macular edema, Ophthalmology 89:902, 1982.

1754. Tso MOM: Pathogenetic factors of aging macular degeneration, Ophthalmology 92:628, 1985.

1755. Usui T and others: Late-infantile type galactosialidosis. Histopathology of the retina and optic nerve, Arch Ophthalmol 109:542, 1991.

1756. Verhoeff F: Histologic findings in a case of angioid streaks, Br J Ophthalmol 32:531, 1948.

1757. Vine AK: Advances in treating cystoid macular edema, Int Ophthalmol Clin 21(3):157, 1981.

1758. Vine AK and Schatz H: Adult-onset foveomacular pigment epithelial dystrophy, Am J Ophthalmol 89:680, 1980.

1759. Vingerling JR and others: The prevalence of age-related maculopathy in the Rotterdam study, Ophthalmology 102:205, 1995.

1760. Vinores SA, Campochiaro PA, and Conway BP: Ultrastructural and electron-immunocytochemical characterization of cells in epiretinal membranes, Invest Ophthalmol Vis Sci 31:14, 1990.

1761. Vinores SA and others: Ultrastructural and electron-immunocytochemical changes in retinal pigment epithelium, retinal glia, and fibroblasts in vitreous culture, Invest Ophthalmol Vis Sci 31:2529, 1990.

1762. Vinores SA and others: Simultaneous expression of keratin and glial fibrillary acidic protein by the same cell in epiretinal membranes, Invest Ophthalmol Vis Sci 33:3361, 1992.

1763. Wallow IL and Miller SA: Preretinal membrane by retinal pigment epithelium, Arch Ophthalmol 96:1643, 1978.

1764. Wang FM, Afran SI, and Goldberg RB: Congenital myopia in Stickler's hereditary arthro-ophthalmology, Am J Ophthalmol 110:435, 1990.

1765. Warburg M: Diagnosis of metabolic eye disease, Copenhagen, 1972, Munksgaard, International Booksellers & Publishers, Ltd.

1766. Watzke RC, Burton TC, and Leaverton PE: Ruby laser photocoagulation therapy of central serous retinopathy. I. A controlled clinical study. II. Factors affecting prognosis, Trans Am Acad Ophthalmol Otolaryngol 78:OP 205, 1974.

1767. Watzke RC and Snyder W: Light coagulation for hemorrhagic disciform degeneration of the macula, Trans Am Acad Ophthalmol Otolaryngol 72:389, 1968.

1768. Weiner A and others: Hydroxychloroquine retinopathy, Am J Ophthalmol 112:528, 1991.

1769. Weingeist TA, Kobrin JL, and Watzke RC: Histopathology of Best's macular dystrophy, Arch Ophthalmol 100:1108, 1982.

1770. Weise E and Yannuzzi L: Ring maculopathies mimicking chloroquine retinopathy, Am J Ophthalmol 78:204, 1974.

1771. Weiss MJ and others: GM1 gangliosidosis type I, Am J Ophthalmol 76:999, 1973.

1772. Weleber RG: Stargardt's macular dystrophy, Arch Ophthalmol 112:752, 1994.

1773. Weller M, Heimann K, and Wiedemann P: Demonstration of mononuclear phagocytes in a human epiretinal membrane using a monclonal antihuman macrophage antibody, Graefes Arch Clin Exp Ophthalmol 226:252, 1988.

1774. Wessing A: Zur Pathogenese und Therapie der sogenannten Retinitis centralis serosa, Ophthalmologica 153:259, 1967.

1775. Wessing A: Central serous retinopathy and related lesions, Mod Probl Ophthalmol 9:148, 1971.

1776. Wessing A: Photocoagulation in the treatment of macular lesions, Acta XXI Congress Ophthalmology, Mexico 1970, Amsterdam, 1971, Excerpta Medica, BV.

1777. West SK and others: Exposure to sunlight and other risk factors for age-related macular degeneration, Arch Ophthalmol 107:875, 1989.

1778. Whitelocke RAF and others: The diabetic maculopathies, Trans Ophthalmol Soc UK 99:314, 1979.

1779. Whitcup SM and others: A randomized, masked, cross-over trial of acetazolamide for cystoid macular edema in patients with uveitis, Ophthalmology 103:1054, 1996.

1780. Wilkes SR, Mansour AM, and Green WR: Proliferative vitreoretinopathy. Histopathology of retroretinal membranes, Retina 7:94, 1987.

1781. Willerson D and Aaberg T: Senile macular degeneration and geographic atrophy of the retinal pigment epithelium, Br J Ophthalmol 62:551, 1978.

1782. Wilson DJ, Weleber RG, and Green WR: Ocular clinicopathologic study of gyrate atrophy, Am J Ophthalmol 111:24, 1991.

1783. Wise G: Clinical features of idiopathic preretinal macular fibrosis, Am J Ophthalmol 79:349, 1975.

1784. Wobmann P: Angioidstreifen und Drusenpapille, Klin Monatsbl Augenheilkd 161:919, 1972.

1785. Wolter J and Falls H: Bilateral confluent drusen, Arch Ophthalmol 68:219, 1962.

1786. Wolter J, Goldsmith R, and Phillips R: Histopathology of the star-figure of the macular area in diabetic and angiospastic retinopathy, Arch Ophthalmol 57:376, 1957.

1787. Wolter J, Phillips R, and Butler R: The star figure of the macular area: histopathologic study of a case of angiospastic (hypertensive) retinopathy, Arch Ophthalmol 60:49, 1958.

1788. Wright BE, Bird AC, and Hamilton AM: Placoid pigment epitheliopathy and Harada's disease, Br J Ophthalmol 62:609, 1978.

1789. Wright PL and others: Angiographic cystoid macular edema after posterior chamber lens implantation, Arch Ophthalmol 106:740, 1988.

1790. Wu G and others: Hereditary hemorrhagic macular dystrophy, Am J Ophthalmol 111:294, 1991.

1791. Yagoda AD, Walsh JB, and Henkind P: Idiopathic preretinal macular gliosis, Int Ophthalmol Clin 21(3):107, 1981.

1792. Yamashita H and others: Glial cells in culture of preretinal membrane of proliferative vitreoretinopathy, Jap J Ophthalmol 29:42, 1985.

1793. Yamashita H and others: Microfilaments in preretinal membrane cells of proliferative vitreoretinopathy, Jap J Ophthalmol 29:42, 1985.

1794. Yannuzzi LA and others: Peripheral retinal detachments and retinal pigment epithelial atrophic tracts secondary to central serous pigment epitheliopathy, Ophthalmology 91:1554, 1984.

1795. Yanoff M and Schwarz GA: The retinal pathology of Lafora's disease: a form of glycoprotein-acid mucopolysaccharide dystrophy, Trans Am Acad Ophthalmol Otolaryngol 69:701, 1965.

1796. Yanoff M, Rahn E, and Zimmerman LE: Histopathology of juvenile retinoschisis, Arch Ophthalmol 79:49, 1968.

1797. Yanoff M and others: Pathology of human cystoid macular edema, Surv Ophthalmol 28(suppl):505, 1984.

1798. Yassur Y and others: Autosomal dominant inheritance of retinoschisis. Am J Ophthalmol 94:338, 1982.

1799. Yooh HS and others: Ultrastructural features of tissue removed during idiopathic macular hole surgery, Am J Ophthalmol 122:67, 1996.

1800. Young RW: Pathophysiology of age-related macular degeneration, Surv Ophthalmol 31:291, 1987.

1801. Young RW: Solar radiation and age-related macular degeneration, Surv Ophthalmol 32:252, 1988.

1802. Yuzawa M and others: Observation of idiopathic full-thickness macular holes. Follow-up observations, Arch Ophthalmol 112:1051, 1994.

1803. Zarbin MA and others: Farber's disease: light and electron microscopic study of the eye, Arch Ophthalmol 103:73, 1985.

1804. Zarbin MA, Michels RG, and Green WR: Epiretinal membrane co-intracture associated with macular prolapse, Am J Ophthalmol 110:610, 1990.

1805. Zhang K and others: Genetic and molecular studies of macular dystrophies; recent developments, Surv Ophthalmol 40:51, 1995 (review).

1806. Zhang K and others: A dominant Stargardt's macular dystrophy locus maps to chromosome 13q34, Arch Ophthalmol 112:752, 1994.

1807. Zrenner E, Nowicki J, and Adamczyk R: Cone function and cone interaction in hereditary degenerations of the central retina, Doc Ophthalmol 62:5, 1986.

1808. Zscheile F: Disciform lesion of the macula simulating a melanoma, Arch Ophthalmol 71:505, 1964.

Histopathologic changes induced by photocoagulation

1809. Apple DJ: Histopathology of xenon-arc and argon laser photocoagulation. In L'Esperance FA Jr, editor: Current diagnosis and management of chorioretinal diseases, St Louis, 1977, The CV Mosby Co.

1810. Apple DJ, Goldberg MF, and Wyhinny GJ: Histopathology and ultrastructure of the argon laser lesion in human retinal and choroidal vasculatures, Am J Ophthalmol 75:595, 1973.

1811. Apple DJ, Goldberg MF, and Wyhinny GJ: Argon laser treatment of von Hippel-Lindau retinal angiomas. II. Histopathology of treated lesions, Arch Ophthalmol 92:126, 1974.

1812. Apple DJ, Wyhinny GJ, and Goldberg MF: Argon laser photocoagulation: limitations and dangers. In Transactions of the Twenty-Second Meeting of the International Congress of Ophthalmology, Paris, May 1974 and 1976.

1813. Apple DJ and others: Argon laser photocoagulation of choroidal malignant melanoma: tissue effects after a single treatment, Arch Ophthalmol 90:97, 1973.

1814. Apple DJ and others: Experimental argon laser photocoagulation. I. Effects on retinal nerve fiber layer, Arch Ophthalmol 94:137, 1976.

1815. Apple DJ and others: Experimental argon laser photocoagulation. II. Effects on the optic disk, Arch Ophthalmol 94:296, 1976.

1816. Apple DJ and others: Experimental argon laser photocoagulation. III. Relative dangers of immediate versus delayed treatment, Arch Ophthalmol 94:309, 1976.

1817. Apple DJ and others: Histopathology of argon and krypton photocoagulation. In Birngruber R and Gabel V, editors: Proceedings of the Internation Symposium on Photocoagulation of the Eye, The Hague, 1983, W Junk Co.

1818. Chopdar A: Retinal telangiectasis in adults: fluorescein angiographic findings and treatment by argon laser, Br J Ophthalmol 62:243, 1978.

1819. Diddie KR and Ernest JT: The effect of photocoagulation on the choroidal vasculature and retinal oxygen tension, Am J Ophthalmol 84:62, 1977.

1820. Folk JC and others: Early retinal adhesion from laser photocoagulation, Ophthalmology 96:1523, 1989.

1821. Frankhauser F and Van der Zypen E: Future of the laser in ophthalmology, Trans Ophthalmol Soc UK 102:159, 1982.

1822. Goldbaum M and others: Acute choroidal ischemia as a complication of photocoagulation, Arch Ophthalmol 94:1025, 1976.

1823. Goldberg MF and others: Macular hole caused by a 589-nanometer dye laser operating for 10 nanoseconds, Retina 3:40, 1983.

1824. Johnson RN, Irvine AR, and Wood IS: Endolaser, cryopexy, and retinal reattachment in the air-filled eye: a clinicopathologic correlation, Arch Ophthalmol 105:231, 1987.

1825. Johnson RN, Irvine AR, and Wood IS: Histopathology of krypton red laser panretinal photocoagulation: a clinicopathologic correlation, Arch Ophthalmol 105:235, 1987.

1826. L'Esperance FA Jr: An ophthalmic argon laser photocoagulation system: design, construction, and laboratory investigations, Trans Am Ophthalmol Soc 6:870, 1968.

1827. L'Esperance FA Jr: The treatment of ophthalmic-vascular disease by argon laser photocoagulation, Trans Am Acad Ophthalmol Otolaryngol 73:1077, 1969.

1828. L'Esperance FA Jr: Ocular photocoagulation: a stereoscopic atlas, St Louis, 1975, The CV Mosby Co.

1829. Lunde MW: Capsulectomy and membranectomy with the argon laser, Am J Ophthalmol 95:794, 1983.

1830. Maguire MG and others: Persistent and recurrent neovascularization after krypton laser photocoagulation for neovascular lesions of ocular histoplasmosis, Arch Ophthalmol 107:344, 1989.

1831. Mango C and others: Cryotherapy and photocoagulation in the management of retinoblastoma: treatment and failure and unusual complication, Ophthalmic Surg 14:336, 1983.

1832. Marshall J, Hamilton AM, and Bird AC: Histopathology of ruby and aragon laser lesions in monkey and human retina. A comparitive study, Br J Ophthalmol 59:610, 1975.

1833. Marshall J and Bird AC: A comparative histopathological study of argon and krypton laser irradiations of the human retina, Br J Ophthalmol 63:657, 1979.

1834. Mensher J: Anterior chamber depth alteration after retinal photocoagulation, Arch Ophthalmol 95:113, 1977.

1835. Meyer-Schwickerath G: Lichtkoagulation, Stuttgart, 1959, Ferdinand Enke Verlag.

1836. Okisaka S, Kuwabara T, and Aiello L: The effects of laser photoagulation in the retinal capillaries, Am J Ophthalmol 80:591, 1975.

1837. Patz A, Maumenee AE, and Ryan S: Argon laser photocoagulation: advantages and limitations, Trans Am Acad Ophthalmol Otolaryngol 75:569, 1971.

1838. Peyman GA, Wyhinny GJ, and Goldberg MF: Optical radiation and Zeiss short-pulsed xenon photocoagulators. I. Clinical considerations of articulation with the Frankhauser slit-lamp delivery system, Arch Ophthalmol 92:341, 1974.

1839. Peyman GA and others: A neodymium-YAG endolaser, Ophthalmic Surg 14:309, 1983.

1840. Pollack A, Heriot WJ, and Henkind P: Cellular processes causing defects in Bruch's membrane following krypton laser photocoagulation, Ophthalmology 93:1113, 1986.

1841. Polley E and Apple DJ: The laser as a research tool in visual system research, Anat Rec 175:415, 1973 (abstract).

1842. Polley E, Apple DJ, and Bizzell J: The laser as a research tool in visual system investigation, Am J Psychol 30:340, 1975.

1843. Powell JO and others: Ocular effects of argon laser radiation. II. Histopathology of choriorretinal lesions, Am J Ophthalmol 71:1267, 1971.

1844. Raymond LA: Neodymium: Yag laser treatment for hemorrhages under the internal limiting membrane and posterior hyaloid face in the macula, Ophthalmology 102:406, 1995.

1845. Sabates FN, Lee KY, and Ziemianski MC: A comparative study of argon and krypton laser photocoagulation in the treatment of presumed ocular histoplasmosis syndrome, Ophthalmology 89:729, 1982.

1846. Singerman LJ: Red krypton laser therapy of macular and retinal vascular diseases, Retina 2:15, 1982.

1847. Smiddy WE and others: Cell proliferation after laser photocoagulation in primate retina: an autoradiographic study, Arch Ophthalmol 104:1065, 1986.

1848. Stratas BA and others: Observations on the microvascular repair process after confluent argon laser photocoagulation, Arch Ophthalmol 104:126, 1986.

1849. Swartz M: Histology of macular photocoagulation, Ophthalmology 93:959, 1986.

1850. Thomas EL and Langhofer M. Closure of experimental subretinal neovascular vessels with dihematoporphirin ether augmented argon green laser photocoagulation, Photochem Photobiol 46:881, 1987.

1851. Thomas EL and others: Histopathology and ultrastructure of krypton and argon laser lesions in a human retina-choroid, Retina 4: 22, 1984.

1852. Thomas MA and Ibanez HE: Subretinal Endophotocoagulation in the treatment of choroidal neovascularization, Am J Ophthalmol 116:279, 1993.

1853. Tso MOM, Wallow IHL, and Elgin S: Experimental photocoagulation of the human retina, Arch Ophthalmol 95:1035, 1977.

1854. van der Zypen E, Fankhauser F, and Raes K: Choroidal reaction and vascular repair after chorioretinal photocoagulation with the free-running neodymium-YAG laser, Arch Ophthalmol 103:580, 1985.

1855. van der Zypen E and others: Morphologic findings in the rabbit retina following irradiation with the free-running neodymium-YAG laser: disruption of Bruch's membrane and its effect on the scarring process in the retina and choroid, Arch Ophthalmol 104:1070, 1986.

1856. Wallo IHL, Tso MOM, and Elgin S: Experimental photocoagulation of the human retina. II. Electron microscope study, Arch Ophthalmol 95:1041, 1977.

1857. Wallow IHL and Davis MD: Clinicopathologic correlation of xenon-arc and argon laser photocoagulation: procedure in human diabetic eyes, Arch Ophthalmol 97:2308, 1979.

1858. Wallow IHL and Skuta GL: Histopathology of focally photocoagulated preretinal new vessels, Arch Ophthalmol 102:1340, 1984.

1859. Weingeist TA: Argon laser photocoagulation of the human retina. I. Histopathologic correlation of chorioretinal lesions in the region of the maculopapillar bundle, Invest Ophthalmol 13:1024, 1974.

1860. Wilson DJ and Green WR: Argon laser panretinal photocoagulation for diabetic retinopathy: scanning electron microscopy of human choroidal vascular casts, Arch Ophthalmol 105:239, 1987.

1861. Yannuzzi LA and others: Analysis of vascularized pigment epithelial detachments using indocyaninee green videoangiography, Retina 14:99, 1994.

1862. Yannuzzi LA: Krypton red laser photocoagulation for subretinal neovascularization, Retina 2:29, 1982.

1863. Yannuzzi LA and Shakin JL: Krypton red laser photocoagulation of the ocular fundus, Retina 2:1, 1982.

1864. Zweng H, editor: Recent advances in photocoagulation, Int Ophthalmol Clin 16(4), 1976.

CHAPTER 9

RETINOBLASTOMA, LEUKOKORIA, AND PHAKOMATOSES

Retinoblastoma

CLINICAL FEATURES

Retinoblastoma, with leukemia and neuroblastoma, is one of the most common childhood malignancies.[1-260] It is responsible for approximately 1% of all deaths from cancer in the pediatric age group.[200] It is third to uveal malignant melanoma and metastatic carcinoma as the most common intraocular malignancy in humans. It occurs with greater frequency today than in previous years because survival rates have improved from about 5% in the 1860s to 80% to 90% or more in favorable cases. In familial cases the disease is, therefore, propagated by gene transmission from survivors to their offspring.

The heritable form of retinoblastoma, which is often bilateral, is transmitted as an autosomal-dominant trait with incomplete (60% to 90%) penetrance.[*] Improved cure rates have resulted in a greater number of survivors of this tumor. Thus, with respect to cases transmitted genetically, there is an ever-increasing incidence of the retinoblastoma-inducing gene distributed throughout the general population. An incidence as high as 1 in 14,000 births has been documented, and this incidence will probably increase in the future.[59,108] Most cases occur before age 3 and are unusual after age 7.[138,216,233] Predilection for race or sex is not significant.

The increase in the number of nonocular or second cancers in survivors of retinoblastoma compared with the general population is statistically significant, especially in inherited cases, in association with other sarcomas, and with pineal tumors.[†] The pineal gland, which represents a "third eye" and contains photoreceptor-like cells in many species, is, therefore, capable of producing a retinoblastoma. The syndrome of bilateral retinoblastoma associated with pineal tumor is termed a *trilateral retinoblastoma.*[‡]

The heredity of retinoblastoma is best explained by the Knudson "two-hit" hypothesis.[118,119] Chromosome 13, specifically region 13q14 the retinoblastoma (R6) gene, is involved.[§] If mutational events occur in a postzygotic somatic cell a noninheritable, unilateral tumor occurs. In the hereditary form two mutations occur, in both a prezygotic cell and a postzygotic cell, resulting in the possibility of multifocal tumors in one or both eyes and other tumors such as pinealoma. Based on present knowledge transmission of

---

[*] References 46–48, 67, 76, 78–82, 85, 87, 88, 93, 109, 125, 126, 127, 144, 154, 161, 187, 205, 206, 210, 220, 235, 245, 249, 254, 258.
[†] References 4, 5, 12, 14, 21, 24–26, 64, 111, 190, 207, 216, 229, 260.
[‡] References 24–26, 41, 133, 169, 178, 190.
[§] References 26, 42, 66, 402, 160, 164, 208.

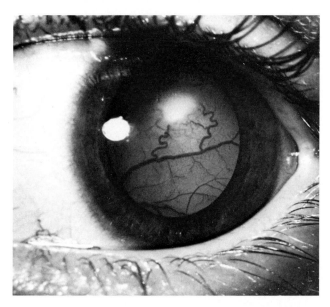

Fig. 9-1. Retinoblastoma. The retrolental white mass (leukokoria, or white pupil) is a common initial sign of the disease. The retinal vessels have been pushed anteriorly by this exophytic growth, which fills the subretinal space. See page 493 for a listing of the differential diagnosis of a white pupil in a child.

Table 9-1. Features differentiating PHPV from retinoblastoma

PHPV	Retinoblastoma
Unilateral	Unilateral, but often (20%–40% bilateral)
No (or very rare hereditary disposition)	May be transmitted as autosomal dominant
Relative microphthalmia	Usually normal-sized eye
Elongated ciliary processes	Ciliary processes not elongated
Retrolental mass early	Retrolental mass usually later when entire globe is filled with tumor
Relatively early cataract	Cataract is rare or occurs in later phases
Relatively microphakia often present	Normal lens size
Hyaloid remnants present (seen with media sufficiently clear)	Hyaloid remnants not characteristic
No calcification seen on radiograph except in very late stages in which phthisis bulbi occurs	Calcification of necrotic tumor foci is common
Normal LDH levels in aqueous	Increased levels of aqueous LDH

From Apple DJ, Hamming NA, and Gieser DK: In Peyman GA, Apple DJ, and Sanders DR, editors: Intraocular tumors, New York, 1977, Appleton-Century-Crofts.

retinoblastoma, recommended genetic counseling is as follows:[255]

1. Healthy parents with one affected child have about a 6% risk of producing more affected children (the parent may be genotypically abnormal but phenotypically normal).
2. If two or more siblings are affected, about a 50% risk exists that each additional child will be affected.
3. A retinoblastoma survivor with the hereditary type has approximately a 50% chance of producing affected children. Phenotypically normal children of an affected parent may be genetically abnormal.
4. A sporadic case has about 12.5% chance of producing affected children.

Leukokoria (white pupil, or "cat eye reflex") (Fig. 9-1; Color Plate 9-1) is a common initial clinical sign of retinoblastoma. The parents may notice a squint, nystagmus, visual loss, or anisocoria.[247] The child may also have rubeosis iridis,[149,223] hyphema, secondary glaucoma (with or without buphthalmos),[257] or signs of intraocular inflammation (uveitis, keratic precipitates, hypopyon, endophthalmitis).[149,223,257] One must always consider a retinoblastoma in any case of childhood intraocular inflammation. After juvenile xanthogranuloma (p. 294), retinoblastoma is probably the second most common cause of spontaneous hyphema in children. In advanced cases, phthisis bulbi may be present, or, after orbital extension of the tumor, the child may develop a proptosis. In contrast to persistent hyperplastic primary vitreous (PHPV), a disease that can mimic retinoblastoma (Table 9-1) and can rarely occur simultaneously in an eye with retinoblastoma,[104,153] the eye is usually normal in size at birth.[104,153] In late stages, however, the eye may become phthisic or buphthalmic. Children with retinoblastoma may have other abnormalities in-

cluding chromosome anomalies, such as the chromosome 13 deletion syndrome or a trisomy.*

Early diagnosis of retinoblastoma is important. The average age of diagnosis is about 1 year. The above-mentioned hereditary factor necessitates that all siblings of patients with retinoblastoma and all children of survivors of retinoblastoma be examined.[23,34] Retinoblastoma is rare in adults, but Mackley has reported its occurrence in a 52-year-old man.[138]

Both clinical examination and gross pathologic examination of a retinoblastoma (Figs. 9-1–9-5; Color Plates 9-1–9-4) typically reveal a white retrolental mass, which may show a smooth surface or may be irregular and lobulated because of areas of necrosis and calcification of the mass. Many retinoblastomas are white or light gray or have a pink-cream color, with formation of new blood vessels over the surface or within the substance of the tumor. This tumor sometimes is confused with Coats' disease (Color Plate 9-5). However, it can generally be differentiated from the clinical or gross appearance of an eye with Coats' syndrome (Fig. 9-23; Color Plate 9-5) or von Hippel–Lindau disease.[29,71,107] The lipid-rich exudate seen in Coats' syndrome (Color Plate 9-6) usually imparts a distinctive yellow rather than white color to the lesion (p. 493). The marked telangiectasia of retinal vessels seen in Coats' syndrome is usually less prominent or is absent in retinoblastoma.

In addition to basic clinical examination, such as ophthalmoscopy under anesthesia and transillumination, several noninvasive laboratory techniques are helpful:[150]

---

* References 54, 115, 129, 171, 180, 230.

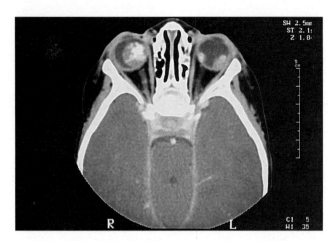

Fig. 9-2. Bilateral retinoblastoma, CT scan showing bilateral intraocular tumor. (Courtesy, Timothy Powers, M.D., Knoxville, TN).

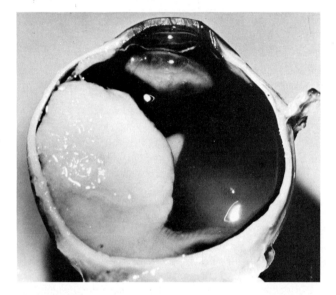

Fig. 9-3. Retinoblastoma, gross photograph. This tumor is typically light gray to white. On cut sections the surface may be smooth or may exhibit an irregular granular or cobblestone appearance because of partial necrosis of areas of the tumor. A white, chalky, granular appearance may be imparted by calcium (Fig. 9-13) and is a useful clinical and pathologic diagnostic finding when present.

1. Retinoblastomas are frequently chalky in appearance because of focal calcification of the tumor (Fig. 9-3).[130] This is an important diagnostic roentgenographic feature (Figs. 9-2 and 9-13, *B*). Calcium is deposited within necrotic foci in the tumor. Necrosis of tumor cells occurs either as a host defense mechanism mediated through an antigen-antibody reaction or because the rapidly growing cells often outgrow their blood supply and undergo ischemic necrosis (Fig. 9-6).
2. Ultrasound computerized tomography (CT) and magnetic resonance imaging (MRI) studies have proved useful in the evaluation of patients with atypical presentations of retinoblastoma.[136] Not only can they reveal calcification but also help differentiate two types: solid and cystic. The solid type may represent the early lesion, while the cystic type may be

characteristic of more advanced tumors with necrosis and free islands of tumor in the vitreous.

3. Anterior chamber paracentesis can be risky because of the potential for tumor seeding. This technique, however, has been successfully performed in the past and in some cases may still be useful in differentiating tumor cells from inflammatory cells in patients whose initial signs included uveitis and hypopyon (Figs. 9-4 and 9-6). This fluid may be processed for direct cytologic examination of aspirated cells within the aqueous, or chemical analysis of aspirated aqueous may be performed.* Several authors have demonstrated elevated lactic dehydrogenase (LDH) levels in the aqueous fluid of patients with retinoblastoma. This test, although still experimental,[6,112] appears to assist in differentiating retinoblastomas from the many other causes of a white pupil.[6,112] (The conditions other than retinoblastoma that give rise to white pupil in infants and young children are commonly referred to collectively as pseudoretinoblastoma (p. 492).
4. The radioactive phosphorus (^{32}P) uptake test, which is sometimes useful in the diagnosis of uveal malignant melanoma, has rarely been used for diagnosis of retinoblastoma because of potential hazardous side effects, which may occur in the developing bones of the child. To date there is no conclusive evidence demonstrating increased urinary excretion of vanillylmandelic acid in patients with retinoblastoma. This is often elevated in adrenal neuroblastoma.
5. Fluorescein angiography has been of little value in differentiating small retinoblastomas from astrocytic hamartomas.[214,218] They both contain a capillary network that is permeable to fluorescein. Angiography may be of some benefit in differentiating large retinoblastomas from highly elevated exudative detachments caused by retinal telangiectasia. Retinoblastomas often contain blood vessels deep within the tumor parenchyma, but in retinal telangiectasia or Coats' syndrome the abnormal retinal vascular network is confined to the inner surface of the large exudative mass.

HISTOGENESIS

Histogenetically the retinoblastoma is derived from cells of the sensory retina, specifically cells that stem from the pars optica retinae (Figs. 1-9, 1-11, and 8-1) of the inner neuroepithelial layer of the embryonic optic cup.[159,167,172] Neoplasms of the outer layer of the optic cup, that is, adenomas or carcinoma of the retinal pigment epithelium, are extremely rare and are not described here. Tumors that arise from both the inner and outer layers at the level of the ciliary epithelium (pars ciliaris retinae; Fig. 1-11) are classified as neuroepithelial tumors of the ciliary body (p. 329). Virchow[244] believed that this tumor was similar in histogenesis to the well-recognized group of intracranial glial tumors, and he concluded that what is now called retinoblastoma was a glioma. Although this concept is now modified, long-standing use of the term *glioma retinae* has been responsible for the evolution of the term *pseudoglioma*.[30,173] Pseudoglioma refers to any of several conditions that usually exhibit a retrolental mass and can produce a leukokoria.[98,99,261] These may clinically mimic a retinoblastoma. It is clear now that the cellular differentiation of the retinoblastoma is neural or mixed neuroglial rather than glial alone.

In 1891 Flexner[77] and in 1897 Wintersteiner[252] described the rosettes that frequently are found in the tumor.

---

* References 6, 15, 60–62, 112, 116, 219, 231, 232.

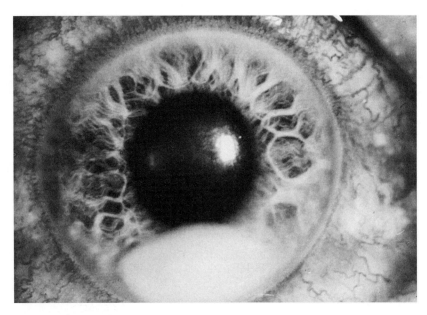

Fig. 9-4. Clinical photograph of a patient with retinoblastoma, showing a tumor hypopyon. This is caused by anterior seeding from the main tumor mass.

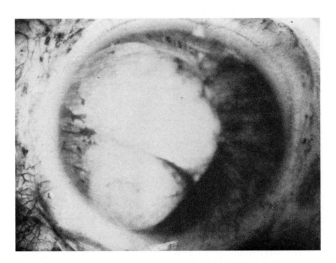

Fig. 9-5. Endophytic retinoblastoma with growth into the anterior chamber. (From Daicker B: Anatomie und Pathologie der menschlichen retino-ziliaren Fundusperipherie, Basel, 1972, S Karger, AG.)

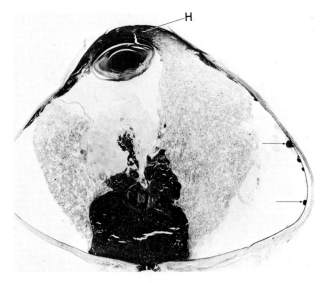

Fig. 9-6. Retinoblastoma. The main tumor mass is situated at the posterior aspect of the globe. Extensive seeding of necrotic tumor cells has occurred throughout the entire globe, including the anterior chamber, where a hypopyon (*H*) composed of exfoliated neoplastic cells is present. Because the presence of a hypopyon caused by the anterior segment seeding may mimic inflammatory diseases, diagnosis may be delayed. *Arrows,* Small deposits of tumor cells away from the main mass. The optic nerve has been invaded by the tumor. (H & E stain; ×4.)

They first demonstrated that the neoplasm arises from precursor cells of the neuroepithelium and forms rods and cones; therefore, they termed it a *neuroepithelioma.* In 1922, Verhoeff first applied the term *retinoblastoma* (cited by Bishop and Madson[34]). He appreciated that the tumor arises from the retina but was unable to further subclassify the particular cell of origin within the retina. The suffix *blastoma* correctly emphasizes the presence of primitive, immature, embryonic-appearing cells that form the tumor. The term *retinoblastoma,* therefore, implies an embryonic tumor but is noncommittal regarding any assessment of the neural versus glial nature of the neoplasm. With acceptance of the term *retinoblastoma* by the American Ophthalmological Society in 1926, the old terms such as *glioma*

retinae, encephaloid tumor, neuroepithelioma, and *fungus hematoides* were discarded.

Neuroblastoma of the peripheral nervous system and medulloblastoma and pinealoma (pinealoblastoma) of the central nervous system have much in common with retinoblastoma. All are highly malignant neuroblastic neoplasms that arise in infants and young children and display similar cytologic characteristics, sometimes even forming rosettes. The optic vesicle from which the retina originates is a derivative of the neural tube. Because the retina and central nervous system are both formed from the same primitive medullary epithelium of the neural tube, any tumors occurring in one can be expected to have similarities to the other.

The possible role of viruses, RNA-directed DNA polymerase ("reverse transcriptase"), immune mechanisms, and tumor angiogenesis factor in the pathogenesis of retinoblastoma is discussed by Sang and Albert[200] and others.[19-21,49,50,109,188]

HISTOPATHOLOGIC FINDINGS

Not only are retinoblastomas frequently bilateral, but they often demonstrate multicentric growth within the same eye (Figs. 9-7 and 9-8; Color Plates 9-3 and 9-4). Such cases involve multiple sites of origin from a single retina. Multiple primary tumors in a single eye differ from multiple deposits of tumor along the retinal surface because of seeding of the tumor (Figs. 9-6 and 9-18). Any seeding into the vitreous connotes a poorer prognosis, while the occurrence of multiple primary tumors is not necessarily an ominous finding.

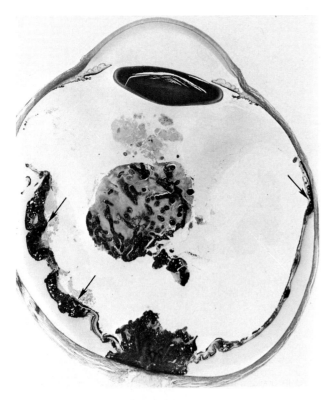

Fig. 9-7. Retinoblastoma showing endophytic growth into the vitreous and diffuse, multicentric growth along large segments of the retina *(arrows)*. The deeply staining areas within the main tumor (in the center of the vitreous cavity) represent viable tumor elements around the vessels. The intervening paler-staining, light gray areas are composed of necrotic tumor cells that are situated in areas more removed from the stromal vascular supply. Therefore the tumor has partially outgrown its blood supply. Deposition of calcium often occurs in the necrotic areas (dystrophic calcification). When present, this is responsible for the diagnostic roentgenographic appearance on orbital radiographs (Fig. 9-13).

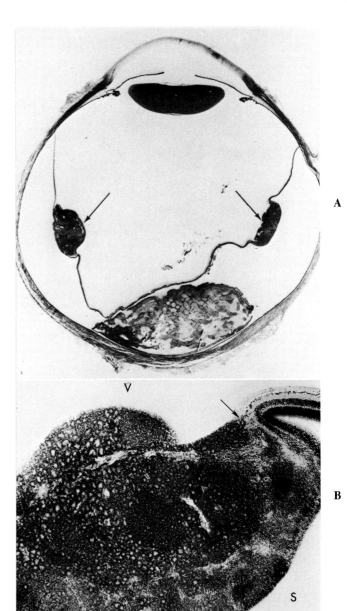

Fig. 9-8. Retinoblastoma. **A,** Both endophytic and exophytic patterns of growth are illustrated in this single globe. The main tumor mass lies beneath the retina and is therefore exophytic. Two smaller endophytic growths *(arrows)* protrude inward (vitreally) from the retina. They are independent of the main mass and illustrate the potential for multicentric growth. Multicentric growth should not be confused with tumor seeding, in which "seedlets" of tumor are deposited throughout the retina, vitreous, or anterior segment. The alternating deep-staining areas (viable tumor cells) and light-staining areas (necrotic tumor cells) within the main tumor mass are caused by focal tumor cell necrosis resulting from outgrowth of the blood supply in some regions of the tumor. (H & E stain; ×7.) **B,** Retinoblastoma, same case as in **A.** This photomicrograph shows the junction of normal retina *(upper right)* and the origin of the tumor *(arrow)*. The growth is mostly directed toward the vitreous (*V*) and is, therefore, classified as endophytic. *S,* Subretinal space. This neoplasm is composed of numerous small hyperchromatic cells, which are reminiscent of embryonic (blastic) neural elements, and numerous Flexner-Wintersteiner rosettes. The cells are arranged in a circular manner around a central clear area. (H & E stain; ×55.)

Hirschberg[96] distinguished two types of retinoblastoma growth: exophytic and endophytic (see also Sang and Albert[201]). An endophytic growth protrudes inward (vitreally) from the retina (Figs. 9-3, 9-5, 9-7, and 9-8; Color Plate 9-3). Because the lesion protrudes anteriorly above the retina, this form of growth is sometimes easier to detect clinically than a subretinal tumor. However, such growths not infrequently eventually seed the vitreous, a factor that can worsen the prognosis. An exophytic growth signifies an outward growth of the tumor toward the subretinal space (Figs. 9-1, 9-8, and 9-9; Color Plate 9-4). This type may be more difficult to diagnose, because it is more likely to mimic a simple nonrhegmatogenous retinal detachment.

An endophytic growth does not necessarily imply an origin from an inner cellular layer (e.g., ganglion cell layer); similarly, an exophytic growth does not necessarily arise from a deeper layer. Inward or outward growth of the tumor is independent of cellular origin. A retinoblastoma may exhibit a diffuse, infiltrating type of growth without a discrete mass (less than 1.5% of cases).[32,152]

A retinoblastoma may arise from any cellular layer of the sensory retina. Designation of growth from any particular layer is arbitrary and is of little value in determining pathogenesis or prognosis. The neoplastic cells are probably derived from embryonic rests of neural stem cells, or retinoblasts, that may be situated in any layer of the retina.[162,172] It is debatable that a mature retina cell, such as a ganglion cell, has the capability to dedifferentiate and commence an active neoplastic growth.

Retinoblastoma involves two major cell types: differentiated cells (including newly described retinomas and retinocytomas) and undifferentiated cells.[13,69,141] In the older literature retinoblastomas showing relative differentiation were sometimes termed *retinal neuroepitheliomas*, and poorly differentiated tumors were named *retinoblastomas*. A differentiated retinoblastoma termed a *retinocytoma* is less common and rarely appears in a pure form. The degree of differentiation is morphologically defined in terms of rosette formation (Fig. 9-10). A general rule of oncology states that the more differentiation a tumor cell exhibits (i.e., the more it resembles its normal, mature counterpart), the less anaplastic and/or metastatic potential is expected. This rule, therefore, suggests a more satisfactory prognosis for retinoblastomas composed primarily of differentiated cells. This rule is true to a limited extent, but, as is noted later, several other criteria are important in determining a prognosis.

The Flexner-Wintersteiner rosette (Figs. 9-10 and 9-11) is the morphologic hallmark of retinoblastoma differentiation. In the 1890s Flexner[77] and Wintersteiner[252] first recognized by light microscopy that the rosettes are composed of newly formed abortive rods and cones, and they postulated a neural origin of this tumor. Tso and coauthors[239–243] confirmed by electron microscopy that the Flexner-Wintersteiner rosette represents a differentiation of tumor cells simulating retinal photoreceptors. Lane and Klintworth[124] and others[146] have recently studied astrocytes in retinoblastomas. Flexner-Wintersteiner rosettes also occur in pineal tumors with or without associated retinoblastoma.[41,178] The Homer-Wright rosette, radial arrangements of tumor cells around a tangle of fibrils, is occasionally seen in retinoblastoma; it is much more characteristic of neuroblastoma and does not reveal photoreceptor differentiation.[253,255]

Histologically a normal rod or cone has as part of its structure an outer segment composed of several layers of discs or plates (Fig. 9-10). The outer segment is connected to the inner segment by a cilium, a tube-like structure that characteristically contains nine smaller microtubules arranged in a circular pattern around a center devoid of tubules. This 9 + 0 pattern is a significant identifying feature of rods and cones. The nucleus of the photoreceptor corresponds to the outer nuclear layer of the retina. The external limiting "membrane" is not a true membrane; instead it is a series of cell junctions (zonula adherens), which by light microscopy resemble a continuous membrane.

All of the aforementioned features of a normal photoreceptor have been identified in cells of retinal rosettes.[20,143,181,242,243] In oversimplified terms the rosette might be considered a row of photoreceptors, which have been molded into a circular pattern. The outer segments are within the lumen; also within the lumen are hyaluronidase-resistant acid mucopolysaccharides similar to those normally surrounding rods and cones. The external limiting membrane lines the outer margin of the lumen; the outer nuclear layer forms the cellular lining of the lumen. In Figure 9-10 a single, enlarged photoreceptor is schematically illustrated in the rosette. Only the nucleus of each

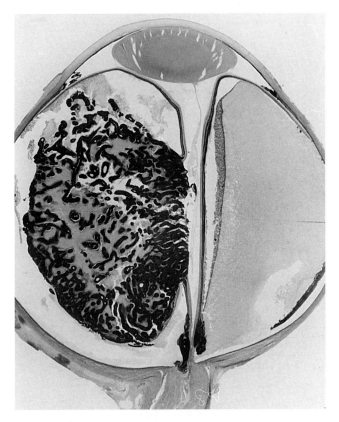

Fig. 9-9. Photomicrograph of retinoblastoma. The major tumor mass is in the subretinal space with total detachment of the sensory retina by the tumor mass and associated subretinal fluid (exophytic tumor). There is anterior displacement of the lens and complete anterior synechiae. The areas of viable tumor cells are deeply basophilic, whereas the intervening gray areas represent areas of tumor cell necrosis. (H & E stain; ×1.)

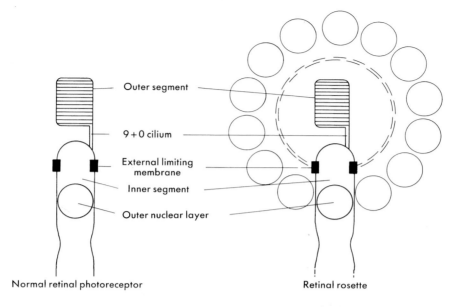

Outer segment

9 + 0 cilium

External limiting membrane

Inner segment

Outer nuclear layer

Normal retinal photoreceptor

Retinal rosette

Malignant: Flexner-Wintersteiner
Congenital: retinal dysplasia

Fig. 9-10. Photoreceptor differentiation of retinal rosettes. Electron microscopic analysis has shown that these structures represent a formation of retinal photoreceptors (rods and cones) from primitive or embryonic neural elements.

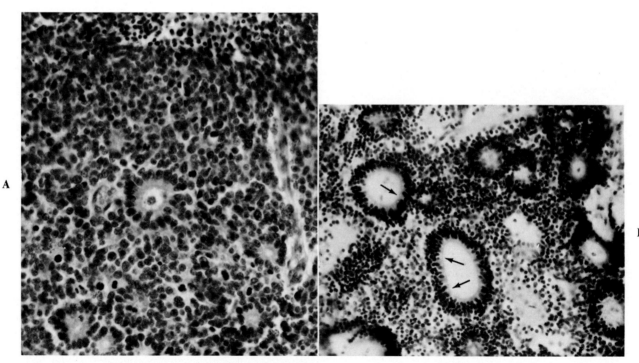

Fig. 9-11. Retinoblastoma, Flexner-Wintersteiner rosettes. **A,** Although several rosettes are present, most of the cells in the section are undifferentiated with numerous mitoses. (H & E stain; ×200.) **B,** The "membrane" *(arrows)* lining the rosette lumen is recognizable. (H & E stain; ×300.)

remaining photoreceptor cell forming the rosette has been drawn.

The cells that form a Flexner-Wintersteiner rosette are characterized by all of the cytologic features of anaplasia that are typically associated with malignant neoplasms. The *fleurette* (little flower) is a term for a microscopic appearance that signifies a degree of retinoblastoma tumor cell maturation of differentiation equivalent to that of the rosette.[209] The cells in a fleurette also show photoreceptor differentiation but are arranged side by side in such a fashion that when studied microscopically, the cellular arrangement resembles a fleur-de-lis rather than a circular rosette. On the other hand, the rosettes seen in retinal dysplasia (p. 401; Figs. 8-57, 8-58, 9-10, and 9-35, *A*) also show analogous differentiation simulating photoreceptor elements but are, of course, not malignant. Dysplastic rosettes represent a developmental or embryopathic aberration rather than true neoplastic differentiation.

True rosettes of the Flexner-Wintersteiner type differ from so-called pseudorosettes (Figs. 9-7, 9-9, 9-13, and 9-15), which are circumferential arrangements around vessels of viable, basophilic tumor cells. These cells can be clearly distinguished from necrotic, eosinophilic-staining, often calcified cells located more distant from the vessel. These cells grow in a circular pattern around the vessel, forming cell cuffs, or cellular mantles. A small group of tumor cells that degenerate and leave a clear space containing cellular debris surrounded by a ring of viable cells may also have a deceptive resemblance to true Flexner-Wintersteiner rosettes. Pseudorosettes, unlike true rosettes, are not considered prognostic factors, and this confusing term should probably be discarded.

An undifferentiated retinoblastoma cell closely resembles a primitive neural stem cell or embryonic retinal cell, with little or no evidence of cell maturation. Histopathologically the undifferentiated cells show a monotonous diffuse distribution of small round-to-polygonal cells with hyperchromatic nuclei and minimal cytoplasm. These neuroblastic tumor cells, or retinoblasts, show nuclear irregularities and atypical intranuclear mitotic figures. They show little or no evidence of differentiation toward rosettes. These cells resemble the cells seen in many other anaplastic, small cell neoplasms, such as lymphoma, neuroblastoma of the adrenal gland, cerebellar medulloblastoma, pinealoblastoma, Ewing's tumor of the bone, or oat cell carcinoma of the lung. Even though the histopathologic differential diagnosis may be difficult, the clinical history usually points to a correct diagnosis.

Special histological staining techniques and/or immunochemistical techniques may help with the diagnosis.° The cells may be positive for neuron-specific enolase.[13,114] They are negative for glial acidic protein and S-100 protein (Chapter 1, Table 1-2).

Retinoblastoma cells are not very cohesive and tend to disseminate throughout the eye. Seedlets of tumor tissue may permeate the vitreous cavity, where they receive sufficient nutrition to remain viable or continue to grow (Fig. 9-18). Implantation growths may occur at any site where nutrition is adequate. The most common sites are the ret-

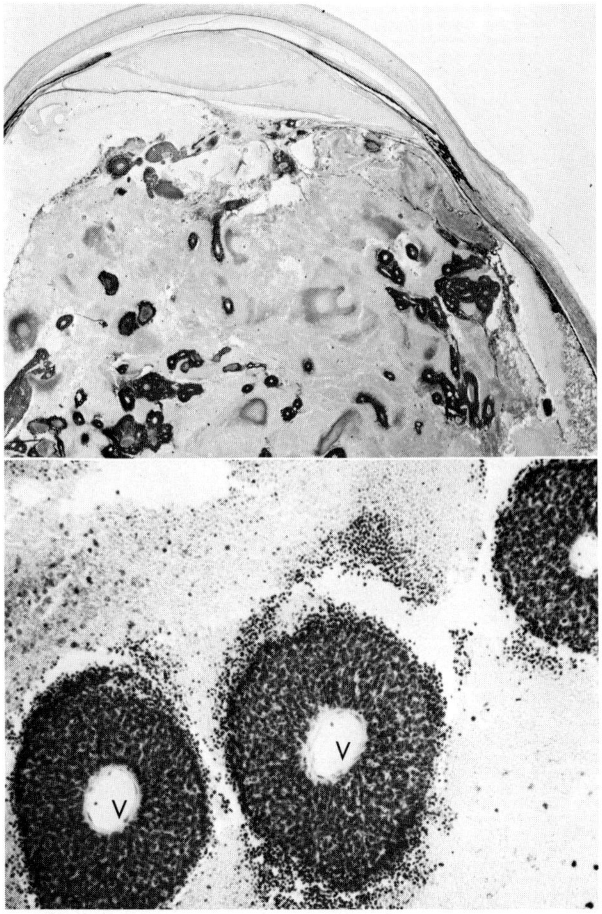

Fig. 9-12. Retinoblastoma. **A,** Extensive vitreous seeding with massive tumor necrosis (light-staining areas) alternating with perivascular viable cells (deeply staining foci), forming so-called pseudorosettes. (H & E stain; ×9.) **B,** High-power photomicrograph within the tumor seen in **A** shows tumor vessels (*V*) surrounded by clusters of viable retinoblastoma cells, with extensive tumor necrosis and ghost cell formation (pale-staining areas) distally. (H & E stain; ×80.) (From Naumann GOH and Apple DJ: In Doerr W, Seifert, G, and Uehlinger E, editors: Handbuch der speziellen pathologischen Anatomie, Band Auge, Berlin, 1980, Springer-Verlag.)

ina, the vitreous, and the choroidal surface; less common sites are the surfaces of the iris, the ciliary body, the posterior surface of the cornea, and the angle. Retinoblastoma cells have been transferred from a donor eye to the eye of a recipient in a corneal transplant operation. Occasionally the entire surface of the iris may be covered by a thin layer of cancer cells. Growths along the surface of the choroid may break through the lamina vitrea and gain access to the choroidal vasculature. When this breakthrough is extensive, the rich blood supply of the choroid offers an excellent medium for rapid growth and dissemination.

In addition to calcification within necrotic areas—a common and important diagnostic feature, which can be detected clinically and radiographically (Fig. 9-13)—basophilic-staining areas may occur in these tumors.[231] These areas are usually seen within blood vessel walls, but they may also lie freely within the tumor. The deposits are com-

---

° References 13, 114, 151, 166, 177, 192, 193, 204.

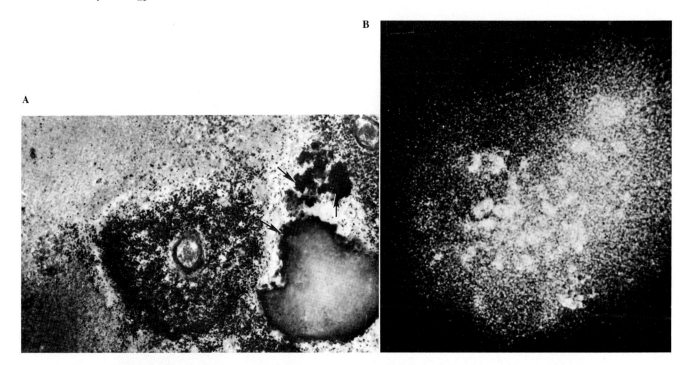

Fig. 9-13. Retinoblastoma. **A,** Dystrophic calcification showing calcific deposits *(arrows)* within necrotic area adjacent to a tumor vessel and perivascular cuff of viable cells (so-called pseudorosette). (H & E stain; ×100.) **B,** Radiograph of an enucleated globe filled with a large retinoblastoma. The radiopacities are created by the diffuse calcification in necrotic areas of the tumor. Orbital radiograph in such cases where calcification is present may be very helpful in establishing the clinical diagnosis. (**A** from Naumann GOH and Apple DJ: In Doerr W, Seifert G, and Uehlinger E, editors: Handbuch der speziellen pathologischen Anatomie, Band Auge, Berlin, 1980, Springer-Verlag.)

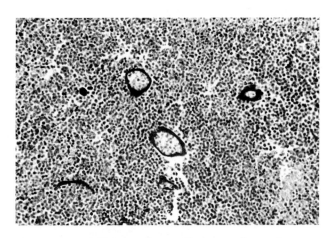

Fig. 9-14. Undifferentiated retinoblastoma with partial necrosis of tumor cells and DNA deposits (densely staining material) in tumor vessel walls. (H & E stain; ×140.)

posed of DNA (Fig. 9-14). They react positively to the Feulgen stain.[43,132,156–158,202] The DNA is derived from breakdown of nucleic acid–rich tumor cells.

In rare instances the tumor may outgrow its stromal blood supply or be destroyed by host defenses to such an extent that the entire tumor undergoes necrosis, leading to spontaneous regression and occasionally to phthisis bulbi (Color Plate 9-7).[*] The mass may become almost totally calcified and transformed into a chalky calcified or bony mass with a cobblestone appearance. The ophthalmoscopic appearance of such spontaneously regressed eyes is often similar to that of tumors destroyed by radiographic or chemotherapeutic agents. In any young child with an atrophic phthisic eye not accounted for by some known pathologic process, such as injury or inflammatory disease, the possibility of a spontaneous regression of a retinoblastoma must be kept in mind.

COURSE AND PROGNOSIS

The prognosis for life has been greatly improved in recent years because of a better understanding of the routes of extension of the tumor, earlier diagnosis, and improved methods of treatment.[†]

In general, undifferentiated retinoblastomas signify a more malignant course because the tumor cells are more anaplastic. The prognosis of retinoblastoma, however, also depends on factors other than cell type:

---

[*] References 22, 31, 37–39, 49–51, 69, 113, 131, 148, 155, 163, 174, 197, 198, 227.
[†] References 3, 5, 7–9, 11, 35, 90, 117, 120, 122, 125, 128, 135, 150.

1. The size of the tumor (see outline following)
2. The amount of seeding into the vitreous and anterior chamber
3. The presence or absence of massive choroidal invasion
4. The degree of tumor invasion of the optic nerve or subarachnoid space.

In some cases, although histologic examination of the intraocular tumor revealed many rosettes, rapid death has occurred. Conversely cures have resulted in cases in which the mass consisted entirely of undifferentiated cells. A retinoblastoma composed *entirely* of differentiated tumor cells does not exist. All retinoblastomas, including those classified as "differentiated," contain large numbers of undifferentiated elements. The classification is, therefore, based more on the ratio or proportion of the two cell types.

Another theoretic consideration suggests that the presence of a highly differentiated tumor is not necessarily as advantageous as would be hoped. The more differentiated cells exhibit a lesser degree of sensitivity to radiation therapy. From this standpoint, then, one might predict that a well-differentiated tumor might be more refractory to treatment.[56]

The clinical prognosis for survival or retention of the eye is determined by the location and size of the tumor according to the following classification of Redler and Ellsworth[183]:

Group 1. Very favorable; solitary tumors less than 4 disc diameters (DD) in size, at or behind equator; multiple tumors, none over 4 DD in size, all at or behind equator
Group 2. Favorable; solitary tumors 4 to 10 DD in size, at or behind equator; multiple tumors 4 to 10 DD in size behind equator
Group 3. Any tumor anterior to equator; solitary tumor larger than 10 DD behind equator
Group 4. Multiple tumors, some larger than 10 DD in size, any lesion extending anteriorly to the ora serrata
Group 5. Massive tumors involving over half the retina, vitreous seeding

In contrast to malignant melanoma of the uvea, in which the tumor often exits from the globe through the scleral emissaria, extraocular extension and subsequent metastasis of the retinoblastoma most commonly occurs after invasion of the optic nerve (Figs. 9-6 and 9-15–9-17).[137,213] As the tumor invades the nerve, tumor cells may directly infiltrate the cranium, may disseminate into the vasculature, or may seed the subarachnoid space by way of the cerebrospinal fluid.[57,226]

The surgeon should attempt to resect at least 10 mm of optic nerve (preferably more) during enucleation. If the optic nerve is invaded as much as 3 to 4 mm posterior to the nerve head, the mortality is 60% to 70% or higher, particularly if surgical excision is inadequate (Fig. 9-17). It is rare for the tumor to extend into the optic nerve beyond the lamina cribrosa for more than a few millimeters and extremely rare for it to extend as far as 8 or 10 mm. If it extends as much as 10 mm, it gains access, at the site where the central vessels leave the nerve, to the subarachnoid space where it rapidly spreads to the chiasm and brain.

When the tumor infiltrate is confined to the superficial aspect of the optic nerve, if the optic nerve is free of tumor and the mass is small, when it has not seeded into the

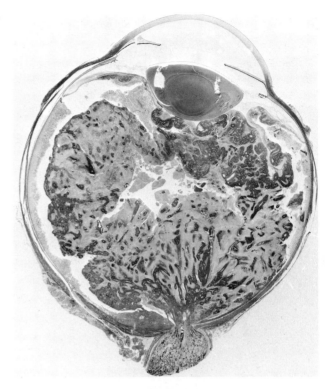

Fig. 9-15. Retinoblastoma filling the globe with tumor (deeply staining infiltrates) invading the optic nerve. (H & E stain; ×2.)

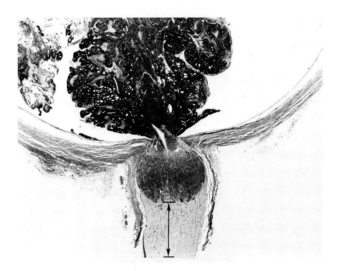

Fig. 9-16. Retinoblastoma filling a large-portion of the posterior aspect of the globe, with extension into the optic nerve. Although such optic nerve involvement is an ominous sign, a tumor-free zone of optic nerve distal to the neoplasm *(lines)* indicates that the surgeon has completely excised the tumor at this site. (H & E stain; ×5.)

vitreous, and when it has not invaded emissaria survival might be as high as 90%. Invasion of the tumor through the lamina cribrosa increases the mortality rate to about 30%. Deep invasion, but not to the surgical margin, decreases the prognosis for survival to about 60%. Invasion into the surgical margin sharply lowers this to a survival rate of 30% to 40%. Seeding of tumor cells into the vitreous humor and anterior segment is an ominous sign and signifies a poor prognosis (Fig. 9-18).

Aqueous humor seeding may simulate a hypopyon and thus mimic an inflammatory process (Fig. 9-6).[189,224] Deposits may appear on the iris and in the anterior chamber angle and produce a secondary open-angle glaucoma. Rubeosis iridis, often but not always associated with such anterior seeding, is also usually indicative of a poor prognosis.

Tumor invasion of the highly vascularized choroid and

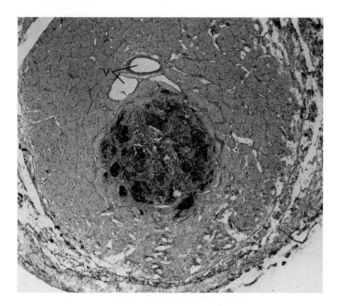

Fig. 9-17. Surgical margin of a cross section of an optic nerve in retinoblastoma. The tumor (deeply staining cells) has penetrated the center of the nerve. *V,* Central retinal vessels. (H & E stain; ×20.)

occasionally of the vortex veins may occur, either associated with or independent of optic nerve involvement.[183,212] Redler and Ellsworth[183] have demonstrated that choroidal involvement, when not massive, is not as ominous a prognostic sign as was previously believed. They found that a large proportion of enucleated eyes in their series had at least some evidence of choroidal invasion without widespread hematogenous dissemination of cancer cells. They write that the prognosis was only affected by massive choroidal invasion, noting that the volume of choroid occupied by tumor correlated better with prognosis than did the presence or absence of choroidal extension.

Retinoblastoma not only invades the cranium but also has a strong propensity for wide dissemination by way of the bloodstream.[45,57] Reese[187] observes that death is caused by intracranial extension in about 50% of cases, by generalized metastasis in about 40%, and by massive invasion of the nose and mouth that makes respiration and deglutition impossible in about 10%. The fatal outcome usually is heralded by an orbital recurrence and occasionally by intracranial manifestation or distal metastases without orbital growth. When therapeutic failure occurs, recurrent tumor may be found locally in the socket and orbit (Fig. 9-19), within the intracranial cavity and/or spinal canal, or within distant foci after hematogenous metastasis. The most commonly involved organs are the bones, lymph nodes, and liver. No tissue in the body is immune to retinoblastoma metastasis. Patients with distal metastasis rarely survive. The histologic pattern of metastases is usually of the undifferentiated type and is difficult to distinguish from other small, round-cell tumors of childhood.

One should always be aware of the possibility of a second tumor such as the above-mentioned pineal tumor (p. 480) when evaluating or following up a patient with retinoblastoma.[24-26,133,169,178,190] Radiation-induced sarcoma is a well-established complication, and in recent years it has

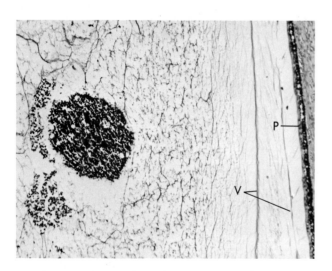

Fig. 9-18. Vitreous seeding by clusters of retinoblastoma cells, an ominous prognostic sign. *P,* Pars plana; *V,* vitreous fibrils at vitreous base. (H & E stain; ×75.) (From Naumann GOH and Apple DJ: In Doerr W, Seifert G, and Uehlinger E, editors: Handbuch der speziellen pathologischen Anatomie, Band Auge, Berlin, 1980, Springer-Verlag.)

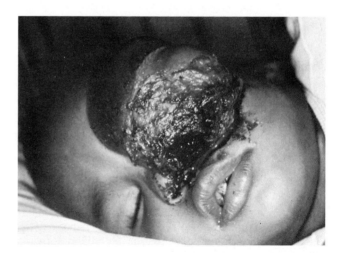

Fig. 9-19. Recurrence of a retinoblastoma despite a previous enucleation. The globe was enucleated immediately after recognition of a white retrolental mass. However, even though 7 mm of optic nerve was resected, the surgical margin of excision of the optic nerve contained tumor that had already reached an advanced state of growth. This orbital tumor recurred within a matter of months.

become evident that these children are also more susceptible to a spontaneous development of nonocular cancer.*

In summary, the major factors influencing prognosis appear less related to the cell type and presence of choroidal invasion than was previously believed. The factors that more accurately reflect the prognosis include rapidity of diagnosis, size or mass of the tumor, degree of vitreous and anterior chamber seeding, with or without rubeosis iridis and secondary glaucoma, degree of invasion of the optic nerve, and the ability of the surgeon to satisfactorily excise sufficient optic nerve to achieve a complete removal of the tumor. In bilateral cases the prognosis is usually no worse than that of monocular cases; the less involved eye is usually amenable to local therapy such as radiation. The prognosis is, therefore, more directly related to the degree of involvement of the eye that contains the larger mass.

TREATMENT

Retinoblastoma was a uniformly fatal neoplasm of childhood until the late nineteenth century. Sang and Albert[200] and Dunphy[68] have reviewed the historical aspects of treatment of retinoblastoma. The recommendations of the Scottish surgeon James Wardrop[248] in 1809 to treat this disease with early enucleation became widely accepted only after the introduction of chloroform and other types of general anesthesia in the 1840s. As von Hemlholtz's ophthalmoscope, which was introduced in 1851, became extensively used, tumors were diagnosed at an earlier stage. Shortly thereafter von Graefe correctly observed that excision of a long segment of optic nerve was advantageous. This, plus Hilgartner's application in 1903 of radiation therapy to retinoblastoma, resulted in an increasing number of survivors.[95] Other sophisticated advances in diagnosis and therapy, such as Reese's classification of retinoblastoma and the institution of protocol therapy and Kupfer's initiation[121] of the use of chemotherapy in addition to radiotherapy, contributed to the progressive decrease in mortality.[11] Current survival rates have been improved from the 5% reported by Hirschberg[96] in 1869 to recent figures of at least 80% in most series and up to 90% or more in favorable cases.[200]

Reese[187] and Ellsworth[72–74] emphasized that the treatment of retinoblastoma is directed toward five types of cases:

1. The unilateral case
2. The bilateral case
3. The case with residual tumor tissue left in the orbit at the time of enucleation
4. The case with later recurrence of tumor in the orbit
5. The case with extension to the brain or with distal metastases.

In the usual far-advanced unilateral case immediate enucleation is usually preferred. At the time of enucleation it is very important that a long portion of optic nerve be obtained so as to place the operative section, if possible, beyond any extension of the tumor into the nerve. Immediately after enucleation the optic nerve should be severed from the globe, flush with the sclera, and prepared as biopsy material. Sections for microscopic study should be cut from the proximal, distal, and central portions to determine if there has been tumor extension and, if so, whether the nerve has been severed beyond it. In recent studies Abramson and coworkers[3,5,9] have shown that both unilateral and bilateral retinoblastoma can be successfully managed by radiation or cryotherapy only, thus obviating enucleation. When the involvement of both eyes is so extensive that no vision can be salvaged, enucleation of both eyes may be warranted. Fortunately this is rare.

Many patients with bilateral retinoblastoma have far-advanced disease in one eye. This eye can be enucleated or irradiated, and it may be possible to arrest the smaller tumor in the other eye by conservative treatment to salvage useful vision.[7]

When enucleation is required and pathologic examination of the optic nerve immediately after enucleation shows residual tumor tissue at the surgical margin of excision, or if the sections of the eye indicate that tumor cells have gained access to the orbit from the choroid through the emissaria, irradiation of the optic nerve or orbit is indicated.

Reese[187] emphasized that a local recurrence in the orbit is in fact a residual focus that escaped notice until it grew enough to become visible or palpable. In such cases treatment consisting of orbital exenteration plus combined chemotherapy and radiotherapy may be indicated.

The treatment of metastasis is palliative; survival after metastasis is extremely rare.[110] The following methods of "conservative," nonenucleation treatment of retinoblastoma are available.

Radiation therapy

Various methods of treating retinoblastoma by radiation have been described by several authors.* Although many retinoblastomas are radiosensitive, the tissue of origin, the retina, is relatively radioresistant—a desirable combination for treatment by radiation. Although normal retinal blood vessels may be affected and lead to a radiation vasculopathy after large doses, many tumors can be completely devitalized by this treatment.

Radon seeds

Moore, Stallard, and Milner (reviewed by Stallard[225]) first conceived the idea of using high-energy isotope radiation from radon seeds for the treatment of retinoblastoma and were pioneers in the development of the technique of placing the seeds in the tumor area.

Chemotherapy combined with radiation

In 1952 Kupfer[121] reported a dramatic regression of a large tumor treated with nitrogen mustard in combination with radiation. This suggested that a combination of radiation with a radiomimetic drug might make it possible to further reduce the radiographic dose for retinoblastoma and perhaps avoid completely the various complications. Triethylenemalamine, methotrexate, doxorubicin, vincristine, and cyclophosphamide have been used in recent years.[74]

* References 4, 5, 12, 21, 64, 65, 75, 92, 190, 207, 214, 221, 229, 238, 252, 256, 260.

* References 7–10, 70, 72–74, 140, 187, 214, 215.

Light coagulation and cryocoagulation

Meyer-Schwickerath[147] showed that light coagulation can effectively destroy small tumors.[97,147] Cryocoagulation applications to the scleral surface adjacent to the tumor are sometimes effective.[3,142,187]

Leukokoria

Three major diagnostic considerations come to mind when evaluating a white (or pink-white or yellow-white) pupillary reflex in a child: retinoblastoma, cataract, and the so-called pseudogliomas, or pseudoretinoblastoma (Fig. 9-20).[261–301] The diagnosis of a congenital cataract is usually relatively easy with adequate history and clinical examination. In general it does not pose a diagnostic problem in the differential diagnosis of retinoblastoma.

The numerous conditions characterized as pseudoretinoblastoma include a wide range of diseases affecting the lens, vitreous, and retina-choroid.[53–203] The clinician must be aware of these diseases to evaluate a child correctly for retinoblastoma. A retrolental white mass (Fig. 9-1; Color Plate 9-1) should always evoke an awareness of this malignant neoplasm, which is, of course, the most serious cause of a white pupil in children, both with respect to vision and to life. This section describes the numerous retrolental and fundus disorders that may mimic a retinoblastoma.

Early investigators, going back to the era of Virchow[244] in the midnineteenth century, considered retinoblastoma to be a glial tumor or glioma. In 1892 Collins,[266] in a clinicopathologic study, first applied the term *pseudoglioma* to a variety of disorders that often cause a white pupil, thereby mimicking the appearance of a retinoblastoma. Although we know that a retinoblastoma is not strictly a glial tumor but more typically shows differentiation emulating neuronal elements, the term *psedoglioma* has persisted in representing the various conditions causing the white retrolental mass that may mimic a retinoblastoma.[77,181,239–243,252] The term *pseudoretinoblastoma* is more accurate, but the older term *pseudoglioma* is firmly entrenched in the literature and, thus, is difficult to dislodge from clinical usage.

There are numerous classifications of pseudoretinoblastoma, most of which are grouped according to a rough approximation of incidence. These include the reports of Sanders,[293] Duke,[267] Kogan and Boniuk,[282] Howard and Ellsworth,[278–280] Naumann,[288] Naumann and Lommatzsch,[289] Sarin and Shields,[296] Puklin and Apple,[291] and Apple, Hamming, and Gieser.[261]

A sufficiently large and statistically significant series that would allow accurate determination of the true incidence of the various conditions is difficult to obtain. One of the better classifications is that of Howard and Ellsworth[279] (Table 9-2), the diseases being listed in order of approximate frequency. They studied 500 patients in whom the diagnostic possibility of retinoblastoma had been raised and who had been referred to their clinic. Of these patients, most of whom had unilateral or bilateral leukokoria, other (nonretinoblastoma) diagnoses were made in 265 cases (53%).

Table 9-2. Two hundred sixty-five patients with suspected retinoblastoma in whom other diagnoses were made

Diagnosis	Number of cases	%
Persistent hyperplastic primary vitreous	51	19.0
Retrolental fibroplasia	36	13.5
Posterior cataract	36	13.5
Coloboma of choroid or optic disc	30	11.5
Uveitis	27	10.0
Larval granulomatosis	18	6.5
Congenital retinal fold	13	5.0
Coats' disease	10	4.0
Organizing vitreous hemorrhage	9	3.5
Retinal dysplasia	7	2.5
Tumor other than retinoblastoma	4	1.5
White-with-pressure sign	3	1.0
Juvenile xanthogranuloma	3	1.0
Retinoschisis	3	1.0
Tapertoretinal degeneration	2	1.0
Endophthalmitis	2	1.0
Persistent tunica vasculosa lentis and pupillary membrane	2	1.0
Miscellaneous:	9	3.5
Anteriorly dislocated lens with secondary glaucoma	1	
Congenital corneal opacity	1	
Incontinentia pigmenti (Bloch-Sulzberger syndrome) with total funnel-shaped retinal detachment	1	
Cyst in remnant of hyaloid artery	1	
Anomalous optic disc	1	
Hematoma under retinal pigment epithelium	1	
High myopia with advanced chorioretinal degeneration	1	
Medullation of nerve fiber layer	1	
Traumatic choroiditis	1	
Total	265	100.0

From Howard GM and Ellsworth RM: Am J Ophthalmol 60:610, 1965.

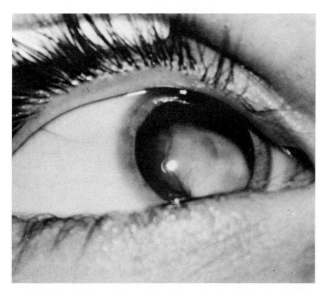

Fig. 9-20. Leukokoria (pseudoglioma, or "amaurotic cat's pupil") in a case of nematode endophthalmitis in a child. Compare with Fig. 9-1. (From Apple DJ, Hamming NA, and Gieser DK: In Peyman GA, Apple DJ, and Sanders DR: Intraocular tumors, New York, 1977, Appleton-Century-Crofts.)

Apple, Hamming, and Gieser considered the differential diagnosis in terms of the cause, pathogenesis, and structural characteristics of each disease[261]:

CLASSIFICATION ACCORDING TO PATHOGENESIS OR STRUCTURAL CHARACTERISTICS

I. Persistence and hyperplasia of embryonic ocular vasculature
   A. Persistent hyperplastic primary vitreous (PHPV)
   B. Posterior PHPV, epipapillary and peripapillary lesions, and congenital falciform fold
II. Retinal vascular anomalies with lipid exudation
   A. Coats' syndrome
   B. Leber's miliary aneurysms
   C. von Hippel–Lindau angiomatosis
III. Toxic retinopathy
   A. Retinopathy of prematurity (retrolental fibroplasia)
IV. Inflammatory conditions
   A. Toxocariasis (nematode endophthalmitis)
   B. Uveitis, pars planitis
   C. Metastatic endophthalmitis
V. Conditions exhibiting abnormal retinal embryogenesis and/or retinal dysplasia as prominent features
   A. Norrie's disease
   B. Trisomy 13 syndrome
   C. Fundus colobomas
   D. Incontinentia pigmenti (Bloch-Sulzberger syndrome)
   E. X-linked retinoschisis
   F. Rhegmatogenous retinal detachment
VI. Prenatal and infantile trauma, organizing vitreous hemorrhage, and massive retinal gliosis
VII. Neoplastic and proliferative lesions

A. Neuroepithelial tumors of the ciliary body (medulloepithelioma)
B. Miscellaneous proliferative lesions, hamartomas, and choristomas of the fundus
C. Leukemia

As is clear from this classification, the differential diagnosis of a white pupil or leukokoria (not including primary opacities of the lens but only retrolental lesions) (Fig. 9-21) in an infant or child includes disturbances of different tissues by different pathologic processes. These include defects in embryogenesis, vascular anomalies, lipid exudations, oxygen toxicity, infectious conditions, genetic aberrations, and neoplasms. Clinical diagnosis is greatly improved by proper genetic history and history of previous oxygen therapy and careful clinical examination under general anesthesia, fluorescein angiography, ultrasonography, electroretinography, and CT scan and MRI.[274] Swartz, Herbst, and Goldberg[231,232] and other authors[15,60–62,112,116,219] found that the determination of LDH levels on aspirated aqueous fluid can assist in differentiating retinoblastoma from other retrolental lesions. Their studies have shown that retinoblastoma is often associated with a high aqueous humor LDH level, while the nonmalignant retrolental masses usually show relatively normal levels of aqueous LDH. Jakobiec, Abramson, and Scher,[319] however, have demonstrated an elevated LDH level in a patient with Coats' disease.

PERSISTENT HYPERPLASTIC PRIMARY VITREOUS

One of the more important and frequent conditions mimicking a retinoblastoma is PHPV.* It and the other diseases with persistence of the embryonic intraocular vasculature have been previously described on p. 28.

RETINAL VASCULAR ANOMALIES WITH LIPID EXUDATION

Coats' syndrome, Leber's miliary aneurysms, and von Hippel–Lindau angiomatosis are retinal vascular diseases that, despite differences in pathogenesis and variations in clinical appearance, are often characterized by the outpouring of lipid exudates.[302–330] It is not simply the vascular anomaly of the former two diseases or the hemangioblastoma of von Hippel disease that is responsible for marked visual loss. The more important factor is the exudation, which leads to retinal detachment, secondary glaucoma, hemorrhage, and eventual phthisis bulbi. Because the lipid exudation can be massive and each disease may mimic a retinoblastoma, those three conditions are described together.

Coats' syndrome

In 1908, when George Coats first described the syndrome that bears his name, he divided it into three groups.[308] Groups 1 and 2 showed massive retinal exudation and lipid deposition (Fig. 9-22) but differed in the clinical appearance of their vessels (see outline, p. 495). Group 1 vessels appeared normal ophthalmoscopically; group 2 vessels exhibited clinically evident changes such

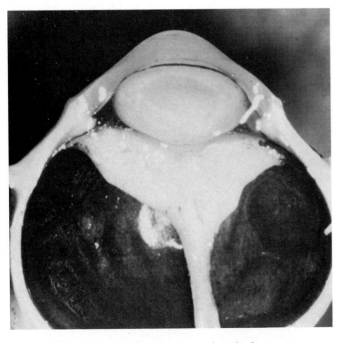

Fig. 9-21. Globe enucleated for a retrolental white mass suspected to be retinoblastoma. The dense white fibrovascular mass behind the lens was found to be a persistent hyperplastic primary vitreous with total funnel-shaped retinal detachment caused by traction from the mass. (From Apple DJ, Hamming NA, and Gieser DK: In Peyman GA, Apple DJ, and Sanders DR, editors: Intraocular tumors, New York, 1977, Appleton-Century-Crofts.)

* References 261, 264, 281, 272, 278–280, 284, 287, 291, 294.

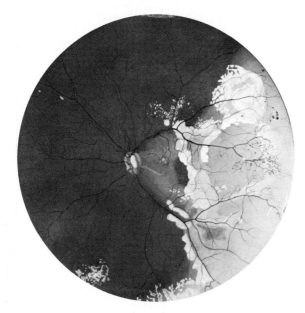

Fig. 9-22. Early artist's fundus drawing from a patient with Coats' disease showing massive outpouring of lipid. Microvascular anomalies are also present. (From the collection of Professor Wolfgang Stock, University of Tübingen, Tübingen, Germany.)

as telangiectasia (Fig. 9-23; Color Plates 9-6–9-10), aneurysms, vascular sheathing, and neovascularization. Coats' group 3 is now recognized as von Hippel–Lindau angiomatosis.

The classic syndrome of Coats consists of a nonfamilial, almost always unilateral, affection primarily occurring in infants or juveniles in the absence of other systemic findings.* Males are more commonly affected. The diagnosis is usually made at a slightly later age than for retinoblastoma, the peak incidence being toward the end of the first decade.[302] Subretinal and intraretinal deposition of cholesterol-containing lipid exudates are clinically and pathologically evident (Figs. 9-24–9-26). The clinical differentiation from retinoblastoma is facilitated by recognition of the characteristic retinal telangiectasia seen in Coats' syndrome (Fig. 9-23). Although vascular engorgement may occur in retinoblastoma, the severe vascular changes listed in the following outline are much more characteristic of Coats' syndrome.

In many cases the exudative retrolental mass assumes a yellow color because of the accumulation of lipids. This contrasts with the usual chalk-white or pink-white appearance of retinoblastoma, which often shows calcification. The yellow, glistening, crystalline deposits of cholesterol within the exudates in Coats' syndrome should not be confused with the chalky white calcium deposits seen in necrotic retinoblastomas. Untreated eyes almost always progress to retinal hemorrhage, retinal detachment (Fig. 9-24), secondary glaucoma, and phthisis bulbi. Photocoagulation is one of the few available means of treatment; it may be successful in early cases in achieving resorption of the exudates.

When considered together, three major histopathologic

---

*References 281, 302–313, 315, 317–321, 325, 326, 330.

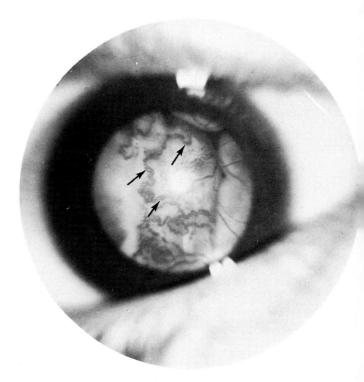

Fig. 9-23. Fundus photograph of a retrolental mass in a young boy. Two clinical features led to the correct clinical diagnosis of Coats' syndrome: (1) marked retinal vascular telangiectasia (*arrows*) and (2) a yellow discoloration of the mass, caused by massive lipid exudation. (From Apple DJ, Hamming NA, and Gieser DK: In Peyman GA, Apple DJ and Sanders DR, editors: Intraocular tumors, New York, 1977, Appleton-Century-Crofts.)

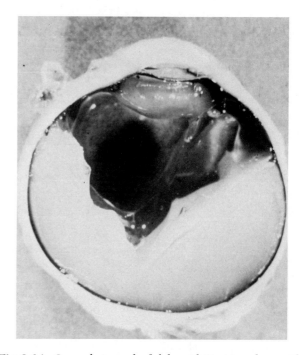

Fig. 9-24. Gross photograph of globe with Coats' syndrome. The retina is totally detached by a milky-white, turbid fluid, which is rich in lipids. (From Apple DJ, Hamming NA, and Gieser DK: In Peyman GA, Apple DJ, and Sanders DR, editors: Intraocular tumors, New York, 1977, Appleton-Century-Crofts.)

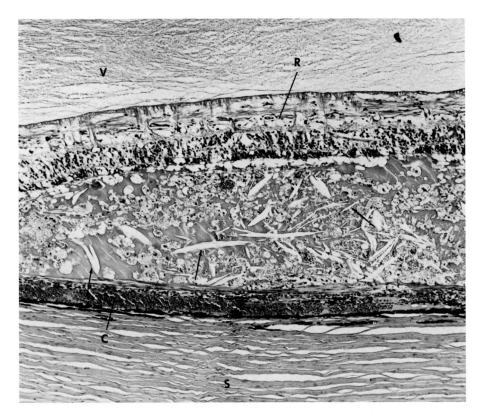

Fig. 9-25. Coats' syndrome. The degenerated retina (*R*) is detached from the underlying choroid by a subretinal exudate of lipid (cholesterol clefts, *arrows*) and hemosiderin and lipid-laden macrophages, all entrapped in a proteinaceous exudate. The macrophages are recognized as round, poorly staining cells, with small punctate nuclei located centrally within the cell. In addition to this characteristic type of subretinal exudate, the two other major features of Coats' syndrome are retinal telangiectasia and the deposition of PAS-positive exudates within the retina. *V*, Vitreous; *C*, choroid; *S*, sclera. (H & E stain; ×69.)

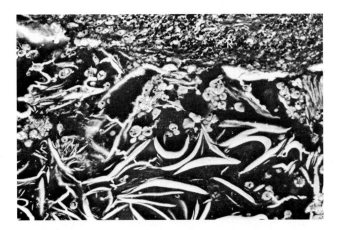

Fig. 9-26. High-power photomicrograph of subretinal fluid in Coats' syndrome showing cholesterol slits or clefts and lipid- and pigment-laden macrophages. *R*, Overlying retina. (PAS stain; ×180.) (Courtesy Professor GOH and Naumann, Tübingen, Germany; from Apple DJ, Hamming NA, and Gieser DK: In Peyman GA, Apple DJ, and Sanders DR, editors: Intraocular tumors, New York, 1977, Appleton-Century-Crofts.)

hallmarks are pathognomonic of Coats' syndrome (modified from Apple and associates[303]):

A. Vascular changes
   1. Coats' type 1: vascular changes not clinically prominent
   2. Coats' type 2
      a. Irregular vessel caliber, including telangiectasia, aneurysms
      b. Hyalinization, sheathing
      c. Arteriovenous anastomoses
      d. Neovascularization
B. Lipid exudation
   1. Intraretinal and subretinal deposits of lipid (cholesterol clefts)
   2. Hemorrhage and gliosis, deposition of hemosiderin laden and lipoidal macrophages
C. Intraretinal periodic acid-Schiff (PAS)-positive deposits

The essential pathogenetic factor is probably a loss of vascular, endothelial cell, tight junctions leading to breakdown of the blood-retinal barrier. Blood fluids and lipids cross this barrier and are deposited within the vessel wall (plasmatic vasculosis) and in the perivascular interstitial tissues.[315,330] The nature of the intraretinal, PAS-positive de-

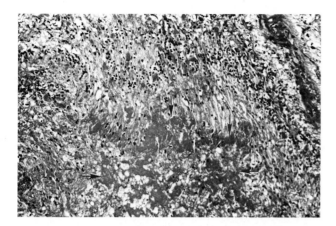

Fig. 9-27. High-power photomicrograph of the retina in Coats' syndrome. In addition to diffuse neuronal degeneration and gliosis with loss of normal architecture, there is a characteristic deposit of amorphous PAS-positive material *(arrows)* within the retinal substance. (PAS stain; ×180.)

posits (Fig. 9-27) is unclear, but these also probably are derived from extravasated serum. They are useful for diagnosis and, if present in large amounts, are highly characteristic of Coats' syndrome.

Similar clinical and pathologic findings may be seen unilaterally in eyes of adults without systemic disease.[315] In such cases the complex of lesions is similar to that seen in the juvenile form, but a unifying cause between the adult and the juvenile forms has not been demonstrated.

Leber's miliary aneurysms

The relationship between Leber's miliary aneurysms and Coats' syndrome continues to cause controversy.[304,314,316,324,329] Some authors consider them to be variations of the same disease with similar etiologic factors and pathogenesis; others consider them totally separate entities. Leber's multiple miliary aneurysms with retinal degeneration most commonly occur in young to middle-aged persons. These patients, therefore, are generally somewhat older than those with typical juvenile Coats' syndrome.

The most distinguishing feature of this disease is a saccular or bulbous dilatation of retinal arterial channels. These aneurysms can be tiny and asymptomatic or mildly symptomatic, producing what are sometimes known as segmental microaneurysms of the macular region. The saccular or bulbous arterial aneurysms can be relatively large, involving discrete foci on the involved vessel. The aneurysmal dilatations of the retinal vessels show perfusion by fluorescein angiography but do not leak and do not represent new vessels. Plasma fluids and lipids can, however, leak into the retina, although not to the extent seen in the classic Coats' syndrome. This leakage apparently is caused by the formation of associated arteriovenous shunts and leaking small vessels rather than by leakage of the larger, dilated arterial channels.

Many of the aneurysmal lesions spontaneously regress, and visual impairment is often minimal if the serum-lipid exudates do not involve the fovea. The most satisfactory treatment of threatening lesions in the macular region is photocoagulation. Obliteration of leaking channels within

and adjacent to the exudative ring can promote resorption of the exudates.

von Hippel–Lindau angiomatosis

von Hippel–Lindau disease (angiomatosis retinae) is considered in the section on phacomatosis (pp. 506–509). When massive intraretinal and subretinal lipid outpouring is a prominent feature, this condition can clinically resemble retinoblastoma or Coats' syndrome.

TOXIC RETINOPATHY (RETINOPATHY OF PREMATURITY)

Palmer and associates[376] have noted that retinopathy of prematurity (ROP), a disease affecting the retina of premature infants, has a key pathologic change, retinal neovascularization, which has several features in common with the other proliferative retinopathies such as diabetic and sickle cell retinopathy.[300,331–402] Each of these proliferative retinal vascular disorders appears to be associated with local ischemia and the subsequent development of neovascularization. The disease is found only in infants with an immature, incompletely vascularized retina. The spectrum of outcome findings in ROP extends from the most minimal sequelae without affecting vision in the mild cases to bilateral, irreversible, and total blindness in more advanced cases. Contemporary neonatology practices in the premature infant nursery have improved the survival rate of the smallest premature infants, who are at the highest risk developing ROP.

In 1942 Terry[401] first described the clinicopathologic characteristics of toxic retinopathy and coined the term *retrolental fibroplasia.* He described the condition as a "fibroplastic overgrowth of persistent vascular tissue behind each crystalline lens." At that time and in subsequent years the role of oxygen administration in the pathogenesis of this disease was unknown. The tendency toward widespread administration of oxygen to premature infants in the 1940s and early 1950s led to a dramatic increase in blindness. The mechanism of oxygen toxicity was elucidated in the 1950s by several investigators (reviewed by several authors[331–400]), and the tendency toward aggressive oxygen therapy was correspondingly reduced.

The observations made by Terry generally dealt with cases showing advanced stages of the disease in which a fibrovascular retrolental mass is the most prominent finding. This mass is caused by the formation of peripheral neovascular buds (Figs. 9-28 and 9-29; Color Plates 9-11 and 9-12) that penetrate the inner membrane of the retina, invade the vitreous, and subsequently undergo exuberant proliferation and fibrous metaplasia.[357] These fibrovascular bands in the vitreous can then induce traction on the retina and optic nerve head (Fig. 9-30), leading to retinal detachment in which the retina is sequestered into a position behind the lens. It is this retrolental involvement (Fig. 9-31) seen in the later stages that produces the leukokoria and is responsible for the term *retrolental fibroplasia.* In the milder clinical form, in which this intravitreal proliferation is minimal, only a small peripheral mass is seen.

The fully developed or mature vasculature of the retina of a full-term infant is relatively insensitive to oxygen damage. The incompletely vascularized retina of an immature newborn, however, is susceptible to toxic damage induced

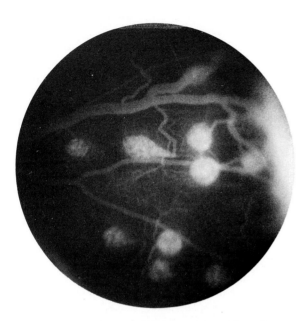

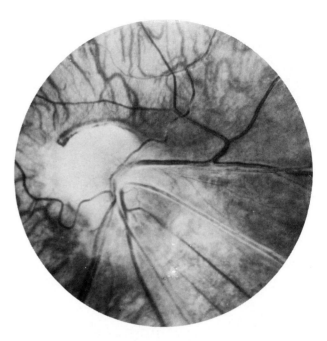

Fig. 9-28. Retrolental fibroplasia. Late venous phase fluorescein angiogram, from the same case as in Color Plate 9-11, showing multiple nonleaking vascular tufts posterior to the arteriovenous shunt. (From Garoon I and others: Ophthalmology 87:1128, 1980.)

Fig. 9-30. Retrolental fibroplasia with "dragged disc" and tenting of retinal tissue coursing from the disc *(lower right)*.

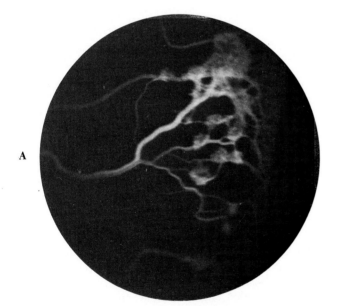

A

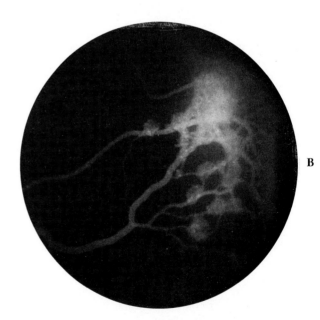

B

Fig. 9-29. Retrolental fibroplasia: fluorescein angiograms from the same case as in Color Plate 9-12. **A,** Early venous phase. No vascular tufts arise from the vessels near the arteriovenous shunt. **B,** Late venous phase. No dye is leaking from the vascular tufts. (From Garoon I and others: Ophthalmology 87:1128, 1980.)

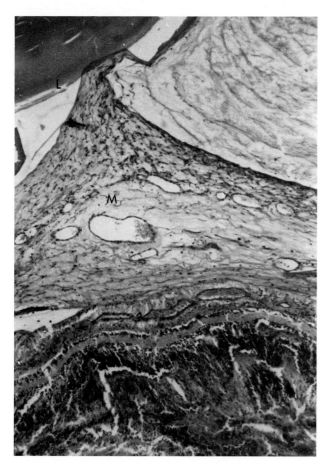

Fig. 9-31. Retrolental fibroplasia. The fibrovascular retrolental mass *(M)*, derived from foci of preretinal neovascularization in the peripheral retina, fills the space between the lens *(L)* and the totally detached retina *(below)*. (H & E stain; ×220.) (From Apple DJ, Hamming NA, and Gieser DK: In Peyman GA, Apple DJ, and Sanders DR, editors: Intraocular tumors, New York, 1977, Appleton-Century-Crofts.)

by high levels of oxygen inhalation. The most peripheral areas of the sensory retina are incompletely vascularized before birth. During normal embryogenesis the vascular buds emanate from the disc and reach the nasal or a serrata at 8 months gestation. The temporal ora serrata is not fully vascularized until several weeks after birth. This delay temporally presumably is the result of the greater distance from the optic disc to the temporal aspect of the eye. This phenomenon, in which immature vessels remain for a longer period temporally, is largely responsible for the greater incidence of damage on the temporal aspect of the fundus seen in retrolental fibroplasia. The fact that the temporal retina is not fully vascularized until several weeks after birth explains why this disease may be seen occasionally in full-term infants.

About two thirds of infants weighing less than 1250 g at birth develop retinopathy of prematurity. The severity is related to the duration and amount of oxygen exposure. When oxygen is administered to the premature infant, the still developing angioblastic tissue of the retinal periphery is stimulated toward an initial primary stage of vasoconstriction. The work of Kretzer and coworkers[368] suggests

that (1) in human retrolental fibroplasia no retinal vasoobliterative phase follows the vasoconstriction and (2) the neovascularization occurs because of lack of formation of adequate gap junctions between the vasoformative spindle cells of the peripheral human retina. Their work suggested a beneficial effect of vitamin E on gap junction formation.[275,349,368] The neovascularization after removal of the oxygen does not arise from the tips of previously lumenized vessels but from the vascular primordium anterior to formed vessels. In the early phase a demarcation line is seen that separates the peripheral avascular retina from the vascular. The neovascularization is exuberant, and glomeruloid buds and tufts of vessels form.[360] These elements proliferate, break through the internal limiting membrane, and eventually invade the vitreous in a manner analogous to that observed in other neovascular conditions such as diabetic retinopathy or sickle retinopathy. The secondary proliferative response following oxygen removal is best explained as an overreaction by the tissue to the relative hypoxia and ischemia.

Retinopathy of prematurity evolves from the stage of early active neovascularization to a cicatricial stage that commonly appears after the third to fifth month of life. Stages of the disease are as follows:

1. Stage 1: demarcation line
   a. The demarcation line separates the avascular neural retina anteriorly from the vascular neural retina posteriorly.
   b. The retinal vessels leading to the line have brush-like endings.
2. State 2: ridge
   a. Extraretinal neovascularization results from growth in width and height of the demarcation.
   b. Small isolated tufts of new vessels may be seen lying on the surface posterior to the ridge.
3. Stage 3: ridge with extraneural retina fibrovascular proliferation
   a. Fibrovascular proliferation occurs posterior to the ridge.
   b. Mild, moderate, and severe grades exist.
4. Stage 4: partial neural retinal detachment
   a. Stage 4a: partial extrafoveal neural retinal detachment
   b. Stage 4b: partial neural retinal detachment involving fovea
5. Stage 5: total neural retinal detachment

Howard and Ellsworth[280] emphasize that a specific form of the cicatricial stage of this disease (grade 3) is particularly noteworthy because of its resemblance to congenital falciform retinal fold (Color Plate 2-14). In this form, often referred to as a "dragged disc" (Fig. 9-30), traction on the retina produces a sharply demarcated, elevated retinal septum that arches forward in to the vitreous body, usually coursing temporally from the disc to the extreme periphery of the fundus.

Ciliary processes can almost invariably be seen in the periphery of the tissue—a feature characteristic of retinopathy of prematurity and never seen in retinoblastoma. The ciliary body is pulled centrally by contracting fibrous tissue.

These latter stages are also characterized by synechiae formation, glaucoma, hemorrhage, scarring and fibrosis, and eventual phthisis bulbi. Although phthisis bulbi is a common sequela, the changes are not necessarily progressive. The disease may become quiescent at any stage.

Several features differentiate retinopathy of prematurity from retinoblastoma and other causes of leukokoria. The relationship of the disease to premature birth and oxygen therapy is obvious (although retinopathy of prematurity may occur rarely in full-term infants in the absence of oxygen therapy).[393] The formation of the retrolental membrane is usually not present immediately at birth but develops subsequently. The condition is usually bilateral, and the eyes are normal in size at birth, although they may show growth retardation with relative microphthalmia later. No calcium is seen clinically or radiographically in retinopathy of prematurity. In later stages the dragged disc may resemble a congenital falciform fold but is usually easily differentiated from retinoblastoma. The centrally displaced ciliary processes of retinopathy of prematurity are not seen in retinoblastoma.

Clinical management of the premature infant requires judgment in the preservation of life by oxygen and the potential for blindness from oxygen toxicity.[363,381] Present emphasis is on a titration of oxygen delivered from the incubator to a level at which systemic complications caused by hypoxia and ocular complications resulting from hyperoxia might be avoided. A multicenter trial has established that cryotherapy for retinopathy of prematurity is efficacious.[342] The retrolental mass may be removed by vitrectomy.[372]

INFLAMMATORY CONDITIONS

Toxocariasis (nematode endophthalmitis)

In 1952 Beaver and coworkers[405] described a syndrome of childhood caused by infection by *Toxocara canis* and coined the term *visceral larva migrans*. Infection of the eye is termed nematode endophthalmitis.[403–426] Typically affecting children in the first decade of life, the ova of *Toxocara* species, usually *T. canis* (canine host), are ingested and hatch in the small intestine.[268,295,408,422,426] One usually can obtain a history of exposure of the child to the family pet, more commonly a puppy rather than an adult dog.[414] The larvae are distributed to the peripheral organs, particularly the liver, lungs, brain, and eye (Figs. 9-32–9-34; Color Plate 9-13) via the arterial circulation, where they are deposited and consumed or encapsulated by an eosinophilic granulomatous response.[405–407] In human beings the life cycle is never completed and ends at this point. Clinically the condition is usually only diagnosed presumptively because, short of finding the worms in the stools, there are few reliable means of identifying them. Because the eye lesion usually manifests itself as a unilateral leukokoria at a time when it is no longer possible to find worms, one must rely on the clinical picture and history.

Intraocular toxocariasis was first described and emphasized by Wilder in 1950.[375] She found larvae in histologic sections of more than half of a selected series of pseudoglioma cases. The leukokoria is usually unilateral. The infection usually takes one of three forms: (1) a retrolental, intravitreal lesion forming a vitreous abscess (Fig. 9-33)[410,411,418,424]; (2) an isolated posterior polar lesion, often confined to the macula or optic nerve head, and creating

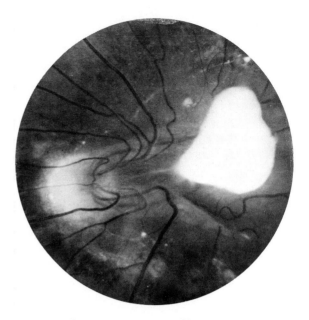

Fig. 9-32. Inflammatory mass caused by *Toxocara canis* (nematode endophthalmitis) showing the formation of a "dragged disc."

a retinal fold or "dragged disc" (Fig. 9-32)[403,409,412,417]; or (3) a well-localized peripheral retinal or ciliary body inflammatory mass.[413,423] Wilkinson and Welsh[425] believe that the initial site of the larva is determined solely by chance. An interesting but puzzling fact is that patients with a systemic form, for example, hepatic infestations, rarely contract the ocular lesion, and vice versa. Similar to most parasitic diseases, eosinophilia of the peripheral blood often occurs; however, the eosinophil count is more consistently elevated in cases of systemic visceral larva migrans than in cases localized to the eye. The enzyme-linked immunosorbent assay (ELISA) is often helpful in establishing the diagnosis.[294,408,419,421]

Demonstration of the organisms in histopathologic sections of enucleated globes is difficult without extensive serial sectioning. There is actually very little inflammatory reaction until after the organism dies. The cellular reaction is then distinct, however, and a tissue diagnosis can be made confidently, even without localization of the actual organism.

The infected intraocular tissues typically show a central focus of necrosis, usually surrounding the worm, accompanied by abundant eosinophils. The eosinophil, characterized by eosinophilic-staining cytoplasm and bilobed nucleus, is usually associated with an accompanying infiltration rich in neutrophils and plasma cells, epithelioid cells, and other nonspecific chronic inflammatory elements. Generally one can safely conclude that this combination of eosinophils and plasma cells within a retinal or vitreous abscess in a child with leukokoria is sufficient for a presumptive diagnosis of nematode endophthalmitis. Extensive fibrosis and organization of the involved tissues and a decrease in cellularity of the lesion occur in very late stages of the disease; however, even these cases usually involve residual cellular infiltrates differentiating this condition from other conditions causing a white pupil.

When a vitreous abscess and severe endophthalmitis

Fig. 9-33. A, Gross photograph of an eye showing a large intravitreal mass subsequently found to be composed of an inflammatory infiltrate consisting primarily of eosinophils and plasma cells, characteristic of nematode endophthalmitis caused by *Toxocara canis.* **B,** Nematode endophthalmitis. The retrolental fibroinflammatory mass *(M)* contains fossilized remnants of a *Toxocara* organism *(arrows). R,* Totally detached retina adherent to the mass. (H & E stain; ×250.) (Courtesy Dr. Jerry Kobrin, University of Iowa.)

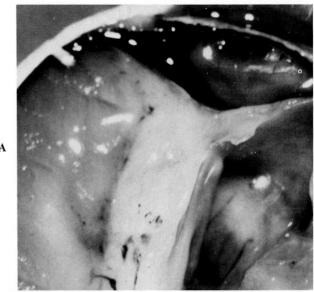

A

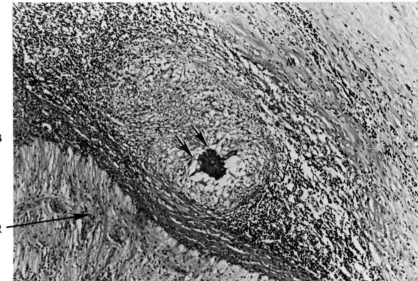

B

R

occur, differentiation from retinoblastoma is often difficult by simple clinical examination. In such cases the aqueous humor LDH assay described by Swartz, Herbst, and Goldberg[299] may prove useful.

Wilkinson and Welsh[425] emphasize the relatively high incidence of peripherally (anteriorly) situated centers of inflammation. In 4 of 10 of their enucleated cases, the lesion was within the peripheral retina or ciliary body. Because this form is often associated with retinal folds, it is more likely to be confused with grade 3 cicatricial retinopathy of prematurity or congenital falciform fold.

Peripheral toxocariasis also may be confused with pars planitis. Indeed, pars planitis has occasionally been observed secondary to proved toxocariasis. Howard and Ellsworth[280] observed pars planitis in 4 of their 265 cases of pseudoglioma. The caked yellow exudate in the lower half of the retina and the large, fluffy exudates within the vitreous may closely resemble retinoblastoma.

Cysticercus cellulosae may also occasionally induce fundus or intravitreal masses that produce a leukokoria. The intensity of the disease ranges from localized masses to advanced cases with complete detachment of the retina caused by cicatricial contracture. The degree of the inflammatory reaction and the extent of the pathologic change seem to depend on whether the cysticercus is alive or dead. The living worm induces a minimal response; the dead worm, a maximal response.

Metastatic endophthalmitis

Before the era of antibiotic therapy, metastatic retinitis was a significant cause of pseudoretinoblastoma. Today this condition is rare and is usually differentiated from retinoblastoma by recognition of the concurrent disease.

CONDITIONS EXHIBITING ABNORMAL RETINAL EMBRYOGENESIS AND/OR RETINAL DYSPLASIA

The concept of faulty retinal embryogenesis and retinal dysplasia[460,461] is defined and discussed on p. 401.[460,461] The following four diseases exhibit, to a greater or lesser

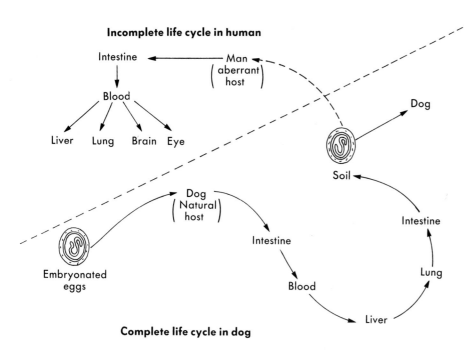

Incomplete life cycle in human

Intestine ← Man (aberrant host)

Blood

Liver Lung Brain Eye

Dog

Soil

Intestine

Dog (Natural host)

Intestine

Blood

Liver

Lung

Embryonated eggs

Complete life cycle in dog

Fig. 9-34. Life cycle of *Toxocara canis.* (From Zinkham W: Johns Hopkins Med J 123:41, 1968.)

degree, some pathologic features that place them in these categories.[427-471]

Norrie's disease

Norrie's disease is a rare syndrome with an X-linked recessive inheritance pattern characterized by bilateral congenital leukokoria, amaurosis, and varying degrees of hearing impairment and mental retardation.[*] Ophthalmoscopically the usual clinical presentation is that of a white, often hemorrhagic, retrolental mass noted at birth or during the first few months of life. A putative gene for this condition has been isolated: 27kb within band p13 of the X chromosomes (Xp11.3). Sons of female carriers have a 50% risk for expressing the gene.

Affected eyes have rarely had histopathologic examination, but the evidence available to date suggests that the basic mechanism of pathogenesis is a defect in the development of the embryonic retina. The changes are primarily neuroectodermal in origin. Not only is there an arrest (hypoplasia) in the development of the inner layer of the optic cup (the sensory retina), but also there is an aberrant growth of some segments of the retina, leading to retinal dysplasia.[442,451] This is evident by the development of rosettes and cords of proliferating embryonic cuboidal epithelium resembling primitive optic cup epithelium that forms within the retrolental mass (Fig. 9-35).

The primary defect in optic cup differentiation offers a pathogenetic explanation as to the origin of the myriad findings of this disease. In addition to the neuroglial proliferation from the retina into the vitreous, extensive secondary changes are largely responsible for the formation of the large preretinal mass that sometimes mimics a retinoblastoma. These include secondary retinal detachment and intraretinal and preretinal hemorrhage. Organization of blood breakdown products with formation of granulation

tissue creates a large fibrous mass that may compose the bulk of the retrolental mass. It is not entirely clear from histopathologic studies whether the intravitreal capillary buds formed in affected globes are derived in greater proportion from pure neovascularization or whether a certain percentage of these vascular elements are derived from persistent hyaloid vasculature.[428]

Trisomy 13 syndrome

Trisomy 13 (Patau's syndrome), which is considered in detail in Chapter 2, is the chromosomal aberration most closely associated with severe intraocular abnormalities.[447] The specific clinical findings characteristic of the disease, the diagnostic pattern seen by karyotypic analysis, and the fact that almost all affected infants die in the first few months of life clearly differentiate this syndrome from retinoblastoma. Therefore, although leukokoria is a prominent feature of trisomy 13, the general aspects of the disease differ sufficiently from retinoblastoma so that leukokoria is not an important factor in the differential diagnosis.[427]

Fundus colobomas

Howard and Ellsworth[280] noted fundus colobomas in 30 of 265 children with suspected retinoblastoma, ranking this entity fourth (after PHPV, retrolental fibroplasia, and posterior cataract) as a cause of leukokoria (Table 9-2). In most cases the colobomas are of the "typical" type, based on malclosure of the embryonic intraocular fissure.[437] These have been described in detail on page 17.

The white color imparted to the fundus by a massive coloboma is primarily caused by maldevelopment of the involved retina and choroid permitting visual observation of the overlying sclera (Fig. 2-11). This is responsible for the white reflex in the pupil, but careful fundus examination usually suffices to differentiate the colobomatous defect from retinoblastoma.

---

[*] References 283, 428, 431–433, 435, 438, 441, 448, 452, 465, 467–469.

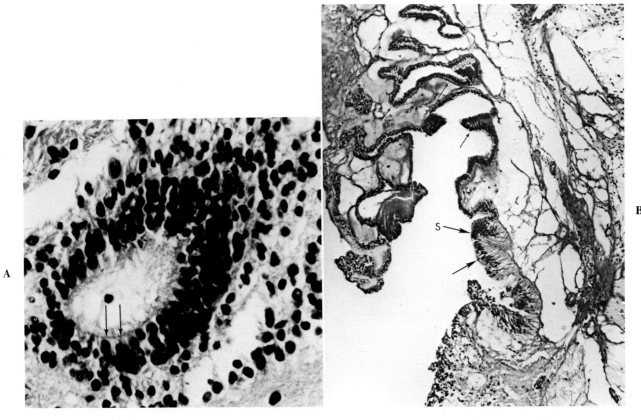

Fig. 9-35. Norrie's disease. **A,** Photomicrograph of retinal tissue showing retinal dysplasia. The rosette present in this field is surrounded by monotonous arrays of retinal neurons, which have developed haphazardly. The nuclei lining the rosette are analogous to the photoreceptor nuclei of the outer nuclear layer of the retina. The membrane lining the lumen of the rosette *(arrows)* represents the outer limiting membrane of the retina, and the delicate fibrillar processes seen within the lumen are abortive attempts to form photoreceptor inner and outer segments. (H & E stain; ×425.) **B,** Same case as **A,** with dysplastic neuroepithelium differentiating toward a cuboidal embryonic ciliary-type epithelium *(arrows)* and primitive sensory retina *(S).* The extensive formation of intertwining fibrils is positively stained by techniques for mucopolysaccharides, including hyaluronic acid. (Alcian blue stain; ×95.) (From Apple DJ, Fishman GA, and Goldberg MF: Am J Ophthalmol 78:196, 1974.)

Incontinentia pigmenti (Bloch-Sulzberger syndrome)

The skin lesions of incontinentia pigmenti (Bloch[431] and Sulzberger[463,464]) are usually present at birth or shortly thereafter. The disease usually occurs in females. Many hereditary cases have been noted, and the disease is probably transmitted by a gene on the **X** chromosome. The skin lesions occur in three stages. In the initial stage, immediately after birth, intraepidermal vesicles are a prominent feature. These develop mainly on the extremities and last several months. The second stage consists of linear, verrucous lesions. In the third stage the characteristic disseminated pigmented skin lesions become evident. They are located mainly on the sides of the trunk (so-called Blascho's lines) and arise de novo.[454] They arise totally independent of the vesicular and verrucous lesions that were primarily located on the extremities.

The histopathologic appearance of these pigmented lesions is responsible for the term *incontinentia pigmenti.* There is loss of melanin from the cells of the basal layer of epithelium with deposition and accumulation of pigment in the dermis. Sulzberger[464] assumed that primary damage to the cells of the basal layer causes them to become incapable of holding and metabolizing melanin. The pigmented skin lesions often fade with aging and may be difficult to observe in later life. Analogous subepithelial melanin deposits have also been described in the conjunctiva.[454] Clinical differentiation of this lesion from retinoblastoma is best attained by localization and biopsy of this skin lesion. In addition to the cutaneous and ocular lesions, other ectodermal structures are often affected, including the nails, hair (alopecia), and teeth. Central nervous system convulsions, paresis, and mental retardation result. Eosinophilia is sometimes present.

Ocular findings occur in one fourth to one third of cases (reviewed by Nix and Apple, Scott and coworkers, Wollensak, Best and Rentsch, and Rosenfeld and Smith).* Relatively unusual findings include myopia, iris hypoplasia, stra-

---

* References 292, 434, 440, 445, 446, 450, 453, 455, 457, 459, 462, 466, 470, 471.

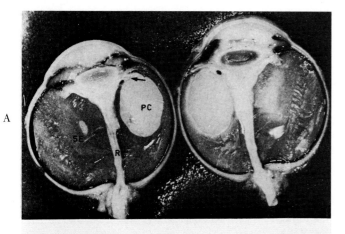

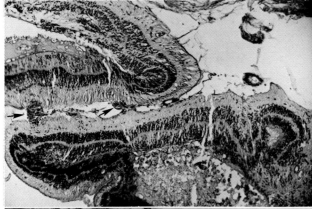

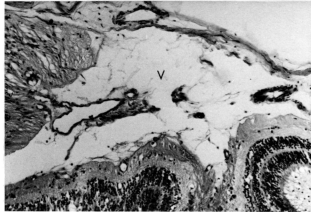

Fig. 9-36. Incontinentia pigmenti. **A,** Gross photograph showing a total funnel-shaped detachment of the retina *(R),* which causes a leukokoria. A peripheral cyst *(PC)* communicates with the retina *(arrow). SE,* Subretinal exudate. **B,** Section through the folded retina of the case in **A** showing glomeruloid preretinal buds of endothelial cells *(arrows).* (H & E stain; ×200 approximately.) **C,** The vitreous *(V)* contains numerous preretinal newly formed vessels derived from the ischemic retina *(below).* (H & E stain; ×250 approximately.) (From Best W and Rentsch F: Klin Monatsbl Augenheilkd 164:19, 1974.)

bismus, nystagmus, microphthalmia, optic atrophy, and blue solera.[458] More common, and more important in relation to the differential diagnosis of retinoblastoma, is the occurrence of posterior and retrolental changes creating a pseudoretinoblastoma (Fig. 9-36). This has been variously

described as resembling an exudative or proliferative retinitis, a falciform retinal fold, metastatic endophthalmitis, or ROP. Many of these cases reveal a cataract, which usually arises as a result of the retrolental mass.

It is extremely difficult to relate the pathogenesis of the intraocular changes leading to a leukokoria to that of the skin lesions. Three major theories of pathogenesis have been proposed:

1. Intraocular inflammation, for example, exudative chorioretinitis.[456,471] However, many cases in which an inflammatory response was absent have been histologically studied.
2. A form of persistent hyperplastic primary vitreous.[429] PHPV has been reported in only a few instances, and more cases must be added before this can be considered a significant etiologic factor.
3. Although the cause of the intraocular changes of incontinentia pigmenti clearly differs from that of retrolental fibroplasia (oxygen toxicity), Findlay,[439] Cole and Cole,[436] Best and Rentsch,[430] and Nix and Apple[457] point out the striking similarity of the pathologic changes in these two diseases and suggest a similar pathogenesis, that is, the formation of new vessels with subsequent proliferative retinopathy as a response to a hypoxic stimulus.

The most recent theory of pathogenesis was proposed by Best and Rentsch.[430] They assert that the primary insult consists of a congenital defect in the development of the retinal vascular system. They reported a case in which the initial fundus findings included what appeared to be a vessel-free zone, that is, an extensive hypoplasia of the peripheral retinal arterial system (analogous to the immature peripheral retinal vessels associated with retinopathy of prematurity). This phenomenon, also observed by other authors and visible by means of fluorescein and angiography, has also been described as an obliterative endarteritis.[457,469] The pseudoglioma probably results from the hypoxic stimulus induced by the arterial insufficiency, in a manner analogous to that seen in retrolental fibroplasia when the oxygen is withdrawn and a state of relative hypoxia is induced. As with many neovascular retinopathies (diabetic retinopathy, sickle retinopathy, and so on), the proliferative process is a nonspecific response to oxygen insufficiency. The histopathologic appearance, consisting of proliferation of buds of newly formed vascular endothelium with eventual preretinal neovascularization and proliferative retinopathy, is similar in all of these diseases (Fig. 9-36, *B* and *C*). These changes are similar to those found in Norrie's disease by Apple, Fishman, and Goldberg,[428] the pathogenesis of which may also relate to a primary defect in development of the retina and/or retinal vessels.

The findings of Best and Rentsch have been supported by Watzke, Stevens, and Carney,[469] whose study of 19 patients with incontinentia pigmenti included 7 with similar bizarre retinal anomalies consisting of a zone of abnormal arteriovenous connections and preretinal fibrous tissue at the temporal equator with no perfusion peripheral to it.

Best and Rentsch found no evidence to support theories that inflammation or PHPV plays a role in the pathogenesis of the pseudoglioma. The atrophy and elongation of the ciliary processes produced by traction from the proliferative retrolental fibrovascular mass may resemble that seen in PHPV and retrolental fibroplasia. The massive retinal detachment that occurs in full-blown cases can also be easily explained by the preretinal proliferative process.

X-linked (juvenile) retinoschisis

X-linked juvenile retinoschisis (congenital vascular veils in the vitreous) is a condition in which ophthalmologic evidence of the disease is ordinarily present at birth. The clinical appearance is usually readily differentiated from retinoblastoma, but cases occasionally have been reported in which leukokoria is a prominent feature. X-linked juvenile retinoschisis is more fully considered on page 422.

PRENATAL AND INFANTILE TRAUMA, ORGANIZING VITREOUS HEMORRHAGE, AND MASSIVE RETINAL GLIOSIS

In 1926 Friedenwald[474] coined the term *massive gliosis of the retina*. Such cases are characterized by massive fibroglial proliferation within the retina and vitreous to such an extent that the lesion resembles a neoplasm (Fig. 9-37). Reese[477] published a similar series of cases in which the eyes were characterized by protrusion from the retina of a gray-white mass, primarily occurring in young persons and caused by the organization of hemorrhage at birth (Fig. 9-37, A) or by trauma after birth.[473] He first emphasized that the picture resembles a retinoblastoma and must be differentiated from it. Moreover, following hemorrhage in the newborn or in infancy, there is contracture of fibrous tissue, with more and more of the retina pulled into the lesion, giving it the appearance of progression, thereby leading all the more to the suspicion of a retinoblastoma.

Howard and Ellsworth[280] observed 9 patients in their series of 265 in whom an organizing vitreous hemorrhage was encountered, which mimicked retinoblastoma. As the large vitreous hemorrhage undergoes organization, it may assume a yellow-white color and produce leukokoria between organizing vitreous hemorrhage and trauma and hemorrhagic disease of the newborn.[472–480] Indirect ophthalmoscopy should indicate the location of the lesion within the vitreous cavity, often in an inferior position, and confusion with retinoblastoma should not occur.

A review at the Armed Forces Institute of Pathology of 38 cases of massive gliosis of the retina indicated that the lesion configuration of massive retinal fibrosis varied from rather obviously reactive proliferations to growths that appeared neoplastic.[480] The authors showed that massive gliosis occurs not only in conjunction with prenatal and infantile trauma and hemorrhage but also occasionally in relation to congenital malformations, chronic inflammatory processes, and vascular disorders such as Coats' syndrome. They emphasized that one problem in the differential diagnosis of retinoblastoma from massive retinal gliosis is the fact that in both diseases tissues may undergo calcification, making radiographic differentiation difficult. However, the calcification in massive retinal glioma usually occurs in later stages and, thus, in an older age group than retinoblastoma. Therefore, the two main features facilitating differentiation from retinoblastoma are a history of trauma or other antecedent disease and the fact that massive gliosis is more commonly manifest in young adulthood rather than in infancy or childhood as in retinoblastoma. Occasionally the differentiation of a posttraumatic phthisis bulbi with mas-

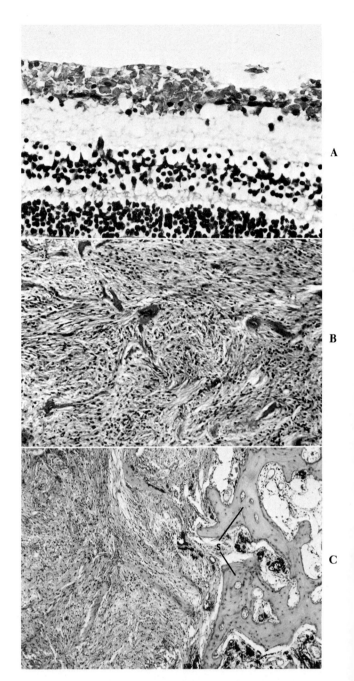

Fig. 9-37. A, Photomicrograph showing retinal hemorrhage in a newborn. *Top,* Erythrocytes within the nerve fiber layer. (H & E stain; ×185.) **B,** Photomicrograph through the vitreous showing a fibrous or glial mass that filled the center of the globe. (H & E stain; ×150.) **C,** Another case of massive retinal fibrosis (gliosis) showing bone formation (*right*) within the mass. *S,* Bone spicules. (H & E stain; ×115.)

sive retinal gliosis from a spontaneously regressed retinoblastoma may be clinically difficult.

NEOPLASTIC AND PROLIFERATIVE LESIONS

Neuroepithelial tumors of the ciliary body, including medulloepithelioma, can be mistaken for retinoblastoma. These are considered on p. 329. Hamartomas and choristomas, which may mimic retinoblastoma, are described with the phakomatoses.

Phakomatoses

The phakomatoses (Greek, *phakos*, a lentil), first classified together by van der Hoeve, constitute a group of heredofamilial diseases characterized by formation of lesions affecting the skin ("mother spots" or birthmarks), the eye, the central and peripheral nervous systems, and the viscera.[481–490] Certain combinations of lesions reappear in families with sufficient consistency to allow categorization of the various symptoms and sign complexes into specific syndromes. The four major phakomatoses are tuberous sclerosis, von Hippel–Lindau angiomatosis, neurofibromatosis (von Recklinghausen's disease), and the Sturge-Weber syndrome. All except Sturge-Weber are dominantly transmitted. Some authors classify the Wyburn-Mason syndrome and ataxia telangiectasia (Louis-Bar syndrome) with the phakomatoses.

Most of the diseases categorized as phakomatoses show widespread formation of tumors and cysts. The cystic growths most frequently affect the viscera, for example, pancreatic or renal cysts. Diverse benign tumorlike tissue growths termed *hamartomas* and *choristomas* characteristically occur.

A hamartoma is an anomalous proliferation of tissue involving only tissues that are normally present at the site of the growth. For example, the vascular malformation of the retina seen in the Wyburn-Mason syndrome is categorized as a hamartoma. Vascular channels are, of course, normally present in the retina. The astrocytic growths seen in the retina in tuberous sclerosis also qualify as hamartomas because astrocytes are normally present in the retina.

A choristoma, on the other hand, is a tumorlike growth composed of tissue not normally present at the site of growth. For example, a bone-forming tumor of limbal conjunctiva (epibulbar osteoma) is a choristoma because bone is not normally present in the conjunctiva.

The proliferative growths in the phakomatoses may be derived from any of the embryonic germ layers. Vascular tumors derived from mesoderm may occur simultaneously with astrocytic growths that are derived from neuroectoderm and/or visceral growths or cysts derived from endoderm. Hamartomas and choristomas seen in the phakomatoses *rarely* undergo malignant change. However, these anomalous growths create side effects or are sometimes seen in association with other tumors that occasionally lead to a more ominous prognosis. For example, the cardiovascular effects of a pheochromocytoma of the adrenal gland may dominate the clinical picture in any of the phakomatoses. Neurofibrosarcomas occasionally occur in von Recklinghausen's disease (Fig. 9-55).

Detailed discussions of the phakomatoses appear elsewhere.[482,483,488] In the following sections the salient features of each condition are illustrated and summarized.

TUBEROUS SCLEROSIS

Tuberous sclerosis (Bourneville's syndrome, epiloia) is characterized by a triad of (1) skin lesions (adenoma sebaceum), (2) epilepsy, and (3) mental deficiency.[491–513] It is inherited as an autosomal-dominant trait with low penetrance and without sexual or racial predilection. The clinical expression is so variable that the severity may range from a single isolated anomaly, or forme fruste, to the complete triad of changes with multiple system involvement. Many cases are fatal by early to middle adulthood because of the intracranial involvement. The signs and symptoms are usually present at birth or appear within the first 3 years of life, but in mild cases the diagnosis may not be apparent until adulthood.

Skin lesions (adenoma sebaceum, Pringle's disease) characteristically appear on the forehead and face (Fig. 9-38). The term *adenoma sebaceum* is erroneous because the condition is neither an adenoma nor a proliferation of sebaceous tissue. It is an angiofibroma composed of fibrous tissue admixed with capillary channels.

Tuberous sclerosis derives its name from the glial hamartomas seen within the central nervous system, including the eye. The nodules in the cerebral cortex superficially resemble peeled potatoes, hence the prefix *tuberous*, or rootlike (Fig. 9-39). The presence of these astrocytic hamartomas partially explains the epilepsy and mental deficiency, which constitute two thirds of the clinical triad. Intracranial calcification is also a common finding and provides a useful radiographic sign. For unexplained reasons, intracranial calcification is usually greater in patients with average intelligence than in patients with mental retardation.

The most common visceral tumors occur in the kidneys, less commonly the heart, lungs, and other organs. Peculiar mixed, soft-tissue growths such as angiomyolipomas are frequently present in these organs.

The intraocular lesions, occurring in about half of all cases, are proliferations of astrocytes similar to those occurring in the brain. The optic disc and fundus lesions seen in Color Plates 9-14 and 9-15 are hamartomas involving the nerve head and retinal nerve fiber layer (Fig. 9-40).[491,497,500,513] The lesions are gray-white and may be-

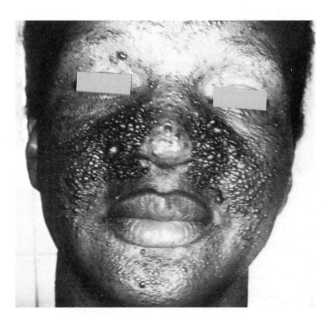

Fig. 9-38. Tuberous sclerosis showing the so-called adenoma sebaceum. This skin lesion is neither an adenoma nor derived from sebaceous glands. It is best classified as an angiofibroma.

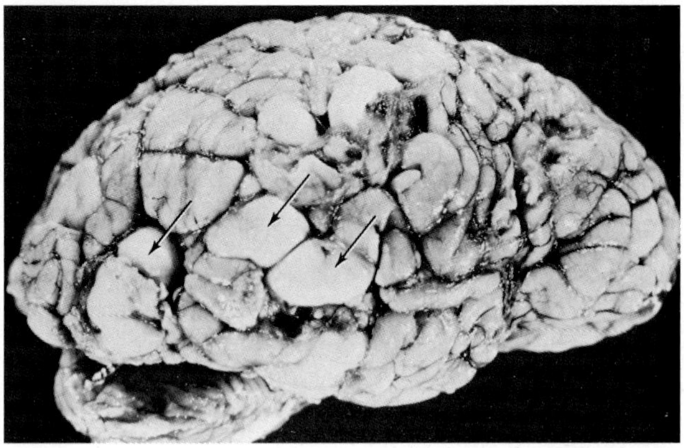

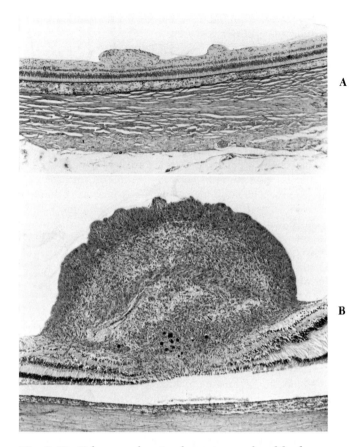

Fig. 9-39. Brain from a patient who died from tuberous sclerosis. *Arrows,* Nodular white protuberances within the cerebral cortex. These white protuberances resemble peeled potatoes and are responsible for the derivation of the term *tuberous sclerosis* (*tuber,* root). (Courtesy Dr. Paul McGarry.)

Fig. 9-40. Tuberous sclerosis, photomicrographs of fundus astrocytic hamartomas. **A,** Small midperipheral nodules. (H & E stain; ×110.) **B,** Larger peripapillary hamartoma with secondary calcification (deeply staining foci at the lower edge of the lesion). (H & E stain; ×180.)

come calcified (Fig. 9-40, *B*); they are frequently multiple and may mimic retinoblastoma in its earliest stages.

Although similar in clinical appearance, the "giant drusen" of the optic nerve head seen as an incidental finding in the general population (Chapter 10) differ from the optic disc lesions observed in patients with tuberous sclerosis.[508] Both may mimic papillitis or papilledema. Simple "giant drusen" of the disc in otherwise normal patients represent a degenerative process in which a "hyaline" material of unknown nature is deposited in the nerve. The lesion of tuberous sclerosis is a true hamartomatous proliferation of astroglia. Both types of "drusen" frequently undergo secondary calcification and in long-standing cases are difficult to differentiate, even at the microscopic level.

Because the retinal and optic nerve lesions are stationary, visual difficulties are relatively unimportant when compared with the life-threatening systemic manifestations of the disease.

VON HIPPEL–LINDAU ANGIOMATOSIS

Von Hippel–Lindau angiomatosis is a disease that is transmitted as an autosomal-dominant trait with incomplete penetrance.[514-552] Von Hippel[544,545] was the first to correctly describe the retinal vascular changes that occur in this disease, and he coined the term *angiomatosis retinae* (Color Plate 9-16). Lindau[532,533] later correlated these retinal changes with the cerebellar angioma that now bears his name (Fig. 9-41). The "Lindau tumor" may also affect the medulla, pons, and spinal cord, causing neurologic defects and early death.[519,526,528,529,535] Cysts of the pancreas and kidney, as well as hypernephroma and pheochromocytoma, may also occur (Table 9-3).[525]

The ocular changes occur in three stages:

1. The early stage of angioma formation, with development of feeder and draining vessels
2. The stage of exudation, hemorrhage, and retinal detachment
3. The final stage of destruction of the eye, secondary glaucoma, and phthisis bulbi

The fundus lesion consists of an afferent feeder arteriole and an efferent draining venule that enter into and exit

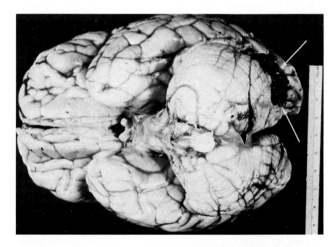

Fig. 9-41. Gross photograph of the base of the brain of a patient who died from complications arising from a cerebellar hemangioblastoma. *Arrows,* Blood-filled mass within the left cerebellum. The cerebellar tumor is known as the Lindau tumor; the retinal tumor is named after von Hippel. The histopathologic appearance of both lesions is similar (Fig. 9-46).

Table 9-3. Major pathologic lesions in von Hippel–Lindau disease

Site	Lesion
Retina	Hemangioblastoma
Cerebral cortex, pons, medulla, and spinal cord	
Cerebellum	Hemangioblastoma
	Ependymoma
Pancreas	Cysts
	Hemangioblastoma
Kidney	Cysts
	Hypernephromas
	Adenoma
	Hemangioblastoma
Adrenal cortex	Hyperplasia
	Adenoma
Adrenal medulla	Cysts
	Pheochromocytoma
Lung and liver	Cysts
	Adenoma
Bladder	Hemangioblastoma
Bones	Cysts

Courtesy Dr. Nick Mamalis.

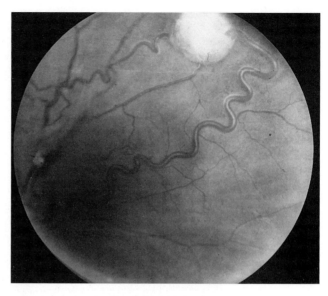

Fig. 9-43. Fundus photograph of a classic von Hippel lesion in a patient with von Hippel–Lindau angiomatosis. Note in this left eye that a tortuous arterial feeder vessel nourishes the actual tumor (retinal hemangioblastoma). The drainage occurs via the large diameter tortuous vein below the mass.

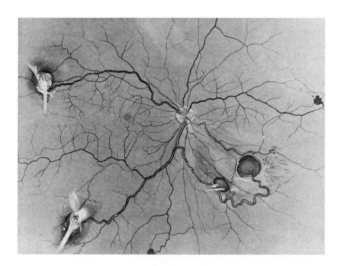

Fig. 9-42. Early artist's drawing of a fundus showing von Hippel–Lindau disease. Multiple hemangiomas affect virtually all quadrants of the fundus. Each tumor is associated with dilated, tortuous feeder and draining vessels. (From the collection of Professor Wolfgang Stock, University of Tübingen, Tübingen, Germany.)

from a well-circumscribed, midperipheral yellow to pink retinal tumor (Figs. 9-42–9-44). The angiomas are frequently multiple in each eye, and about half of the cases are bilateral. The disease affects both sexes. The onset of symptoms generally occurs during the teens or early 20s. Although clinical symptoms and signs are rarely evident at birth, intraretinal microvascular abnormalities that are not clinically evident are present very early in life in host-affected patients (Fig. 9-45). These lesions evolve into the clinically evident progressive vascular anomalies present in later life.[522,530] The retinal lesions represent only a local

manifestation of an extensive systemic anomalous development of vascular units.

In addition to the vascular anomalies and the retinal angioma, there is characteristically a massive outpouring of lipid into and beneath the retina. The angiomatous tumor itself is capable of forming lipid, but exudation of serum and lipid also occurs in areas *remote* from the primary angioma, particularly in the macular region. A macular star figure (Fig. 8-9) or circinate figure may be the presenting symptom. When serum transudation, lipid exudation, or hemorrhage is profuse, the fundus pictures of retinal angiomatosis and Coats' syndrome are similar. Indeed, in his original description Coats' classified what we now designate von Hippel–Lindau disease as type 3 of Coats' syndrome.[304]

Several features differentiate the two diseases. Coats' syndrome is usually unilateral; von Hippel's retinal angiomatosis is often bilateral. Coats' syndrome is usually diagnosed at a much earlier age. The clinical appearance of the diffuse retinal vascular telangiectasia seen in Coats' syndrome differs significantly from the clinical picture of the vascular anomalies seen in retinal angiomatosis. The clinical appearance of the intraretinal and subretinal exudates, however, may be identical.

The angioma can occur adjacent to the optic nerve head instead of the midperipheral or peripheral retina.[517,520,534,540–543,548] When this occurs it may mimic a papilledema, papillitis, or other epipapillary or peripapillary tumors. The characteristic afferent and efferent retinal vessels are absent in this variant.

The retinal-optic nerve tumor, like its counterpart in the cerebellum of the brain, is designated a *hemangioblastoma* (Fig. 9-46).[537] This term reflects the cytologic appearance of the proliferating endothelial cells, which are embryonic (blastlike) in appearance. In comparison, simple hemangio-

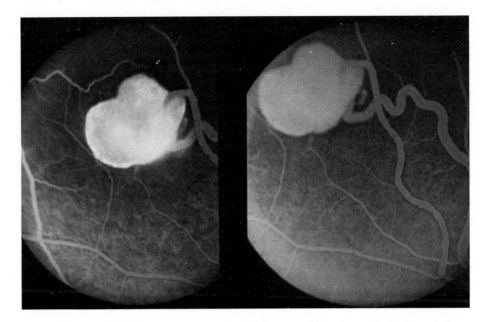

Fig. 9-44. Fluorescein angiograms of von Hippel hemangioblastomas with feeder and drainer vessels.

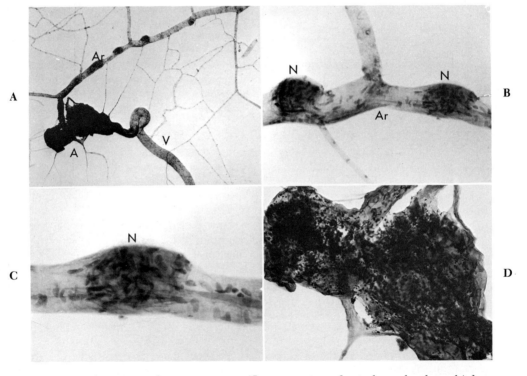

Fig. 9-45. These trypsin digest preparations (flat preparations of retinal vascular channels) demonstrate the earliest stages of angioblastic proliferation in von Hippel–Lindau angiomatosis. **A,** Feeder on the arteriolar *(Ar)* side of the angioma *(A)*. *V*, Venous drainer. **B** to **D,** Foci of nodular *(N)* proliferation of endothelial cells. Such early lesions eventually enlarge and form the typical retinal tumors. (From Goldberg MF and Duke JR: Am J Ophthalmol 66:693, 1968.)

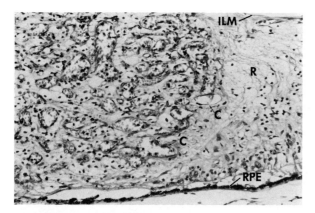

Fig. 9-46. von Hippel–Lindau disease. This photomicrograph of an affected segment of the sensory retina shows complete replacement of retinal elements by this vascular hamartoma. The hemangioblastoma is composed of proliferating endothelial cells, which line blood-filled lumens. The thin-walled channels are similar in structure and size to capillaries. Although it is not visible in this section, these growths are capable of forming lipid. *C*, Capillary-sized channel; *R*, sensory retina; *ILM*, internal limiting membrane; *RPE*, retinal pigment epithelium. (H & E stain; ×200.) (From Nicholson DH, Green WR, and Kenyon KR: Published with permission from The American Journal of Ophthalmology 82:193–204, 1976. Copyright by The Ophthalmic Publishing Company.)

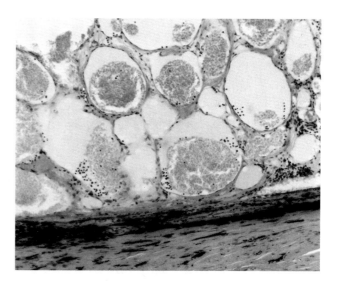

Fig. 9-47. Retinal hemangioma with large cavernous spaces. (H & E stain; ×140.)

mas are composed of mature endothelial cells and are not usually associated with von Hippel–Lindau disease (Fig. 9-47).* The hemangioblastoma not only comprises vascular endothelial cells but also shows varying degrees of differentiation toward fibrous tissue. Lipid (foam cells) and abundant glial tissue are often dispersed throughout the angiomatous lesion. It is not entirely clear whether this glial component reflects a primary component of the tumor or merely represents a reactive gliosis of normal retinal glial tissue in response to the hamartomatous vascular growth.

The presence of the anomalous blood vessels and tumors per se is not the immediate cause of the blindness; the vascular proliferation is in fact relatively slow. The exudation from the leaking channels actually induces the tragic secondary complications that lead to visual loss. If the tumor is not destroyed, the subsequent subretinal and preretinal hemorrhage, outpouring of serum and lipid, and hypoxia result in retinal folds and detachment, rubeosis iridis, peripheral anterior synechiae, secondary glaucoma, and ultimately to phthisis bulbi.

The retinal hemangioblastoma can be obliterated by cryotherapy[514–516,523,537,547–549] or photocoagulation. Cryotherapy is convenient for treating peripheral lesions and tumors in eyes with opaque media. It is particularly advantageous in eyes with a thick and large tumor mass, for the entire depth of the tumor can be affected by freezing. Photocoagulation is advantageous because by altering the size of the photocoagulation beam one may treat only the angioma and reduce the scarring of surrounding retina to a minimum. Both xenon arc and argon laser photocoagulation are extremely effective for small- to medium-sized flat

tumors that do not have a surrounding secondary detachment.

NEUROFIBROMATOSIS

Neurofibromatosis (neurofibromatosis type I, peripheral neurofibromatosis, von Recklinghausen's disease) is inherited as an autosomal-dominant trait with highly variable expressivity, irregular penetrance, and an extremely high rate of genetic mutation (Figs. 9-48–9-55; Color Plates 9-17 and 9-18).[553–612] The definitive nonocular features of this disorder include multiple café-au-lait spots, axillary freckling, and multiple, often cosmetically disfiguring tumors involving the skin and the central, peripheral, and sympathetic nervous systems (Figs. 9-48–9-50; Color Plates 9-17 and 9-18). The central nervous system hamartomas may cause increased intracranial pressure, blindness, deafness, epilepsy, motor and sensory disturbances, and mental retardation.

Although the primordia of many of the tumor elements are probably present at birth, the onset of symptoms generally occurs in late childhood. Neurofibromas are hamartomas derived from neural crest stem cells.[607]

Patients with neurofibromatosis have a higher than normal incidence of optic glioma (p. 553), meningioma[560] (p. 522), acoustic neuroma (neurofibromatosis type II, central neurofibromatosis), pheochromocytoma, and multiple hamartomas of the viscera, and multiple endocrine neoplasia (type II b).* Many lesions associated with neurofibromatosis (neuroma, café-au-lait spots, enlarged corneal nerves) may also occur in the general category of multiple endocrine neoplasia.[561] Malignant neurogenic sarcomas (neurofibrosarcomas, malignant schwannoma) may form, but they are unusual.[553,563,571,574,609] Thomas, Schwartz, and Gragoudas[606] have reported a simultaneous occurrence of von Hippel–Lindau disease and neurofibromatosis.

Almost all tissues of the eye and adnexa may be involved.

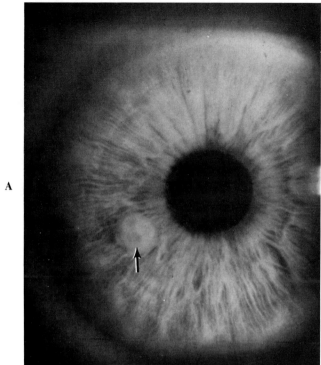

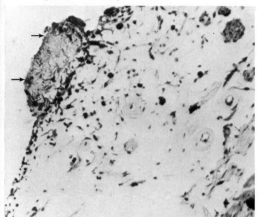

Fig. 9-52. Neurofibromatosis with iris involvement. **A,** Neurofibroma, or Lisch nodule, on iris surface *(arrow).* **B,** Photomicrograph of **A** *(arrows).* (H & E stain; ×300.) (Courtesy Dr. Thomas Weingeist, University of Iowa.)

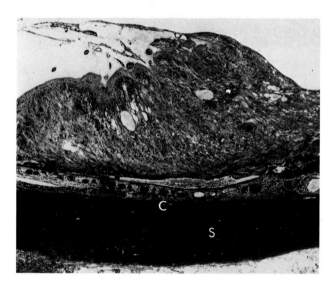

Fig. 9-53. Neurofibromatosis with a large neurofibroma protruding into the vitreous. *C,* Choroid; *S,* underlying sclera. (H & E stain; ×80.)

Common eye findings in neurofibromatosis are (courtesy Dr. Nick Mamalis):

A. Face, ocular adnexae, and orbit
    1. Facial asymmetry or homolateral hemihypertrophy
    2. Enlarged bony orbit and optic canal
    3. Exophthalmos
    4. Pulsating encephalocele
B. Eyelids
    1. Café-au-lait spots
    2. Solitary or plexiform neurofibroma and elephantiasis
    3. S-shaped ptosis
C. Conjunctiva, cornea, and sclera
    1. Thickened and myelinated corneal nerves
    2. Neurofibromas of conjunctiva[575]
    3. Episcleral and scleral hamartomas
D. Iris
    1. Lisch nodules[559,585,593]
E. Trabecular meshwork
    1. Glial hamartomas
    2. Increased incidence of congenital glaucoma
F. Uveal tract
    1. Hamartomas[580]
    2. Choroidal nevi and malignant melanoma
G. Retina
    1. Pigment epithelial glial hamartomas[557,565,581,588]
    2. Medullated retinal nerve fibers
H. Optic nerve[579]
    1. Optic nerve glioma[600,602,605]
    2. Meningioma

The hamartomas may cause facial asymmetry (Fig. 9-54, *A*) or homolateral hemihypertrophy involving bone and soft tissue.[558] Orbital changes include an enlarged bony orbit and optic canal and pulsating exophthalmos associated with sphenoid bone defects.[577,589,601,603] The eyelids may have café-au-lait spots, and the lid margins may attain an S-shaped configuration resulting from distortion by subcutaneous tumors (Fig. 9-54, *A*; Color Plate 9-17).[553,604] The eyelid skin, the conjunctiva, and the soft tissues of the orbit may contain solitary neurofibromas (Color Plate 9-18), neurilemomas, or plexiform neurofibromas. This plexiform

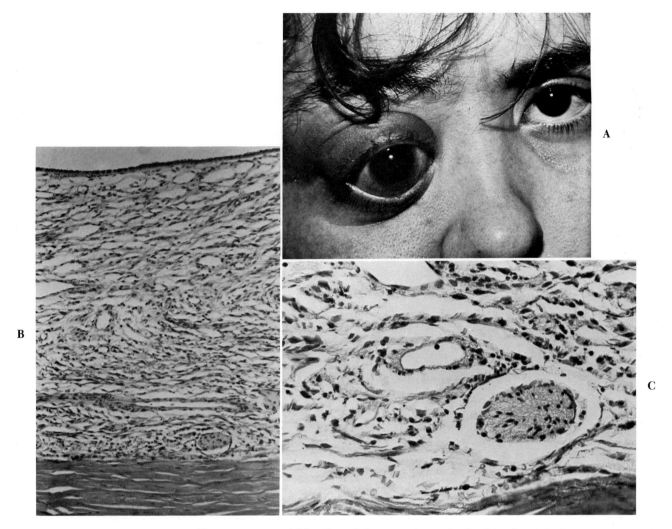

Fig. 9-54. Neurofibromatosis in a child with eyelid, intraocular, and orbital involvement. **A,** External photograph showing ptosis and proptosis of the right eye. **B,** Photomicrograph of the choroid of the enucleated globe showing marked thickening of this layer by a neurofibroma. This lesion clinically resembled a moderately elevated amelanotic malignant melanoma of the choroid by ophthalmoscopy. *RPE,* Overlying retinal pigment epithelium; *S,* sclera. (H & E stain; ×120.) **C,** Higher power photomicrograph through the choroidal hamartoma in **B** showing numerous small cells with spindle-shaped nuclei arranged in a diffuse manner with one solitary nest. (H & E stain; ×25.)

pattern is caused by an intertwining of cords of tumor cells around each other forming a "bag of worms" (Fig. 9-50).

Intraocular changes include prominent thickened and myelinated corneal nerves (Fig. 9-51) and characteristic hamartomatous iris growths called *Lisch nodules* (Fig. 9-52). Uveal tract involvement in neurofibromatosis includes glial hamartomas of the trabecular meshwork and choroid (Figs. 9-53 and 9-54, *B* and *C*), as well as an increased incidence of choroidal nevi and malignant melanomas.[553,569,591,610,612] The simultaneous occurrence of "schwannian" hamartomas and melanocytic nevi should not be surprising when one recalls that both cell lines share a common embryologic source, the neural crest (p. 9). Glial hamartomas of the retina and optic nerve head, which resemble those of tuberous sclerosis, may develop. Children with neurofibromatosis have a higher incidence of congenital glaucoma (p. 272).[569]

STURGE-WEBER SYNDROME

The Sturge-Weber syndrome (encephalotrigeminal angiomatosis) is a congenital syndrome characterized by two major components: a facial hemangioma (port wine stain, nevus flammeus) and a homolateral intracranial hemangioma often associated with a homolateral choroidal hemangioma and glaucoma.[613–628] The syndrome differs from the other phakomatoses in that no well-defined pattern of hereditary transmission exists.

The facial lesion is generally unilateral and limited to the area of distribution of the first and second divisions of the trigeminal nerve (Fig. 9-56). The skin lesion is present at birth and is composed of dilated telangiectatic, proliferating vessels within the dermis. The intracranial hemangioma is usually of the racemose type; the vessels are dilated, tortuous, and wormlike. It most commonly occurs in the meninges overlying the occipital lobe. Calcification of the

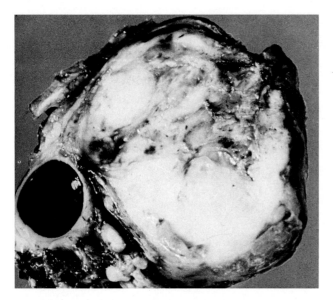

Fig. 9-55. Unusual transformation of a neurofibroma into malignant neurofibrosarcoma. This gross, sagittal section of an exenterated eyeball *(left)* and orbital tissue from a man with von Recklinghausen's disease shows the very large, necrotic orbital malignancy.

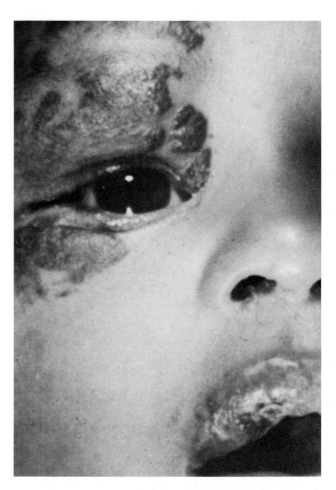

Fig. 9-56. Port-wine stain (nevus flammeus) on the right side of the face of a patient with Sturge-Weber syndrome. The intracranial and intraocular vascular malformations and hamartomas that often occur in this syndrome are typically ipsilateral to this skin lesion.

underlying cortex can be demonstrated radiographically. The so-called railroad track appearance, in which the calcified flecks are deposited in a double-line pattern resembling a railroad track, is highly characteristic of this disease. Epilepsy is frequently seen; however, unlike the retardation associated with tuberous sclerosis, mental retardation is less common in Sturge-Weber disease than would be expected, considering the severity of many of the intracranial lesions.

The most significant intraocular lesion is a cavernous hemangioma of the choroid (Figs. 9-57 and 9-58), which almost always occurs on the same side of the head as the skin lesions and intracranial vascular anomalies. The hemangioma is composed of dilated endothelial-lined spaces that cause slight-to-moderate elevation of the involved choroid.[619,628] In general the choroidal mass seen in patients with the Sturge-Weber syndrome is less elevated than choroidal hemangiomas not associated with this syndrome.[628] Visual difficulties may occur as a result of degeneration of the overlying retinal or serous retinal detachment above and adjacent to the tumor. The mechanism of the homolateral glaucoma seen in most patients with Sturge-Weber syndrome is not entirely clear; Font and Ferry[682] have itemized several hypotheses. Some authors believe that episcleral hemangiomas can lead to elevated episcleral venous pressure and, therefore, to an increase in the intraocular pressure. This may be the primary cause of the glaucoma (Fig. 9-59). Most cases that have been examined histopathologically reveal formation of peripheral anterior synechiae, but these are probably secondary changes.

WYBURN-MASON SYNDROME

The Wyburn-Mason syndrome (racemose, serpentine, plexiform, or cavernous hemangioma; cirsoid aneurysms; retinal varices; arteriovenous aneurysms) is an association of intracranial angiomatous malformations with similar

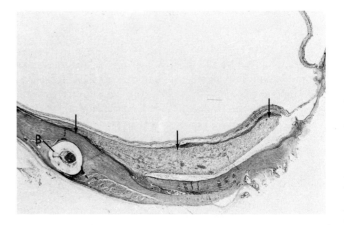

Fig. 9-57. Sturge-Weber syndrome with a choroidal hemangioma *(arrows)*. The "retinal detachment" was treated surgically with an encircling band *(B)*. The deeply cupped optic disc *(right)* signifies glaucoma. (H & E stain; ×12.)

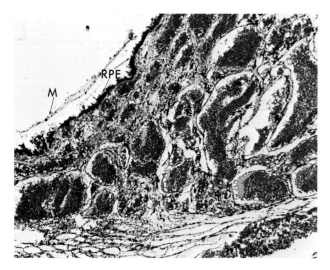

Fig. 9-58. Sturge-Weber syndrome, choroidal hemangioma. The edge of the tumor and the beginning of the normal choroid are toward the left. The choroid is greatly thickened by this cavernous hemangioma composed of dilated, endothelium-lined channels. The overlying retina is detached and not present in this section. The retinal pigment epithelium *(RPE)* is adjacent to the inner (vitreal) aspect of the tumor. Normal choroidal vascular channels, easily differentiated from the dilated channels seen in the tumor, are present at the bottom of the micrograph. *M,* Vascular membrane within the subretinal space. (H & E stain; ×100.)

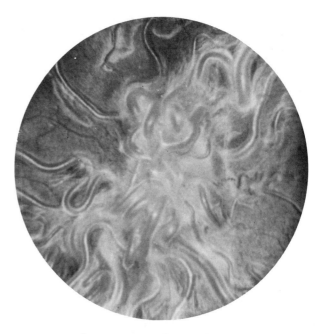

Fig. 9-60. Wyburn-Mason syndrome. This racemose angioma of the retina is sometimes associated with a similar tumor of the homolateral midbrain.

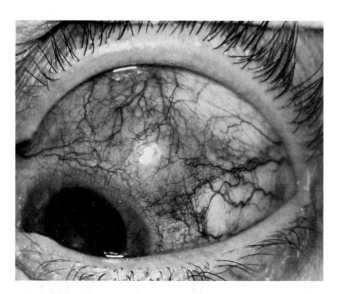

Fig. 9-59. External photograph showing dilated episcleral channels associated with raised episcleral venous pressure and increased intraocular pressure.

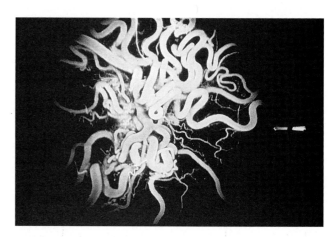

Fig. 9-61. Fluorescein angiogram of Wyburn-Mason syndrome. Note hyperfluorescence of vessels but no leakage (see Color Plate 9-19).

racemose angiomas of the homolateral retina.[629–644] The intracranial lesions, which sometimes are calcified, have been found in the orbit and optic nerve, the maxillary sinuses, the basofrontal area, and the posterior fossa, including the rostral midbrain. The most important clinical manifestations of this disease are epilepsy, neurologic defects created by the space-occupying lesions, and intracranial hemorrhage caused by the intracranial vascular malformations. Rarely there are associated facial hemangiomas.

In some cases retinal arteriovenous aneurysmal communication can be demonstrated. The retinal lesions are congenital, but the signs and symptoms evolve very slowly, usually appearing before age 30. Important symptoms include squint and visual loss. Orbital involvement may produce proptosis. The dilated, wormlike retinal vessels formed from dilated, tortuous small vessels (Figs. 9-60 and 9-61; Color Plate 9-19) do not pulsate. This lesion is not a retinal tumor (such as the hemangioblastoma of von Hippel–Lindau disease). In contrast to von Hippel–Lindau disease, Coats' disease, or Leber's miliary aneurysms, lipid exudation does not occur.

ATAXIA TELANGIECTASIA

Ataxia telangiectasia (Louis-Bar syndrome) is considered by some authors to be a member of the phacomatosis group.[631] This autosomal-recessive condition has its onset in infancy and consists of progressive cerebellar ataxia, recurrent pulmonary infarctions, and drying of the skin. The lung involvement probably results from simultaneous occurrence of immunologic defects or lymphocytic abnormalities, which often accompany the disease. The main ocular lesion is a telangiectasia of conjunctival capillaries and nystagmus caused by presumed cerebellar involvement.

REFERENCES

1. Abramson DH, Ellsworth RM, and Kitchin PD: Osteogenic sarcoma of the lumerus after cobalt plaque treatment for retinoblastoma, Am J Ophthalmol 90:374, 1980.
2. Aaby AA, Price RL, and Zakov ZN: Spontaneously regressing retinoblastomas, retinoma, or retinoblastoma Group O, Am J Ophthalmol 96:315, 1983.
3. Abramson DH, Ellsworth RM, and Rozakis GW: Cryotherapy for retinoblastoma, Arch Ophthalmol 100:1253, 1982.
4. Abramson DH, Ellsworth RM, and Zimmerman LE: Nonocular cancer in retinoblastoma survivors, Trans Am Acad Ophthalmol Otolaryngol 81:454, 1976.
5. Abramson DH, Ronner HJ, and Ellsworth RM: Second tumors in nonirradiated bilateral retinoblastoma, Am J Ophthalmol 87:624, 1979.
6. Abramson DH and others: Lactate dehydrogenase levels and isozyme patterns. Measurements in the aqueous humor and serum of retinoblastoma patients, Arch Ophthalmol 97:870, 1979.
7. Abramson DH and others: Simultaneous bilateral radiation for advanced bilateral retinoblastoma, Arch Ophthalmol 99:1763, 1981.
8. Abramson DH and others: Treatment of bilateral groups I through III retinoblastoma with bilateral radiation, Arch Ophthalmol 99:1761, 1981.
9. Abramson DH and others: Retreatment of retinoblastoma with external beam irradiation, Arch Ophthalmol 100:1257, 1982.
10. Abramson DH and others: The management of unilateral retinoblastoma without primary enucleation, Arch Ophthalmol 100:1249, 1982.
11. Abramson DH and others: Retinoblastoma treated in infants in the first six months of life, Arch Ophthalmol 101:1362, 1983.
12. Abramson DH and others: Second nonocular tumors in retinoblastoma survivors: are they radiation-induced? Ophthalmology 91:1351, 1984.
13. Abramson DH and others: Neuron-specific enolase and retinoblastomas, retinoma, or retinocytoma, Retina 9:148, 1989.
14. Aherne G: Retinoblastoma associated with primary malignant tumors, Trans Ophthalmol Soc UK 94:938, 1974.
15. Aksu G: Aqueous humor lactic dehydrogenase activity in normal and diseased eyes, Ann Ophthalmol 13:1067, 1981.
16. Albert DM: Historic review of retinoblastoma, Ophthalmology 94:654, 1987.
17. Albert DM and Rabson AS: The role of viruses in the pathogenesis of ocular tumors, Int Ophthalmol Clin 12(1):195, 1972.
18. Albert DM, Rabson AS, and Dalton AJ: In vitro neoplastic transformation of uveal and retinal tissue by oncogenic DNA viruses, Invest Ophthalmol 7:357, 1968.
19. Albert DM and Reid TW: RNA-directed DNA polymerase activity in retinoblastoma: report of its presence and possible significance, Trans Am Acad Ophthalmol Otolaryngol 77:630, 1973.
20. Albert DM and others: Recent observations regarding retinoblastoma. I. Ultrastructure, tissue culture growth, incidence, animal models, Trans Ophthalmol Soc UK 94:909, 1974.
21. Albert DM and others: Development of additional primary tumors after 62 years in the first patient with retinoblastoma cured by radiation therapy, Am J Ophthalmol 97:189, 1984.
22. Anderson SR and Jensen OA: Retinoblastoma with necrosis of central retinal artery and vein and partial spontaneous regression, Acta Ophthalmol 52:183, 1974.
23. Apple DJ and Puklin JE: Leukokoria. In Peyman CA, Sanders DR, and Goldberg MF, editors: Principles and practice of ophthalmology, Philadelphia, 1980, WB Saunders Co.
24. Bach LE and others: Trilateral retinoblastoma—incidence and outcome: a decade of experience, Int J Radiat Oncol Biol Phys 29:729, 1994.
25. Bader JL and others: Bilateral retinoblastoma with ectopic intracranial retinoblastoma: trilateral retinoblastoma, Cancer Genet Cytogenet 5:203, 1982.
26. Bader JL and others: Trilateral retinoblastoma, Lancet 2:582, 1980.
27. Barr FG and others: Molecular assays for chromosomal translocation in the diagnosis of pediatric soft tissue sarcomas, JAMA 273:553, 1995.
28. Bedford MA, Bedotto C, and MaeFaul PA: Retinoblastoma: a study of 139 cases, BR J Ophthalmol 55:19, 1971.
29. Bedford MA and MacFaul PA: Retinal vascular changes in untreated retinoblastoma: resemblance to von Hippel–Lindau disease, Br J Ophthalmol 53:382, 1969.
30. Benedict WL and Parkhill EM: Glioma of the retina in successive generations, Am J Ophthalmol 26:511, 1943.
31. Benson WE and others: Presumed spontaneously regressed retinoblastoma, Ann Ophthalmol 10:897, 1978.
32. Bhatnagar R and Vine AK: Diffuse infiltrating retinoblastoma, Ophthalmology 98:1657, 1991.
33. Binder PS: Unusual manifestations of retinoblastoma, Am J Ophthalmol 77:674, 1974.
34. Bishop JO and Madson FC: Retinoblastoma: review of the current status, Surv Ophthalmol 19:342, 1975.
35. Blodi FC: Zur Prognose des Retinoblastomas, Graefes Arch Clin Exp Ophthalmol 164:78, 1961.
36. Blodi FC and Watzke R: A clinicopathologic report on treated retinoblastoma, Am J Ophthalmol 71:193, 1971.
37. Boniuk M and Girard LJ: Spontaneous regression of bilateral retinoblastoma, Trans Am Acad Ophthalmol Otolaryngol 73:194, 1969.
38. Boniuk M and Zimmerman LE: Spontaneous regression of retinoblastoma, Int Ophthalmol Clin 2:525, 1962.
39. Brockhurst RJ and Donaldson DD: Spontaneous resolution of probable retinoblastoma, Arch Ophthalmol 84:388, 1970.
40. Brown DH: The clinicopathology of retinoblastoma, Am J Ophthalmol 61:508, 1966.
41. Brownstein S, de Chadarevian J-P, and Little, JM: Trilateral retinoblastoma: report of two cases, Arch Ophthalmol 102:257, 1984.
42. Bunin GR and others: Frequency of 13q abnormalities among 203 patients with retinoblastoma, J Natl Cancer Inst 18:370, 1989.
43. Bunt AH and Tso MOM: Feulgen-positive deposits in retinoblastoma: incidence, composition, ultrastructure, Arch Ophthalmol 99:145, 1981.
44. Burnier MN and others: Retinoblastoma, Invest Ophthalmol Vis Sci 31:2037, 1990.
45. Carbajal UM: Metastasis in retinoblastoma, Am J Ophthalmol 48:47, 1959.
46. Carlson FA and others: Factors for improved genetic counseling for retinoblastoma based on a survey of 55 families, Am J Ophthalmol 87:449, 1979.
47. Cavenee WK and others: Genetic origin of mutations predisposing to retinoblastom, Science 228:501, 1985.
48. Chan HSL and others: Multidrug-resistant phenotype in retinoblastoma correlates with P-glycoprotein expression, Ophthalmology 98:1425, 1991.
49. Char DH and Herberman RB: Cutaneous delayed hypersensitivity responses of patients with retinoblastoma to standard recall antigens and crude membrane extracts of retinoblastoma tissue culture cells, Am J Ophthalmol 78:40, 1974.
50. Char DH and others: Cell-mediated immunity to a retinoblastoma tissue culture line in patients with retinoblastoma, Am J Ophthalmol 78:5, 1974.
51. Char DH and others: Immune complexes in retinoblastoma, Am J Ophthalmol 86:395, 1978.
52. Char DH, Hedges TR III, and Norman D: Retinoblastoma, CT diagnosis. Ophthalmology 91:1347, 1984.
53. Cibis GW and others: Bilateral choroidal neonatal neuroblastoma, Am J Ophthalmol 109:445, 1990.
54. Cross HE and others: Retinoblastoma in a patient with a 13qXp translocation, Am J Ophthalmol 84:548, 1977.
55. Daicker B: Anatomic and Pathologic der menschlichen retinoziliaren Fundusperipherie, Basel, 1972, Karger.
56. Daoud A and others: Late ocular recurrence of retinoblastoma after external radiation, J Pediatr Ophthalmol Strabismus 15:282, 1978.
57. de Buen S: Retinoblastoma, with spread by direct continuity to the

contralateral optic nerve: report of a case, Am J Ophthalmol 49:815, 1960.

58. Detrick B and others: Cytokine-induced modulation of cellular proteins in retinoblastoma, Invest Ophthalmol Vis Sci 32:1714, 1991.

59. Devesa SS: The incidence of retinoblastoma, Am J Ophthalmol 80: 263, 1975.

60. Dias PLR: Correlation of aqueous humour lactic acid dehydrogenase activity with intraocular pathology, Br J Ophthalmol 63:574, 1979.

61. Dias PLR: Prognostic significance of aqueous humour lactic dehydrogenase activity, Br J Ophthalmol 63:571, 1979.

62. Dias PLR, Shanmuganathan SS, and Rajaratnam M: Lactic dehydrogenase activity of aqueous humor in retinoblastoma, Br J Ophthalmol 55:130, 1971.

63. Dollfus M and Auvert B: Le gliome de la rétine (retinoblastome) et les pseudogliomes, Paris, 1953, Masson et Cie, Editeurs.

64. Donoso LA and others: Intracranial malignancy in patients with bilateral retinoblastoma, Retina 1:67, 1981.

65. Donoso LA and others: Rhodopsin and retinoblastoma: a monoclonal antibody histopathologic study, Arch Ophthalmol 104:111, 1986.

66. Dryja TP and others: Homozygosity of chromosome 13 in retinoblastoma, N Eng J Med 310:550, 1984.

67. Dunn JM and others: Identification of germline and somatic mutations affecting the retinoblastoma gene, Science 241:1797, 1988.

68. Dunphy EB: The story of retinoblastoma, Trans Am Acad Ophthalmol Otolaryngol 68:249, 1964.

69. Egbert PR and others: Posterior ocular abnormalities after irradiation for retinoblastoma: a histopathological study, Br J Ophthalmol 64:660, 1980.

70. Eagle RC and others: Malignant transformation of spontaneously regressed retinoblastoma, retinoma/retinocytoma variant, Ophthalmology 96:1389, 1989.

71. Egerer I, Tasman W, and Tomer TL: Coats' disease, Arch Ophthalmol 92:109, 1974.

72. Ellsworth RM: Treatment of retinoblastoma, Am J Ophthalmol 66: 49, 1968.

73. Ellsworth RM: The practical management of retinoblastoma, Trans Am Ophthalmol Soc 67:462, 1969.

74. Ellsworth RM: Current concepts in the treatment of retinoblastoma. In Peyman GA, Apple DJ, and Sanders DR, editors: Intraocular tumors, New York, 1977, Appleton-Century-Crofts.

75. Eng C and others: Mortality from second tumors among long-term survivors of retinoblastoma, Cancer Inst 85:1121, 1993.

76. Falls HF and Neel JV: Genetics of retinoblastoma, Arch Ophthalmol 46:367, 1951.

77. Flexner S: A peculiar glioma (neuroepithelioma?) of the retina, Bull Johns Hopkins Hosp 2:115, 1891.

78. François J, DeBie S, and Matton-Van Leuven MT: The Costenbader memorial lecture: genesis and genetics of retinoblastoma J Pediatr Ophthalmol Strabismus 19:85, 1979.

79. François J and Matton-Van Leuven MT: Recent data on the heredity of retinoblastoma. In Boniuk M, editor: Ocular and adnexal tumors, St Louis, 1964, The CV Mosby Co.

80. François J and others: Genesis and genetics of retinoblastoma, Ophthalmologica 170:405, 1975.

81. Friendly DS and Parks MM: Concurrence of hereditary congenital cataracts and hereditary retinoblastoma, Arch Ophthalmol 84:525, 1970.

82. Fung Y-KT and others: Structural evidence for the authenticity of the human retinoblastoma gene, Science 236:1657, 1987.

83. Gallie BL and Phillips RA: Retinoblastoma: a model of oncogenesis, Ophthalmology 91:666, 1984.

84. Gallie BL and others: Significance of retinoma and phthisis bulbi for retinoblastoma, Ophthalmology 89:1393, 1982.

85. Gass P and other: Antigenic expression of neuron-associated class 111 beta-tubulin isotype (hB4) and microtubule-associated protein 2 (map2) by the human retinoblastoma cell line WERI-Rb1, Ophthalmic Res 22:57, 1990.

86. Grinker RR: Gliomas of the retina: including the results of studies with silver impregnations, Arch Ophthalmol 5:920, 1931.

87. Halloran SL and others: Accuracy of detection of the retinoblastoma gene by esterase D linkage, Arch Ophthalmol 103:1329, 1985.

88. Harbour JW and other: Abnormalities in structure and expression of the human retinoblastoma gene in SCLC, Science 241:353, 1988.

89. Haik BG and others: Retinoblastoma with anterior chamber extension, Ophthalmology 94:367, 1987.

90. Heinrich T and other: Das Metastasierungsrisiko beim retinoblastom (the metastatic risk in retinoblastoma), Monatsbl. Augenheilkd 199:319, 1991.

91. He W and other: A reassessment of histologic classification and an immunohistochemical study of 88 retinoblastomas. A special reference to the advent of bipolar-like cells, Cancer 70:2901, 1992.

92. Helton KJ and other: Bone tumors other than osteosarcoma after retinoblastoma, Cancer 71:2847, 1993.

93. Hemmes GD: Untersuchung nach dem Vorkommen von Glioma retinae bei Verwandten von mit dieser Krankheit Behafteten, Klin Monatsbl Augenhcilkd 86:331, 1931.

94. Herm RJ and Health P: A study of retinoblastoma, Am J Ophthalmol 41:22, 1956.

95. Hilgartner H: Report of a case of double glioma treated with x-ray, Texas Med J 18:322, 1903.

96. Hirschberg J: Der Markschwamm der Nctzhaut, Berlin, 1869, Hirschwald.

97. Hopping W and Meyer-Schwickerath C: Light coagulation treatment in retinoblastoma. In Boniuk M, editor: Ocular and adnexal tumors, St Louis, 1964, The CV Mosby Co.

98. Howard GM and Ellsworth RM: Differential diagnosis of retinoblastoma: a statistical survey of 500 children. I. Relative frequency of the lesions which simulate retinoblastoma, Am J Ophthalmol 60: 610, 1965.

99. Howard GM and Ellsworth RM: Differential diagnosis of retinoblastoma: a statistical survey of 500 children. II. Factors relating to the diagnosis of retinoblastoma, Am J Ophthalmol 60:618, 1965.

100. Howard GM and Ellsworth RM: Findings in the peripheral fundi of patients with retinoblastoma, Am J Ophthalmol 62:243, 1966.

101. Howard MA and others: Identification and significance of multinucleate tumor cells in retinoblastoma, Arch Ophthalmol 107:1025, 1989.

102. Howard RO and others: Retinoblastoma and chromosome abnormality, Arch Ophthalmol 92:490, 1974.

103. Howarth C and other: Stage-related combined modality treatment of retinoblastoma: results of a prospective study. Cancer 45:851, 1980.

104. Irvine AR, Albert DM, and Sang DN: Retinal neoplasia and dysplasia. II. Retinoblastoma occurring with persistence and hyperplasia of the primary vitreous, Invest Ophthalmol Vis Sci 16:403, 1977.

105. Jain IS, Mohan K, and Jain S: Retinoblastoma: clinical and pathologic correlations, J Ocul Ther Surg 4:86, 1985.

106. Jain IS and other: Retinoblastoma: modes of presentation, J Ocul Ther Surg 4:83, 1985.

107. Jaffe MS and other: Retinoblastoma simulating Coats' disease; a clinicopathologic report, Ann Ophthalmol 9:863, 1977.

108. Jensen RD and Miller RW: Retinoblastoma: epidemiologic characteristics, N Engl J Med 285:307, 1971.

109. Jones AL: Immunogenetics of retinoblastoma, Trans Ophthalmol Soc UK 94:945, 1974.

110. Judisch GF, Apple DJ, and Fratkin J: Retinoblastoma: a survivor 12 years after treatment for metastatic disease, Arch Ophthalmol 98: 711, 1980.

111. Judisch GF and Patil SR: Concurrent heritable retinoblastoma, pincaloma, trisomy X, Arch Ophthalmol 99:1767, 1981.

112. Kabak J and Romano PE: Aqueous humor lactic dehydrogenase isoenzymes in retinoblastoma, Br J Ophthalmol 59:26S, 1975.

113. Karsgaard AT: Spontaneous regression of retinoblastoma: a report of two cases, Can J Ophthalmol. 6:218, 1971.

114. Katsetos CD and others: Neuron-associated class 111 sB-tubulin isotype, microtubule-associated protein 2, synaptophysin in human retinoblastomas in situ, Lab Invest 64:45, 1991.

115. Keith CG and Webb GC: Retinoblastoma and retinoma occurring in a child with a translocation and deletion of the long arm of chromosome 13, Arch Ophthalmol 103:941, 1985.

116. Keneko A: Lactic acid dehydrogenase activity and isoenzyme in the retinoblastoma, Acta Soc Ophthalmol Jpn 76:672, 1972.

117. Kobrin JL and Blodi FC: Prognosis in retinoblastoma: influence of histopathologic characteristics, J Pediatr Ophthalmol Strabismus 15: 278, 1978.

118. Knudson AG Jr and others: Chromosomal deletion and retinoblastoma, N Eng J Med 295:1120, 1976.

119. Knudson AG Jr: Persons at high risk of cancer, N Engl J Med 301: 606, 1979.

120. Kopelman JE, McLean IW, and Rosenberg SH: Multivariate analysis of risk factors for metastasis in retinoblastoma treated by enucleation, Ophthalmology 94:371, 1987.

121. Kupfer C: Retinoblastoma treated with intravenous nitrogen mustard, Am J Ophthalmol 36:1721, 1953.

122. Lam BL and others: Visual prognosis in macular retinoblastoma, Am J Ophthalmol 110:229, 1990.

123. Lamping KA and others: Melanotic neuroectodermal tumor of infancy (retinal anlage tumor), Ophthalmology 92:143, 1985.

124. Lane JC and Klintworth CK: A study of astrocytes in retinoblastomas using the immunoperoxidase technique and antibodies to glial fibrillary acidic protein, Am J Ophthalmol 95:197, 1983.

125. Lcclawong N and Regan CDJ: Retinoblastoma: a review of ten years, Am J Ophthalmol 66:1050, 1968.

126. Lee WH and others: Human retinoblastoma susceptibility gene: cloning, identification, sequence, Science 235:1394, 1987.

127. Lemieux J and others: First cytogenetic evidence of homozygosity for the retinoblastoma deletion in chromosome 1, Cancer Genet Cytogenet 43:73, 1989.

128. Lenox EL, Draper GJ, and Saunders BM: Retinoblastoma: a study of natural history and prognosis of 268 cases, Br Med J 3:731, 1975.

129. Liberfarb RM and others: Incidence and significance of a deletion of chromosome band 13q14 in patients with retinoblastoma and in their families, Ophthalmology 91:1695, 1984.

130. Lin CCL and Tso MOM: An electron microscopic study of calcification of retinoblastoma, Am J Ophthalmol 96:765, 1983.

131. Lindley J and Smith S: Histology and spontaneous regression of retinoblastoma, Trans Ophthalmol Soc UK 94:953, 1974.

132. Loeffler KU and McMenamin PG: An ultrastructural study of DNA precipitation in the anterior segment of eyes with retinoblastoma, Ophthalmology 94:1160, 1987.

133. Leuder GR, Judisch GF, and Wen BC: Heritable retinoblastoma and pinealoma, Arch Ophthalmol 109:1707, 1991.

134. Machemer R: Closed vitrectomy for severe retrolental fibroplasia in the infant, Ophthalmology 90:436, 1983.

135. MacKay CJ, Abramson DH, and Ellsworth RM: Metastatic patterns of retinoblastoma, Arch Ophthalmol 102:391, 1984.

136. Mafee MF and others: Magnetic resonance imaging versus computed tomography of leukoric eyes and use of in vitro proton magnetic resonance spectroscopy of retinoblastoma, Ophthalmology 96: 965, 1989.

137. Magramm I, Ambramson DH, and Ellsworth RM: Optic nerve involvement in retinoblastoma, Ophthalmology 96:217, 1989.

138. Makley TA: Retinoblastoma in a 52-year-old man, Arch Ophthalmol 69:325, 1963.

139. Manthey R, Apple DJ, and Kivlin JD: Iris hypoplasia in incontinentia pigmenti, J Pediatr Ophthalmol Strabismus 19:279, 1982.

140. Marcus DM, Craft JL, and Albert DM: Histopathologic verification of Verhoeff's 1918 irradiation cure of retinoblastoma, Ophthalmology 97:221, 1990.

141. Margo C and others: Retinocytoma. A benign variant of retinoblastoma, Arch Ophthalmol 101:1519, 1983.

142. Margo C and others: Cryotherapy and photocoagulation in the management of retinoblastomas: treatment failure and unusual complication, Ophthalmic Surg 14:336, 1983.

143. Mashiah M and Barishak YR: Photoreceptor differentiation in retinoblastomas and its significance in prognosis, Br J Ophthalmol 61: 417, 1977.

144. Mendoza AE and others: A case of synovial sarcoma with abnormal expression of the human retinoblastoma susceptibility gen, Hum Pathol 19:487, 1988.

145. Merriam GR: Retinoblastoma: analysis of 17 autopsies, Arch Ophthalmol 44:71, 1950.

146. Messmer EP and others: Immunohistochemical demonstration of neuronal and astrocytic differentiation in retinoblastoma, Ophthalmology 92:167, 1985.

147. Meyer-Schwickerath G: The preservation of vision by treatment of intraocular tumors with light coagulation, Arch Ophthalmol 66:458, 1961.

148. Midgal C: Spontaneous regression of retinoblastoma in identical twins, Br J Ophthalmol 66:691, 1982.

149. Moazed K, Albert DM, and Smith TR: Rubeosis iridis in "pseudogliomas," Surv Ophthalmol 25:85, 1980.

150. Mohney BG and Robertson DM: Ancillary testing for metastasis in patients with newly diagnosed retinoblastoma, Am J Ophthalmol 118:707, 1994.

151. Molnar ML and others: Immunohistochemistry of retinoblastomas in humans, Am J Ophthalmol 97:301, 1984.

152. Morgan G: Diffuse infiltrating retinoblastoma, Br J Ophthalmol 55: 600, 1971.

153. Morgan KS and McLean IW: Retinoblastoma and persistent hyperplastic vitreous occurring in the same patient, Ophthalmology 88: 1087, 1981.

154. Morgan SS and Blair HL: Hereditary retinoblastoma: report of a family with retinoblastoma occurring in three successive generations, Am J Ophthalmol 65:43, 1968.

155. Morris WE and La Piana FG: Spontaneous regression of bilateral multifocal retinoblastoma with preservation of normal visual acuity, Ann Ophthalmol 6:1192, 1974.

156. Mullaney J: DNA in retinoblastoma, Lancet 2:918, 1968.

157. Mullaney J: Retinoblastoma: a review and some new aspects, Ir J Med Sci 8:57, 1969.

158. Mullaney J: Retinoblastoma with DNA precipitation, Arch Ophthalmol 82:454, 1969.

159. Murphree AL and Benedict WF: Retinoblastoma: clues to human oncogenesis, Science 223:1028, 1984.

160. Naumova A and others: Concordance between parental origin of chromosome 13q loss and chromosome 6p duplication in sporadic retinoblastoma, Am J Hum Genet 54:274, 1994.

161. Naumova A and Sapienza C: The genetics of retinoblastoma, revisited. Am J Hum Genet 54:264, 1994.

162. Naves AE and Gaisiner PD: Different cell populations in retinoblastoma, Ann Ophthalmol 13:1073, 1981.

163. Nehen JH: Spontaneous regression of retinoblastoma, Acta Ophthalmol 53:647, 1975.

164. Nichols WW and others: Further observations on a 13qXp translocation associated with retinoblastoma, Am J Ophthalmol 89:621, 1980.

165. Nicholson DH and Green WR: Pediatric ocular tumors, New York, 1981, Masson Publishing USA, Inc.

166. Nork TM, Millecchia LL, and Poulsen G: Immunolocalization of the retinoblastoma protein in the human eye and in the retinoblastoma, Invest Ophthalmol Vis Sci 35:2682, 1994.

167. Nork TM and others: Retinoblastoma. Cell of origin, Arch Ophthalmol 113:791, 1995.

168. Nyboer JH, Robertson DM, and Gomez MR: Retinal lesions in tuberous sclerosi, Arch Ophthalmol 94:1277, 1976.

169. O'Brien J and others: Trilateral retinoblastoma in transgenic mice, Trans Am Ophthalmol Soc 87:301, 1989.

170. Oeller J: Atlas seltener ophthalmoskopischer Befunde, Wiesbaden, 1903, JF Bergmann.

171. O'Grady RB, Rothstein TB, Romano PE: D-group deletion syndromes and retinoblastoma, Am J Ophthalmol 77:40, 1974.

172. Olnishi Y: The histogenesis of retinoblastoma, Ophthalmologica 174: 129, 1977.

173. Parkhill EM and Benedict WL: Gliomas of the retina: a histopathologic study, Am J Ophthalmol 24:1354, 1941.

174. Pearce WG and Gillan JG: Bilateral spontaneous regression of retinoblastoma, Can J Ophthalmol 7:234, 1972.

175. Pe'er J: Calcification in Coats' disease, Am J Ophthalmol 106:742, 1988.

176. Pendergrass TW and Davis S: Incidence of retinoblastoma in the United States, Arch Ophthalmol 98:1204, 1980.

177. Perentes E and others: Immunohistochemical characterization of human retinoblastomas in situ with multiple markers, Am J Ophthalmol 103:647, 1987.

178. Pesin SR and Shields JA: Seven cases of trilateral retinoblastoma, Am J Ophthalmol 107:121, 1989.

179. Peyman GA, Apple DJ, and Sanders DR, editors: Intraocular tumors, New York, 1977, Appleton-Century-Crofts.

180. Pruett RC and Atkins L: Chromosome studies in patients with retinoblastoma, Arch Ophthalmol 82:177, 1969.

181. Radnot M: Synaptic lamellar in retinoblastoma, Am J Ophthalmol 79:393, 1975.

182. Ramirez LC and de Buen S: Clinical and pathologic findings in 100 retinoblastoma patients, J Pediatr Ophthalmol 10:12, 1973.

183. Redler LD and Ellsworth RM: Prognostic importance of choroidal invasion in retinoblastoma, Arch Ophthalmol 90:294, 1973.

184. Reese AB: Frequency of retinoblastoma in the progeny of parents who have survived the disease, Arch Ophthalmol 52:815, 1954.

185. Reese AB: Atlas of tumor pathology section 10, fascicle 38, Washington, DC, 1956, Armed Forces Institute of Pathology.

186. Reese AB: Retinoblastoma: past, present and future, editorial, Arch Ophthalmol 77:293, 1967.

187. Reese AB: Tumors of the eye, ed 3, New York, 1976, Harper & Row, Publishers.

188. Reid TW and Russell P: Recent observations regarding retinoblastoma. II. An enzyme study of retinoblastoma, Trans Ophthalmol Soc UK 94:929, 1974.

189. Richards WW: Retinoblastoma simulating uveitis, Am J Ophthalmol 65:427, 1968.

190. Roarty JD, McLean IW, and Zimmerman LE: Incidence of second neoplasms in patients with bilateral retinoblastoma, Ophthalmology 95:1583, 1988.

191. Roberts CW, Iwamoto M, and Haik BC: Ultrastructural correlation of specular microscopy in retinoblastoma, Am J Ophthalmol 102:182, 1986.

192. Rodrigues MM and others: Retinoblastoma: a clinical, immunohistochemical and electron microscopic case report, Ophthalmology 93:1010, 1986.

193. Rodrigues MM and others: Retinoblastoma: immunohistochemistry and cell differentiation, Ophthalmology 94:378, 1987.

194. Rosenfeld SI and Smith ME: Ocular findings in incontinentia pigmenti, Ophthalmology 92:543, 1985.

195. Roth AM: Retinoblastoma seen after surgery for traumatic cataract, Ann Ophthalmol 10:1561, 1978.

196. Rubenfeld M and others: Unilateral vs bilateral retinoblastoma: correlations between age at diagnosis and stage of ocular disease, Ophthalmology 93:1016, 1986.

197. Rubin ML and Kaufman HE: Spontaneously regressed probable retinoblastoma: report of a case, Arch Ophthalmol 81:442, 1969.

198. Sanborn GE, Augsburger JJ, and Shields JA: Spontaneous regression of bilateral retinoblastoma, Br J Ophthalmol 66:685, 1982.

199. Sanders BM, Draper GJ, and Kingston JE: Retinoblastoma in Great Britain 1969-80: incidence treatment, survival, Br J Ophthalmol 72:576, 1988.

200. Sang DN and Albert DM: Recent advances in the study of retinoblastoma, (p.285) In Peyman GA, Apple DJ, and Sanders DR, editors: Intraocular tumors, New York, 1977, Appleton-Century-Crofts.

201. Sang DN and Albert DM: Recent advances in the study of retinoblastoma, (p.295) In Peyman GA, Apple DJ, and Sanders DR, editors: Intraocular tumors, New York, 1977, Appleton-Century-Crofts.

202. Sang DN and Albert DM: Recent advances in the study of retinoblastoma, (p.316) In Peyman GA, Apple DJ, and Sanders DR, editors: Intraocular tumors, New York, 1977, Appleton-Century-Crofts.

203. Sang DN and Albert DM: Retinoblastoma: Clinical and histopathologic features, Hum Pathol 13:133, 1982.

204. Sawaguchi S and others: An immunopathologic study of retinoblastoma protein, Trans Am Ophthalmol Soc 88:51, 1990.

205. Schappert-Kimmijser J, Hemmes GD, and Nijland R: The heredity of retinoblastoma, Ophthalmologica 151:197, 1966.

206. Scheff H and others: Linkage analysis of families with hereditary retinoblastoma: nonpenetrance of mutation revealed by combined use of markers within and flanking the RBI gene, Am J Hum Genet 45:252, 1989.

207. Schimke RM, Lowman JT, and Cowan GAB: Retinoblastoma and osteogenic sarcoma in siblings, Cancer 34:2077, 1974.

208. Seidman DJ and others: Early diagnosis of retinoblastoma based on dysmorphic features and karyotype analysis, Ophthalmology 94:663, 1987.

209. Sevel D, Rohm GF, and Sealy R: Clinical significance of the fleurette in retinoblastoma, Br J Ophthalmol 58:687, 1974.

210. Shields CL, Shields JA, and Shah P: Retinoblastoma and p53 gene expression related to relapse and survival in human breast cancer. An immunohistochemical study, J Pathol 168:23, 1992.

211. Shields CL, Shields JA, and Pankajkumar S: Retinoblastoma in older children, Ophthalmology 98:395, 1991.

212. Shields CL and others: Choroidal invasion of retinoblastoma. Metastic potential and clinical risk factors, Br J Ophthalmol 77:544, 1993.

213. Shields CL and others: Optic nerve invasion of retinoblastoma. Metastatic potential and clinical risk factors, Cancer 73:692, 1994.

214. Shields JA: Diagnosis and management of intraocular tumors, St Louis, 1983, The CV Mosby Co.

215. Shields JA and Augsburger JJ: Current approaches to the diagnosis and management of retinoblastoma, Surv Ophthalmol 25:347, 1981.

216. Shields JA and others: Retinoblastoma in an 18-year-old male, J Pediatr Ophthalmol 13:274, 1976.

217. Shields JA and others: Retinoblastoma manifesting as orbital cellulitis, Am J Ophthalmol 112:442, 1991.

218. Shields JA and others: Fluorescein angiography of retinoblastoma, Trans Am Ophthalmol Soc 80:98, 1982.

219. Singh R, Rohatgi AK, and Shukla PK: Lactate dehydrogenase activity in ocular tumors, Ann Ophthalmol 15:317, 1983.

220. Smith SM and Sorsby A: Retinoblastoma: some genetic aspects, Ann Hum Genet 23:50, 1958.

221. Soloway HB: Radiation-induced neoplasms following curative therapy for retinoblastoma, Cancer 19:1984, 1966.

222. Spaulding AC and Naumann G: Unsuspected retinoblastoma, Arch Ophthalmol 76:575, 1966.

223. Spaulding AG: Rubeosis iridis in retinoblastoma and pseudoglioma, Trans Am Ophthal Soc 76:584, 1978.

224. Stafford WR, Yanoff M, and Parnell BL: Retinoblastoma initially misdiagnosed as primary ocular inflammations, Arch Ophthalmol 82:771, 1969.

225. Stallard HB: The conservative treatment of retinoblastoma. In Boniuk M, editor: Ocular and adnexal tumors, St Louis, 1964, The CV Mosby Co.

226. Stannard C and others: Retinoblastoma: correlation of invasion of the optic nerve and choroid with prognosis and metastases, Br J Ophthalmol 63:560, 1979.

227. Stewart JK, Smith JLS, and Arnold EL: Spontaneous regression of retinoblastoma, Br J Ophthalmol 40:449, 1956.

228. Stowe GC III others: Vascular basophilia in ocular and orbital tumors, Invest Ophthalmol 18:1068, 1979.

229. Strong LC and Knudson AG Jr: Second cancers in retinoblastoma, Lancet 2:1086, 1973.

230. Strong LC and others: Familial retinoblastoma and chromosome 13 deletion transmitted via an insertional translocation, Science 213:1501, 1981.

231. Swartz M: Aqueous humor lactic acid dehydrogenase in retinoblastoma. In Peyman GA, Apple DJ, and Sanders DR, editors: Intraocular tumors, New York, 1977, Appleton-Century-Crofts.

232. Swartz M, Herbst RW, and Goldberg MF: Aqueous humor lactic acid dehydrogenase in retinoblastoma, Am J Ophthalmol 78:612, 1974.

233. Takahashi T and others: Retinoblastoma in a 26-year-old adult, Ophthalmology 90:179, 1983.

234. Tamboli A, Podgor MJ, and Horm JW: The incidence of retinoblastoma in the United States: 1974 through 1985, Arch Ophthalmol 108:128, 1990.

235. T'Ang A and others: Structural rearrangement of the retinoblastoma gene in human breast carcinoma, Science 242:263, 1988.

236. Taylor HR and others: A scanning electron microscope examination of retinoblastoma in tissue culture, Br J Ophthalmol 63:551, 1979.

237. Thompson RW, Small RC, and Stein JJ: Treatment of retinoblastoma, Am J Roentgenol Radium Ther Nucl Med 114:16, 1972.

238. Traboulsi EI, Zimmerman LE, and Manz HJ: Cutaneous malignant melanoma in survivors of heritable retinoblastoma, Arch Ophthalmol 106:1059, 1988.

239. Tso MOM, Fine BS, and Zimmerman LE: The Flexner-Wintersteiner rosettes in retinoblastoma, Arch Pathol 88:664, 1969.

240. Tso MOM, Fine BS, and Zimmerman LE: The nature of retinoblastoma. II. Photoreceptor differentiation: an electron microscopic study, Am J Ophthalmol 69:350, 1970.

241. Tso MOM, Zimmerman LE, and Fine BS: The nature of retinoblastoma. I. Photoreceptor differentiation: a clinical and histopathological study, Am J Ophthalmol 69:339, 1970.

242. Tso MOM and others: Photoreceptor elements in retinoblastoma: a preliminary report, Arch Ophthalmol 82:57, 1969.

243. Tso MOM and others: A cause of radioresistance in retinoblastoma: photoreceptor differentiation, Trans Am Acad Ophthalmol Otolaryngol 74:959, 1970.

244. Virchow R: Die krankhaften Geschwülste, Berlin, 1864–1865, Hirschwald.

245. Vogel F: Genetics of retinoblastoma, Hum Genet 52:1, 1979.

246. Vrabec T and others: Rod cell-specific antigens in retinoblastoma, Arch Ophthalmol 107:1061, 1989.

247. Walton DS and Grant WM: Retinoblastoma and iris neovascularization, Am J Ophthalmol 65:598, 1968.

248. Wardrop J: Observations on fungus haematodes, or soft cancer, in several of the most important organs of the human body, Edinburgh, 1809, Constable (Translated from German by CC Kühn and A Van der Hout, Amsterdam, 1819, Sulpke.)

249. Weller CV: The inheritance of retinoblastoma and its relationship to practical eugenics, Cancer Res 1:517, 1941.

250. Wiggs DL and Dryja TP: Predicting the risk of hereditary retinoblastoma, Am J Ophthalmol 106:346, 1988.

251. Wiggs J and others: Prediction of the risk of hereditary retinoblastoma using DNA polymorphisms within the retinoblastoma gene, N Engl J Med 318:151, 1988.

252. Wintersteiner H: Das Neuroepithelioma Retinae: Eine anatomische und klinische Studie, Leipzig, 1897, Franz Deuticke.

253. Wright JH: Neurocytoma or neuroblastoma, a kind of tumor not generally recognized, J Exp Med 12:556, 1910.

254. Yandell DW and others: Oncogenic point mutations in the human retinoblastoma gene: their application to genetic counseling, N Engl J Med 321:1689, 1989.

255. Yanoff M: The rosettes of James Homer Wright, Arch Ophthalmol 108:1761, 1981 (letter).

256. Yoneyama T and Greenlaw RH: Osteogenic sarcoma following radiotherapy for retinoblastoma, Radiology 93:1185, 1969.

257. Yoshizumi MD, Thomas JV, and Smith TR: Glaucoma-inducing mechanisms in eyes with retinoblastoma, Arch Ophthalmol 96:105, 1978.

258. Zhu X and others: Preferential germline mutation of the paternal allele in retinoblastoma, Nature 340.312, 1989.

259. Zimmerman LE: Retinoblastoma, Med Ann DC 38:366, 1969.

260. Zimmerman LE and others: Trilateral retinoblastoma: ectopic intracranial retinoblastoma associated with bilateral retinoblastoma, J Pediatr Ophthalmol Strabismus 19:320, 1982.

Leukokoria

261. Apple DJ, Hamming NA, and Gieser DK: Differential diagnosis of leukocoria. In Peyman GA, Apple DJ, and Sanders DR, editors: Intraocular tumors, New York, 1977, Appleton-Century-Crofts.

262. Apple DJ and Puklin JE: Leukokoria. In Peyman GA, Sanders DR, and Goldberg MF, editors: Principles and practice of ophthalmology, Philadelphia, 1980, WB Saunders Co.

263. Apple DJ and others: Anomalous intraocular and periocular formation of adipose tissue, Am J Ophthalmol 94:344, 1982.

264. Awan KJ and Humayun M: Changes in the contralateral eye in uncomplicated persistent hyperplastic primary vitreous, Ophthalmology 92:1153, 1985.

265. Ben Sira I, Nissenkorn I, and Kremer I: Retinopathy of prematurity, Surv Ophthalmol 33:1, 1988.

266. Collins ET: Pseudoglioma, R Lond Ophthalmol Hosp Rep 13:361, 1892.

267. Duke J: Pseudoglioma in children, South Med J 51:754, 1958.

268. Ellis GS and others: *Toxocara canis* infestation: clinical and epidemiological associations with seropositivity in kindergarten children, Ophthalmology 93:1032, 1986.

269. Foos RY: Chronic retinopathy of prematurity, Ophthalmology 92:563, 1985.

270. Fryczkowksi AW and others: Scanning electron microscopy of the ocular vasculature in retinopathy of prematurity, Arch Ophthalmol 103:224, 1985.

271. Gieser DK and others: Persistent hyperplastic primary vitreous in an adult: case report with fluorescein angiography finds, J Pediatr Ophthalmol Strabismus 15:213, 1978.

272. Goldberg MF and Mafee M: Computed tomography for diagnosis of persistent hyperplastic primary vitreous (PHPV), Ophthalmology 90:442, 1983.

273. Haddad R, Font RL, and Reeser F: Clinical pathological review: persistent hyperplastic primary vitreous—a clinicopathologic study of 62 cases and review of the literature, Surv Ophthalmol 23:123, 1978.

274. Haik BG and others: Magnetic resonance imaging in the evaluation of leukocoria, Ophthalmology 92:1143, 1985.

275. Hamming NA and others: Ultrastructure of the hyaloid vasculature in primates, Invest Ophthalmol Vis Sci 16:408, 1977.

276. Hermsen VM and others: Persistent hyperplastic primary vitreous associated with protein C deficiency, Am J Ophthalmol 109:608, 1990.

277. Hittner HM, Rudolph AJ, and Kretzer FL: Suppression of severe retinopathy of prematurity with vitamin E supplementation: ultrastructural mechanisms of clinical efficacy, Ophthalmology 91:1512, 1984.

278. Howard GM: Erroneous clinical diagnoses of retinoblastoma and uveal melanoma, Trans Am Acad Ophthalmol Otolaryngol 73:199, 1969.

279. Howard GM and Ellsworth RM: Differential diagnosis of retinoblastoma: a statistical survey of 500 children. I. Relative frequency of the lesions which simulate retinoblastoma, Am J Ophthalmol 60:610, 1965.

280. Howard GM and Ellsworth RM: Differential diagnosis of retinoblastoma: a statistical survey of 500 children. II. Factors relating to the diagnosis of retinoblastoma, Am J Ophthalmol 60:618, 1965.

281. Khan JA, Ide CH, and Strickland MP: Coats-type retinitis pigmentosa, Surv Ophthalmol 32:317, 1988.

282. Kogan L and Boniuk M: Causes of enucleation in childhood with special reference to pseudogliomas and unsuspected retinoblastomas, Int Ophthalmol Clin 2:507, 1962.

283. Liberfarb RM and others: Norrie's disease: a study of two families, Ophthalmology 92:1445, 1985.

284. Meisels HI and Goldberg MF: Vascular anastomoses between the iris and persistent hyperplastic primary vitreous, Am J Ophthalmol 88:179, 1979

285. Moazed K, Albert DM, and Smith TR: Rubeosis iridis in "pseudogliomas," Surv Ophthalmol 25:85, 1980.

286. Morgan KS and McLean LW: Retinoblastoma and persistent hyperplastic vitreous occurring in the same patient, Ophthalmology 88:1087, 1981.

287. Nankin SJ and Scott WE: Persistent hyperplastic primary vitreous, Arch Ophthalmol 95:240, 1977.

288. Naumann GOH: Intraoculäre Tumoren bein Kinder. In Bericht über die 69 Zusammenkunft der Deutschen Ophthalmologischen Gesellschaft in Heidelberg 1968, Munich, 1969, JF Bergmann.

289. Naumann GOH and Lommatzsch P: Tumoren der Augenund Augenhohle. In Opitz II and Schmid F, editors: Handbuch der Kinderheilkunde: Tumoren in Kindesalter, vol 8, part 2, Berlin, 1972, Springer-Verlag.

290. Peyman GA, Apple DJ, and Sanders DR, editors: Intraocular tumors, New York, 1977, Appleton-Century-Crofts.

291. Puklin JE and Apple DJ: Retinoblastoma and leukokoria. In Peyman GA, Sanders DR, Goldberg MF, editors: Principles and practice of ophthalmology, Philadelphia, 1980, WB Saunders Co.

292. Rosenfeld SI and Smith ME: Ocular findings in incontinentia pigmenti, Ophthalmology 92:543, 1985.

293. Sanders TE: Pseudoglioma, Trans Am Ophthalmol Soc 48:575, 1950.

294. Shields JA: Diagnosis and management of intraocular tumors, St Louis, 1983, The CV Mosby Co.

295. Shields JA: Ocular toxocariasis: a review, Surv Ophthalmol 28:361, 1984.

296. Shields JA, Stephens RF, and Sarin LK: The differential diagnosis of retinoblastoma. In Harley RD, editor: Pediatric ophthalmology, ed 2, vol 2, Philadelphia, 1983, WB Saunders Co.

297. Shields JA and others: Lesions simulating retinoblastoma, J pediatr Ophthalmol Stabismus 28:338, 1991.

298. Shields JA, Shields CL, and Parson HM: Differential diagnosis of retinoblastoma, Retina 11:232, 1991.

299. Swartz M, Herbst R, and Goldberg MF: Aqueous humor lactic acid dehydrogenase in retinoblastoma, Am J Ophthalmol 78:612, 1974.

300. Tasman W: The natural history of active retinopathy of prematurity, Ophthalmology 91:1499, 1984.

301. Yanoff M: Pseudogliomas differential diagnosis of retinoblastoma, Ophthalmol Dig 34:9, 1997.

Retinal vascular anomalies with lipid exudation

302. Apple DJ, Geiser DK, and Goldberg MF: Pathologische Befunde bei einem Erwachsenen mit Morbus Coats, Klin Monatsbl Augenheilkd 179:336, 1981.

303. Apple DJ, Hamming NA, and Gieser DK: Differential diagnosis of leucocoria. In Peyman GA, Apple DJ, and Sanders DR, editors: Intraocular tumors, New York, 1977, Appleton-Century-Crofts.

304. Archer DB: Leber's miliary aneurysms, Ophthalmol Dig 33:8, 1971.

305. Campo RV and Reeser FH: Retinal telangiectasia secondary to bilateral carotid artery occlusion. Arch Ophthalmol 101:1211, 1983.

306. Cameron JD, Yanoff M, and Frayer WC: Coats' disease and Turner's syndrome, Am J Ophthalmol 78:852, 1974.

307. Chang M, McLean IW, and Merritt JC: Coats' disease. A study of 62 histologically confirmed cases, J Pediatr Ophthalmol Strabismus 21:163, 1984.

308. Coats G: Forms of retinal disease with massive exudation, R Lond Ophthalmol Hosp Rep 17:440, 1908.

309. Egerer I, Tasman W, and Tomer TL: Coats' disease, Arch Ophthalmol 92:109, 1974.

310. Elwyn H: Coats' disease. In Diseases of the retina, Philadelphia, 1946, The Blakiston Company.

311. Farkas TC, Potts AM, and Boone C: Some pathologic and biochemical aspects of Coats' disease, Am J Ophthalmol 75:289, 1973.

312. Folk JC, Genovese FN, and Biglan AW: Coats' disease in a patient with Cornelia De Lange syndrome, Am J Ophthalmol 91:607, 1981.

313. Fuchs E: Aneurysma arterio-venosum retinae, Arch Augenheilkd 11:440, 1882.

314. Gass JDM: A fluorescein angiographic study of macular dysfunction secondary to retinal vascular disease. V. Retinal telangiectasis, Arch Ophthalmol 80:592, 1968.

315. Gieser DK, Apple DJ, and Goldberg MF: Pathologic findings of adult Coats' syndrome, Paper presented at a meeting of the Central Section of the Association for Research in Vision and Ophthalmology, Milwaukee, 1973.

316. Gold DH, La Piana FG, and Zimmerman LE: Isolated retinal arterial aneurysms, Am J Ophthalmol 82:848, 1976.

317. Harris CS: Coats' disease, diagnosis and treatment, Mod Probl Ophthalmol 10:277, 1972.

318. Horn G, Rabb MF, and Lewicky AO: Retinal telangiectasis of the macula; a review and differential diagnosis. Int Ophthalmol Clin 21(3):139, 1981.

319. Jakobiec FA, Abramson DH, and Scher R: Increased aqueous lactate dehydrogenase in Coats' disease, Am J Ophthalmol 85:686, 1978.

320. Judisch GF and Apple DJ: Acute orbital cellulitis secondary to Coats' syndrome, Arch Ophthalmol 98:2004, 1980.

321. Meythaler H: Zur pathologischen Anatomie der Retinitis exsudativa externa, Klin Monatsbl Augenheilkd 156:644, 1970.

322. Moazed K, Albert D, and Smith TR: Rubeosis iridis in "pseudogliomas," Surv Ophthalmology 25:85, 1980.

323. Pe'er J: Calcification in Coats' disease, Am J Ophthalmol 106:742, 1988.

324. Perry HD, Zimmerman LE, and Benson WE: Hemorrhage from isolated aneurysm of a retinal artery, Arch Ophthalmol 95:281, 1977.

325. Reese AB: Telangiectasia of the retina and Coats' disease, Am J Ophthalmol 42:1, 1956.

326. Ridley ME and others: Coats' disease: evaluation of management, Ophthalmology 89:1381, 1982.

327. Senft SH, Hidayat AA, and Cavender JC: Atypical Coats' disease, Retina 14:36, 1994.

328. Shields JA and others: Coats' disease as a cause of anterior chamber cholesterolosis, Arch Ophthalmol 113:975, 1995.

329. Shults WT and Swan KC: Pulsatile aneurysms of the retinal arterial tree, Am J Ophthalmol 77:304, 1974.

330. Tripathi R and Ashton N: Electron microscopical study of Coats' disease, Br J Ophthalmol 55:289, 1971.

Toxic retinopathy (retinopathy of prematurity)

331. Adamkin DH and others: Nonhyperosic retrolental fibroplasia, Pediatrics 60:828, 1977.

332. Ashton N, Ward B, and Serpell G: Role of oxygen in the genesis of retrolental fibroplasia: a preliminary report, Br J Ophthalmol 37:513, 1953.

333. Ashton N, Ward B, and Serpell G: Effect of oxygen on developing retinal vessels with particular reference to the problem of retrolental fibroplasia, Br J Ophthalmol 38:397, 1954.

334. Barr CC, Ride TA, and Michels RG: Angioma-like mass in a patient with retrolental fibroplasia, Am J Ophthalmol 89:647, 1980.

335. Blodi FC: Prematurity in the causation of ocular anomalies. In Sorsby A, editor: Systemic ophthalmology, ed 2, London, 1958, Butterworth & Co, Ltd.

336. Blodi FC: Vascular anomalies of the fundus. In Duane T, editor: Clinical ophthalmology, New York, 1976, Harper & Row, Publishers.

337. Blodi FC, Reese AB, and Locke J: The pathology of early retrolental fibroplasia: with an analysis of the histologic findings in the eyes of newborn and stillborn infants, Am J Ophthalmol 35:1407, 1952.

338. Chan-Ling T and others: Vascular changes and their mechanisms in the feline, Invest Ophthalmol Vis Sci 33:2128, 1992.

339. Committee for the Classification of Retinopathy of Prematurity: An international classification of retinopathy of prematurity, Br J Ophthalmol 68:690, 1984.

340. Committee for the Classification of Retinopathy of Prematurity: An international classification of retinopathy of prematurity, Arch Ophthalmol 102:1130, 1984.

341. Committee for the Classification of Retinopathy of Prematurity: An international classification of retinopathy of prematurity, Pediatrics 74:127, 1984.

342. Cryotherapy for Retinopathy of Prematurity Cooperative Group: Multicenter trial of cryotherapy for retinopathy of prematurity: $3\frac{1}{2}$ year outcome—structure and function, Arch Ophthalmol 111:334, 1993.

343. Darlow BA, Horwood LJ, and Clement RS: Retinopathy of prematurity: risk factors in a prospective population-based study, Paed Perinatal Epiderm 6:62, 1992.

344. de Juan E, Gritz DC, and Machemer R: Ultrastructural characteristics of proliferative tissue in retinopathy of prematurity, Am J Ophthalmol 104:149, 1987.

345. Dias PLR: Correlation of aqueous humour lactic acid dehydrogenase activity with intraocular pathology, Br J Ophthalmol 63:574, 1979.

346. Duc B: Retinopathy of prematurity/idiopathic fibroplasia: editorial correspondence, J Pediatr 98:662, 1981.

347. Eller AW and others: Retinopathy of prematurity. The association of a persistent hyaloid artery, Ophthalmology 94:444, 1987.

348. Fetter WP and others: Visual acuity and visual field development after cryocoagulation in infants with retinopathy of prematurity, Acta Paediatrica 81:25, 1992.

349. Finer NN and others: Vitamin E and retrolental fibroplasia: improved visual outcome with early vitamin E, Ophthalmology 90:428, 1983.

350. Flower RW and Patz A: Oxygen studies in retrolental fibroplasia. IX. The effects of elevated arterial oxygen tension on retinal vascular dynamics in the kitten, Arch Ophthalmol 85:197, 1971.

351. Flynn JT and others: Retrolental fibroplasia. I. Clinical observations, Arch Ophthalmol 95:217, 1977.

352. Flynn JT and others: Retinopathy of prematurity. Diagnosis, severity, natural history, Ophthalmology 94:620, 1987.

353. Flynn JT and others: A cohort study of transcutaneous oxygen tension and the incidence and severity of retinopathy of prematurity, N Engl J Med 326:1078, 1992.

354. Foos RY: Acute retrolental fibroplasia, Albrecht Von Graefes Arch Klin Exp Ophthalmol 195:87, 1975.

355. Foos RY: Retinopathy of prematurity, Pathologic correlation of clinical stages. Retina 7:260, 1987.

356. Fryczkowski AW and others: Scanning electron microscopy of the ocular vasculature in retinopathy of prematurity, Arch Ophthalmology 103:224, 1985.

357. Garoon I and others: Vascular tufts in retrolental fibroplasia, Ophthalmology 87:1128, 1980.

358. Glass P and others: Effect of bright light in the hospital nursery on the incidence of retinopathy of prematurity, N Engl J Med 313:401, 1985.

359. Greven C and Tasman W: Scleral buckling in stages 4B and 5 retinopathy of prematurity, Ophthalmology 97:817, 1990.

360. Henkind P: If experts agree, life might be dull, Ophthalmology 90(5):31A, 1983 (editorial).

361. Jabour NM and others: Stage 5 retinopathy of prematurity. Prognostic value of morphologic findings, Ophthalmology 94:1640, 1987.

362. James LS and Lanman JT, editors: The early history of oxygen use for premature infants, Pediatrics 57:591, 1976.

363. Kalina RE: Treatment of retrolental fibroplasia, Surv Ophthalmol 24:229, 1980.

364. Kalina RE and Forrest GL: Proliferative retrolental fibroplasia in infant retinal vessels, Am J Ophthalmol 76:811, 1973.

365. Karlsberg RC, Green WR, and Patz A: Congenital retrolental fibroplasia, Arch Ophthalmol 89:122, 1973.

366. Keith CG and Kitchen WH: Retinopathy of prematurity in extremely low birth weight infants, Med J Aust 141:225, 1984.

367. Kingham JD: Acute retrolental fibroplasia, Arch Ophthalmol 95:39, 1977.

368. Kretzer FL and others: Vitamin E and retrolental fibroplasia: ultrastructural support of clinical efficiency, Ann. N. Y. Acad. Sci. 393:145, 1982.

369. Kretzer FL, McPherson AR, and Hittner HM: An interpretation of retinopathy of prematurity in terms of spindle cells: relationship of vitamin E prophylaxis and cryotherapy, Graefes Arch Clin Exp Ophthalmol 224:205, 1986.

370. Kushner BJ and others: Retrolental fibroplasia, Arch Ophthalmol 95:29, 1977.

371. Kushner BJ and Gloeckner E: Retrolental fibroplasia in full-term infants without exposure to supplemental oxygen, Am J Ophthalmol 97:148, 1984.

372. Machemer R: Closed vitrectomy for severe retrolental fibroplasia in the infant, Ophthalmology 90:436, 1983.

373. Naiman J, Green WR, and Patz A: Retrolental fibroplasia in hypoxic newborn, Am J Ophthalmol 88:55, 1979.

374. Newman NM: Retinopathy of prematurity and vitamin E, Med J Aust 141:209, 1984.

375. Owens WC and others: Symposium: retrolental fibroplasia (retinopathy of prematurity), Trans Am Acad Ophthalmol Otolaryngol 59:7, 1955.

376. Palmer EA and others: Incidence and early course of retinopathy of prematurity, Ophthalmology 98:1628, 1991.

377. Patz A: Oxygen studies in retrolental fibroplasia. IV. Clinical and experimental observations, Am J Ophthalmol 38:291, 1954.

378. Patz A: New role of the Ophthalmologist in prevention of retrolental fibroplasia, Arch Ophthalmol 78:565, 1967.

379. Patz A: Retrolental fibroplasia, Trans Am Ophthalmol Soc 66:940, 1968.

380. Patz A: Retrolental fibroplasia, Surv Ophthalmol 14:1, 1969.

381. Patz A: Current therapy of retrolental fibroplasia: retinopathy of prematurity, Ophthalmology 90:425, 1983.

382. Patz A: An international classification of retinopathy of prematurity. II. The classification of retinal detachment, Arch Ophthalmol 105:906, 1987.

383. Patz A: Observations on the retinopathy of prematurity, Am J Ophthalmol 100:164, 1985.

384. Phelps DL: Retinopathy of prematurity. An estimate of vision loss in the United States—1979, Pediatrics 67:924, 1981.

385. Prendiville A and Schlenberg WE: Clinical factors associated with retinopathy of prematurity, Arch Dis Child 63:522, 1988.

386. Quinn GE, Schaffer DB, and Johnson L: A revised classification of retinopathy of prematurity, Am J Ophthalmol 94:744, 1982.

387. Reese AB: Retrolental fibroplasia, Am J Ophthalmol 34:1, 1951.

388. Reese AB and Blodi FC: Retrolental fibroplasia. In: Acta XVI Concilium Ophthalmologicum Britannia 1950, London, 1951, British Medical Association.

389. Reese AB and Blodi FC: The relation of prematurity to ocular anomalies in post-natal-development. In Sorsby A, editor: Systemic ophthalmology, London, 1951, Butterworth & Co, Ltd.

390. Reese AB, King MJ, and Owens WC: A classification of retrolental fibroplasia, Am J Ophthalmol 36:1333, 1953.

391. Reese AB, Stepanik J: Cicatricial stage of retrolental fibroplasia, Am J Ophthalmol 38:308, 1954.

392. Schaeffer DB and others: Vitamin E and retinopathy of prematurity. Follow-up at one year, Ophthalmology 92:1005, 1985.

393. Schulman J, Jampol LM, and Schwartz H: Peripheral proliferative retinopathy without oxygen therapy in a full-term infant, Am J Ophthalmol 90:509, 1980.

394. Shohat M and others: Retinopathy of prematurity. Incidence and risk factors, Pediatric 72:159, 1983.

395. Sira IB, Nissenkorn I, and Kremer I: Retinopathy of prematurity, Surv Ophthalmol 33:1, 1988.

396. Stefani FH and Heidi E: Non-oxygen induced retinitis proliferans and retinal detachment in full-term infants, Br J Ophthalmol 58:490, 1974.

397. Tasman W: Vitreoretinal changes in cicatricial retrolental fibroplasia, Trans Am Ophthalmol Soc 68:548, 1970.

398. Tasman W: Retinal detachment in retrolental fibroplasia, Graefes Arch Clin Exp Ophthalmol 195:129, 1975.

399. Tasman W: Exudative retinal detachment in retrolental fibroplasia, Trans Am Acad Ophthalmol Otolaryngol 83:535, 1977.

400. Tasman W: Late complications of retrolental fibroplasia, Ophthalmology 86:1724, 1979.

401. Terry TL: Extreme prematurity and fibroplastic overgrowth of persistent vascular sheath behind each crystalline lens. I. Preliminary report, Am J Ophthalmol 25:203, 1942.

402. Tyner GS and Frayer WC: Clinical and autopsy findings in early retrolental fibroplasia, Arch Pathol 46:647, 1954.

Inflammatory conditions

403. Ashton N: Larval granulomatosis of the retina due to *Toxocara*, Br J Ophthalmol 44:129, 1960.

404. Baldone JA, Clark WB, and Jung RC: Nematode ophthalmitis, Am J Ophthalmol 57:763, 1964.

405. Beaver PC and others: Chronic eosinophilia due to visceral larva migrans: report of three cases, Pediatrics 9:7, 1952.

406. Beaver PC: Larva migrans, Exp Parasitol 5:587, 1956.

407. Beaver PC: The nature of visceral larva migrans, J Parasitol 55:3, 1969.

408. Berrocal J: Prevalence of *Toxocara canis* in babies and in adults as determined by the ELISA test, Trans Am Ophthalmol Soc 78:376, 1980.

409. Bird A, Smith JLS, and Curtin VT: Nematode optic neuritis, Am J Ophthalmol 69:72, 1970.

410. Brown DH: Ocular *Toxocara canis*, J Pediatr Ophthalmol 7:182, 1970.

411. Duguid IM: Chronic endophthalmitis due to *Toxocara*, Br J Ophthalmol 45:705, 1961.

412. Duguid IM: Features of ocular infestation by *Toxocara*, Br J Ophthalmol 45:789, 1961.

413. Irvine WC and Irvine AR Jr: Nematode endophthalmitis: *Toxocara canis*—report of one case, Am J Ophthalmol 47:185, 1959.

414. Leopold IH: Is the dog really man's best friend? Am J Ophthalmol 59:717, 1965.

415. Molk R: Ocular toxocariasis: a review of the literature, Ann Ophthalmol 15:216, 1983.

416. Nichols RL: The etiology of visceral larva migrans. I. Diagnostic morphology of infective second-stage *Toxocara* larvae, J Parasitol 42:349, 1956.

417. Raistrick ER and Hart JCD: Adult toxocaral infection with focal retinal lesion, Br Med J 3:416, 1975.

418. Rey A: Nematode endophthalmitis due to *Toxocara*, Br J Ophthalmol 46:616, 1962.

419. Rockey JH and others: Immunopathology of *Toxocara canis* and *Ascaris SUUM* infections of the eye; the role of the eosinophil, Invest Ophthalmol Vis Sci 18:1172, 1979.

420. Rubin ML and others: An intraretinal nematode: a case report, Trans Am Acad Ophthalmol Otolaryngol 72:855, 1968.

421. Searl SS and others: Ocular toxocariasis presenting as leucocoria in a patient with low ELISA titer to *Toxocara canis*, Ophthalmology 88:1302, 1981.

422. Watzke RC, Oaks JA, and Folk JC: *Toxocara canis* infection of the eye: correlation of clinical observations with developing pathology in the primate model, Arch Ophthalmol 102:282, 1984.

423. Welsh RB, Maumenee AE, and Wahlen HE: Peripheral posterior segment inflammation, vitreous opacities, edema of the posterior pole; pars planitis, Arch Ophthalmol 64:540, 1960.

424. Wilder HC: Nematode endophthalmitis, Trans Am Acad Ophthalmol Otolaryngol 55:99, 1950.

425. Wilkinson CP and Welsh RB: Intraocular *Toxocara*, Am J Ophthalmol 71:921, 1971.

426. Zinkham WH: Visceral larva migrans due to *Toxocara* as a cause of eosinophilia, Johns Hopkins Med J 123:41, 1968.

Conditions exhibiting abnormal retinal embryogenesis and/or retinal dysplasia

427. Apple DJ: Chromosome-induced ocular disease. In Goldberg MF, editor: Genetic and metabolic eye disease, Boston, 1974, Little, Brown & Co.

428. Apple DJ, Fishman GA, and Goldberg MF: Ocular histopathology of Norrie's disease, Am J Ophthalmol 78:196, 1974.

429. Benedikt O and Ehalt H: Familiär auftretendes Bloch-Sulzberger-Syndrom (Incontinentia pigmenti) mit Augenbeteiligung, Klin Monatsbl Augenheilkd 157:652, 1970.

430. Best W and Rentsch F: Über das "Pseudogliom" bei der Incontinentia pigmenti, Klin Monatsbl Augenheilkd 164:19, 1974.

431. Bloch B: Eigentümliche bisher nicht beschriebene Pigmentaffektion, Schweiz Med Wochenschr 56:404, 1926.

432. Blodi FC and Hunter W: Norrie's disease in North America, Doc Ophthalmol 26:434, 1969.

433. Brini A, Sacrez P, and Levy JP: Maladie de Norrie, Ann Oculist 205:1, 1972.

434. Catalano RA: Incontinentia pigmenti, Am J Ophthalmol 110:696, 1990.

435. Chen ZY and others: A mutation in the Norre disease gene (NDP) associated with X-linked familial exudative vitreoretinopathy, Nature genet 5:180, 1993.

436. Cole JC and Cole HG: Incontinentia pigmenti, Am J Ophthalmol 47:321, 1959.

437. De Buen S and Fenton RH: Coloboma of the optic disc mistaken for retinoblastoma, Surv Ophthalmol 10:7, 1965.

438. Enyedi LB, de Juan E Jr, and Gaitan A: Ultrastructural study of Norrie's disease, Am J Ophthalmol 111:439, 1991.

439. Findlay GH: On the pathogenesis of incontinentia pigmenti, Br J Dermatol 64:141, 1952.

440. Fowell SM and others: Ocular findings of incontinentia pigmenti in a male infant with Klinefelter syndrome, J Pediatr Ophthalmol Strabismus 29:180, 1992.

441. Fradkin AH: Norrie's disease: congenital progressive oculo-acoustico-cerebral degeneration, Am J Ophthalmol 72:947, 1971.

442. Friendly DS and Parks MM: Concurrence of hereditary congenital cataracts and hereditary retinoblastoma, Arch Ophthalmol 84:525, 1970.

443. Fulton AB and others: Human retinal dysplasia, Am J Ophthalmol 85:690, 1978.

444. Godel V and others: Primary retinal dysplasia transmitted as X-chromosome-linked recessive disorder, Am J Ophthalmology 86:221, 1978.

445. Goldberg MF: The blinding mechanism of incontentia pigmenti, Trans Am Ophthalmol Soc 92:167, 1994.

446. Goldberg MF and Custis PH: Retinal and other manifestations of incontinentia pigmenti (Bloch-Sulzberger syndrome), Ophthalmology 100:1645, 1993.

447. Hoepner J and Yanoff M: Spectrum of ocular abnormalities in trisomy 13-15, Am J Ophthalmol 74:729, 1972.

448. Holmes LB: Norrie's disease—an X-linked syndrome of retinal malformation, mental retardation and deafness, N Engl J Med 284:367, 1971.

449. Jacklin HN: Falciform fold, retinal detachment, Norrie's disease, Am J Ophthalmol 90:76, 1980.

450. Jain RB and Willetts GS: Fundus changes in incontinentia pigmenti (Bloch-Sulzberger syndrome): a case report, Br J Ophthalmol 62:622, 1978.

451. Lahav M and Albert DM: Clinical and histopathologic classification of retinal dysplasia, Am J Ophthalmol 75:648, 1973.

452. Liberfarb RM and others: Norrie's disease: a study of two families, Ophthalmology 92:1445, 1985.

453. Manthey R, Apple DJ, and Kivlin JD: Iris hypoplasia in incontinentia pigmenti, J Pediatr Ophthalmol Strabismus 19:279, 1982.

454. McCrary JA and Smith JL: Conjunctival and retinal incontinentia pigmenti, Arch Ophthalmol 79:417, 1968.

455. Mensheha-Manhart O and others: Retinal pigment epithelium in incontinentia pigmenti, Am J Ophthalmol 111:614, 1993.

456. Miller RJ and Anderson RE: A retrolental mass in incontinentia pigmenti, Surv Ophthalmol 11:41, 1966.

457. Nix RR and Apple DJ: Proliferative retinopathy associated with incontinentia pigmenti, Retina 1:156, 1981.

458. Peyman GA, Apple DJ, and Sanders DR, editors: Intraocular tumors, New York, 1977, Appleton-Century-Crofts.

459. Raab EL: Ocular lesions in incontinentia pigmenti, J Pediatr Ophthalmol Strabismus 20:42, 1983.

460. Reese AB and Blodi FC: Retinal dysplasia, Am J Ophthalmol 33:23, 1950.

461. Reese AB and Straatsma BR: Retinal dysplasia, Arch Ophthalmol 45:199, 1958.

462. Scott JG and others: Ocular changes in the Bloch-Sulzberger syndrome (incontinentia pigmenti), Br J Ophthalmol 39:276, 1955.

463. Sulzberger MB: Über cine bisher nicht beschriebene congenitale Pigmentanomalie (Incontinentia pigmenti), Arch Dermatol Syphilol 154:19, 1928.

464. Sulzberger MB: Incontinentia pigmenti (Bloch-Sulzberger), Arch Dermatol Syphilol 38:57, 1938.

465. Townes PL and Roca PD: Norrie's disease (hereditary oculo-acoustic-cerebral degeneration): report of a United States family, Am J Ophthalmol 76:797, 1973.

466. Wald KJ and others: Retinal detachments in incontinentia pigmenti, Arch Ophthalmol 94:743, 1976.

467. Warburg M: Norrie's disease and falciform detachment of the retina. In Goldberg MF, editor: Genetic and metabolic eye disease, Boston, 1974, Little, Brown & Co.

468. Warburg M and others: Norrie's disease: delineation of carriers among daughters of obligate carriers by linkage analysis, Trans Ophthalmol Soc UK 105:88, 1986.

469. Watzke RG, Stevens TS, and Carney RG Jr: Retinal vascular changes of incontinentia pigmenti, Arch Ophthalmol 94:743, 1976.

470. Watzke RG: Incontinentia pigmenti, Arch Ophthalmol 96:1922, 1978 (letter to the editor).

471. Wollensak J: Charakteristische Augenbefunde beim Syndroma Bloch-Sulzberger (Incontinentia pigmenti), Klin Monatsbl Augenheilkd 134:692, 1959.

Prenatal and infantile trauma, organizing vitreous hemorrhage, and massive retinal gliosis

472. Arnold AC and others: Solitary retinal astrocytoma, Surv Ophthalmol 30:173, 1985.

473. Baum JD and Bulpitt CJ: Eye hemorrhage incidence in newborns, Arch Dis Child 45:344, 1970.

474. Friedenwald JS: Massive gliosis of the retina. In Contributions to ophthalmic science, Menasha, Wis, 1926, Banta Publishing Co.

475. Hobach L and Volcker HE: Introkularer pseudotumor dutch massive gliose der retina-nachweis des sauren gliafaserprotein, Klin Mbl augenbeilk 185:518, 1984.

476. Planten J and von der Schaaf PC: Retinal hemorrhage in the newborn, Ophthalmologica 162:213, 1971.

477. Reese AB: Massive retinal fibrosis in children, Am J Ophthalmol 19:576, 1936.

478. Sezaen F: Retinal hemorrhages in newborn infants, Br J Ophthalmol 55:248, 1971.

479. von Barsewisch B: Perinatal retinal haemorrhages: morphology, aetiology and significance, Berlin, 1979, Springer-Verlag.

480. Yanoff M, Davis RL, and Zimmerman LE: Massive gliosis of the retina, Int Ophthalmol Clin 11:211, 1971.

Phakomatoses

481. Brazel SM and others: Iris sector heterochromia as a marker for neural crest disease, Arch Ophthalmol 110:233, 1992.

482. Font RL and Ferry AP: The phakomatoses, Int Ophthalmol Clin 12(1):1, 1972.

483. Gass JDM: The phakomatoses. In Smith JL, editor: Neuroophthalmology, vol 2, St Louis, 1965, The CV Mosby Co.

484. Harwig P and Robertson D: von Hippel-Lindau disease: a familial, often lethal, multi-system phakomatosis, Ophthalmology 91:263, 1984.

485. Hofeldt AJ and others: Orbitofacial angiomatosis, Arch Ophthalmol 94:484, 1979.

486. Mansour AM and others: Ocular choristomas, Surv Ophthalmol 33:339, 1989.

487. Nerad JA, Kersten RC, and Anderson RL: Hemangioblastoma of the optic nerve: report of a case and review of literature, Ophthalmology 95:398, 1988.

488. Tasman W: The phakomatoses. In Tasman W, editor: Retinal diseases in children, New York, 1971, Harper & Row, Publishers.

489. van der Hoeve J: Eye symptoms in phakomatoses, Trans Ophthalmol Soc UK 52:380, 1932.

490. van der Hoeve J: Phakomatoses. In Ridley F and Sorsby A, editors: Modern trends in ophthalmology, vol 1, New York, 1940, Paul B Hoeber, Inc, Medical Book Dept of Harper & Brothers.

Tuberous sclerosis

491. Appiah A and Hirose T: Secondary causes of premacular fibrosi, Ophthalmology 96:389, 1989.

492. Arnold AC and others: Solitary retinal astrocytom, Surv Ophthalmol 30:173, 1985.

493. Boniuk MM and Friedman AH: Vitreous hemorrhage complicating retinal astrocytic hamartoma, Surv Ophthalmol 26:31, 1981.

615. Ballantyne AJ: Buphthalmos with facial nevus and allied conditions, Br J Ophthalmol 14:481, 1930.
616. Blodi FC: Naevus flammeus faciei und Glaukoma ohne Vergrösserung des Bulbus, Ophthalmologica 117:82, 1949.
617. Cibis GW, Tripathi RC, and Tripathi BJ: Glaucoma in Sturge-Weber syndrome, Ophthalmology 91:1061, 1984.
618. Iwach AG and others: Analysis of surgical and medical management of glaucoma in Sturge-Weber syndrome, Ophthalmology 97:904, 1990.
619. Jones IS and Cleasby GW: Hemangioma of the choroid: a clinicopathologic analysis, Am J Ophthalmol 48:612, 1959.
620. Joy HH: Nevus flammeus associated with glaucoma, Am J Ophthalmol 33:1401, 1950.
621. Lindsey PS and others: Bilateral choroidal hemangiomas and facial nevus flammeus, Retina 1:88, 1981.
622. MacLean AL and Maumenee AF: Hemangioma of the choroid, Am J Ophthalmol 50:3, 1960.
623. Norton EWD and Gutman F: Fluorescein angiography and hemangiomas of the choroid, Arch Ophthalmol 78:121, 1967.
624. O'Brien CS and Porter WC: Glaucoma and nevus flammeus, Arch Ophthalmol 9:715, 1933.
625. Shin GS and Demer JL: retinal arteriovenous communications associated with features of Sturge-Weber syndrome, Am J Ophthalmol 117:115, 1994.
626. Stokes JJ: The ocular manifestations of the Sturge-Weber syndrome, South Med J 50:82, 1957.
627. Susae JO, Smith JL, and Scelfo RJ: The "tomato catsup" fundus in Sturge-Weber syndrome, Arch Ophthalmol 92:69, 1974.
628. Witschel II and Font R: Hemangioma of the choroid: a clinicopathologic study of 71 cases and a review of the literature, Surv Ophthalmol 20:415, 1976.

Wybrun-Mason syndrome; ataxia telangiectasia

629. Archer DB and others: Arteriovenous communications of the retina, Am J Ophthalmol 75:224, 1973.
630. von Baurmann H, Meyer F, and Oberhoff P: Komplikationen bei der arteriovenösen Anastomose der Netzhaut, Klin Monatsbl Augenheilkd 153:562, 1968.
631. Boder E and Sedgwick RP: Ataxia-telangiectasia: a familial syndrome of progressive cerebellar ataxia, oculocutaneous telangiectasia and frequent pulmonary infections, Pediatrics 21:526, 1958.
632. Bonnet P, Dechaume J, and Blanc E: L'anëurysme cirsoïde de la rétine (anéurysme racémeux): ses relations avee l'anéurysme cirsoïde de la face et avee l'anérysme cirsoïde du cerveau, J Med Lyon 18:165, 1937.
633. Brown DC, Hilal SH, and Tenner HS: Wyburn-Mason syndrome, Arch Neurol 28:67, 1973.
634. Danis R and Appen RE: Optic atrophy and the Wyburn-Mason syndrome, J Clin Neuro Ophthalmol 4:91, 1984.
635. Éffron I, Zakov ZN, and Tomask RI: Neovascular glaucoma as a complication of the Wyburn-Mason syndrome, J. Clin Neuro Ophthalmol 5:95, 1985.
636. Gatti RA and others: Localization of an ataxia-telangiectasia gene to chromosome 11q22-2, Nature 336:577, 1988.
637. Gatti RA and others: Ataxia-telangietasia: and interdisciplinary approach to pathogenesis, Medicine 70:99, 1991.
638. Hopen G and others: The Wyburn-Mason syndrome; concomitant chiasmal and fundus vascular malformation, J Clin Neuro Ophthalmol 3:53, 1983.
639. Hoyt WF and Cameron RB: Racemose angioma of the mandible, face, retina and brain, J Oral Surg 26:596, 1968.
640. Mansour AM, Walsh JB, and Henkind P: Arteriovenous anastomoses of the retina, Ophthalmology 94:35, 1987.
641. Mansour AM and others: Ocular complications of arteriovenous communication of the retina, Arch Ophthalmol 17:232, 1989.
642. Perry TL and others: Neurochemical abnormalities in a patients with ataxia-telangiectasi, Nerol 34:187, 1984.
643. Schalch DS, Mc Farlin DE, and Barlow MH: An unusual form of diabetes mellitus in ataxia telangiectasi, N Engl J Med 282:136, 1970.
644. Wyburn-Mason R: Arteriovenous aneurysm of midbrain and retina: facial nevi and mental changes, Brain 66:163, 1943.

Embryology and anatomy[1-33]

The optic nerve (Figs. 10-1–10-9) differs in several respects from a peripheral nerve.[1-33] It is an anteriorly protruding white-matter tract of the brain, which links the ganglion cells of the sensory retina with the visual centers of the brain.[2,4,33] A peripheral nerve possesses a neurilemmal sheath; this provides the nerve with some degree of regenerative capability after it is severed. Nerve fibers within the central nervous system, including the optic nerve, do not possess a neurilemmal sheath and, therefore, do not have regenerative capability.

The optic nerve also more closely resembles brain rather than peripheral nerve because it is ensheathed by meninges (Figs. 10-6 and 10-7). Cross-sections of the optic nerve show a compartmental arrangement (Fig. 10-8) resulting from a network of pial septae, which grow into the parenchyma from the surrounding pia mater. This is lacking in peripheral nerves.

The optic nerve develops from the embryonic optic stalk (Fig. 1-7). During the earliest stages of development the cavity of the optic vesicle maintains an open communication with the ventricle of the diencephalon through the stalk (Fig. 1-7, *A*). The first nerve fibers form as buds from the retinal ganglion cells at about 6 weeks and course centripetally through the embryonic fissure and optic stalk toward the brain (Figs. 1-7, *A*, 1-8, 1-9, and 1-11). The lumen of the stalk is gradually filled by the nerve parenchyma. Myelination proceeds in the opposite direction; it begins centrally and progresses in a centrifugal direction toward the eye, usually terminating at the level of the lamina cribrosa. The myelin sheath is elaborated by oligodendroglial cells.

The depth of the physiologic cup at the optic nerve head probably depends partly on the degree of development and regression of the trunk of the hyaloid artery and its glial sheath, the papilla of Bergmeister (Figs. 2-23, 2-24, 2-27, 2-28, and 10-1).[6,28] This artery enters the substance of the optic nerve before closure of the embryonic fissure and forms the forerunner of the mesodermal vessels of the central retinal artery system. The artery and its sheath normally regress at birth or shortly thereafter. The more extensive the regression, the greater resorption of epipapillary tissue and, consequently, the deeper the physiologic cup (Figs. 10-2, *B*, and 10-3).

The optic disc, or papilla, lies nasal to the geometric axis of the globe and measures approximately 1.5 mm in horizontal diameter and 1.7 mm in vertical diameter. Clinically its outer margins are sharply circumscribed, even though the nerve fibers course gradually over the borders into the surrounding retina (Figs. 10-2 to 10-4).

The fibers are nonmyelinated and transparent within the retina and at the optic nerve head but are myelinated[1,27] and, therefore, white behind the lamina cribrosa (Fig. 10-5).[1,27] The slightly pink-yellow color of the normal optic

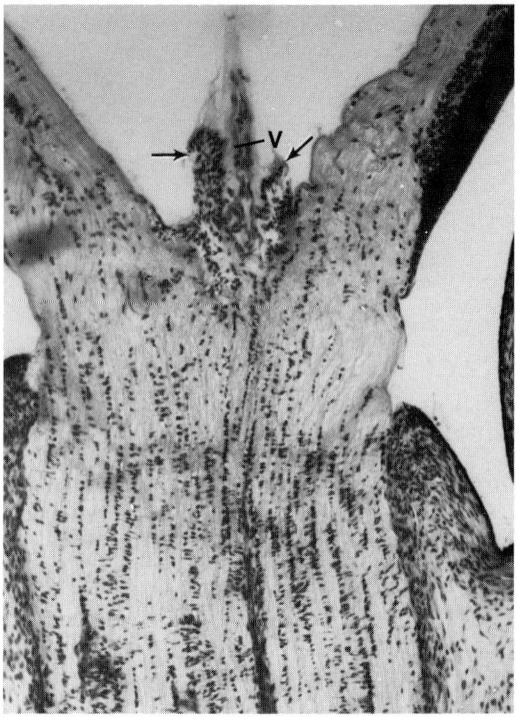

Fig. 10-1. Fetal optic nerve showing Bergmeister's papilla with central vascular core (*V*) and glial sheath (*arrows*) encircling the vessel. The vertically parallel glial columns in the nerve parenchyma are especially prominent.

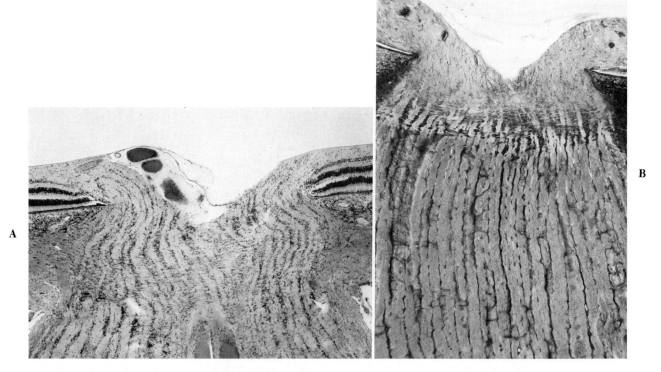

Fig. 10-2. Optic nerve. **A,** Junction of retina and optic nerve showing the continuity between the nerve fiber layer and optic nerve axons. The physiologic cup is of average depth, and the central vessels are seen in cross-section below and as they reappear, emerging at the left of the optic cup in this section. (H & E stain; ×120.) **B,** Slightly deeper but normal optic cup. The lamina cribrosa is prominent and shows slight posterior bowing. (H & E stain; ×100.) (**B** from Naumann GOH and Apple DJ: In Doerr W, Seifert G, and Uehlinger E, editors: Handbuch der speziellen pathologischen Anatomie, Band Auge, Berlin, 1980, Springer-Verlag.)

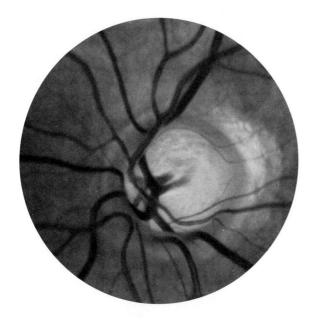

Fig. 10-3. Fundus photograph of a normal optic disc with a relatively large and deep physiologic cup and a cup-disc ratio of 0.7 : 0.8. The depth of the physiologic cup depends on several factors, including genetic factors and degree of resorption of the physiologic optic cup. (From Apple DJ, Rabb MF, and Walsh PM: Surv Ophthalmol 27:3, 1982.)

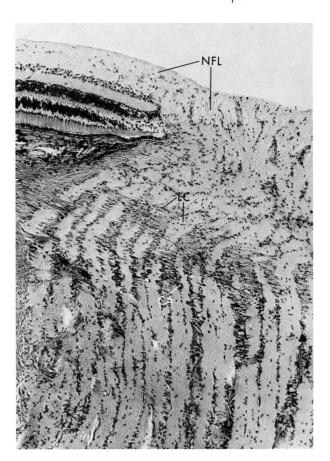

Fig. 10-4. Normal optic nerve, with a relatively shallow physiologic cup *(upper right)* and slight posterior bowing of the lamina cribrosa *(LC)*. The optic nerve axons are continuations of the retinal nerve fiber layer *(NFL)*. The astrocytic (glial) nuclei are arranged in parallel rows. The small hyaline body (corpora amylacea, *CA*) situated within the nerve parenchyma is probably a degenerated glial cell. (H & E stain; ×90.)

disc seen ophthalmoscopically can be explained by the presence of numerous capillaries within the nerve substance. When the optic nerve atrophies, usually some of the capillaries are destroyed and it may, therefore, assume a white or gray discoloration.[116] On the other hand in some pathologic states—for example, inflammatory conditions—the red hue of the nerve may actually be increased by dilatation of optic nerve vessels.

The central retinal artery and vein lie directly adjacent to each other as they emerge from the physiologic cup (Fig. 8-7).[8] The artery most commonly lies nasal to the vein. The four major branches of the central vessels usually form by branching immediately at the optic nerve head.[20-23]

Temporal crescents, caused by unequal termination of the borders of the retina-pigment epithelium-choroid at the margins of the disc, are often seen as a physiologic variation and are common in myopia (Figs. 2-43 and 2-45).

Between the disc and the chiasm the optic nerve is not taut but reveals a slight S-shaped curvature. It is, therefore, capable of elongation during extreme movement of the globe and during injuries to the orbit. The nasal retinal fibers cross at the optic chiasm, forming, with the uncrossed temporal fibers, the optic tracts. The fibers of the optic tract terminate in the lateral geniculate body of the thalamus. They then synapse to link with the optic radiations, which terminate in the visual cortex in the region of the calcarine fissure.

The nerve fiber layer is the most superficial layer at the disc, containing the compact optic nerve fibers as they converge from all parts of the retina and bend backward (Figs. 10-2 and 10-3). The surface nerve fiber layer is covered by the inner limiting membrane of Elschnig, which is com-

posed of astrocytes and which separates the nerve fiber layer from the vitreous.[3,11]

The prelaminar region lies between the superficial nerve fiber layer and the lamina cribrosa. At its peripheral edge, the prelaminar region is sometimes separated from the adjacent deeper layers of the retina by a layer of glial tissue, the intermediary tissue of Kuhnt. The border tissue of Jacoby, a marginal layer of astroglia, separates the prelaminar region from the adjacent choroid.[3]

The sclera is perforated in a sievelike manner at the optic nerve head forming the lamina cribrosa.[117,119] The physiologic posterior bowing of the lamina cribrosa (Figs. 10-2, 10-3, and 10-6) is minimal and should not be confused with the pathologic posterior bowing caused by a glaucomatous excavation (Figs. 6-30–6-34). The anterior portion of the lamina cribrosa (the lamina choroidalis) is composed mostly of glial fibers that form oval-to-round compartments through which the axons pass. The posterior aspect (the lamina scleralis) consists largely of connective tissue, which merges with the adjacent scleral collagen. The diameter of the nerve increases from about 1.5 to 3.6 mm immediately behind the lamina cribrosa because of the myelination of the fibers.

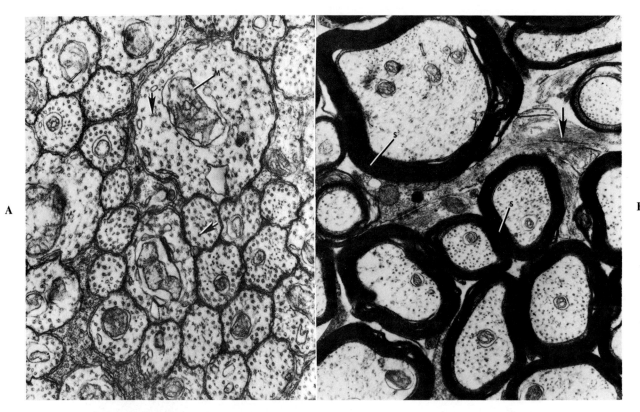

Fig. 10-5. A, Electron micrograph of prelaminar optic nerve fibers showing cross-sections of normal visual axons and their two major components: (1) numerous mitochondria *(M),* the presence of which underscores the large energy requirements of visual impulse transmission, and (2) the intraaxonal microtubules *(arrows),* which are believed to function as pathways for transmission of the neural impulse. A myelin sheath is absent in these prelaminar layers. (Uranyl acetate and lead citrate stain; ×72,400.) **B,** The optic nerve posterior to the lamina cribrosa shows myelinated axons. The individual axons appearing in this cross-section are similar to those seen in **A** but are now surrounded by a myelin envelope or sheath *(S),* which appears electron-dense in this photograph. It is seen to be laminated if observed at higher magnification. The fibrillar processes *(arrow)* between the individual axons are components of the supportive glial cells (astrocytes) of the optic nerve. (Uranyl acetate and lead citrate stain; ×37,000.)

Fig. 10-6. Drawing of the optic nerve showing the meninges and their intravaginal faces.

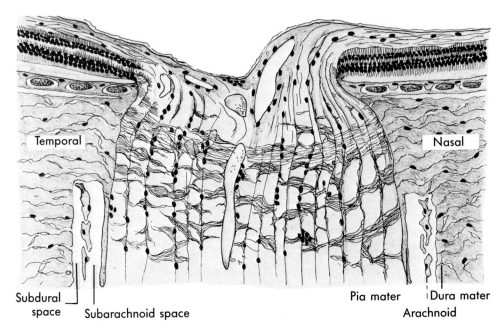

The border tissue of Elschnig, which is more strongly developed on the temporal than on the nasal side, separates the sclera from the nerve fibers at the level of the lamina cribrosa. It is composed of dense collagenous tissue, with many glial and elastic fibers and some pigment. It continues forward to separate the choroid from nervous tissue.[3]

The optic nerve is ensheathed by three meningeal layers: the dura mater, the arachnoid, and the pia mater (Figs. 10-6 and 10-7). They are continuous posteriorly with the meninges of the brain, and anteriorly they terminate abruptly at the globe, where the dura mater merges with the sclera.

The dura mater consists of dense collagenous tissue and is similar in structure to the sclera. It forms the outer lining of the subdural space. Commonly occurring subdural hematomas usually result from hemorrhage from venous channels.

The middle layer, the arachnoid, consists of meningothelial cells (Fig. 10-7) and a network of fine, delicate fibrils. The meningothelial cells are of clinical significance because they are the cells of origin of the most important tumor arising from the meninges, the meningioma (Figs. 10-5, 10-6, 10-7, and 10-36). The subarachnoid space is the intervaginal space between the arachnoid and pia mater; it contains cerebrospinal fluid and is continuous with the cerebrospinal fluid–containing spaces within the brain. The subarachnoid space ends blindly at the eye; therefore, there is normally no communication between the cerebrospinal fluid and the subretinal space within the eye. Subarachnoid hemorrhages are thus confined within the meninges without direct communication within the eye. The simultaneous occurrence of intraocular hemorrhage and subarachnoid hemorrhage cannot be explained by direct

extension of the hemorrhage from the meninges but must be a result of the pressure buildup within the meninges, which causes secondary intraocular bleeding.

Subarachnoid hemorrhages occur most commonly after traumatic rupture of the cerebral arteries or after rupture of cerebral (berry) aneurysms. These hemorrhages, therefore, are typically arterial, in contrast to subdural hemorrhages, which are usually venous.

Nests of meningothelial cells within the arachnoid often proliferate in a concentric manner, forming onionlike structures, the so-called psammoma bodies, or corpora aranacea. These are sometimes seen in meningiomas (Fig. 10-36, *B*). In cases of retinoblastoma one should not confuse these small nests of meningothelial cells with infiltration of tumor cells within the optic nerve meninges.

The psammoma bodies, or corpora arenacea, differ from corpora amylacea.[9] Psammoma bodies are periodic acid-Schiff (PAS)-positive, hyaline structures situated within the optic nerve parenchyma and probably represent degenerative remnants of glial cells (Fig. 10-4). Corpora amylacea are seen in increased numbers in optic nerves of the elderly. These homogeneous structures are easily distinguished from psammoma bodies in that they are within the optic nerve substance; the laminated psammoma bodies are outside the nerve substance within the meninges.

The pia mater lies flush on the surface of the nerve and sends septae into the substance of the nerve (Fig. 10-7). The pial septae contain vessels that enter the optic nerve; they are separated from the surrounding nervous tissue by the foot processes of the glial cells, primarily the astrocytes. The septae are continuous with the collagenous adventitial sheaths of the central retinal artery and vein within the optic nerve (Fig. 10-8).

There are three distinct types of glial cells in the optic nerve: astrocytes, oligodendrogliocytes, and microglia.[29-33] In sagittal sections of the nerve (Figs. 10-1, 10-2, and

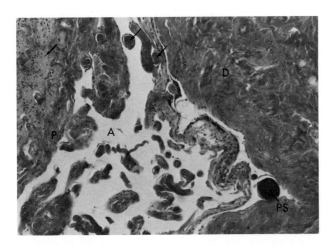

Fig. 10-7. The optic nerve meninges are identical to those of the brain. The nerve parenchyma *(upper left)* contains axons and nuclei of astrocytes *(arrow)*. Fibrous pial septae pass through the nerve as branches of the pia mater *(P)*. The middle layer, or arachnoid *(A)*, consists of delicate proliferations of meningothelial cells, which in many instances grow in a circular formation *(arrows)* and may become calcified (forming the psammoma body, *PS*, also termed corpora arenacea). The outer layer, or dura *(D)*, is composed of dense collagen resembling the sclera. The dura is continuous centrally with the periosteum of the cranial bones. (H & E stain; ×250.)

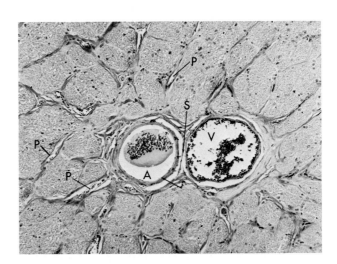

Fig. 10-8. Photomicrograph of an optic nerve cross-section demonstrating the central retinal artery *(A)* and vein *(V)*. The artery is characterized by a thick muscular coat *(arrow)*. The vessels contain erythrocytes and serum and are in a common adventitial sheath *(S)*, which becomes continuous with the pial septae *(P)*. The vascular channels that supply the nerve course through the pial septae. (H & E stain; ×200.)

10-4) one observes astrocytes within vertically oriented columns or rows of cells. Their nuclei are only moderately basophilic. Heavy metal stains are useful to demonstrate the dendritic processes and vascular foot-plates that characterize these cells (Fig. 10-39). The astrocytes provide structural support to the retina and optic nerve and also contribute to the nourishment of the neuron as an intermediary of metabolism. The foot processes of the astrocytes ensheathe the blood vessels within the nerve and form a barrier between the nerve fibers and the vessels.[32] This barrier plays a large role in regulation of fluid exchange between the nervous compartments and the vascular compartments, contributing at least in part to the blood-brain (blood-optic or blood-retinal) barrier.[6,25,32]

Oligodendroglial cells elaborate the myelin sheaths of the axons. These cells grow into the nerve from the brain before and at the time of birth. The oligodendroglia are analogous to the Schwann cells of the peripheral nervous system, which similarly manufacture myelin. The nuclei of the oligodendroglia are smaller and more intensely basophilic by hematoxylin and eosin staining than are the nuclei of astrocytes. Oligodendroglia are located almost exclusively posterior to the lamina cribrosa; therefore, typically no myelin forms anterior to the lamina or within the retina.

Oligodendroglia in front of the lamina and in the retina occur only when there are myelinated (medullated) retinal nerve fibers (Fig. 10-11). Medullated nerve fibers in the retina appear as conspicuous, white, shiny, feathery, or flame-like projections from the papilla. They are sometimes of clinical importance in that they create an enlargement of the blind spot by covering over the peripapillary photoreceptors.

The individual optic nerve axons are most readily demonstrated by electron microscopy (Fig. 10-5) or by heavy-metal stains such as the gold and silver stains of the classic Cajal and Hortega methods. Myelin is a lipid-rich chemical most visible in sections stained specifically for lipids. After routine paraffin embedding and hematoxylin and eosin staining, it is not demonstrable because the lipid material is extracted during technical processing; therefore, in routine stains a large part of the optic nerve is normally unstained. The resultant foamy or spongy appearance is characteristic of the normal optic nerve. Loss of the spongy appearance signifies a loss of myelin and possible optic atrophy (Figs. 10-25–10-30).

The third type of glial cell, the microglial cell, is the primary phagocyte or macrophage of the central nervous system. They are significant and increase in number only during pathologic insult to the optic nerve or retina.[29,30]

Hayreh[16,17] has shown that with the exception of the superficial nerve fiber layer of the optic disc, which receives most of its supply from retinal arterioles, the major blood supply to the disc in the prelaminar, lamina cribrosa, and retrolaminar regions is derived from the ciliary vascular system through the choroid and posterior ciliary arteries (Fig. 10-9).

Usually two posterior ciliary arteries (also designated long posterior ciliary arteries) arise from the ophthalmic artery and supply the choroid and optic nerve head. Smaller divisions of the main posterior and short posterior ciliary arteries supply smaller sectors.

Although the surface nerve fiber layer is supplied mainly

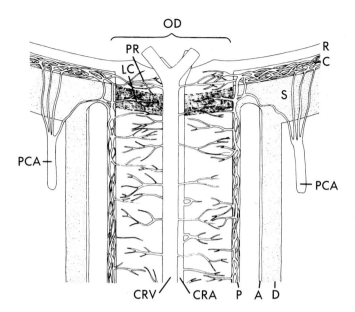

Fig. 10-9. Blood supply of the optic nerve. *A,* Arachnoid; *C,* choroid; *CRA,* central retinal artery; *CRV,* central retinal vein; *D,* dura; *LC,* lamina cribrosa; *OD,* optic disc; *P,* pia; *PCA,* posterior ciliary artery; *PR,* prelaminar region; *R,* retina; *S,* sclera. (Redrawn by Dr. Steven Vermillion, University of Iowa, from Hayreh SS: Anterior ischemic optic neuropathy, New York, 1975, Springer-Verlag.)

by branches of the retinal arterioles, it is not uncommon to also find vessels of choroidal origin derived from the adjacent prelaminar part of the disc in this layer. These vessels occur most often in the temporal sector of the disc, and one may enlarge to form a cilioretinal artery (Fig. 8-41).

The prelaminar region is supplied mainly by centripetal branches from the peripapillary prechoriocapillaris choroidal vessels, with no communication between the capillaries in the optic nerve head and peripapillary choriocapillaris. The temporal part of this region is the most vascular and receives maximum contribution from the adjacent peripapillary choroid. The central retinal artery does not contribute branches to this region.

Centripetal branches from the short posterior ciliary arteries and, in a few cases, by the so-called circle of Zinn and Haller, supply the lamina cribrosa region in its entirety. A typical well-formed circle of Zinn-Haller is uncommon and, when present, is often an incomplete circle. The blood vessels lie in the fibrous pleural septa and form a dense capillary plexus. The central retinal artery gives no branch in this region.

The retrolaminar region of the optic nerve is supplied mainly by centripetal branches from the pial vessels, which most often are recurrent pial branches from the peripapillary choroid, although some are from the circle of Zinn-Haller (or usually its substitute, that is, direct branches from the short posterior ciliary arteries). Although in 75% of optic nerves the central retinal artery gives out centrifugal branches during its intraneural course in the optic nerve, in many instances there may be no branch from the artery in the region immediately behind the lamina cribrosa. In such cases the pial supply from the posterior ciliary arteries may be the only or the major source of blood to the retrolaminar region.

Posteriorly the central retinal artery and the ophthalmic artery send small branches directly into the substance of the nerve.

Developmental abnormalities

The optic disc is the principal site of many congenital diseases. Colobomas, optic pits, disc changes in hyperopia and myopia, tilted disc syndromes, and morning glory syndrome are discussed in Chapter 2. Congenital hamartomas and tumors of the optic nerve are described with the phakomatoses (pp. 505).° Anomalies affecting the optic nerve are usually clinically innocuous; however, they can sometimes cause significant symptoms and lead to visual loss.[34-146] Recognition of even the relatively benign lesions is important, because the physician must differentiate them from other, more threatening lesions or disease processes that they may clinically resemble. Both anomalous development and damage to the optic nerve produce clinical signs that are evident by ophthalmoscopy, fluorescein angiography, and perimetry, and the appearance of the disc has become a major criterion in the diagnosis of many diseases, particularly glaucoma. A knowledge of the appearance of the normal disc and an appreciation of its anomalies are especially required to distinguish between the healthy and the glaucomatous eye.† There are a number of anomalies that may be confused with glaucomatous disc changes. Some anomalies may cause various types of visual field loss, which, if the actual optic disc lesion is not recognized, may lead to unnecessary neurologic evaluation or even to intracranial surgery.[121]

PHYSIOLOGIC VARIATIONS IN SIZE AND SHAPE

Minor congenital malformations in shape, such as oval (vertically, horizontally, or obliquely) elongated discs, are common and, in the absence of other anomalies such as coloboma, coni, or myopic changes are of little clinical significance.‡

For years, investigators have devised various classifications based on the ophthalmoscopic appearance of the optic nerve head as a means of making comparisons between normal and pathologic discs. In 1900 Elschnig[56] provided one of the first clinical classifications defining the various types of physiologic excavations (Table 10-1). This classification is interesting for historic reasons, and it forms the basis for the important, well-known criteria used today in judging the status of the optic nerve head—for example, cup-disc ratios, size and shape of the cup, and presence or absence of a conus. Since most clinicians have developed their own systems of disc evaluation, a detailed discussion of formal clinical classifications is not included in this section; however, excellent classifications and descriptions of the normal optic nerve head have been published by Armaly,[36] Ford and Sarwar,[58] Hayreh,[71] Snydacker,[132] and Tomlinson and Phillips.[137] Numerous normal variants and transitional forms are intermediate between the major nor-

Table 10-1. Summary of Elschnig's classification of optic nerve cupping

Category	Description
Type I	Small cup with a cup-disc ratio of 0.2. The lamina cribosa is usually not visible and no conus is present.
Type II	Cylindrical cup with a cup-disc ratio usually less than 0.5. The nasal wall is usually steeper than the temporal, and the lamina cribosa is often visible. Usually no conus is present
Type III	The cup is usually disc- or bowl-shaped with a cup-disc ratio of 0.5–0.6. The nasal wall is steeper and the lamina cribosa is usually visible. Conus formation is variable; often none is present
Type IV	The cup usually shows a gradually sloping temporal wall, producing a −cup-disc ratio of 0.5 or greater. A conus is almost always present. The vessel are usually displaced nasally.
Type V	Anomalous cups: the cup is usually directed toward the greatest width of associated conus, if present; the central vessels are often anomalous, e.g., situs inversus

Modified from Elschnig A: Graefes Arch Ophthalmol. 51:391, 1900; from Apple DJ, Rabb MF, and Walsh PM: Surv Ophthalmol 27(1):3, 1982.

mal types described in any formal classification, and these can cause difficulty in interpretation.[87]

Congenital "excavation" of the optic disc is an exaggeration of the physiologic cup. The degree of excavation depends on the space available in the optic foramen, in the sclera, and partly on the degree of atrophy of the tissues of Bergmeister's papilla (p. 30; Figs. 2-27, 2-28, and 10-1). The more glial tissue that is resorbed, the deeper the physiologic cup. A small central depression is the rule, frequently allowing the stippling of the lamina cribosa to be seen on its floor, but occasionally this tendency is increased to form a physiologic cup of great size and depth, which ophthalmoscopically may resemble a coloboma of the nerve head or a glaucomatous excavation. The differential diagnosis between physiologic and pathologic cupping rests with the fact that in the former the cup usually does not extend as far as the periphery and, therefore, leaves a healthy-appearing rim. In a glaucomatous cup the excavation may extend to the disc edge.

Pseudoneuritis, or pseudopapilledema, is the opposite of congenital excavation; the cup is shallow, or the anterior surface may be bowed forward (p. 537). Some cases may result from the relative persistence of the glial elements of Bergmeister's papilla. The major importance of this nonprogressive lesion is in the differential diagnosis of papilledema and optic neuritis. Congenital inferior crescents and acquired temporal crescents (often seen in myopia) are considered on page 41.

APLASIA

Aplasia is a rare anomaly characterized clinically by a totally blind eye with an afferent pupillary defect, an absent disc, and an absent retinal vasculature.° Meissner[96] (1911)

° References 35, 39, 42, 60, 64, 68, 86, 92, 103, 106.
† References 36, 48-52, 58, 64, 71, 85, 87, 99, 117-119, 132, 148.
‡ References 35, 36, 56, 64, 96, 129.

° References 63, 65, 88, 96, 125, 142.

was one of the first to document the microscopic appearance of this condition.

HYPOPLASIA

Hypoplasia (Fig. 10-10) is relatively rare° but has been investigated thoroughly in recent literature because of important intracranial anomalies that often accompany it. Zion's tabulation[146] of 104 cases of disc hypoplasia revealed that hypoplasia usually is sporadic; familial transmission is rare. He noted a bilateral-unilateral ratio of approximately 1.5:1 and a significant predilection for males, with no racial bias, for this anomaly. The affected eye may be microphthalmic or of normal size and usually exhibits a spectrum of visual impairment ranging from normal vision to severe visual loss with strabismus or nystagmus in bilateral cases.[41,61,112] The disc is usually gray, is one third to one half of normal size, and can be confused with optic atrophy. This disc is often surrounded by a peripapillary halo, the so-called double-ring sign. Radiographic examination often demonstrates size disparity of the optic foramina in unilateral cases.

Several intracranial and facial anomalies, often in midline structures, have been reported in association with optic nerve hypoplasia. These include septooptic dysplasia, congenital hypopituitarism, hydranencephaly, arrhinencephaly, aniridia, homonymous hemioptic hypoplasia associated with congenital hemispheric aplasia, cyclopia, orbital encephalomeningocele, and hypotelorism.†

VASCULAR REMNANTS

Anomalies resulting from persistence of the embryonic disc vessels are considered in Chapter 2. Persistence of Bergmeister's papilla and the hyaloid artery, anomalous distribution of the central retinal vessels, epipapillary vascular loops, abnormal chorioretinal anastomoses, and epipapillary membranes fall into this category.

MEDULLATED (MYELINATED) RETINAL NERVE FIBERS

Medullation, or myelination, of the optic nerve (Fig. 10-11; Color Plate 10-1) begins during fetal life and progresses from the lateral geniculate body toward the globe. Thus, the optic tracts are the first portions of the visual pathway to be ensheathed by myelin; the chiasm and the optic nerve are the last portions to be myelinated. Normally myelination is completed shortly after birth, at which time the myelin sheaths extend to the posterior aspect of the lamina cribrosa.

Myelination of nerve fibers of the peripapillary retina occurs in approximately 0.3% to 1.0% of individuals as a developmental variation.[1,27,40,91,134-136] This anomaly is twice as common in males as in females and is unilateral in 80% of the cases. A familial tendency occurs occasionally. This anomaly is usually easily differentiated from intraocular neoplasms or remnants of Bergmeister's papilla. Because the superficial retina is opacified by these fibers, a scotoma subtends the affected area.

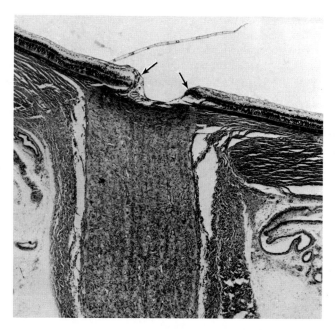

Fig. 10-10. Optic nerve hypoplasia. Retinal ganglion cells and the nerve fiber layer are absent, and there is no passage of axons from the retina into the nerve *(arrows)*, (compare with Figs. 6-34, *B*, and 10-2). The retina often partially overlies the nerve head in optic nerve hypoplasia. This is particularly prominent on the left side in this case. The optic nerve parenchyma contains myriad, diffuse arrays of glial nuclei rather than ordered, vertical columns. The retrolaminar nerve is not thicker than the anterior portion because there is no myelin. (H & E stain; ×90.)

Affected eyes are usually otherwise normal in structure and function; however, variably decreased visual acuity, visual field defects, amblyopia, strabismus, and nystagmus have been associated with extensive medullation of retinal nerve fibers. Myopia accompanies the condition in up to 50% of cases.[134] Coloboma, polycoria, keratoconus, oxycephaly, and neurofibromatosis have been reported with medullated fibers. Figure 10-11 shows the typical clinical appearance of medullated retinal nerve fibers. In most cases the macula is uninvolved.

Myelin[91] is a product of oligodendroglial cells, which normally are present only in the myelinated portion of the nerve, that is, behind the lamina cribrosa. Predictably, however, in cases of medullated nerve fibers these glial cells are present in the involved regions of the optic nerve head and retina. The medullated fibers are demonstrated well histopathologically by specific special stains for myelin (Table 1-1).

DRUSEN

Drusen of the optic disc were first described clinically by Liebreich in 1868.[86] Lorentzen[89] reported an incidence of optic disc drusen of 0.75 per 1000 in a clinical study of 3200 people. Other terms for drusen include *hyaline bodies* and *colloid bodies* of the optic disc.

The deposition of a hyaline-like, calcified material within the substance of the nerve head° (Fig. 10-12; Color Plates

---

° References 45, 72, 116, 119, 121.

† References 34, 37, 38, 41, 44, 49, 61, 63, 66, 67, 72-75, 82, 83, 93, 94, 97, 102, 122, 128.

° References 35, 46, 47, 59, 60, 70, 79, 81, 89, 95, 106, 110, 113-115, 120, 133, 145, 285.

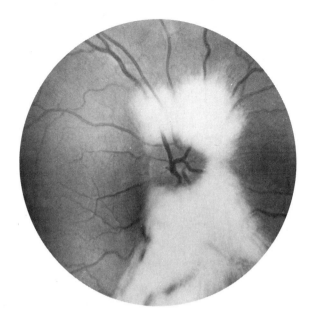

A

B

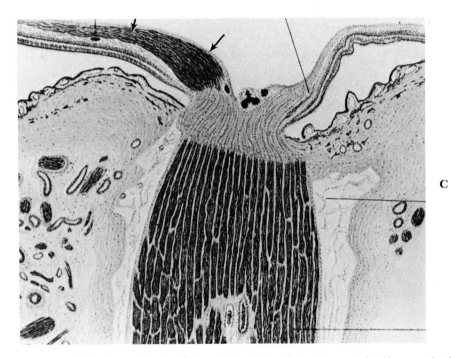

C

Fig. 10-11. Medullated retinal nerve fibers. **A,** Small focus located superiorly. The superficial fibers cover the retinal vessels. **B,** More extensive medullated (myelinated) retinal nerve fibers. A "feathery" border separates the white myelinated area from the normal retina. **C,** Reproduction of a preparation of J von Michel (1878) showing histopathologic features of medullated retinal nerve fibers *(arrows).* This Weigert preparation stains myelin black. The retrolaminar myelin is normal. Lipid-rich erythrocytes and intramural lipids in posterior ciliary vessels also stain positively. (From Schieck F: In Henke F and Lubarsch O, editors: Handbuch der speziellen pathologischen Anatomie und Histologie, Berlin, 1928, Julius Springer.)

10-2 and 10-3) may lead to an enlargement and prominence of the disc that can be mistaken for papilledema. This is especially true in cases in which the deposits are situated deeply (Fig. 10-12, *B*). Such "buried drusen" are sometimes difficult to diagnose by ophthalmoscopy. Although drusen of the retinal pigment epithelium and of the optic nerve have the same name, they differ in cause and structure. Drusen that are products of pigment epithelium differ in cause and structure. Drusen, which are products of pigment epithelium, form excrescences on Bruch's membrane. Optic disc drusen can be divided into three main groups[51]:

1. Idiopathic cases in otherwise normal eyes, sometimes showing an autosomal-dominant transmission[57]
2. Cases associated with acquired diseases of the globe or optic nerve, including hypertensive retinopathy, vascular occlusions, chorioretinitis, papillitis, optic atrophy, long-standing glaucoma, angioid streaks, chronic papilledema, and old injuries
3. Cases associated with heredodegenerative affections, such as retinitis pigmentosa (p. 402)

Although rarely seen in early childhood, some optic nerve drusen may be present at birth and become clinically apparent in later life as they enlarge and encroach on the disc surface. Examination of the discs of family members is warranted in doubtful cases. Approximately 75% of ophthalmoscopically visible drusen are bilateral. Drusen and the myriad ocular and neurologic disorders described in association with them have no consistent relationship. No relationship to refractive error has been shown. For the most part, white children are affected; disc drusen are rarely seen in black and Oriental persons.

Clinical examination frequently reveals an irregular, nodular, mulberrylike appearance of the surface of the disc.

The physiologic cup may be absent, but a venous pulse is usually seen. The vessels are usually unobscured and course from the central apex of the disc. Drusen normally do not cause venous and capillary dilatation or exudates. Disc hemorrhages and peripapillary subretinal neovascularization occur in a small percentage of cases; however, there may be an abnormally large number of tortuous, anomalously branching vessels.[70] These tortuous vessels may be of some importance in pathogenesis.[123,139] Aberrant axoplasmic transport through optic nerve axons may also be a cause. A summary of the literature on this topic has been provided by Spencer.[133]

The disc itself does not usually show pallor but may have an irregular margin. Many drusen (90%) exhibit autofluorescence.[42] Sometimes they can be differentiated from papilledema by fluorescein angiography. High-definition computed tomography (CT) scanning may be useful in detecting buried drusen.[62]

Histopathologically, disc drusen are composed of concentric laminations with no cellular structure or capsule. They frequently become calcified (Fig. 10-12, *B*). Clinically unrecognized drusen sometimes are found incidentally in tissue sections.

Drusen may persist for years with little change and, in general, if they are situated superficially, are less likely to cause significant symptoms. If they lie deeply in the sclerochoroidal canal, however, they may produce a pressure atrophy of the contiguous nerve fibers with resultant changes in the visual fields. Central visual acuity is usually unaffected.

Although similar in clinical appearance, the simple optic nerve drusen described here differ from the optic disc lesions observed in patients with tuberous sclerosis or neurofibromatosis. Simple drusen of the disc represent a devel-

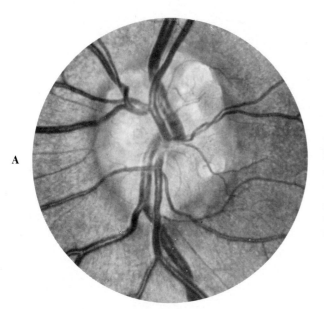
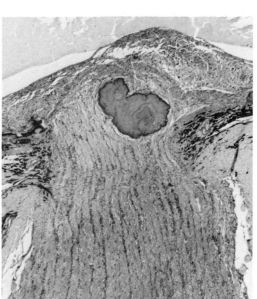

Fig. 10-12. A, Drusen of optic nerve head in an otherwise healthy individual. The optic disc is elevated, the borders are irregular, and it appears lobulated and glistening because of calcification. **B,** Optic disc drusen in an eye enucleated for other causes. A solitary, laminated calcified focus is present centrally. (H & E stain; ×90.)

opmental or degenerative process in which a "hyaline" material of unknown nature is deposited in the nerve. The lesion of tuberous sclerosis (which often resembles a mulberry, tapioca, or salmon eggs) is a true harmartomatous proliferation of astroglia. Both types of drusen frequently undergo secondary calcification and, in long-standing cases, can be difficult to differentiate, even at the microscopic level.

CONGENITAL AND HEREDITARY OPTIC ATROPHY

Hereditary retinal and optic atrophy is classified according to pattern of inheritance, age of onset, severity of symptoms, and presence or absence of associated hereditary and neurologic abnormalities:*

A. Usually unassociated with other known anomalies
   1. Congenital or infantile hereditary optic atrophy
      a. Recessive
      b. Dominant
   2. Juvenile hereditary optic atrophy
      a. Recessive
      b. Dominant
   3. Leber's optic atrophy of unclarified heredity (sometimes with other anomalies); not to be confused with Leber's congenital amaurosis of retinal origin.†
B. Associated with other hereditary neurologic anomalies
   1. Infantile recessive optic atrophy of Behr
   2. With hereditary cerebellar ataxia's
      a. Marie's ataxia (optic atrophy common)
      b. Friedreichs' ataxia (optic atrophy rare)
   3. Familial spastic paraplegia
   4. Lipidosis (cerebromacular degeneration)
C. Associated with the hereditary craniostenosis
   1. Osteopetrosis
   2. Oxycephaly

Details of congenital and hereditary optic atrophy are reviewed by Caldwell, Howard, and Riggs.[45] The cause of these conditions remains uncertain, and pathologic reports detailing the early stages of the disease are unavailable. The basic lesion is a primary destruction of retinal and optic nerve fibers and their cell bodies (the retinal ganglion cells), but no firm clues to pathogenesis have been derived from pathologic studies.

Papilledema

Papilledema is a swelling of the optic nerve head caused by a variety of disorders, occurring without primary inflammatory changes and often, at least in the earliest stages, without disturbance of function.[147-187] Papillitis (optic neuritis) indicates an inflammatory swelling of the nerve head, usually associated with functional loss.[161] It is often impossible to differentiate the two ophthalmoscopically. In both conditions there is a disc swelling, which manifests itself as a prominent nerve head with blurred margins, an apparent increased disc diameter, and varying amounts of hemorrhage. In optic neuritis there is usually profound loss of vision, often disproportionately severe. Dense central scotomas are also present. Papilledema is most commonly

bilateral; optic neuritis is usually unilateral. The terms *pseudopapilledema* and *pseudoneuritis* refer to ophthalmoscopic pictures, which must be considered in the differential diagnosis of papilledema.[175]

CLINICAL SYMPTOMS AND SIGNS

In contrast to optic neuritis, papilledema is usually not associated with severely impaired visual acuity. Sometimes, however, premonitory transient attacks of blurred vision may occur. There is gradual concentric enlargement of the blind spot because of an increase in size of the edematous nerve head and lateral displacement of the retina. Following are the main ophthalmoscopic criteria of fully developed papilledema (Fig. 10-13; Color Plate 10-4)[122,161]:

1. Increase in disc diameter; formation of Paton's concentric lines
2. Indistinctness and blurring of the disc margins
3. Elevation of the disc and mushrooming of the nerve head into the vitreous (the disc tissues often lose their transparency and become increasingly opaque)
4. Reddish discoloration of the disc (capillary stasis)
5. Venous congestion and tortuosity of the veins, with relatively normal arteries (increase of ratio in caliber of veins and arteries); optociliary shunt formation[152]
6. Deflection of the vessels over the disc margin
7. Hemorrhages at the disc margin and within the disc
8. White exudates and cytoid body formation over the surface and at the margin of the disc
9. No primary disturbances of sensory function initially

A papilledema may fully resolve if the underlying cause is corrected early enough, but sooner or later any persistent papilledema leads to a secondary optic atrophy. The time required for the progression of a severe, fully developed papilledema to complete atrophy is variable but can range from 6 to 9 months, occasionally up to more than a year.[161]

The most common cause of papilledema is increased intracranial pressure. An impairment of the return flow

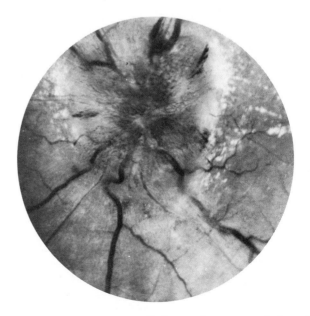

Fig. 10-13. More severe papilledema with prominent "splinter" hemorrhages.

---

* References 45, 55, 78, 116, 131, 138, 141.
† References 54, 76, 77, 80, 90, 100, 104, 105, 108, 109, 111, 127, 259.

of venous blood from the optic nerve as a result of increased intracranial pressure or other causes plays a major role.[157-159,161,182,183] Interruption of axoplasmic flow, which normally occurs from the retina into the disc and optic nerve, may cause axonal swelling.*

The lamina cribrosa separates the optic nerve into its intraocular and retroocular portions. This anatomic subdivision is of physiologic significance, because under normal circumstances the tissue pressure within the intraocular portion of the optic nerve is much higher than that posterior to the lamina. This normal pressure gradient at the level of the lamina reflects the influence of the intraocular pressure, which exceeds the cerebrospinal fluid pressure. Lowering the tissue pressure in the prelaminar area or elevating the pressure in the retrolaminar area of the optic nerve disrupts axoplasmic flow gradients and results in disc swelling. Not all cases may be explained this easily. Edema of the disc may occur when prelaminar tension is abruptly *elevated* in acute glaucoma; therefore, other factors must be considered.

The majority of cases of passive swelling of the optic disc may be, therefore, classified as (1) prelaminar (intraocular) or (2) retrolaminar (resulting from intraorbital, intracranial, or spinal cord disease):

I. Prelaminar (usually unilateral papilledema), caused by intraocular disease
   A. Hypotony
      1. External fistula, for example, trauma
      2. Inflammations, for example, uveitis
      3. Retinal detachment
   B. Acute glaucoma
   C. Local and systemic vascular disease[154,162]
      1. Malignant hypertension
      2. Venous stasis and hemorrhagic retinopathy (occlusion of the central retinal vein)
      3. Anterior ischemic optic neuropathy
      4. Collagen diseases
         a. Sarcoid
         b. Giant cell arteritis
         c. Lupus erythematosus
         d. Polyarteritis nodosa
      5. Hematologic disorders
         a. Anemia
         b. Polycythemia vera
         c. Leukemia
         d. Macroglobulinemia
      6. Cardiopulmonary diseases
         a. Emphysema
         b. Congenital heart defects. Cystic fibrosis
II. Retrolaminar (usually bilateral papilledema), caused by intraorbital, intracranial, or spinal cord disease
   A. Tumor or pseudotumor or endocrine ophthalmopathy
      1. Increased intracranial pressure secondary to space-occupying lesions
      2. Inflammations (meningitis, encephalitis, abscess)
      3. Increased viscosity of the cerebrospinal fluid
      4. Trauma with meningeal or intracerebral hemorrhage

      5. Vascular lesions or malformations (e.g., aneurysms)
   B. Internal hydrocephalus (idiopathic)
      1. Secondary to decreased volume of intracranial space (craniostosis, oxycephaly, Crouzon's disease, Paget's disease)
   C. Pseudotumor cerebri (papilledema with idiopathic increase in intracranial pressure)[148]

PRELAMINAR (INTRAOCULAR) DISEASE

Hypotony

A sudden lowering of the intraocular pressure is commonly followed by disc edema. The papilledema of hypotony is clinically and histologically indistinguishable from that associated with other disease processes. It often follows ocular inflammation or is caused by accidental or surgical trauma, particularly when a fistula is created. Ocular hypotony apparently not only lowers the prelaminar tissue pressure but also slows axoplasmic transport.[170] The effects of stagnation of the axoplasm are most significant in the prelaminar area, where focally distended axons contain prominent accumulations of mitochondria. This axonal distention secondary to obstruction of axoplasmic transport increases the volume of the optic disc and leads to the clinical and histologic features that characterize papilledema.

Acute increase in intraocular pressure

Edema of the optic disc may occur as part of the generalized edema that affects the ocular tissues when the tension of the eye is acutely raised, for example, in an acute attack of angle-closure glaucoma. This may be a result of obliteration of the peripapillary vessels by the rise in pressure, which produces congestion and hypoxia.

Intraocular effects of local or systemic disease

The local and systemic vascular or pulmonary diseases that produce papilledema are listed in the preceding outline.[166] Venous stasis retinopathy (occlusion of the central retinal vein; p. 390) and hypertensive retinopathy (p. 370) are the most important diseases in this group. Papilledema in patients with malignant systemic hypertension is one of the most important entities to be considered in the differential diagnosis of a swollen disc. This may be confused with edema resulting from increased intracranial pressure, because both are usually bilateral.

RETROLAMINAR (INTRAORBITAL, INTRACRANIAL, OR SPINAL CORD) DISEASE

Although there are many etiologic factors of increased intracranial pressure and papilledema, tumors of the brain are the most common cause in 75% to 80% of cases.[161,165] According to Huber and Blodi,[161] the presence of bilateral papilledema is pathognomonic for increased intracranial pressure, if an ocular or orbital factor can be ruled out.

Modern diagnostic methods have advanced to the point that recognition of increased intracranial pressure, and its cause and therapy, is usually made well before papilledema appears. As a result, papilledema is becoming a less common initial finding of increased intracranial pressure. A relatively early onset of papilledema can be expected, how-

---

*References 149-151, 155, 156, 164, 167-170, 172, 174, 180.

ever, from lesions that interfere with the circulation of the cerebrospinal fluid, producing an internal hydrocephalus. Thus, tumors arising in the posterior fossa are more likely to produce papilledema because of early encroachment on the cerebral aqueduct and fourth ventricle, after which internal hydrocephalus and papilledema rapidly develop. Papilledema resulting from tumors occurs frequently in children because of the special character of infantile cerebral tumors. These tumors are often rapid growing and infratentorial, with early blockage of cerebrospinal fluid circulation.

Unilateral papilledema is rare and usually results from localized ocular or orbital causes. A unilateral papilledema in cases of increased intracranial pressure can be explained only by noting the presence of other local factors, such as unilateral optic atrophy, which prevents the increased intracranial pressure from producing swelling of the disc on the corresponding side. An atrophic optic nerve is incapable of developing a papilledema. This explains why pituitary tumors, which commonly produce optic atrophy by direct pressure on the nerve, usually do not cause papilledema, even though there might be a large, space-occupying lesion.

The Foster Kennedy syndrome (Fig. 10-28) connotes unilateral optic atrophy on the side of a tumor (caused by direct pressure on the intracranial part of the optic nerve) and a papilledema on the opposite side. This form of Kennedy syndrome was thought to be tumor induced. It is now believed that the primary process in many instances is actually an anterior ischemic optic neuropathy (p. 544), in which a previously involved atrophic optic nerve in one eye is associated with an acutely swollen acute lesion in the opposite eye. Myopia is a second example of a factor that may retard the development of papilledema in cases of increased intracranial pressure. The anatomic characteristics of a myopic optic nerve head (p. 37) are such that papilledema will not develop despite increased intracranial pressure. A unilateral myopic disc may, therefore, be associated with a contralateral papilledema; papilledema rarely occurs in bilaterally severely myopic globes.

Although papilledema and increased cerebrospinal fluid pressure usually have an expanding intracranial mass as the common denominator, there are occasionally cases in which neither mass nor specific cause can be found.[153] This entity, called pseudotumor cerebri, is characterized by bilateral elevation of the disc and negative findings during neurologic examination. Except for the unexplainable pressure increase (Fig. 10-14), the ventricular system is anatomically normal, and the composition of the cerebrospinal fluid is normal. This disease occurs in young to middle-aged adults and generally has a good prognosis. According to Huber and Blodi,[161] the pathogenesis of the syndrome is either a hypersecretion or an obstruction of resorption of cerebrospinal fluid.

HISTOPATHOLOGIC FINDINGS[161,169,170,173,181,184,187]

Permeation of transudate occurs within the optic nerve head axons themselves and extracellularly within the interstitial spaces between axons (Figs. 10-15 and 10-16). The nonmyelinated axons are widely separated from each other by edema fluid. Because of alterations in axoplasmic flow,

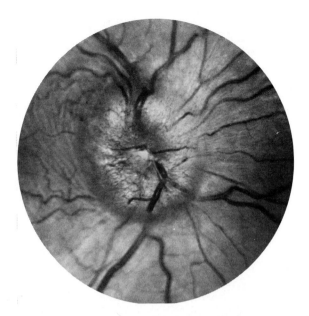

Fig. 10-14. Pseudotumor cerebri in a case of benign intracranial hypertension. Despite the papilledema-like appearance seen in this young woman, extensive systemic and neurologic findings were otherwise negative.

mitochondria and fluids accumulate in the swollen axons anterior to the lamina cribrosa.[169,170,185]

Often an anterior bowing of the lamina cribrosa forms an anterior convexity. The normal lamina shows a slight posterior bowing, a feature that is greatly exaggerated in glaucomatous optic atrophy. The anterior mushroomlike protrusion of disc tissue may cause a shallowing of the physiologic optic cup.

The fluid deposits can cause a displacement of the sensory retina away from the outer edge of the disc (hence the enlarged blind spot).[176] The outer layers of the retina are buckled or folded. These folds are recognized ophthalmoscopically as arcuate stripes concentric with the disc (Paton's concentric lines). The peripapillary retina may be slightly detached from the pigment epithelium by fluid effusion—an additional contribution to the enlargement of the blind spot (Fig. 10-16, *B*). The subarachnoid space of the optic nerve may contain edema fluid.

The veins and capillaries in the area of the disc are markedly dilated. Hemorrhages on the disc or at the margin appear predominantly in the nerve fiber layer. Ophthalmoscopically, these produce the flame-shaped configuration (Fig. 10-15).

The nerve fibers show characteristic changes as a result of the edema and stagnation of axoplasmic flow. The edema and subsequent atrophy first involve the periphery of the optic nerve and gradually progress toward the axial area. This process has its functional equivalent in the progressive concentric constriction of the visual field. With papilledema of long duration the nerve fibers develop varicosities or cytoid bodies (Fig. 8-18, *B* and *C*) and undergo degeneration leading to secondary optic atrophy. In the final stages of chronic papilledema there is an ascending and descending degeneration and microglial phagocytosis of the nerve fibers with associated glial proliferation.[161] Ophthalmo-

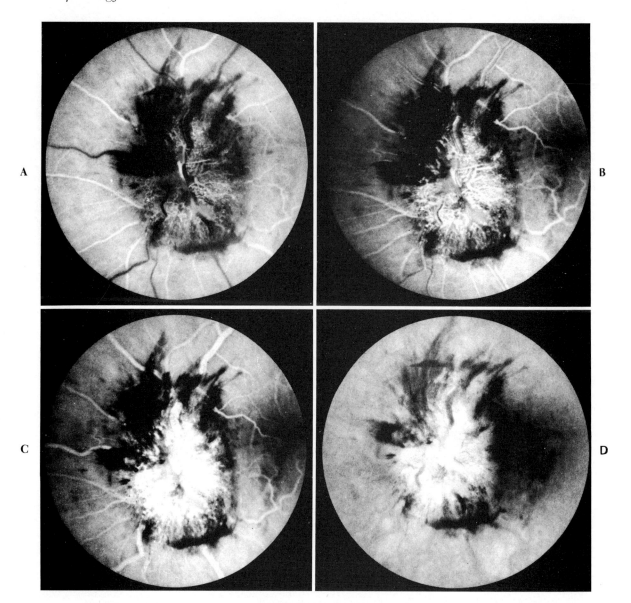

Fig. 10-15. Fluorescein angiograph in papilledema. **A,** Arterial phase, 16 seconds. Noteworthy is the dense network of vessels on the optic nerve head. The hemorrhages in the upper temporal quadrant obscure observation of the deeper structures. **B,** The retinal veins show laminar flow at 19 seconds, and the vascular network on the disc is even more visible. **C,** Full arteriovenous phase, 26 seconds. The disc acquires a diffuse glow because of permeation of extravasated transudates. **D,** Diffuse staining of the optic nerve head 7 1/2 minutes after injection, as the dye penetrates the tissues. Only the large vessels and the dense hemorrhages on the disc obscure the fluorescence. (From Blodi FC, Allen L, and Frazier O: Stereoscopic manual of the ocular fundus in local and systemic disease, vol II, St. Louis, 1970, The CV Mosby Co.)

scopically, this corresponds to the grayish-white discoloration of the disc.

DIFFERENTIAL DIAGNOSIS

The following lesions, which cause an elevation of the nerve head clinically mimicking a papilledema (pseudopapilledema), are individually described in this and other chapters[160,161,175,184]:

1. Papillitis optic neuritis
2. Pseudotumor cerebri or benign intracranial hypertension
3. Proliferation of epipapillary fibrous tissue (epipapillary membranes), persistence of Bergmeister's papilla (Chapter 2)
4. Hyperopia (Chapter 2)
5. Drusen of the optic disc
6. Medullated retinal nerve fibers
7. Epipapillary hamartomas and tumors (Chapter 9)

Unfortunately, these lesions, many of which are harmless congenital anomalies, are sometimes misdiagnosed. The suspicion of a brain tumor may lead to unnecessary and unjustified diagnostic procedures and even neurosurgical intervention.

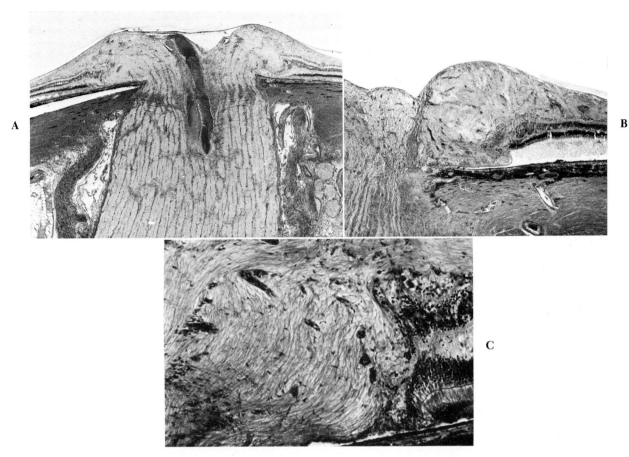

Fig. 10-16. Histopathologic features of papilledema. **A,** Low-power micrograph showing disc elevation but retention of the physiologic cup. (H & E stain; ×90.) **B,** Another case showing marked bulging of the nerve fiber bundles as they course from the nerve. The peripapillary retina is slightly detached *(right)*. (H & E stain; ×125.) **C,** High-power micrograph demonstrating marked separation of nerve fibers by interstitial edema. The retina *(right)* is distorted and pushed toward the right by the bulging, edematous peripapillary nerve fiber layer. (H & E stain; ×250.) (**B** from Naumann GOH and Apple DJ: In Doerr W, Seifert G, and Uehlinger E, editors: Handbuch der speziellen pathologischen Anatomie, Band Auge, Berlin, 1980, Springer-Verlag.)

Optic neuritis and postneuritic atrophy

The term *optic neuritis (papillitis)* signifies an optic nerve disease that hinders nerve conductivity (papillitis) producing decreased visual acuity and changes in the field of vision (Figs. 10-17–10-30).[88-328] The term *neuritis* does not necessarily imply an inflammation.[288] Through common usage the term has come to include a diverse group of entities caused by (1) inflammation, (2) vascular disease, or (3) degeneration.

A. True inflammatory processes
  1. Direct spread from neighboring structures
    a. Perineuritis, meningitis, intraorbital and nasal sinus infections, cellulitis
    b. Intraocular processes: uveitis, retinitis, endophthalmitis, panophthalmitis, keratitis, sympathetic ophthalmia, sarcoidosis
  2. Infections of the brain substance (encephalitis)
    a. Bacterial infections (syphilis, tuberculosis, pyogenic infections)
    b. Viral infections[326]
    c. Fungal infections

B. Vascular disease (ischemic optic neuropathy)
  1. Stenosis or embolization of posterior ciliary arteries, ophthalmic artery, or carotid artery
    a. Arteriosclerosis
    b. Giant cell arteritis
    c. Pulseless disease (Takayasu's disease)
    d. Hypertension[254]
    e. Diabetes
    f. Collagen diseases
    g. Vasculitis and thrombophlebitis[197-251]
    h. Raynaud's disease
  2. Elevated intraocular pressure (imbalance between perfusion pressure in the posterior ciliary arteries and the intraocular pressure)
  3. Systemic arterial hypotension
    a. Shock
    b. Myocardial infarction
  4. Hematologic disorders
    a. Polycythemia
    b. Sickle cell disease
    c. Thrombocytopenic purpura
    d. Leukemia

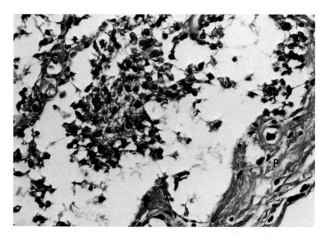

Fig. 10-17. Toxic optic neuritis. High-power photomicrograph of a sagittal section at the margin of an optic nerve. *P,* Pia mater. The optic nerve shows acute necrosis and degeneration after methyl alcohol ingestion. A significant loss of substance in the optic nerve parenchyma and pyknosis of virtually all cellular nuclei have occurred. (H & E stain; ×220.) (Courtesy Dr. Elizabeth Cheah.)

    5. Compression of optic nerve blood vessels
      a. Peripapillary malignant melanoma
      b. Glioma of the optic nerve
      c. Meningioma
      d. Orbital masses[298]
      e. Long-standing massive papilledema
      f. Drusen of the disc
C. Degenerative optic neuritis
    1. Demyelinating diseases
      a. Multiple sclerosis
      b. Acute disseminated encephalomyelitis
      c. Neuromyelitis optica of Devic
      d. Diffuse cerebral sclerosis of Schilder
    2. Toxic optic neuritis
      a. Tobacco, ethyl alcohol toxicity
      b. Methyl alcohol toxicity[201,239]
      c. Lead poisoning (plumbism)
      d. Medication toxicity[255]
    3. Systemic disease
      a. Sarcoidosis[202,214,232]
      b. Blood disorders
      c. Collagen diseases
      d. Endocrine (hyperthyroidism and diabetes mellitus)
      e. Malignant tumors
      f. Allergy
      g. Starvation (nutritional)

The disc in papillitis (or neuroretinitis when there is associated retinal involvement) becomes swollen and hyperemic, its vessels dilated and congested, and its margin blurred and indistinct.

The loss of vision is usually sudden in onset and is often accompanied by abnormal pupillary reactions, central scotomas, a lowering of dark adaptation, defects in color discrimination, and ocular pain that worsens with eye movements. These functional findings may precede significant observable disc changes. As a general rule, the symptoms

develop suddenly and last only 1 to 4 weeks; recovery may be complete. In cases in which the involvement of the nerve has been sufficiently severe to cause destruction of nerve fibers, some degree of degeneration follows, which in severe cases may result in an atrophy with a corresponding permanent visual defect.[227]

While the functional symptoms of papillitis are usually disproportionately greater than the disc changes would suggest, the reverse is true regarding papilledema. With papilledema there is usually only moderate visual impairment with an enlarged blind spot. In addition, ocular pain and tenderness are uncommon findings in papilledema. The differential diagnosis of pseudoneuritis and pseudopapilledema is discussed on page 540.

Papillitis signifies involvement of the optic disc; retrobulbar neuritis implies that the pathologic process has attacked a portion of the optic nerve behind the globe, sparing the intraocular segment. Although the optic disc is normal in appearance in retrobulbar neuritis, there is usually functional impairment resembling that of papillitis, which may be extremely profound.

In some cases the retrobulbar process may extend forward into the optic disc, producing a combined process.

Optic neuritis and atrophy can be classified according to the topographic location of the involvement within or around the nerve:

    1. Perineuritis: involvement of leptomeninges around the nerve, usually caused by extension from adjacent orbital or ocular structures
    2. Periaxial neuritis: involvement of the peripheral portions of the nerve, usually caused by spread from the leptomeninges
    3. Axial neuritis: involvement of the central portion of the optic nerve (Figs. 10-26, *A*, and 10-27)
    4. Transverse neuritis: characterized by a complete, massive cross-sectional destruction (Fig. 10-26, *B*)
    5. Patchy neuritis: random foci of the optic nerve involved, without specific topographic orientation

Although the ophthalmoscopic distinction between papillitis and retrobulbar neuritis and the anatomic or topographic histologic classifications are descriptively useful, they do not emphasize pathogenetic mechanisms. The classification on page 451 is based on pathogenesis and lends itself more to an understanding of the major disease mechanisms.

The general histopathology of optic neuritis varies widely because of the wide variety of causes, and the pathologic response depends on whether the cause is inflammatory (in which inflammatory cell infiltration predominates) (Fig. 10-18), ischemic (Figs. 10-19 to 10-25), or degenerative (Figs. 10-25–10-30). In long-standing progressive or untreated cases, however, all forms of optic neuritis can be expected to progress to optic atrophy the histopathologic features of which are described on page 548.

TRUE INFLAMMATORY PROCESSES

True inflammations of the optic nerve may be divided into two classes:

    1. Inflammation primarily within structures adjacent to the nerve, that is, within the meninges (perineuritis) or globe, which spreads secondarily into the optic nerve

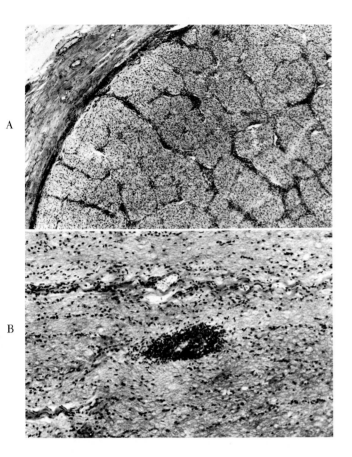

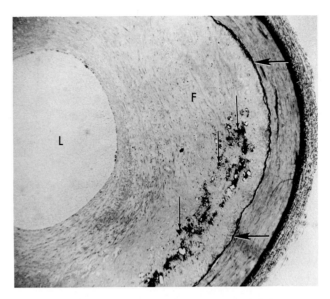

Fig. 10-19. Cross section of an atherosclerotic ophthalmic artery in a case of anterior ischemic optic neuropathy. This 37-year-old woman had long-standing diabetes mellitus. A thick, calcified fibrous plaque *(F)* has greatly compromised the vessel lumen *(L)*. *Small arrows,* Deeply staining calcium; *large arrows,* internal elastic lamina. (Verhoeff-van Gieson stain for elastic tissue, ×75.)

Fig. 10-18. Probable viral optic neuritis, associated with encephalitis. **A,** Diffuse permeation of peripheral optic nerve substance by lymphocytes. (H & E stain; ×20.) **B,** Focus of perivascular lymphocytic cuffing, characteristic of virus-induced inflammation. (H & E stain; ×180.) (From Naumann GOH and Apple DJ: In Doerr W, Seifert G, and Uehlinger E, editors: Handbuch der speziellen pathologischen Anatomie, Band Auge, Berlin, 1980, Springer-Verlag.)

2. Inflammation within the substance of the nerve itself (optic neuritis)

Perineuritis is an inflammation primarily involving the sheaths of the optic nerve, which frequently coexists with a periaxial neuritis or involvement of the periphery of the nerve itself. Orbital cellulitis resulting from sinusitis, trauma with the introduction of foreign bodies into the orbit, and extension of a viral encephalitis into the optic nerve sheaths and parenchyma (Fig. 10-18) are common causes of perineuritis. The pyogenic bacteria, tuberculosis bacillus, and fungi, particularly *Cryptococcus, Aspergillus,* and species of the order Mucoroles, are the most common infective agents.[280] The organisms or inflammatory infiltrates enter the substance of the nerve through the pial septa and vessels. Because the peripheral zone of the optic nerve is more intensely involved with relative sparing of the papillomacular bundle centrally, there may be considerable loss of the peripheral field but retention of central vision.

The presence of intraocular inflammation not uncommonly incites a reactive type of inflammatory response within the optic nerve. For example, inflammatory cell infiltration of the optic disc often accompanies many forms of anterior and posterior uveitis and endophthalmitis. Optic nerve involvement in sarcoidosis is well documented (see also p. 293).* Clinically the disc changes in endophthalmitis are seldom clearly seen because of the clouded media that accompany most cases of endophthalmitis of fungal or bacterial origin. On the other hand, in cases of focal toxoplasmic retinochoroiditis, which often causes only partial vitreal clouding, an inflammatory papillitis is frequently present. Toxoplasmosis (p. 395) is a particularly well-known cause of neuroretinitis. *Toxocara,* or nematode, endophthalmitis, better known as a cause of leukokoria (p. 492), may produce a neuroretinitis. Neuroretinitis is also common in Behçet's disease. Retinal vasculitis and necrosis combined with papillitis have been observed histologically and clinically. In some cases these inflamed vessels may eventually initiate new vessel formation emanating from the disc into the vitreous.

VASCULAR DISEASE

The vascular occlusive processes that produce optic nerve ischemia fall into two groups: vascular occlusion caused by noninflammatory degenerative changes in the vessels, the most important being arteriosclerosis (Fig. 10-19), and vascular occlusion caused by an inflammatory process, typified by temporal arteritis (Figs. 10-20 to 10-22, Color Plates 10-5 and 10-6).[212,233,240-245] Hayreh[194] summarizes the salient features of this subject. Although commonly classified as optic "neuritis," these are not true inflammations of the nerve and are properly termed *neuropathies.*

---

* References 202, 214, 232, 257, 265, 312.

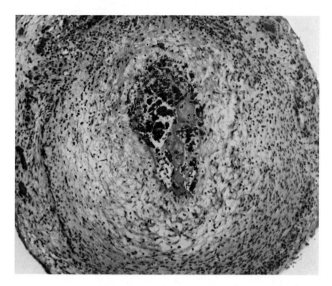

Fig. 10-20. Temporal (giant cell) arteritis. This temporal artery is thickened, the wall is edematous, and the lumen is almost obliterated by an inflammatory cell infiltrate. The internal elastic lamina has been totally destroyed. No giant cells were seen in this case, a frequent occurrence in "giant cell" arteritis. (H & E stain; ×100.)

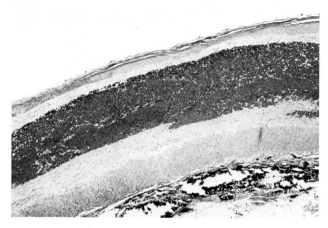

Fig. 10-22. Some authors have suggested the histologic examination of longitudinal rather than cross-sections of the temporal artery as seen in this illustration. One obtains an overview of the entire length of the artery and theoretically avoids the trap of missing the diagnosis as a result of overlooking a "skip area." In this particular case, there were no inflammatory infiltrates; the patient did not have temporal arteritis. The efficacy of this method requires further study. (H & E stain; ×20.)

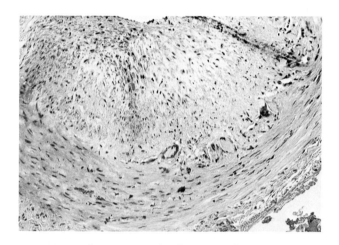

Fig. 10-21. Photomicrograph of a temporal artery showing a scant number of giant cells and a few surrounding round cell infiltrates that confirm a diagnosis of temporal arteritis. The initial pathologic findings in this case were reported as "negative." However, the clinical index of suspicion was so high that multiple serial sections were requested. Because of the presence of so-called skip lesions, the inflammatory response seen here was only present in 1 of more than 75 sampled microslides. (H & E stain; ×175.)

Anterior ischemic optic neuropathy resulting from atherosclerosis

Atherosclerotic narrowing and occlusion (Figs. 10-19 to 10-22), usually affecting the posterior ciliary arteries, is the most common cause of anterior ischemic optic neuropathy.* These arteries provide the main blood supply to the

---

* References 199, 203, 219, 226, 236, 237, 245, 263, 266, 269, 270, 291, 295, 297.

laminar, prelaminar, and retrolaminar regions of the nerve. Usually there is a partial occlusion that reduces the perfusion pressure. The pressure may also fall because of significant systemic arterial hypotension, for example, in shock or hemorrhage. As the perfusion pressure falls to a critical level, the optic disc circulation is compromised.

In more severe cases the peripapillary choroid and even the rest of the choroid may be affected. This explains why anterior ischemic optic neuropathy can occur with or without a chorioretinal lesion, usually the latter. Because a cilioretinal artery or even a branch of the central retinal artery can arise from the ciliary circulation, infarction of a sector of retina or the entire retina may be associated with anterior ischemic optic neuropathy. Associated anterior segment ischemia has also been reported.[328]

Anterior ischemic optic neuropathy associated with temporal arteritis is seen most often in patients over the age of 70 years.[245] In arteriosclerosis it usually occurs in a comparatively younger age group.

Transient blurring or loss of vision (amaurosis fugax) as a prodromal symptom occurs in about three fourths of the temporal arteritis cases and in about one fourth of the nonarteritic cases. This condition can proceed to complete loss of vision.

The main ocular abnormality is a swelling of the optic disc, which resembles that of papilledema. The swelling usually starts to subside in about 7 to 10 days, and the optic atrophy, often of the cavernous type (p. 547; Fig. 10-23), develops after a month or two. The edema and atrophy may involve the entire disc or only a sector of it. Most optic discs with anterior ischemic optic neuropathy caused by temporal arteritis develop cupping of the disc; this is less common in nonarteritic cases.

A variety of visual field defects are seen, mainly of nerve fiber bundle patterns that include altitudinal field defects, central scotomas, segmental defects, arcuate scotomas, ver-

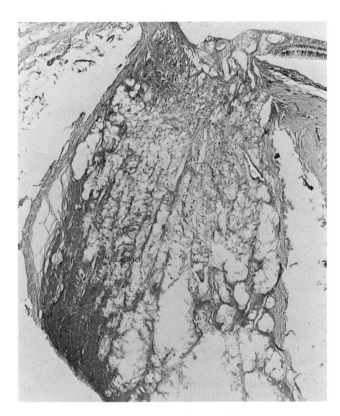

Fig. 10-23. Cavernous optic atrophy in ischemic anterior optic neuropathy. Note the "Swiss cheese" degeneration of the nerve substance. (H & E stain; ×75.)

tical defects, and peripheral contraction. These are a result of interference with the posterior ciliary supply to the optic nerve head, which is sectoral in distribution.

The electrooculogram and electroretinogram are usually normal unless there is associated retinal infarction.

Visual prognosis is worse in patients with anterior ischemic optic neuropathy resulting from temporal arteritis than in patients without temporal arteritis.[245,281,305] When the latter are treated with systemic corticosteroids, the prognosis for vision may be comparatively better.

Because arteriosclerotic anterior ischemic optic neuropathy is often associated with other cardiovascular disorders, the neuropathy may be a warning signal of a poor systemic prognosis. Patients with temporal arteritis, on the other hand, suffer no long-term systemic ill effects.

Anterior ischemic optic neuropathy resulting from temporal arteritis

Temporal arteritis (giant cell arteritis) is an uncommon disease of the elderly, most often affecting women over 55.[252] It is often associated with headaches, scalp pain and jaw claudication. The ocular complications result from the participation of the ciliary arteries in an occlusive inflammatory process that also involves the ophthalmic artery, the cranial arteries, the aorta, and the subclavian and coronary arteries.* The involvement of the ciliary artery leads to an

---

* References 189, 191-194, 205-207, 209-211, 215, 216, 218, 221, 222, 224, 230, 231, 245-250, 253, 258, 260, 261, 264, 268, 272, 277-279, 282, 285, 286, 292, 294, 299, 301, 302, 304, 305, 309, 311, 313, 320, 321, 323-325.

anterior ischemic optic neuropathy similar to that described previously.

The optic nerve ischemia can affect vision in various ways. Amaurosis fugax and the various type of scotomas described previously may occur. Not uncommonly, vision is totally extinguished, and as a rule this visual is irreversible. In the typical case a characteristic feature is the prominence and knottiness of the superficial temporal artery, which is tortuous, thickened, exquisitely tender, and shows no pulsation. From this the clinical diagnosis can be made.

An erythrocyte sedimentation rate estimation is important to determine the presence or absence of temporal arteritis. A Westergren finding higher than 40 mm the first hour suggests this cause, and a temporal artery biopsy is indicated.[210,211,221,245,315]

The pathologic changes in the temporal artery (Fig. 10-20), when present, are likely to mirror the changes in the ciliary arteries.[322] The arterial wall is thickened by a granulomatous inflammatory process. The lumen of the artery is narrowed, and the inner elastic lamina becomes thickened and fragmented. When these occlusive lesions simultaneously involve the vessels supplying the eye, that is, the ophthalmic artery, the posterior ciliary arteries, or the central retinal artery, they induce an ischemic necrosis of the optic nerve and retina. The inflammatory infiltrates may be spotty (skip lesions), and several sections may be necessary to find the lesion.[193,222,261]

Corticosteroids are given with the intent of suppressing the granulomatous vasculitis, restoring vision in the involved eye by relieving optic nerve swelling, normalizing the sedimentation rate, and preventing involvement of the other eye.

Histopathologic sections of the optic nerve show zones of ischemic necrosis.[158,159] Severe cases involve a destruction of optic nerve parenchyma identical to Schnabel's cavernous atrophy (p. 278; Figs. 6-35 and 10-23).[273] The cavernous spaces have been shown to contain hyaluronic acid derived from the vitreous.[250] Therefore, the histopathologic findings of optic nerve ischemia in giant cell arteritis and those caused by acute glaucoma have many similarities.

Pulseless disease

Ocular ischemia and amaurosis fugax are also features of Takayasu's disease (pulseless disease, aortic arch syndrome), in which there is narrowing of the large arteries that branch from the aortic arch.[217,228,289,298,314] Atherosclerosis, the collagen diseases, and giant cell arteritis produce the aortic arch syndrome. It is characterized by diminished arterial pulsations in the upper extremity. There is *decreased* blood pressure in the upper extremity and an *elevation* of the blood pressure in the lower extremity. Chronic ocular ischemia may be associated with a pallid swelling or atrophy of the optic disc similar to that described above, retinal and/or iris neovascularization, venous stasis retinopathy, and cataract.

DEGENERATIVE (DEMYELINATING) DISEASE

The highly specialized central (axial) zone of the optic nerve is particularly vulnerable to various demyelinating, toxic, and nutritional disorders; therefore, most degenerative processes preferentially attack the axial portion of the optic nerve (Figs. 10-26, *A*, and 10-27).[190] Loss of central vision and associated central scotomas characterize this group, frequently unaccompanied by any observable optic disc abnormality. Eventually, however, the retrobulbar axial neuritis progresses and results in temporal pallor of the disc, reflecting the atrophy of axons within the papillomacular bundle.

Although demyelination ultimately occurs in all degenerated or atrophic optic nerves, in one group of diseases it is the most conspicuous abnormality. In this group of demyelinating disorders one initially observes a loss of myelin, whereas the other elements of the nerve such as axons, astrocytes, and associated blood vessels remain relatively well preserved in the initial stages.

Multiple sclerosis

Multiple sclerosis, the most common demyelinating disease, is a disabling, crippling, and often blinding affliction of middle life (Figs. 10-25 to 10-27). It may persist for decades and is characterized by spontaneous remissions and exacerbations.*

Because the axons of the optic nerve posterior to the lamina cribrosa acquire a myelin sheath, the retrobulbar portion of the nerve, like the white matter elsewhere throughout the central nervous system, is vulnerable to the demyelinating process that characterizes multiple sclerosis.[306] Vision loss is typically unilateral and often profound, being associated with a dense central scotoma (although involvement of the eye may occur) marked impairment of color perception, abnormal pupillary reflexes, ocular muscle palsies, nystagmus, and/or internuclear ophthalmoplegia. The risk of developing multiple sclerosis after optic neuritis is much greater in women than men.

The ophthalmoscopic appearance may be abnormal; there may be retinal vascular sheathing or a papillitis.[198] The optic disc, however, initially usually appears normal because the site of myelin degeneration is within the axial zone of the retrobulbar portion of the optic nerve (retrobulbar neuritis). Retrobulbar neuritis is characterized by a sudden loss of vision in one eye with a tendency to recover vision in a few weeks or months. Impaired conductivity, without disruption of the central axons within this demyelinated axial zone, accounts for the visual loss in these cases. In late stages the atrophic white optic disc is indistinguishable from optic atrophy caused by other factors (Fig. 10-25).

Multiple sclerosis occurs more commonly in temperate climates. Reports of the occurrence of more than one case in a family have not been interpreted in terms of genetic passage but suggest that multiple sclerosis may have an infectious basis. The revival of the viral theory also stems from the recent interest in slow-virus disease, that is, a disease in which a virus is acquired in childhood with symptoms appearing later in life.[229,276] A variety of viruses have been implicated in multiple sclerosis, in particular the measles and vaccinia viruses. The elevation of gamma globulin in the cerebrospinal fluid, which is frequently observed in patients with multiple sclerosis, has also been observed in slow-virus diseases of the central nervous system. Multiple sclerosis may be an immune-mediated disease, either a specific autoimmune response to myelin or a viral-induced immune response against the oligodendrocyte-myelin sheath complex.

The demyelinating lesions of multiple sclerosis are termed *plaques* because of their focal distribution and circumscribed borders (Figs. 10-26 and 10-27). The firm glial scars that characterize old plaques prompted the name multiple "sclerosis."

There are three successive histologic changes: demyelination, microglial reaction, and astrocytic proliferation.[190,327] Histopathologically the early lesions are characterized by the simultaneous degeneration of oligodendrocytes and myelin sheaths, leaving the axons relatively intact. These degenerative changes are associated with vascular congestion and a mild perivascular infiltrate of lymphocytes and plasma cells.

The microglia phagocytize the myelin debris in response to the release and breakdown of myelin. The myelin debris stimulates an intense gliosis, and the older lesions are characterized by a dense glial network. In general, the age of the lesion can be determined by the presence or absence of inflammation and swelling, the location and number of lipid-bearing microglial cells, and the degree of gliosis.

Acute disseminated encephalomyelitis

Acute disseminated encephalomyelitis may be seen after viral infections, vaccination, or inoculations. A similar symptom complex occurs spontaneously without any previous illness and has not been associated with any specific organism. Young adults are usually affected, and it may occur in children, in whom it assumes an acute and frequently fatal form.

Neuromyelitis optica of Devic

Devic's disease (neuromyelitis optica) is an acute, particularly virulent form of multiple sclerosis.[225] It is characterized by a rapid, bilateral loss of vision followed by an equally rapid onset of paraplegia resulting from spinal cord demyelination. Sometimes the disease begins by an attack of blindness or paraplegia that improves temporarily only to relapse when the other component makes its appearance. The age of onset ranges from childhood to late adult life. Remissions and relapses may occur.

Histopathologically the lesions, largely confined to the optic nerve, optic chiasm, optic tract, and spinal cord, reflect an intensely destructive process characterized by profound demyelination, loss of astrocytes and axons, and an influx of acute inflammatory cells. Tissue necrosis may actually lead to cavitary changes. A transverse retrobulbar neuritis similar to that demonstrated in Fig. 10-26, *B*, virtually transects the nerve and generally leads to optic atrophy.

Schilder's disease

Schilder's disease (diffuse periaxial encephalitis) is a sudanophilic leukodystrophy. Other leukodystrophies include Krabbe's disease, metachromatic leukodystrophy, adenoleukodystrophy and Pelizaeus-Merzbacher syndrome.[238]

Schilder's disease is genetically transmitted as a sex-linked recessive trait. Its onset is in childhood, with pro-

---

*References 204, 208, 257, 271, 274, 296, 319.

gressive ataxia, slurred speech, and loss of hearing and vision. Low serum cortisol levels lead to addisonian tanning of the skin. Histopathologically throughout the white matter of the central nervous system, including the optic nerve and the optic radiations, there are large symmetric zones that demonstrate loss of myelin and oligodendrocytes, degeneration of nerve fibers, and gliosis. Because of the presence of foamy, lipid-positive sudanophilic substances in affected tissues, it is sometimes referred to as a sudanophilic leukodystrophy.

Optic atrophy

PATHOGENETIC CLASSIFICATION

The ultimate sequela of progressive optic nerve disorders is optic atrophy (Figs. 10-24–10-30).[188-328] Optic atrophy is defined in terms of loss of conductive function of the optic nerve, usually with an increase in pallor of the disc as a result of gliosis and a decrease or loss of the minute capillaries that normally impart a pink color to the nerve head.[290] In addition to ophthalmoscopy and visual examination, fluorescein angiography of the disc may be helpful; the normal disc shows an early fluorescence preceding filling of the vessels; in optic atrophy this glow is often decreased or absent. The type of optic atrophy depends on the pathogenetic factors involved. Important categories of optic atrophy are listed as either a descending or ascending process.[195]

A. Descending optic atrophy (the primary lesion is intracranial or in the retrobulbar optic nerve; the atrophic process proceeds toward the eye)
  1. Primary, within the nerve substance
    a. Demyelinating diseases
    b. Following encephalitis or neuritis
    c. Optic nerve tumors, for example, glioma or metastatic tumors
    d. Following trauma
  2. Caused by disease outside and adjacent to the nerve parenchyma
    a. Neoplasms, particularly pituitary tumors and meningiomas
    b. Following inflammation, for example, meningitis or perineuritis
    c. Following any process that leads to increased intracranial pressure
    d. Trauma, for example, compression at the optic canal
B. Ascending optic atrophy (the primary lesion begins at the optic nerve head or retina-choroid; the atrophic process proceeds toward the brain)
  1. Optic nerve head
    a. Caused by papilledema
    b. Caused by optic neuritis (inflammatory, ischemic, or degenerative)
    c. Glaucomatous optic atrophy
  2. Primary lesion in retina-choroid (degenerations, inflammations, and dystrophies)
    a. Central retinal artery occlusion
    b. Anterior ischemic optic neuropathy
    c. Syphilis (tabes dorsalis)
    d. Chorioretinitis
    e. Uveitis and endophthalmitis
    f. Retinitis pigmentosa syndromes

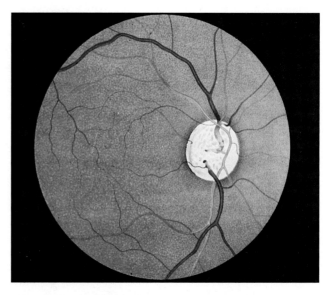

Fig. 10-24. Schematic illustration of an ocular fundus showing advanced optic atrophy.

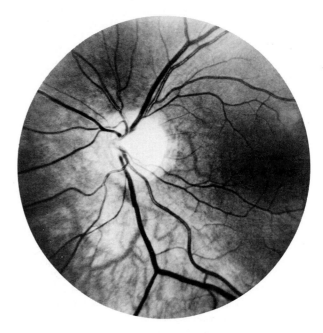

Fig. 10-25. "Primary" optic atrophy in multiple sclerosis. White discoloration is prominent.

    g. Cerebromacular degenerations
    h. Toxic or nutritional degenerations[201]
    i. Myopic optic atrophy
    j. Ocular trauma

Although the ultimate tissue changes in optic atrophy reveal the five common features listed in the next section, cases of optic atrophy can show specific changes indicative of the underlying disease. For example, in various diseases in which neural tissue resorption without excessive superficial glial replacement often occurs, such as in glaucoma, the demyelinating diseases, methyl alcohol poisoning (Fig.

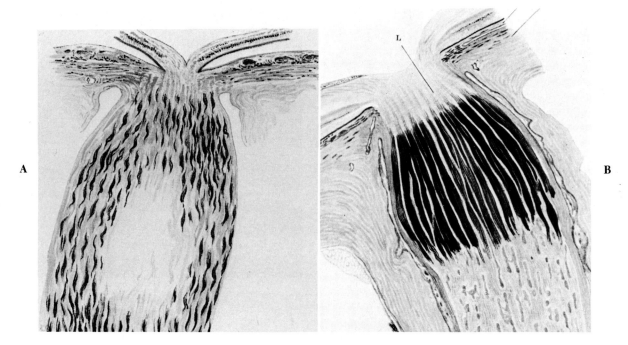

Fig. 10-26. Reproductions of drawings of myelin-stained optic nerves showing foci of demyelination of axons in multiple sclerosis. The Weigert stains normal myelin black; the nonstained areas are demyelinated plaques. **A,** Focal plaque of demyelination. **B,** Diffuse myelin loss posteriorly *(below). L,* Lamina cribrosa. (**A** from Greeff R: In Orth J, editor: Lehrbuch der speziellen pathologischen Anatomie, Berlin, 1902, Hirschwald; **B** from Abelsdorff G: In Henke F and Lubarsch O, editors: Handbuch der speziellen pathologischen Anatomie und Histologie, Berlin, 1928, Julius Springer.)

10-17), or tabes dorsalis, a deepening of the optic cup may be prominent. In contrast, the optic atrophy following papilledema and some forms of papillitis reveals an anterior bowing of the lamina cribrosa, with a buckling and elevation of the retina and marked separation of individual axons. The postpapilledema and postneuritic atrophic nerve may, therefore, reveal morphologic evidence of the distortions that characterized the acute stages of the disease.

Optic atrophy caused by infectious processes such as bacterial or fungal optic neuritis would likely cause intense postinflammatory tissue destruction that could be pathologically distinguished from a simple optic neuritis. Microorganisms also may be demonstrated in such cases.

Glaucomatous optic atrophy is easily distinguished by the typical pathologic cup (Chapter 6). A special form of optic atrophy, Schnabel's cavernous atrophy (p. 278), is occasionally associated with glaucoma, particularly in cases in which acute pressure increases have been documented. It also occurs following anterior ischemic optic neuropathy (p. 544). Cavernous atrophy differs from most other types of optic atrophy in that a reactive gliosis does not closely follow or parallel the loss of neural substance. The tissue loss results in the formation of hyaluronic acid-containing lacunar spaces, which resemble those formed in the cerebral cortex after ischemic, nonhemmorrhagic cerebral vascular accidents.

HISTOPATHOLOGIC FINDINGS

Several histopathologic criteria taken singly or collectively are characteristic of optic atrophy. These changes are relatively constant regardless of the underlying disease process. Five histopathologic indications of optic atrophy are noteworthy:

1. Loss of myelin
2. Loss of the parallel architecture of the glial columns that are normally seen in sagittal sections of the optic nerve (these columns are obliterated by the three factors listed next)
3. Glial proliferation (gliosis)
4. Widening of the space separating the optic nerve and the meninges
5. Thickening of the pial septa of the nerve

As optic atrophy progresses, there is a continuous loss of functioning neural tissue; both the myelin sheath (Figs. 10-26 and 10-27) and the central axonal component of the involved nerve fiber ultimately disappear. The neural parenchyma shrinks, with eventual thickening of pial septa and replacement gliosis (Figs. 10-29 and 10-30). The latter two processes compensate for the tissue loss, but this is usually not sufficient to prevent a decrease in diameter of the nerve. This decreased diameter explains the phenomenon of widening of the space between the nerve and the dura mater (Fig. 10-30).

The tissue loss also explains the deepening of the optic cup that frequently occurs, particularly in glaucoma, often with baring or exposure of the lamina cribrosa. Less commonly, in some forms of atrophy the glial proliferation of the nerve head may actually flatten or obliterate the physiologic cup.

When demyelination occurs, the microglia assume their phagocytic function and ingest the degenerate neural ele-

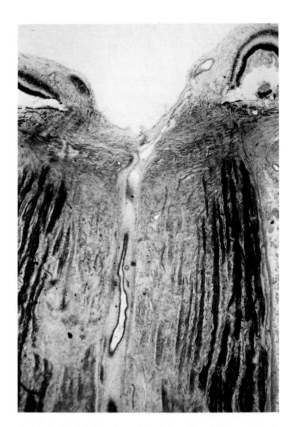

Fig. 10-27. Multiple sclerosis. Weigert's myelin stain of optic nerve cross-sections. The loss of myelin is great centrally. (Weigert's stain; ×90.) (From the collection of Professor Wolfgang Stock, University of Tübingen, Tübingen, Germany, and from Naumann GOH and Apple DJ: In Doerr W, Seifert G, and Uehlinger E, editors: Handbuch der speziellen pathologischen Anatomie, Band Auge, Berlin, 1980, Springer-Verlag.)

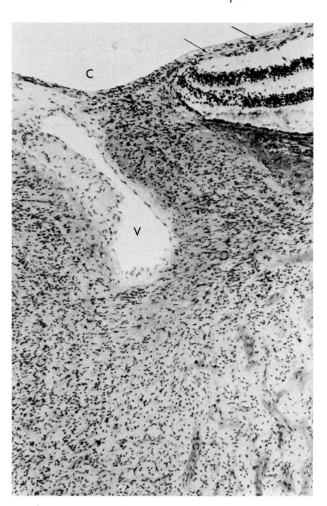

Fig. 10-29. Optic atrophy resulting from Tay-Sachs disease. There is primary degeneration of the retinal ganglion cell cytoplasm. In this terminal stage the ganglion cells are absent, having long since been replaced by glia *(arrows)*. Following ganglion cell loss, the nerve fibers of the optic nerve degenerate. This section illustrates an extreme degree of gliosis. Myriad glial nuclei are dispersed throughout the entire cross-section of the nerve. Compare this figure with that of a normal sagittal section of optic nerve (Figs. 9-2 and 9-4). *V,* Lumen of central retinal vein; *C,* base of optic cup. (H & E stain; ×170.)

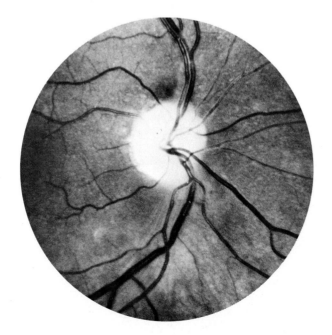

Fig. 10-28. Optic atrophy in Foster Kennedy syndrome. This nerve was compressed by an intracranial tumor; the other optic disc showed papilledema.

ments, forming lipid-laden macrophages, which eventually remove the myelin and axonal residues. Demyelination is indicated in hematoxylin and eosin tissue sections by the more compact nature of the nerve parenchyma. In routinely prepared sections of a normally myelinated, intact nerve, the nerve substance appears spongy or foamy because myelin is a lipid that does not stain in such preparations. When myelin is lost by disease, the tissue of the optic nerve appears to become more compact and dense as the foamy-appearing myelin is depleted. Demyelination is even more obvious when special stains such as the myelinophilic Luxol fast blue or Weigert's stain are applied. Demyelinated areas appear poorly stained in such preparations (Figs. 10-26 and 10-27).

Gliosis of the optic nerve is probably the change most easily recognized during histopathologic examination. The normally parallel columns of glial nuclei are replaced by proliferating glial cells, which replace the previously functioning neural tissue and assume a random distribution throughout the optic nerve parenchyma. These proliferating cells appear to become sprinkled or peppered throughout the entire thickness of the nerve (Figs. 10-29 and 10-30).

Tumors

A clinically useful means of classifying growths or tumors affecting the optic nerve is according to location, that is, (1) at the optic nerve head, where they are ophthalmoscopically visible, or (2) posterior to the lamina cribrosa, where they are secluded from direct inspection[329-432]:

A. Intraocular origin (epipapillary and peripapillary)
  1. Pigmented
    a. Melanocytoma
    b. Malignant melanoma of the choroid extending onto the optic nerve
    c. Pigment epithelial proliferation and neoplasia
  2. Miscellaneous nonpigmented tumors
    a. Drusen
    b. Hamartomas, usually associated with the phakomatoses
    c. Retinoblastoma, invasive from the adjacent retina
B. Tumors usually originating or deposited in the retrobulbar optic nerve or its sheaths
  1. Meningioma
  2. Optic glioma
  3. Metastatic tumors to the optic nerve

INTRAOCULAR ORIGIN (EPIPAPILLARY AND PERIPAPILLARY)

Melanocytoma

The melanocytoma is a benign pigmented tumor that usually arises at the optic nerve head or from the adjacent peripapillary region (Fig. 10-31 to 10-33; Color Plates 10-7 and 10-8).* This tumor was frequently misdiagnosed as a malignant melanoma, and many unnecessary enucleations were carried out. Today its clinical features are well recognized, and specimens of melanocytoma are fortunately rarely received in the ocular pathology laboratory. In contrast to uveal malignant melanoma, which is unusual in black patients, melanocytoma is seen with greater frequency in blacks than in whites.[373,430,431]

Like uveal nevi and malignant melanomas, the melanocytoma is derived from uveal dendritic melanocytes.[362,367,430,431] Although this lesion, which is a special form of uveal nevus, usually arises on or adjacent to the optic disc, it may also occur at any site within the uvea.

Choroidal nevi composed of spindle cells are in most cases impossible to differentiate clinically from identical-appearing choroidal melanocytomas. Although a cytologic evaluation cannot be made on a clinical basis with methods currently available, this cell type distinction is significant.

---

* References 348, 360, 366, 384, 385, 396, 398, 409, 410, 416, 428, 430, 431.

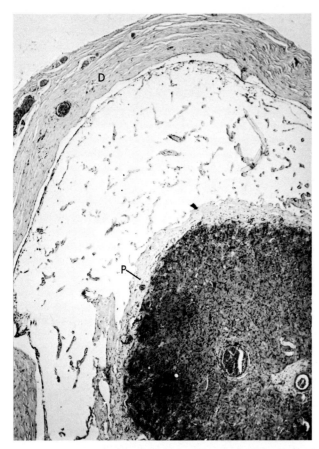

Fig. 10-30. Cross section of an atrophic optic nerve and surrounding meninges. Diffuse sprinkling of nuclei throughout the optic nerve parenchyma *(lower right)* is indicative of marked gliosis. Because of a decrease in size of the atrophic nerve, there is a marked widening of the meningeal space, the space between the dura *(D)*, and the pia mater *(P)*. The cells in the widened space consist of delicate tufts of the meningothelial cells that form the arachnoid layer. (H & E stain; ×25.)

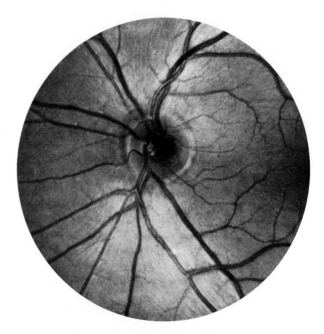

Fig. 10-31. Melanocytoma, optic nerve head. This pigmented tumor is deep within the base of the optic cup.

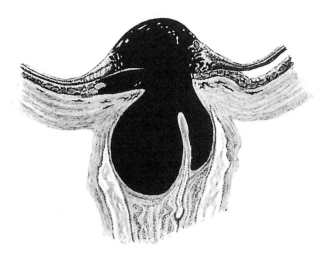

Fig. 10-32. Schematic illustration showing a typical growth pattern of melanocytoma (magnocellular nevus). Note that the tumor involves the choroid, the pavenchyma of the optic nerve and the prelaminar region of the nerve head. This is a tumor of uveal origin arising from neural crest melanocytic cells.

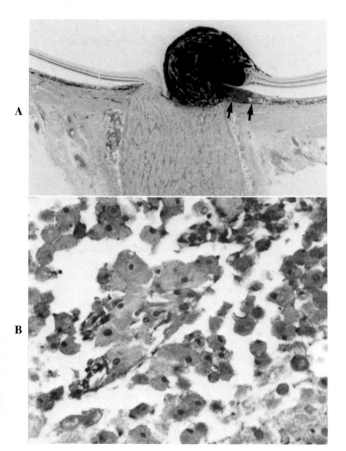

Fig. 10-33. Melanocytoma, optic nerve head. **A,** The deeply pigmented tumor is slightly elevated and is noninvasive, being confined to the anteriolaminar region and peripapillary choroid (*arrows*). (H & E stain; ×50.) **B,** Bleached preparation of tumor cells in melanocytoma. The cells are round to polygonal in shape, and the nuclei are small and normochromatic, with no characteristics suggesting malignancy. (H & E stain; bleached preparation; ×350.)

Spindle cell nevi may occasionally progress to malignant melanomas. A melanocytoma only rarely undergoes a malignant transformation.[331,332,401]

The epipapillary and peripapillary melanocytoma must be distinguished from hyperplastic, hamartomatous, or neoplastic growth of the peripapillary pigment epithelium, as well as from uveal melanomas arising in the region of the optic disc (Fig. 10-34 and 10-35).[331,354,418] The absence

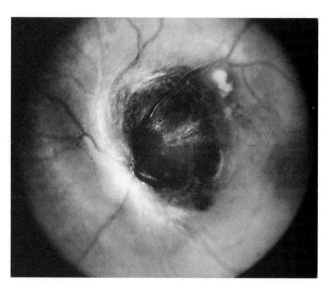

Fig. 10-34. Photograph of an elevated, deeply pigmented epipapillary lesion. This picture fits into the differential diagnosis of epipapillary malignant melanoma versus benign melanocytoma. In many instances it is sometimes possible to arrive at the diagnosis only by careful follow-up of the patient.

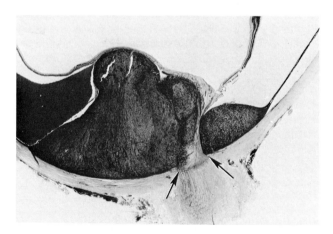

Fig. 10-35. Epipapillary and peripapillary choroidal malignant melanoma, the most important tumor in the differential diagnosis of melanocytoma. Although melanocytomas and pigment epithelial proliferative lesions and neoplasms may also be elevated, the degree of elevation and the surface irregularity in this case are very strongly indicative of the true nature of the tumor. The arrows indicate the margins of the optic nerve head. The focus of tumor to the right of the nerve represents an extension around the nerve from the main tumor on the left. A proteinaceous fluid is present in the subretinal space to the left of the main tumor mass. (H & E stain; ×25.)

of significant loss of visual acuity or severe field loss in melanocytoma helps differentiate it from malignant melanoma.

Most disc melanocytomas do not protrude more than 1 mm forward toward the vitreous. The jet-black pigmentation is the most characteristic feature; this blocks fluorescence by fluorescein angiography. Diagnostic differentiation, however, is complicated by the fact that a disc melanocytoma may also reveal only mild-to-moderate pigmentation (Color Plate 10-8). While most optic nerve melanocytomas are comparatively black, uveal melanocytomas away from the optic nerve exhibit a wide variation in pigmentation.

Although most melanocytomas have a clinical course similar to that of other uveal nevi and the tumor cells are derived from a similar embryologic source, the cytologic appearance of individual cells in melanocytoma is distinct from the usual spindle cell type seen in most uveal nevi. The melanin pigment must be chemically bleached from the tissue before adequate microscopic examination is possible. Melanocytoma cells are large and usually round or slightly polyhedral, with distinct cell borders (Fig. 10-33, *B*; Color Plate 10-9). The nucleus within each tumor cell is small and round, and there is no variation in nuclear size and shape. The nuclei are normochromic, and mitotic activity is minimal in these slowly growing or stationary tumors. Spindle cells are rare, and there is little evidence of cellular pleomorphism, giant cell formation, or other features suggestive of an epithelioid cell differentiation.

Malignant melanoma of the choroid extending onto the optic disc

Choroidal malignant melanomas are described in detail in Chapter 7. Those arising as primary tumors of the optic disc are rare, but juxtapapillary melanomas[353,418] of the choroid are not uncommon and constitute the most important tumor in the differential diagnosis of melanocytoma (Fig. 10-35; Color Plate 10-10). The tumor may grow over the disc and project into the vitreous or may invade posteriorly through the lamina cribrosa into the nerve substance.

Pigment epithelial proliferation and hyperplasia

Another cause for pigmentation of the optic disc, and a factor in the differential diagnosis of malignant melanoma and melanocytoma, is proliferation of the juxtapapillary retinal pigment epithelium.[418] As in melanocytoma, the main goal is to ensure that the globe is not unnecessarily enucleated. True carcinoma of the retinal pigment epithelium is very rare.

Miscellaneous nonpigmented tumors

Drusen of the nerve head are described on page 534; epipapillary and peripapillary growths associated with the phakomatoses and retinoblastoma are considered in Chapter 9.[334,395,417]

TUMORS USUALLY ORIGINATING IN THE RETROBULBAR OPTIC NERVE

Meningioma

Optic nerve meningioma is usually considered in the differential diagnosis of orbital tumors but is described here because of its occasional close association with the optic nerve.*

Karp and coworkers[379] have emphasized that there are two forms of meningiomas in the orbit. In most cases the primary site is within the cranium, and the meningioma invades the orbit secondarily. Less commonly the tumors may arise directly from the intraorbital or intracanalicular meninges of the optic nerve. In the brain gliomas occur much more frequently than meningiomas, but in the orbit meningiomas are slightly more common. It is estimated that meningiomas account for 3% to 10% of expanding lesions of the orbit that produce unilateral proptosis.[379]

Orbital meningiomas occur much more commonly in females. The median age of diagnosis is 38 years, but 40% of the patients are under 20 years of age at the time of surgery.[379] This differs from intracranial meningiomas, which are rarely observed in children. Loss of vision and progressive exophthalmos are the two most common presenting symptoms. Some cases reveal visual field loss, optic atrophy, optociliary shunt vessel formation, lid edema, ocular muscle palsies, retinal striae, and hypertrophy or hyperostosis of the bony walls of the orbit.[427] Like optic nerve glioma, meningioma has a higher than normal incidence in patients with von Recklinghausen's disease.

A meningioma may grow as an eccentric lump on one side of the optic nerve, and it may spread forward or backward along the nerve. The lesion may also surround and compress the nerve like a collar.

In the older literature meningiomas were termed *dural endotheliomas*. They arise from the meningoendothelial cells of the arachnoid. Also termed *meningiocytes* or *cap cells*, these cells are located in clusters at the tip of the arachnoid villi (Fig. 10-7). They are thought to be of neuroectodermal, neural crest origin. This partially explains their close relationship to neurofibromas, which also are derived from the neural crest.

Histopathologically the same patterns of growth seen with the more common intracranial meningiomas are also seen in the orbit. Most meningiomas fall into the following histologic categories.[349,392,404]

1. Meningotheliomatous or syncytial (solid sheets of cells rather than a whorled pattern)
2. Psammonatous (whorled pattern of cells containing abundant psammoma bodies)
3. Fibroblastic
4. Angioblastic
5. Mixed or transitional—a combination of any of the above

Most primary intraorbital meningiomas are either meningotheliomatous or the mixed type. The cells of a *meningotheliomatous meningioma* are arranged in a syncytium rather than in whorls. The nuclei of these cells are large and vesicular and have a rather uniform distribution. The cell boundaries are indistinct. In a *psammomatous meningioma* the tumor cells are arranged in a whorled pattern consisting of concentric layers of cells, with or without a

---

* References 330, 332, 333, 338, 339, 345, 356, 357, 359, 364, 371, 377, 379, 382, 388, 400, 402, 407, 411, 412, 419, 400, 422-424, 427.

central vascular channel (Fig. 10-36). The central core of some of the cell nests becomes hyalinized and calcified, forming psammoma bodies (Figs. 10-7 and 10-36; Color Plate 10-11).

In analyzing biopsy tissue from a suspected case of primary orbital meningioma, one must remember that a common feature of primary optic gliomas is a marked hyperplasia of the surrounding meninges. This can resemble the cellular pattern of a true meningioma. Adequate tissue sampling must, therefore, be obtained to rule out this possibility.

Symptomatic orbital meningiomas usually require surgical intervention. Irradiation is of no value. Orbital meningiomas in childhood are more aggressive than those occurring in older persons. The differential diagnosis always includes optic nerve glioma, particularly in children. Any time an optic nerve meningioma is present, one must consider a possible associated neurofibromatosis.

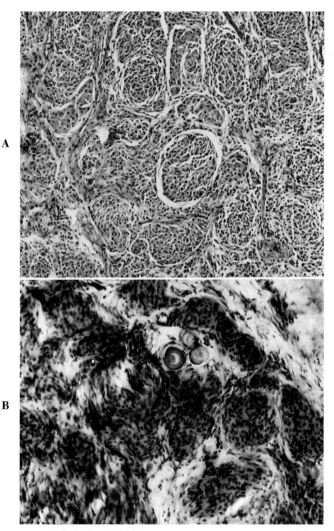

Fig. 10-36. Optic nerve meningioma. **A,** Prominent "whorled" pattern with meningothelial cells arranged in nests. (H & E stain; ×250.) **B,** Similar case with additional formation of a cluster of psammoma bodies (see also Color Plate 10-11). (H & E stain; ×250.)

Optic glioma

This discussion is primarily concerned with glioma of the optic nerve arising within its intraorbital portion, although this tumor may arise more centrally in the chiasm and optic tracts.

Gliomas of the optic nerve usually appear during the first decade of life, the median age of onset being about 5 years.* Most cases are probably congenital and are only diagnosed later when the ocular signs become chronic. There may be a slight prepondance of glioma in females.[374]

The clinical signs relate directly to the presence of an intraorbital space-occupying mass. The most common initial signs are unilateral proptosis (usually straight forward or temporal), loss of vision, and strabismus. Papilledema and a later optic atrophy are common, and an occlusion of the central retinal vein resulting from pressure exerted by the tumor may complicate the clinical picture. A major diagnostic sign is roentgenographic evidence of enlargement of the optic foramen. When there is combined involvement of the orbital, chiasmal, and intracranial regions, or the intracranial region alone, the most prominent clinical signs are referable to brain involvement, for example, headaches, seizures, nystagmus, ataxia, mental changes, hydrocephalus, precocious puberty, and diabetes insipidus.

Like orbital meningiomas, a significant percentage of optic glioma cases are associated with von Recklinghausen's disease. Apparently, the same catalyst that initiates the growth of peripheral neurofibromas may affect the glial elements of the optic nerve. Both cell lines share a common derivation from the neural crest.

Gliomas of the optic nerve lead to an enlargement of the nerve with visual loss. There are five different stages in the evolution of optic nerve gliomas:

1. Generalized hyperplasia of the glial cells within the nerve
2. Extension of the growth through the pial sheath, with hyperplasia of the arachnoid cells forming a tumorlike growth
3. Extension of the tumor cells further into the sheath of the optic nerve, with penetration and infiltration of the mass into the subarachnoid space (the two tissue elements—glial and arachnoidal—become so intermingled that it is difficult to distinguish one from the other)
4. Destruction of most of the landmarks of the sheath by a haphazard intermixture of glial and arachnoid cells
5. Loss of landmarks within *both* the nerve stem and sheath

Grossly the tumor usually causes a smooth-surfaced, fusiform enlargement of the optic nerve between the eyeball and optic foramen (Fig. 10-37). Occasionally, growth of the tumor is asymmetric in relation to the nerve. In such cases the nerve, almost normal in appearance, passes tangentially along one surface of the mass. Such configuration may mislead a surgeon into believing the nerve has been pushed aside by an independent tumor (Fig. 10-38).

The mass often extends directly into the optic nerve meninges. The reactive meningeal hyperplasia may extend far beyond the reaches of the tumor itself. It may be exuberant, and it is sometimes difficult to differentiate a glioma of the nerve from a meningioma. Because of this, when tissue sampling at the time of exploratory surgery is inade-

* References 329, 335-337, 340, 351, 355, 361, 368, 369, 372, 374, 376, 383, 386, 389-391, 403, 412, 413, 415, 418, 425, 426.

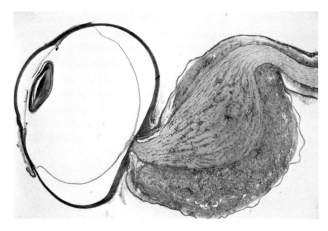

Fig. 10-37. Optic glioma. The tumor has caused marked thickening of the nerve, and massive meningeal proliferation around the nerve has occurred as a secondary reaction. (Masson trichrome stain; ×1.) (From Stock W: Pathologische Anatomie des Auges, Stuttgart, 1939, Ferdinand Enke Verlag.)

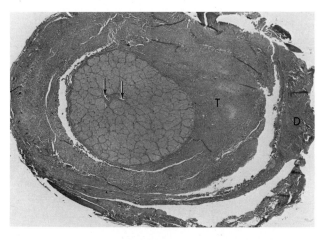

Fig. 10-38. Glioma of the optic nerve. The optic nerve proper is recognizable by the presence of the numerous pial septae, which divide the nerve into small bundles. *Arrows,* Central vessels. The dura (*D*) is widely separated from the circumference of the nerve by a massive infiltrate of tumor (*T*). The tumor in this plane of section has involved the arachnoid and surrounds the nerve; it is most prominent in the upper right portion of the photomicrograph. (H & E stain; ×160.)

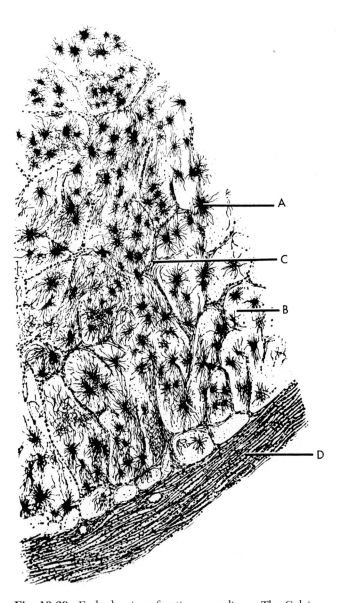

Fig. 10-39. Early drawing of optic nerve glioma. The Golgio-impregnated dendritic or star-shaped glial cells (*A*, demonstrates the true nature of the tumor. *B*, Bundles of axons between glial cells; *C*, pial septae; *D*, pia mater. (From Fischer F: Arch Augenheilkd 59:181, 1908.)

quate, and only the hyperplastic meninges at the edge of the lesion are reached, a false diagnosis may be made. Meningeal hyperplasia should be differentiated from direct infiltration of the glioma through the pia mater into the meningeal spaces.[342]

According to the Cushing-Bailey classification of glial tumors of the brain, the optic glioma is grade I astrocytoma (also sometimes referred to as a juvenile pilocytic astrocytoma). These tumors are slow growing and show almost no tendency to metastasize, in distinct contrast to the most malignant tumors within this classification. For example, the so-called grade IV glioma, the glioblastoma multiforme,

is invariably fatal, but fortunately it rarely affects the optic nerve.

Microscopically the tumor is composed of round to spindle-shaped cells that somewhat resemble the glial nuclei of the normal optic nerve.[392] The tumor often merges with the adjacent normal optic nerve parenchyma and may actually resemble a reactive gliosis. Some observers have considered this lesion to be a form of degenerative gliomatosis rather than an actual tumor. The glial cells, characterized by the presence of multiple dendritelike, fibrillar cytoplasmic processes, are markedly increased in numbers and arranged in a random fashion rather than the ordered, parallel arrangement characteristic of normal optic nerve glia (Figs. 10-36 and 10-37). Pleomorphism is minimal, and mitoses are rare; accordingly, metastases are exceptional.

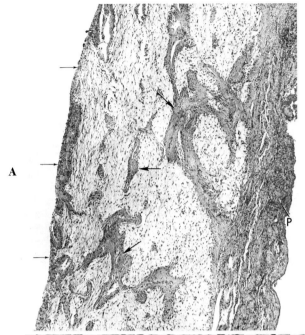

A

Fig. 10-40. Optic glioma (juvenile astrocytoma, grade 1). **A,** The pia mater *(P)* forms a sheath around the enlarged nerve. The pial septae *(large arrows)* are separated by numerous neoplastic glial cells, which are recognized in this section by increased numbers of nuclei. There is little evidence of anaplasia, and the glial proliferation appears similar to the process of reactive gliosis illustrated in Figs. 10-29 and 10-30. The left border *(small arrows)* represents the surgical margin of excision. (H & E stain; ×63.) **B,** This photomicrograph reveals spindle-shaped cells derived from astrocytes. The deeply staining, eosinophilic structures *(arrows)* are termed *Rosenthal fibers.* When present, they assist in diagnosis. (H & E stain; ×350.)

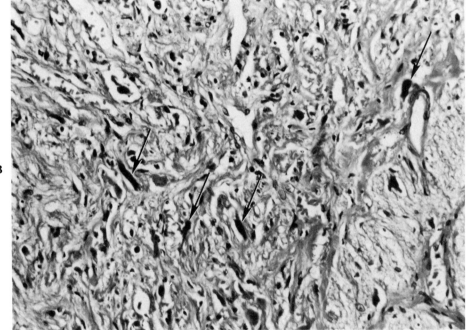

B

Tumor cells may stain positively for glial fibriallary protein, S-100, and vimentin (see Table 1-2, p. 6)

Locating the so-called Rosenthal fibers may greatly assist in the histopathologic diagnosis (Fig. 10-40, *B*). These are fusiform, elongated, or cigar-shaped, deeply eosinophilic-staining structures that when present are highly characteristic, although not diagnostic, of this tumor. As commonly occurs with intracerebral astrocytomas, mucopolysaccharide-containing microcystoid spaces form within the tumor, probably as a result of tumor cell necrosis.

With rare exceptions optic gliomas are clinically indolent tumors, which have features of congenital hamartomas.[273,369,391] They tend to enlarge and cause symptoms in life and then remain static. Visual impairment, present at the time of diagnosis, does not usually change appreciably. Childhood gliomas do not undergo malignant degeneration. Two mechanisms account for their growth: (1) collateral hyperplasia of adjacent glia, connective tissue, and meninges and (2) production of intracellular and extracellular mucopolysaccharides. The absence of mitoses is evidence that these tumors do not enlarge by cell division or invasion.

A wide variety of therapeutic approaches to optic glioma are available. Gliomas confined to the intraorbital region are usually relatively benign with regard to histologic cell type; therefore, surgery is not indicated if severe, intolerable symptoms referable to the space-occupying lesion are not present. Transcranial operations or irradiation on more centrally located and dangerous tumors do not prolong life.[374] In fact, excision or manipulation of a chiasmal mass during biopsy may increase morbidity and mortality. Excision of the tumor is justified only for the relief of recurrent increases in intracranial pressure, severe proptosis, or when the eye is blind. Incomplete excision of a tumor by way of a lateral or medial orbitotomy is adequate if symptoms are relieved.[374]

Metastatic tumors to the optic nerve

Metastatic tumors in the optic nerve are extremely rare.[365,380,393,394] Because of the high frequency of these tumors, carcinomas from the lung or breast are the most common. The tumor infiltrates are deposited in the substance of the nerve, and destruction of nerve fibers and their septa may result in optic nerve atrophy.

REFERENCES

Embryology and Anatomy

1. Aaby AA and Kushner BJ: Acquired and progressive myelinated nerve fibers, Arch Ophthalmol 103:542, 1985.
2. Abramov I and others: The retina of the newborn infant, Science 217:265, 1982.
3. Anderson DR: Circulation and axonal transport in the optic nerve, Trans Ophthalmol Soc UK 96:3-15, 1976.
4. Anderson DR and Hoyt WF: Ultrastructure of intraorbital portion of human and monkey optic nerve, Arch Ophthalmol 82:506, 1969.
5. Balazsi AG and others: The effect of age on the nerve fiber population of the human optic nerve, Am J Ophthalmol 97:760, 1984.
6. Beck RW and others: Is there a racial difference in physiologic cup size? Ophthalmology 92:873, 1985.
7. Cant JS, editor: The optic nerve: proceedings of the second William Mackenzie Memorial Symposium held in Glasgow, Sept 7-10, 1971, St. Louis, 1972, The CV Mosby Co.
8. Cunha-Vaz JG: The blood-ocular barriers, Surv Ophthalmol 23:279, 1979.
9. Dolman CL, McCormick AQ, and Drance SM: Aging of the optic nerve, Arch Ophthalmol 98:2053, 1980.
10. Ernest JT: Optic disc blood flow, Trans Ophthalmol Soc UK 96:3-18, 1976.
11. Fantes FE and Anderson DR: Clinical histologic correlation of human peripapillary anatomy, Ophthalmology 96:20, 1989.
12. Fine BS and Yanoff M: Ocular Histology. A text and atlas, ed 2, Hagerstown, Harper & Row, 1979.
13. Glaser J: Neuro-ophthalmology, New York, 1978, Harper & Row, Publishers.
14. Goldbaum MH and others: The extracellular matrix of the human optic nerve, Arch Ophthalmol 107:1225, 1989.
15. Hart MH Jr: Clinical perimetry and topographic diagnosis in disease of the afferent visual system, In Slamovits TL and Burde R, editors: Neuro-ophthalmology, vol 6, In Podos AM and Yanoff M, editors: Textbook of ophthalmology, London, 1994, Mosby-Year Book.
16. Hayreh, SS: Blood supply of the optic nerve head and its role in optic atrophy, glaucoma and edema of the optic disc, Br J Ophthalmol 53:721, 1969.
17. Hayreh SS: Anatomy and physiology of the optic nerve head, Trans Am Acad Ophthalmol Otolaryngol 78:240, 1974.
18. Hernandez MR and others: Age-related changes in the extracellular matrix of the human optic nerve head, Am J Ophthalmol 107:476, 1989.
19. Joffe L and others: Varix of the optic disk, Am J Ophthalmol 86:520, 1978.
20. Lieberman M, Maumenee A, and Green W: Histologic studies of the vasculature of the anterior optic nerve, Am J Ophthalmol 82:105, 1976.
21. Neetens A: Autoregulation of the blood supply to the anterior optic nerve and lamina cribrosa, Trans Ophthalmol Soc UK 97:168, 1977.
22. Oeller JH: Atlas seltener ophthalmoskopischer Befunde, Wiesbaden, 1903, JF Bergmann.
23. Onda E and others: Microvasculature of human optic nerve, Am J Ophthalmol 120:92, 1995.
24. Peyman GA and Apple DJ: Peroxidase diffusion in optic nerve, Arch Ophthalmol 88:650, 1972.
25. Peyman GA, Apple DJ, and Sanders DR, editors: Intraocular tumors, New York, 1977, Appleton-Century-Crofts.
26. Repka MX and Quigley HA: The effect of age on normal human optic nerve fiber number and diameter, Ophthalmology 96:26, 1989.
27. Straatsma BR and others: Myelinated retinal nerve fibers, Am J Ophthalmol 91:25, 1981.
28. Trobe JD and others: Nonglaucomatous excavation of the optic disc, Arch Ophthalmol 98:1046, 1980.
29. Wolter J: Astroglia of the human retina and other glial elements of the retina under normal and pathologic conditions, Am J Ophthalmol 40:88, 1955.
30. Wolter J: Reactions of elements of retina and optic nerve in common morbid entities of the human eye, Am J Ophthalmol 42:10, 1956.
31. Wolter J: The human optic papilla: a demonstration of new anatomic and pathologic findings, Am J Ophthalmol 44:48, 1957.
32. Wolter J: Pervascular glia of the blood vessels of the human retina, Am J Ophthalmol 44:766, 1957.
33. Wolter J: Glia of the human retina, Am J Ophthalmol 48:370, 1959.

Developmental abnormalities

34. Acers TE: Optic nerve hypoplasia: septo-optic-pituitary dysplasia syndrome, Trans Am Ophthalmol Soc 79:425, 1981.
35. Apple DJ, Rabb MF, and Walsh PM: Congenital anomalies of the optic disc, Surv Ophthalmol 27:3, 1982.
36. Armaly MF: The optic cup in the normal eye. I. Cup width, depth, vessel displacement, ocular tension and outflow facility, Am J Ophthalmol 68:401, 1969.
37. Awan KJ: Hypotelorism and optic disc anomalies: an ignored ocular syndrome, Ann Ophthalmol 9:771, 1977.
38. Awan KJ: Association of Duane's retraction and hypoplasia of optic nerve, J Pediatr Ophthalmol Strabismus 17:206, 1980 (letter to the editor).
39. Barber A: Embryology of the human eye, St Louis, 1955, The CV Mosby Co.
40. Bellhorn RW and others: Schwann cell proliferations mimicking medullated retinal nerve fibers, Am J Ophthalmol 87:469, 1979.
41. Bjork A, Laurell CG, and Laurell U: Bilateral optic nerve hypoplasia with normal visual acuity, Am J Ophthalmol 86:524, 1978.
42. Bonnin P, Passot E, and Triolaire-Cotton T: L'autofluorescence des drüsen papillaires dans le diagnostic des faux cedèmes de la papille, Bull Soc Ophthalmol Fr 76:331, 1976.
43. Brodsky MC and others: Optic nerve hypoplasia, Arch Ophthalmol 108:1562, 1990.
44. Brown GC: Optic nerve hypoplasia and colobomatous defects, J Pediatr Ophthalmol Strabismus 19:90, 1982.
45. Caldwell J, Howard R, and Riggs I: Dominant juvenile optic atrophy, Arch Ophthalmol 85:133, 1971.
46. Chambers J and Walsh F: Hyaline bodies in the optic discs: report of ten cases exemplifying importance in neurological diagnosis, Brain 74:95, 1951.
47. Chamlin M and Davidoff LM: Drusen of optic nerve simulating papilledema, J Neurosurg 7:70, 1950.
48. Craythorn JM, Swartz M, and Creel DJ: Clofazimine-induced bull's-eye retinopathy, Retina 6:50, 1986.
49. de Morsier G: Etudes sur les dystrophies cranioencephaliques. III. Agenesie du septum lucidum avec malformation du tractus optique, Arch Suisses Neurol Psychiatr 77:267, 1956.
50. Duke-Elder S: System of ophthalmology, vol III, Normal and abnormal development, part 2, Congenital deformities, St Louis, 1963, The CV Mosby Co.
51. Duke-Elder S: System of ophthalmology, vol XII, Neuro-ophthalmology, St Louis, 1971, The CV Mosby Co.
52. Duke-Elder S and Abrams D: System of ophthalmology, vol V, Ophthalmic optics and refraction, St Louis, 1970, The CV Mosby Co.
53. Edwards W and Layden W: Optic nerve hypoplasia, Am J Ophthalmol 70:950, 1970.
54. Edwards W, Price W, and Macdonald R: Congenital amaurosis of retinal origin (Leber), Am J Ophthalmol 72:724, 1971.
55. Elliot D, Traboulsi EI, and Maumenee IH: Visual prognosis in autosomal dominant optic atrophy, Am J Ophthalmol 115:360, 1993.
56. Elschnig A: Das Colobom am Schnervencintritte und der Conus nach unten, Graefes Arch Ophthalmol 51:391, 1900.
57. Erkkilä H: Clinical appearance of optic disc drusen in childhood, Graefes Arch Clin Exp Ophthalmol 193:1, 1975.

58. Ford M and Sarwar M: Features of a clinically normal optic disc, Br J Ophthalmol 47:50, 1963.

59. Friedman A and Beckerman B, Gold D: Drusen of the optic disc, Surv Ophthalmol 21:375, 1977.

60. Friedman A, Gartner S, and Modi S: Drusen of the optic disk: a retrospective study in cadaver eyes, Br J Ophthalmol 59:413, 1975.

61. Frisén L, Holmegaard L: Spectrum of optic nerve hypoplasia, Br J Ophthalmol 62:7, 1978.

62. Frisén L, Schöldström G, and Svendsen P: Drusen in the optic nerve head: verification by computerized tomography, Arch Ophthalmol 96:1611, 1978.

63. Ginsberg J, Bove KE, and Cuesta MG: Aplasia of the optic nerve with aniridia, Ann Ophthalmol 12:433, 1980.

64. Glaser JS: Neuro-ophthalmology, New York, 1978, Harper & Row, Publishers.

65. Graefe A, cited in Duke-Elder S and Abrams D: System of ophthalmology, vol V, Ophthalmic optics and refraction, St Louis, 1970, The CV Mosby Co.

66. Greenfield PS and others: Hypoplasia of the optic nerve in association with porencephaly, J Pediatr Ophthalmol Strabismus 17:75, 1980.

67. Grüner HJ and Fechner PU: Optic nerve hypoplasia, J Pediatr Ophthalmol Strabismus 15:222, 1978.

68. Harcourt B: Developmental abnormalities of the optic nerve, Trans Ophthalmol Soc UK 96:395, 1976.

69. Harley RD, editor: Pediatric ophthalmology, vols 1 and 2, ed 2, Philadelphia, 1983, WB Saunders Co.

70. Harris MJ, Fine SL, and Owens SL: Hemorrhagic complications of optic nerve drusen, Am J Ophthalmol 92:70, 1981.

71. Hayreh SS: Blood supply of the optic nerve head and its role in optic atrophy, glaucoma, and oedema of the optic disc, Br J Ophthalmol 53:721, 1969.

72. Hotchkiss ML and Green WR: Optic nerve aplasia and hypoplasia, J Pediatr Ophthalmol Strabismus 16:225, 1979.

73. Hoyt CS and Billson FA: Maternal anticonvulsants and optic nerve hypoplasia, Br J Ophthalmol 62:3, 1978.

74. Hoyt WF and others: Septo-optic dysplasia and pituitary dwarfism, Lancet 1:893, 1970.

75. Hoyt WF and others: Homonymous hemiopic hypoplasia, Br J Ophthalmol 56:537, 1972.

76. Johns DR and others: Leber's hereditary optic neuropathy, Arch Ophthalmol 111:495, 1993.

77. Johns DR and others: Leber's hereditary optic neuropathy, Ophthalmology 100:981, 1993.

78. Johnston PB and others: A clinicopathologic study of autosomal dominant optic atrophy, Am J Ophthalmol 88:868, 1979.

79. Kamin DF, Hepler RS, and Foos RY: Optic-nerve drusen, Arch Ophthalmol 89:359, 1973.

80. Keller-Wood H and others: Leber's hereditary optic neuropathy mitochondrial DNA mutations in multiple sclerosis, Ann Neurol 36:109, 1994.

81. Kelley J: Autofluorescence of drusen of the optic nerve head, Arch Ophthalmol 92:263, 1974.

82. Kingham JD and Fox MJ: Bilateral optic nerve hypoplasia with unilateral retinal vessel abnormality, Ann Ophthalmol 12:377, 1980.

83. Krause-Brucker W and Gardner DW: Optic nerve hypoplasia associated with absent septum pellucidum and hypopituitarism, Am J Ophthalmol 89:113, 1980.

84. Lambert SR, Hoyt CS, and Narahara MH: Optic nerve hypoplasia, Surv Ophthalmol 32:1, 1987.

85. Landers MB III, Bradbury MJ, and Sydnor CF: Retinal vascular changes in retrograde optic atrophy, Am J Ophthalmol 86:177, 1978.

86. Leibrich R: in discussion of Iwanoff, A: Ueber neuritis optica, Klin Monatsbl Augenheilkd 6:426, 1868.

87. Lichter PR: Variability of expert observers in evaluating the optic disc, Trans Am Ophthalmol Soc 74:532, 1976.

88. Little LE, Whitmore PV, and Wells TW Jr: Aplasia of the optic nerve, J Pediatr Ophthalmol Strabismus 13:84, 1976.

89. Lorentzen SE: Drusen of the optic disk: a clinical and genetic study, Acta Ophthalmol (suppl) 90:1, 1966.

90. Lott MT, Voljavec AS, and Wallace DC: Variable genotype of Leber's hereditary optic neuropathy patients, Am J Ophthalmol 109:625, 1990.

91. Magoon E II and Robb RM: Development of myelin in human optic nerve and tract: a light and electron microscopic study, Arch Ophthalmol 99:655, 1981.

92. Mann IC: Developmental abnormalities of the eye, Philadelphia, 1957, JB Lippincott Co.

93. Manschot WA: The optic nerve in hydranencephaly and anencephaly. In Cant JS, editor: The optic nerve, St Louis, 1972, The CV Mosby Co.

94. McKinna AJ: Quinine induced hypoplasia of the optic nerve, Can J Ophthalmol 1:261, 1966.

95. McPherson S: Primary drusen (hyaline bodies) of the optic nerve, Am J Ophthalmol 39:294, 1955.

96. Meissner W: Colobom der Aderhaut und Netzhaut mit Aplasie des Sehnerven, Graefes Arch Ophthalmol 79:308, 1911.

97. Miller JW and others: A specific congenital brain defect (arrhinencephaly) in 13-15 trisomy, N Eng J Med 268:120, 1963.

98. Miller NR and others: Giant cell (temporal) arteritis: the differential diagnosis, Surv Ophthalmol 23:259, 1979.

99. Minckler DS: The organization of nerve fiber bundles in the primate optic nerve head, Arch Ophthalmol 98:1630, 1980.

100. Mizuno K and others: Leber's congenital amaurosis, Am J Ophthalmol 83:32, 1977.

101. Morrison JC and others: Ultrastructural location of extracellular matrix components in the optic nerve head, Arch Ophthalmol 107:123, 1989.

102. Mosier MA and others: Hypoplasia of the optic nerve, Arch Ophthalmol 96:1437, 1978.

103. Naumann GO II and Apple DJ: Pathology of the eye, New York, 1986, Springer-Verlag (Translation, modification, and update of Pathologic des Auges by DJ Apple).

104. Newman NJ, Lott MT, and Wallace DC: The clinical characteristics of pedigrees of Leber's hereditary optic neuropathy with the 11778 mutation, Am J Ophthalmol 111:750, 1991.

105. Newman NJ and Wallace DC: Mitochondria and Leber's hereditary optic neuropathy, Am J Ophthalmol 109:726, 1990.

106. Nicholson DH: Tumors of the optic disc. Trans Am Acad Ophthalmol Otolaryngol 83:751, 1977.

107. Nikoskelainen E and others: The early phase in Leber hereditary optic atrophy, Arch Ophthalmol 95:969, 1977.

108. Nikoskelainen E, Hoyt WF, and Nummelin K: Ophthalmoscopic findings of Leber's hereditary optic neuropathy, I. Fundus findings in asymptomatic family members, Arch Ophthalmol 100:1597, 1982.

109. Nikoskelainen EK and others: Leber's hereditary optic neuroretinopathy, a maternally inherited disease. A genealogic study in four pedigrees, Arch Ophthalmol 105:665, 1987.

110. Okun E: Chronic papilledema simulating hyaline bodies of the optic disc: a case report, Am J Ophthalmol 53:922, 1963.

111. Oostra RJ and others: Leber's hereditary optic neuropathy, Correlations between mitochondrial genotype and visual outcome. J Med Genet 31:280, 1994.

112. Petersen RA and Walton DS: Optic nerve hypoplasia with good visual acuity and visual field defects: a study of children of diabetic mothers, Arch Ophthalmol 95:254, 1977.

113. Pollack I and Becker B: Hyaline bodies (drusen) of the optic nerve, Am J Ophthalmol 54:651, 1962.

114. Puck A, Tso MOM, and Fishman GA: Drusen of the optic nerve associated with retinitis pigmentosa, Arch Ophthalmol 103:231, 1985.

115. Purcell J Jr and Goldberg R: Hyaline bodies of the optic papilla and bilateral acute vascular occlusions, Ann Ophthalmol 6:1069, 1974.

116. Quigley A II and Anderson DR: The histologic basis of optic disc pallor in experimental optic atrophy, Am J Ophthalmol 83:709, 1977.

117. Radius RL: Regional specificity in anatomy at the lamina cribrosa, Arch Ophthalmol 99:478, 1981.

118. Radius RL and Anderson DR: The course of axons through the retina and optic nerve head, Arch Ophthalmol 97:1154, 1979.

119. Radius RL and Gonzales M: Anatomy of the lamina cribrosa in human eyes, Arch Ophthalmol 99:2159, 1981.

120. Rucker CW: Defects in visual fields produced by hyaline bodies in optic disks, Arch Ophthalmol 32:56, 1944.

121. Rucker CW: Bitemporal defects in the visual fields resulting from developmental anomalies of the optic disks, Arch Ophthalmol 35:546, 1946.

122. Rush JA and Bajandas FJ: Septo-optic dysplasia (de Morsier syndrome), Am J Ophthalmol 86:202, 1978.

123. Sacks JG and others: The pathogenesis of optic nerve drusen: a hypothesis, Arch Ophthalmol 95:425, 1977.

124. Scheie H and Adler F: Aplasia of the optic nerve, Arch Ophthalmol 26:61, 1941.

125. Schieck F: Netzhaut. In Henke F and Lubarsch O, editors: Handbuch der speziellen pathologischen Anatomie and Histologie, Berlin, 1928, Julius Springer.

126. Schwarz GA and Yanoff M: Lafora bodies, corpora amylacea, and Lewy bodies, A morphologic and histochemical study, Arch Neurobiol (Madr) 28:803, 1965.

127. Seedorff T: Leber's disease, Acta Ophthalmol 48:186, 1970.

128. Sheridan SJ and Robb RM: Optic nerve hypoplasia with diabetes insipidus, J Pediatr Ophthalmol Strabismus 15:82, 1978.

129. Shields MB: Gray crescent in the optic nerve head, Am J Ophthalmol 89:238, 1980.

130. Skarf B and Hoyt CS: Optic nerve hypoplasia in children. Association with anomalies of the endocrine and CNS, Arch Ophthalmol 102:62, 1984.

131. Smith J, Hoyt W, and Susae J: Ocular fundus in acute Leber optic neuropathy, Arch Ophthalmol 90:349, 1973.

132. Snydacker D: The normal optic disc: ophthalmoscopic and photographic studies. Am J Ophthalmol 58:958, 1964.

133. Spencer WH: Drusen of the optic disc and aberrant axoplasmic transport. Am J Ophthalmol 85:1, 1978.

134. Straatsma BR and others: Myelinated retinal nerve fibers associated with ipsilateral myopia, amblyopia, and strabismus, Am J Ophthalmol 88:506, 1979.

135. Straatsma BR and others: Myelinated retinal nerve fibers: clinicopathological study and clinical correlations. In Shimizu K, editor: XXIII Concilium Ophthalmologicum, Kyoto, 1978, Amsterdam, 1979, Excerpta Medica.

136. Straatsma BR and others: Myelinated retinal nerve fibers, Am J Ophthalmol 91:25, 1931.

137. Tomlinson A and Phillips CI: Ratio of optic cup to optic disc: in relation to axial length of eyeball and refraction, Br J Ophthalmol 53:765, 1969.

138. Treft RL and others: Dominant optic atrophy, deafness, ptosis, ophthalmoplegia, dystaxia, and myopathy. A new syndrome, Ophthalmology 91:908, 1984.

139. Tso MOM: Pathology and pathogenesis of drusen of the optic nerve head, Ophthalmology 88:1066, 1981.

140. Van Dyk J II and Morgan KS: Optic nerve hypoplasia and young maternal age, Am J Ophthalmol 89:879, 1980 (letter to the editor).

141. Wallace DC: Leber's optic atrophy: a possible example of vertical transmission of a slow virus in a man, Australas Ann Med 19:259, 1970.

142. Weiter J, McLean I, and Zimmerman LE: Aplasia of the optic nerve and disc, Am J Ophthalmol 83:569, 1977.

143. Whinery RD and Blodi FC: Hypoplasia of the optic nerve, Trans Am Acad Ophthalmol Otolaryngol 67:733, 1963.

144. Woodford B and Tso MOM: An ultrastructural study of the corpora amylacea of the optic nerve head and retina, Am J Ophthalmol 90:492, 1980.

145. Yanoff M, Rorke LB, and Allman MI: Bilateral optic system aplasia with relatively normal eyes, Arch Ophthalmol 96:97, 1978.

146. Zion V: Optic nerve hypoplasia, Ophthalmic Semin 1:171, 1976.

Papilledema

147. Blodi, FC, Allen L, and Frazier O: Stereoscopic manual of the ocular fundus in local and systemic disease, vol II, St Louis, 1970, The CV Mosby Co.

148. Carter SR and Seiff SR: Macular changes in pseudotumor cerebri before and after optic nerve sheath fenestration, Ophthalmology 102:937, 1995.

149. Cartlidge NEF, Ng RCY, and Tilley PJB: Dilemma of the swollen optic disc: a fluorescein retinal angiography study. Br J Ophthalmol 61:385, 1977.

150. Collins ML, Traboulsi EI, and Maumenee IH: Optic nerve head swelling and optic atrophy in the systemic mucopolysaccharidoses, Ophthalmology 97:1445, 1990.

151. Collins ML, Traboulsi EL, and Maumenee IH: Optic nerve head swelling and optic atrophy in the systemic mucopolysaccharidoses, Ophthalmology 98:502, 1980.

152. Eggers HM and Sanders MD: Acquired opticociliary shunt vessels in papilledema, Br J Ophthalmol 64:267, 1980.

153. Friedman M: Bilateral papilledema in otherwise well patients, Arch Ophthalmol 58:59, 1957.

154. Galvin R and Sanders MD: Peripheral retinal haemorrhages with papilledema, Br J Ophthalmol 64:262, 1980.

155. Hayreh MS and Hayreh SS: Optic disc edema in raised intracranial pressure, Arch Ophthalmol 95:1237, 1977.

156. Hayreh SS: Pathogenesis of the optic disc edema in raised intracranial pressure, Trans Ophthalmol Soc UK 96:404, 1976.

157. Hayreh SS: Optic disc edema in raised intracranial pressure. V. Pathogenesis, Arch Ophthalmol 95:1553, 1977.

158. Hayreh SS: Fluids in the anterior part of the optic nerve in health and disease, Surv Ophthalmol 23:1, 1978.

159. Hedges T: Papilledema: its recognition and relation to increased intracranial pressure, Surv Ophthalmol 19:201, 1975.

160. Hoyt W and Pont M: Pseudopapilledema: anomalous elevations of optic disc, pitfalls in diagnosis and management, JAMA 181:191, 1962.

161. Huber A and Blodi FC: Eye signs and symptoms in brain tumors, ed 3, St Louis, 1976, The CV Mosby Co.

162. Klaver CCW, Hoyng CB, and Dejong PTVM: Pigmentary irregularities and optic disc edema after heart transplantation, Archives of Ophthalmology 113:1281, 1995.

163. Laibovitz RA: Presumed phlebitis of the optic disc, Ophthalmology 86:313, 1979.

164. Leinfelder P: Choked disc and other types of edema of the nerve head, JAMA 144:919, 1950.

165. Leinfelder PJ: Choked discs and low intrathecal pressure occurring in brain tumor, Am J Ophthalmol 26:1294, 1943.

166. Leinfelder P and Paul W: Papilledema in general diseases, Arch Ophthalmol 28:983, 1942.

167. McLeod D: Retinal ischaemia, disc swelling and axoplasmic transport, Trans Ophthalmol Soc UK 96:313, 1976.

168. McLeod D, Marshall J, and Kohner EM: Role of axoplasmic transport in the pathophysiology of ischaemic disc swelling, Br J Ophthalmol 64:247, 1980.

169. Minckler D and Tso MOM: A light microscopic, autoradiographic study of axoplasmic transport in the normal rhesus optic nerve head, Am J Ophthalmol 82:1, 1976.

170. Minckler D, Tso MOM, and Zimmerman LE: A light microscopic, autoradiographic study of axoplasmic transport in the optic nerve head during ocular hypotony, increased intraocular pressure, and papilledema, Am J Ophthalmol 82:741, 1976.

171. Morris AT and Sanders MD: Macular changes resulting from papilledema, Br J Ophthalmol 64:211, 1980.

172. Morris AT and Dwek RA: Some recent applications of the use of paramagnetic centres to probe biological systems using nuclear magnetic resonance, Q Rev Biophys 10:421, 1977.

173. Paton L, and Holmes G: The pathology of papilledema: a histological study of sixty eyes, Brain 33:389, 1910.

174. Radius RL and Anderson DR: Fast axonal transport in early experimental disc edema, Invest Ophthalmol 19:158, 1980.

175. Rosenberg MA, Savino PJ, and Glaser JS: A clinical analysis of pseudopapilledema. I. Population, Arch Ophthalmol 97:65, 1979.

176. Rush JA: Hard retinal exudates and visual loss due to papilledema, Ann Ophthalmol 14:168, 1982.

177. Sanders MD: Diagnostic difficulties in optic nerve disease and in papilledema and disc edema, Trans Ophthalmol Soc UK 96:386, 1976.

178. Sanders MD and Sennhenn R II: Differential diagnosis of unilateral optic disc edema, Trans Ophthalmol Soc UK 100:123, 1980.

179. Sher NA and others: Unilateral papilledema in "benign" intracranial hypertension (pseudotumor cerebri), JAMA 250:2346, 1983.

180. Tso MOM: Axoplasmic transport in experimental papilledema, Trans Ophthalmol Soc UK 96:399, 1976.

181. Tso MOM and Fine B: Electron microscopic study of human papilledema, Am J Ophthalmol 82:424, 1976.

182. Tso MOM and Hayreh SS: Optic disc edema in raised intracranial pressure, Arch Ophthalmol 95:1448, 1977.

183. Tytell M and others: Axonal transport: each major rate component reflects the movement of distinct macromolecular complexes. Sciences 214:179, 1981.

184. Walsh F and Hoyt W, editors: Pseudopapilledema, pseudoneuritis, and drusen of the optic disc: disc anomalies frequently confused with papilledema. In Hoyt W and Walsh F: Clinical neuro-ophthalmology, ed 3, Baltimore, 1969, The Williams & Wilkins Co.

185. Wirtschafter J, Rizzo F, and Smiley B: Optic nerve axoplasm and papilledema, Surv Ophthalmol 20:157, 1975.
186. Wolter J: Reactions of elements of retina and optic nerve in common morbid entities of the human eye, Am J Ophthalmol 42:10, 1956.
187. Wolter J and Butler R: Zur Pathologic des Papilleödems des menschlichen Auges, Klin Monatsbl Augenheilkd 130:154, 1957.

Optic neuritis; optic atrophy

188. Abelsdorff G: Schnerv. In Henke F and Lubarsch O, editors: Handbuch der speziellen pathologischen Anatomic und Histologie, Berlin, 1928, Julius Springer.
189. Achkar AA and others: How does previous corticosteroid treatment affect the biopsy findings in giant cell (temporal) arteritis? Ann Inter Med 120:987, 1994.
190. Adams R and Kubik C: The morbid anatomy of the demyelinative diseases, Am J Med 12:510, 1952.
191. Aiello PD and others: Visual prognosis in giant cell arteritis, Ophthalmology 100:550, 1993.
192. Albert DM and Hedges TR III: The significance of negative temporal artery biopsies, Trans Am Ophthalmol Soc 80:143, 1982.
193. Albert DM, Ruchman M, and Keltner J: Skip areas in temporal arteritis, Arch Ophthalmol 94:2072, 1976.
194. Albert DM, Searl SS, and Craft JL: Histologic and ultrastructural characteristics of temporal arteritis: the value of the temporal artery biopsy, Ophthalmology 89:1111, 1982.
195. Anderson D: Ascending and descending optic atrophy produced experimentally in squirrel monkeys, Am J Ophthalmol 76:693, 1973.
196. Appen RE and Allen J: Optic neuritis under 60 years of age, Ann Ophthalmol 6:143, 1974.
197. Appen RE, De Venecia G, and Ferwerda J: Optic disc vasculitis, Am J Ophthalmol 90:352, 1980.
198. Arnold AC and others: Retinal periphlebitis and retinitis in multiple sclerosis. I Pathologic characteristics, Ophthalmology 91:255, 1984.
199. Arnold AC and Hepler RS: Fluorescein angiography in acute nonarteritic anterior ischemic optic neuropathy. Am J Ophthalmol 117:222, 1994.
200. Awan KJ: Hypotelorism and optic disc anomalies: an ignored ocular syndrome, Ann Ophthalmol 9:771, 1977.
201. Baumbach GL and others: Methyl alcohol poisoning, IV. Alterations of the morphological findings of the retina and optic nerve, Arch Ophthalmol 95:1859, 1977.
202. Beardsley TL and others: Eleven cases of sarcoidosis of the optic nerve, Am J Ophthalmol 97:62, 1984.
203. Beck RW and others: Acute ischemic optic neuropathy in severe preeclampsia, Am J Ophthalmol 90:342, 1980.
204. Beck RW and others: The effect of corticosteroids for acute optic neuritis on the subsequent development of multiple sclerosis, N Engl J Med 329:1764, 1993.
205. Bengtsson BA and Malmvall BE: Prognosis of giant cell arteritis including temporal arteritis and polymyalgia rheumatica, Acta Med Scand 209:337, 1981.
206. Beri RW and others: Anterior ischemic optic neuropathy. VII, Incidence of bilaterality and various influencing factors, Ophthalmology 94:1020, 1987.
207. Bevan AT, Dunmil MS, and Harrison MJG: Clinical and biopsy findings in temporal arteritis, Ann Rheum Dis 27:271, 1968.
208. Birch MK and others: Retinal venous sheathing and the blood-retinal barrier in multiple sclerosis, Arch Ophthalmol 114:34, 1996.
209. Biller J and others: Temporal arteritis associated with sedimentation rate, JAMA 247:486, 1982.
210. Blodi FC: Die Bedeutung der Temporalarterie in der Augenheikunde, Klin Monatsbl Augenheilkd 155:318, 1969.
211. Blodi FC: The temporal artery biopsy as a diagnostic procedure in ophthalmology, Trans Aust Coll Ophthalmol 1:26, 1969.
212. Boone MI and others: Visual outcome in bilateral nonarteritic anterior ischemic optic neuropathy, Ophthalmology 103:1223, 1996.
213. Brown GC and others: Radiation optic neuropathy, Ophthalmology 89:1489, 1982.
214. Brownstein S and Jannotta F: Sarcoid granulomas of the retina and optic nerve, Can J Ophthalmol 9:372, 1974.
215. Brownstein S, Nicolle DA, and Codere F: Bilateral blindness in temporal arteritis with skip areas, Arch Ophthalmol 101:388, 1983.
216. Brownstein S and others: Optic nerve in globoid leukodystrophy (Krabbe's disease), Arch Ophthalmol 96:864, 1978.
217. Caccamise W and Okuda K: Takayasu's or pulseless disease: unusual

218. Chess J and others: Serologic and immunopathologic findings in temporal arteritis, Am J Ophthalmol 96:283, 1983.
219. Chung SM, Gay CA, and McCrary JA: Nonarteritic ischemic optic neuropathy, Ophthalmology 101:779, 1994.
220. Cogan DG: Neurology of the visual system, Springfield, Ill, 1966, Charles C Thomas, Publisher.
221. Cohen D: Temporal arteritis: an improvement in visual prognosis and management with repeat biopsies, Trans Am Acad Ophthalmol Otolaryngol 77:74, 1973.
222. Cohen D and Smith T: Skip areas in temporal arteritis: myth versus fact, Trans Am Acad Ophthalmol Otolaryngol 78:772, 1974.
223. Cohen SMZ and others: Ocular histopathologic studies of neonatal and childhood adrenoleukodystrophy, Am J Ophthalmol 95:82, 1983.
224. Cullen L and Coleiro J: Ophthalmic complications of giant cell arteritis, Surv Ophthalmol 20:233, 1976.
225. Dennis R and Calkins L: Optic neuroencephalomyelopathy (Devic's disease): report of a case, Arch Ophthalmol 42:768, 1949.
226. Drance SM: Ischemic optic neuropathy, Trans Ophthalmol Soc UK 96:415, 1976.
227. Fleishman JA and others: Deficits in visual function after resolution of optic neuritis, Ophthalmology 94:1029, 1987.
228. Font R and Naumann G: Ocular histopathology in pulseless disease, Arch Ophthalmol 82:784, 1969.
229. Fratkin J, Smith A: Slow virus infections, Surv Ophthalmol 21:356, 1977.
230. Friedman J: Occult temporal arteritis, Am J Ophthalmol 60:333, 1965.
231. Fulton A and others: Active giant cell arteritis with cerebral involvement, Arch Ophthalmol 94:2068, 1976.
232. Gass J and Olson C: Sarcoidosis with optic nerve and retinal involvement: a clinicopathologic case report, Trans Am Acad Ophthalmol Otolaryngol 77:739, 1973.
233. Giarelli L, Melato M, and Campos E: Fourteen cases of cavernous degeneration of the optic nerve, Ophthalmologica 174:316, 1977.
234. Glasgow BJ and others: Ocular pathologic findings in neonatal adrenoleukodystrophy, Ophthalmology 94:1054, 1987.
235. Greeff R: Die pathologische Anatomie des Auges. In Orth J, editor: Lehrbuch der speziellen pathologischen Anatomie, Berlin, 1902, Hirschwald.
236. Guyer DR and others: The risk of cerebrovascular and cardiovascular disease in patients with anterior ischemic optic neuropathy, Arch Ophthalmol 103:1136, 1985.
237. Guyer DR and others: Bilateral ischemic optic neuropathy and retinal vascular occlusions associated with lymphoma and sepsis, clinicopathologic correlation, Ophthalmology 97:882, 1990.
238. Harcourt B and Ashton N: Ultrastructure of the optic nerve in Krabbe's leukodystrophy, Br J Ophthalmol 57:885, 1973.
239. Hayreh MS and others: Methyl alcohol poisoning, III, Ocular toxicity, Arch Ophthalmol 95:1851, 1977.
240. Hayreh SS: Optic disc vasculitis, Br J Ophthalmol 56:652, 1972.
241. Hayreh SS: Occlusion of the posterior ciliary arteries, Trans Am Acad Ophthalmol Otolaryngol 77:300, 1973.
242. Hayreh SS: Anterior ischemic optic neuropathy. I. Terminology and pathogenesis, Br J Ophthalmol 58:955, 1974.
243. Hayreh SS: Anterior ischemic optic neuropathy. II. Fundus on ophthalmoscopy and fluorescein angiography, Br J Ophthalmol 58:964, 1974.
244. Hayreh SS: Anterior ischemic optic neuropathy. III. Treatment, prophylaxis and differential diagnosis, Br J Ophthalmol 58:981, 1974.
245. Hayreh SS: Anterior ischemic optic neuropathy. New York, 1975, Springer-Verlag.
246. Hayreh SS: Anterior ischemic optic neuropathy, IV, Occurrence after cataract extraction. Arch Ophthalmol 98:1410, 1980.
247. Hayreh SS: Anterior ischemic optic neuropathy, V, Optic disc edema and early sign, Arch Ophthalmol 99:1030, 1981.
248. Hedges T III, Gieger GL, and Albert DM: The clinical value of negative temporal artery biopsy specimens. Arch Ophthalmol 101:1251, 1983.
249. Herkind P, Charles N, and Pearson J: Histopathology of ischemic optic neuropathy, Am J Ophthalmol 69:78, 1970.
250. Hinzpeter E and Naumaan G: Ischemic papilledema in giant-cell

arteritis, mucopolysaccharide deposition with normal intraocular pressure, Arch Ophthalmol 94:624, 1976.

251. Hollenhorst R: Ocular manifestations of insufficiency or thrombosis of the internal carotid artery, Am J Ophthalmol 47:753, 1959.

252. Horton B, Magath T, and Brown G: An undescribed form of arteritis of the temporal vessel, Proc Mayo Clin 7:700, 1932.

253. Hupp SL, Nelson GA, and Zimmerman LE: Generalized giant-cell arteritis with coronary artery involvement and myocardial infarction, Arch Ophthalmol 108:1385, 1990.

254. Johnson MW, Kincaid MC, and Trobe JD: Bilateral retrobulbar optic nerve infarctions after blood loss and hypotension: a clinicopathologic case study, Ophthalmology 94:1577, 1987.

255. Kazarian EL and Gager WE: Optic neuritis complicating measles, mumps and rubella vaccination, Am J Ophthalmol 86:504, 1978.

256. Keast-Butler J and Taylor D: Optic neuropathies in children, Trans Ophthalmol Soc UK 100:111, 1980.

257. Kelley J and Green W: Sarcoidosis involving the optic nerve head, Arch Ophthalmol 89:486, 1973.

258. Keltner JL: Giant-cell arteritis: signs and symptoms, Ophthalmology 89:1101, 1982.

259. Kerrison JB and others: Leber hereditary optic neuropathy—electron microscopy and molecular genetic analysis of a case, Ophthalmology 102:1509, 1995.

260. Kimmelstiel P, Gilmour MT, and Hodges HH: Degeneration of elastic fibers in granulomatous giant cell arteritis (temporal arteritis), Arch Pathol 59:157, 1952.

261. Klein R and others: Skip lesions in temporal arteritis, Mayo Clin Proc 51:504, 1976.

262. Kline LB, Kim JY, and Ceballos R: Radiation optic neuropathy, Ophthalmology 92:1118, 1985.

263. Knox D and Duke J: Slowly progressive ischemic optic neuropathy: a clinicopathologic case report, Trans Am Acad Ophthalmol Otolaryngol 75:1065, 1971.

264. Kuwabara T and Reinecke RD: Temporal arteritis. II. Electron microscopic study on consecutive biopsies, Arch Ophthalmol 83:692, 1970.

265. Laties A and Scheic H: Evolution of multiple small tumors in sarcoid granuloma of the optic disc, Am J Ophthalmol 74:60, 1972.

266. Levin LA and Louhab A: Apoptosis of retinal ganglion cells in anterior ischemic optic neuropathy, Arch Ophthalmol 114:488, 1996.

267. Levin PS and others: A clinicopathologic study of optic neuropathies associated with intracranial mass lesions with quantification of remaining axons, Am J Ophthalmol 95:295, 1983.

268. Liang GC, Simkin PA, and Manrik M: Immunoglobulins in temporal arteries: an immunofluorescent study, Ann Intern Med 81:19, 1974.

269. Lichter PR and Henderson JW: Optic nerve infarction, Am J Ophthalmol 85:302, 1978.

270. Lieberman MF, Shabi A, and Green WR: Embolic ischemic optic neuropathy, Am J Ophthalmol 86:206, 1978.

271. Lim JI, Tessler HH, and Goodwin JA: Anterior granulomatous uveitis in patients with multiple sclerosis, Ophthalmology 98:142, 1991.

272. Liu GT and others: Visual morbidity in giant cell arteritis, Clinical characteristics and prognosis for vision, Ophthalmology 101:1779, 1994.

273. Loewenstein A: Cavernous degeneration, necrosis and other regressive processes in optic nerve with vascular disease of the eye, Arch Ophthalmol 34:220, 1945.

274. Lucarelli MJ and others: Immunopathologic features of retinal lesions in multiple sclerosis, Ophthalmology 98:1652, 1991.

275. Margo CE, Levy MH, and Beck RW: Bilateral idiopathic inflammation of the optic nerve sheaths: light and electron microscopic findings, Ophthalmology 96:200, 1989.

276. Marx J: Slow viruses: role in persistent disease, Science 180:1351, 1973.

277. McDonnell PJ: Ocular manifestations of temporal arteritis, Current opinion in Ophthalmology 1:158, 1990.

278. McLeod D and others: Fundus signs in temporal arteritis, Br J Ophthalmol 62:591, 1978.

279. Melberg NS and others: Cotton-wool spots and the early diagnosis of giant cell arteritis, Ophthalmology 102:1611, 1995.

280. Miller B and Frankel M: Report of a case of tuberculous retrobulbar neuritis and osteomyelitis, Am J Ophthalmol 71:751, 1971.

281. Miller NR: Walsh and Hoyt's clinical neuro-ophthalmology, ed 4, Baltimore, 1982, Williams & Wilkins.

282. Miller NR and others: Giant cell (temporal) arteritis: the differential diagnosis, Surv Ophthalmol 23:259, 1979.

283. Mowat AG and Hazleman BL: Polymyalgia rheumatica: a clinical study with particular reference to arterial disease, J Rheumatol 1:190, 1974.

284. Newman NJ and others: Neuro-ophthalmic manifestations of meningocerebral inflammation from the limited form of Wegener's granulomatosis, Am J Ophthalmol 120:613, 1995.

285. Novack RL and Foos RY: Drusen of the optic disk in retinitis pigmentosa, Am J Ophthalmol 103:44, 1987.

286. Parker F and others: Light and electron microscopic studies on human temporal arteries with special reference to alterations related to senescence, atherosclerosis and giant cell arteritis, Am J Pathol 79:57, 1975.

287. Percy A, Nobregan F, and Kurland L: Optic neuritis and multiple sclerosis: an epidemiologic study, Arch Ophthalmol 87:135, 1972.

288. Perkins CD and Rose FC: Optic neuritis and its differential diagnosis, New York, 1979, Oxford University Press, Inc.

289. Pinkham R: The ocular manifestations of the pulseless syndrome, Acta of the XVII International Congress of Ophthalmology, Toronto, 1955, University of Toronto Press.

290. Quigley H and Anderson D: The histologic basis of optic disc pallor in experimental optic atrophy, Am J Ophthalmol 83:709, 1977.

291. Quigley H and Anderson DR: Cupping of the optic disc in ischemic optic neuropathy, Trans Am Acad Ophthalmol Otolaryngol 83:755, 1977.

292. Quillen DA and others: Choroidal nonperfusion in giant cell arteritis, Am J Ophthalmol 116:171, 1993.

293. Radius RL and Anderson DR: Retinal ganglion cell degeneration in experimental optic atrophy, Am J Ophthalmol 86:673, 1978.

294. Reinecke RD and Kuwabara T: Temporal arteritis. I. Smooth muscle cell involvement, Arch Ophthalmol 82:446, 1969.

295. Repka MX and others: Clinic profile and long-term implications of anterior ischemic optic neuropathy, Am J Ophthalmol 93:478, 1983.

296. Rizzo JF and Lessel S: Risk of developing multiple sclerosis after uncomplicated optic neuritis, Neurology 38:185, 1988.

297. Rootman J and Butler D: Ischaemic optic neuropathy—a combined mechanism, Br J Ophthalmol 64:826, 1980.

298. Ross R and McKusick V: Aortic arch syndromes: diminished or absent pulses in arteries arising from arch of aorta, Arch Intern Med 92:701, 1953.

299. Roth AM, Milsow I, and Keltner JL: The ultimate diagnoses of patients undergoing temporal artery biopsies, Arch Ophthalmol 102:901, 1984.

300. Sadun AA and Bassi CJ: Optic nerve damage in Alzheimer's disease, Ophthalmology 97:9, 1990.

301. Salvin ML and Barondes MJ: Visual loss caused by choroidal ischemia preceding anterior ischemic optic neuropathy in giant cell arteritis, Am J Ophthalmol 117:81, 1994.

302. Sandok B: Temporal arteritis, JAMA 222:1405, 1972.

303. Schatz H and others: Clinicopathologic correlation of retinal to choroidal venous collaterals of the optic nerve head, Ophthalmology 98:1287, 1991.

304. Schmidt D and L ffler KU: Temporal arteritis, Comparison of histologic and clinical findings, Acta Ophthalmol 72:319, 1994.

305. Schneider H, Weber A, and Ballen P: The visual prognosis in temporal arteritis, Ann Ophthalmol 3:1215, 1971.

306. Sergott RC and Brown MJ: Current concepts of the pathogenesis of optic neuritis associated with multiple sclerosis, Surv Ophthalmol 33:108, 1988.

307. Shields CL and Eagle CE: Pseudo-Schnabel's cavernous degeneration of the optic nerve secondary to intraocular silicone oil, Arch Ophthalmol 107:714, 1989.

308. Siätkowski RM and others: Optic Neuropathy in Hodgkin's disease, Am J Ophthalmol 114:625, 1992.

309. Simmons J and Cogan D: Occult temporal arteritis, Arch Ophthalmol 68:8, 1962.

310. Slavin ML and Barondes MJ: Visual loss caused by choroidal ischemia preceding anterior ischemic optic neuropathy in giant cell arteritis, Am J Ophthalmol 117:265, 1994.

311. Spencer W and Hoyt W: A fatal case of giant cell arteritis (temporal or cranial arteritis) with ocular involvement, Arch Ophthalmol 64:862, 1960.

312. Stratton R, Blodi F, and Hanigan J: Sarcoidosis of the optic nerve, Arch Ophthalmol 71:834, 1964.

313. To KW, Enzer YR, and Tsiaras WG: Temporal artery biopsy after one month of corticosteroid therapy. Am J Ophthalmol 117:265, 1994.

314. Tour R and Hoyt W: The syndrome of the aortic arch: ocular manifestations of "pulseless disease" and a report of a surgically treated case, Am J Ophthalmol 47:35, 1959.

315. Townes D and Blodi F: The diagnostic value of temporal artery biopsy, Trans Am Ophthalmol Soc 66:33, 1968.

316. Traboulsi EI and Maumenee IH: Ophthalmologic manifestations of X-linked childhood adrenoleukodystrophy, Ophthalmology 94:47, 1987.

317. Ubert J and others: Ocular findings in metachromatic leukodystrophy: an electron microscopic and enzyme study in different clinical and genetic variants, Arch Ophthalmol 97:1495, 1979.

318. Ulrich GG and others: Cat scratch disease associated with neuroretinitis in a 6-year-old girl, Ophthalmology 99:246, 1992.

319. Vine AK: Severe periphlebitis, peripheral retinal ischemia, and preretinal neovascularization in-patients with multiple sclerosis, Am J Ophthalmol 113:28, 1992.

320. Wang FM and Henkind P: Visual system involvement in giant cell (temporal) arteritis, Surv Ophthalmol 23:264, 1979.

321. Wegener H and Hollenhorst R: Ocular lesions of temporal arteritis, Am J Ophthalmol 45:617, 1958.

322. Wells KK and others: Temporal artery biopsies: correlation of light microscopy and immunofluorescence microscopy, Ophthalmology 96:1058, 1989.

323. Whitfield A, Bateman M, and Trevar C: Temporal arteritis, Br J Ophthalmol 47:555, 1963.

324. Wilkinson IMS and Russell PWR: Arteries of the head and neck in giant cell arteritis: a pathologic study to show the pattern of arterial involvement, Arch Neurol 27:378, 1972.

325. Wilske KR and Healy LA: Polymyalgia rheumatica: a magnification of systemic giant-cell arteritis, Ann Intern Med 66:77, 1967.

326. Yau TH and others: Unilateral optic neuritis caused by histoplasma capsulatum in a patient with the acquired immunodeficiency syndrome, Am J Ophthalmol 121:324, 1996.

327. Zimmerman H and Netsky M: The pathology of multiple sclerosis: Proc Assoc Res Nerv Ment Dis 28:271, 1950.

328. Zion V and Goodside V: Anterior segment ischemia with ischemic optic neuropathy, Surv Ophthalmol 19:19, 1974.

Tumors

329. Alvord EC Jr and Lofton S: Gliomas of the optic nerve or chiasm, Outcome by patients age, tumor site, and treatment, J Neurosurg 68:85, 1988.

330. Anderson D and Khalil M: Meningioma and the ophthalmologist: a review of 80 cases, Ophthalmology 88:1004, 1981.

331. Apple DJ: Malignant melanoma arising from a melanocytoma (abstract). In Proceedings of the XII International Pigment Cell Conference, Sept 18-22, 1983, Giessen, Germany, 1984, Justus-Liebig Universität.

332. Apple DJ and others: Malignant transformation of an optic nerve melanocytoma, Can J Ophthalmol 19:30, 1984.

333. Arnold AC and others: Metastasis of adenocarcinoma of the lung to optic nerve sheath meningioma, Arch Ophthalmol 113:346, 1995.

334. Beck RW and others: Decreased visual acuity from optic disc drusen, Arch Ophthalmol 103:155, 1985.

335. Bergin DJ and others: Ganglioglioma of the optic nerve, Am J Ophthalmol 105:146, 1988.

336. Blodi FC and Braley A: Primäre und sekundäre Meningiome der Augenhöhle. In François J, editor: Die Tumoren des Auges und seiner Adnexe, Proceedings of the Second Congress of the European Ophthalmology Society held in Vienna, Austria, 1964, Basel, 1966, S Karger, AG.

337. Boles W, Naugle T, and Samson C: Glioma of the optic nerve: report of a case arising from the optic disc, Arch Ophthalmol 59:229, 1958.

338. Boniuk M, Messmer EP, and Font RL: Hemangiopericytoma of the meninges of the optic nerve: a clinicopathologic report including electron microscopic observations, Ophthalmology 92:1780, 1985.

339. Borit A and Richardson EP: The biological and clinical behavior of pilocytic astrocytomas of the optic pathways, Brain 105:161, 1982.

340. Brandt D and Beisner D: Meningioma of the optic nerve, Arch Ophthalmol 84:177, 1970.

341. Brown GC and Shields JA: Tumors of the optic nerve head, Surv Ophthalmol 29:239, 1985.

342. Charles NC and others: Pilocytic astrocytoma of the optic nerve with hemorrhage and extreme cystic degeneration, Am J Ophthalmol 92:691, 1981.

343. Christmas NJ and others: Secondary optic nerve tumors, Surv Ophthalmol 36:196, 1991.

344. Christmas NJ and others: Clinical pathological review: secondary optic nerve tumors, Surv Ophthalmol 36:196, 1991.

345. Cibis GW, Whittaker CK, and Wood WE: Intraocular extension of optic nerve meningioma in a case of neurofibromatosis. Arch Ophthalmol 103:404, 1985.

346. Cooling RJ and Wright JE: Arachnoid hyperplasia in optic nerve glioma: confusion with orbital meningioma, Br J Ophthalmol 63:596, 1979.

347. Coons SW, Davis JR, and Way DL: Correlation of DNA content and histology in prognosis of astrocytomas, Am J Clin Pathol 90:289, 1988.

348. Croxatto JO and others: Angle closure-glaucoma as initial manifestation of melanocytoma of the optic disc, Ophthalmology 90:830, 1983.

349. Cushing H and Eisenhardt L: Meningiomas, their classification, regional behaviour, life history, and surgical end results, Springfield, IL, 1938, Charles C Thomas, Publisher.

350. Cutarelli PE and others: Immunohistochemical properties of human optic nerve glioma, Invest Ophthalmol Vis Sci 32:2521, 1991.

351. de Keizer RJW and others: Optic glioma with intraocular tumor and seeding in a child with neurofibromatosis. Am J Ophthalmol 108:717, 1989.

352. de Potter P and others: Malignant melanoma of the optic nerve, Arch Ophthalmol 114:608, 1996.

353. de Veer J: Juxtapapillary malignant melanoma of the choroid and so-called malignant melanoma of the optic disc, Arch Ophthalmol 51:147, 1954.

354. de Veer J: Melanotic tumors of the optic nerve head, Arch Ophthalmol 65:536, 1961.

355. Dossetor FM, Landau K, and Hoyt WF: Optic disk glioma in neurofibromatosis type 2, Am J Ophthalmol 602, 1989.

356. Dutton JJ: Optic nerve sheath meningiomas, Surv Ophthalmol 38:427, 1994.

357. Dutton JJ: Optic nerve sheath meningiomas, Surv Ophthalmol 37:167, 1992.

358. Eggers H, Jakobiec F, and Jones I: Tumors of the optic nerve, Doc Ophthalmol 41:43, 1976.

359. Ellenberger C Jr: Perioptic meningiomas, Arch Neurol 33:671, 1976.

360. Erzurum SA and others: Primary malignant melanoma of the optic nerve simulating a melanocytoma, Arch Ophthalmol 110:684, 1992.

361. Fischer F: Uber gliomatöse Entartung der Optikusbahn, Arch Augenheilkd 59:181, 1908.

362. Frangieh GT and others: Melanocytoma of the ciliary body: presentation of four cases and review of nineteen reports, Surv Ophthalmol 29:328, 1985.

363. Fratkin J and Smith A: Slow virus infections, Surv Ophthalmol 21:356, 1977.

364. Frisén L, Royt WF, and Tengroth BM: Opticociliary veins, disc pallor and visual loss: a triad of signs indicating spheno-orbital meningioma, Acta Ophthalmol 51:241, 1973.

365. Gallie BL, Graham JE, and Hunter WS: Optic nerve head metastasis, Arch Ophthalmol 93:983, 1975.

366. Garcia-Arumi J and others: Neuroretinitis associated with a melanocytoma of the optic disc, Retina 14:173, 1994.

367. Haas BD and others: Diffuse choroidal melanocytoma in a child: a lesion extending the spectrum of melanocytic hamartomas, Ophthalmology 93:1632, 1986.

368. Haik BG and others: Magnetic resonance imaging in the evaluation of optic nerve glioma, Ophthalmology 94:709, 1987.

369. Hamilton A and others: Malignant optic nerve glioma: report of a case with electron microscopic study, Br J Ophthalmol 57:253, 1973.

370. Henkind P and Benjamin JV: Vascular anomalies and neoplasms of the optic nerve head, Trans Ophthalmol Soc UK 96;:418, 1976.

371. Hollenhorst RW Jr, Hollenhorst RW Sr, and MacCarty CS: Visual prognosis of optic nerve sheath meningiomas producing shunt vessels of the optic disk: the Hoyt-Spencer syndrome, Trans Am Ophthalmol Soc 75:141, 1977.

372. Holman RE and others: Magnetic resonance imaging of optic gliomas, Am J Ophthalmol 100:596, 1985.

373. Howard G and Forrest A: Incidence and location of melanocytomas, Arch Ophthalmol 77:61, 1967.

374. Hoyt WF and Baghdassarian SA: Optic glioma of childhood: natural history and rationale for conservative management, Br J Ophthalmol 53:793, 1969.

375. Imes RK and others: Evolution of opticociliary veins in optic nerve sheath meningioma, Arch Ophthalmol 103:59, 1985.

376. Jakobiec FA and others: Combined clinical and computed tomographic diagnosis of orbital glioma and meningioma, Ophthalmology 91:137, 1984.

377. Joffe L and others: Clinical and follow-up studies of melanocytomas of the optic disc, Ophthalmology 86:1067, 1979.

378. Juarez CP and Tso MOM: An ultrastructural study of melanocytomas (magnocellular nevi) of the optic disk and uvea, Am J Ophthalmol 90:48, 1980.

379. Karp LA and others: Primary intraorbital meningiomas, Arch Ophthalmol 91:24, 1974.

380. Kattah JC and others: Metastatic prostate cancer to the optic canal, Ophthalmology 100:1711, 1993.

381. Kazim M and others: Choristoma of the optic nerve and chiasm, Arch Ophthalmol 110:236, 1992.

382. Kennerdell JS and others: The management of optic nerve sheath meningiomas, Am J Ophthalmol 1066:450, 1988.

383. Koenig SB, Naidich TP, and Zaparackas Z: Optic glioma masquerading as spasmus nutans, J Pediatr Ophthalmol Strabismus 19:20, 1982.

384. Lauritzen K, Augsburger JJ, and Timmes J: Vitreous seeding associated with melanocytoma of the optic disc, Retina 10:60, 1990.

385. Lee JS, Smith RF, and Minckler DS: Scleral melanocytoma, Ophthalmology 89:178, 1982.

386. Lewis RA and others: Von Recklinghausen neurofibromatosis, II, Incidence of optic gliomata, Ophthalmology 91:929, 1984.

387. Lichter PR and Henderson JW: Optic nerve infarction, Am J Ophthalmol 85:302, 1978.

388. Lindblom B, Truwit CI, and Hoyt WF: Optic nerve sheath meningioma. Ophthalmology 99:560, 1992.

389. Listernick R, Charrow J, and Greenwald MJ: Emergence of optic pathway gliomas in children with neurofibromatosis type 1 after normal neuroimaging results, J Pediatr 121:584, 1992.

390. Lloyd L: Gliomas of the optic nerve and chiasm in childhood, Trans Am Ophthalmol Soc 71:488, 1973.

391. Manor R, Israeli J, and Sandbank U: Malignant optic glioma in a 70-year-old patient, Arch Ophthalmol 94:1142, 1976.

392. Marquardt MD and Zimmerman LE: Histopathology of meningiomas and gliomas of the optic nerve. Hum Pathol 13:226, 1982.

393. Newman NJ, Grossniklaus HE, and Wojno TH: Breast carcinoma metastatic to the optic nerve, Arch Ophthalmol 114:102, 1996.

394. Newman NM and DiLoreto DA: Metastasis of primary osteogenic sarcoma to the eyelid, Am J Ophthalmol 104:659, 1987.

395. Novack RL and Foos RY: Drusen of the optic disk in retinitis pigmentosa. Am J Ophthalmol 103:44, 1987.

396. Raichand M and others: Resection of uveal melanocytoma: clinicopathological correlation, Br J Ophthalmol 67:236, 1983.

397. Reese A: Tumors of the eye, ed 3, New York, 1976, Harper & Row, Publishers.

398. Reidy JJ and others: Melanocytoma: Nomenclature, pathogenesis, natural history and treatment, Surv Ophthalmol 29:319, 1985.

399. Rodgers R, Weiner M, and Friedman AH: Ocular involvement in congenital leukemia, Am J Ophthalmol 101:730, 1986.

400. Rodrigues M, Savino P, and Schatz N: Spheno-orbital meningioma with opticociliary veins, Am J Ophthalmol 81:666, 1976.

401. Roth AM: Malignant change in melanocytomas of the uveal tract, Surv Ophthalmol 22:404, 1978.

402. Rucker C and Kearns T: Mistaken diagnoses in some cases of meningioma, Am J Ophthalmol 51:15, 1961.

403. Rush JA and others: Optic glioma: long-term follow-up of 85 histopathologically verified cases, Ophthalmology 89:1213, 1982.

404. Russell D and Rubinstein L: Pathology of tumors of nervous system, London, 1959, Edward Arnold (Publishers), Ltd.

405. Schatz H and others: Clinicopathologic correlation of retinal to choroidal venous collaterals of the optic nerve head, Ophthalmology 98:1287, 1991.

406. Scheie HG and Yanoff M: Pseudomentanoma of ciliary body, report of a patient, Arch Ophthalmol 77:81, 1967.

407. Schuangshoti S: Meningioma of the optic nerve, Br J Ophthalmol 57:265, 1973.

408. Seiff SR and others: A morphologic and histochemical study, Arch Ophthalmol 105:1689, 1987.

409. Shammas HJF and others: Melanocytoma of the ciliary body, Ann Ophthalmol 13:1381, 1981.

410. Shields JA and others: Malignant melanoma associated with melanocytoma of the optic disc, Ophthalmology 97:225, 1990.

411. Sibony PA and others: Optic nerve sheath meningiomas: Clinical manifestations, Ophthalmology 91:1313, 1984.

412. Spencer W: Primary neoplasms of the optic nerve and its sheaths: clinical features and current concepts of pathogenetic mechanism, Trans Ophthalmol Soc UK 70:490, 1972.

413. Spoor TC and others: Malignant gliomas of the optic nerve pathways, Am J Ophthalmol 89:284, 1980.

414. Stock W: Pathologische Anatomic des Auges, Stuttgart, 1939, Ferdinand Enke Verlag.

415. Taphoorn MJB and others: Malignant optic glioma in adults, J Neurosurg 70:277, 1989.

416. Thomas C and Purnell E: Ocular melanocytoma, Am J Ophthalmol 67:79, 1969.

417. Tso MOM: Pathology and pathogenesis of drusen of the optic nerve head, Ophthalmology 88:1066, 1981.

418. Verhoeff F: Tumors of the optic nerve. In Penfield W, editor: Cytology and cellular pathology of the nervous system, New York, 1932, Paul B Hoeber, Inc, Medical Book Dept of Harper & Brothers.

419. Wilson WB: Meningiomas of the anterior visual system, Surv Ophthalmol 26:109, 1981.

420. Wineck RR, Scheithauer BW, and Wick MR: Meningioma, meningeal hemangiopericytoma (angioblastic hemangiopericytoma), peripheral hemangiopericytoma, and acoustic schwannoma: a comparative immunohistochemical study, Am J Ophthalmol 13:251, 1989.

421. Wiznia R and Price J: Recovery of vision in association with a melanocytoma of the optic disc. Am J Ophthalmol 78:236, 1974.

422. Wolter F and Benz S: Ectopic meningioma of the superior orbital rim, Arch Ophthalmol 94:1920, 1976.

423. Wright JE: Primary optic nerve meningiomas: clinical presentation and management, Trans Am Acad Ophthalmol Otolaryngol 83:617, 1977.

424. Wright JE, Call NB, and Liaricos S: Primary optic nerve meningioma, Br J Ophthalmol 64:553, 1980.

425. Wulc AE and others: Orbital optic nerve glioma in adult life, Arch Ophthalmol 107, 1013, 1989.

426. Yanoff M, Davis R, and Zimmerman LE: Juvenilepilocytic astrocytoma ("glioma") of optic nerve: clinicopathologic study of 63 cases, In Jakobiec FA, editor: Ocular and adnexal tumors, Birmingham, 1978, Aesculpius Publishing Co.

427. Zakka KA and others: Opticociliary veins in a primary optic nerve sheath meningioma, Am J Ophthalmol 87:91, 1979.

428. Zimmerman CF, Schatz NJ, and Glaser JS: Magnetic resonance imaging of optic nerve meningiomas. Ophthalmology 97:585, 1990.

429. Zimmerman LE and others: A rare choristoma of the optic nerve and chiasm, Arch Ophthalmol 101:766, 1983.

430. Zimmerman LF: Melanocytes, melanocytic nevi and melanocytomas, Invest Ophthalmol 4:11, 1965.

431. Zimmerman LF and Carron L: Melanocytoma of the optic disc, Int Ophthalmol Clin 2:431, 1961.

432. Zimmerman RA and others: Orbital magnetic resonance imaging, Am J Ophthalmol 100:312, 1985.

CHAPTER 11

CONJUNCTIVA AND EYELIDS

Histology of the conjunctiva

The conjunctiva is a mucous membranelike covering divided into three portions (Figs. 1-1 and 11-1, 11-2, 11-3).[1–30] The palpebral, or tarsal, conjunctiva begins anteriorly at the posterior aspect of the eyelid margin and covers the rear surface of the eyelids. It is then reflected on itself at the fornix (fornix conjunctiva) and continues over the anterior segment of the globe, forming the bulbar and limbal conjunctivae. The limbal conjunctiva merges with the stroma and epithelium of the cornea (Fig. 11-1).[12] At the nasal aspect of the eye the conjunctiva is modified by the formation of the caruncle (Fig. 11-2, B) and the plica semilunaris, a remnant of the nictitating membrane of animals. The bulbar conjunctiva is loosely connected to the underlying sclera and episclera to allow the eye free movement in all directions.

All conjunctival tissue consists of an epithelium and underlying substantia propria, or stroma. The conjunctival epithelium is embryologically derived from the surface ectoderm, which also forms the epidermis of the skin, the cornea epithelium, and the lens (Figs. 1-7, A, 1-9, and 4-1). Because the cornea, conjunctiva, and lid epithelium form a geographic continuum on the body surface and share a common embryologic origin with the lens, certain anomalies and diseases that are prone to affect structures derived from this embryologic source could simultaneously affect all of these tissues.

PALPEBRAL AND FORNIX CONJUNCTIVA

At the posterior end of the lid margin, the mucocutaneous junction, the skin epidermis of the lid gradually transforms into the palpebral conjunctiva (Fig. 11-3). The epithelium of the palpebral conjunctiva is a moist mucous membrane rather than a keratinized, dry covering like the eyelid skin.[1,2,4] It is a nonkeratinized stratified squamous epithelium, the thickness of which decreases as it proceeds further from the lid margin. The superficial cells become less flattened in character and eventually contain a more cuboidal or transitional shape in the midregions of the palpebral conjunctiva. There are numerous mucin-containing goblet cells, particularly near the fornix (Fig. 11-2, A).

The underlying stroma is composed of delicate connective tissue and vessels with scattered accumulations of lymphocytes, lymphoid follicles, and plasma cells.* These cellular elements may proliferate extensively in many pathologic processes, for example, inflammatory or allergic conjunctivitis. The conjunctiva also contains Langerhans' cells (dendritic-appearing cells expressing class II antigens.

The conjunctival epithelium is thinner in the region of

---

* References 3, 5–9, 20–22, 25, 27, 45, 46.

reseparate until late in the last trimester (see "kissing nevus," p. 589; Fig. 11-40).

From anterior to posterior there are four main layers (Fig. 11-3):

1. Skin, or cutaneous, layer
2. Muscular layer
3. Tarsal layer
4. Conjunctival layer

The major glands of the eyelids are listed in Table 11-1.

EPIDERMAL LAYER

The anterior skin is characterized by a very thin, slightly keratinized epidermis composed of stratified squamous epithelium, which overlies a loose connective tissue dermis, or corium (Figs. 11-3 and 11-4). Numerous rete ridges (finger-like projections of epithelium toward the dermis) and dermal papillae (upward extensions of dermal connective tissue between the rete ridges) are present. The typical appendages of the skin include hair follicles (cilia) and sebaceous and sweat glands.

The epidermis consists of four layers (Fig. 11-4):

Table 11-1. Eponymic designation of the eyelid gland

Gland	Type of gland	Location
Meibomian	Holocrine, sebaceous gland (oily secretion)	Tarsus
Zeis	Holocrine, sebaceous gland of the cilia	Lid margin
Moll	Apocrine sweat gland (oily secretion)	Lid margin
Krause	Accessory lacrimal gland	Fornix
Wolfring	Accessory lacrimal gland	Upper margin of the tarsus

1. Basal cell layer (stratum germinativum)
2. Squamous cell layer (stratum spinosum or stratum malpighi)
3. Granular layer (stratum granulosum)
4. Layer of keratin (stratum corneum)

The basal layer is composed of tall, columnar cells that differentiate into prickle or squamous cells as they grow into the malpighian layer. As they grow toward the surface, they contain basophilic droplets (granular layer), and their nuclei become pyknotic and disappear. The epithelial cells degenerate and are transformed into acellular keratin when they reach the stratum corneum. This final process of degeneration of the epithelial cells is termed *keratinization*.

In many dermatologic diseases the main clinicopathologic features of the lesion are caused by abnormal, often accelerated growth of the epithelial layers. The following microscopic pathologic terms are used to describe these basic changes:

1. Hyperkeratosis: thickening of the keratin layer or stratum corneum.
2. Acanthosis: thickening of the squamous cell layer.
3. Parakeratosis: retention of the nuclei in the keratin layer, caused by rapid cell growth.
4. Increased thickness of granular layer: caused by slow cell growth.
5. Acantholysis: loss of cohesion between cells of the epidermis as a result of breakdown of the intercellular bridges (desmosomes), which can cause vesicles and bullae. Bullae may form at many levels throughout the epithelium, including subcorneal, intraepithelial and subepithelial (junctional).
6. Atrophy: thinning of epithelium with smoothing of rete ridges, decrease in appendages and degeneration and elastosis of subepithelial connective tissue. It is often caused by aging and solar radiation.
7. Dyskeratosis: abnormal maturation of the epidermis, often resulting in abnormal keratinization within individual cells

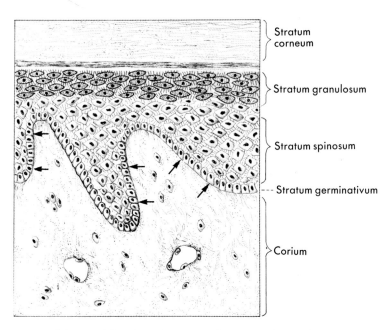

Fig. 11-4. Normal layers of the skin. The arrows denote the basement membrane separating the epithelium from the underlying corium or dermis. (Drawn by Dr Steven Vermillion, University of Iowa.)

anywhere in the squamous layer; keratin is normally absent in this layer.

In addition to the columnar basal cells, the basal cell layer contains pigment cells (melanocytes, clear cells of Masson), which determine the color of the skin. The melanocyte may be the primary cell of origin of the many types of melanotic tumors of the skin. Undifferentiated "stem cells" are also present in the basal cell layer.[17] These are primitive embryonic epithelial cells that have pluripotential developmental capability. It is believed that these cells may develop into hyperplastic or neoplastic epithelial tumors of the skin, particularly basal cell carcinoma (p. 590).[17] Langerhans' cells expressing class II antigen are also present.

The cilia are situated at the anteroinferior lid margin. The glands of Zeis (Fig. 11-3; Table 11-1) are the sebaceous glands of the cilia. Together they form the pilosebaceous apparatus.

The skin of the eyelids is one of the thinnest and most delicate of the body, and the epidermis is loosely bound to the underlying dermis; therefore fluid deposits such as edema and chemosis may be considerable. The subcutaneous layer of the lids is free of fat; adipose tissue is generally confined to the area superior or inferior to the lids in the orbital region.

At the lid margin the epidermis is more firmly attached to the dermis. The most anterior aspect of the lid margin is relatively round, and the posterior margin is more right-angled. At the posterior margin, the mucocutaneous junction, the keratinized epithelium of the lid gradually is transformed into the moist nonkeratinized conjunctival epithelium. The mucocutaneous junction and the gray line are *not* synonymous (Fig. 11-3). The former is situated slightly posterior to the orifices of the meibomian glands. The gray line corresponds to the plane immediately anterior to the tarsal plate and the meibomian glands.[24] The gray line is important in eyelid surgery as a cleavage plane between the two major anterior layers of the lids (skin and muscle) and the two posterior layers (tarsus and conjunctiva).

MUSCULAR LAYER

The second layer of the lid is the muscular layer, which consists of orbicularis oculi muscle and the tendinous processes of levator palpebrae muscle.[16] The orbicularis is a skeletal muscle consisting of four parts: pretarsal, preseptal, orbital, and Riolan's muscle. The fibers of Riolan's muscle (Fig. 11-3) are situated near the lid margin. They may function to hold the posterior border of the eyelid snug against the globe to prevent overflow of tears.

The muscular portion of the levator palpebrae lies under the roof of the orbit and sends its tendinous processes into the lid. These insert into the pretarsal connective tissue and onto the anterior surface of the tarsus. Only the collagenous aponeurosis of the levator muscle is found in the eyelid; the actual skeletal muscle bundles occur only within the orbit. The sympathetically innervated smooth muscle of Müller lies posterior to the levator and influences the tonus and width of the palpebral fissure. In Horner's syndrome, loss of tonus of this muscle may lead to ptosis.

TARSAL LAYER

The third layer of the lids, the tarsus, consists of a plate of dense fibrous connective tissue with a thickness of approximately 0.8 to 1.0 mm.[11] As a rule there is no cartilage within the human tarsus; a cartilaginous tarsal plate is often present in lower animals (Fig. 11-5). The tarsus provides structural support and stiffens the eyelid. The tarsus is slightly concave, corresponding to the slight arching caused by the globe itself.

The meibomian glands (Table 11-1), the largest glandular complex in the lids, consist of elongated glands with their long axes vertical to the free lid margins (Fig. 11-50). The upper lid contains about 40 tarsal or meibomian glands, and the lower lid has approximately 20. They consist of branching tubuloalveolar sebaceous glands, which have their skin orifices immediately posterior to the gray line, and produce a lipid secretion, which forms a component of the tear film.

In contrast to other sebaceous glands of the skin, for example, the Zeis glands of the eyelids, the meibomian glands have no association with adjacent hair follicles or erector pili muscles. In contrast, the Zeis glands are situated anterior to the tarsus at the lid margin and combine with the cilia, forming a true pilosebaceous apparatus. The glands of Zeis drain at the sites of the hair follicles.

Because of the relatively high concentration of sebaceous glands within the eyelid, sebaceous carcinoma of the lid occurs more frequently than in other parts of the skin. The fact that approximately twice as many meibomian glands occur in the upper lids as in the lower may partially

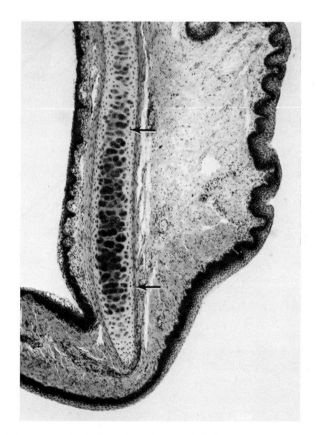

Fig. 11-5. Sagittal section of rat eyelid showing cartilaginous tarsal plate *(arrows)*. The tarsal plate in humans is composed of dense fibrous tissue rather than cartilage. (H & E stain; ×5.)

explain the fact that sebaceous tumors are more common on the upper lid.

The glands of Moll are located near the lid margin (Figs. 11-3 and 11-38, *A;* Table 11-1). These are apocrine sweat glands, which are characterized by apical or "decapitation" secretion.

The accessory lacrimal glands of Krause are located within the substantia propria of the fornix conjunctiva; the accessory lacrimal glands of Wolfring are situated at the upper margin of the tarsus (Fig. 11-3).

CONJUNCTIVAL LAYER

The fourth and most posterior layer of the eyelids, the palpebral conjunctiva, has been described on page 587.

Conjunctiva

CORNEAL AND CONJUNCTIVAL DERMOIDS AND CYSTS

Dermoids and epibulbar hamartomas and choristomas are congenital growths that most commonly occur at the temporal limbus (Figs. 11-6 and 11-7; Color Plate 11-1).[31-42,84] They are often present in the Goldenhar-Gorlin syndrome (oculoauriculovertebral dysplasia).[37,40]

The degree of the growth's involvement of the cornea varies greatly, and the clinical appearance varies with the tissue makeup of the lesion.[34,42] Most dermoids are solid, but some may be cystic.[35] In contrast to potentially malignant or carcinomatous growths at the limbus, which tend to be more irregular and invasive (Fig. 11-21; Color Plates 11-1 and 11-2), dermoids commonly exhibit a regular, smooth surface with more rounded margins.

Dermoids are hamartomatous or choristomatous growths that are composed of derivatives of epithelial or connective tissue elements believed to have become entrapped within facial clefts during embryogenesis (Fig. 11-6).[31,32,36,37,41] Subsequent proliferation of this tissue creates the solid or cystic masses seen at birth. Because the dermoid growth usually remains dormant throughout life, the major indications for surgical intervention are cosmetic considerations or minimization of possible visual impairment if corneal involvement occurs.

These solid or cystic congenital dermoid tumors of the conjunctiva differ from the simple acquired conjunctival epithelial cyst and the epidermoid and dermoid cysts of the skin (p. 587).[33,39] An acquired conjunctival epithelial cyst is usually derived from an inclusion of conjunctival epithelium into the substantia propria (Fig. 11-7). As the nests of epithelial cells proliferate, a central cavity forms, creating a cyst. The epithelial lining of the cyst wall is usually composed of the nonkeratinized conjunctival epithelium from which it is derived. The cyst may contain mucin if goblet cells in the lining epithelium are present. Small and often multiple conjunctival epithelial inclusion cysts commonly occur in association with conjunctival nevi (Fig. 11-28). A malignant lymphoma sometimes resembles a cyst and should be considered in the differential diagnosis (Fig. 11-8).[64]

INFLAMMATORY CONDITIONS

Follicles and papillae

The hallmarks of many types of subacute and chronic conjunctivitis are follicles and papillae.[43-110] There are dis-

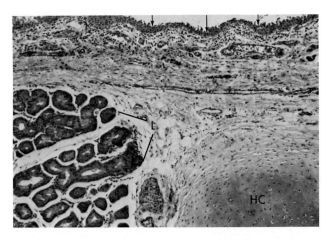

Fig. 11-6. Photomicrograph of a limbal dermoid (see also Color Plates 11-1 and 11-2). This choristomatous growth contains lacrimal gland (L) and hyaline cartilage (HC). The arrows indicate overlying corneal-conjunctival epithelium. (H & E stain; ×200.)

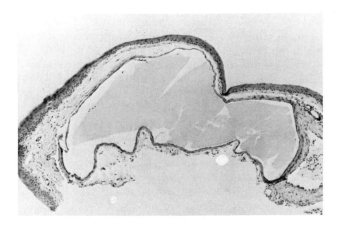

Fig. 11-7. Benign simple cyst of conjunctiva, lined with cuboidal epithelium and filled with transudate. (H & E stain; ×5.)

tinct clinical and histopathologic differences that distinguish them.

A follicle (Figs. 11-9 to 11-11) is a hyperplasia of lymphoid tissue, probably derived from lymphoid tissue, which is normally present in the substantia propria, particularly near the fornices. Follicles are a common reaction to virus infection. Clinically they appear as gray or white lobular elevations (Fig. 11-11, *A*). The central portion of the follicle, which is avascular, contains germinal cells (immature lymphocytes) and macrophages, which are surrounded by more mature lymphocytes toward the periphery of the follicle.

A papilla is a small projection or elevation that occurs in many acute and chronic inflammatory diseases (Fig. 11-9, *B*).[69,71] The hyperplastic conjunctival epithelium is thrown into numerous folds or projections. A small vessel enters the center of each papilla and branches beneath the conjunctival surface. The papillary projections of epithelium and underlying stroma often give the affected surface a velvety appearance. In addition to the central vessel, a typical papilla contains a diffuse infiltration of various types

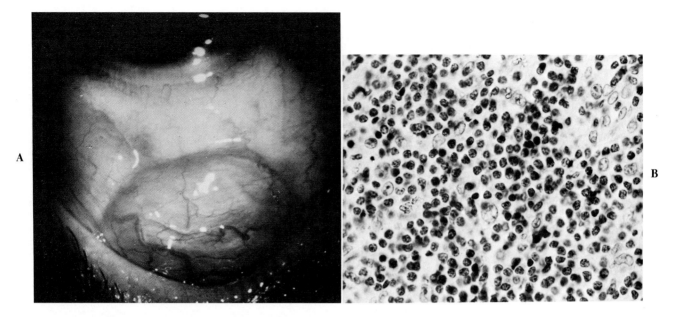

Fig. 11-8. Lymphoma of conjunctiva. **A,** Clinical cystlike appearance. **B,** Typical histopathologic appearance of lymphoma with myriad arrays of enlarged, atypical lymphocytes. (H & E stain; ×150.) (**A** courtesy Dr. Ernst Martin Meyner, formerly of University of Tübingen, Tübingen, Germany.)

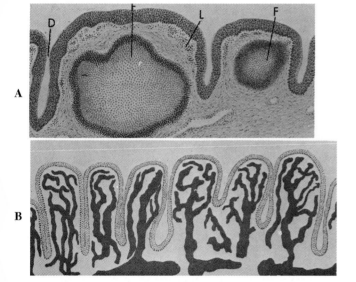

Fig. 11-9. Classic artist's drawings showing differences between follicles and papillae. **A,** The lymphoid follicle *(F)* is composed of a central germinal center rimmed by mature lymphocytes. *L,* Scattered subepithelial lymphocytes; *D,* depressions between follicles. **B,** Papillae. Vessels *(black arborizing projections in this drawing)* typically fill the core of the papillary projections. (From Greeff R: In Orth J: Lehrbuch der speziellen pathologischen Anatomie, Berlin, 1902, Hirschwald.)

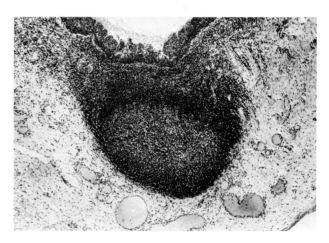

Fig. 11-10. Lymphoid follicle in conjunctival stroma. (H & E stain; ×175.)

of chronic inflammatory cells, including lymphocytes, plasma cells, and eosinophils.

The myriad inflammatory conditions and the variety of microorganisms affecting the conjunctiva are discussed in detail in standard textbooks of external diseases and micro-

biology.* This section is limited to a discussion of trachoma, still a leading cause of blindness in the world; sarcoidosis, a commonly observed form of granulomatous inflammation; rhinosporidiosis, an example of fungal conjunctivitis that is rare in the United States but is endemic in areas such as India; and vernal conjunctivitis.

Trachoma

Trachoma is one of the world's most common ocular diseases.[67,103] It is caused by a member of the lymphogranuloma-psittacosis group of agents.† This organism is a gram

---

* References 3, 5, 6, 8, 9, 18, 21, 106, 107.
† References 54, 55, 63, 75, 80, 81, 82, 90, 91, 98, 109.

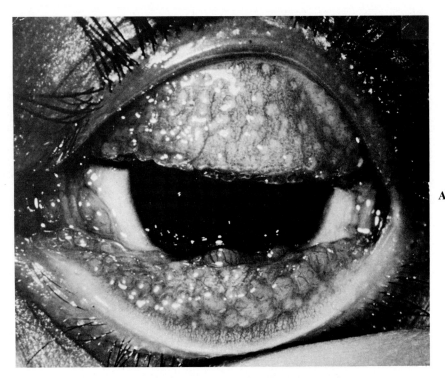

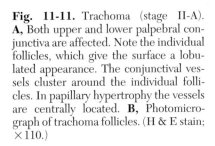

Fig. 11-11. Trachoma (stage II-A). **A,** Both upper and lower palpebral conjunctiva are affected. Note the individual follicles, which give the surface a lobulated appearance. The conjunctival vessels cluster around the individual follicles. In papillary hypertrophy the vessels are centrally located. **B,** Photomicrograph of trachoma follicles. (H & E stain; ×110.)

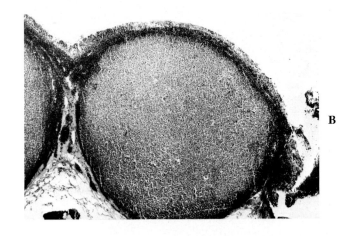

negative, basophilic bacteria. The trachoma and inclusion conjunctivitis agents are almost identical in appearance in culture.[102] The organisms causing trachoma, inclusion conjunctivitis, and lymphogranuloma venereum are all closely related antigenically but can be differentiated by microimmunofluorescent techniques. These organisms, and those of psittacosis and related diseases, are classified generically as *Chlamydia*.

Tracoma is caused by *Chlamydia trachomatis.* Clinically the most commonly accepted staging of trachoma infection of the cornea and conjunctiva is that of MacCallan.[81,82,91]

1. *Stage I:* Minute conjunctival follicles and subepithelial infiltrates give the conjunctiva a velvety appearance.
2. *Stage II:* The conjunctiva becomes thickened and roughened, and two substages may be seen:
   A. A follicular reaction predominates.
   B. A papillary reaction predominates.
3. *Stage III:* Cicatrization and contraction is widespread.
4. *Stage IV:* The disease is completely arrested.

Stage I, the earliest stage of trachoma in adults, is usually relatively asymptomatic. It is characterized by small, immature follicles on the upper tarsal plate, minimal papillary hypertrophy, edema and hyperemia of the stroma, and little if any conjunctival exudate. Slitlamp examination almost always reveals minimal epithelial keratitis. Stage I may last for several months to years. Conjunctival thickening eventually ensues. An increasingly severe follicular conjunctivitis may develop as the involvement progresses toward Stage II.

Follicular hypertrophy is the hallmark of stage II-A (Fig. 11-11). The conjunctival infection is well established, and limbal keratitis, limbal follicular hypertrophy, and vascular pannus frequently occur at this stage. These follicles are described as "sagograins" and are easy to express because

of central necrosis. Stage II-A can last from months to years, and the symptoms vary depending on the presence and severity of secondary bacterial infection. Furthermore, a superimposed bacterial conjunctivitis is often responsible for the most severe inflammatory reactions clinically evident.

Stage II-A and particularly stage II-B are characterized by a dense submucosal infiltrate of lymphocytes that leads to conjunctival thickening and stromal fibrosis. Leber cells are large debris-laden macrophages within the subepithelial stroma. Stage II-B may resolve to stage II-A, or it may progress directly to stage III if the intense reaction persists.

Pannus formation may occur in stage I or II. Corneal involvement usually begins early in the course of the disease, with the upper half initially affected. Breakdown of the trachoma inflammatory infiltrates may form corneal ulcers. Herbert's pits, pathognomonic of trachoma, form after rupture and/or cicatrization of contiguous limbal follicles, which become filled with translucent epithelial cells.

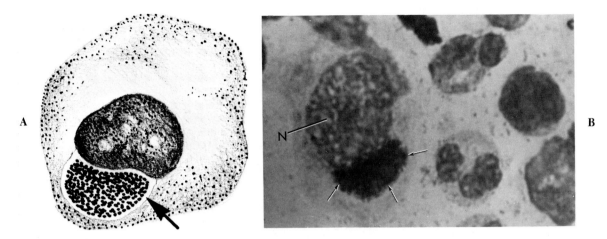

Fig. 11-12. Halberstaedter-Prowazek inclusion body, characteristic of trachoma and inclusion conjunctivitis. **A,** Schematic drawing of inclusion *(arrow)* seen within a conjunctival epithelial cell obtained from a conjunctival scraping. The basophilic, granular-appearing inclusion is situated in the cell cytoplasm immediately adjacent to the nucleus. **B,** Photomicrograph of the cytoplasmic inclusion *(arrows).* The other cells in this field are inflammatory cells, mostly polymorphonuclear neutrophils. *N,* Nucleus of conjunctival epithelial cell. (Giemsa stain, oil immersion; ×600.) (Courtesy Dr. David Vastine, University of Illinois.)

In stages I and II the characteristic Halberstaedter-Prowazek inclusion bodies may be visible by examination of Giemsa-stained conjunctival epithelial scrapings (Fig. 11-12). This inclusion, which occurs within infected epithelial cells, consists of a granula, basophilic body situated immediately adjacent to the cell nucleus and is identical to that in inclusion conjunctivitis. Inclusion conjunctivitis, caused by *Chlamydia oculogenitale,* characteristically occurs in newborn infants, although it sometimes affects adults.[93] In the acute phases inclusion conjunctivitis reveals similar, but usually less severe, changes of papillary and follicular conjunctivitis. The severe sequelae of trachoma generally are not encountered in inclusion conjunctivitis, although in unusually severe cases a residual vascular pannus may appear.

Stage III (Fig. 11-13) is the stage of progression to cicatrization. Dense fibrous tissue progressively replaces the diffuse inflammatory infiltrate. There is widespread loss of mucin-secreting goblet cells, with eventual xerophthalmia, and scarring of the lymphoid follicles. Shrinkage of the conjunctiva leads to trichiasis and entropion, then to symblepharon. Arlt's line is one manifestation of the scarring process that occurs at this stage. This linear scar lies 2 mm from the lower margin of the upper lid and extends parallel with the lid margin across the entire length of the eye.

The trachoma pannus initially consists of an infiltrate of inflammatory cells situated between the limbal epithelium and Bowman's layer. However, by the latter cicatricial stages (III and IV), most or all of the inflammatory infiltrate is replaced by dense fibrovascular tissue that often creates a permanent opacity.

Stage IV represents healed or burned-out trachoma. The disease is inactive, and histopathologic analysis demonstrates that the original inflammatory infiltrate affecting the cornea and conjunctiva is replaced by scar tissue.[73]

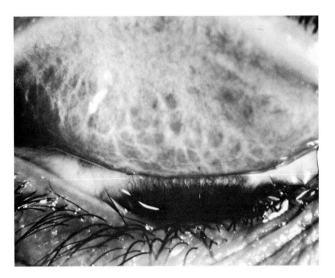

Fig. 11-13. Trachoma (stage III). Development of scarring in the upper tarsal conjunctiva denotes the progression from stage II to stage III trachoma. The interlacing linear and stellate scarring is typical of trachoma. No definite Arlt's line (a linear scar coursing across the lid 2 mm from the lid margin) is noted in this case. (Courtesy Dr. David Vastine.)

Sarcoidosis

The uvea (p. 293), retina optic nerve (p. 542), and conjunctiva are often affected in Boeck's sarcoid.* Histopathologically the conjunctival lesions are no different from those in any other region of the body. A diagnosis of sarcoidosis is indicated when (1) noncaseating granulomas composed of epithelioid cells and giant cells are seen in biopsy sec-

---

* References 50, 61, 62, 67, 78, 86, 95, 99, 108, 110.

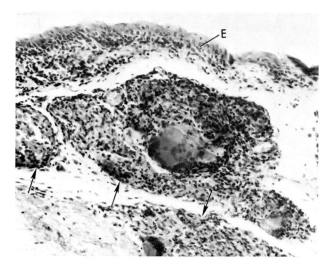

Fig. 11-14. Sarcoidosis of the bulbar conjunctiva. The conjunctival epithelium is recognizable as a nonkeratinized stratified squamous epithelium *(E)*. *Arrows,* Individual noncaseating granulomas in the subepithelial substantia propria. The granulomas are composed of epithelioid cells and occasional giant cells. (H & E stain; ×120.)

tions (Figs. 3-7, 7-15, and 11-14); (2) special staining techniques identify no specific microorganisms; and (3) no historical or systemic findings suggest other specific causes of granulomatous inflammation.[92] The outline on page 64 lists several other diseases characterized by a granulomatous inflammatory process, which should be considered in the differential diagnosis of sarcoidosis.[51,52,58,59]

The conjunctiva provides a relatively accessible site of diagnostic biopsy in possible cases of systemic sarcoidosis.[66,76] In our experience only 10% to 20% of blind conjunctival biopsies reveal a positive diagnosis; however, because this is a relatively benign procedure, it is warranted as a diagnostic procedure when other systemic findings are equivocal.

Rhinosporidiosis

Fungal diseases of the conjunctiva are rare. One fungal disease, rhinosporidiosis, only occasionally seen within the United States but endemic in India and other regions, provides a morphologic example of a sporulating, encapsulated fungus.* This fungus, *Rhinosporidium seeberi,* exemplifies a group of fungi that form sporangia (Fig. 11-15). In endemic areas *R. seeberi* commonly causes fleshy, papillary, conjunctival growths that occasionally lead to episcleral necrosis, thinning, and sometimes scleral perforation. The organisms may infect the nasolacrimal drainage apparatus, impeding tear outflow. It is recurrent and may represent a major threat to vision. With increased intercontinental travel, this condition is now being seen with greater frequency in Western countries.

Each sporangium is encapsulated by a fibrous wall or envelope and is filled with numerous spherule-containing endospores. The morphology of this encapsulated fungus

can be compared with that of those demonstrating hyphae in tissue sections (Fig. 3-10, *B*). The latter include *Candida albicans* and *Aspergillus* organisms, well known in the United States because of their potential effect on the eye and ocular adnexa.

Vernal conjunctivitis

Vernal conjunctivitis (vernal catarrh) occurs primarily in the spring, most often affecting young boys.* The most clinical manifestation is a bilateral, often recurrent but self-limiting, papillary hypertrophy caused by subepithelial inflammatory infiltrates. In the more severe cases massive infiltration leads to the typical cobblestone appearance. Horner-Trantas spots (Color Plate 11-3) are inflammatory foci composed predominantly of eosinophils.

The conjunctival stroma in affected cases contains abundant eosinophils. An eosinophil never contains more than two lobes in the nucleus, in contrast to the polymorphonuclear neutrophil, which often contains four or five lobes. The cytoplasmic eosinophilic granules are best seen with the Giemsa technique applied to conjunctival smears or with special staining techniques such as the azure-eosin technique.

MUCOCUTANEOUS ERUPTIONS

The conjunctival epithelium and the epidermis of the skin are continuous. They are derived from the original surface ectoderm of the embryo, and both undergo similar pathologic processes. Important examples of this skin-conjunctiva interrelation are the disorders collectively termed *mucocutaneous eruptions*. These include pemphigus, pemphigoid, and Stevens-Johnson syndrome.[111–140]

Pemphigus

Pemphigus (pemphigus vulgaris) is a potentially fatal disease characterized by intraepithelial bullae within the skin and mucous membranes of the body, including the conjunctiva.[114,129,137] Fortunately this condition is rare. The histopathologic hallmark of true pemphigus is intraepithelial breakdown of squamous cells (acantholysis). Separation of the squamous epithelial cells caused by rupture of the intercellular bridges or desmosomes creates the bullous cavity.[128]

Pemphigoid and Stevens-Johnson syndrome

Benign mucosal pemphigoid† (ocular pemphigoid, chronic cicatrizing conjunctivitis, essential shrinkage of the conjunctiva) usually occurs in the absence of systemic skin changes. It is a T-cell mediated disease. Small subepithelial bullae form (Fig. 11-16), but the primary destructive process involves marked inflammation of the subepithelial tissue with formation of thick, contracting bundles of scar tissue (Fig. 11-17).[122,138] This cicatricial process leads to shrinkage of the conjunctiva and symblepharon formation.

In addition to solitary involvement of the conjunctiva, ocular lesions closely resembling those of pemphigoid may occur in association with oral, genital, and skin lesions (erythema multiforme). This complex of lesions is sometimes

---

* References 44, 48, 49, 74, 79, 94.

* References 43, 53, 56, 57, 83, 105.

† References 111, 113, 115–117, 120, 121, 125, 130–132, 135–137, 140.

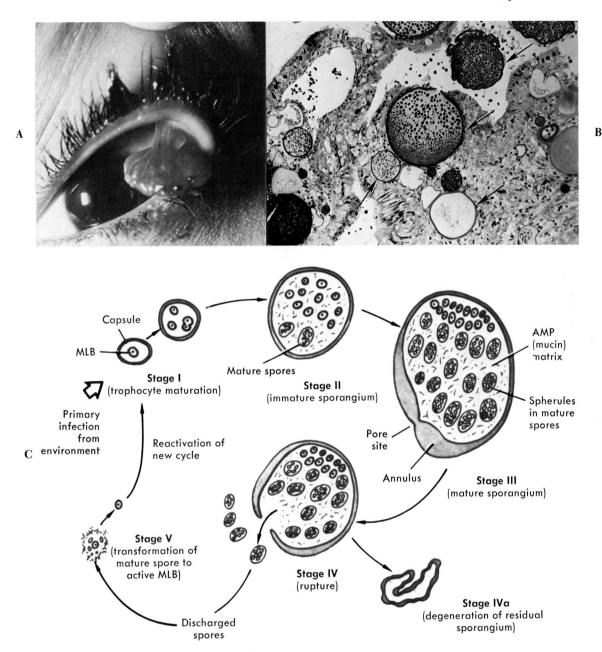

Fig. 11-15. Conjunctival rhinosporidiosis. **A,** Polypoid inflammatory mass induced by the fungus. **B,** *Rhinosporidium seeberi* is an example of a sporulating fungus that may affect the conjunctiva or lacrimal drainage apparatus. The lesions are usually polypoid **(A);** in rare instances the organism may induce scleral necrosis, thinning, and staphyloma formation. Each organism (sporangium) is seen at varying stages of maturation *(arrows)*. Note the large ruptured sporangium centrally. The morphology of this class of fungi, characterized by endospores within the sporangial envelope *(arrows)*, can be contrasted with that of other fungi that form hyphae (Fig. 3-10, *B*). (Mallory blue stain; ×100.) **C,** Life cycle of *Rhinosporidiosis*. *MLB*, Multilamellar body, the nucleic acid core of the organism. (From Apple DJ: Fortschr Ophthalmol 79:571, 1983.)

termed *dermatostomatitis* or Stevens-Johnson syndrome and usually occurs in young adults, especially men.[112,122,126] Systemic findings include general malaise, headaches, fever, and acute infections of the respiratory tract. Maculopapular or vesiculobullous eruptions occur on the skin, usually the dorsum of the hands and feet, and mucous membranes. The oral cavity, nasal epithelium, and the conjunctiva may be affected. In instances of vulvovagi-

nitis, cystitis, urethritis, or balanitis the clinical picture may resemble that of Reiter's disease.

Although some cases undoubtedly represent an allergic reaction to drugs (such as sulfonamides), most cases of Stevens-Johnson syndrome are idiopathic.[88,133] The conjunctival findings are usually identical to those of uncomplicated benign mucous membrane pemphigoid. The papulovesicular type is characterized by the diagnostic

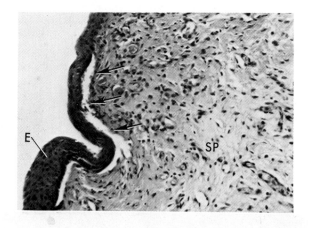

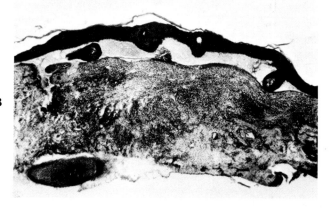

Fig. 11-16. Ocular pemphigoid. **A,** Conjunctiva. *Arrows,* Subepithelial cleft between the nonkeratinized conjunctival stratified squamous epithelium *(E)* and the underlying substantial propria *(SP).* This subepithelial cleavage is characteristic of benign mucous membrane pemphigoid. The subepithelial stroma contains dense fibrous tissue. Cicatrization creates conjunctival shrinkage and symblepharon. (H & E stain; ×200.) **B,** Eyelid skin. The case is similar to **A,** but the separation of the epidermis from the underlying inflamed dermis is more extensive (H & E stain; ×85.)

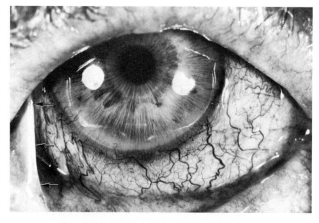

Fig. 11-17. Benign mucous membrane pemphigoid, right eye. The cornea remains clear. *Arrows,* Symblepharon formation from the lower palpebral conjunctiva extending upward onto the temporal aspects of the bulbar conjunctiva. (Courtesy Dr Carole West.)

subepithelial bullae. The fibromembranous type, usually seen in late stages of the disease, represents the cicatricial stage identical to that seen in essential shrinkage of the conjunctiva.

Histopathologic findings

The intraepithelial blisters of pemphigus should be clearly distinguished from the subepithelial bullae characteristic of pemphigoid and Stevens-Johnson syndrome (Fig. 11-16). The histopathologic differentiation between pemphigus and these other two diseases is not of mere academic interest, because pemphigus can be fatal. Pemphigoid and Stevens-Johnson syndrome are much more common than pemphigus but typically are not fatal.[134]

Pemphigoid and Stevens-Johnson syndrome are characterized by bullae derived from a cleavage between the basal layer of the epithelium and the underlying stroma or dermis. The bullae in pemphigoid often contain lymphocytes including T cells, Langerhans' cells, and plasma cells. If a mucous membrane such as the conjunctiva is involved, the epithelium is separated from the underlying stroma or substantia propria. If the skin is involved, the epidermis is separated from the underlying dermis.

ENVIRONMENTAL DEGENERATIONS
Pingueculae and pterygia

Growths of the conjunctiva are often a reactive or proliferative response to environmental influences, including dust, wind, particulate and chemical air pollution, and most important, solar radiation. Pingueculae and pterygia (Fig. 11-18, *A* and *B*) represent the most benign end of the spectrum of solar-induced lesions; solar-induced carcinomas comprise the opposite end.[141–159]

Pingueculae, which do not encroach on the cornea, and pterygia, which do involve the cornea, are distinguishable clinically but for the most part are identical in histologic sections because they reflect similar degenerative and proliferative processes. Both conditions* are characterized by degeneration of the subepithelial bulbar conjunctival stroma similar to that observed in the dermis of the skin in solar ("senile") keratosis (p. 593). This stromal degeneration (Fig. 11-18, *C*) is described by such varying terms as *senile elastosis, solar elastosis, elastotic degeneration,* and *basophilic degeneration of subepithelial collagen.* The subepithelial connective tissue occasionally becomes secondarily calcified.

Although the subepithelial changes of pingueculae and of pterygia and the solar keratoses of the skin are similar, the epithelial changes must be clearly differentiated. The epithelium of a pinguecula or pterygium is alternately thinned (as a result of atrophy) or thickened (as a result of reactive proliferation). There is seldom any evidence of cellular atypism, and these conditions are not premalignant. In contrast the epithelium in solar keratosis of the skin usually exhibits varying degress of cellular atypism, which may suggest malignant growth.

Keratinoid degeneration

Keratinoid degeneration (spheroidal or Labrador keratopathy, Bietti's nodular keratopathy, climatic droplet kerato-

---

* References 142, 145, 146, 148, 150, 151, 154, 155, 159.

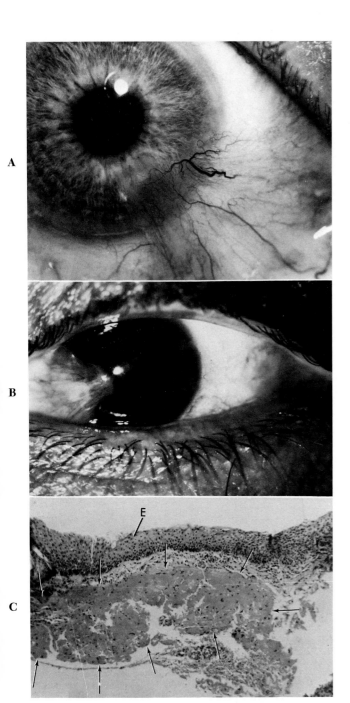

A

B

C

Fig. 11-18. Pterygium. **A,** and **B,** Clinical photographs of two patients showing encroachment onto the cornea. **C,** The most important histopathologic feature of a pinguecula or pterygium is the subepithelial degeneration of collagen and elastic tissue (basophilic degeneration of collagen or solar elastosis). The homogeneous or structureless appearance of the substantia propria *(arrows)* is similar to the degenerative process occurring in solar keratosis of the skin. Both the conjunctival and skin lesions result from noxious influences from the environment, particularly the sun. **E,** Conjunctival epithelium showing minimal thickening. (H & E stain; ×100.)

pathy, elastotic degeneration) consists of yellow-brown, droplike, hyaline deposits in the superficial corneal-conjunctival stroma, which are often associated with pingueculae. Like pingueculae, they are induced by exposure to sun, wind, dust, and other environmental influences° (Fig. 11-19). They usually occur bilaterally and affect elderly persons with a long history of outdoor exposure. The granules are probably composed of degenerated collagen (so-called elastotic degeneration of collagen).

PAPILLOMAS, PROLIFERATIVE LESIONS, AND NONPIGMENTED TUMORS

This section considers several common and benign lesions that must be differentiated from malignant tumors.[160–228]

Papillomas

Most papillomas of the conjunctiva, particularly those occurring in children, are probably induced by viruses, for example, the human papillomavirus types 16 and 18.† In Fig. 11-15 is an example of a rare fungal-induced papilloma.

They are frequently multiple (Color Plate 11-4). The surface of the lesion is composed of irregularly proliferating squamous epithelium, which creates a lobulated, cauliflower-like appearance. The epithelial surface typically overlies a fibrovascular core that forms a stalk leading to the base of the growth. Papillomas are often recurrent and difficult to eradicate. Cryotherapy in addition to excision is sometimes useful.

Occasionally a papilloma can exhibit a marked hypercellularity and may show features of cellular atypism, nuclear hyperchromatism, or atypical mitoses, which resemble those of true neoplasms. For this reason differentiation of a simple benign papilloma from a new growth is sometimes difficult.

Inflammatory lesions of the conjunctiva, particularly in children, sometimes produce an exuberant proliferation of fibrovascular and inflammatory tissue to such a degree that a papilloma-like lesion forms. The polypoid lesion in Fig. 11-20 is identical in shape to many squamous papillomas; however, the lesion is composed of fibrovascular tissue and inflammatory elements (inflammatory polyp) rather than acanthotic, hyperplastic, epithelial components typical of squamous papilloma.

Sometimes such inflammatory polyps are classified as pyogenic granuloma; however, this can be misleading because this lesion does not represent granulomatous inflammation. Pyogenic granulomas are inflammatory lesions composed of granulation tissue similar to that seen in wound healing. Granulation tissue consists of proliferating connective tissue (fibroblasts and fibrocytes) and newly formed capillary channels. Acute and chronic inflammatory cells are often interspersed between the fibrovascular elements.

Proliferative lesions and nonpigmented tumors

The differentiation of sessile or irregularly raised growths of the bulbar conjunctiva, particularly at the lim-

° References 141, 143, 144, 147, 149, 152, 153, 157.
† References 188, 193, 194, 205–207, 214, 221.

A

B

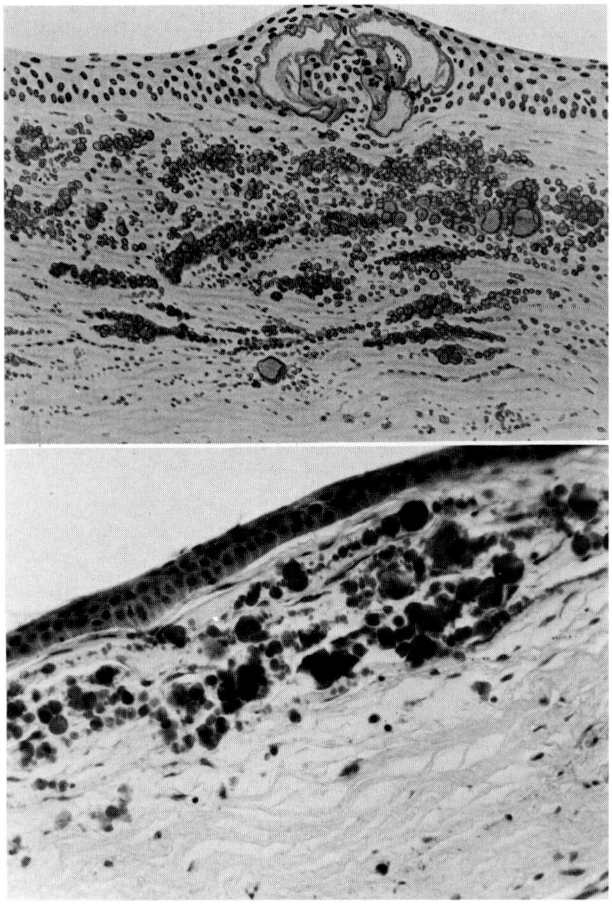

Fig. 11-19. Elastotic degeneration (keratinoid degeneration, Labrador keratopathy) of cornea. **A,** Artist's drawing. **B,** Photomicrograph showing droplets in superficial corneal-conjunctival stroma. (H & E stain; ×250.) (**A** from von Hippel E: In Henke F and Lubarsch O, editors: Handbuch der speziellen pathologischen Anatomie und Histologie, Berlin, 1928, Julius Springer.)

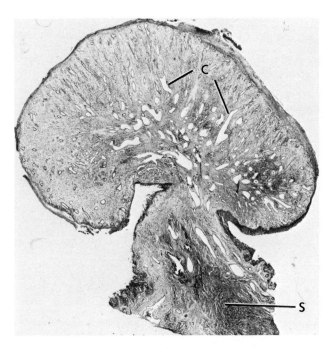

Fig. 11-20. Polypoid lesion of the lower eyelid. *S,* Elongated stalk at the base of the lesion. The histopathologic picture is similar to that of pyogenic granuloma, in which buds of proliferating capillaries (*C*) and fibroblasts are admixed with chronic inflammatory cells. (H & E stain; ×30.)

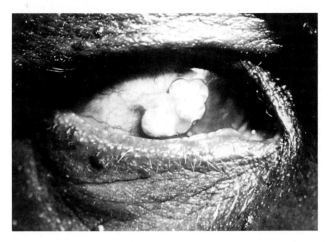

Fig. 11-21. Hyperkeratotic (leukoplakic) squamous cell carcinoma in situ of the conjunctiva.

bus, poses a difficult diagnostic problem (Fig. 11-21; Color Plate 11-5).* Determination of the true nature of a limbal growth almost always requires histopathologic examination of excised tissue. The limbal dermoid has been previously discussed in this chapter. Other limbal lesions range in degree of severity from benign pingueculae and pterygia to benign epithelial hyperplasia with or without cellular atypism, to carcinoma in situ, to invasive, potentially metastatic squamous cell carcinoma.[163] These lesions are all characterized by abnormal proliferation or neoplastic transformation of the conjunctival squamous epithelium.[195,196] A definitive categorization of each lesion depends on the degree of cellular dedifferentiation and atypism seen microscopically.

If keratinization of the involved squamous epithelium is absent (Fig. 11-22), the lesion generally is transparent or translucent. Extensive keratinization at the epithelial surface of the lesion produces a white plaque, or leukoplakia (Fig. 11-21; Color Plate 11-5). Regardless of the degree

of malignancy of the squamous epithelial growth, clinical examination may reveal any degree of transparency, translucency, or leukoplakia. This consideration, therefore, is of little value in clinically determining the nature of the lesion.

As a general rule, limbal lesions such as those illustrated in Color Plate 11-5, which are associated with dilated and/or tortuous conjunctival vessels, should evoke suspicion of carcinoma in situ or may actually signify a squamous cell carcinoma. Various modes of therapy are discussed in references 161, 169, 172, 176, 177, 178, 200, and 228.

---

* References 120, 160, 162, 168, 170, 173-175, 179, 182-184, 192, 203, 209, 211, 220, 223.

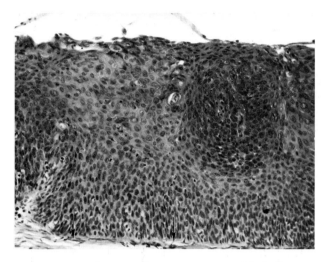

Fig. 11-22. Nonkeratinized carcinoma in situ of the bulbar conjunctiva. The epithelium, which is normally only five to six layers thick (Fig. 11-1), is extremely thickened and hypercellular. The cells are small and exhibit a loss of the polarity that they normally demonstrate. Many of the cells are elongated in an abnormal vertical direction rather than parallel with the epithelial basement membrane in the normal horizontal direction. There are several mitotic figures. The base of the tumor appears smooth *(arrows)* because of an intact basement membrane separating the epithelium from the underlying substantia propria. The basement membrane itself is difficult to see in routinely stained sections, but the presence of an intact membrane is confirmed by the smooth contour of the base of the tumor. No islands of tumor invade below the membrane. (H & E stain; ×200.)

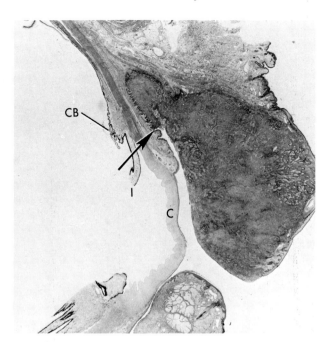

Fig. 11-23. Squamous cell carcinoma of the conjunctiva invading and destroying a portion of the upper eyelid. Note the transition from the normal bulbar conjunctival epithelium into the thickened epithelium of the tumor *(arrow)*. Such conjunctival carcinomas may be locally invasive, but they rarely undergo significant metastasis. C, Cornea; CB, ciliary body; I, iris. (H & E stain; ×5.)

PREMALIGNANT AND MALIGNANT NEOPLASMS

Carcinoma in situ

Carcinoma in situ, or intraepithelial epithelioma, of the conjunctiva is frequently called Bowen's disease (Color Plate 11-5).° Bowen's original description referred only to lesions of the integument; therefore, this designation should not be applied to mucous membrane growths, such as those of the conjunctiva, oral cavities, or uterine cervix.

In microscopic sections carcinoma in situ of the conjunctiva (Fig. 11-22) exhibits epithelial changes similar to those of squamous cell carcinoma. Characteristically an increase occurs in the number of cells, with formation of atypical, large nuclei. An important diagnostic feature relates to the loss of polarity of the squamous epithelial cells. Normally these cells are flattened, and the long axis is parallel to the conjunctival surface. Loss of polarity indicates that the cells have assumed a random orientation. Many of the cells are actually rotated 90 degrees, causing the long axis of the cell to be abnormally oriented perpendicular to the mucous membrane surface. Usually the epithelium shows acanthosis (thickening of the epithelial layer), and the neoplastic cells are generally smaller than normal. The nuclei are typically hyperchromatic, and increased numbers of mitotic figures signify active cellular proliferation. Leukoplakic tumors show hyperkeratosis in microscopic sections. Transparent or translucent tumors are devoid of keratin on the surface.

The most important and definitive histopathologic criterion of a carcinoma in situ is the presence of an intact subepithelial basement membrane confining the tumor to the epithelial layer. The intact basement membrane between the epithelium and stroma indicates a lack of invasion of tumor cells into the stroma (Fig. 11-22). When the large limbal growths are removed, it is wise to obtain multiple sections through several areas of the tumor. Microscopic examination of the underlying basement membrane throughout the extent of the tumor is necessary to rule out the presence of focal breaks in the membrane. Deep stromal penetration is a feature of true squamous cell carcinoma.

Squamous cell carcinoma

Squamous cell carcinoma of the conjunctiva (Fig. 11-23) is seen less frequently than carcinoma in situ (Color Plates 11-6 and 11-7).° Premalignant lesions often are quickly noted by the patient because of the exposed site of growth, and prompt surgical intervention usually prevents progression of the lesion to invasive carcinoma. Basal cell carcinoma, the most common tumor of the eyelid skin, rarely, if ever, arises from conjunctival epithelium.[185,216,218]

Most carcinomas of the conjunctiva are only locally invasive (Color Plate 11-7) and rarely metastasize if treated promptly (Figs. 11-23 and 11-24).[222] In untreated cases or after delayed treatments, local invasion into the anterior segment of the globe through the sclera may oc-

° References 145, 171, 189, 202, 208, 210, 224.

° References 163, 165, 167, 180, 181, 186, 191, 197-199, 201, 204, 212.

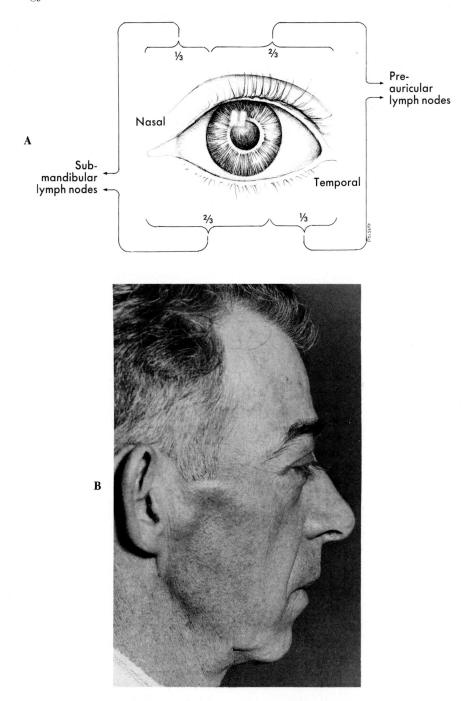

Fig. 11-24. A, Lymphatic drainage of the conjunctiva and eyelids. **B,** Enlarged preauricular node caused by conjunctival squamous cell carcinoma (the primary tumor is not visible in this profile photograph). (**A** drawn by Dr. Steven Vermillion, University of Iowa.)

cur.[164,213,219,226] Lymphatic spread to the preauricular or sumbaxillary lymph nodes occurs (Fig. 11-24) but is unusual. Diffuse carcinomatosis of squamous cell carcinoma of the conjunctiva is extremely rare. The relatively benign course of this lesion is consistent with the tendency of carcinomas of sun-exposed surfaces to behave in a much less malignant manner than similar carcinomas arising de novo in internal organs.

The histopathologic features of squamous cell carcinoma of the conjunctiva are similar to those of carcinoma in situ,

with the critical exception that the underlying stroma or substantia propria beneath the epithelial basement membrane shows invasion of tumor cells. When the tumor shows extensive keratinization of individual cells or clusters of tumor cells, epithelial pearls, similar to those in skin carcinomas (Fig. 11-48), are prominent in microscopic sections.

PIGMENTED TUMORS

Pigmented lesions of the conjunctiva exhibit a wide range of malignancy or malignant potential.[229-284] For this reason it is important to be able to differentiate the various types of melanotic lesions. Although adequate excision or destruction of a disfiguring or malignant lesion is necessary, one should avoid over-treatment and unnecessarily aggressive surgery.[233,253–255,262,264,268]

In addition to simple freckles (ephelis) and lentigo, exogenously acquired pigmentations, and metabolic disorders, three important categories of conjunctival pigmented lesions are noteworthy: congenital and acquired melanosis, nevi, and malignant melanoma.

Congenital and acquired melanosis

Melanosis oculi is an increase in absolute numbers of melanocytes that are distributed diffusely throughout a tissue.[273,274,284] This differs from a nevus, which is composed of abnormal nevus cells, which are often more localized into a discrete mass.

We emphasize the *congenital* nature of congenital melanosis oculi (Color Plate 11-8) because this is not often associated with malignant melanoma of the skin, conjunctiva, or uvea.[245–247] The pigment cells are situated in the deep layers of the substantia propria of the conjunctiva or in the episclera and sclera. Clinically the involved regions appear as diffuse broad patches of brown to light blue discoloration.[231] The foci of pigmentation sometimes appear blue because the dark brown color of the melanin pigment is slightly modified by the fibrous tissue and epithelium overlying the deeply placed pigmented cells in the conjunctiva, sclera, or skin (if involved).

The nevus of Ota (oculodermal melanocytosis; Fig. 2-50) is a specific form of congenital melanosis characterized by a hyperpigmentation of the affected tissue produced by increased numbers of heavily pigmented melanocytes within the tissue. Not only are the conjunctiva, sclera, and episclera involved, but there is a diffuse thickening of the uveal tract by relatively normal-appearing uveal melanocytes and similar pigmentation of the eyelid and of the facial skin. The nevus of Ota is commonly observed in Oriental persons. Uveal malignant melanoma occasionally occurs in patients with nevus of Ota but is unusual.

Acquired melanosis oculi connotes a pigmented epibulbar lesion that may or may not be similar in appearance to congenital melanosis oculi.[239,242,260,281] Such lesions usually appear only after the second or third decade of life. In contrast to the congenital form of melanosis oculi, which generally exhibits benign behavior, the lesions classified as acquired melanosis may show variation in the extent of cellular anaplasia, and some are frankly malignant.[284]

1. *Stage I:* Benign acquired melanosis
   A. Minimal junctional activity
   B. Marked junctional activity
2. *Stage II:* Cancerous acquired melanosis
   A. With minimal invasion
   B. With marked invasion

Histopathologically the lesion of acquired melanosis of the conjunctiva shows a proliferation of pigmented cells situated at the junction of the conjunctival epithelial cells with the underlying substantia propria (junctional activity) (Fig. 11-25). In its most benign form (stage I) the histopathologic pattern is similar to that of a junctional nevus. In stage II there is a marked increase in cellular anaplasia, and it may progress toward a frank, invasive malignant melanoma of the conjunctiva (stage II-B).

The history of onset and duration of the lesion is of utmost importance in calculating the prognosis, because an acquired melanosis is more likely to progress toward malignant melanoma than is congenital melanosis; however, it is equally important to avoid over-treatment. Clinically most cases fall into stage I-A, I-B, or II-A (stage II-B is relatively unusual). Extensive surgery is warranted only when the lesion is categorized as a cancerous acquired melanosis, particularly stage II-B (Fig. 11-26).

Nevi

Nevi of the conjunctiva are common and usually, but with many exceptions, differ clinically from a melanosis by being more localized and forming relatively discrete foci (Fig. 11-27; Color Plate 11-9).[238,258,278] These traits contrast with the more diffuse, blotchy pigmentation over broad areas that characterizes the lesions classified as melanosis oculi. Nevi are categorized as (1) junctional, (2) compound, or (3) subepithelial.

When the cellular proliferation is localized at the junction or interface of the surface epithelium and substantia propria, the nevus is junctional. When a nevus with junctional activity also shows extensive melanocytic cellular proliferation into the underlying connective tissue stroma, it is a compound nevus (Fig. 11-28, *A*). The latter is the most common type.

Nevi of the conjunctiva are often solid; however, in many cases epithelial inclusion cysts form and are mixed with the nests of nevus cells. These small, frequently multiple inclusions are lined by an epithelium containing mucin-secreting goblet cells. Occasionally the cystic proliferation is so extensive that the nevus cells remain unnoticed, and an incorrect diagnosis of multiple simple cysts may result.

In a subepithelial nevus, the nevus cells lie entirely within the substantia propria (Fig. 11-28, *B*). This is analogous to the dermal nevus of the skin (Fig. 11-41). Nevi of mucous membranes and the skin that do not exhibit junctional activity rarely, if ever, become malignant.

Malignant melanoma

Malignant melanomas of the conjunctiva may arise secondary to cancerous acquired melanosis (Fig. 11-26), from junctional or compound nevi of the conjunctiva, or de novo.[260] They may also appear as secondary growths from intraocular uveal melanomas (Fig. 7-50). Most occur at the limbus (Fig. 11-29). They may spread superficially or grow in a nodular pattern. They are often locally infiltrative and show only local metastatic spread (Fig. 11-24). Metastasis to distant foci is not as common as in primary skin melanomas. Conjunctival malignant melanomas are, therefore, considered less malignant than their counterparts arising from the skin of the eyelids or from the skin elsewhere (Fig. 11-20; Color Plate 11-10).[*]

---

[*] References 230, 232, 243, 248, 259, 261, 264, 265, 266, 271, 272, 275, 276, 280.

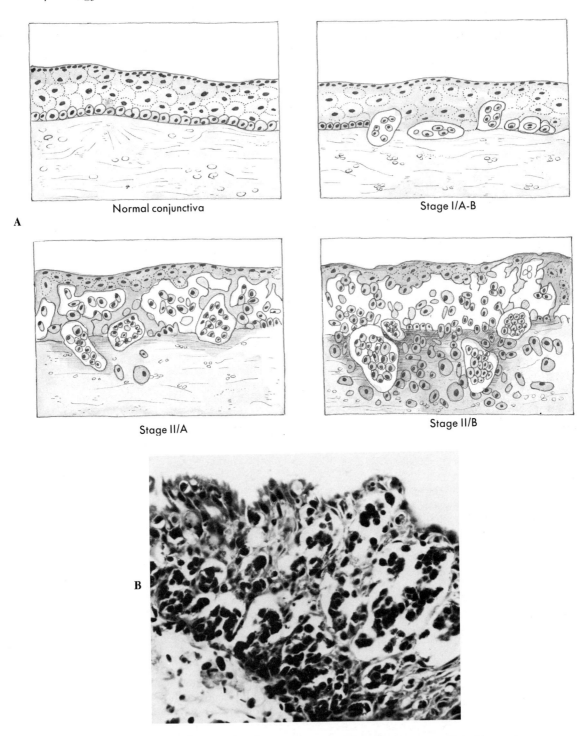

Normal conjunctiva

Stage I/A-B

A

Stage II/A

Stage II/B

B

Fig. 11-25. A, Stages of acquired melanosis. **B,** Acquired melanosis, stage II-A. The entire thickness of epithelium is involved, and melanin-containing cells are beginning to permeate the epithelial-stromal junction. (H & E stain; ×300.) (**A** drawn by Dr. Steven Vermillion, University of Iowa; **B** from Naumann GOH and Apple DJ: Doerr W, Seifert G, and Uehlinger E, editors: Handbuch der speziellen pathologischen Anatomie, Band Auge, Berlin, 1980, Springer-Verlag.)

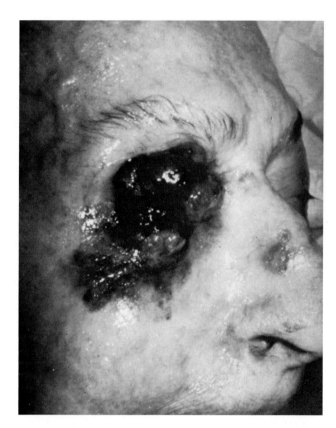

Fig. 11-26. Elderly woman with 8-year history of acquired melanosis. Six surgical excisions of multiple recurrent lesions were performed during this period, but the lesion slowly progressed toward frank malignant melanoma, and the patient died with widespread metastasis.

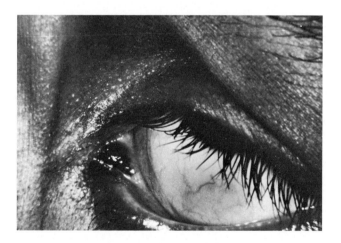

Fig. 11-27. Benign nevus of the caruncle.

The cellular pattern of conjunctival melanomas can be similar to that seen in spindle cell melanomas of the uvea (Figs. 7-53 to 7-55). More commonly, however, the predominant cell type is a large, irregularly shaped cell that resembles or is identical to the epithelioid cell seen in uveal malignant melanomas (Figs. 7-57 and 7-58).

Kaposi's sarcoma

Kaposi's sarcoma (Color Plates 11-11 and 11-12) is an uncommon multicentric vascular neoplasm, which affects the skin, mucous membranes, lymph nodes and viscera, usually of elderly males of Eastern European or Mediterranean origin.[225] It begins in the lower extremities and may spread elsewhere, usually in an indolent fashion. The eyelids or conjunctiva are rarely involved. It has assumed greater importance in recent years because of its association with the acquired immune deficiency syndrome (AIDS). It is known to occur in several clinical settings including the classic type, which is primarily mucocutaneous, a lymphadenopathic/visceral form which occurs in equatorial Africans and a mixed cutaneous/visceral type, which is found in patients with AIDS. Presentation, behavior, treatment, and response to therapy differs among types. Histopathologically, although Kaposi's sarcoma lesions are often clinically and grossly similar, they can be grouped into three types based on a system that unites their pathologic and clinical features.

Type I lesions are flat, violaceous patches, which contain thin vascular channels lined with flat endothelial cells and filled with erythrocytes. Type II lesions are likened more to plaques that contain more fusiform, plump endothelial cells with occasional hyperchromatic nuclei, foci of spindle cells, and sporadic small vessels. Type III lesions are nodular (0.3 mm in height) and feature increased numbers of packed spindle cells with hyperchromatic nuclei, mitotic figures, and numerous small vessels. All types may contain a varying infiltrate of lymphocytes, plasma cells, and histiocytes. Chronologically type I and type II lesions are considered to be less than 4 months duration while type III lesions are usually older than 4 months. Biopsy sites may contain features of all three types. Different staged lesions may also be more responsive to different therapeutic modalities.

Clinical differential diagnosis of Kaposi's sarcoma lesions of the eyelid and conjunctiva includes pyogenic granuloma, cavernous hemangioma, subconjunctival hemorrhage and malignant melanoma. Because Kaposi's sarcoma lesions of the eyelid and conjunctiva affect roughly 5% of patients with AIDS, the ophthalmologist is faced with increasing challenges in the diagnosis of Kaposi's sarcoma.

A variety of treatment options for Kaposi's sarcoma have been investigated, including radiation therapy, chemotherapy, cryotherapy, immunotherapy, and excision. The tumor appears to be radiosensitive, especially in immunocompetent individuals. Recurrences are common with all treatment modalities and Kaposi's sarcoma is usually multifocal, so unless either ocular complications such as entropion, trichiasis, or exposure develop, or unless the patient is extremely concerned with cosmetics, conservative management is indicated.

Eyelids

In addition to changes that are generally amenable to plastic surgical procedures and are unimportant from the histopathologic standpoint (e.g., changes associated with growth and aging such as blepharochalasis, orbital fat prolapse, and dehiscence skin atrophy, ectropion and entropion in the orbital septum), the eyelids may suffer from any dermatologic condition that one might expect elsewhere in

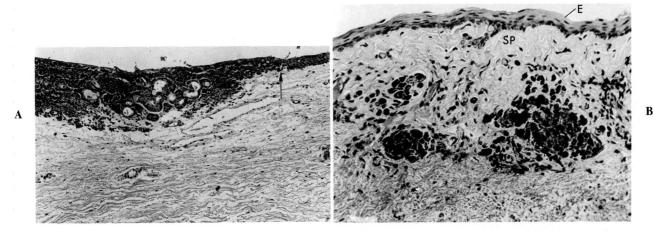

Fig. 11-28. A, Compound nevus of the conjunctiva with diffuse infiltration of nevus cells, which are adherent to and merge with the overlying conjunctival epithelium (junctional activity). The arrow indicates the junction of the normal epithelium (on the right) and the nevus. Small mucin-filled cysts are present within the nevus, a characteristic finding in many cases. The loose substantia propria *(below)* is characteristic of the bulbar conjunctiva. (H & E stain; ×71.) **B,** Bulbar conjunctiva showing a benign subepithelial nevus analogous to a dermal nevus of the skin. The individual nevus nests contain huge amounts of melanin pigment. No junctional activity is apparent. *E,* Epithelium; *SP,* substantia propria. (H & E stain; ×250.)

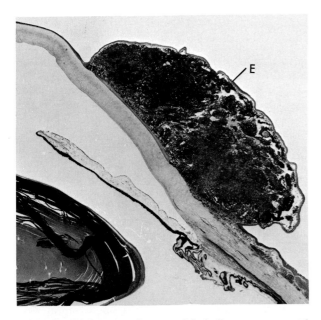

Fig. 11-29. Malignant melanoma of the bulbar conjunctiva. The pigmented tumor straddles the cornea and conjunctiva. No deep invasion into the sclera or globe has occurred. *E,* Conjunctival epithelium. Compare this primary conjunctival melanoma with Fig. 7-50, in which a small ciliary body melanoma extended and created a similar secondary conjunctival mass. (H & E stain; ×12.)

the skin.[285–400] Commonly observed inflammatory entities that require no further mention include the numerous chronic nonspecific dermatitides, seborrheic blepharitis, and acute staphylococcal blepharitis (sty or hordeolum).[288,289]

INCIDENCE AND CLASSIFICATION OF EYELID DISORDERS

In a review of 1403 eyelid lesions studied histopathologically at Charity Hospital in New Orleans, the relative incidence of these lesions was tabulated (Table 11-2).

This series included only cases submitted for pathologic examination. It is noteworthy, although not desirable, that many excised eyelid lesions are discarded by the surgeon rather than sent to the pathologist. This tabulation, therefore, does not represent the true percentage of all lesions observed clinically. It does, however, represent a cross-section of the more worrisome lesions requiring histopathologic confirmation. Obviously such lesions as cysts, nevi, papillomas, xanthelasma, and molluscum contagiosum are seen clinically more frequently than this table suggests. In addition, obvious chalazia were not included in this study, because most are not submitted to the laboratory. Nevertheless, the recurrent granulomatous lesions (Table 11-2) consisted almost entirely of recurrent chalazia, many of which turned out to be meibomian (sebaceous) carcinoma (p. 564).

As would be expected, a large proportion of lesions the ophthalmologist chooses to submit for pathologic diagnosis are malignant tumors. Approximately a third of the cases itemized in Table 11-2 were categorized as malignant. Table 11-3 lists, according to frequency, the important malignant tumors.

To simplify and provide a usable summary of these data, it is useful to formulate an estimation of the incidence of eyelid lesions submitted for pathologic analysis (Table 11-4).

This classification applies only to (1) lesions in which an unequivocal positive clinical diagnosis is not possible by clinical inspection alone but requires histopathologic analysis and (2) lesions that are obviously malignant and that

Table 11-2. Incidence of eyelid lesions submitted for pathologic analysis

Lesion	Percent
Basal cell carcinoma	27
Squamous cell growths ranging from benign hyperplasia to frank carcinoma	16
Papillomas (veruccae, polyps)	11
Epithelial cysts	11
Nevi	9
Seborrheic keratoses	6
Recurrent granulomatous lesions: predominantly chalazion and sebaceous (meibomian) carcinoma	5
Xanthelasma	2
Hemangioma	1
Miscellaneous	12

Unpublished data obtained by DJ Apple and L Stewart from 1403 consecutive cases studied at Charity Hospital of New Orleans. Reproduced with permission of the Tumor Registry, Charity Hospital of New Orleans and Dr. Jack P Strong, Chairman, Department of Pathology, Louisiana State University, New Orleans

Table 11-3. Relative incidence of malignant tumor of the eyelids

Tumor	Percent
Basal cell carcinoma	79
Squamous cell carcinoma, low-grade malignancy (including carcinoma in situ and microinvasive carcinoma)	18
Frankly invasive squamous cell carcinoma	2
Malignant melanoma	1
Sebaceous (meibomian) carcinoma	<1
Miscellaneous	<1

Unpublished data obtained by DJ Apple and L Stewart. Reproduced with permission of the Tumor Registry, Charity Hospital of New Orleans and Dr. Jack P Strong, Chairman, Department of Pathology, Louisiana State University, New Orleans

Table 11-4. Major categories of eyelid lesions: a simplified approximation of incidence of lesions submitted for histopathologic analysis

Lesions	Percent
Miscellaneous benign condition	40
Papillomas	
Epithelial cysts	
Nevi	
Seborrheic keratoses	
Hemangiomas	
Basal cell carcinoma	25
Squamous cell lesions ranging from benign to relatively low-grade malignancy	20
Epithelial hyperplasia, including pseudoepitheliomatous hyperplasia	
Keratoacanthoma	
Inverted follicular keratosis	
Atypical epithelial hyperplasia and senile keratosis	
Carcinoma in situ (Bowen's disease)	
Low-grade or microinvasive squamous cell carcinoma	
Frankly invasive malignant neoplasms	11
Squamous cell carcinoma	
Meibomian or sebaceous carcinoma	
Malignant melanoma	
Miscellaneous	
Miscellaneous benign dermatoses	4

Based on unpublished data obtained DJ Apple and L Stewart. Reproduced with permission of the Tumor Registry, Charity Hospital of New Orleans and Dr Jack P Strong, Chairman, Department of Pathology, Louisiana State University, New Orleans

must be subjected to histopathologic study. Table 11-4 does not include clinically "obvious" lesions that in the surgeon's estimation do not require tissue analysis. It represents, therefore, an approximation, based on statistics summarized in Tables 11-2 and 11-3, of the incidence of eyelid lesions for which the clinician would seek histopathologic confirmation of clinical impressions.

These statistics were obtained from a limited study in a single hospital in one locality and, thus, are considered guidelines to assist the ophthalmologist in differential diagnosis. This listing is not intended to provide an accurate statistical analysis of the true *clinical* incidence of all eyelid lesions. In this series almost a third of the 1403 clinical diagnoses for the submitted specimens were found to be incorrect.

BENIGN LESIONS

Several benign conditions are commonly encountered clinically but are submitted only occasionally for pathologic examination.[285–326]

Chalazion

The chalazion is the most frequently observed granulomatous inflammatory lesion of the eyelid. It sometimes confuses the general pathologist unfamiliar with ocular pathology, because it is easily mistaken for other potentially more serious causes of granulomatous inflammation. Sometimes the microscopist unnecessarily uses batteries of special stains searching for microorganisms in cases subsequently identified as chalazia.

Histopathologically the essential reaction is that of an epithelioid and giant cell response to liberated fat from the major sebaceous gland of the eye, the meibomian gland. The finding of nonstainable lipid droplets within the tissue (Fig. 11-30) is the most reliable indicator of a chalazion. These droplets usually occur within a ring of inflammatory cells. In addition to this typical pattern of granulomatous inflammation, a young, active lesion may show acute inflammation and may actually form an abscess. An old, inactive lesion may have extensive fibrosis and scarring, with minimal inflammatory infiltrate.

The diagnostic fat droplets differentiate a chalazion from other less common granulomatous conditions, such as sarcoidosis, fungal disease, leprosy, tuberculosis, and syphilis. These specific diseases can be diagnosed only by demonstration of a causative organism or by correlation with the history and clinical observations. Sarcoidosis should be diagnosed only after ruling out the other numerous causes of granulomatous inflammation affecting the eyelid.

Molluscum contagiosum

Molluscum contagiosum appears as raised skin nodules, often with unbilicated centers.[312,314,317] The skin lesion is

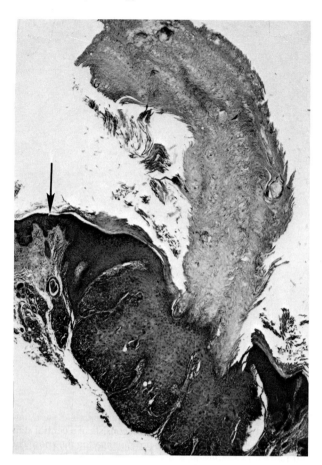

Fig. 11-35. Cutaneous horn, another variant of squamous papilloma. There is a benign hypercellularity and thickening (acanthosis) of the epidermis. Compare the acanthotic epithelium with the normal epithelium to the left *(arrow)*. However, the prime distinguishing feature is the extreme degree of hyperkeratosis, elevating the keratin (horny) layer to a great degree. (H & E stain; ×25.)

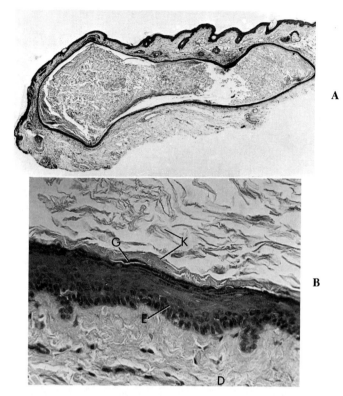

Fig. 11-36. Epidermoid cyst. **A,** The cyst is lined by a stratified squamous epithelium and is filled with keratin. (H & E stain; ×50.) **B,** Higher-power photomicrograph through the wall of an epidermoid cyst. Because all layers that are normal components of the skin are present, this cyst wall mimics the appearance of the normal skin (Fig. 11-4). The lumen of the cyst is filled with keratin *(K)* derived from the epithelium. The epithelial lining *(E)* of the cyst contains (1) a basal layer (bottom row of cells bordering the dermis *(D)*; (2) several layers of prickle cells (the malpighian layer) composed of stratified squamous epithelium with intercellular bridges; (3) a granular layer *(G)*, which contains deeply staining prekeratin, or keratohyaline, granules and is the transitional layer between the cellular epithelium; and (4) the keratin. The cheesy or oily material visible by clinical or gross examination of most "sebaceous" cysts is actually keratin derived from the skinlike epithelial lining. (H & E stain; ×200.)

however, a malignant or potentially malignant lesion may have the clinical appearance of an innocuous squamous papilloma. Such a lesion could invade the dermis deeply or invade lymphatics before the diagnosis is made; therefore, biopsy is certainly indicated for enlarging or progressing squamous papillomas.

Cysts

Eyelid cysts are usually easily diagnosed by clinical examination (Figs. 11-36 to 11-38; Color Plate 11-14).[257,305] However, more threatening lesions, such as basal cell carcinoma, may occasionally cavitate or contain fluid, thereby assuming a cystlike appearance and masking the true lesion (Fig. 11-44, *A*). This point underscores the desirability of obtaining histopathologic confirmation on every excised lesion possible, regardless of its apparently innocuous nature.

Most eyelid cysts submitted for pathologic examination are designated by the surgeon as *sebaceous cysts*. This clinical term is firmly entrenched in common usage and is a satisfactory term referring to the clinical appearance of the cyst; however, if adhering to strict dermatopathologic criteria, diagnosis of a true simple sebaceous cyst is extremely

rare. Skin cysts are named according to the derivation and type of epithelium that lines the lumen. Although skin cysts are sometimes lined by a derivatives of the pilosebaceous apparatus, they are seldom lined by a pure sebaceous epithelium and, therefore, do not fit into the category of the true sebaceous cyst.

Most skin cysts are lined by one of two types of epithelium derived from the skin and its adnexa: (1) keratinizing squamous epithelium forms the lining of the epidermoid cyst (or epidermal inclusion cyst), and (2) sweat gland-derived cuboidal epithelium forms the wall of a sudoriferous cyst.[319]

Epidermoid and dermoid cysts. An epidermoid cyst (milium) is characterized clinically by its content of cheesy (erroneously termed *sebaceous*) material, which is in fact keratin derived from the hyperkeratotic squamous epithelial lining of the cysts (Fig. 11-36). Most of these cysts are derived from plugged hair follicles or inclusions of squa-

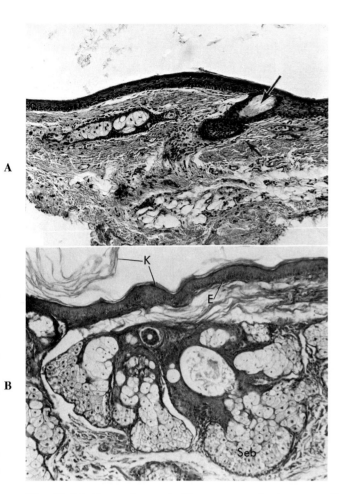

Fig. 11-37. Dermoid cyst. **A,** Photomicrograph of a cyst wall showing a skin appendage *(arrows).* (H & E stain; ×40.) **B,** The dermoid cyst possesses a squamous epithelial lining *(E)* identical to that of the epidermoid cyst (Fig. 11-36) but is distinguished from the latter type by the presence of skin appendage structures associated with the cyst wall. As is true of epidermoid cysts, the cyst cavity *(above)* is filled with keratin *(K)* derived from the epithelium. However, because a skin appendage (the sebaceous gland, *Seb*) is an integral part of the cyst wall, this lesion is defined as a dermoid cyst. (H & E stain; ×100.)

mous epithelial cells that have penetrated deep into the dermis. Some authors reserve the term *epidermal inclusion cyst* for traumatic cases in which nests of epithelial cells are deposited within the dermis following injury to the epithelium. The cells initially grow in solid clusters. The center eventually undergoes cavitation, and a true cyst is formed. Rupture of an epidermoid cyst may incite a foreign body granulomatous inflammatory reaction in the surrounding tissues.

The dermoid cyst (Fig. 11-37) consists of a squamous epithelium–lined, keratin-filled cyst that in most respects is identical to the simple epidermoid cyst.[298] It is further characterized, however, by the presence of skin appendage structures, such as hair, sweat glands, or sebaceous glands derived from the lining epithelium of the cyst. Dermoid cysts are sometimes present at birth. One should not confuse the dermoid cyst of the skin with the solid dermoid tumors of the conjunctiva (Fig. 11-6).

In addition, one should not confuse congenital dermoid cysts and dermoid tumors from a specific lesion termed a *phakomatous choristoma.* This is a unique tumor composed of cells of apparent crystalline lens deviation. They contain lens epithelium, cells resembling bladder cells, and a periodic acid-Schif (PAS) positive, basement membrane material simulating lens capsule. This tumor stains positive with S-100 protein and lens-specific antigens.[294,295,318,325]

Sweat gland cysts (hydrocystomas). Sweat gland cysts of the lid are derived from eccrine glands or from the apocrine glands of Moll (Fig. 11-38).[297] The sweat gland-derived cyst, or sudoriferous cyst, usually contains a watery fluid within the lumen. This contrasts with the cheese-like keratin within epidermoid cysts. Sudoriferous cysts are usually lined by one or two layers of tall or flattened cuboidal epithelium, which mimics the epithelium of the parent gland or duct.

Hemangioma

Hemangiomas are frequently congenital and often appear as soft, pale blue masses in infants' eyelids (Color Plate 11-15). Many such legions regress spontaneously without treatment or excision. Larger lesions require excision. Capillary hemangiomas, the most common type (Fig. 11-39), are composed of endothelial-lined vascular channels equivalent in diameter to normal capillaries. In contrast, cavernous hemangiomas contain vascular channels that may be as large as a medium-sized artery or vein.

Nevi

Although the clinical appearance of nevi is variable, these lesions rarely pose a major diagnostic problem to the clinician. The so-called "kissing nevus" (Fig. 11-40) is interesting from an embryologic or developmental standpoint. It is characterized by simultaneous involvement of the upper and lower lids. The edges of the tumor usually involve the lid margins, and the tumor edges touch, or "kiss," when the lids are closed. Apparently the primordial cells destined to later form a nevus were present in the eyelids during gestation when the eyelids were transiently fused. Fusion of the eyelids during midgestation is a normal phenomenon. When the eyelids separate before birth, nevus cells, which previously overlapped the two fused lids, become randomly distributed onto each separate lid.

Skin nevi are classified in a manner similar to those of the conjunctiva (p. 581). To classify and correctly predict the behavior of nevi, the pathologist studies the position of the nevus cells in the skin layers and looks for the presence or absence of junctional activity, that is, growth or proliferation of nevus cells within the deeper layers of the epithelium and at the epidermal-dermal junction. When the rows or clusters of nevus cells that exhibit junctional activity are only one layer to a few layers thick and do not extend deep within the dermis, the growth is designated a junctional nevus. A compound nevus is one that not only exhibits junctional activity but also extends deep into the dermis. Malignant change can, albeit rarely, occur in junctional and compound nevi.

When junctional activity is absent and when the growth of nevus cells or nests is totally confined to the dermis, the lesion is a dermal or intradermal nevus. The tumor cells

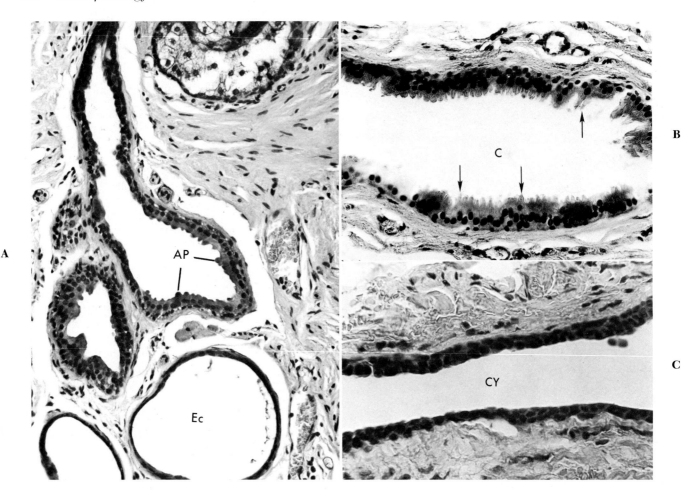

Fig. 11-38. A, Normal glands of the eyelid. The eccrine sweat glands *(Ec)* are composed of a single layer of low cuboidal epithelium. The apocrine gland of Moll *(AP)* is composed of acini lined by tall columnar cells that usually exhibit a brightly eosinophilic cytoplasm. Long apical processes extend into the lumen of the gland. These apices, or caps, are extruded during the normal secretory process (decapitation secretion). Note the adjacent sebaceous gland of Zeis at the top of the figure. (H & E stain; ×200.) **B,** Photomicrograph of an eyelid cyst lined by tall columnar epithelium that shows apocrine-type differentiation *(arrows).* Compare this epithelial lining with that seen in the normal gland of Moll in **A.** Cysts of this type, which demonstrate a direct origin from apocrine elements, are probably less common than sudoiferous cysts that are derived from the unnamed eccrine sweat glands *(C).* (H & E stain; ×275.) **C,** Eccrine-derived eyelid cyst *(Cy)* lined by simple cuboidal epithelium and an outer flattened layer of cells derived from myoepithelial cells. (H & E stain; ×275.)

are totally separated from the epidermis by a band of collagen (Fig. 11-41). Dermal nevi are totally benign and possess no malignant potential.

Two major criteria histopathologically differentiate a malignant melanoma from a compound nevus. Malignant cells show more extensive cellular anaplasia. These cells often resemble the epithelioid cells characteristic of uveal melanomas (Figs. 7-57 and 7-58). Malignant melanomas show individual tumor cells and nests invading deeper into the dermis than would be expected from a benign compound nevus. Furthermore, the neoplastic cells often exhibit permeation of lymphatic channels, a characteristic that clearly indicates the malignant nature of the tumor. True malignant melanomas of the eyelid skin are relatively uncommon.

Seborrheic keratosis

Seborrheic keratoses are common benign lesions of the eyelid and often appear in the pathology laboratory with an incorrect clinical diagnosis (Fig. 11-42). Clinically these lesions are hyperkeratotic, usually hyperpigmented, and often have a greasy appearance. The mass is typically raised above the normal level of the skin and is often referred to as being "tacked" onto the skin surface. Because the growth is generally confined on or above the skin surface, there is rarely evidence of downward invasion into the dermis. There is considerable overlap with seborrheic keratoses in the appearance of many squamous papillomas, but the distinction is academic because each lesion is entirely benign.

The histopathologic appearance of seborrheic keratosis

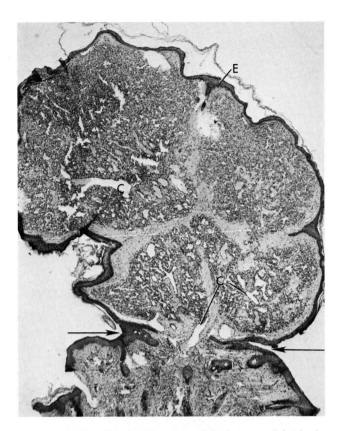

Fig. 11-39. Capillary hemangioma of the lower eyelid. The lesion appeared clinically as a pale blue polypoid lesion protruding above the skin surface *(arrows)*. It contains multiple small endothelial-lined channels. The vascular channels are roughly equivalent to capillaries in diameter. *C,* Capillary lumen; *E,* skin epithelium overlying the lesion. (H & E stain; ×30.)

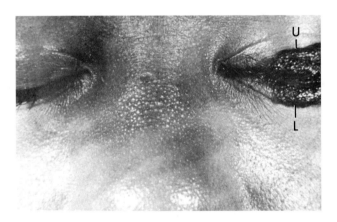

Fig. 11-40. Benign deeply pigmented nevi involving both the upper *(U)* and lower *(L)* eyelids on the left, so-called "kissing nevi." The anlage, or primordial, cells responsible for the tumors existed during the embryonic period when the lids were fused. After separation of the two eyelids during the latter half of the gestational period, clusters of nevus cells (or cells destined to form the nevus) are sequestered in both lids.

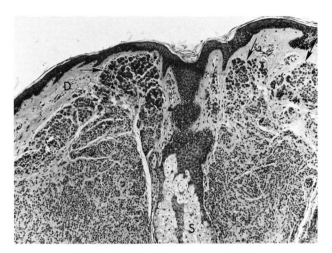

Fig. 11-41. Intradermal nevus. The nevus cells are arranged in a diffuse pattern in the deep dermis but are more pigmented and form discrete nests *(arrows)* superficially. Note the uninvolved band of collagen in the dermis *(D)* separating the tumor from the overlying epidermis. This feature distinguishes an intradermal nevus from a nevus with junctional activity at the level of the epidermal-dermal junction. A conjunctival nevus with junctional activity is illustrated in Fig. 11-28, *A. S,* Sebaceous apparatus associated with a hair follicle (gland of Zeis). (H & E stain; ×80.)

can be confusing to an inexperienced microscopist. Because the proliferative epithelial cells that comprise the bulk of the mass superficially resemble the cells of basal cell carcinoma, this tumor is sometimes termed a *basal cell papilloma;* however, such designation is confusing, particularly in view of the differences in prognosis between a basal cell carcinoma and a simple seborrheic keratosis. The most characteristic structures are the small keratin-containing cysts entrapped among the proliferating cells. These cysts are called pseudohorn cysts (Fig. 11-42). They should not be confused with the epithelial pearls of squamous cell carcinoma.

MALIGNANT TUMORS
Basal cell carcinoma

Satisfactory control of a basal cell carcinoma (epithelioma) depends largely on early diagnosis and treatment.[327–345] Usually, this tumor can be adequately treated by any of several modes of therapy, including excision, irradiation, and chemotherapy.[330,331] Distant metastasis is seldom seen; morbidity and mortality are more closely related to the neoplasm's potential for local invasion, particularly the so-called morphealike or sclerosing form (Fig. 11-45).* With prompt treatment and adequate follow-up of the patient, recurrence and more severe problems resulting from facial and orbital invasion by this tumor may be minimized.[330,331,340] Indeed, some authors prefer the term *basal cell epithelioma,* a designation that tends to deemphasize the more ominous prognosis suggested by the term *carcinoma.* Basal cell carcinoma of the eyelid is by far the most common malignant tumor involving the ocular adnexa. Because early treatment is a prime factor in ensuring

---

* References 307, 310, 327, 328, 336, 339, 344.

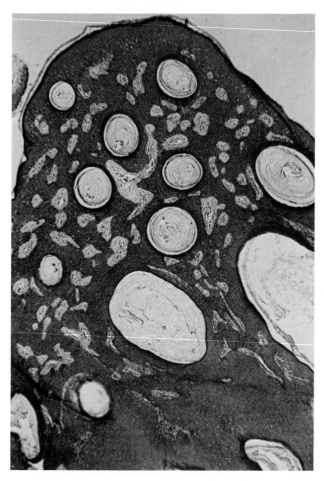

Fig. 11-42. Seborrheic keratosis. This elevated lesion is composed of sheets of small hyperchromatic cells resembling those of basal cell carcinoma. The large keratin-filled "pseudohorn cysts" are characteristic. (H & E stain; ×12.)

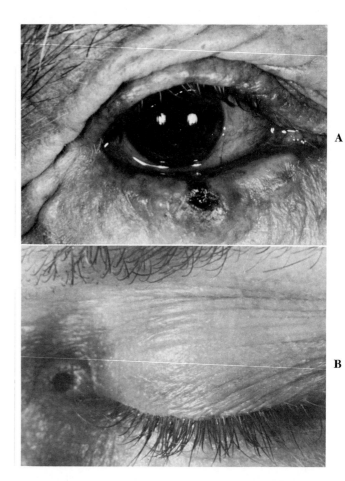

Fig. 11-43. Basal cell carcinoma. **A,** Lower eyelid. The central ulcer is surrounded by a raised pearly border. Most basal cell carcinomas originate in the lower or medial aspect of the eyelids. **B,** Ulcerated lesion at the inner canthus.

a good prognosis, the ability of the ophthalmologist to recognize this tumor and initiate prompt therapy is important.

Clinical features. Basal cell carcinoma is a tumor affecting the sun-exposed areas of the body. Of the one-half million skin cancers diagnosed annually in the United States, 75% are basal cell carcinoma. The sun is a major predisposing factor not only in the genesis of basal cell carcinoma but also in most other epithelial tumors of the skin, particularly in fair-skinned persons. Basal cell carcinoma is seen only occasionally in black persons. In the series described in Table 11-3 only 2 of 381 patients with basal cell carcinoma were black. The tumor rarely, if ever, occurs on the conjunctiva or other mucous membranes; only the integument is involved.

The basal cell carcinoma may assume a wide variety of clinical appearances (Fig. 11-43; Color Plates 11-16 and 11-17). The noduloulcerative type consists of a central ulcer (rodent ulcer) that slowly enlarges and is surrounded by a pearly, often shiny, rolled border. Basal cell carcinomas, however, may assume other forms that can cause confusion in formulating a differential diagnosis. For example, the cystic type of basal cell carcinoma (Fig. 11-44) was mistaken for an innocuous, benign simple cyst during clinical inspection.

In our series 45% of basal cell carcinomas of the eyelids occurred on the lower lid and 24% at the medial canthus. The upper lid was less frequently involved. The ratio of frequency of basal cell carcinoma to squamous cell carcinoma of the eyelid is greater than 9 : 1.

Squamous cell carcinoma and sebaceous carcinoma of the eyelid may occur on the upper or the lower lid; however, involvement of the upper lid by a malignant-appearing growth should provoke the suspicion that it is a squamous cell or sebaceous carcinoma rather than the basal cell type. This reflects the relative infrequency of basal cell carcinoma of the upper lid compared with that of the lower and inner quadrants. Furthermore, a sebaceous carcinoma arising from the meibomian gland is much more common in the upper lid than in the lower. This probably reflects, at least in part, the fact that roughly twice as many meibomian glands are present in the upper lid than in the lower.

The basal cell nevus syndrome inherited as an autosomal dominant consists of multiple basal cell carcinomas associated with defects in other tissues such as odontogenic cysts of the jaw, ribs, vertebrae, and hands.°

° References 332, 333, 337, 338, 342, 343.

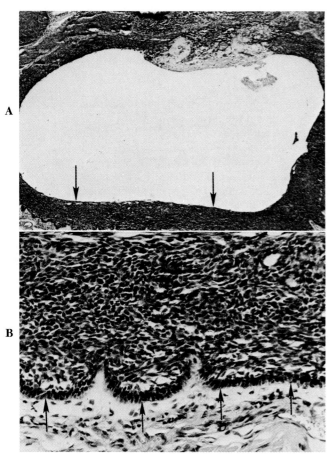

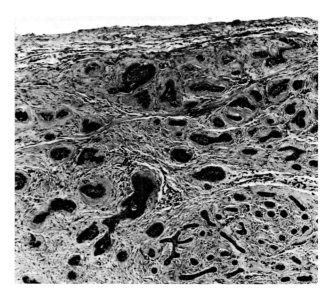

Fig. 11-45. Basal cell carcinoma, sclerosing or morphea-like. This type shows a tendency for more aggressive growth than most other forms of basal cell carcinoma. The tumor cells are packed into small nests and have evoked an intense fibrous or schirrous reaction of the surrounding dermis, hence the term *morphealike* or *scleroderma-like.* Morphea is a localized form of scleroderma that clinically resembles this type of basal cell. (H & E stain; ×40.)

Fig. 11-44. Cystic basal cell carcinoma of the eyelid. **A,** This lesion was removed after a clinical diagnosis of a simple benign cyst. The hypercellularity of the cyst wall *(arrows)* and the palisading arrangement of the peripheral row of cells (the so-called picket fence) are diagnostic. (H & E stain; ×35.) **B,** High-power photomicrograph of the basal cell carcinoma in **A.** The main portion of this tumor is composed of a monotonous array of small cells with hyperchromatic nuclei. The major distinguishing feature of this tumor is the palisading or "picket fence" formation of the peripheral or outer row of cells *(arrows)*. D, Surrounding dermis. (H & E stain; ×325.)

Histopathologic findings. The histogenesis of basal cell carcinoma is disputed; however, it is probably not derived from mature "basal cells," as the name would imply, but from the primary epithelial germ cells in the deepest layer of the epidermis.[307]

The basal layer of epidermis normally contains three cellular components: the basal cells, melanocytic cells (cells that possess the potential to develop into nevi and malignant melanoma), and primary epithelial germ cells, which are believed to possess the potential to develop into basal cell carcinoma and other tumors. The germ cells is a primordial cell derived from the surface ectoderm. During embryogenesis most of these cells mature and from the skin epithelium and skin appendages, but some of these pluripotential embryonal cells remain within the epidermis throughout life. Transformation into tumor cells occurs after appropriate stimulation, such as solar radiation. This theory of origin of basal cell carcinomas is supported by the propensity of this tumor to differentiate toward a wide

variety of skin and skin appendage-like structures, all of which are known to originate from such embryonal germ cells. For example, basal cell carcinomas commonly exhibit morphologic features that reflect a differentiation toward adnexal structures such as hair follicles or glands.

Most basal cell carcinomas grow in lobules that contain monotonous arrays of small, regularly shaped cells with scanty cytoplasm and hyperchromatic nuclei. Figure 11-44 illustrates a basal cell carcinoma in which, although a central cavity is formed, the typical tumor growth forms an outer lining around the cavity. The most distinctive histopathologic feature of this tumor is the so-called picket fence caused by palisading of the peripheral row of nuclei at the edge of the mass. Because the tumor is derived from a pluripotential germ cell, it can differentiate along many cellular lines (e.g., toward hair follicles, sebaceous elements, or adnexal glands). It is not surprising, therefore, that a bewildering number of histopathologic patterns might lead to great difficulty in correct diagnosis. However, the palisading of peripheral nuclei present in most basal cell carcinomas is often the final clue to correct diagnosis. For example, even in cases in which keratin formation is prominent (thus suggesting a squamous cell carcinoma), in cases in which sweat gland differentiation might suggest an adenocarcinoma, or when a dense fibrous reaction around the tumor nests occurs (morphealike basal cell carcinoma, Fig. 11-45), recognition of the "picket fence" appearance is an invaluable indicator of the neoplasm's true nature.[146] The morpheaform (fibrosis) type of basal cell carcinoma tends to be more aggressive with deep invasion and reoccurrence being more common than with the nodular or superficial type.[345]

Squamous epithelial proliferative and neoplastic lesions

Squamous cell growths of the skin are acanthotic proliferative or neoplastic lesions in which the predominant cell type resembles the squamous or prickle cell of the malpighian layer of the epidermis.[346-370] These cause much confusion in terminology and classification. They range in severity from totally benign lesions to growths showing cellular atypism with malignant potential, to low-grade malignant neoplasms, to unequivocal malignant carcinomas.

A. No or minimal cellular atypism (not considered premalignant)
   1. Squamous papillomas (polyps, skin tags, warts, verrucous growths)
   2. Nonspecific epithelial hyperplastic lesions or keratoses, which arise as a result of underlying inflammations, infection, or environmental influence
B. Apparent or real cellular atypism
   1. Pseudoepitheliomatous hyperplasia, not premalignant
      a. Keratoacanthoma
      b. Inverted follicular keratosis
   2. Solar (senile, actinic) keratosis, premalignant
   3. Carcinoma in situ (Bowen's disease)
   4. Squamous cell carcinoma, low-grade malignancy (microinvasive)
   5. Invasive squamous cell carcinoma
   6. Xeroderma pigmentosum

Invasive squamous cell carcinoma of the lids is rare. In the past it has been repeatedly overdiagnosed, frequently resulting in unnecessarily aggressive surgery.[356] Clinical and pathologic studies have demonstrated that most eyelid tumors exhibiting microscopic criteria normally applied to squamous cell carcinomas of internal organs do not show the degree of malignant behavior expected. With few exceptions, a squamous cell carcinoma of the skin is clearly less malignant than its counterpart in such organs as the esophagus or lung. This probably reflects the principle that solar-induced skin lesions possess a much lower potential for malignant behavior than do carcinomas of a similar cell type that arise from other carcinogenic factors.

Lesions exhibiting no or minimal cellular atypism. A large percentage of squamous epithelial growths are proliferative lesions without cellular anaplasia. They are benign and not progressive or premalignant.

Although squamous papillomas and other hyperplastic lesions and nonspecific keratoses are completely benign, malignant skin tumors can occasionally assume a clinical or gross pathologic appearance that mimics these benign growths. These exceptions emphasize the point that the ultimate diagnosis of all skin growths rests with the cytologic pattern of the lesion rather than its general clinical or gross morphologic appearance.

Lesions exhibiting apparent or real cellular atypism, pseudoepitheliomatous hyperplasia. Pseudoepitheliomatous hyperplasia signifies a nonmalignant lesion that appears deceptively malignant by clinical or histopathologic examination. It is so named because it represents an epithelial hyperplasia that may mimic a carcinoma (epithelioma). Inflammatory processes in the underlying dermis often stimulate the hyperplastic epithelial proliferation. In the past many of these lesions have been mistakenly diagnosed as squamous cell carcinomas, but it is now recognized that the natural course of such lesions is self-limiting. Histopathologically the diagnosis is difficult because the extensive cellular proliferation and epithelial acanthosis associated with cytologic features of anaplasia often strongly suggest a cancer.

Two specific examples are keratoacanthoma and inverted follicular keratosis.

Keratoacanthoma, sometimes termed *self-healing squamous cell carcinoma*, is a lesion that formerly was diagnosed as basal cell carcinoma or squamous cell carcinoma.[238,358] It is typically dome shaped, and a large central keratotic plug, or crater, sometimes projects from the center of the mass. It is also sometimes termed *molluscum sebaceum* because of superficial resemblance to molluscum contagiosum (p. 583), which also usually has a central umbilication containing a keratotic plug. The label of *self-healing squamous cell carcinoma* underscores the lesion's natural tendency to involute within weeks to several months (Fig. 11-46).

Inverted follicular keratosis is a second form of pseudoepitheliomatous hyperplasia.[347,364-366] Although clinical and histopathologic details of this condition are beyond the scope of this chapter, a second term describing this condition—*basosquamous epithelial tumor*—is indicative of the characteristic histopathologic pattern. So-called squamous cell eddies, or clusters of squamous cells, are deposited within the deeper layers of the acanthotic mass, which is otherwise composed of cells resembling those of basal cell lesions. Some authors believe that this lesion is a variety of verruca vulgaris.[367,370]

Solar keratosis. Solar keratosis ("senile" keratosis, actinic keratosis) is considered a premalignant skin lesion.[363] Most affected persons are elderly, fair-skinned, and frequently exposed to the sun and other environmental irritants. Multiple lesions can occur on the sun-exposed areas of the skin. With passage of time, as many as 25% of untreated lesions may progress toward squamous cell carcinoma; however, in keeping with the general concept regarding solar-induced skin neoplasms, squamous cell carcinomas arising from solar keratosis rarely metastasize.

The morphologic changes seen in solar keratosis occur in both the epithelium and the dermis. The surface epithelium often reveals acanthosis, hyperkeratosis, parakeratosis, and dyskeratosis (p. 585). Individual cell dyskeratosis is an excellent indicator of propensity toward premalignancy or malignancy. It occurs when random epithelial cells in the deeper layers of the epithelium begin to form abnormal keratin and pearlike structures. Keratin is normally found only on the surface of the epidermis during physiologic maturation of the epithelial cells. Epithelial pearls seen in squamous cell carcinoma represent a similar pathologic process (Fig. 11-48).

The superficial dermis in solar keratosis shows varying degrees of chronic inflammation secondary to irritation by solar radiation and other environmental irritants. A second dermal change, so-called basophilic degeneration of collagen or solar elastosis, is almost pathognomonic of sun-induced degeneration of dermal collagen and elastic tissue. These changes are similar to those occurring in the subepithelial stroma of the bulbar conjunctiva in pingueculae and pterygia (Fig. 11-18, *C*). This is not surprising if one recalls that all of these lesions generate in response to solar radiation and other irritative environmental influences.

Carcinoma in situ (Bowen's disease).[349,351] Carcinoma in situ of the skin, in contrast to most other squamous epithelial proliferative and neoplastic lesions, occurs with a relatively high frequency in nonexposed and sunexposed areas of the skin.[349,351] It has a relatively common association with internal or visceral malignancies in affected patients. It is not clear whether this association merely reflects the fact that most affected persons are elderly and fall within the age group in which internal neoplasms are more common or whether the skin lesion is directly associated with carcinogenic factors that also produce the internal tumors.

The condition produces a wide variety of clinical appearances. Hyperkeratotic lesions produce a leukoplakia and are often nodular or ulcerated. The epithelial cytologic changes, which resemble those of squamous cell carcinoma, include loss of polarity by the immature, neoplastic epithelial cells. The cells are arranged with their long axes in the vertical direction, as opposed to the normal state in which the long axis is parallel to the surface. Epithelial cellular atypism is a consistent finding.

As noted in the section on conjunctival carcinoma is situ (p. 577), the histopathologic hallmark of this condition is the lack of penetration of the cancerous cells into the underlying dermis. The basement membrane, which is formed by the basal layer of epidermal cells and separates the epithelium from the dermis, remains intact (Fig. 11-47). This membrane is difficult to observe in hematoxylin and eosin preparations but is clearly seen with the PAS technique (p. 3). Regardless of the thickness or apparent degree of cellular anaplasia of the tumor, the intact basement membrane represents the definitive diagnostic criterion. Excision is usually curative.

Squamous cell carcinoma, low-grade malignancy (microinvasive) type. Although unequivocal invasive squamous cell carcinoma of the eyelid skin occurs in a small percentage of cases (Table 11-2–11-4), it has been demonstrated clearly that such a diagnosis has been made too often in the past.[356]

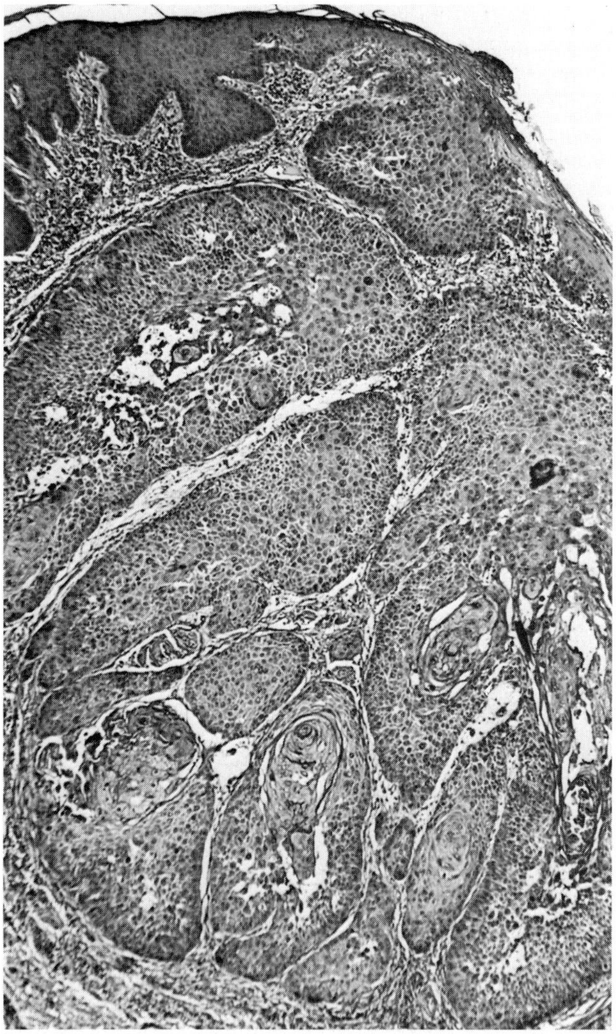

Fig. 11-46. Keratoacanthoma. This is the left half of a highly dysplastic, acanthotic mass. The underlying basement membrane was not penetrated, and the lesion regressed spontaneously. (H & E stain; ×22.)

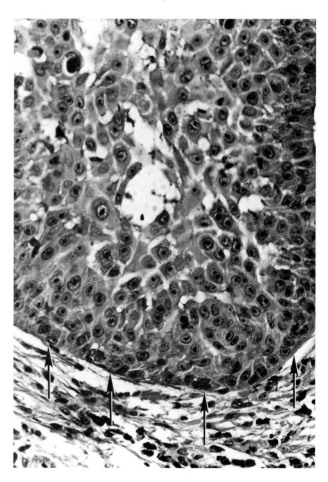

Fig. 11-47. In situ squamous cell carcinoma of the eyelid. The intraepithelial tumor cells exhibit marked pleomorphism and nuclear atypism. This lesion was originally considered to be an invasive squamous cell carcinoma. However, the clinical course was benign, and reexamination revealed no invasion through the underlying epithelial basement membrane *(arrows)*. (H & E stain; ×275.)

A significant percentage of excised squamous epithelial tumors show evidence of penetration of the underlying basement membrane and tumor invasion of the superficial dermis. By standard histopathologic criteria, these lesions qualify as true "squamous cell carcinomas." Experience has shown, however, that most patients affected by this type of growth suffer less morbidity and mortality than expected. Such lesions might be considered "intermediate" between intraepithelial carcinoma and deeply invasive squamous cell carcinoma.

For want of better terms, we designate this type of growth as low grade, or *microinvasive*, squamous cell carcinoma to avoid the stigma associated with the more ominous, unequivocal invasive squamous cell carcinoma. During a review of the microslides of the cases listed in Table 11-2, recognition of this group of microinvasive carcinomas was primarily responsible for a reclassification of previously diagnosed invasive carcinomas to a more benign position on the spectrum of squamous cell neoplasms. These lesions exhibiting low-grade malignant behavior occur with much greater frequency than unequivocal invasive squamous cell carcinoma. Follow-up evaluation of patients in whom the lesion was reclassified revealed little tendency toward recurrence of metastasis.

Invasive squamous cell carcinoma. The previous discussions have emphasized that deep invasion and metastatic spread of a squamous cell carcinoma of the eyelid is rare and that less malignant lesions such as pseudoepitheliomatous hyperplasia or microinvasive squamous cell carcinoma are much more common.[330,352,362] In cases of advanced, deeply invasive squamous cell carcinoma of the lid (Fig. 11-48; Color Plate 11-18), the advanced state of the lesion usually reflects the patient's delay in seeking medical attention or the physician's delay in diagnosis. However, even large, fungating, ulcerated lesions do not have a hopeless prognosis because these solar-induced tumors do not usually metastasize to distant organs. When metastasis occurs, it is in most cases confined to regional lymph nodes, such as the preauricular and submandibular groups (Fig. 11-24, *A*).

The cytologic changes of squamous cell carcinoma represent similar but more extensive anaplastic changes than those of the premalignant and low-grade malignant lesions described previously. The primary microscopic features of squamous cell carcinoma include pleomorphism (variation in size and shape of the tumor cells), formation of tumor cells with hyperchromatic nuclei and scanty cytoplasm, atypical mitotic figures, deep invasion of tumor cell nests into the dermis (Fig. 11-48), and abnormal keratinization.

Keratinization normally occurs only in the superficial layer of the epidermis during maturation of each squamous epithelial cell. Abnormal keratinization (dyskeratosis) seen in neoplasia represents abortive attempts by the neoplastic squamous epithelial cell to form this product. In a sense the tumor cell attempts to form the secretory product normally formed by the cell line. This is analogous to formation of melanin pigment by a malignant melanoma or formation of lipid by a sebaceous (meibomian) carcinoma. These attempts at keratinization provide the pathologist with a readily identifiable morphologic criterion for classification of the lesion. Individual cell dyskeratosis represents abnormal keratin formation within individual cells of the epithelium. Formation of squamous epithelial pearls by nests of tumor cells is a second type of abnormal keratinization. Pearls may be situated intraepithelially or may occur within foci of deep invasion in the dermis (Fig. 11-48).

Xeroderma pigmentosum. In xeroderma pigmentosum (Fig. 11-49), a disorder inherited in an autosomal-

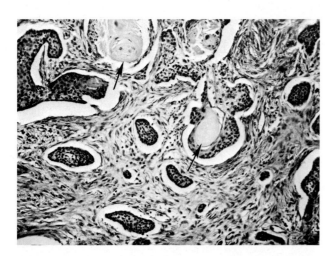

Fig. 11-48. Invasion of deep dermis of eyelid skin by nests of infiltrative squamous cell carcinoma cells. The clusters of malignant cells permeate the subepidermal lymphatic channels of the eyelid and occasionally may metastasize to the regional lymph nodes (Fig. 11-24, *A*). Lesions involving the upper lid commonly spread to preauricular lymph nodes. The lower lid lymphatics drain to the submandibular and preauricular lymph nodes. The epithelial "pearls" *(arrows)* arise from abnormal keratinization of individual cell nests. The pearl is the most distinguishing feature permitting definitive diagnosis of squamous cell carcinoma. (H & E stain; ×100.)

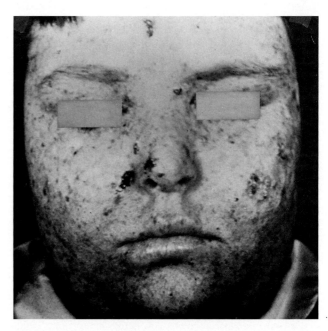

Fig. 11-49. Xeroderma pigmentosum. Family members affected with this condition may suffer from almost every variety of skin tumor.

recessive manner, the skin exhibits a marked sensitivity to sunlight.[346,353-355,368] Multiple skin lesions become manifest in childhood, and the major hope of prevention rests in secluding the child from exposure to the sun. In early stages the lesions are identical to those of solar (actinic) keratosis. The sun-exposed skin and conjunctiva ultimately develop multiple malignant tumors that may lead to metastasis and death. Virtually all categories of skin tumors have been reported in this condition. Malignant melanoma of the iris has been reported.[335] For example, a single patient may simultaneously develop basal cell carcinoma, squamous cell carcinoma, and malignant melanoma.

Malignant melanoma

During the past few decades, the incidence of cutaneous malignant melanoma has risen 3 to 5 fold, probably attributable to increased voluntary exposure to sun. Malignant melanoma involves the lower lid two thirds more often than the upper lid and is not infrequently associated with nevi, solar elastosis, nevus, and basal cell carcinoma. Malignant melanoma may arise from a preexisting junctional, compound, or (rarely) a large or giant congenital melanocytic nevus. It may arise de novo.

Skin melanomas are not classified according to cell type as are uveal melanomas. Lentigo maligna melanoma develops in a preinvasive lesion called melanotic freckle of Hutchinson. Following a radial growth phase (intraepidermal spread), a vertical growth phase (dermal invasion), may occur, elevating the lesion. Superficial spreading malignant melanoma involves the epithelium and has a prolonged radial growth phase before the vertical growth phase. Clinically, the lesion appears as a nodule or plaque with variable pigmentation and has a "surround component," caused by the intradermal spread. Nodular malignant melanoma has only a vertical growth phase, involves the dermis early and has the worst prognosis. Clinically, the lesion appears as a nodule or plaque without a surround component because no radial growth phase occurs.

Sebaceous gland tumors

Sebaceous glands occur throughout the skin in association with hair follicles. This complex is called a pilosebaceous apparatus. The eyelid sebaceous glands contribute the lipid (oily) layer to the tear film. The meibomian glands[376] (Fig. 11-50), the glands of Zeis, the unnamed sebaceous glands associated with the small hairs on the anterior integument of the lid, and the sebaceous glands of the caruncle are potential sources of abnormal sebaceous growths.[391-394,396,397,399,400] These lipid-secreting glands occasionally undergo hyperplastic or neoplastic dedifferentiation, with development of either a sebaceous cell hyperplasia (Fig. 11-51), adenoma, or adenocarcinoma (Figs. 11-52 and 11-53). The eyelid is the most common site of sebaceous carcinoma in the body.

Most sebaceous tumors arise from the meibomian glands. They occur most frequently on the upper lids because there are approximately twice as many meibomain gland-duct complexes on the upper lid as on the lower. The most common sign of a growth derived from the meibomian glands is a mass affecting the tarsal plate or the lid margin. Lesions originating from the glands of Zeis are always at the lid margin.

Sebaceous cell growths (Color Plates 11-19–11-21) commonly exhibit varying degrees of yellow coloration because of the presence of lipid material within the mass. Hyperplastic or neoplastic sebaceous growths continue to some extent to perform the lipid-secreting function of the normal sebaceous gland; therefore, the yellow color of the mass may exclude other tumors, such as squamous cell or basal cell carcinoma, in which yellow lipid is characteristically absent.

Sebaceous hyperplasias, adenomas, and many carcinomas often form well-circumscribed nodules surrounded by a capsule or pseudocapsule. A sebaceous carcinoma may look like a fungating infiltrative or ulcerated growth. The latter are easily mistaken for basal cell carcinomas.

Sebaceous growths are often mistaken clinically for chalazia.* The location of the tarsus, the yellow color, and the

---

* References 332, 374, 375, 378, 381, 382, 391.

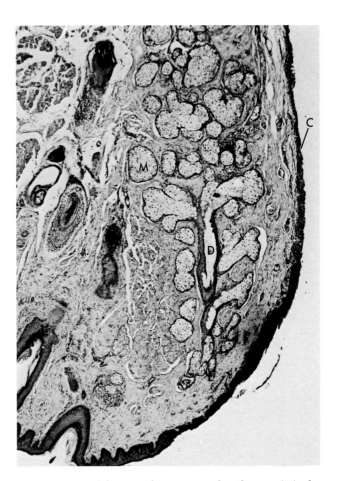

Fig. 11-50. Eyelid margin showing normal meibomian (*M*) sebaceous glands composed of clear lipid-secreting cells that empty into a single duct (*D*). This duct opens at the lid margin posterior to the gray line. This duct orifice is not present in the plane of section demonstrated here. Either the meibomian glands or the glands of Zeis may undergo a benign hyperplasia, form a benign adenoma, or undergo malignant differentiation with the development of a sebaceous carcinoma (Figs. 11-51–11-53). The eyelid is the most common site of sebaceous carcinoma in the body. The orbicularis muscle is present on the left, the palpebral conjunctival epithelium (*C*), on the right (see also Fig. 11-3). (H & E stain; ×35.)

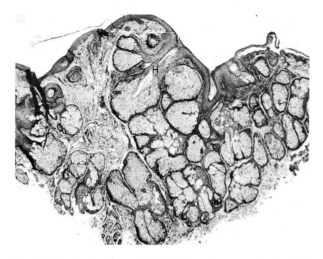

Fig. 11-51. Benign hyperplasia of the sebaceous glands of the lid margin. This lesion probably arose from the glands of Zeis because of the close association with hair follicles (*H*). The lobular proliferation of well-differentiated sebaceous glands is characteristic of a benign sebaceous gland proliferation. (H & E stain; ×30.)

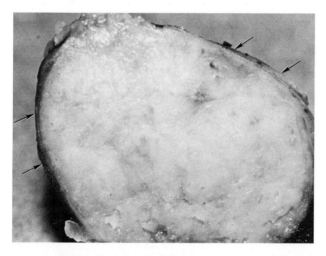

Fig. 11-52. Gross photograph of an encapsulated (*arrows*) sebaceous carcinoma of the eyelid. The tumor, which involved the tarsus and was yellow, was originally considered to be a chalazion. The yellow color of the mass resulted from the lipid formed by the tumor cells.

nodular appearance of the lesion may closely resemble the appearance of a chalazion. When a "chalazion" recurs, the lesion should be studied histopathologically to rule out sebaceous carcinoma or other serious tumors.

Sebaceous cell hyperplasia (Fig. 11-51) is a benign proliferation of lobules of normal-appearing sebaceous gland tissue. Although increased in number, there is no tendency toward anaplastic dedifferentiation of the involved cells. Like normal lipid-secreting sebaceous glands, the proliferating cells reveal an apparently empty cytoplasm after routine processing in paraffin and staining with hematoxylin and eosin. Intracellular lipid is visible only after frozen sections are prepared and specially stained for lipid.

A sebaceous adenoma is a benign neoplastic prolifera-

tion that is typically smooth, round, and well demarcated.[379] Such lesions are composed of lobules of normal-appearing sebaceous elements mixed with lobules of cells closely resembling immature sebaceous cells, which are precursors to typical, normal, adult lipid-laden cells. These cells exhibit more basophilia than the mature sebaceous cell but show no evidence of frank anaplasia indicative of carcinomatous change. When the growth is composed predominantly of the more basophilic-staining germinative cells, it may resemble basal cell carcinoma. However, observation of cystoplasmic lipid within the proliferating lobules easily confirms the nature of the growth.

Adenocarcinoma of the sebaceous glands of the eyelid is a tumor affecting middle-aged and elderly persons.[371–400] It is more common in females, and the median age at diagnosis is 65 years.

Boniuk and Zimmerman[372,373] have determined that relatively common eyelid tumors, such as basal cell carcinomas, are correctly diagnosed clinically in a large percentage of the cases. Because such tumors are common and have certain characteristic clinical features, the ophthalmologist is well aware of these and considers them in the differential diagnosis. In contrast, the incidence of sebaceous carcinomas is much less, and this tumor may present a wide spectrum in clinical appearance. These tumors frequently mimic other tumors or inflammatory conditions. This tumor may be misdiagnosed as a chalazion or chronic blepharitis and is termed the *great masquerader*; therefore, the index of suspicion is low, and errors in diagnosis and management of these malignant tumors sometimes occur.

As noted before, the sebaceous carcinoma may grow as a well-circumscribed, sometimes encapsulated mass (Fig. 11-52) or as an ulcerated or fungating infiltrative growth (Fig. 11-53). Tumor cells may invade the overlying epidermis, resulting in a "pagetoid change" with intraepithelial growth and frequent extension to the adjacent conjunctiva.[392] Predictably the carcinoma exhibits a significantly greater degree of cellular anaplasia than that seen in a sebaceous adenoma. Nuclear hyperchromatism and abundant normal and abnormal mitotic figures are seen in the carcinomatous cells. The degree of differentiation of the individual neoplastic cell varies considerably in different cases. In tumors with considerable sebaceous differentiation, identification is not difficult. The more differentiation a given tumor exhibits, the more closely the neoplastic cells resemble the normal sebaceous cell, which exhibits an apparently empty or foamy cytoplasm. The tumor illustrated in Fig. 11-53, *B*, contains many such cells. The lipid was leached from the cytoplasm during processing in paraffin; however, frozen sections of formalin-fixed slices of this tumor stained with the oil red O technique demonstrated the presence of intracytoplasmic lipid.

In more poorly differentiated tumors, categorization of the neoplastic cells is sometimes difficult because routine staining techniques do not show distinctive lipid-laden cells.[377] Such tumors are occasionally mistaken for squamous cell carcinomas or basal cell carcinomas; however, in almost all cases frozen sections and lipid stains reveal lipid droplets in the tumor cells, a finding that confirms the diagnosis (Fig. 11-53, *C*).

In a study of 88 patients with sebaceous carcinoma of the eyelids, Boniuk and Zimmerman[372,373] reviewed the behavior of this neoplasm. They determined that orbital

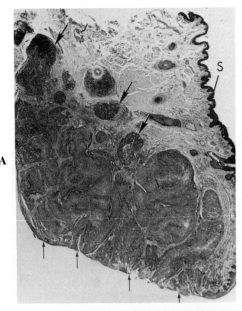

A

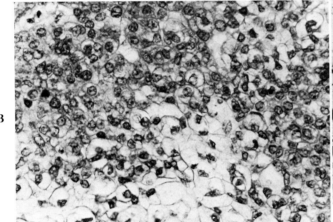

B

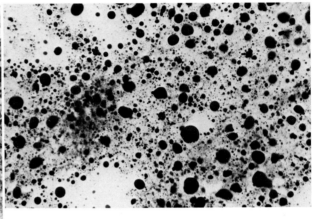

C

Fig. 11-53. Sebaceous carcinoma. **A,** Carcinoma involving the inferior and posterior aspects of the upper eyelid. It is not always possible to determine whether such tumors arise from the meibomian glands or the glands of Zeis. The lower margin is ulcerated and, therefore, devoid of epithelium *(small arrows)*. Lobules of dark-staining tumor cells penetrate deeply into the lid substance *(large arrows)*. The tarsus is totally destroyed in this plane of section. S, Anterior skin of the eyelid. (H & E stain; ×135.) **B,** High-power photomicrograph of the meibomian carcinoma seen in **A**. A sebaceous cell differentiation is apparent in that many of the cells exhibit a clear, poorly staining, empty-appearing cytoplasm. The cells secrete a lipid product much as a normal meibomian (or Zeis) gland acinus might. The lipid in the cell cytoplasm does not stain because of leaching during technical processing. (H & E stain; ×350.) **C,** Sebaceous carcinoma, frozen section lipid stain. The lipid droplets manufactured by the tumor cells stain brilliantly. (Sudan stain; ×250.) (Courtesy Dr. Michael Fajoni.)

invasion occurred in 17% of affected patients, and lymph node metastasis (in most instances involving regional spread to the preauricular nodes or the submandibular lymph nodes) occurred in 28.4% of the patients on whom follow-up information was available; 13.5% of the patients in this series died of provable or proved metastasis.

In a more recent series Rao and coworkers[389] studied 104 cases with at least 5 years follow-up information after diagnosis of sebaceous carcinoma that arose from the ocular adnexa. Twenty-three patients (22%) died of metastatic disease. The various clinicopathologic features that indicated a bad prognosis were vascular, lymphatic, and orbital invasion; involvement of both upper and lower eyelids; poor differentiation; multicentric origin; duration of symptoms greater than 6 months; a tumor diameter exceeding 10 mm; a highly infiltrative pattern; and pagetoid invasion of the overlying epithelia of the eyelids. Tumors of the apocrine gland of moll are very rare.[395]

REFERENCES

Histology of the conjunctiva

1. Abdel-Khalek LMR, Williamson J, and Lee WR: Morphological changes in the human conjunctival epithelium. I. In the normal elderly population, Br J Ophthalmol 62:792, 1978.

2. Abdel-Khalek LMR, Williamson J, and Lee WR: Morphological changes in the human conjunctival epithelium. II. In keratoconjunctivitis sicca, Br J Ophthalmol 62:800, 1978.

3. Abrahamson JA: Color atlas of anterior segment eye diseases, New York, 1964, McGraw-Hill Book Co.

4. Chin GN, Chi EY, and Bunt AH: Ultrastructural and histochemical studies on conjunctival concretions, Arch Ophthalmol 98:720, 1980.

5. Donaldson DD: Atlas of external diseases of the eye, vol 2, Orbit, lacrimal apparatus, eyelids, and conjunctiva, St Louis, 1968, CV Mosby Co.

6. Donaldson DD: Atlas of external diseases of the eye, vol 3, Cornea and sclera, St Louis, 1971, CV Mosby Co.

7. Donshik PC and others: Conjunctival resection treatment and ultrastructural histopathology of superior limbic keratoconjunctivitis, Am J Ophthalmol 85:101, 1978.

8. Duke-Elder S: System of ophthalmology, vol VIII, Diseases of the outer eye, part 1, Conjunctiva, St Louis, 1965, CV Mosby Co.

9. Fedukowicz H: External infections of the eye: bacterial, viral and mycotic, New York, 1963, Appleton-Century-Crofts.

10. Greef R: Die pathologische Anatomie des Auges. In Orth J, editor: Lehrbuch der speziellen pathologischen Anatomie, Berlin, 1902, Hirschwald.

11. Greiner JV, Covington HI, and Allansmith MR: Surface morphology of the human upper tarsal conjunctiva, Am J Ophthalmol 83:892, 1977.

12. Greiner JV, Covington HI, and Allansmith MR: The human limbus: a scanning electron microscopic study, Arch Ophthalmol 97:1159, 1979.

13. Greiner JV and others: Goblet cells of the human conjunctiva, Arch Ophthalmol 99:2190, 1981.

14. Henke F and Lubarsch O: Handbuch der speziellen pathologischen Anatomie und Histologie, vols 1 to 3, Berlin, 1928, Julius Springer.

15. Hornblass A: Tumors of the ocular adnexa and orbit, St Louis, 1979, CV Mosby Co.

16. Kuwabara T, Cogan DG, and Johnson CC: Structure of the muscles of the upper eyelid, Arch Ophthalmol 93:1189, 1975.

17. Lever WF and Schaumburg-Lever G: Histopathology of the skin, ed 7, Philadelphia, 1990, JB Lippincott.

18. Locatcher-Khorazo D and Seegal BC: Microbiology of the eye, St Louis, 1972, CV Mosby Co.

19. Luthra CL, Doxanas MT, and Green WR: Lesions of the caruncle: a clinicohistopathologic study, Surv Ophthalmol 23:183, 1978.

20. McCallum RM, Cobo LM, and Haynes BF: Analysis of corneal and conjunctival microenvironments using monoclonal antibodies, Invest Ophthalmol Vis Sci 34:1793, 1993.

21. Meyner E: Atlas der Spaltlampenphotographic, Stuttgart, 1976, Ferdinand Enke Verlag.

22. Rao NA and Font RL: Plasmacytic conjunctivitis with crystalline inclusions: immunohistochemical and ultrastructural studies, Arch Ophthalmol 98:836, 1980.

23. Reeh M: Treatment of lid and epibulbar tumors, Springfield, Il, 1963, Charles C Thomas, Publisher.

24. Sacks EH and others: Lymphocytic subpopulations in the normal human conjunctiva: a monoclonal antibody study, Ophthalmology 93:1276, 1986.

25. Sigelman J and Jakobiec FA: Lymphoid lesions of the conjunctiva: relation of histopathology to clinical outcome, Ophthalmology 85:818, 1978.

26. Sisler HA, Labay GR, and Finlay JR: Senile ectropion and entropion: a comparative histopathological study, Ann Ophthalmol 8:319, 1976.

27. Spinak M: Cytological changes of the conjunctiva in immunoglobulin-producing dyscrasias, Ophthalmology 88:1207, 1981.

28. Steiglitz LN and Crawford JS: Blepharochalasism, Am J Ophthalmol 77:100, 1974.

29. Wulc AE, Dryden RM, and Khatchaturian T: Where is the gray line? Arch Ophthalmol 105:1092, 1987.

30. Yanoff M and Fine BS: Ocular pathology, A color atlas, ed 2 New York, 1996, Gower Medical Publishing.

Conjunctiva

Corneal and conjunctival dermoids and cysts

31. Benjamin SN and Allen HF: Classification for limbal dermoid choristomas and brachial arch anomalies, presentation of an unusual case, Arch Ophthalmol 87:305, 1972.

32. Ellis FJ and others: Phakomatous choristoma (Zimmerman's tumor) immunohistochemical confirmation of lens-specific proteins, Ophthalmology 100:955, 1993.

33. Ferry AP and Hein HF: Epibulbar osseous choristoma within an epibulbar dermoid, Am J Ophthalmol 70:764, 1970.

34. Henkind P and others: Bilateral corneal dermoids, Am J Ophthalmol 76:972, 1973.

35. Jakobiec FA, Bonanno PA, and Sigelman J: Conjunctival adnexal cysts and dermoids, Arch Ophthalmol 96:1404, 1978.

36. Lucarelli MJ and others: Complex choristoma, Arch Ophthalmol 114:498, 1996.

37. Mandelcorn MS, Merin S, and Cardarelli J: Goldenhar's syndrome and phocomelia: case report and etiologic considerations, Am J Ophthalmol 72:618, 1971.

38. Mansour AM and others: Ocular choristomas, Surv Ophthalmol 33:339, 1989 (review).

39. Srinivasan BD and others: Epibulbar mucogenic subconjunctival cysts, Arch Ophthalmol 96:857, 1978.

40. Sugar HS: The oculoauriculovertebral dysplasia syndrome of Goldenhar, Am J Ophthalmol 62:678, 1966.

41. Young TL and others: Respiratory epithelium in a cystic choristoma of the limbus, Arch Ophthalmol 108:1736, 1990.

42. Zaidman GW, Johnson B, and Brown SI: Corneal transplantation in an infant with corneal dermoid, Am J Ophthalmol 93:78, 1982.

Inflammatory conditions

43. Abuelasrar AM and others: An immunohistochemical study of topical cyclosporine in vernal keratoconjunctivitis, Am J Ophthalmol 121:156, 1996.

44. Agrawal S, Sharma KD, and Shrivastava JB: Generalized rhinosporidiosis with visceral involvement, Arch Dermatol 80:22, 1959.

45. Allansmith MR: The eye and immunology, St Louis, 1982, CV Mosby Co.

46. Allansmith MR, Greiner JV, and Baird RS: Number of inflammatory cells in the normal conjunctiva, Am J Ophthalmol 86:250, 1978.

47. Al-Rajhi AA and others: The histopathology and the mechanism of entropion in patients with trachoma, Ophthalmology 100:1293, 1993.

48. Apple DJ: Papillome der Conjunctive debingt durch *Rhinosporidium seeberi*. Fortschr Ophthalmol 79:571, 1983.

49. Apple DJ and Natchiar G: The life cycle of *Rhinosporidium seeberi*: an ultrastructural analysis, Lab Invest 32:442, 1975.

50. Asdourian GK, Goldberg MF, and Busse BJ: Peripheral retinal neovascularization in sarcoidosis, Arch Ophthalmol 93:787, 1975.

51. Ashton N and Cook C: Allergic granulomatous nodules of the eyelid and conjunctiva: the XXXV Edward Jackson Memorial Lecture, Am J Ophthalmol 87:1, 1978.

52. Ashton N and Cook C: The XXXV Edward Jackson Memorial Lecture: allergic granulomatous nodules of the eyelid and conjunctiva, Ophthalmology 86:8, 1979.

53. Beigelman MN: Vernal conjunctivitis, Los Angeles, 1950, University of Southern California Press.

54. Bialasiewicz AA and Joahn GJ: Evaluation of diagnostic tools for adult chlamydial keratoconjunctivitis, Ophthalmology 94:532, 1987.

55. Bobo L and others: Diagnosis of chlamydia trachomatis eye infection in Tanzania by polymerase chain reaction/enzyme immunoassay, Lancet 338:847, 1991.

56. Bonini S and others: Estrogen and progesterone receptors in vernal keratoconjunctivitis, Ophthalmology 102:1374, 1995.

57. Butrus SI and others: Vernal conjunctivitis in the hyperimmunoglobulinemia E syndrome, Ophthalmology 91:1213, 1984.

58. Cameron JA, Al-Rajhi AA, and Badr IA: Corneal ectasia in vernal keratoconjunctivitis, Ophthalmology 96:1615, 1989.

59. Cameron ME and Greer H: Allergic conjunctival granulomas, Br J Ophthalmol 64:494, 1980.

60. Chang SW, Hou PK, and Chen MS: Conjunctival concretions, Arch Ophthalmol 108:405, 1990.

61. Chumbley LC and Kearns TP: Retinopathy of sarcoidosis, Am J Ophthalmol 73:123, 1972.

62. Cohen KL, Peiffer RL Jr, and Powell DA: Sarcoidosis and ocular disease in a young child, Arch Ophthalmol 99:422, 1981.

63. Conference on Trachoma and Allied Diseases, Am J Ophthalmol 63:1027, 1967.

64. Ellis JH and others: Lymphoid tumors of the ocular adnexa: clinical correlation with the working formulation classification and immunoperoxidase staining of paraffin sections, Ophthalmology 92:1311, 1985.

65. Friedlaender MH: Immunologic aspects of diseases of the eye, JAMA 268:2869, 1992.

66. Fulton A, Jampol L, and Albert DM: Gastrointestinal sarcoidosis diagnosed by conjunctival biopsy, Am J Ophthalmol 82:102, 1976.

67. Gass JDM and Olson CL: Sarcoidosis with optic nerve and retinal involvement, Arch Ophthalmol 94:941, 1976.

68. Gilbert WR, Smith JL, and Nylan WL: The Sjögren-Larsson syndrome, Arch Ophthalmol 80:308, 1968.

69. Greiner JV, Covington HI, and Allansmith MR: Surface morphology of giant papillary conjunctivitis in contact lens wearers, Am J Ophthalmol 85:242, 1978.

70. Heerfordt CF: Ueber eine Febris uveo-parotidea subchronica an der Glandula parotis und der Uvea des Auges lokalisiert und haüfig mit Paresen cerebrospinaler Nerven kompliziert, Arch Ophthalmol 70:254, 1909.

71. Henriquez AS, Kenyon KR, and Allansmith MR: Mast cell ultrastructure comparison in contact lens-associated giant papillary conjunctivitis and vernal conjunctivitis, Arch Ophthalmol 99:1266, 1981.

72. Hidayat AA and Riddle PJ: Ligneous conjunctivitis: a clinicopathologic study of 17 cases, Ophthalmology 94:949, 1987.

73. Holland MJ and others: Conjunctival scarring in trachoma is associated with depressed cell-immune responses to chlamydial antigens, J Infect Dis 168:1528, 1993.

74. Jimenez JF, Young DE, and Hough AJ: Rhinosporidosis, A report of two cases from Arkansas, Am J Clin Pathol 82:611, 1984.

75. Jones BR: Changing concepts of trachoma and its control, Trans Ophthalmol Soc UK 100:25, 1980.

76. Karcioglu ZA and Brear R: Conjunctival biopsy in sarcoidosis, Am J Ophthalmol 99:68, 1985.

77. Lawson JM, David JK, and McCartney AC: Conjunctival nodule associated with the Splendore-Hoeppli phenomenon, Arch Ophthalmol 109:285, 1991.

78. Letocha C, Shields JA, and Goldberg RE: Retinal changes in sarcoidosis, Can J Ophthalmol 10:184, 1975.

79. Levy MG, Meuten DJ, and Breitschwerdt EB: Cultivation of rhinosporidium seeberi in vitro: interaction with epithelial cells, Science 234:474, 1986.

80. Lindner Le and others: Identification of chlamydia in cervical smears by immunofluorescence, technic, sensitivity, and specificity, Am J Clin Pathol 85:180, 1986.

81. MacCallan AF: The epidemiology of trachoma, Br J Ophthalmol 15:369, 1931.

82. MacCallan AF: Trachoma, London, 1936, Butterworth & Co, Ltd.

83. Mackie IA and Wright P: Giant papillary conjunctivitis (secondary vernal) in association with contact lens wear, Trans Ophthalmol Soc UK 98:3, 1978.

84. Mansour AM and others: Bilateral total corneal and conjunctival choristomas associated with epidermal nevus, Arch Ophthalmol 104:245, 1986.

85. Naumann GO and others: Autologous nasal mucosa transplantation in severe bilateral conjunctival mucus deficiency syndrome, Ophthalmology 97:1011, 1990.

86. Obenauf CD and others: Sarcoidosis and its ophthalmic manifestations, Am J Ophthalmol 86:648, 1978.

87. Peyman GA, Sanders DR, and Goldberg MF, editors: Principles and practice of ophthalmology, Philadelphia, 1980, WB Saunders Co.

88. Pouliquen Y and others: Drug-induced cicatricial pemphigoid affecting the conjunctiva: light and electron microscopic features, Ophthalmology 93:775, 1986.

89. Purcell JJ, Birkenkamp R, and Tsai CC: Conjunctiva lesions in periarteritis nodosa: a clinical and immunopathologic study, Arch Ophthalmol 102:736, 1984.

90. Reacher MH and others: T cells and trachoma, Ophthalmology 98:334, 1991.

91. Roy FH: Trachoma, Ann Ophthalmol 6:1167, 1974.

92. Saer JB, Karchioglu GL, and Karcioglu ZA: Incidence of granulomatous lesions in postmortem conjunctival biopsy specimens, Am J Ophthalmology 104:605, 1987.

93. Sandstrom I, Kallings I, and Melen B: Neonatal chlamydial conjunctivitis, Acta Pediatr Scand 77:207, 1988.

94. Savino DR and Margo CE: Conjunctival rhinosporidiosis, light and electron microscopic study, Ophthalmology 90:1482, 1983.

95. Schaumann J: On nature of certain peculiar corpuscles present in tissue of lymphogranulomatosis benigna, Acta Med Scand 106:239, 1941.

96. Schuman JS and others: Toxoplasmic scleritis, Ophthalmology 95:1399, 1988.

97. Sen KD: Granuloma pyogenicum of the palpebral conjunctiva, J Pediatr Ophthalmol Strabismus 19:11, 1982.

98. Sheppard JD and others: Immunodiagnosis of adult chlamydial conjunctivitis, Ophthalmology 95:434, 1988.

99. Siltzbach LE, editor: Seventh International Conference on Sarcoidosis and Other Granulomatous Disorders, Ann NY Acad Sci 278 (entire issue), 1976.

100. Sjögren H: Zur Kenntnis der Keratoconjunctivitis sicca (Keratitis Filiformes bei Hypofunktion der Tränendrüsen), Acta Ophthalmol Suppl 2:1, 1933.

101. Sjögren H and Bloch KK: Keratoconjunctivitis sicca and the Sjögren syndrome, Surv Ophthalmol 16:145, 1971.

102. Stenson S: Adult inclusion conjunctivitis, Clinical characteristics and corneal changes, Arch Ophthalmol 99:605, 1981.

103. Taylor HR and others: The epidemiology of infection in trachoma, Invest Ophthalmol Vis Sci 30:1823, 1989.

104. Toda I, Shimazaki J, and Tsubota K: Dry eye with only decreased tear break-up time is sometimes associated with allergic conjunctivitis, Ophthalmology 102:302, 1995.

105. Trocme SD and others: Eosinophil granule major basic protein deposition in corneal ulcers associated with vernal keratoconjunctivitis, Am J Ophthalmol 115:640, 1993.

106. Ullman S, Roussel TJ, and Forster RK: Gonococcal keratoconjunctivitis, Surv Ophthalmol 32:199, 1987.

107. Ullman S and others: *Neisseria gonorrhoeae* keratoconjunctivitis, Ophthalmology 94:525, 1987.

108. Walsh FB: Ocular importance of sarcoid: its relation to uveoparotid fever, Arch Ophthalmol 21:421, 1939.

109. Wilhelmus KR and others: Conjunctival cytology of adult chlamydial conjunctivitis, Arch Ophthalmol 104:691, 1986.

110. Woods AC: Sarcoidosis: the systemic and ocular manifestations, Trans Am Acad Ophthalmol Otolaryngol 53:333, 1949.

Mucocutaneous eruptions

111. Anderson SR and others: Benign mucous membrane pemphigoid. III. Biopsy, Acta Ophthalmol 52:282, 1974.

112. Arstikaitis MJ: Ocular aftermath of Stevens-Johnson syndrome: review of 33 cases, Arch Ophthalmol 90:376, 1973.

113. Bernauer W and others: The conjunctiva in acute and chronic mucous membrane pemphigoid, An immunohistochemical analysis, Ophthalmology 100:339, 1993.

114. Carroll JM and Kuwabara T: Ocular pemphigus: an electron microscopic study of the conjunctival and corneal epithelium, Arch Ophthalmol 80:683, 1968.

115. Chan LS and others: Ocular cicatricial pemphigoid occurring as a sequela of Stevens-Johnson syndrome, JAMA 266:1543, 1991.

116. Chan LS and others: Immune-mediated subepithelial blistering diseases of mucous membranes, pure ocular cicatricial pemphigoid is a unique clinical and immunopathological entity distinct from bullous pemphigoid and others subsets identified by antigenic specificity of autoantibodies, Arch Dermatol 129:448, 1993.

117. Church RE and Sneddon IB: Ocular pemphigus, Br J Dermatol 70:361, 1958.

118. Custodis E: Die essentielle Bindehautschrumpfund des menschlichen Auges, Arch Ophthalmol 137:364, 1937.

119. Foster CS and Allansmith MR: Chronic unilateral blepharoconjunctivitis caused by sebaceous carcinoma, Am J Ophthalmol 86:218, 1978.

120. Foster CS: Cicatricial pemphigoid, Trans Am Ophthalmol Soc 84:527, 1986.

121. Foster SC and others: Episodic conjunctival inflammation after Steven's-Johnson syndrome, Ophthalmology 95:453, 1988.

122. Foster CS, Shaw CD, and Wells PA: Scanning electron microscopy of conjunctival surfaces in patients with ocular cicatricial pemphigoid, Am J Ophthalmol 102:584, 1986.

123. Foster CS and others: Episodic conjunctival inflammation after Stevens-Johnson syndrome, Ophthalmology 95:453, 1988.

124. Glasson WJ and others: Invasive squamous cell carcinoma of the conjunctiva, Arch Ophthalmol 112:1342, 1994.

125. Hood CI: Essential shrinkage of conjunctiva, chronic cicatrizing conjunctivitis, and benign mucous membrane pemphigoid, Invest Ophthalmol 12:308, 1973.

126. Howard GM: The Stevens-Johnson syndrome, Am J Ophthalmol 55:893, 1963.

127. Jakobiec FA and others: Dacryoadenoma: A unique tumor of the conjunctival epithelium, Ophthalmology 96:1014, 1989.

128. Lam S and others: Paraneoplastic pemphigus, cicatricial conjunctivitis, and acanthosis nigricans with pachydermatoglyphy in a patient with bronchogenic squamous cell carcinoma, Ophthalmology 99:108, 1992.

129. Lever WF: Pemphigus: histopathologic study, Arch Dermatol 64:727, 1951.

130. MacVicar DN and Graham JH: Localized chronic pemphigoid: clinicopathologic and histochemical study, Am J Pathol 48:52, 1966.

131. Mondino BJ and Brown SI: Ocular cicatricial pemphigoid, Ophthalmol 88:95, 1981.

132. Mondino BJ and others: Autoimmune phenomena in ocular cicatricial pemphigoid, Am J Ophthalmol 83:443, 1977.

133. Pouliquen Y and others: Drug-induced cicatricial pemphigoid affecting the conjunctiva, Light and electron microscopic features, Ophthalmology 93:775, 1986.

134. Power WJ: Increasing the diagnostic yield conjunctival biopsy in patients with suspected ocular cicatricial pemphigoid, Ophthalmology 102:1158, 1995.

135. Rice BA and Foster CS: Immunopathology of cicatricial pemphigoid affecting the conjunctiva, Ophthalmology 97:1476, 1990.

136. Rice BA and Foster CS: Immunopathology of cicatricial pemphigoid affecting the conjunctiva, Ophthalmology 97:1476, 1990.

137. Roat MI and others: Hyperproliferation of conjunctival fibroblasts

from patients with cicatricial pemphigoid, Arch Ophthalmol 107: 1064, 1989.
138. Rook A and Waddington E: Pemphigus and pemphigoid, Br J Dermatol 65:425, 1953.
139. Sacks EH and others: Immunophenotypic analysis of the inflammatory infiltrate in ocular cicatricial pemphigoid: further evidence for a T cell–mediated disease, Ophthalmology 96:236, 1989.
140. Tauber J, Melamed S, and Foster CS: Glaucoma in patients with ocular cicatricial pemphigoid, Ophthalmology 96:33, 1989.

Environmental degenerations

141. Ahmad A and others: Climatic droplet keratopathy in a 16-year-old boy, Arch Ophthalmol 95:149, 1977.
142. Austin P, Jakobiec FA, and Iwamoto T: Elastodysplasia and elastodystrophy as the pathologic bases of ocular pterygia and pinguecula, Ophthalmology 90:96, 1983.
143. Brownstein S and others: The elastotic nature of hyaline corneal deposits: a histochemical, fluorescent and electron microscopic examination, Am J Ophthalmol 75:799, 1973.
144. Christensen GR: Proteinaceous corneal degeneration: A histochemical study, Arch Ophthalmol 89:30, 1973.
145. Clear AS, Chirambo MC, and Hutt MRS: Solar keratosis, pterygium and squamous cell carcinoma of the conjunctiva in Malawi, Br J Ophthalmol 63:102, 1979.
146. Cogan DG, Kuwabara T, and Howard J: The nonelastic nature of pingueculas, Arch Ophthalmol 61:388, 1959.
147. Fraunfelder FT and Hanna C: Spheroidal degeneration of cornea and conjunctiva. 3. Incidences, classification, and etiology, Am J Ophthalmol 76:41, 1973.
148. Fuchs E: Zur Anatomie der Pinguecula, Arch Ophthalmol 37:143, 1891.
149. Garner A, Morgan G, and Tripathi RC: Climatic droplet keratopathy. II. Pathologic findings, Arch Ophthalmol 89:198, 1973.
150. Hilgers J: Pterygium: its incidence, heredity, and etiology, Am J Ophthalmol 50:635, 1960.
151. Hogan MJ and Alvarado J: Pterygium and pinguecula: electron microscopic study, Arch Ophthalmol 78:174, 1967.
152. Jwamoto T, DeVoe AG, and Farris RL: Electron microscopy in cases of marginal degeneration of the cornea, Invest Ophthalmol 14:241, 1972.
153. Klintworth GK: Chronic actinic keratopathy: a condition associated with conjunctival elastosis (pingueculae) and typified by characteristic extracellular concretions, Am J Pathol 67:327, 1972.
154. Levine RA and Rabb MF: Bitot's spot overlying a pinguecula, Arch Ophthalmol 86:525, 1971.
155. Li ZY and others: Elastic fiber components and protease inhibitors in pinguecula, Invest Ophthalmol Vis Sci 32:1573, 1991.
156. Lund HZ and Sommerville RL: Basophilic degeneration of the cutis: data substantiating its relation to prolonged solar exposure, Am J Clin Pathol 27:183, 1957.
157. Rodrigues MM, Laibson PR, and Weinreb S: Corneal elastosis, appearance of band-like keratopathy and spheroidal degeneration, Arch Ophthalmol 93:111, 1975.
158. Schöninger L: Über Pterygium, Klin Monatsbl Augenheilkd 77:805, 1936.
159. Taylor HR: Aetiology of climatic droplet keratopathy and pterygium, Br J Ophthalmol 64:154, 1980.

Papillomas, proliferative lesions, and nonpigmented tumors

160. Ash JE and Wilder HC: Epithelial tumors of the limbus, Trans Am Acad Ophthalmol Otolaryngol 46:215, 1942.
161. Bech K and Jensen OA: External ocular tumors, Eastbourne, England, 1978, Holt-Saunders, Ltd.
162. Biggs SL and Font RL: Oncocytic lesions of the caruncle and other ocular adnexa, Arch Ophthalmol 95:474, 1977.
163. Blodi FC: Squamous cell carcinoma of the conjunctiva, Doc Ophthalmol 34:93, 1973.
164. Brownstein S: Mucoepidermoid carcinoma of the conjunctiva with intraocular invasion, Ophthalmology 88:1226, 1984.
165. Buuns DR, Tse DT, and Folberg R: Microscopically controlled excision of conjunctival squamous cells carcinoma, Am J Ophthalmol 117:97, 1994.
166. Cameron JD and Wick MR: Embryonal rhabdomyosarcoma of the conjunctiva: a clinicopathologic and immunohistochemical study, Arch Ophthalmol 104:1203, 1986.
167. Cameron JA and Hidayat AA: Squamous cell carcinoma of the cornea, Am J Ophthalmol 111:571, 1991.
168. Carroll JM and Kuwabara T: A classification of limbal epitheliomas, Arch Ophthalmol 73:545, 1965.
169. Char DH: The management of lid and conjunctival malignancies, Surv Ophthalmol 24:679, 1980.
170. Cohen BH and others: Spindle cell carcinoma of the conjunctiva, Arch Ophthalmol 98:1809, 1980.
171. Dark AJ and Streeten BW: Preinvasive carcinoma of the cornea and conjunctiva, Br J Ophthalmol 64:506, 1980.
172. Divine RD and Anderson RL: Nitrous oxide cryotherapy for intraepithelial epithelioma of the conjunctiva, Arch Ophthalmol 104:782, 1983.
173. Elsas FJ and Green WR: Epibulbar tumors in childhood, Am J Ophthalmol 79:1001, 1975.
174. Erie JC, Campbell RJ, and Liesegang TJ: Conjunctival and corneal intraepithelial and invasive neoplasia, Ophthalmology 93:176, 1986.
175. Font RL, Mackay B, and Tang R: Acute monocytic leukemia recurring as bilateral perilimbal infiltrates: immunohistochemical and ultrastructural confirmation, Ophthalmology 92:1681, 1985.
176. Fraunfelder FT and Wingfield D: Management of intraepithelial conjunctival tumors and squamous cell carcinoma, Am J Ophthalmol 95:359, 1983.
177. Fraunfelder FT and others: Results of cryotherapy for eyelid malignancies, Am J Ophthalmol 97:184, 1984.
178. Freedman J and Röhm G: Surgical management and histopathology of invasive tumours of the cornea, Br J Ophthalmol 63:632, 1979.
179. Gamel JW, Eiferman RA, and Guibor P: Mucoepidermoid carcinoma of the conjunctiva, Arch Ophthalmol 102:730, 1984.
180. Glass AG and Hoover RN: The emerging epidemic of melanoma and squamous cell skin cancer, JAMA 262, 2097, 1989.
181. Glasson WJ and others: Invasive squamous cell carcinoma of the conjunctiva, Arch Ophthalmol 112:1342, 1994.
182. Grossniklas HE and others: Hemangiopericytoma of the conjunctiva: two cases, Ophthalmology 93:265, 1986.
183. Grossniklaus HE and others: Conjunctival lesions in adults, A clinical and histopathologic review, Cornea 6:78, 1987.
184. Huntington AC, Langloss JM, and Hidayat AA: Spindle cell carcinoma of the conjunctiva, Ophthalmology 97:711, 1990.
185. Husain SE and others: Primary basal cell carcinoma of the limbal conjunctiva, Ophthalmology 100:1720, 1993.
186. Irvine AR Jr: Epibulbar squamous cell carcinoma and related lesions, Int Ophthalmol Clin 12(1):71, 1972.
187. Jakobiec FA, Iwamoto T, and Knowles DM II: Ocular adnexal lymphoid tumors, Arch Ophthalmol 100:84, 1982.
188. Jakobiec FA, Harrison W, and Aronian D: Inverted mucoepidermoid papillomas of the epibulbar conjunctiva, Ophthalmology 94: 283, 1987.
189. Karp CL and others: Conjunctival intraepithelial neoplasia—a possible marker for human immunodeficiency virus infection, Arch Ophthalmol 114:257, 1996.
190. Knowles DM, Jakobiec FA, and Halper JP: Immunologic characterization of ocular adnexal lymphoid neoplasms, Am J Ophthalmol 87: 603, 1979.
191. Kohn R, Nofsinger K, and Freedman SI: Rapid recurrence of papillary squamous cell carcinoma of the canaliculus, Am J Ophthalmol 92:363, 1981.
192. Lahoud S, Brownstein S, and Laflamme MY: Fibrous histiocytoma of the corneoscleral limbus and conjunctiva. Am J Ophthalmol 106: 579, 1988.
193. Lauer SA, Malter JS, and Meier JR: Human papillomavirus type 18 in conjunctival intraepithelial neoplasia, Am J Ophthalmol 110:23, 1990.
194. Lass JH and others: Papillomavirus in human conjunctival papillomas, Am J Ophthalmol 95:364, 1983.
195. Lee GA, Williams G, and Hirst LW: Risk factors in the development of ocular surface epithelial dysplasia, Ophthalmology 101:360, 1994.
196. Lee GA and Hirst LW: Ocular surface squamous neoplasia, Surv Ophthalmol 39:429, 1995.
197. Lewallen S and others: Aggressive conjunctival squamous cell carcinoma in three young African, Arch Ophthalmol 114:215, 1996.
198. Li WW, Pettit TH, and Zakka KA: Intraocular invasion by papillary squamous cell carcinoma of the conjunctiva, Am J Ophthalmol 90: 697, 1980.
199. Lindenmuth KA and others: Invasive squamous cell carcinoma of

the conjunctiva presenting as necrotizing scleritis with scleral perforation and uveal prolapse, Surv Ophthalmol 33:50, 1988.

200. Lommatzsch P: Beta-ray treatment of malignant epithelial tumors of the conjunctiva, Am J Ophthalmol 81:198, 1976.

201. Maclean H, Dhillon B, and Ironside J: Squamous cell carcinoma of the eyelid and the acquired immunodeficiency syndrome, Am J Ophthalmol 121:219, 1996.

202. Margo CE and Groden LR: Intraepithelial neoplasia of the conjunctiva with mucoepidermoid differentiation, Am J Ophthalmol 600, 1989.

203. Margo CE and Weitzenkorn DE: Mucoepidermoid carcinoma of the conjunctiva: report of a case in a 36 year-old with paranasal sinus invasion, Ophthalmic Surg 17:151, 1986.

204. Margo CE, Mack W, and Guffey JM: Squamous cell carcinoma of the conjunctiva and human immunodeficiency virus infection, Am J Ophthalmol 114:349, 1996.

205. McDonnell JM, Mayr AJ, and Martin WJ: DNA of human papillomavirus type 16 dysplastic and malignant lesions of the conjunctiva and cornea, N Engl J Med 320:1442, 1989.

206. McDonnell JM and others: Demonstration of papillomavirus capsid antigen in human conjunctival neoplasia, Arch Ophthalmol, 104:1801, 1986.

207. McDonnell JM, McDonnell PJ, and Sun YY: Human papillomavirus DNA in tissues and ocular surface swabs of patients with conjunctival epithelial neoplasia, Arch Ophthalmol 33:184, 1992.

208. McGavic JS: Intraepithelial epithelioma of cornea and conjunctiva (Bowen's disease), Am J Ophthalmol 25:167, 1942.

209. Morgan G and Harry J: Lymphocytic tumours of indeterminate nature: a 5 year follow-up of 98 conjunctival and orbital lesions, Br J Ophthalmol 62:381, 1978.

210. Morsman DC: Spontaneous regression of a conjunctival intraepithelial neoplastic tumor, Arch Ophthalmol 107:1490, 1989.

211. Munro S, Brownstein S, and Liddy B: Conjunctival keratoacanthoma, Am J Ophthalmol 116:654, 1993.

212. Muccioli C and others: Squamous cell carcinoma of the conjunctiva in a patient with acquired immunodeficiency syndrome, Am J Ophthalmol 121:94, 1996.

213. Nicholson DH and Herschler J: Intraocular extension of squamous cell carcinoma of the conjunctiva, Arch Ophthalmol 95:843, 1977.

214. Odrich MG and others: A spectrum of bilateral squamous conjunctival tumor associated with human papillomavirus type 16, Ophthalmology 98:628, 1991.

215. Ortiz JM and Yanoff M: Epipalpebral conjunctival osseous choristoma, Br J Ophthalmol 63:173, 1979.

216. Quillen DA and others: Basal cell carcinoma of the conjunctiva, Am J Ophthalmol 116:244, 1993.

217. Rennie IG: Oncocytomas (oxyphil adenomas) of the lacrimal caruncle, Br J Ophthalmol 64:935, 1980.

218. Salisbury JA, Szpak CA, and Klintworth GK: Pigmented squamous cell carcinoma of the conjunctiva, a clinicopathologic ultrastructural study, Ophthalmology 90:1477, 1983.

219. Searl SS and others: Invasive squamous cell carcinoma with intraocular mucoepidermoid features: conjunctival carcinoma with intraocular invasion and diphasic morphology, Arch Ophthalmol 100:109, 1982.

220. Seddon JM and others: Solitary extramedullary plasmacytoma of the palpebral conjunctiva, Br J Ophthalmol 66:450, 1982.

221. Streeten BW and others: Inverted papilloma of the conjunctiva, Am J Ophthalmol 88:1062, 1979.

222. Tabbara KF and others: Metastatic squamous cell carcinoma of the conjunctiva, Ophthalmology 95:318, 1988.

223. Urdiales-Viedma M, Moreno-Prieto M, and Martos-Padilla S: Pleomorphic fibrous histiocytoma of the corneoscleral limbus, Am J Ophthalmol 95:560, 1983.

224. Waring GO III, Roth AM, and Ekins MB: Clinical and pathologic description of 17 cases of corneal intraepithelial neoplasia, Am J Ophthalmol 97:547, 1984.

225. Weiter JJ, Jakobiec FA, and Iwamoto T: The clinical and morphologic characteristics of Kaposi's sarcoma of the conjunctiva, Am J Ophthalmol 89:546, 1980.

226. Wexler SA and Wallow IHL: Squamous cell carcinoma of the conjunctiva presenting with intraocular extension, Arch Ophthalmol 103:1175, 1985.

227. Wright P, Collin RJO, and Garner A: The masquerade syndrome, Trans Ophthalmol Soc UK 104:244, 1981.

228. Yeatts RP and others: Topical 5-fluorouracil in treating epithelial neoplasia of the conjunctiva and cornea, Ophthalmology 102:1338, 1995.

Pigmented tumors

229. Abramson DH, Rodriguez-Sains RS, and Rubmaa R: B-K mole syndrome: cutaneous and ocular malignant melanoma, Arch Ophthalmol 98:1397, 1980.

230. Bernardino VB, Naidoff MA, and Clark WH: Malignant melanomas of the conjunctiva, Am J Ophthalmol 82:383, 1976.

231. Blicker JA, Rootman J, and White VA: Cellular blue nevus of the conjunctiva, Ophthalmology 99:1714, 1992.

232. Blodi FC and Widner RR: The melanoma freckle (Hutchinson) of the lids, Surv Ophthalmol 13:23, 1968.

233. Brownstein S and others: Cryotherapy for precancerous melanosis (atypical melanocytic hyperplasia) of the conjunctiva, Arch Ophthalmol 99:1224, 1981.

234. Buckman G and others: Melanocytic nevi of the palpebral conjunctiva: an extremely rare location usually signifying melanoma, Ophthalmology 95:1053, 1988.

235. Charles NC, Stenson, and Taterka HB: Epibulbar malignant melanoma in a black patient, Arch Ophthalmol 97:316, 1979.

236. Crawford JB: Conjunctival melanomas: prognostic factors—a review and an analysis of a series, Trans Am Ophthalmol Soc 78:467, 1980.

237. Croxatto JO and others: Malignant melanoma of the conjunctiva: report of a case, Ophthalmology 94:1281, 1987.

238. Dhermy P and Barry R: Naevus naevocellulaire à cellules ballonnisantes de la conjunctiva: à propos de trois nouveaux eas, Arch Ophthalmol (Paris) 34:303, 1974.

239. Elsas FJ, Green WR, and Ryan SJ: Benign pigmented tumors arising in acquired conjunctival melanosis, Am J Ophthalmol 78:229, 1974.

240. Folberg R, McLean IW, and Zimmerman LE: Conjunctival melanosis and melanoma, Ophthalmology 91:673, 1984.

241. Folberg R and others: Benign conjunctival melanocytic lesions: clinicopathologic features, Ophthalmology 96:436, 1989.

242. Folberg R, McLean IW, and Zimmerman LE: Primary acquired melanosis of the conjunctiva, Hum Pathol 16:129, 1985.

243. Folberg R, McLean IW, and Zimmerman LE: Conjunctival malignant melanoma, Hum Pathol 16:136, 1985.

244. Glasgow BJ, McCall LC, and Foos RY: HMB-45 antibody reactivity in pigmented lesions of the conjunctiva, Am J Ophthalmol 109:696, 1990.

245. Gonder JR and others: Bilateral ocular melanocytosis with malignant melanoma of the choroid, Br J Ophthalmol 65:843, 1981.

246. Gonder JR and others: Ocular melanocytosis: a study to determine the prevalence rate of ocular melanocytosis, Ophthalmology 89:950, 1982.

247. Gonder JR and others: Uveal malignant melanoma associated with ocular and oculodermal melanocytosis, Ophthalmology 89:953, 1982.

248. Gow JA and Spencer WH: Intraocular extension of an epibulbar malignant melanoma, Arch Ophthalmol 90:57, 1973.

249. Henkind P and Benjamin JV: Conjunctival melanocytic lesions: natural history, Trans Ophthalmol Soc UK 97:373, 1977.

250. Henkind P and Friedman AH: External ocular pigmentation, Int Ophthalmol Clin 11:87, 1971.

251. Jakobiec FA: The ultrastructure of conjunctival melanocytic tumors, Trans Am Ophthalmol Soc 82:599, 1984.

252. Jakobiec FA, Folberg R, and Iwamoto T: Clinicopathologic characteristics of premalignant and malignant melanocytic lesions of the conjunctiva, Ophthalmology 96:147, 1989.

253. Jakobiec FA and Iwamoto T: Cryotherapy for intraepithelial conjunctival melanocytic proliferations: ultrastructural effects, Arch Ophthalmol 101:904, 1983.

254. Jakobiec FA and others: Adjuvant cryotherapy for focal nodular melanoma of the conjunctiva, Arch Ophthalmol 100:115, 1982.

255. Jakobiec FA and others: The role of cryotherapy in the management of conjunctival melanoma, Ophthalmology 89:502, 1982.

256. Jakobiec FA and others: Unusual melanocytic nevi of the conjunctiva, Am J Ophthalmol 100:100, 1985.

257. Jakobiec FA and others: Metastatic melanoma within and to the conjunctiva, Ophthalmology 96:999, 1989.

258. Jay B: Naevi and melanomata of the conjunctiva, Br J Ophthalmol 49:169, 1965.

259. Jeffrey IJM and others: Malignant melanomas of the conjunctiva, Histopathology 10:363, 1986.

260. King W and others: Neurofibromatosis and neural crest neoplasms: Primary acquired melanosis and malignant melanoma of the conjunctiva, Surv Ophthalmol 33:373, 1989.

261. Ko KW and others: Malignant melanomas of the conjunctiva, Histopathology 10:363, 1986.

262. Leisegang TJ and Campbell RJ: Mayo Clinic experience with conjunctival melanomas, Arch Ophthalmol 98:1385, 1980.

263. Lewis PM and Zimmerman LE: Delayed recurrences of malignant melanomas of the bulbar conjunctiva, Am J Ophthalmol 45:536, 1958.

264. Lomnnatzsch PK: Beta irradiation of conjunctival melanomas, Trans Ophthalmol Soc UK 97:378, 1977.

265. Margo CE: Conjunctival melanoma with balloon cell transformation, Arch Ophthalmol 106:1653, 1988.

266. McCarthy JM and others: Conjunctival and uveal melanoma in the dysplastic nevus syndrome, Surv Ophthalmol 37:377, 1993.

267. McDonnell JM and others: Conjunctival melanocytic lesions in children, Ophthalmology 96:986, 1989.

268. McDonnell JM, Sun YY, and Wagner D: HMB-45 Immunohistochemical staining of conjunctival melanocytic lesions, Ophthalmology 98:453, 1991.

269. Morris DA and others: Recurrent conjunctival melanoma with neuroidal spindle cell features, Ophthalmology 94:56, 1987.

270. Naidoff MA, Bernardino VB, and Clark WH: Melanocytic lesions of the eyelid skin, Am J Ophthalmol 82:371, 1976.

271. Paridaens ADA and others: Prognostic factors in primary malignant melanoma of the conjunctiva, A clinicopathological study of 256 cases, Br J Ophthalmol 78:252, 1994.

272. Puk De and others: Conjunctival malignant melanoma, Arch Ophthalmol 114:100, 1996.

273. Reese AB: Precancerous and cancerous melanosis of conjunctiva, Am J Ophthalmol 39:96, 1955.

274. Reese AB: Precancerous and cancerous melanosis, Am J Ophthalmol 61:1272, 1966.

275. Robertson DM, Hungerford JL, and McCartney A: Malignant melanomas of the conjunctiva, nasal cavity, and paranasal sinuses, Am J Ophthalmol 108:440, 1989.

276. Robertson DM, Hungerford JL, and McCartney A: Pigmentation of the eyelid margin accompanying conjunctival melanoma, Am J Ophthalmol 108:435, 1989.

277. Saornil MA and others: Nucleolar organizer regions in determining malignancy of pigmented conjunctival lesions, Am J Ophthalmol 115:800, 1993.

278. Sekundo W and others: Hemangiopericytoma of the inner canthus, Am J Ophthalmol 121:445, 1996.

279. Seregard S: Cell proliferation as a prognostic indicator in conjunctival malignant melanoma, Am J Ophthalmol 116:93, 1993.

280. Saornil MA and others: Nucleolar organizer regions in determining malignancy of pigmented conjunctival lesions, Am J Ophthalmology 115:800, 1993.

281. Scott KR, Jakobiec FA, and Font RL: Peripunctal melanocytic nevi, Distinctive clinical findings and differential diagnosis, Ophthalmology 96:994, 1989.

282. Seregard S and others: Prevalence of primary acquired melanosis and nevi of the conjunctiva and uvea in the dysplastic nevus syndrome-a case-control study, Ophthalmology 102:1524, 1995.

283. Wilkes TDI and others: Malignant melanoma of the orbit in a black patient with ocular melanocytosis, Arch Ophthalmol 102:904, 1984.

284. Zimmerman LE: Criteria for management of melanosis, Arch Ophthalmol 76:307, 1966 (letter to the editor).

Eyelids

Benign lesions

285. Allington HV and Allington JH: Eyelid tumors, Arch Dermatol 97:50, 1968.

286. Aurora AL and Blodi FC: Lesions of the eyelids: a clinicopathological study, Surv Ophthalmol 15:94, 1970.

287. Aurora AL and Blodi FC: Benign epithelial cysts of the eyelids, In Blodi FC: Current concepts in ophthalmology, vol III, St Louis, 1972, The CV Mosby Co.

288. Bartley GB: Blastomycosis of the eyelid, Ophthalmology 102:2020, 1995.

289. Blackman HJ, Rodriguez MM, and Peck GL: Corneal epithelial lesions in keratosis follicularis (Darier's disease), Ophthalmology 87:931, 1980.

290. Blodi FC and Widner RR: The melanotic freckle (Hutchinson) of the lids, Surv Ophthalmol 13:23, 1968.

291. Cohen KL, Peiffer RL, and Lipper S: Mucinous sweat gland adenocarcinoma of the eyelid, Am J Ophthalmol 92:183, 1981.

292. Depot MJ and others: Bilateral and extensive xanthelasma palpebrarum in a young man, Ophthalmology 91:522, 1984.

293. Doxanas MT and others: Lid lesions of childhood: a histopathologic survey at the Wilmer Institute, J Pediatr Ophthalmol 13:7, 1976.

294. Ellis FJ and others: Phakomatous choristoma (Zimmerman's tumor), Ophthalmology 100:955, 1993.

295. Eustis HS and others: Phakomatous choristoma: clinical histopathologic and ultrastructural findings in a 4-month-old-boy, J Ped Ophthalmol Strab 27:208, 1990.

296. Font RI and others: Apocrine hidrocystomas of the lids, hypodontia, palmar-plantar hyperkeratosis, and onychodystrophy, a new variant of ectodermal dysplasia, Arch Ophthalmol 104:1811, 1986.

297. Gordon AJ and others: Complex choristoma of the eyelid containing ectopic cilia and lacrimal gland, Ophthalmology 98:1547, 1991.

298. Gordon AJ and others: Complex choristoma of the eyelid containing ectopic cilia and lacrimal gland, Ophthalmology 98:1547, 1991.

299. Graham JH, Johnson WC, and Helwig EB: Dermal pathology, New York, 1972, Harper & Row, Publishers.

300. Grossniklaus HE and Knight SH: Eccrine acrospiroma (clear cell hidradenoma) of the eyelid. Immunohistochemical and ultrastructural features, Ophthalmology 98:347, 1991.

301. Jakobiec FA and others: Primary infiltrating signet ring carcinoma of the eyelids, Ophthalmology 90:291, 1983.

302. Jakobiec FA and others: Lymphoid tumor of the lid, Ophthalmology 87:1058, 1980.

303. Kivela T and Tarkkanen A: The merkel cell and associated neoplasms in the eyelids and periocular region, Surv Ophthalmol 35:171, 1990.

304. Korting GW: The skin and the eye: a dermatologic correlation of diseases of the periorbital region, Philadelphia, 1974, WB Saunders Co (Translated by W Curth, HO Curth, FF Urbach, and DM Albert).

305. Kronish JW, Sneed SR, and Tse DT: Epidermal cysts of the eyelid, Arch Ophthalmol 106:270, 1988.

306. Leshin B and others: Management of periocular basal cell carcinoma: Moh's micrographic surgery versus radiotherapy, Surv Ophthalmol 38:193, 1993.

307. Lever WF: Histopathology of the skin, ed 5, Philadelphia, 1977, JB Lippincott Co.

308. Lisman RD, Jakobiec FA, and Small P: Sebaceous carcinoma of the eyelids, Ophthalmology 96:1021, 1989.

309. Lu LW, Bansal RK, and Katzman B: Primary congenital eversion of the upper lids, J Pediatr Ophthalmol Strabismus 16:149, 1979.

310. Lund HZ: Tumors of the skin. In Atlas of tumor pathology, section I, fascicle 2, Washington, DC, 1957, Armed Forces Institute of Pathology.

311. Lund HZ and Kraus JM: Melanotic tumors of the skin. In Atlas of tumor pathology, section 1, fascicle 3, Washington, DC, 1962, Armed Forces Institute of Pathology.

312. Lutzner MA: Molluscum contagiosum, verruca and zoster viruses: electron microscopic studies in skin, Arch Dermatol 87:436, 1963.

313. Mansour AM and Hidayat AA: Metastatic eyelid disease, Ophthalmology 94:667, 1987.

314. Middlekamp JN and Munger BL: Ultrastructure and histogenesis of molluscum contagiosum, J Pediatr 64:888, 1964.

315. Ni C and Albert DM, editors: Tumors of the eyelid and orbit: a Chinese-American collaborative study, Int Ophthalmol Clin 22(1) (entire issue), 1982.

316. Reeh MJ: Treatment of lid and epibulbar tumors, Springfield, IL, 1963, Charles C Thomas, Publisher.

317. Robinson MR and others: Molluscum contagiosum of the eyelids in patients with acquired immune deficiency syndrome, Ophthalmology 99:1745, 1992.

318. Rosenbaum PS and others: Phakomatous choristoma of the eyelid: immunohistochemical and electron microscopic observations, Ophthalmology 99:1779, 1992.

319. Sacks E and others: Multiple bilateral apocrine cystadenomas of the lower eyelids: light and electron microscopic studies, Ophthalmology 94:65, 1987.

320. Shields JA and Guibor P: Neurilemoma of the eyelid resembling a recurrent chalazion, Arch Ophthalmol 102:1650, 1984.

321. Tessler HH, Apple DJ, and Goldberg MF: Ocular findings in a kindred with Kyrle disease: hyperkeratosis follicularis et parafollicularis en cutem penetrans, Arch Ophthalmol 90:278, 1973.

322. Thall E and others: Acute monocytic leukemia presenting in the eyelid: an immunohistochemical and electron microscopic study, Ophthalmology 93:1628, 1986.

323. Thygeson P: Dermatoses with ocular manifestations. In Sorsby A, editor: Systemic ophthalmology, St Louis, 1958, CV Mosby Co.

324. Tillawi I, Katz R, and Pellettiere EV: Solitary tumors of meibomian gland origin and Torre's syndrome, Am J Ophthalmol 104:179, 1987.

325. Zimmerman LE: Phakomatous choristoma of the eyelid: a tumor of lenticular anlage, Am J Ophthalmol 71:169, 1971.

326. Zug KA, Palay DA, and Rock B: Dermatologic diagnosis and treatment of itchy red eyelids, Surv Ophthalmol 40:293, 1996 (review).

Malignant tumors; basal cell carcinoma

327. Aldred WV, Ramirez VG, and Nicholson DH: Intraocular invasion by basal cell carcinoma of the lid, Arch Ophthalmol 98:1821, 1980.

328. Aurora AL and Blodi FC: Reappraisal of basal cell carcinoma of the eyelids, Am J Ophthalmol 70:329, 1970.

329. Caya JG, Hidayat AA, and Weiner JM: A clinicopathologic study of 21 cases of adenoid squamous cell carcinoma of the eyelid and periorbital region, Am J Ophthalmol 99:291, 1985.

330. Chalfin J and Putterman AM: Frozen section control in the surgery of basal cell carcinoma of the eyelid, Am J Ophthalmol 87:802, 1979.

331. Doxanas MT, Green WR, and Iliff CE: Factors in the successful surgical management of basal cell carcinoma of the eyelids, Am J Ophthalmol 91:726, 1981.

332. Feman SS, Apt L, and Roth AM: The basal cell nevus syndrome, Am J Ophthalmol 78:222, 1974.

333. Hornblass A and Stefano JA: Pigmented basal cell carcinoma of the eyelid, Am J Ophthalmol 92:193, 1984.

334. Husain SE and others: Primary basal cell carcinoma of limbal conjunctiva, Ophthalmol 100:1720, 1993.

335. Margo CE and Waltz K: Basal cell carcinoma of the eyelid and periocular skin, Surv, Ophthalmol 38:169, 1993.

336. Margo CE and Waltz K: Basal cell carcinoma of the eyelid and periocular skin, Surv Ophthalmol 38:169, 1993.

337. Markovits AS and Quickert MH: Basal cell nevus, Arch Ophthalmol 88:397, 1972.

338. Mason JK and Helwig FB: Nevoid basal cell carcinoma syndrome, Arch Pathol 79:401, 1965.

339. Payne JW and others: Basal cell carcinoma of the eyelids: a long-term follow-up study, Arch Ophthalmol 81:553, 1969.

340. Perlman GS and Hornblass A: Basal cell carcinoma of the eyelids a review of patients treated by surgical excision, Ophthalmol Surg 7:23, 1976.

341. Resnick KI, Sadun A and Albert DM: Basal cell epithelioma: an unusual case, Ophthalmology 88:1182, 1981.

342. Schlieter F: Basal cell nevus syndrome associated with multiple skeletal, cerebral and mesenteric abnormalities: the "fifth phakomatosis," Klin Monatsbl Augenheilkd 163:184, 1973.

343. von Nover A and Korting GW: Zur Kenntnis des familiaren Basalzellnaevus, Klin Monatsbl Augenheilkd 156:621, 1970.

344. Wesley RE and Collins JW: Basal cell carcinoma of the eyelid as an indicator of multifocal malignancy, Am J Ophthalmol 94:591, 1982.

345. Wiggs EO: Morphea-form basal cell carcinomas of the canthi, Trans Am Acad Ophthalmol Otolaryngol 79:649, 1975.

Squamous epithelial proliferative and neoplastic lesions

346. Bellows RA and others: Ocular manifestations of xeroderma pigmentosum in a black family, Arch Ophthalmol 92:113, 1974.

347. Boniuk M and Zimmerman LE: Eyelid tumors with reference to lesions confused with squamous cell carcinoma. II. Inverted follicular keratosis, Arch Ophthalmol 69:698, 1963.

348. Boniuk M and Zimmerman LE: Eyelid tumors with reference to lesions confused with squamous cell carcinoma. III. Keratoacanthoma, Arch Ophthalmol 77:29, 1967.

349. Braverman IM: Bowen's disease and internal cancer, JAMA 266:842, 1991.

350. Breuninger H, Black B and Rassner G: Microstaging of squamous cell carcinomas, Am J Clin Pathol 59:306, 1973.

351. Chute CG and others: The subsequent risk of internal cancer with Bowen's disease, JAMA 266:816, 1991.

352. Doxanas MT and others: Squamous cell carcinoma of the eyelids, Ophthalmology 94:538, 1987.

353. Gaasterland DE, Rodrigues MM, and Moshell AN: Ocular involvement in xeroderma pigmentosum, Ophthalmology 89:980, 1982.

354. Hadida E, Marill FG, and Sayag J: Xeroderma pigmentosum: à propos de 48 observations personnelles, Ann Dermatol Syph 90:467, 1963.

355. Johnson MW and others: Malignant melanoma of the iris in xeroderma pigmentosum, Arch Ophthalmol 107:402, 1989.

356. Kwitko ML, Boniuk M, and Zimmerman LE: Eyelid tumors with reference to lesions confused with squamous cell carcinoma. I. Incidence and errors in diagnosis, Arch Ophthalmol 69:693, 1963.

357. McDonnell JM and others: Human papillomavirus DNA in a recurrent squamous carcinoma of the eyelid, Arch Ophthalmol 107:1631, 1989.

358. Munro S, Brownstein S, and Liddy B: Conjunctival keratoacanthoma, Am J Ophthalmol 116:654, 1993.

359. Nelson CC and Kincaid MC: Breast carcinoma metastatic to the eyelids, Arch Ophthalmol 105:1724, 1987.

360. Nerad JA and Whitaker DC: Periocular basal cell carcinoma in adults 35 years of age and younger, Am J Ophthalmol 106:723, 1988.

361. Randall MB and others: DNA content and proliferative index in cutaneous squamous cell carcinoma and keratoacanthoma, Am J Clin Pathol 93:259, 1990.

362. Reifler DM and others: Squamous cell carcinoma of the eyelid, Surv Ophthalmol 30:349, 1986.

363. Salama SD and Margo CE: Large pigmented actinic keratosis of the eyelid, Arch Ophthalmol 113:977, 1995.

364. Sassani JW and Yanoff M: Inverted follicular keratosis, Am J Ophthalmol 87:810, 1979.

365. Scheie HG, Yanoff M, and Sassani JW: Inverted follicular keratosis clinically mimicking malignant melanoma, Ann Ophthalmol 9:949, 1977.

366. Schweitzer JG and Yanoff M: Inverted follicular keratosis: a report of two recurrent cases, Ophthalmology 94:1465, 1987.

367. Spielvogel RL, Austin C, and Ackerman AB: Inverted follicular keratosis is not a specific keratosis but a verruca vulgaris (or seborrheic keratosis) with squamous eddies, Am J Dermatopathol 5:427, 1983.

368. Stenson S: Ocular findings in xeroderma pigmentosum: report of two cases, Ann Ophthalmol 14:580, 1982.

369. Stern RS, Bourdreaux KC, and Arndt KA: Diagnostic accuracy and appropriateness of care for seborrheic keratoses, JAMA 104:179, 1987.

370. Yanoff M: Most inverted follicular keratoses are probably verruca vulgaris, Am J Dermatopathol 5:475, 1983.

Sebaceous gland tumors

371. Albert DM and others: the dysplastic nevus syndrome, A pedigree with primary malignant melanomas of the choroid and skin, Ophthalmology 92:1728, 1985.

372. Boniuk M and Zimmerman LE: Sebaceous gland carcinoma of the eyelid, eyebrow, caruncle, and orbit, Tran Am Acad Ophthalmol Otolaryngol 72:619, 1968.

373. Boniuk M and Zimmerman LE: Sebaceous carcinoma of the eyelid, eyebrows, caruncle, and orbit, Int Ophthalmol Clin 12(1):225, 1972.

374. Condon GP, Brownstein S, and Codere F: Sebaceous carcinoma of the eyelid masquerading as superior limbic keratoconjunctivitis, Arch Ophthalmol 103:1525, 1985.

375. Domarus D, Hinzpeter E, and Naumann G: Klinische Fehldiagnose "Chalazion," Klin Monatsbl Augenheilkd 168:175, 1976.

376. Gutgesell VJ, Stern GA, and Hood CI: Histopathology of meibomian gland dysfunction, Am J Ophthalmol 94:383, 1982.

377. Herman DC and others: Immunohistochemical staining of sebaceous cell carcinoma of the eyelid, Am J Ophthalmol 107:127, 1989.

378. Hollwich F, Schiffer HP, and Busse H: Fehldiagnose Chalazion, Klin Monatsbl Augenheilkd 168:591, 1976.

379. Jakobiec FA: Sebaceous adenoma of the eyelid and visceral malignancy, Am J Ophthalmol 78:952, 1974.

380. Jakobeic FA and others: Primary infiltrating signet ring carcinoma of the eyelids, Ophthalmology 90:291, 1983.

381. Jakobiec FA and others: Unusual eyelid tumors with sebaceous differentiation in the Muir-Torre syndrome: rapid clinical regrowth

and frank squamous transformation after biopsy, Ophthalmology 95: 1543, 1988.

382. Kass LG and Hornblass A: Sebaceous carcinoma of the ocular adnexa, Surv Ophthalmol 33:477, 1989.

383. Khalil M and others: Eccrine sweat gland carcinoma of the eyelid with orbital involvement, Arch Ophthalmol 98:2210, 1980.

384. Margo CE and Grossniklaus He: Intraepithelial sebaceous neoplasm without underlying invasive carcinoma, Surv Ophthalmol 39:293, 1995.

385. Margo CE and Grossniklaus HE: Intraepithelial sebaceous neoplasia without underlying invasive carcinoma, Surv Ophthalmol 39:293, 1995.

386. Margo CE, Lessner A, and Stern GA: Intraepithelial sebaceous carcinoma of the conjunctiva and skin of the eyelid, Ophthalmology 99:227, 1992.

387. Maclean H, Dillion B, and Ironside J: Squamous cell carcinoma of the eyelid and the acquired immunodeficiency syndrome, Am J Ophthalmol 121:219, 1996.

388. Perlman E and McMahon RT: Sebaceous gland carcinoma of the eyelid, Am J Ophthalmol 86:699, 1978.

389. Rao NA and others: Sebaceous carcinomas of the ocular adnexa: a clinicopathologic study of 104 cases, with five-year follow-up data, Hum Pathol 13:113, 1982.

390. Rao NA and others: Bilateral carcinomas of the eyelid, Am J Ophthalmol 101:480, 1986.

391. Ross JJ, Lass JH, and Grossniklaus HE: Sebaceous gland carcinoma, Arch Ophthalmol 106:119, 1988.

392. Russell WG and others: Sebaceous carcinoma of meibomian gland origin, The diagnostic importance of pagetoid spread of neoplastic cells, Am J Clin Pathol 73:504, 1980.

393. Scheie HG, Yanoff M, and Frayer WC: Carcinoma of sebaceous glands of the eyelid, Arch Ophthalmol 72:800, 1964.

394. Schlernitzauer DA and Font RL: Sebaceous gland carcinoma of the eyelid, Arch Ophthalmol 94:1523, 1976.

395. Seregard S: Apocrine adenocarcinoma arising in moll gland cystadenoma, Ophthalmology 100:1716, 1993.

396. Straatsma BR: Meibomian gland tumors, Arch Ophthalmol 56:71, 1956.

397. Tenzel RR and others: Sebaceous adenocarcinoma of the eyelid, Arch Ophthalmol 95:2203, 1977.

398. Thomas JW, Fu YS, and Levine MR: Primary mucinous sweat gland carcinoma of the eyelid simulating metastatic carcinoma, Am J Ophthalmol 87:29, 1979.

399. Tillawai I, Katz R, and Pellettiere EV: Solitary tumors of meibomian gland origin and Torre's syndrome, Am J Ophthalmol 104:179, 1987.

400. Wagoner MD and others: Common presentations of sebaceous gland carcinoma of the eyelid, Ann Ophthalmol 14:159, 1982.

SELF-ASSESSMENT

QUESTIONS

CHAPTER 1

1. The main feature that renders the cornea (as opposed to the sclera) transparent to incoming light is:
   A. rich mucopolysaccharide content
   B. relatively thick Descemet's membrane
   C. geometric arrangement of stromal collagen lamellae and a constant state of relative dehydration of the stroma
   D. ability of the surface epithelium and overlying tear film to keep the corneal surface smooth
   E. high density of keratocyte nuclei within the stroma

2. This is a photomicrograph showing multiple cholesterol clefts that typically accumulate in the subretinal space of eyes affected with Coats' syndrome (see Chapter 9). This is classified as an exudative retinal detachment. Transudates and/or exudates often contain deposits that may stain positively with the following stains:

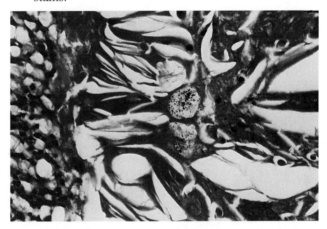

   A. periodic acid-Schiff (PAS)
   B. Oil red O
   C. eosin
   D. all of the above
   E. none of the above

3. Basement membranes in the eye include all of the following *except*:
   A. outer (external) limiting membrane of the retina
   B. Descemet's membrane
   C. Bruch's membrane
   D. lens capsule
   E. internal limiting membrane of the retina

4. The following statements regarding melanocytes and the various melanin-containing pigment cells in the eye are correct *except*:
   A. They function to keep stray light rays that enter the eye from interfering with image formation.
   B. The pink color of the iris of an albino is due to the reflection of incident light from the blood vessels of the iris.
   C. Stromal melanocytes are neural crest-derived cells that represent the cell of origin for uveal nevi and melanomas.

D. Pigmentation of the middle and anterior aspects of the uvea (uveal stroma) is completed only after birth during the first few days of life.

E. The pigment epithelium of the iris is responsible for eye color.

5. Which of the following is used as a fixative for electron microscopy?

A. Bouin's fixative

B. 10% buffered neutral formalin

C. glutaraldehyde

D. PAS

E. none of the above

6. The posterior or nasal end of which muscle insertion almost overlies the macula?

A. superior oblique

B. inferior oblique

C. lateral rectus

D. superior rectus

E. inferior rectus

7. In this photomicrograph of an embryonic human eye the inner and outer layers of the neuroectodermal optic cup are well portrayed. Which of the following statements about the optic cup is *not* correct?

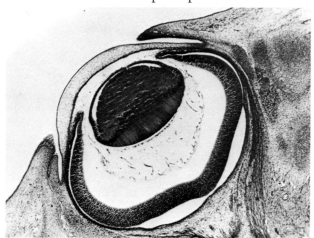

A. It forms the primordia of sensory retina, pigment epithelium, and portions of the optic nerve.

B. The original inner layer of the optic cup forms the pigment epithelium, and the outer layer forms the sensory retina.

C. Cells at the most anterior aspect will develop into the epithelial component of the iris.

D. Some cells represent the primordium, or anlage, of cells that secrete aqueous humor.

E. It develops embryologically as an anterolateral evagination of the forebrain.

8. Which of the following statements about the gross examination of the eye is *not* correct?

A. The cornea, which occupies approximately the anterior sixth of the globe, has a lesser radius of curvature than the sclera.

B. Identification of major landmarks on the exterior of the unopened enucleated globe allows the pathologist to differentiate the right from the left eye and to determine the horizontal-vertical orientation of the globe.

C. The normal adult cornea appears to measure approximately 12 × 11 mm; however, it actually is round although it appears slightly oval because of an overhanging of the conjunctiva.

D. The nasal horizontal long posterior ciliary vessel almost always is more prominent than the temporal vessel.

E. The inferior oblique muscle has a tendinous insertion into the sclera.

9. The following statements regarding the vitreous are correct *except*:

A. The most important use of a vitreous-like substance (hyaluronic acid obtained from other biologic sources such as rooster combs) is as a surgical adjunct in anterior segment surgery (viscoelastic agent).

B. The tertiary vitreous forms the suspensory ligament of the lens (zonules of Zinn) during the fourth month of gestation.

C. Secondary vitreous, which begins to form during the second month of gestation, is composed of 99% water bound with collagen and hyaluronic acid, forming a hydrogel of high viscosity.

D. Primary vitreous is the definitive adult vitreous.

E. Primary vitreous, formed during the first month of gestation, consists of both mesodermally derived tissue, including the hyaloid vasculature, and a fibrillar meshwork of uncertain origin.

10. Which of the following tumors may be differentiated, using electron microscopy, by the presence of myofibrils and cross striations?

A. cavernous hemangioma

B. optic nerve glioma

C. dermoid cyst

D. rhabdomyosarcoma

E. leiomyoma

11. Following is a photomicrograph of the equatorial region of the lens showing the zonules and the lens bow. The histologic stain that has an affinity for certain mucopolysaccharides and glycoproteins and that is especially useful in demonstrating ocular basement membranes such as the lens capsule is:

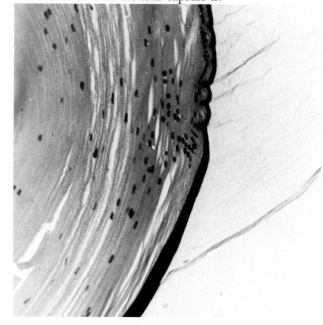

A. Alcian blue
B. Prussian blue
C. PAS
D. Mason trichrome
E. Sudan

12. A retinal detachment is an opening of the potential space that was formerly the cavity of the embryonic optic vesicle. The following histopathologic findings generally are present in retinal detachments *except*:
    A. degeneration of photoreceptors
    B. cystoid degeneration in the nerve fiber layer and the inner plexiform layer with eventual coalescence of cystoid spaces
    C. filling of the subretinal space with fluid that may be serous in nature or also may contain inflammatory cells, blood, or tumor cells, depending on the cause of the detachment
    D. degeneration and atrophy of cells that lined the cavity of the embryonic optic vesicle
    E. atrophy of the retinal pigment epithelium beneath the detachment

13. The corneal dystrophy shown in this transillumination photograph of the cornea exhibits linear opacities. The best stain to demonstrate these opacities histopathologically is:

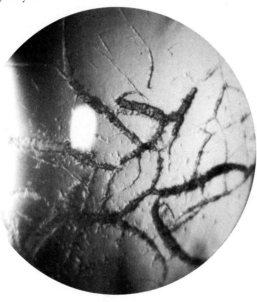

A. methylene blue
B. hematoxylin and eosin (H & E)
C. Sudan
D. PAS
E. Congo red

14. Which muscle is of neuroectodermal rather than mesodermal derivation?
    A. inferior oblique muscle
    B. superior oblique muscle
    C. fibrae meridionales
    D. iris sphincter muscle
    E. lateral rectus muscle

15. This photograph shows the histopathologic appearance of an acute purulent endophthalmitis with a vitreous abscess. The best special stain to identify the etiologic agent would be:

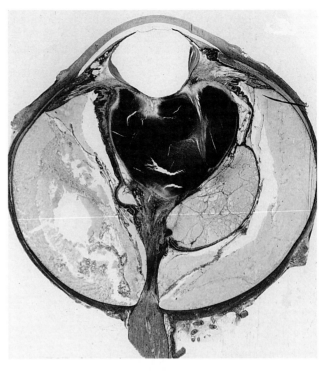

A. gram stain, anerobic culture
B. acid fast stain
C. Gomori methamine silver (GMS) stain
D. gram stain, standard aerobic culture
E. von Kossa stain

16. All of the following are derived from neuroectoderm *except*:
    A. iris dilator muscle
    B. retinal vascular endothelium
    C. sympathetic ganglion cells
    D. lateral geniculate body
    E. sensory retina

17. Embryonic surface ectoderm gives rise to all of the following *except*:
    A. corneal epithelium
    B. Schlemm's canal
    C. eyelid epidermis
    D. glands of Moll
    E. conjunctival epithelium

18. The weakest spot in the tunica fibrosa (sclera) of the eye is at the
    A. macula
    B. equator
    C. ora serrata
    D. lamina cribrosa
    E. insertion of the extraocular muscles

19. The anterior chamber angle filtration structures and its boundaries include all of the following *except*:
    A. major iris circle
    B. scleral spur
    C. trabecular meshwork
    D. Schlemm's canal
    E. Schwalbe's line

20. With the exception of eyes enucleated because of intraocular tumors, the majority of the eyes sent to a pathology laboratory are removed because of blindness, pain, and disfigurement. An eye with long-stand-

ing glaucoma, in which the dimensions of the eye often are greater than the average of 24 to 25 mm in each diameter, usually would fall into which of the following classifications of "end-stage" blind eyes?

A. phthisis bulbi
B. atrophy with shrinkage and disorganization
C. atrophy with shrinkage
D. atrophy without shrinkage
E. phthisis bulbi without shrinkage

21. Embryonic mesoderm (or mesectoderm) gives rise to all of the following *except*:

A. retinal blood vessels
B. portions of the choroid and ciliary body
C. extraocular muscles
D. pigment granules
E. sclera

22. Immunofluorescent methods have been used to detect the following:

A. cell-surface receptors
B. tumor-specific antigens
C. bacteria
D. viruses
E. all of the above

23. The ciliary body is derived embryologically from

A. surface ectoderm, neuroectoderm, and mesectoderm
B. neuroectoderm
C. neuroectoderm, mesectoderm, and mesoderm
D. mesectoderm and mesoderm
E. mesectoderm, neuroectoderm, and surface ectoderm

24. Which of the following statements about the newborn eye is *not* correct?

A. The iris is almost always gray-blue.
B. The pigment epithelium is poorly pigmented.
C. The sclera usually has a bluish hue.
D. The development of the definitive iris color may require several weeks or months.
E. The stroma of the uveal tract is very cellular.

25. The following photomicrograph shows a subepithelial corneal foreign body resulting from shrapnel penetration during a military conflict. Which stain would prove that this material is composed of iron?

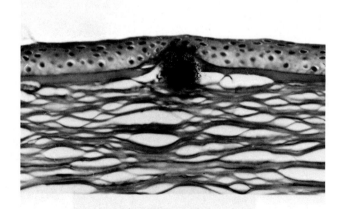

A. methylene blue
B. Prussian blue

C. toluidine blue
D. Fontana
E. Alcian blue

26. Which of the following statements is *not* correct?

A. The pathologist often can histologically examine the ciliary body and estimate the age of the patient.
B. The lens of a newborn is more spheric (has a greater anteroposterior diameter) than that of an adult.
C. Development of the fovea usually requires 4 or more weeks after birth.
D. The optic nerve head of the newborn may show a deceptively exaggerated cupping because the nerve fibers posterior to the lamina cribrosa are incompletely myelinated at birth.
E. Remnants of the trunk of the hyaloid artery and its sheath on the optic nerve head are pathologic if present at birth and often cause persistent hyperplastic primary vitreous (PHPV).

27. This photomicrograph shows the discreet deposits, separated from each other by relatively normal cornea, that are characteristic of granular corneal dystrophy (G type). Which of the following special stains is most useful to detect the presence of the hyaline proteinaceous deposits in this form of corneal dystrophy?

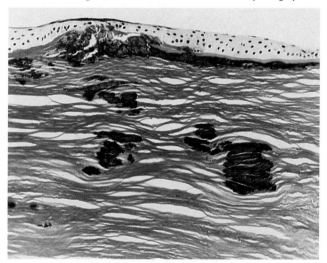

A. Masson's trichrome
B. Luxol fast blue
C. Alizarin red
D. Oil red O
E. Congo red

28. Which of the following growth or aging processes of the eye is most likely to be associated with potentially severe systemic disease?

A. Fuchs' adenoma
B. hyperplasia and proliferation of the ciliary epithelium
C. corneal arcus in a child or an adolescent
D. clear or "teardrop" cysts of the pars plana and pars plicata
E. peripheral microcystoid degeneration of the retina without schisis

29. Which of the following aging processes is most likely to be associated with visual impairment?

A. Fuchs' adenoma
B. Keratinoid degeneration of the cornea
C. Drusen
D. Peripheral microcystoid degeneration of the retina
E. Hassall-Henle warts

30. Which of the following are used to detect the presence of amyloid?
A. Congo red
B. crystal violet
C. thioflavine T
D. polarizing filters
E. all of the above

31. Which of the following statements is *not* correct?
A. Pinguecula and pterygia occur in persons exposed to extremes in environmental influences.
B. Keratinoid degeneration of the cornea or conjunctiva usually is a nonspecific degenerative change caused by environmental influences such as sun rays, wind, and dust.
C. Hassall-Henle warts represent a pathologic process and may affect vision.
D. The retina of almost all persons older than 40 years of age reveals a constant gradual decrease in the amount of nervous elements with corresponding replacement by glial tissue.
E. Chorioretinal adhesions and pigmentary lesions are common aging processes in the retinal periphery and at the ora serrata.

32. Histologically Blessig-Iwanoff cysts are located in which layer of the retina?
A. outer nuclear layer
B. outer plexiform layer
C. inner nuclear layer
D. inner plexiform layer
E. superficial nerve fiber layer

33. Phthisis bulbi is a common sequela of many eye diseases, including inflammation and trauma. It is characterized by changes such as (1) a dense fibrous membrane running across the ciliary body (cyclitic membrane), (2) intraocular bone formation without cartilage as a result of osseous metaplasia of the retinal pigment epithelium, (3) cataractous changes of the lens, often with calcium deposition, (4) gliotic scarring of the detached retina, and (5) marked shrinkage of the globe. Which of the following histologic stains would be most likely to be positive?
A. alpha-1 antitrypsin
B. von Kossa and/or alizarin red
C. calcofluor white
D. Ziehl-Neelsen

34. A patient has an obvious malignant melanoma affecting the macular region. The eye was enucleated, and the pathologist located the mass in the macular region by transillumination. Gross sectioning of the globe would be in which of the following planes?
A. horizontal
B. vertical
C. oblique
D. coronal or frontal
E. none of the above

35. Which of the following components of the eye and adnexa are *not* derived from neural crest cells?

A. vascular endothelium
B. uveal melanocytes
C. sympathetic ganglion cells
D. peripheral nerves related to eye function
E. meningothelial cells

36. This photomicrograph of a cross-section of an optic nerve shows several structures, including the central vessels with their common sheath, pial septae, nuclei of glial scattered throughout the nerve parenchyma, and cross-sections of axons. During development of the eye and adnexa the embryonic ocular fissure passes through the nerve. All of the following statements regarding the embryonic ocular fissure are *false* except:

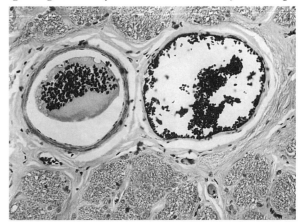

A. The term Achoroidal-fissure is more appropriate than Aembryonic-fissure because the cleft actually is formed from the choroid.
B. Its formation is necessary to create a dorsal groove through which the trunk of the hyaloid vessel (the forerunner of the vessels seen in this photograph) is able to grow into the eye.
C. Its formation is necessary to provide a pathway for the axons of the ganglion cells to grow into the brain.
D. Closure occurs at approximately 12 weeks of gestation and is initiated in the anterior and posterior regions.
E. Failure of closure of the fissure results in the formation of congenital falciform fold.

37. The most important reason for locating the vortex veins during gross examination of the globe is to:
A. determine the presence of phlebitis
B. determine the presence of thrombotic vascular occlusions
C. determine whether an intraocular tumor has extended into the epibulbar region
D. rule out the presence of atherosclerotic vascular disease
E. estimate the viability of the status of the ciliary vascular system

38. The closure of the embryonic ocular fissure normally occurs at which week of gestation?
A. 4
B. 6
C. 9
D. 12
E. 20

39. Which of the following diseases is *not* best analyzed with crossed polarizing filters?
    A. lattice dystrophy of the cornea
    B. conjunctival amyloidosis
    C. suture granulomas
    D. intraocular vegetable foreign body
    E. iron foreign body

40. The lens capsule is thinnest at the
    A. Anterior pole of the lens
    B. Area directly inferior and superior to the anterior pole of the lens
    C. Posterior pole of the lens
    D. Equator of the lens inferiorly
    E. Equator of the lens superiorly

41. A 65-year-old patient has an ulcerated, slightly yellow lesion affecting the midportion of the lid margin of the right upper eyelid. The lesion has grown slowly over a period of several months and has a somewhat fungating appearance. After biopsy of the lesion, a paraffin-embedded hematoxylin and eosin stain revealed the pattern in the following photomicrograph. Numerous "empty" vacuoles are present. Which special technique would probably help most in determining the nature of this tumor?

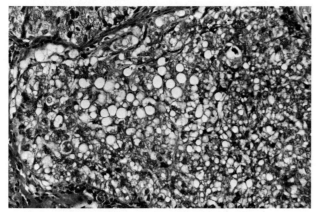

    A. paraffin section with PAS stain
    B. paraffin section with Oil red O stain
    C. frozen section with Oil red O stain
    D. frozen section with PAS stain
    E. freeze-dry technique with H & E stain

42. Lange's fold represents:
    A. an artifact at the ora serrata in a fetal eye
    B. a precursor of retinal detachment
    C. a fold at the pupillary margin
    D. a fold where the retina courses into the optic nerve
    E. a transient fold of the embryonic lens capsule near the tunica vasculosa lentis

43. When preparing an enucleated eye for subsequent microscopy, it is best to:
    A. open the globe immediately so that the fixative can freely permeate the tissue
    B. freeze the globe before immersion in fixative
    C. immediately immerse the globe in fixative (usually 10% buffered formaldehyde) for several hours before sectioning
    D. remove the vitreous via a needle, entering through the pars plana to enhance retinal fixation
    E. none of the above

44. All of the following layers of the retina and choroid have a corresponding structural layer as each continues forward and forms the pars plana *except* the:
    A. internal limiting membrane
    B. pigment epithelium of the retina
    C. sensory retina
    D. Bruch's membrane
    E. choriocapillaris

45. A retinal detachment connotes a separation of the retina from the underlying pigment epithelium. The fluid-containing subretinal space thus created represents a reopening of which embryonic space?
    A. cavity of the optic vesicle
    B. space between the inner and outer layers of the optic cup
    C. space between the apices of the retinal pigment epithelium and the apices of the embryonic photoreceptors
    D. space that very early in gestation was the cavity of the neural tube
    E. all of the above

46. The most important extraocular muscles used to orient the globe from behind during gross examination are:
    A. the inferior and superior oblique muscles
    B. the inferior oblique and lateral rectus muscles
    C. the inferior oblique and medial rectus muscles
    D. the superior oblique and lateral rectus muscles
    E. the superior oblique and medial rectus muscles

47. The following statements regarding intraocular neoplasms are correct *except*:
    A. Melanocytic tumors may reveal positive 5–100 protein staining.
    B. In women, breast carcinoma is a common cause of choroidal metastasis. In some cases the Alcian-blue stain is helpful in diagnosing a mucin-secreting adenocarcinoma.
    C. In men, lung carcinoma is the most common origin of metastatic lesions. Alcian blue also is helpful in diagnosing most cases of this tumor.
    D. Metastatic intraocular tumors, bilateral in 25% of cases, are sometimes difficult to differentiate from primary uveal malignant melanoma.
    E. Immunohistochemistry may be a useful diagnostic tool.

48. Following is a photomicrograph of the vitreous cavity of an eye. The abnormal structures are best demonstrated histologically by:

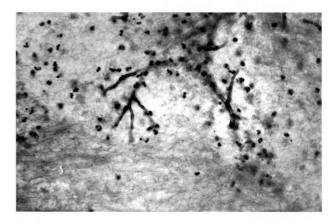

A. trichrome stain
B. Alcian blue stain
C. GMS stain
D. methylene blue dye
E. oil red O stain

49. A thorough histologic and histochemical examination of a globe enucleated from a patient who has multiple sclerosis with optic nerve involvement includes use of, among others, the following stain:
   A. Prussian blue
   B. Luxol fast blue
   C. Mallory blue
   D. Alcian blue
   E. Masson trichrome

50. Hematoxylin is specific for what component of the cell?
   A. mucopolysaccharides
   B. nucleic acids within nuclei
   C. mitochondria
   D. calcium
   E. smooth muscle

CHAPTER 2

Questions

1. Concerning keratoconus, all of the following are true *except*:
   A. Keratoconus is seen more frequently in Down syndrome than in chromosomally normal individuals.
   B. Acute keratoconus is characterized by corneal hydrops.
   C. It is hypothesized that keratoconus is a defect at the level of the epithelial basement membrane and Bowman's layer.
   D. Thinning of the corneal stroma typically occurs, but corneal edema also may be present.
   E. Keratoconus occasionally is seen Patau's in syndrome.

2. Following is a turn-of-the-century drawing showing an eye lesion. Currently this congenital anomaly is called:

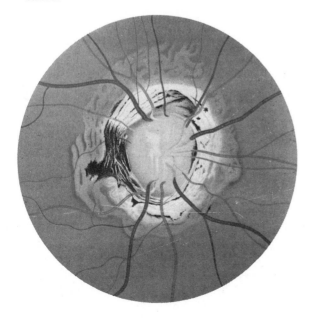

A. tilted disc syndrome
B. optic nerve aplasia
C. optic nerve dysplasia
D. morning glory syndrome
E. optic glioma

3. Apical forebrain lesions such as synophthalmia are sometimes associated with each of the following *except*:
   A. arrhinencephaly
   B. proboscis
   C. optic nerve glioma
   D. ethmocephaly
   E. trisomy 13

4. Any significant abnormality in the evagination process of the optic vesicle produces all of the following ocular malformations *except*:
   A. anophthalmia
   B. cyclopia (synophthalmia)
   C. congenital cystic eye
   D. anterior chamber cleavage syndrome
   E. congenital nonattachment of the retina

5. Following is a photomicrograph of an iris. This iris:

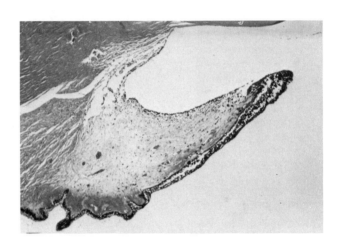

A. exhibits a typical coloboma
B. exhibits an atypical coloboma
C. exhibits aniridia
D. exhibits Miller syndrome
E. may represent all of the above

6. Macular colobomas are characterized by all of the following *except*:
   A. They are always unilateral.
   B. They usually are associated with severely decreased visual acuity.
   C. They can be familial.
   D. They often are white, craterlike depressions of the fundus with a pigmented border.
   E. They sometimes are postinflammatory (secondary to maternal infectious disease).

7. The following fundus photograph shows a typical coloboma. Such a typical coloboma is caused by:

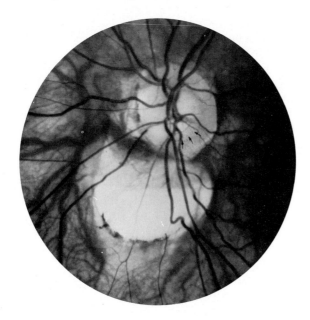

A. defective optic vesicle formation
B. defective closure of the embryonic ocular fissure
C. failure of evagination of the optic vesicle
D. lens vesicle malformation
E. PHPV

8. Trisomy 13 syndrome may involve all of the following *except*:
   A. ciliary body coloboma
   B. arrhinencephaly
   C. microphthalmia
   D. medulloepithelioma
   E. intraocular cartilage

9. Closure of the embryonic ocular tissue along the length of the optic cup begins:
   A. anteriorly and extends posteriorly
   B. posteriorly and extends anteriorly
   C. at the margin and extends to the midzone
   D. in the midzone and later extends posteriorly and anteriorly
   E. none of the above

10. Optic pits
    A. can be thought of as atypical colobomatous defects of the optic nerve head
    B. usually are blue or gray in color
    C. have an approximate incidence of 1 in 10,000
    D. have a strong correlation with serous maculopathy
    E. can be described by all of the above

11. Which of the following statements about optic pits is *least* correct?
    A. They are congenital defects of the optic nerve head.
    B. They sometimes are considered to be atypical colobomas.
    C. When temporally located, they often are associated with a serous detachment of the macula.
    D. They can be associated with visual field defects.
    E. They often reveal a direct connection with the adjacent subarachnoid space around the optic nerve, leading to influx of cerebrospinal fluid.

12. Sporadically occurring aniridia has a statistically significant coexistence with which of the following?

A. Wilms' tumor (nephroblastoma: Miller syndrome)
B. pheochromocytoma
C. Wilms' tumor (neuroblastoma)
D. solitary neuroblastoma
E. Sturge-Weber syndrome

13. Patients with the morning glory syndrome:
    A. occasionally have good vision
    B. always have poor vision
    C. have bilateral lesions
    D. usually have affected siblings
    E. rarely suffer a retinal detachment

14. This is a schematic illustration of a congenital tilted disc.[120] The designations 1, 2, and 3 respectively connote:

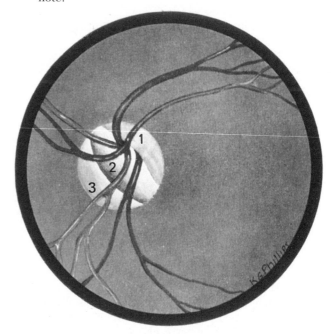

A. temporal supertraction, disc excavation, inferior-nasal conus
B. temporal excavation, disc elevation, inferior-nasal conus
C. temporal excavation, normal disc surface, inferior-nasal conus
D. normal temporal disc, disc excavation, inferior-nasal conus
E. temporal supertraction, normal disc surface, inferior-nasal conus

15. Which of the following statements about the primary vitreous is *not* correct?
    A. It is formed by the hyaloid vascular system.
    B. It eventually is replaced by secondary vitreous.
    C. It is confined to Cloquet's canal in the adult.
    D. It gives rise to the tertiary vitreous.
    E. It is necessary for growth and development of the total eye.

16. Albinism is typified by all of the following *except*:
    A. most commonly a metabolic disturbance of deficient tyrosinase
    B. a relative lack of pigment cells
    C. a component of Chediak-Steinbrinck-Higashi syndrome, when associated with neuropathy and leukopenia

D. photophobia, strabismus, and nystagmus

E. refractive error and visual loss caused by aplasia or hypoplasia of the macular region

17. This fundus photograph shows a delicate epipapillary veil derived from the glial sheath of Bergmeister. This sheath:

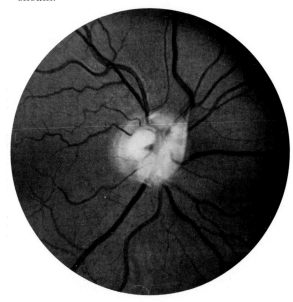

A. ultimately is responsible for a persistent pupillary membrane

B. envelops the posterior third or trunk of the embryonic hyaloid artery

C. covers the posterior half of the primary lens capsule

D. arises from elements of the circle of Zinn-Haller surrounding the optic nerve region

E. persists throughout adult life as the Mittendorf dot

18. A congenital tilted disc is associated most often with which optical abnormality?

A. nystagmus

B. myopic astigmatism

C. hyperopia

D. premature presbyopia

E. metamorphopsia

19. This is a photograph of an eye with a remnant of Bergmeister's papilla. This may be thought of as:

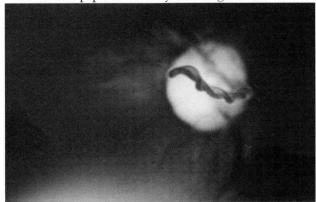

A. a persistence of the hyaloid canal

B. such a common phenomenon that it can be considered an anatomic variant

C. clinically manifesting as peripapillary membranes that should be differentiated from small retinoblastomas

D. structures with a central vascular core surrounded by a fibroglial sheath

E. all of the above

20. Which of the following statements about PHPV is *not* correct?

A. It is unilateral in most cases.

B. It has no apparent predisposition for race or sex.

C. Leukokoria is the most common initial sign.

D. It is inherited as an autosomal-dominant characteristic.

E. The affected eye usually is microphthalmic.

21. Temporally located optic pits may be associated with:

A. serous macular detachment

B. retinopathy of prematurity

C. cavernous hemangioma

D. iris coloboma

E. rubella embryopathy

22. All of the following statements about congenital falciform fold are true *except*:

A. It is believed to be similar in pathogenesis to retinopathy of prematurity (retrolental fibroplasia), occurring in low-birthweight, mostly premature babies.

B. It is a cause of leukocoria.

C. It is an elongated fold of retinal tissue coursing from the optic nerve head toward the peripheral retina.

D. It is often bilateral.

E. It is believed to be a variant of PHPV.

23. Leukokoria in PHPV is most commonly caused by:

A. persistent Bergmeister's papilla

B. a fibrovascular mass of tissue in the retrolental space

C. a hyperplastic pupillary membrane

D. coloboma of the fundus

E. none of the above

24. PHPV may be associated with:

A. adipose tissue metaplasia

B. peripheral retinal folds

C. cataracts

D. elongated ciliary processes

E. all of the above

25. Heterochromia irides is *not* defined as a condition in which:

A. The two irides are different colors.

B. A portion of an iris differs in color from other areas of the same iris.

C. Focal melanosis or partial albinism may be encountered.

D. Transmission as a dominant trait is the rule.

E. People are affected more often than animals.

26. An internist calls for advice on the treatment of PHPV in his young daughter. You inform him that untreated cases of PHPV can have all of the following consequences *except*:

A. sympathetic ophthalmia

B. glaucoma

C. repeat hemorrhage

D. phthisis bulbi

E. retinal detachment and atrophy

27. Persistent hyperplastic primary vitreous (PHPV) usually is:
    A. bilateral
    B. associated with systemic abnormalities
    C. associated with leukokoria
    D. easily cured with lensectomy
    E. rarely seen in the trisomy 13
28. Concerning aniridia, all of the following are true *except*:
    A. It may represent a severe form of atypical iris coloboma.
    B. It has two modes of occurrence, sporadic and autosomal dominant.
    C. It is a misnomer because it represents iris hypoplasia, not aplasia.
    D. It invariably is associated with congenital glaucoma
    E. Its sporadic form is associated with Wilm's tumor.
29. So-called posterior PHPV may include which of the following?
    A. corkscrew vessels
    B. persistent Bergmeister's papilla
    C. persistent hyaloid trunk
    D. epipapillary membrane
    E. all of the above
30. The following photomicrograph shows a posterior embryotoxon (enlarged, anteriorly displaced Schwalbe's line) associated with abnormal iris processes adherent to the cornea. This is an example of an anterior chamber cleavage syndrome. All of the following are considered anterior chamber cleavage syndromes *except*:

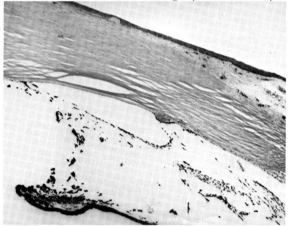

    A. Axenfeld's anomaly
    B. Rieger's syndrome
    C. Peter's anomaly
    D. mesodermal dysgenesis of the anterior segment
    E. Schnabel's syndrome
31. Which of the following statements is *false* regarding Axenfeld's anomaly?
    A. It is autosomal dominant.
    B. It is associated with glaucoma.
    C. It is associated with corectopia and colobomas.
    D. It is associated with posterior embryotoxon.
    E. It may occur in the absence of glaucoma.
32. As compared with simple myopia, high pathologic myopia is characterized by all of the following *except*:
    A. degenerative changes of the posterior segment
    B. restrained myopic tendency after puberty
    C. greater lengthening of the anteroposterior axis of the globe

D. greater tendency toward posterior staphyloma formation
    E. vitreoretinal changes with propensity toward retinal detachment
33. Persistent hyperplastic primary vitreous is characterized by all of the following *except*:
    A. It may present as a leukocoria.
    B. It can be differentiated from retinoblastoma (RB) because an eye with RB usually is microphthalmic.
    C. It may contain a remnant of the hyaloid artery.
    D. It is composed of richly vascularized tissue, and spontaneous hemorrhage is a significant complication.
    E. There is an initially clear lens that eventually become cataractous.
34. All of the following are common peripapillary changes in pathologic myopia *except*:
    A. tilted disc
    B. myopic (temporal) crescent
    C. nasal supratraction
    D. deepened physiologic excavation
    E. temporal flattening
35. All of the following are complications of pathologic myopia *except*:
    A. atrophy of the choroid
    B. macular degeneration Förster-Fuchs' spot
    C. cataract
    D. rhegmatogenous retinal detachment
    E. neovascularization of the optic nerve head
36. The nevus of Ota is associated with:
    A. primary acquired melanosis
    B. precancerous melanosis
    C. Chédiak-Higashi syndrome
    D. posterior pole staphyloma
    E. concurrent involvement of the eye (uveal or conjunctival involvement) and skin
37. All the following changes occur in highly myopic eyes with increased axial length *except*:
    A. Scleral thinning with posterior staphyloma
    B. Epiperipapillary changes such as tilted disc and myopic crescent
    C. Degenerative changes in the vitreous and vitreous detachment
    D. Retinal microcystoid degeneration and peripheral retinal break formation
    E. Förster-Fuchs' spot due to excessive stretching of the retina-choroid at the pars plana
38. Following is a photomicrograph of the ocular fundus. The condition illustrated is best interpreted as:

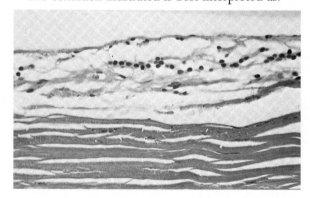

A. the retina of an albino
B. myopic retinal degeneration
C. a typical coloboma of the fundus
D. the retina in trisomy 13
E. a congenital falciform fold

39. Ocular albinism may be characterized by all of the following *except*:
    A. a decrease in the absolute number of retinal and uveal pigment epithelial cells
    B. a decrease in the number of pigmented melanin granules within pigment cells
    C. photophobia
    D. poor vision
    E. nystagmus

40. Which of the following is not true of morning glory syndrome?
    A. Retinal detachment is not a significant complication.
    B. It may be associated with a failure of closure of the embryonic fissure because it fails to "zipper shut" around the optic nerve.
    C. This disc is abnormally excavated, with vessels arcading toward periphery.
    D. It is characterized by visual acuity ranging from reasonably good to poor.
    E. It usually is bilateral.

41. Congenital melanosis oculi can be characterized by all of the following *except*:
    A. an increase in the absolute number of normal melanocytes in various ocular tissues
    B. an increased incidence of conjunctival malignant melanomas
    C. pigmentation of the sclera and episclera
    D. pigmentation of both ocular tissues and skin
    E. a darkened appearance of the fundus

42. White spots on the iris may be found in all of the following *except*:
    A. patients with Down syndrome
    B. healthy individuals
    C. patients with Brushfield's spots
    D. individuals with Wolfflin-Kruckmann spots
    E. none of the above

43. Microphthalmia is *not*
    A. associated with corectopia
    B. associated with colobomas
    C. associated with infectious disease, such as maternal rubella
    D. a less extreme form of nanophthalmia
    E. a possible side effect of maternal thalidomide use

44. The most common and diagnostic finding(s) of trisomy 13 is (are):
    A. primary anophthalmia
    B. intraocular cartilage within a coloboma of the ciliary body
    C. cyclopia and ethmocephaly
    D. congenital cystic eye
    E. congenital nonattachment of the retina

45. Common ocular findings of trisomy 13 include all of the following *except*:
    A. microphthalmia
    B. colobomas of the ciliary body and iris
    C. PHPV
    D. retinal dysplasia
    E. melanosis oculi

46. The most commonly observed clinically significant intraocular lesions in trisomy 21 (Down syndrome) include all of the following *except*:
    A. cataracts
    B. iris lesions (Brushfield's spots)
    C. iris hypoplasia
    D. congenital cystic eye
    E. keratoconus

47. Peters' anomaly is characterized by all of the following *except*:
    A. It generally is considered to be the most severe of the anterior chamber angle cleavage syndromes.
    B. It usually is transmitted as an X-linked recessive condition.
    C. It is associated with corectopia.
    D. It can be described as a defect caused by delayed separation of lens vesicle and surface ectoderm.
    E. It differs from Axenfeld's and Rieger's anomalies because they are autosomal dominant.

48. This fundus drawing was made in 1898, when the lesion was believed to represent an atypical coloboma of the macula. Current thinking on the cause of this lesion in many instances is:

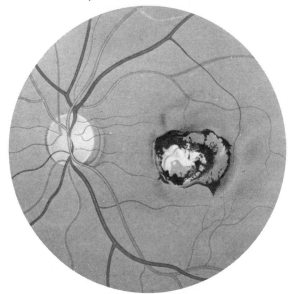

    A. postinflammatory (e.g., congenital toxoplasmosis)
    B. PHPV
    C. failure of optic fissure closure
    D. persistent hyaloid vasculature
    E. pathologic myopia

49. Which of the following forms of albinism may be associated with septicemia and pyogenic infections?
    A. Chédiak-Stainbrinck-Higashi syndrome
    B. Waardenburg-Klein syndrome
    C. tyrosinase-negative (complete) albinism
    D. iris heterochromia
    E. congenital melanosis oculi

50. Ocular findings in Down Syndrome include all of the following *except*:
    A. Almond-shaped palpebral fissures.
    B. Blepharitis

C. Convergent strabismus in one third of patients
D. Cataracts in two thirds of patients.
E. Increased incidence of anterior uveitis.

CHAPTER 3

1. Which of the following statements regarding the nerve loop of Axenfeld are true?
   A. It is a pathologic outward bowing of the anterior ciliary nerves just behind the limbus.
   B. The nerve courses from the sclera superficially into the conjunctiva before reentering the sclera.
   C. It is of clinical significance only because it may be painful.
   D. It must be included in the differential diagnosis of primary or metastatic malignant melanoma of the uvea or of the ocular surface supine.
   E. All of the above.

2. The phthisic eye shown in this photograph was lost because of perforation during routine strabismus surgery. The adult sclera is thinnest:

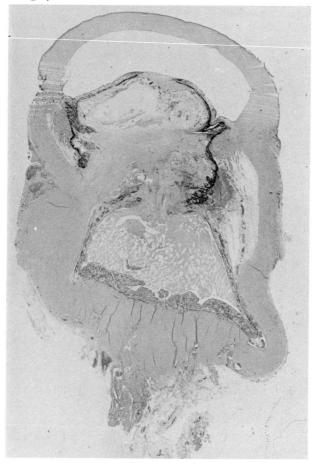

   A. posterior to the insertion of the extraocular (rectus) muscles
   B. anterior to insertion of the extraocular (rectus) muscles
   C. at the macula
   D. just anterior to the equator
   E. at the limbus

3. Which of the following statements concerning the tear-forming apparatus is *not* correct?
   A. The tear film is composed of three layers.
   B. The inner layer consists of a mucopolysaccharide film.
   C. The middle layer of the tear film consists of a watery fluid secreted primarily by the lacrimal glands.
   D. Meibomian and Zeis glands are sebaceous glands that secrete the oily outer layer of the tear film.
   E. The conjunctiva is not involved in the production of the tear film.

4. Which of the following statements concerning Bowman's layer is true?
   A. Bowman's layer is the anterior-most basement membrane of the cornea.
   B. Hassall-Henle warts are histologicaly identical in appearance to guttata and represent membrane thickenings of Bowman's layer.
   C. Unlike Descemet's membrane, damaged portions of Bowman's layer do not have the ability to regenerate.
   D. Bowman's layer is produced by the corneal epithelial cells.
   E. Bowman's layer is best demonstrated histologically by PAS staining.

5. Which of the following is *not* characteristic of Bowman's layer?
   A. It is a basement membrane.
   B. It covers the entire cornea, terminating near the corneoscleral junction.
   C. It is basically acellular, composed of delicate collagen fibrils and ground substance.
   D. Delicate collagen fibrils normally are distributed randomly within Bowman's layer.
   E. Portions of Bowman's layer that are destroyed by trauma cannot regenerate; the defects often are filled in by epithelium (facet).

6. Band keratopathy due to metastatic calcification of a normal Bowman's layer may be caused by:
   A. renal insufficiency
   B. Fanconi syndrome
   C. milk-alkali syndrome
   D. hyperparathyroidism
   E. all of the above

7. Which of the following statements about Descemet's membrane is *not* correct?
   A. It is a true PAS-positive basement membrane.
   B. It covers, with the endothelium, the entire posterior aspect of the cornea, terminating at Schwalbe's line peripherally.
   C. It is elaborated by the corneal endothelium.
   D. It shows no tendency to regenerate after trauma-induced breakage.
   E. When broken, it shows a tendency to coil or roll into a scroll shape or form excrescences (e.g., Haab's striae in congenital glaucoma or after forceps birth injury).

8. All of the following exemplify a granulomatous inflammation affecting the eye *except*:
   A. sympathetic ophthalmia
   B. acute fungal keratitis
   C. chalazion
   D. toxoplasmosis
   E. orbital pseudotumor with epithelioid cells

9. Hassall-Henle warts:
   A. are major lesions associated with Fuchs' dystrophy
   B. have a viral cause
   C. cause significant corneal edema and visual impairment in elderly patients
   D. consist of focal excrescences on Descemet's membrane in the central cornea
   E. are a normal aging phenomenon

10. Which statement regarding ectasia and staphyloma is incorrect?
    A. Any condition that creates a focal weakness of the cornea or sclera predisposes their formation.
    B. Major causes include trauma, corneoscleral inflammatory and melting disease, and advanced glaucoma.
    C. By definition, ectasia refers to a protrusion of the cornea whereas staphyloma consists of protruding sclera.
    D. Many cases of congenital anterior staphyloma are thought to occur secondary to intrauterine corneal inflammatory processes.
    E. They may occur in the presence of a coloboma, resulting in a colobomatous cyst that occasionally replaces the eye within the orbit during fetal development.

11. Following is a photomicrograph of cell aggregates. Aggregates of cells of this general type may be seen in all of the following lesions *except:*

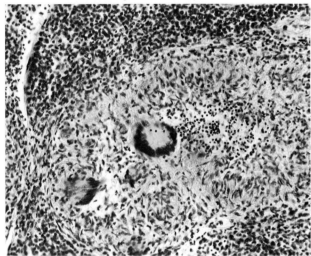

    A. keratic precipitates
    B. chalazion
    C. acute vitreous abscess
    D. Koeppe and Busacca nodules on the iris
    E. sarcoid granulomas (e.g., candle-wax lesions)

12. The term *anterior embryotoxon* refers to:
    A. hypertrophic scar formation in the area of Bowman's layer
    B. normally thickened Bowman's layer seen in the peripheral cornea
    C. arcus juvenilis (composed of lipid infiltrates)
    D. epithelial facet
    E. Schwalbe's line

13. Note the cornea in the following photomicrograph. This cornea most likely represents:

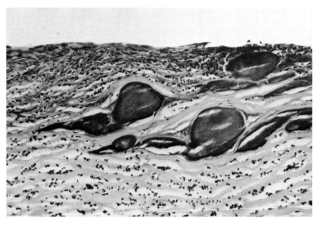

    A. Salzmann's nodular degeneration
    B. superficial keratoconjunctivitis
    C. syphilitic interstitial keratitis
    D. herpes simplex keratitis
    E. acute bacterial ulcer

14. This photomicrograph show two common sequelae of long-standing; corneal disorders. These are:

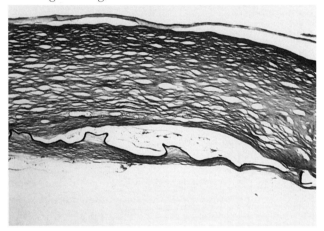

    A. band keratopathy and endothelial hyperplasia
    B. bullous keratopathy and macular dystrophy
    C. bullous keratopathy and retrocorneal fibrous membrane
    D. retrocorneal fibrous membrane and macular dystrophy
    E. macular dystrophy and epithelial erosion

15. Choose the *incorrect* statement. Fungal corneal ulcers:
    A. have become more prevalent because of widespread use of corticosteroids and immunosuppressive agents
    B. often occur after trauma involving vegetative material
    C. will sometimes be associated with an immune ring of Wessely, a ring-shaped infiltration of polymorphonuclear neutrophils and plasma cells deposited around the central lesion
    D. often have a rapid onset of 1 to 2 days after the initial injury
    E. are caused by agents that can be best demonstrated by the GMS stain

16. Which statement regarding Fuchs' endothelial dystrophy is false?
    A. Most cases are, X-linked recessive, affecting men.

B. The clinical hallmark consists of corneal guttata, which begins centrally and spreads peripherally with age.

C. Corneal edema is the most significant clinical finding and results from a decreased pumping and barrier function of the disordered endothelium.

D. Histopathologic studies reveal variation in endothelial cell size and an absolute decrease in the number of endothelial cells.

E. Fuchs' combined dystrophy implies epithelial edema that may lead to repeated attacks of pain because of rupture of epithelial bullae.

17. This photomicrograph is from a case of chronic iridocyclitis. The illustration shows the presence of:

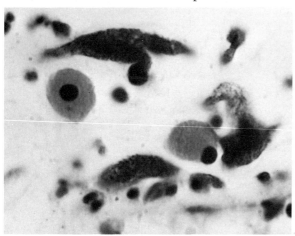

A. plasma cells
B. eosinophils
C. Russell bodies
D. plasmacytoid cells
E. densely staining intracellular viral inclusions

18. In interstitial keratitis (IK), which statement is correct?

A. It is characterized by an inflammation that usually involves the epithelium but not the endothelium.

B. It is always bilateral if acquired.

C. It is pathognomonic for syphilis.

D. If caused by congenital syphilis, it typically occurs in late childhood or the teen years.

E. It is sometimes caused by the virus *Onchocerca volvulus*.

19. Which of the following statements concerning inflammatory cell infiltrates is incorrect?

A. The polymorphonuclear neutrophil has a three- to five-lobed nucleus and is the hallmark of acute inflammation.

B. Eosinophils are bilobed cells with pink-staining granules in the cytoplasm and typically are seen in hypersensitive states and parasitic infestations.

C. The lymphocyte has a deep-staining, discrete, round nucleus with scanty cytoplasm and is the hallmark of chronic inflammation.

D. The plasma cell is an elliptical cell with an eccentric nucleus, a clock face pattern of nuclear chromatin, and cytoplasm that is lightly stained adjacent to the nucleus and deeply basophilic elsewhere; its development into plasmacytoid cells and Russell bodies indicates chronicity.

E. The Langhans, foreign body, and Touton giant cells all are derivatives of the epithelioid cell, and though each display a characteristic arrangement of nuclei, they all are indicators of nongranulomatous chronic inflammation.

20. Which of the following statements about Mooren's ulcer is *not* correct?

A. The majority of cases are unilateral.

B. It is associated with much pain.

C. It erodes centrally from the periphery, with excavation of the epithelium and stroma.

D. Sometimes it involves the scleral portion of the limbus leading to perforation.

E. It is usually associated with *Staphylococcus aureus*.

21. Which statement concerning a corneal pannus is *false*?

A. It may be inflammatory or degenerative.

B. The ingrowth of tissue occurs between the corneal epithelium and Bowman's layer.

C. Bowman's layer often is destroyed.

D. The pannus may occur by ingrowth from the limbus or by in situ fibrosis and degeneration.

E. Fatty plaques often are deposited within the substance of a degenerative pannus.

22. Which statement concerning the epithelial microcystic dystrophies is not true?

A. Meesmann's, Cogan's, and Reis-Bucklers' dystrophies are all classic examples.

B. They are due to congenital absence of desmosomes between epithelial cells and hemidesmosomes between the epithelial basement membrane and Bowman's layer.

C. The inheritable form of the recurrent erosion syndrome is autosomal dominant and is histopathologically identical to Cogan's microcystic dystrophy, otherwise known as map, dot, fingerprint dystrophy.

D. The occurrence is thought to be totally independent of corneal hydration, with rare exceptions.

E. Although often clinically symptomatic because of recurrent attacks of pain, lacrimation, and photophobia secondary to late erosions, they do not affect visual acuity.

23. This photomicrograph shows the posterior aspect of the cornea. It demonstrates:

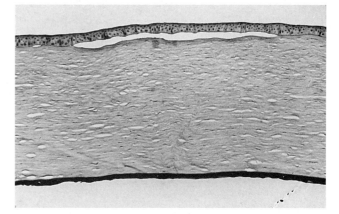

A. keratic precipitates
B. seedlets of retinoblastoma
C. hypopyon

D. bloodstaining

E. a Krukenberg spindle

24. Which of the following statements is *not* correct?

    A. Corneal edema and bullous keratopathy usually are caused by pathologic changes in the endothelium.

    B. The best way to confirm corneal edema microscopically is by observing the stroma for separation of collagen lamellae.

    C. Bullous keratopathy consists of a blisterlike elevation of the corneal epithelium associated with damaged hemidesmosomes.

    D. The late stages of bullous keratopathy may result in formation of a fibrovascular pannus.

    E. Fuchs' dystrophy may lead to corneal edema and bullous keratopathy in its advanced stages.

25. Which of the following statements concerning viral keratitis is incorrect?

    A. Herpes simplex type I virus is the most frequent cause of viral induced corneal ulcers.

    B. Although less common, herpes zoster can cause a dendritic ulcer.

    C. If uveitis is associated with very mild keratitis, another etiologic agent also must be present.

    D. Multinucleated giant cells and type A Cowry intranuclear inclusions in the involved epithelium and superficial keratocytes provide histopathologic confirmation.

    E. Chronic inflammation and vascularization of the deep stromal lamellae may develop without concurrent epithelial ulceration.

26. Which of the following is classically attributed to adenovirus type 8?

    A. epidemic keratoconjunctivitis

    B. superficial punctate keratitis

    C. interstitial keratitis

    D. disciform keratitis

    E. superficial keratitis associated with Reiter's syndrome

27. Krukenberg's spindle:

    A. frequently results in diminished vision

    B. is an intrascleral nerve loop

    C. is a normal anatomic variant

    D. is four times more prevalent in females

    E. depends on anterior chamber convection currents for its formation

28. All of the following statements are characteristic of granular dystrophy *except*:

    A. It is autosomal dominant.

    B. It usually presents at puberty.

    C. Discrete crumblike white to gray opacities appear in the anterior stromal layers axially and extend to the limbus.

    D. Because the intervening cornea between granular opacities is clear, the visual prognosis is much better than in macular and lattice dystrophies.

    E. The granular material is hyaline and stains a brilliant red with Masson trichrome stain.

29. Which statement about a Krukenberg's spindle is *false?*

    A. It usually results in a moderate decrease in vision.

    B. It is caused by deposition of uveal pigment granules on the posterior corneal surface.

    C. It may occur in pigment dispersion syndrome.

    D. It usually is caused by trauma if unilateral.

    E. It may be associated with glaucoma.

30. The Kayser-Fleischer ring:

    A. may be caused by an intraocular foreign body

    B. is a deposit of copper in Bowman's layer

    C. is an iron line seen at the cone base in keratoconus

    D. usually appears initially as an acute pigmentation

    E. usually is associated with pigmentary glaucoma

31. Keratoconus is most commonly:

    A. unilateral

    B. X-linked recessive

    C. autosomal dominant

    D. autosomal recessive

    E. not associated with a clearly demonstrable inheritance pattern

32. Regarding the three major corneal stromal dystrophies, which answer is *not* correct?

    A. Macular dystrophy is inherited as an autosomal-recessive trait.

    B. Recurrent epithelial erosions occur most commonly with lattice dystrophy.

    C. Lattice dystrophy has the best visual prognosis.

    D. Macular dystrophy involves both the central and peripheral cornea.

    E. Lattice dystrophy, although usually an isolated disorder, can be associated rarely with primary or secondary systemic amyloidosis.

33. Choose the incorrect statement regarding corneal dystrophies:

    A. They usually are bilateral spontaneous occurrences.

    B. They often are accompanied by systemic disease.

    C. Neovascularization and inflammation often are late sequelae.

    D. They are classified most conveniently by the primary layer of involvement.

    E. Salzmann's nodular corneal dystrophy is a classic example of dystrophy involving the epithelium and superficial stroma.

34. The photomicrograph shows H & E staining of a cornea with macular dystrophy. Deposits are faintly visible within the space in the superficial stroma just below Bowman's layer. Which of the following statements about this disease and this illustration is *not* correct?

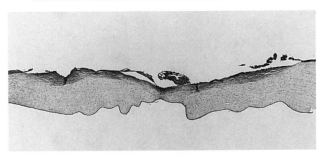

A. It is possible that this patient may have been susceptible to recurrent corneal erosions.

B. This patient probably would lose vision more rapidly than a patient with granular or lattice dystrophy.

C. The deposits would be more apparent in this slide if stained with Masson trichrome stain.

D. The deposits would be more apparent in this slide if stained by the Alcian blue technique.

E. Microscopy with polarizing filters would not have rendered the deposits much more visible.

35. Keratoconus has been associated with all of the following *except*:

A. trisomy 21

B. tapetoretinal degeneration

C. iatrogenic (e.g., topical steroids or contact lens over-wear)

D. aniridia

E. Marfan's syndrome

36. A carelessly thrown dart enters through the central visual axis of a patient's eye, and the tip becomes lodged within the substance of the crystalline lens. Which of the following best describes the wound?

A. This is a corneal penetration and an ocular perforation.

B. This is a corneal perforation and an ocular perforation.

C. This is a corneal perforation and an ocular penetration.

D. This is a corneal penetration and an ocular penetration.

E. None of the above are true.

37. Which of the following statements regarding amyloidosis is true?

A. The eyelid is the most commonly involved site in the body in primary systemic amyloidosis, and involvement warrants a general examination to search for the disease.

B. Secondary systemic amyloidosis primarily affects the kidneys, spleen, liver, and adrenal glands and tends to spare the ocular tissues.

C. Plasma cell myeloma mimics primary systemic amyloidosis in its pattern of amyloid deposition.

D. Secondary localized amyloidosis associated with previous eyelid and conjunctival disease is the most common form with ocular involvement.

E. All of the above.

38. This slide shows a classic example of:

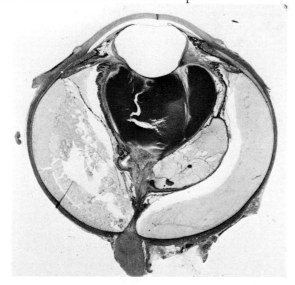

A. chronic granulomatous inflammation

B. acute purulent inflammation

C. subretinal abscess

D. chronic nongranulomatous inflammation

E. acute granulomatous reaction

39. In which of the following systemic mucopolysaccharidoses is the cornea characteristically least involved?

A. Hunter

B. Hurler

C. Morquio

D. Scheie

E. Maroteaux-Lamy

40. Which of the following is not a sequela of a contusion injury of the cornea or sclera?

A. secondary cataract

B. full-thickness corneal rupture

C. hyphema leading to corneal blood staining

D. iridocyclodialysis

E. commotio retina leading to macular hole

41. More than 75% of all globes processed in ocular pathology laboratories are enucleated because of:

A. melanoma

B. retinoblastoma

C. keratoconus

D. trauma

E. surgical complications

42. Which statement concerning *Acanthamoeba* keratitis is false?

A. A ring-shaped corneal stromal infiltrate is a characteristic sign.

B. The calcofluor white stain is useful in detecting cysts in direct smear or biopsy material.

C. Most cases of *Acanthamoeba* keratitis occur in patients wearing daily-wear soft contact lenses.

D. The definitive treatment of *Acanthamoeba* keratitis is neomycin sulfate and propamidine isethionate.

E. The organism exists in two forms: (1) a trophozoite (ectocyst) form that is highly resistant to freezing, desiccation, standard chlorination of water supplies, and a variety of antimicrobial agents and (2) an endocyst form.

43. All of the following are causes of corneal clouding in childhood *except*:

A. congenital glaucoma

B. anterior chamber cleavage syndromes

C. Sanfilippo's systemic mucopolysaccharidosis

D. congenital hereditary endothelial corneal dystrophy

E. hereditary Bowman's layer dysplasia

44. The eye of a 27-year-old male mechanic was injured while he worked on a car door with a metal hammer. Slitlamp examination revealed a massive protrusion of intraocular contents at the site of a wound, and the eye had to be enucleated. The following microslide was prepared. The extruded contents were discovered to be retina. Apart from the corneal defect, the outer tunic of the globe was found to be intact. This is an example of:

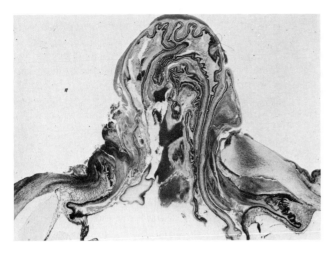

A. corneal penetration
B. corneal perforation and ocular perforation
C. corneal perforation and ocular penetration
D. ocular perforation and corneal penetration
E. none of the above

45. Which of the following statements concerning alkali burns of the cornea is *not* correct?
   A. Alkali burns of the cornea are much more destructive than acid burns.
   B. Collagenase production increases with administration of topical steroids and can be very harmful to the cornea, particularly in the acute phase.
   C. The intraocular pressure may increase within minutes but may decrease after hours to days.
   D. Serious complications are very uncommon after the final cicatricial stage.
   E. A retrocorneal membrane may form.

46. This photomicrograph of a cornea shows:

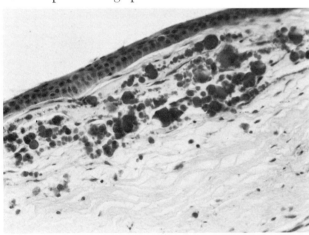

A. Labrador keratopathy
B. Bietti's hyaline degeneration
C. climatic keratopathy
D. keratinoid degeneration
E. all of the above

47. Regarding corneal iron lines, the following statements are true *except:*
   A. Routinely stained histopathologic sections reveal faint light-brown to yellow granules deposited in Descemet's membrane.
   B. The Ferry line appears in front of a filtering bleb.

C. The Hudson-Stahli line is seen horizontally just inferior to the center of the palpebral fissure in the aging cornea.
   D. The Stocker line appears in front of the apex of a pterygium.
   E. The Fleisher line is seen at the base of the cone in keratoconus.

48. Materials that exhibit birefringence when viewed through polarizing lenses include all of the following *except:*
   A. wood
   B. the "bread-crumb" deposits of granular dystrophy
   C. amyloid
   D. calcium oxalate crystals
   E. many types of suture material

49. Which of the following stains is most useful in diagnosing ocular siderosis?
   A. Alcian blue
   B. colloidal iron
   C. Luxol fast blue
   D. Prussian blue
   E. Mallory blue

50. This photomicrograph shows an epithelial ingrowth, a disastrous sequela of perforating trauma. Regarding perforating trauma, the following statements are true *except:*

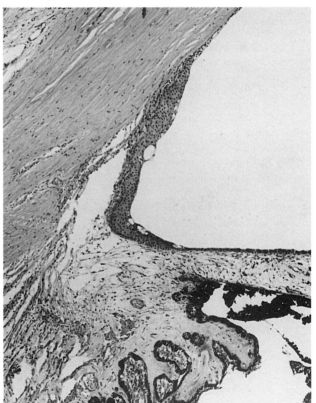

A. Corneoscleral laceration is the most common form of trauma that leads to enucleation.
   B. Prolapse of uveal tissue into the wound predisposes to sympathetic ophthalmia.
   C. Prolapse of retinal tissue is a grave prognostic sign because it almost always is untreatable and leads the phthisis bulbi as a rule.

D. Histopathologically, rupture of Descemet's membrane with a wrinkled and coiled appearance is pathognomonic for previous perforating injury.
E. Epithelial ingrowth with retrocorneal membrane formation is an ominous sign that may lead to severe glaucoma.

CHAPTER 4

1. Which of the following statements about lens fibers is *not* correct?
   A. They have a high protein content.
   B. They contain abundant mitochondria.
   C. They are formed near the equatorial margin (lens bow).
   D. They can survive for long periods without a nucleus.
   E. They are hexagonal on cross section.

2. Which of the following statements about lens sutures is *not* correct?
   A. They account for the characteristic biconvex "disclike" flattening of the lens.
   B. They originate because of unequal growth of newly formed lens fibers.
   C. They appear during the second month of gestation.
   D. The anterior Y suture is inverted, and the posterior Y suture is upright.
   E. They are molded together by ground substance.

3. The embryonal nucleus develops by:
   A. elongation and migration of the anterior epithelial cells toward the posterior capsule
   B. elongation and migration of the posterior epithelial cells toward the anterior capsule
   C. proliferation and migration of epithelial cells and their extension from the equatorial lens bow
   D. protein deposition from the equatorial epithelial cells
   E. mitotic division of old anterior and equatorial epithelial cells

4. Which of the following statements about the lens capsule is *not* correct?
   A. It has an inherent elasticity or pliability that facilitates accomodation.
   B. It is thinnest anteriorly.
   C. It stains positively with PAS.
   D. It is secreted by the epithelium.
   E. It completely ensheathes the lens.

5. This photomicrograph shows a Soemmering's ring. Which of the following statements is *not* correct?

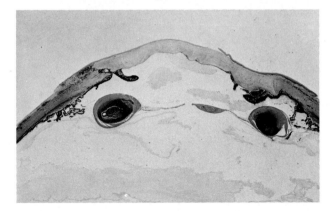

A. It usually indicates that the lens capsule has ruptured.
B. It may be seen associated with an adherent leukoma because they share a similar pathogenesis.
C. A Soemmering's ring may be seen after extracapsular cataract extraction (ECCE).
D. It is doughnut shaped on gross examination.
E. It consists of a lens nucleus and lens capsule remnants.

6. The lens capsule is created.
   A. early in embryonal life (lens vesicle stage)
   B. after embryonal nucleus formation is completed
   C. by junction of the lens fibers, creating the Y sutures
   D. after birth, as part of the adult lens
   E. only as a sequela to pathologic situations

7. Mittendorf dots:
   A. are associated with Wilson's disease
   B. frequently cause significant visual loss
   C. consist of deposits of melanin on the lens capsule
   D. consist of remnants of the tunica vasculosa lentis
   E. often are associated with glaucoma

8. The main clinical types of age-related cataracts include all of the following *except*:
   A. cupuliform (posterior subcapsular)
   B. perinuclear punctate
   C. reduplication
   D. cuneiform (cortical spokes)
   E. nuclear sclerosis

9. The differential diagnosis of "toxic lens syndrome" includes:
   A. phacoanaphylaxis
   B. localized (*P. acnes*) infectious endophthalmitis
   C. tissue irritation caused by sharp edges of poorly made intraocular lens chafing against uveal tissue
   D. residual polishing components on lens surfaces
   E. all of the above

10. The classic cataract seen with juvenile diabetes is:
    A. snowflake
    B. sunflower
    C. morgagnian
    D. embryonal
    E. zonular

11. Cataracts usually are not associated with:
    A. tetany
    B. hypoparathyroidism
    C. Hurler's syndrome (gargoylism)
    D. renal ricketts (e.g., Lowe's syndrome)
    E. Down syndrome

12. Marfan's syndrome includes all of the following *except*:
    A. skeletal abnormalities
    B. cardiovascular abnormalities
    C. lens subluxation
    D. microspherophakia and anterior chamber cleavage syndrome
    E. retinal degeneration (e.g., "salt-and-pepper" fundus)

13. Hirschberg-Elschnig pearls signify:
    A. a congenital cataract
    B. wartlike excrescences on the lens capsule
    C. aggregates of basement membrane fragments after capsular rupture

D. abnormally proliferating epithelial cells, usually seen after capsular rupture

E. abnormally proliferating cortical material in the anterior chamber

14. Cell nuclei in the center of the normal crystalline lens:
    A. show rapid mitotic rates
    B. show slow mitotic rates
    C. are round with abundant cytoplasm
    D. stain basophilic with H & E stain
    E. are absent

15. Which of the following statements about the zonules of Zinn is *not* correct?
    A. The posterior border of insertion of the zonules onto the lens is at or near the lens–vitreous interface.
    B. They radiate from the ciliary body to the equatorial surface of the lens.
    C. They tighten during accommodation.
    D. They are derived from the tertiary vitreous.
    E. They form at approximately the fourth month of gestation.

16. A Vossius' ring may indicate:
    A. a persistence of the embryonic tunica vasculosa lentis
    B. the presence of phacolytic glaucoma
    C. the presence of pigmentary glaucoma
    D. that trauma to the eye has occurred, which may have caused some pigment dispersion
    E. a high probability that a patient has diabetes

17. Cataracts caused by prolonged use of steroids usually are:
    A. hypermature
    B. a result of nuclear sclerosis
    C. of the morganian type
    D. of the posterior subcapsular type or diffuse in nature
    E. of the central anterior subcapsular type

18. The thinnest portion of the lens capsule is located at:
    A. anterior capsule
    B. posterior capsule
    C. equator
    D. midway between the equator and center—anteriorly
    E. midway between the equator and center—posteriorly

19. The most common complication of a closed-loop anterior chamber intraocular lens (IOL) is:
    A. cystoid macular edema (CME)
    B. retinal detachment
    C. uveitis-glaucoma-hyphema (UGH) syndrome
    D. infectious endophthalmitis
    E. pseudophakic corneal decompensation

20. This photomicrograph shows an eye from an embryo with multiple congenital anomalies. The inner layer of the optic cup (future sensory retina, *R*) is present on the right. The lens (*L*) shows early cataractous change as manifested by posterior migration of the epithelial cell nucleus. The abnormal retrolental mass (*M*) probably represents:

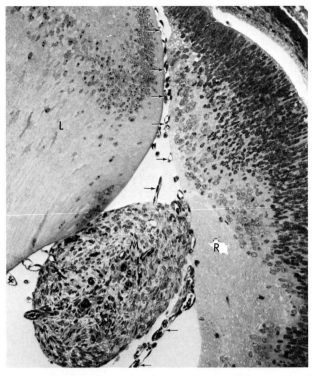

A. preretinal neovascularization caused by maternal diabetes
B. an early stage of PHPV
C. retrolental fibroplasia
D. Lange's fold formation
E. formation of a persistent Bergmeister papilla caused by persistence of the tunica vasculosa lentis

21. Dislocation of the lens is *not* associated with:
    A. Marfan's syndrome
    B. homocystinuria
    C. Weill-Marchesani syndrome
    D. Lowe's syndrome (aminoaciduria)
    E. hyperlysinemia

22. In maternal rubella syndrome all of the following can occur *except:*
    A. a necrotizing iridocyclitis
    B. nuclear-type cataract
    C. microphthalmia
    D. a "salt-and-pepper" fundus
    E. abnormal electroretinogram

23. Following is a photomicrograph of an anterior subcapsular fibrous plaque. Such a plaque forms:

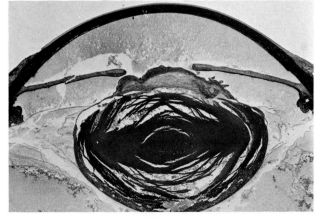

A. as a result of fibrous metaplasia (or pseudometaplasia) of the anterior lens cortex, often secondary to trauma or uveitis
B. as a result of fibrous metaplasia (or pseudometaplasia) of the anterior lens epithelium, often secondary to trauma or uveitis
C. because of fibrous metaplasia (or pseudometaplasia) of the lens cortex after rupture of the lens capsule
D. after organization of anterior subcapsular hemorrhage caused by trauma
E. as a sequela to bladder (Wedl) cell formation

24. Following is a gross photograph of an iris-supported IOL. Which of the following complications may have necessitated its removal:

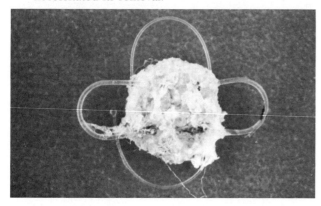

A. cocoon membrane
B. UGH syndrome
C. cyclitic membrane
D. retrocorneal fibrous membrane
E. all of the above

25. This slide is a section through the nucleus of the lens of a female child with maternal rubella syndrome.

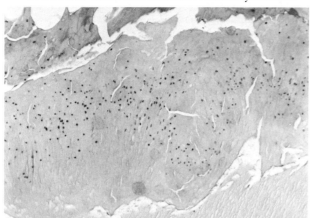

Which of the following is *not* correct regarding this patient and her disease?
A. She also may have necrotizing iridocyclitis.
B. She probably had pigmentary abnormalities of the fundus ("salt-and-pepper" fundus).
C. The pyknotic nuclei seen in this slide may contain virus particles.
D. The retention of lens fiber nuclei within the lens center, as seen in this slide, may have been caused by disturbance of lens fiber formation at the equa-

tor caused by a ciliary body coloboma and defective zonules.
E. Congenital or infantile glaucoma may be seen in eyes afflicted with this syndrome.

26. Sampaolesi's line represents:
A. a pigmented vertical line on the central posterior corneal endothelium seen in pigmentary glaucoma
B. a pigmented line on the posterior corneal endothelium caused by uveitis
C. a pigmented line on the posterior peripheral cornea seen in siderosis
D. a pigmented line on the anterior surface of the lens seen after trauma
E. a pigmented line that may be visible by gonioscopy on the trabecular meshwork in pseudoexfoliation syndrome

27. Which of the following statements about phacoanaphylactic endophthalmitis is *not* correct?
A. It indicates probable rupture of the lens capsule.
B. It is an autosensitization phenomenon.
C. It often is characterized by a zonal granulomatous inflammatory reaction.
D. It may be associated with a sympathetic response.
E. The histopathologic hallmark is a large (40 μm) foamy macrophage containing denatured lens protein.

28. Which of the following is *not* a cause of or related to posterior chamber IOL decentration:
A. "sunrise" syndrome secondary to asymmetric IOL loop implantation (one loop in the ciliary region and one loop in the lens capsular bag)
B. intraoperative or postoperative escape of a loop from the lens capsular sac ("pea-pod" effect)
C. ciliary sulcus fixation
D. fibrous or myoepithelial metaplasia of residual lens epithelial cells causing contraction of the capsular sac
E. "sunset" syndrome caused by zonular-capsular dehiscence

29. The condition seen in this photomicrograph:

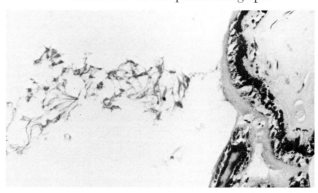

A. is classically described in glassblowers
B. does not cause glaucoma
C. is considered by many authorities to be a disease of basement membranes
D. represents a splitting of the lens capsule with resultant "scroll" formation
E. is associated with exposure to infrared radiation

30. A 65-year-old woman has a posterior subcapsular cata-

ract. Histologic examination of the lens is *most* likely to show:
- A. a fibrous plaque in the posterior subcapsular region
- B. thinning of the posterior capsule
- C. posterior migration of equatorial lens epithelium with bladder cell formation
- D. morgagnian globules in the posterior capsule
- E. Hirschberg-Elschnig pearls

31. Currently the most common cataract operation performed in the world is:
- A. intracapsular extraction (ICCE) with aphakic spectacles
- B. anterior chamber lens implantation
- C. rigid posterior (PMMA) chamber lens implantation after extracapsular cataract extraction (ECCE)
- D. implantation of a foldable IOL after a small incision and phacoemulsification
- E. intracapsular lens extraction (ICCE) with implantation of a rigid (PMMA) posterior chamber lens

32. Which of the following factors had a favorable impact on cataract therapy and visual rehabilitation during the 1980s:
- A. viscosurgery
- B. increased use of closed-loop anterior chamber IOLs
- C. publication of scientific proof that complete cortical cleanup during ECCE is not particularly necessary or desirable because retained epithelial cells rarely cause complications
- D. introduction of medical therapies designed to prevent lens opacification or to prevent progression of cataract, thus lessening the need for surgical intervention
- E. none of the above

33. Intraocular lenses with loops (haptics) may be placed so that the loops are implanted in either the ciliary sulcus or the capsular bag. This scanning electron micrograph shows the curve of an IOL loop that had been implanted "in the bag." In this photograph the lens capsular bag that ensheathed the loop (curved structure below, coursing horizontally) has been ripped artifactitiously and detached from the loop and is seen above the lens loop at the top of the figure.

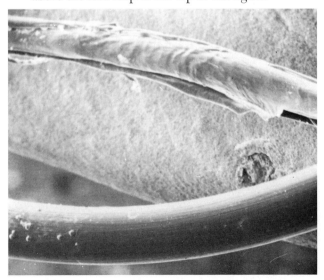

Following are theoretic advantages of placement of both loops in the capsular bag:
- A. There is a potential for posterior iris chafing and erosion of the loop into the ciliary body if placed in the sulcus.
- B. If uveitis ensues, there appears to be much more direct contact of the surface of active metabolism tissue of a loop that is implanted in the sulcus and thus not protected by the surrounding capsular bag.
- C. The lens capsule surrounding the loop after bag implantation seems to provide a protective cover around the loop, a theoretic advantage thus being the prevention of possible alterations of the loop.
- D. Loops implanted within the capsular bag generally remain well centered.
- E. All of the above.

34. This IOL was removed from a patient who had postoperative uveitis. (Note the pigmented uveal tissue on portions of the lens, especially at the far right).

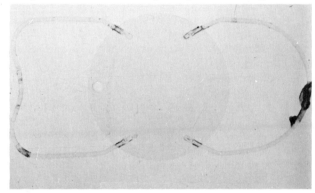

This lens is an example of:
- A. a closed-loop anterior chamber lens
- B. an anterior chamber lens with footplate
- C. a posterior chamber lens designed for implantation in the ciliary sulcus
- D. a posterior chamber lens designed for implantation in the capsular bag
- E. an iris-supported lens

35. Following is a scanning electron micrograph of the optic of an anterior chamber lens.

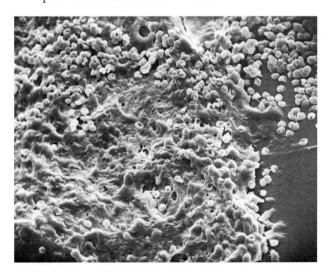

An important complication of IOL implantation that has been documented by Ellingson and others is:
- A. hyphema
- B. glaucoma
- C. uveitis
- D. anterior chamber reaction
- E. all of the above

36. Which of the following applies to continuous curvilinear capsulorhexis (CCC)?
- A. It reduces the incidence of radial tears of the anterior capsule.
- B. It permits efficacious hydrodissection.
- C. It reduces the incidence of IOL decentration.
- D. It reduces the incidence of the "pea-podding" syndrome.
- E. All of the above.

37. The most important factor in decreasing the incidence of posterior capsular opacification is:
- A. complete removal of anterior lens epithelial cells
- B. intraoperative infusion of antilens epithelium antibodies
- C. copious hydrodissection, including cortical cleavage hydrodissection
- D. placement of a slow release pellet of an antimetabolite cytotoxic to lens epithelium within the lens capsular bag
- E. none of the above

38. Modern capsular lenses are of two types: rigid PMMA and foldable designs. Which of the following is *not* characteristic of a modern PMMA capsular IOL?
- A. 14 mm total length.
- B. Modified (short C) configuration.
- C. tumble polishing.
- D. biconvex optics.
- E. use of high molecular weight PMMA (Perspex CQ or equivalent)

39. State of art pediatric IOL implantation is characterized by:
- A. IOL stabilization by suture to the iris
- B. return to well-tested practice of lensectomy and contact lens rehabilitation
- C. implantation of a one-piece all-PMMA IOL into the capsular bag, including 12.5-mm designs for children older than 2 years of age
- D. avoid primary posterior capsulectomy if possible, until vision is severely reduced at a later date
- E. implant a three-piece polypropylene haptic IOL, preferably in the ciliary sulcus

40. In terms of safety, the greatest advantage of a foldable IOL is:
- A. a reduction in postoperative astigmatism
- B. more rapid visual rehabilitation
- C. reduced incidence of intraoperative and postoperative complications
- D. allows use of topical anesthesia
- E. allows use of temporal incision

41. Silicone oil sometimes is used in selected severe vitreoretinal diseases. If an IOL has to be implanted in such a patient, either before or after the time of the vitreoretinal procedure, what would be the IOL of choice?
- A. standard PMMA
- B. soft acrylic material
- C. silicone
- D. IOL with a hydrophilic surface such as hydrogel or heparin surface modified IOL
- E. polypropylene

42. Asymmetric fixation of posterior chamber IOL loops is to be avoided because it often creates decentration. Under which circumstance would decentration be most likely to occur?
- A. placement of both loops in the ciliary sulcus after performing a large can opener capsulectomy
- B. placement of both loops in the capsular bag after performance of a large can opener capsulectomy
- C. placement of both loops in the capsular bag after the performance of medium-sized continuous curvilinear capsulorhexis
- D. placing both loops in the ciliary sulcus after performing a medium sized continuous CCC

43. In the developing world implantation of a modern one-piece PMMA IOL is now possible because:
- A. One-piece PMMA lenses can be made with high quality at low costs in developing world countries and therefore do not have to be imported; these can be easily inserted into the eye using simple surgical techniques.
- B. Spectacle aphakia should be avoided because visual rehabilitation can be impaired severely if the spectacles are lost or broken, and the optic results of aphakic spectacles are very poor.
- C. Inexpensive equipment such as operating microscopes are becoming more available.
- D. Anterior chamber lenses provide a viable alternative when the surgeon only has the intracapsular (ICCE) procedure as an alternative.
- E. All of the above are correct.

44. The most important factor in ensuring a good result after implantation of a foldable IOL is:
- A. keeping the incision size smaller than 4 mm.
- B. keeping the number of closing sutures to a minimum
- C. hydrodissection
- D. performing a relatively small (less than 5 mm) CCC
- E. use clear topical anesthesia and a temporal clear corneal incision in every case

45. The lesion illustrated in this clinical photograph is a complication of pediatric implantation. Various means to avoid or circumvent this complication might include:

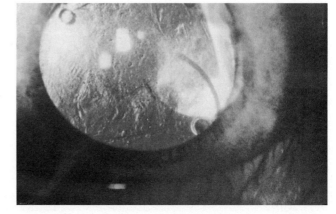

A. copious hydrodissection
B. use of one-piece all-PMMA IOLs
C. perform primary posterior capsulectomy
D. use biconvex IOL optics and IOLs that enhance the "barrier effect"
E. all of the above

46. The implant seen in this gross photograph of a human eye obtained postmortem shows an almost perfect result. From this photograph we can discern with very high probability that:

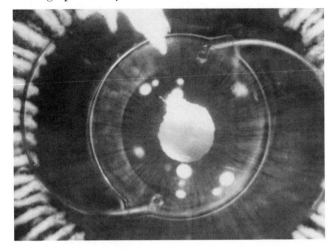

A. a CCC was performed
B. symmetric fixation of the IOL haptics was achieved
C. copious hydrodissection was performed
D. foldable IOL materials (in this case, silicone) can demonstrate excellent biocompatibility
E. all of the above

47. Surgical exchange of a defective IOL from a complicated case or secondary implantation of an IOL into an aphakic eye is best accomplished by:
A. Choyce-Kelman style anterior chamber IOL
B. iris-fixated sutured posterior chamber IOL
C. scleral fixated sutured IOL
D. ciliary sulcus fixated IOL
E. all of the above

48. The best IOL haptic material in terms of appropriate rigidity and retention of haptic memory is:
A. polypropylene
B. extruded PMMA
C. high molecular weight monoblock PMMA
D. hydrogel
E. silicone

49. Which of the following is not a characteristic of modern capsular surgery:
A. can opener capsulectomy
B. CCC
C. hydrodissection
D. cortical cleaving hydrodissection
E. phacoemulsification

50. Complications of Nd:YAG laser posterior capsulotomy include:
A. damage (pitting) to the IOL
B. increased incidence of posterior capsular opacification
C. corneal decompensation

D. closed-angle glaucoma
E. phacoanaphylactic endophthalmitis

CHAPTER 5

1. All of the following statements regarding photorefractive keratectomy (PRK) are true *except:*
A. the greater the attempted correction, the higher the risk of postoperative haze
B. the larger the ablation zone diameter, the greater the depth of ablation required to produce the same refractive correction
C. postoperative pain, peaking at 4 to 6 hours postoperatively, usually resolves within 12 hours corresponding with the duration of the epithelial defect
D. despite the accuracy of the Argon-Floride laser, there still is a considerable interpatient variability in regard to wound healing, and therefore, in response to treatment
E. interpatient variability in regard to wound healing in photorefractive keratectomy increases as the amount of attempted correction increases

2. This histopathologic picture could have been produced by which of the following surgical procedures?

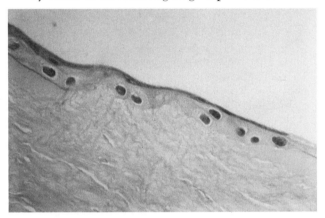

A. automated in situ keratomileus
B. myopic cryokeratomileusis
C. laser in situ keratomileusis
D. all of the above
E. none of the above

3. Which of the following statements is (are) true:
A. After complete wound healing in radial keratotomy, the structural integrity of the cornea is restored to normal.
B. Complete wound healing in radial keratotomy occurs within 6 months of the original surgery.
C. "Miniradial keratotomy (RK)" incisions offer a significantly stronger structural integrity than classical RK incisions.
D. Radial keratotomy and mini RK are no longer viable options in the treatment of myopia.
E. The American technique has a greater effect than the Russian technique.

4. Complications and side effects of radial keratotomy include all of the following *except:*
A. starburst/glare
B. endothelial cell loss
C. progressive hyperopia

D. diurnal fluctuation

E. progressive myopia

5. Intrastromal corneal rings:

A. may be used to correct hyperopia

B. may be used to correct myopia

C. do not alter the structure of the central cornea

D. are reversible

E. all of the above

6. Which of the following factors are shown to be present in the early postoperative healing phase (1 week to 4 months) after PRK?

A. type VII collagen

B. type III collagen

C. hyaluronic acid

D. fibronectin

E. all of the above

7. Which of the following statements regarding long-term healing after PRK is false?

A. A rudimentary Bowman's layer is easily seen in the treatment zone beginning as early as 8 months postoperatively.

B. Although minor irregularities persist as late as 18 months postoperatively, the epithelial basement membrane is largely reestablished.

C. With the exception of a small degree of irregularity in the immediate subepithelial stromal fibers, stromal morphology is preserved.

D. The reestablished corneal epithelial basement membrane often shows fragmentation, thickening, and decreased amounts of anchoring fibrils.

E. Clinically "haze" is the pathologic equivalent of subepithelial scar tissue, which scatters incident light.

8. Which of the following corresponds best with a poorly healed radial keratotomy incision:

A. disrupted surface epithelium

B. large epithelial plug

C. iron deposition

D. calcium deposition

E. all of the above

9. Multizone ablation, rotating masks, scanning slit beams, wobbling mirrors, and scanning "flying spot" beams are all techniques introduced into the hardware of PRK in an attempt to:

A. increase efficiency of Argon-Floride laser

B. decrease cost of laser production

C. increase accuracy of ablation amount per pulse

D. create smoother ablation profiles

E. reduce endothelial cell damage

10. Deposition of scar tissue may occur in the subepithelial zone of a cornea after PRK. This can cause which of the following clinical correlates:

A. infectious keratitis

B. iron deposition

C. dellen formation

D. subepithelial haze

E. overcorrection

11. Complete wound healing in radial keratotomy typically occurs:

A. within 6 months of the original surgery

B. within 2 months of the original surgery

C. within 1 year of the original surgery

D. only 2 or more years after the original surgery

E. only after 5 or more years of the original surgery; sometimes complete healing never occurs

12. Which of the following agents have been used to moderate healing after PRK?

A. topical corticosteroids

B. topical mitomycin C

C. topical interferon-α 2b

D. neolactoglycosphingolipids

E. all of the above

13. The first known published systemic laboratory studies on incisional keratotomy were carried out in:

A. Russia

B. Japan

C. Holland

D. United States

E. South America

14. Keratophakia with synthetic corneal inlays:

A. can be used to correct hyperopia or aphakia

B. can be used to correct presbyopia

C. demands the use of an extremely biocompatible synthetic compound

D. may cause toxic keratitis, aseptic necrosis, corneal edema, lipid deposition, epithelial thinning, and/or lens—cornea interface abnormalities

E. all of the above

15. A common complication of PRK is:

A. undercorrection

B. overcorrection

C. epithelial erosion

D. endothelial cell loss

E. subepithelial ingrowth or deposition of a Weck sponge

16. The use of epikeratophakia:

A. eliminates the complexity and expense of the cryolathe used for keratomileusis

B. is based on laying corneal tissue (lenticles) onto deepithelialized anterior corneal surface

C. is now rare because of variability of outcome

D. all of the above

E. none of the above

17. Early attempts at implantation of phakic IOLs failed for the most part because:

A. this procedure is incompatible with long-term acceptable results

B. the quality of design and manufacture of most IOLs was very poor

C. patients would lose accommodation after this procedure

D. visionary surgeons in the 1950s and 1960s proved that keratorefractive surgery was the only correct method for refractive surgery

E. none of the above

18. Following are pre- and postoperative pictures showing successful phototherapeutic keratectomy (PTK). This procedure:

A. is not effective in the removal of opacities involving the epithelial layer, subepithelial scars, Bowman's layer, and subepithelial anterior stromal scars

B. is not useful for removal of opacities caused by corneal dystrophies

C. may remove a scar or opacity, but a new scar pro-

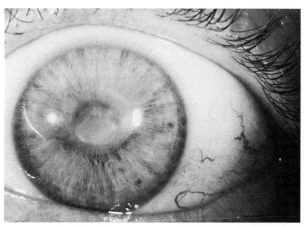 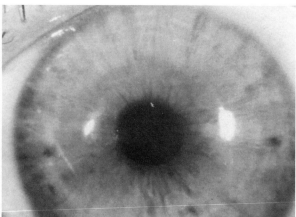

duced by the wound healing response to the laser occasionally may lead to continuing visual problems

D. is ideal for treatment of herpes simplex scaring because treatment has not been found to reactivate the keratitis

E. has shown promising results for improvement of Fuchs' dystrophy

19. Development and implementation of laser refractive surgery has been relatively slow in the United States because:
   A. much overall satisfaction with radial keratectomy has been claimed by some surgeons and patients
   B. the Food and Drug Administration (FDA) has required careful and thorough oversight of this procedure
   C. outfitting a facility for the procedure is costly and the procedure is perceived as relatively expensive by patients
   D. automated lamellar keratoplasty (ALK) initially provided an alternative to the laser
   E. all of the above

20. The complication depicted in this photomicrograph is most compatible with:

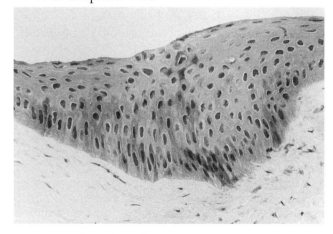

   A. no clinical significance
   B. early bacterial keratitis
   C. excessive stromal haze
   D. poorly performed radial keratotomy
   E. sterile infiltrate

21. "Haze" associated with PRK:
   A. is not related to scattering of transmitted light
   B. typically peaks at 1 week postoperatively
   C. is believed to arise as a result of the decrease in the number of keratocytes
   D. is more common with higher attempted corrections
   E. all of the above

22. Dr. L. J. Lans in 1898 was the first to identify all of the following features of corneal refractive surgery *except:*
   A. The cornea flattens in the meridian of the incision.
   B. Coupling occurs when a transverse incision is made in the cornea, and a compensatory steepening occurs in the perpendicular meridian.
   C. Corneal incisions for refractive surgery can be made via posterior keratotomy (incisions through endothelium and Descemet's membrane via limbal incisions). He later concluded the anterior corneal incisions were superior.
   D. There is more effect with deeper incisions.
   E. Healing results in some loss of effect.

23. Potential or actual complications of RK include:
   A. abnormal wound healing
   B. wound gape
   C. susceptibility to corneal rupture, especially after blunt trauma to the eye
   D. bacterial keratitis
   E. all of the above

24. Transverse keratotomy:
   A. is an incisional procedure designed to correct astigmatism
   B. is not useful in combination with phacoemulsification
   C. is contraindicated in cases of PRK
   D. should not be used in lieu of tried-and-true wedge resection
   E. can be used in lieu of radial keratotomy in cases of myopia above −6.0 diopters (D)

25. All of the following are true regarding incisional corneal refractive surgery *except:*
   A. The original PERK study was one of the first to measure outcomes after refractive surgery.
   B. Greater than 90% of effect of RK is obtained with the first eight incisions.

C. The wound healing response of the cornea is not a significant factor in the refractive outcome of RK.

D. Progressive hyperopia with time is a major concern with classic RK.

E. Mini RK offers greater structural integrity while providing good refractive correction.

26. Success with IOLs implanted as a refractive surgical procedure has been reported with all of the following *except:*

A. Baikoff and Kelman-Clemente style anterior chamber IOLs

B. clear lens extraction with posterior chamber IOLs

C. phakic posterior chamber IOLs

D. closed loop anterior chamber IOLs

E. foldable IOLs

27. Laser thermal keratoplasty:

A. functions by placing radial thermal burns in the central cornea

B. is a nonincisional treatment for myopia

C. may be useful in the treatment of hyperopia

D. creates its effect by causing flattening of the central cornea

E. may turn out to be more effective than standard PRK because it appears to undergo less long-term regression

28. All of the following are possible advantages of the intrastromal corneal ring *except:*

A. It is of relatively low cost.

B. It may be used to correct both hyperopia and myopia.

C. It does not alter the central curvature of the cornea.

D. It does not alter the normal asphericity of the cornea and is reversible.

E. Complicated mathematical models to predict the best means to achieve emmetropia are not necessary.

29. The most significant complication of clear lens extraction that must be overcome if the procedure is to be used extensively includes:

A. retinal detachment

B. posterior capsule opacification

C. postoperative endophthalmitis

D. pseudophakic bullous keratopathy

E. cystoid macular degeneration

30. The major advantage offered by laser-automated in situ keratomileusis (LASIK) over automated in situ lamella keratomileusis (ALK) is:

A. LASIK is capable of treating a much broader range of myopia.

B. In LASIK the refractive excision is made with the accuracy and flexibility of the excimer laser.

C. LASIK is much less dependable on the quality and duration of epithelial-Bowman's layer wound healing than ALK.

D. The microkeratine required for LASIK is much less expensive than that required for ALK.

E. Complications such as epithelial ingrowth and deposition of debris from Weck sponges that have been seen with ALK do not occur with LASIK.

31. Which pair of refractive procedures best meets the following criteria of a) stable refractions and b) least dependence on corneal epithelial-Bowman's layer wound healing?

A. a. RK, b. RK

B. a. phakic IOL, b. RK

C. a. epikeratophakia, b. phakic IOL

D. a. PRK, b. PRK

E. a. phakic IOL, b. LASIK

32. This is a transmission electron micrograph of:

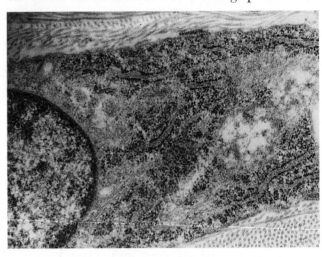

A. a cell containing abundant cytoplasmic endoplasmic reticulum

B. a cell situated between bundles of collagen

C. a cell that commonly exists at the interface of anterior and posterior stroma after LASIK

D. a cell that is compatible with upregulation of protein synthesis

E. all of the above

33. An advantage of phakic IOLs as a refractive procedure is:

A. retention of accommodation

B. less weakening of the cornea than after keratorefractive procedure

C. reversibility if a complication ensues

D. stable long-term refraction usually is attained

E. all of the above

34. The major advantage(s) of standard PRK over LASIK is (are):

A. PRK is effective over a much larger dioptric range.

B. The success of PRK is less dependent on the corneal wound healing response.

C. PRK requires less-specialized surgical expertise.

D. PRK is characterized by wound healing at the level of epithelium-Bowman's layer, which is much safer and more efficacious than the search of the deeper stromal interfaces that occurs with LASIK.

E. PRK causes less pain.

35. The excimer laser:

A. is a pulsed ultraviolet laser with a wave length of 193 nm that ablates corneal tissue via generation of thermal energy

B. is not only efficient in precision removal of corneal tissue as in PRK, but also other is used as a "laser knife" to do laser RK

C. emits photons that are absorbed strongly by corneal tissue and penetrate less than the depth of a cell

   D. is a solid state laser with a wave length of 193 nm

   E. is successful in treating myopia in the range of − 1 or − 12 D

36. The wound healing response that occurs after an anterior keratectomy (e.g., PRK) includes:

   A. initial loss of Bowman's layer

   B. formation of new epithelial basement membrane

   C. formation of hemidesmosomes and fibrils during reepithelialization

   D. unpredictable interaction between the corneal epithelium and the stromal keratocyte; for example, corneas with PRK often show histopathologic evidence of stromal remodeling

   E. all of the above

37. The development of the automated micro keratome was motivated by the idea that:

   A. The automated system would allow inexperienced eye care providers to perform this difficult surgical procedure.

   B. The thickness of the cornea was a major predictor of accuracy of the refractive cut.

   C. The speed of the pass of the microkeratome creating the refractive cut was a major predictor of accuracy of the refractive cut.

   D. The intraocular pressure was a major predictor of accuracy of the refractive cut.

   E. None of the above.

38. All of the following statements are true *except:*

   A. Epikeratoplasty can be used to correct both myopia and aphakia.

   B. Epikeratophakia has shown some success in treatment of keratoconus.

   C. Donor lenticule keratocytes are destroyed in the process of lenticule preparation.

   D. Survival of the lenticule in epikeratoplasty is dependent on repopulation of the graft by recipient keratocytes.

   E. Epikeratophakia is not reversible.

39. The Worst-Fechner lobster claw IOL is used for phakic implantation. This IOL:

   A. is positioned in the anterior chamber and is fixated in the midperiphery of the anterior iris stroma

   B. does not make contact with the iridocorneal angle

   C. has been associated with development of cataract and breakdown of the blood aqueous barrier

   D. has potential disadvantage in that it is in contact with a motile tissue (the iris)

   E. all of the above

40. Advantages of RK over PRK include:

   A. less expensive equipment required for RK

   B. less postoperative pain after RK

   C. less long-term fluctuation and variability of vision and fewer required reoperations with RK

   D. fewer regulatory hurdles with RK

   E. marked improvements in instrumentation and techniques have rendered RK a reasonably satisfactory procedure for corrections less than − 4.00 D

41. Lamellar refractive procedures:

   A. involve incisions that are perpendicular to the anterior surface of the cornea

   B. alter the corneal curvature by either removing existing tissue, adding new tissue, or creating a controlled cornea ectasia

   C. are most commonly performed for hyperopia

   D. are most useful for low changes of refractive error

   E. were pioneered in Japan by Sato

42. The intrastromal wound healing process at the interface of the anterior flap and the stromal bed after LASIK:

   A. consists of minimal fibrosis that is not detrimental to free passage of light

   B. is regulated by mediators derived from the epithelium

   C. consists of a dense fibrosis and scarring of lamellae that nevertheless does not affect passage of light

   D. proceeds rapidly and is complete at 1 month

   E. often heals too rapidly and exhuberantly, thus creating haze

43. A promising method to treat irregular astigmatism:

   A. application of ablatable gels

   B. cryokeratomileusis

   C. LASIK

   D. ALK

   E. Barraquer-Kornmehl-Swinger noncryokeratomileusis

44. The American style RK incision has which of the following advantages:

   A. less risk of continuing the incision into the central clear zone

   B. is more effective than the Russian style incision

   C. is safer because the incisions are made from the limbus toward the central clear zone centripetal

   D. provides more of the desired flattening of the cornea than the Russian method

   E. there are no particular advantages to the American style incision

45. Homoplastic keratomileusis:

   A. is a form of therapeutic lamellar keratoplasty

   B. can be used to treat anterior corneal scarring that is too deep to treat with PTK

   C. donor tissue is used to replace the excised corneal scar tissue

   D. is best performed with a microkeratome

   E. all of the above

46. The treatment of choice for a 12-year-old − 10 D myope is:

   A. RK

   B. LASIK

   C. PRK

   D. epikeratophakia

   E. none of the above

47. The treatment of choice for a 30-year-old − 10 D myope is:

   A. radial keratotomy

   B. LASIK

   C. PRK

   D. epikeratophakia

   E. none of the above

48. This is a scanning electron micrograph of:

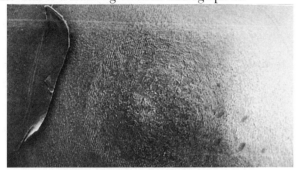

   A. a cornea removed after failed RK
   B. corneal stromal bed obtained following ALK
   C. anterior surface of a one-piece foldable silicone posterior chamber IOL removed after completion of phakic IOL implantation
   D. lenticule prepared of epikeratophakia
   E. endothelial corneal surface obtained after penetrating keratoplasty for pseudophakic bullous keratopathy

49. Measurement of cytokine activation after a) PRK and b) LASIK would show which of the following:
   A. PRK: elevation in the early postoperative stages and decrease in the late postoperative period
   B. LASIK: elevations in the early postoperative stage and decrease in the late postoperative period
   C. LASIK: elevation in the early postoperative stage and elevation in the late postoperative period
   D. PRK: elevation in the early postoperative stage and LASIK: no elevation
   E. LASIK: elevation in the early postoperative stage and PRK: no elevation

50. Which of the following estimates is false?
   A. In the United States approximately a quarter of the population is myopic.
   B. In some regions of the world, the prevalence of myopia is as high as 70%.
   C. More than 70 million Americans have myopia from −1.5 to −7.0 D.
   D. During the past 15 years, more than one million PRKs and 400,000 RKs have been performed.
   E. Although refractive surgery has been available for more than the 110 years, fewer than 10% of myopes have elected to have surgery to relieve their handicap.

CHAPTER 6

1. The following photomicrograph shows an anterior chamber angle. Which of the following types of glaucoma is *not* often unilateral?

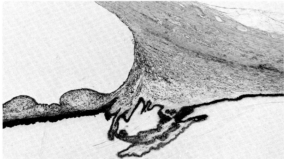

   A. glaucoma that may relate to the lesion in the illustration
   B. glaucoma caused by PHPV
   C. glaucoma associated with Sturge-Weber syndrome
   D. primary open-angle glaucoma
   E. glaucoma caused by ciliary body malignant melanoma

2. Blockage of the trabecular meshwork in phacolytic glaucoma is caused by accumulation of:
   A. epitheloid cells
   B. lipid-laden macrophages
   C. protein-laden macrophages
   D. large monocytic inflammatory cells
   E. macrophages containing Alcian blue-positive material

3. All of the following are true concerning the anterior segment tissues and compartments *except*:
   A. the adult anterior chamber volume is approximately 1 to 2 ml
   B. the iris stroma differentiates from mesectoderm
   C. a definitive filtration apparatus first appears just before birth
   D. failure of fetal iris processes to recede is partially responsible for the various anterior cleavage syndromes
   E. the iris pigment epithelium differentiates from neuroectoderm and forms one compound of the blood-aqueous barrier

4. This photomicrograph shows the trabecular meshwork from a patient with chronic open-angle glaucoma, obtained after a trabeculectomy procedure. This type of glaucoma ranks with diabetes as one of the most common causes of blindness. This blindness is attributed most directly and frequently to:

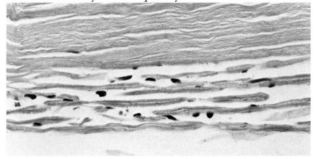

   A. opacification of the cornea
   B. atrophy of retinal photoreceptors
   C. atrophy of the retina and optic nerve
   D. Schnabel's cavernous atrophy of the optic nerve
   E. hemorrhage in the retina

5. The layer of the retina most affected by increased intraocular pressure is:
   A. Bruch's membrane
   B. pigment epithelium
   C. rod and cone layer
   D. inner nuclear layer
   E. nerve fiber layer

6. The intraocular pressure in most people is maintained at a range between approximately 10 and 20 mm Hg. A constant secretion of aqueous will maintain this pressure. This is necessary for all of the following functions *except*:

A. maintaining a regular corneal curvature

B. providing nourishment for relatively avascular structures such as the lens and cornea

C. promoting a constant apposition between the retina, pigment epithelium, ciliary body, and choroid

D. maintaining the spheric form of the globe

E. maintaining a continuous relative dehydration of the cornea

7. Which of the following is true of the aqueous humor?

A. Aqueous reaches the systemic circulation only through the episcleral collecting channels.

B. Aqueous secretion is via passive transport across the inner basement membrane of the ciliary epithelium of the pars plicata.

C. Aqueous normally contains high levels of protein.

D. Aqueous is produced by the inner pigmented layer of the ciliary epithelium.

E. Aqueous is a dialysate of blood that may be considered somewhat analogous to cerebrospinal fluid secreted by the choroid plexus.

8. A 50-year-old man reports a gradual loss of vision. You examine his fundus and find significant cupping of the optic nerve head and arcuate scotoma. Using a tonometer, you find that his pressure is normal. This patient may have:

A. ocular hypertension

B. low-tension glaucoma

C. hypersecretion glaucoma

D. secondary angle-closure glaucoma

E. malignant glaucoma

9. Causes, contributing factors, or sequelae of angle-closure glaucoma with pupillary block include:

A. phacomorphic (lens-swelling) glaucoma

B. occlusion of the pupil

C. iris-supported intraocular lenses

D. rubeosis iridis

E. all of the above

10. The small, irregular opacities seen in the eye in this illustration appeared after an attack of acute glaucoma. They represent punctate foci of necrosis in or near the:

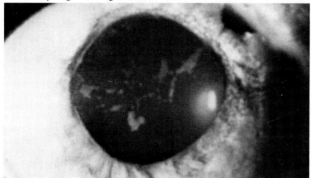

A. posterior surface of the cornea

B. papillary margin of the iris

C. posterior surface of the lens

D. anterior surface of the lens

E. optic nerve head

11. Which of the following factors does *not* contribute to a shallow anterior chamber?

A. ocular hypertension

B. hyperopia

C. swollen lens

D. seclusion of the pupil by posterior synechiae

E. iris bombaccutee

12. One may paradoxically find papilledema associated with which of the following types of glaucoma?

A. congenital glaucoma

B. Sturge-Weber glaucoma

C. iridocorneal endothelial (ICE) syndrome

D. acute glaucoma

E. primary open-angle glaucoma

13. The type of glaucoma in which the anterior chamber volume is typically greatest (at least in early stages) is most likely:

A. phacomorphic glaucoma

B. primary plateau iris

C. congenital glaucoma

D. iris bombaccutee glaucoma

E. mydriatic-induced acute glaucoma

14. In describing glaucoma, correct statements include all of the following *except:*

A. Glaucoma is not a discrete disease entity.

B. It is synonymous with ocular hypertension.

C. Most cases result from impaired aqueous outflow.

D. Hypersecretion of aqueous humor is an uncommon cause.

E. Degeneration of the retina and optic nerve is the ultimate cause of visual loss.

15. The anterior (or central) termination of the trabecular meshwork is at:

A. Schwalbe's line

B. Schlemm's canal

C. Bowman's layer

D. the internal scleral sulcus

E. the scleral spur

16. Regarding the aqueous outflow system, which is correct?

A. The pores of the meshwork decrease in size as one approaches Schlemm's canal.

B. The anterior termination of the trabecular meshwork is at Schwalbe's line.

C. A prominent Schwalbe's line is not always pathologic.

D. The trabecular meshwork is lined by endothelium (mesothelium).

E. All of the above.

17. This photomicrograph shows the ciliary body (pars plicata) of a patient suffering from neovascular glaucoma. Which of the following statements is most likely true?

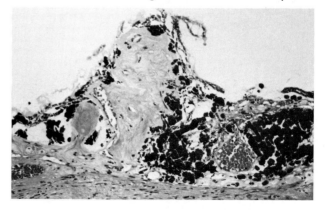

A. The photomicrograph shows a Dalaccuteen-Fuchs nodule caused by sympathetic ophthalmia resulting from overaggressive electrocautery and perforation of the globe.

B. This patient had an incidental finding of a Fuchs' adenoma of the ciliary body.

C. In this end-stage eye, a shutdown of aqueous formation and subsequent atrophy of the ciliary epithelium have occurred.

D. Cryocoagulation has been attempted.

E. This is an end-stage pigmentary glaucoma with marked clumping of the pigment readily visible in the photomicrograph.

18. The ICE syndrome:

A. encompasses multiple entities with various eponyms and overlapping tissue alterations that probably represent different subgroups of the same disease process

B. is characterized by fundamental abnormalities of the corneal endothelium, including thickening and proliferation of a membrane similar to Descemet's membrane

C. is found in patients who report blurred vision and chronic angle-closure glaucoma that develops over several years

D. is characterized by iris lesions that may range from essential iris atrophy to through-and-through iris defects to diffuse nevi

E. all of the above

19. Which of the following statements concerning the outflow of aqueous is *not* correct?

A. The facility of aqueous outflow depends primarily on the outflow resistance of the juxtacanalicular pores.

B. The collecting channels flow into the anterior ciliary veins and into the veins of the extraocular muscles.

C. The aqueous humor passes through Schlemm's canal to reach the trabecular meshwork.

D. The aqueous turnover time is approximately 80 minutes.

E. Intraocular pressure depends on a balance between aqueous formation and outflow.

20. This photomicrograph demonstrates:

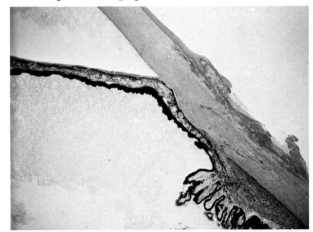

A. normal anatomy of the angle

B. narrow-angle glaucoma

C. angle-closure glaucoma

D. a reversible process

E. primary plateau iris

21. Which of the following is not associated with secondary angle-closure glaucoma?

A. corticosteroid therapy

B. tumor

C. ciliary body swelling

D. anterior chamber hemorrhage

E. phacomorphic glaucoma

22. Which of the following statements most accurately describes the condition seen in this photograph?

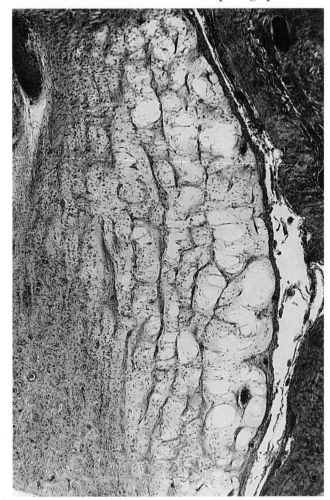

A. It is a term describing the cupping of the optic nerve head and can be observed clinically.

B. The cystoid spaces in the optic nerve are filled with a serous fluid derived from by-products of destroyed axons.

C. The spaces contain lipid derived from degenerated myelin of optic nerve fibers; these can be demonstrated with the Luxol fast blue technique.

D. It may occur because of an imbalance between perfusion pressure in the posterior ciliary arteries and intraocular pressure.

E. It often is inherited as an autosomal-dominant trait.

23. Primary open-angle glaucoma:

A. affects at least 1% of adults

B. is a condition in which it is best to avoid implantation of an anterior chamber IOL after cataract removal
C. may be inherited as an autosomal dominant
D. in its late or terminal stages is characterized by a nonspecific sclerosis or fibrosis of the trabecular meshwork
E. all of the above

24. A liplike protrusion of scleral collagen forms a 360° ring and delimits the posterior margin of the filtration apparatus. It is visible in this Masson trichrome stain of a normal anterior chamber angle. It is termed:

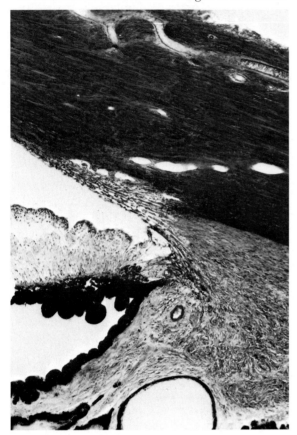

A. Schwalbe's line
B. pectinate ligament or ligament of Fontana
C. internal scleral sulcus
D. external scleral sulcus
E. scleral spur (roll)

25. Which of the following complications is *not* characteristic of buphthalmos?
A. staphyloma formation
B. rupture of the suspensory ligaments of the lens
C. angle recession
D. thin sclera
E. atrophia bulbi

26. True statements concerning the pathogenesis of congenital glaucoma include all of the following *except:*
A. Abnormally situated and persistent fetal iris processes may impair aqueous flow.
B. Faulty cleavage of mesectoderm during chamber angle development may be causative.
C. Some authorities have described a membrane that

covers the anterior chamber angle and presumably impedes aqueous outflow.
D. The most prominent factor is that the endothelium lining the trabecular meshwork may undergo a hypertrophy.
E. The pathogenesis is not well understood.

27. The iris may undergo necrosis after acute or longstanding glaucoma. Which of the following lesions of the iris could *not* be caused by glaucoma?
A. iridodialysis
B. rarefaction of the iris stroma
C. hyalinization of iris stroma
D. atrophy of iris pigment epithelium
E. atrophy of the iris muscles leading to clinical pupillary defects

28. Which of the following statements about primary congenital glaucoma is *not* correct?
A. It can be bilateral.
B. It often is inherited as an autosomal-recessive trait.
C. It must be differentiated from congenital myopia.
D. It is characterized by an open angle.
E. It may be caused partially by faulty cleavage of the differentiating surface ectoderm.

29. The major obstruction of outflow in cases of primary open-angle glaucoma usually is:
A. in Schlemm's canal
B. at the scleral spur
C. in the episcleral veins
D. in the trabecular meshwork bordering the anterior chamber
E. in the trabecular meshwork bordering Schlemm's canal

30. A 35-year-old man comes to see you after he has been hit in the eye with a baseball. You examine his eye and find that his lens is subluxated. The substance of his lens also assumes a peculiar appearance, and when you review the literature, you come across this early artist's drawing that shows a configuration strikingly similar to that seen in your patient. The patient has developed, or has the potential risk of developing, which of the following?

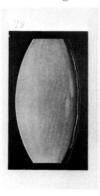 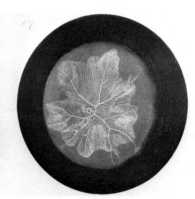

A. angle-recession glaucoma
B. open-angle glaucoma
C. closed-angle glaucoma
D. contusion angle deformity
E. all of the above

31. Sequelae of glaucoma include:
A. buphthalmos

B. diminution or obliteration of the pores of the trabecular meshwork secondary to an ill-defined sclerosis
C. epithelial and stromal corneal edema
D. glaukomflecken
E. all of the above

32. A 55-year-old woman with a mature cataract whom you have been following comes to the office with an acutely painful eye and greatly increased intraocular pressure. An anterior chamber paracentesis is done. The cytologic preparation is poorly done but reveals two cells that measure approximately 40 μm in greatest diameter. The most likely diagnosis is:

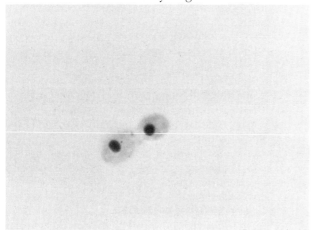

A. phacoanaphylactic endophthalmitis
B. phacolytic glaucoma
C. pigmentary glaucoma
D. pseudoexfoliation (glaucoma capsular)
E. true exfoliation

33. Which of the following statements about phacolytic glaucoma is *not* correct?
A. It occurs in the presence of a mature cataract.
B. Peripheral iridectomy often is palliative for months.
C. Paracentesis of the anterior chamber yields macrophages.
D. Lens removal usually is curative.
E. The trabecular outflow passages are blocked by macrophages.

34. Retina and optic nerve changes in glaucoma include all of the following *except:*

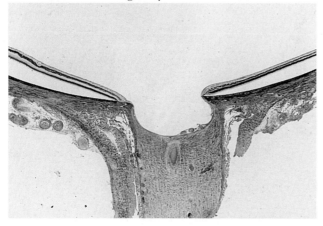

A. degeneration and disappearance of ganglion cells
B. attenuation of the vessels of the outer half of the retina
C. papilledema and/or Schnabel's atrophy in early acute glaucoma
D. the lesion illustrated in the photomicrograph
E. dropout of cells of the inner nuclear layer

35. One must be concerned with the possibility of secondary glaucoma with all of the following *except:*
A. pseudoexfoliation
B. phacoanaphylactic endophthalmitis
C. true exfoliation
D. traumatic anterior lens dislocation
E. phacolytic reaction

36. All of the following statements about the embryology of the anterior segment are true *except:*
A. The future anterior chamber is the space between two endothelial layers.
B. The anterior chamber remains narrow and cleft-shaped until the fifth month of gestation.
C. The final differentiation of the filtration apparatus occurs shortly before birth.
D. A cleavage of the angle occurs, resulting in unequal growth of tissues and a gradual resorption of a portion of the uveal meshwork.
E. Important malformations caused by faulty differentiation and/or cleavage of the anterior chamber angle include congenital glaucoma and anterior chamber cleavage syndromes.

37. All of the following statements about the anterior chamber angle are true *except:*
A. The anterior termination of the trabecular meshwork is at Schwalbe's line.
B. The scleral spur is the peripheral termination of Descemet's membrane.
C. The meshwork is a spongelike, porous tissue with walls of collagen and elastic tissue lined by endothelium.
D. The endothelium of the trabecular meshwork is a continuation of the corneal endothelium.
E. Aqueous passes through juxtacanalicular pores, the smallest pores of the meshwork, before leaving in Schlemm's canal.

38. Causes of secondary open-angle glaucoma include all of the following *except:*
A. corticosteroids
B. inflammation
C. pseudoexfoliation
D. diabetes mellitus
E. increased episcleral venous pressure

39. True statements about angle-closure glaucoma with pupillary block include all of the following *except:*
A. Hyperopic eyes are especially vulnerable.
B. The sudden rise in intraocular pressure results from apposition of peripheral iris to trabecular meshwork after pupillary block.
C. Secondary angle-closure glaucoma with pupillary block most commonly follows trauma or inflammation.
D. Occlusion of the pupil is secondary to formation of a membrane across the pupillary aperture.

E. Seclusion of the pupil is created by peripheral anterior synechiae.

40. Characteristics of ICE syndrome include:
    A. nonfamilial, occurring mainly in young middle-aged women
    B. most often uniocular
    C. angle-closure glaucoma
    D. corneal endothelial proliferation and iris stromal abnormalities
    E. all of the above

41. Sequelae of glaucoma include all of the following *except*:

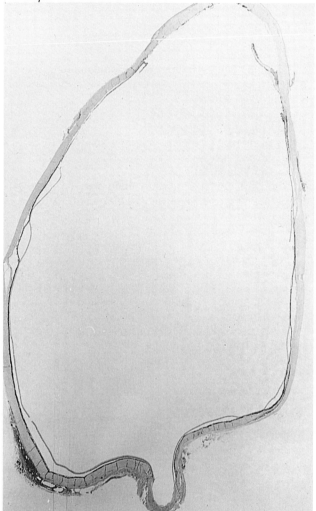

A. the condition illustrated in the photomicrograph
B. "sclerotic" appearance to the trabecular meshwork on histologic examination
C. breaks in Bowman's layer, also known as Haab's striae
D. corneal changes, including bullous keratopathy, band keratopathy, and corneal scarring
E. glaukomflecken

42. Congenital anomalies of the optic disk that may mimic glaucomatous optic atrophy include:
    A. optic pit
    B. tilted disc
    C. morning glory syndrome
    D. optic nerve coloboma
    E. all of the above

43. Changes associated with glaucoma include all of the following *except*:
    A. segmental iris atrophy
    B. transillumination defects of the mid iris
    C. shortened, blunted, hyalinized ciliary processes
    D. thickening of the ciliary body basement membrane
    E. white, punctate opacities in the subcapsular cortex of the lens

44. True statements about ICE include:
    A. The common pathogenesis appears to be a fundamental abnormality of the corneal endothelium.
    B. Essential iris atrophy shows peripheral anterior synechia displacement of the pupil toward the synechia with ectropion uvea, iris stromal atrophy, and iris hole formation.
    C. Iris nevus syndrome (Cogan-Reese) is characterized by a diffuse nevus of the anterior iris that is an effacement of the normal pattern of the iris surface.
    D. Chandler's syndrome is thought to lie on a spectrum midway between essential iris atrophy and Cogan-Reese syndrome.
    E. All of the above.

45. The most common inheritance pattern of primary open-angle glaucoma is:
    A. autosomal dominant
    B. autosomal recessive
    C. X-linked recessive
    D. maternal mitochondrial DNA
    E. paternally derived haplotypes

46. The borders of the anterior chamber include all of the following *except*:
    A. posterior surface of the cornea
    B. anterior chamber angle recess
    C. anterior surface of the iris
    D. ciliary processes
    E. anterior surface of the lens across the pupillary aperture

47. True statements about the anterior segment include:
    A. The anterior chamber volume is approximately 0.2 to 0.3 ml.
    B. The anterior chamber is continuous with the posterior chamber through the pupil.
    C. The posterior chamber volume is much smaller than that of the anterior chamber.
    D. Borders of the posterior chamber include posterior surface of the iris and zonular fibers.
    E. All of the above.

48. True statements about the ciliary body include:
    A. Aqueous is produced in the approximately 70 to 80 fingerlike projections of the pars plicata.
    B. The stroma, of mesectodermal origin, lies immediately adjacent to the two-layered cuboidal epithelium.
    C. The outer layer of the epithelium is pigmented.
    D. The inner, nonpigmented layer of the epithelium is largely responsible for aqueous production.
    E. All the above.

49. Open-angle glaucoma can result from blunt trauma and recession of the angle (contusion angle deformity).

True statements about this condition include all of the following *except:*

A. Actual symptomatic glaucoma develops in a majority of cases.

B. Increased intraocular pressure may be manifest within a short period of time.

C. Glaucoma can develop after a delay of many years.

D. Contusion angle deformity can be associated with iridodialysis, hemorrhage, secondary cataract, and lens dislocation.

E. Glaucoma after blunt trauma cannot always be easily explained, but the presence of a membrane similar to Descemet's membrane has been reported.

50. True statements concerning the inheritance, pathogenesis, and course of congenital glaucoma include:

A. Primary congenital glaucoma usually is bilateral and usually is autosomal recessive.

B. Faulty cleavage of differentiating mesoderm may occur during anterior chamber angle embryogenesis.

C. Abnormal, persistent fetal iris processes may block aqueous outflow.

D. Atrophia bulbi is a common end-stage sequela.

E. All of the above are true.

CHAPTER 7

1. Following is a photomicrograph of a bleached section of a normal iris showing the stroma, posterior epithelial layers, and dilator muscle. Which of the following statements about pigmented cells in the iris (which, of course, are bleached in this section) is *not* correct?

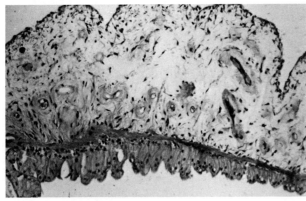

A. The pigmentation of the stromal chromatophores (dendritic melanocytes) becomes complete only after birth.

B. The pigment epithelium of the iris shows less variability in degree of pigmentation in various races than the chromatophores of the stroma.

C. The pigmentation of the epithelium of the iris becomes complete only after birth.

D. In albinism extreme variations in degree of pigmentation of uveal cells can be seen.

E. Dendritic melanocytes probably arise from neural crest cells.

2. Which of the following is least characteristic of sympathetic ophthalmia?

A. It often is seen in association with phacoanaphylactic endophthalmitis.

B. The granulomatous uveitis in the sympathizing eye

is similar to that seen pathologically in the exciting eye.

C. A diffuse-to-nodular granulomatous inflammation of the uvea usually occurs.

D. Histopathologic (routine light microscopic) examination reveals little-to-no involvement of sensory retina.

E. Dalén-Fuchs nodules often are present.

3. The preponderant inflammatory cell type seen in chronic nonsuppurative and chronic nongranulomatous uveitis is the:

A. giant cell

B. epithelioid cell

C. polymorphonuclear cell

D. lymphocyte

E. eosinophil

4. Chronic, long-standing, nongranulomatous uveitis (e.g., chronic iridocyclitis) is characterized by infiltration of:

A. plasmacytoid cells (Russell bodies)

B. polymorphonuclear cells

C. Langhans-type giant cells

D. eosinophils

E. epithelioid cells

5. Endophthalmitis is an acute inflammation severely affecting all of the following tissues *except:*

A. vitreous

B. ciliary body

C. choroid

D. aqueous

E. sclera

6. The following characteristic(s) is (are) common to both Vogt-Koyanagi-Harada syndrome and sympathetic ophthalmia:

A. central nervous system involvement

B. involvement of one eye only

C. association with alopecia

D. granulomatous uveitis

E. increased incidence in Asians and blacks

F. all of the above

7. Following is an illustration of various cells. These cells usually are present in skin and ocular lesions of which disease?

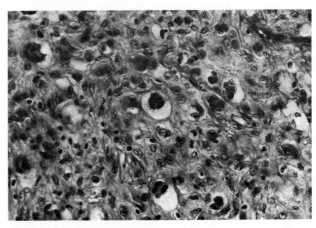

A. toxoplasmic retinochoroiditis

B. juvenile xanthogranuloma

C. sympathetic ophthalmia

D. tuberculosis

E. sarcoidosis

8. Sympathetic ophthalmia typically causes a diffuse uveal thickening as is seen in the following photomicrograph. This granulomatous response may be identical in both eyes. The *classic* theory of pathogenesis of sympathetic ophthalmia (which recently has been questioned) includes the initiation of a hypersensitivity reaction elicited by:

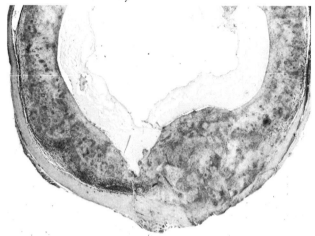

A. exogenous toxic agents

B. liberated lens substance

C. uveal pigment

D. exogenous infectious agents

E. exfoliated lens capsule

9. A patient comes to the office with a primary complaint of "dry eyes." He has numerous maculopapular skin eruptions and bilateral anterior uveitis. Examination of the fundus shows "candle-wax lesions." The condition most consistent with these findings is:

A. Langerhans' cell histiocytosis (histiocytosis X)

B. sarcoidosis

C. juvenile xanthogranuloma

D. presumed histoplasmosis syndrome

E. toxoplasmic retinochoroiditis

10. Which of the following statements is true regarding pigmented cells of the uveal tract?

A. Dendritic melanocytes are derived from the embryonic neural crest.

B. Dendritic melanocytes are derived from the embryonic neural ectoderm of the optic cup epithelium.

C. Dendritic melanocytes are the cells of origin of pigmented medulloepitheliomas of the ciliary body.

D. Dendritic melanocytes seldom play a role in the pathogenesis of uveal malignant melanoma.

E. None of these answers is correct.

11. Which of the following conditions should *not* be considered when evaluating an eye with a thickened choroid?

A. metastatic carcinoma

B. sympathetic opthalmia

C. phacoanaphylactic endophthalmitis

D. diffuse flat malignant melanoma

E. optic glioma

12. Dalén-Fuchs nodules contain clusters of:

A. modified pigment epithelial cells and/or epithelioid cells

B. Langhans-type giant cells

C. lymphocytes and mast cells

D. plasmacytoid cells and/or Russell bodies

E. polymorphonuclear cells and eosinophils

13. Secondary changes seen in the lens following uveitis include all of the following *except:*

A. anterior subcapsular cataract

B. posterior subcapsular cataract

C. liquefaction of lens cortex

D. nuclear cataract

E. posterior migration of lens epithelium

14. A 60-year-old white woman presents with a slightly pigmented lesion on fundus examination. Findings that would prompt a working diagnosis of a malignant lesion would include:

A. a history of adenocarcinoma of the breast

B. 6-mm elevation of the lesion

C. mushroom (collar-button) shape of the lesion

D. a darkly pigmented, discrete lesion elevated 0.5 mm with a total diameter of 0.5 disc diameter situated on the optic nerve head

E. "double" circulation with numerous intraneoplastic vessels seen by fluorescein angiography

15. Following is a photomicrograph of a choroidal mass. The lesion shown is most consistent with:

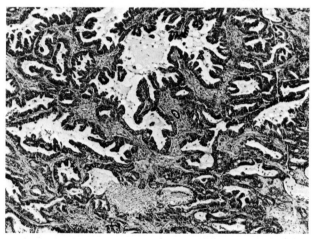

A. nongranulomatous choroiditis

B. sympathetic ophthalmia

C. histiocytosis

D. metastatic carcinoma

E. diffuse flat malignant melanoma

16. Which of the following does *not* contribute to the formation of a cyclitic membrane in uveitis and phthisis bulbi?

A. metaplastic ciliary epithelium

B. organized inflammatory residua

C. lens capsule

D. organized blood in the retrolental region

E. fibrous organization involving the anterior vitreous face

17. The most common metastasizing neoplasm to the uveal tract is:

A. malignant melanoma of the skin

B. bronchogenic carcinoma
C. prostate carcinoma
D. breast carcinoma
E. adenocarcinoma of the ovary

18. Tissue changes indicative of phthisis bulbi include all of the following *except:*
    A. hypotony
    B. marked thickening of the sclera
    C. intraocular bone formation arising from choroidal mesoderm (mesectoderm)
    D. high incidence of detachment and disorganization of the sensory retina
    E. high incidence of calcareous degeneration of the lens

19. Malignant melanomas usually arise from:
    A. pigment epithelium derived from the posterior layer of the embryonic optic cup
    B. mesenchymal (mesectodermal) cells
    C. hyperplastic pigmented epithelium of the ciliary body
    D. melanocytes of neural crest origin
    E. hyperplastic pigmented epithelium of the retina

20. The following generally is true regarding iris malignant melanomas:
    A. may be cured by simple excision
    B. have a poor prognosis
    C. usually are composed of epithelioid cells
    D. usually require a wide block excision (e.g., an iridocyclectomy)
    E. commonly metastasize to the liver

21. This photomicrograph shows a choroidal malignant melanoma in which diagnosis was delayed and massive extraocular extension had occurred. All of the following characteristics of pigmented lesions and ancillary diagnostic studies may help in the diagnosis of malignant melanoma (and ideally avoid such a catastrophe) *except:*

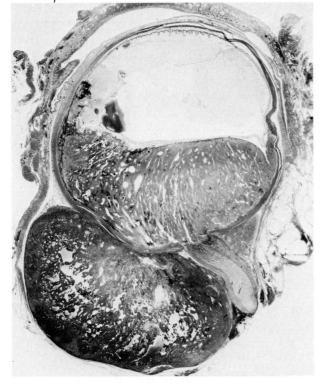

A. ultrasound
B. contour of the lesion
C. rate of growth
D. fluorescein angiogram
E. electroretinogram

22. A 30-year-old patient presents with eye pain; examination reveals flare, cells, and keratic precipitates along with bilateral painless parotid gland swelling. Which of the following statements regarding this condition is *false?*
    A. Bilateral anterior uveitis is a well-established intraocular manifestation of this disease.
    B. Biopsy of conjunctival tissues may reveal noncaseating granulomas.
    C. Candle-wax lesions sometimes are noted in this disease.
    D. The Kviem test is a helpful diagnostic tool.
    E. The lack of a hilar mass on chest radiograph rules out this disease.

23. The most common site of metastasis of a primary melanoma of the uvea is the:
    A. lung
    B. liver
    C. brain
    D. other eye
    E. one

24. A 60-year-old woman comes to the office reporting decreased visual acuity in her left eye. On ophthalmoscopic examination a solid retinal detachment is seen. Fluorescein angiography shows diffuse leakage of dye from the subretinal mass and a vascular network within the mass distinct from the overlying retinal vessels. A-scan ultrasound shows low-medium reflectivity. B-scan ultrasound shows an outline of the tumor similar in appearance to that seen in this photomicrograph of an enucleated eye from another patient. The most likely diagnosis is:

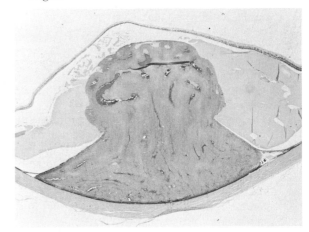

A. malignant melanoma
B. hemangioma
C. melanocytoma
D. chorioretinal inflammatory processes
E. metastatic carcinoma

25. Major criteria to be assessed when attempting to estimate a prognosis for a patient with uveal malignant melanoma include:

A. length of time between discovery of the lesion and excision or enucleation

B. cell typing according to Callender's or McClean's classification

C. size of tumor

D. presence or extent of epibulbar extension

E. all of the above

26. The differential diagnosis of uveitis in which the biopsy reveals epithelioid and giant cells includes:

    A. sarcoidosis
    B. sympathetic ophthalmia
    C. tuberculosis
    D. leprosy
    E. all of the above

27. Which of the following statements about prognosis of malignant melanoma after enucleation is *not* correct?

    A. Patients with a mixed cell type have a worse prognosis than those with a pure epithelioid cell type.
    B. Patients with a pure epithelioid cell type have a 5-year survival rate of less than 30%.
    C. Patients with diffuse flat melanomas have a poor prognosis.
    D. Patients with spindle cell A lesions have a 5-year survival rate of approximately 95%.
    E. Patients with necrotic lesions often have a poor prognosis.

28. Tumors that have shown metastasis to the choroid include:

    A. renal cell carcinoma
    B. bronchogenic carcinoma
    C. malignant melanoma of the skin
    D. adenocarcinoma of the breast
    E. all of the above

29. The disease represented by this photomicrograph may show all of the following features *except:*

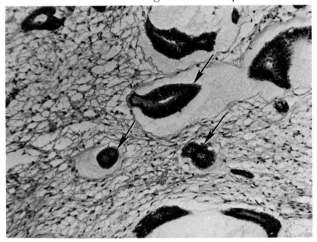

    A. rosettelike and/or neural tubelike structures
    B. structures resembling a two-layered, crescent-shaped optic cup
    C. stroma that may represent an attempt to form embryonic vitreous
    D. cuboidal epithelial cells
    E. organized lens substance

30. A 5-year-old presents with granulomatous uveitis and a spontaneous hyphema. Which of the following is *false?*

    A. The diagnosis may be established with skin biopsy.

B. Giant cells containing a lipoid material may be present in the inflammatory lesions.

C. Candle-wax lesions are pathognomic.

D. Neoplasms (e.g., retinoblastoma) should be considered in the differential diagnosis.

E. This condition is probably cause by a nematode (*Toxocara canis*).

31. Which of the following statements about teratoid medulloepitheliomas is *not* correct?

    A. They usually occur at the posterior pole, not at the ciliary body.
    B. These lesions differ from simple medulloepitheliomas because of the presence of one or more heteroplastic elements.
    C. The microscopic appearance of some of these tumors may resemble a rhabdomyosarcoma.
    D. Brain tissue is seen occasionally.
    E. Hyaline cartilage is seen occasionally.

32. Which of the following statements about acquired primary adenomas or carcinomas of the ciliary body is *not* correct?

    A. The tumor usually arises from neuroepithelial cells.
    B. The tumor shows only moderate propensity to metastasize.
    C. The tumor usually is seen in children.
    D. When the tumor is small, local excision is considered the treatment of choice.
    E. Tumor cells usually show differentiation toward more mature epithelium when compared with cells of a medulloepithelioma.

33. The following condition is not associated with intraocular cartilage:

    A. phthisis bulbi
    B. teratoid medulloepithelioma
    C. trisomy 13
    D. diktyoma
    E. malignant neuroepithelial tumor of the ciliary body in childhood

34. Following is a photomicrograph of a uveal lesion. It is most consistent with:

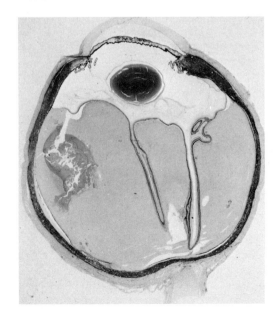

A. leukemic infiltrate
B. medulloepithelioma
C. adenocarcinoma
D. diffuse flat melanoma
E. melanocytoma

35. Following is a photomicrograph of a uveal malignant melanoma. Which major cell type and/or cellular pattern is present?

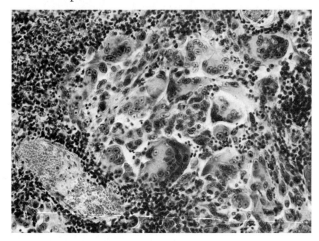

A. spindle cell A
B. spindle cell B
C. fascicular
D. mixed spindle cell and epithelioid
E. necrotic

36. The best way to prevent sympathetic ophthalmia after a penetrating globe injury with vision loss is:
A. high potency topical steroids
B. external beam irradiation to the injured eye
C. prompt enucleation of the injured eye
D. anti-Retinal S antiserum therapy
E. repositioning of prolapsed uvea

37. Sarcoid chorioretinitis is characterized by all of the following *except*:
A. sheathing of the retinal vessels
B. potential neovascularization
C. candle wax lesions
D. caseating granulomas
E. association with other evidence of central nervous system involvement

38. Neural crest cells give rise to all of the following *except*:
A. skin melanocytes
B. Schwann cells
C. cells that determine iris color
D. retinal vasculature
E. various hamastomas and/or choristomas seen in the phakomatoses

39. Complications of Langerhans' cell histiocyrosis (histiocytosis X) include all of the following *except*:
A. intraocular infiltrates
B. diabetes and intraorbital insipidus
C. nevoxanthoendothelioma
D. exophthalmos
E. bone infiltrates

40. This is an intraoperative photograph of a local resection of a choroidal malignant melanoma. The following conditions generally are contradictions to local resection:

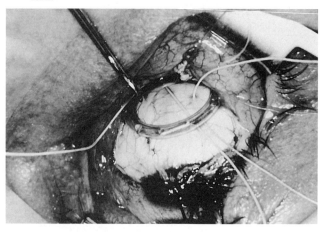

A. diffuse flat melanoma
B. episcleral peripapillary melanoma
C. metastatic choroidal masses
D. choroidal melanoma with emissarial extension
E. all of the above

41. Concerning the vascular supply of the eye:
A. The short posterior ciliary arteries from the circle of Zinn-Haller.
B. Anterior and posterior ciliary arteries contribute to a plexus of channels that converge at the major iris circle.
C. Both retinal pigment epithelium (RPE) and outer retinal layers depend on the choriocapillaris for nutritional support.
D. The ciliary vessels are important in the pathogenesis of anterior ischemic optic neuropathy (AION).
E. All of the above.

42. According to the classification of melanocytic neoplasms by Apple and Blodi:
A. Phase A malignant melanoma tumors have extended outside the globe.
B. Phase B malignant melanoma tumors show more anaplastic features than Phase A.
C. Both Phase A and Phase B tumors have near equal metastatic potential.
D. Collar button morphology is a hallmark of Phase A tumors and is a good prognostic sign.
E. All of the above are true.

43. Concerning Vogt-Koyanagi-Harada (VKH) syndrome:
A. It is most common in northern Europeans > 50 years old.
B. It usually presents as bilateral uveitis.
C. It seldom affects the retina.
D. It is inherited in an autosomal dominant pattern.
E. The histopathologic picture of the uveal infiltrates is differentiated readily from that of apathetic ophthalmia.

44. The angiographic finding of a "double circulation" suggests:
A. phthisis with shrinkage
B. endophthalmitis
C. malignant melanoma
D. retinal hemangioma
E. choroidal nevus

45. The globe illustrated in this photomicrograph was subjected to a corneal-scleral laceration with complete perforation of the cornea-sclera and uveal prolapse. The most likely diagnosis is:

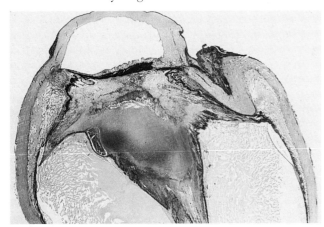

   A. sympathetic ophthalmia
   B. hemophthalmos
   C. *P. acnes* endophthalmitis
   D. phacoanaphylactic endophthalmitis
   E. acute purulent endophthalmitis

46. Phthisis bulbi is associated with all of the following changes *except*:
   A. scleral thickening
   B. disorganization of intraocular contents
   C. intraocular osseous metaplasia of RPE and/or ciliary epithelium
   D. intraocular cartilage formation
   E. cyclitic membrane

47. During the development of the iris:
   A. Both dilator and sphincter muscles arise from ectoderm analagous to formation of the erector pili muscle.
   B. Final color is determined shortly after birth by the melanin content of the pigmented epithelial bilayer.
   C. Stromal components develop from the ectoderm of the optic cup.
   D. All of the above.
   E. None of the above.

48. Segmental iris atrophy and necrosis suggest:
   A. phthisis bulbi
   B. the pressure of a medulloepithelioma (diktyoma) in the anterior chamber
   C. ongoing anterior segment ischemia syndrome
   D. denervation of the iris
   E. heterochromia iridis

49. Langerhans' cells can be identified by all of the following *except*:
   A. Birbeck granules
   B. antigens, including HLA-DR antigens
   C. positive for vimentin
   D. positive S-100 markers
   E. all of the above

50. The cell type illustrated in the following photomicrograph of an intraocular tumor is:

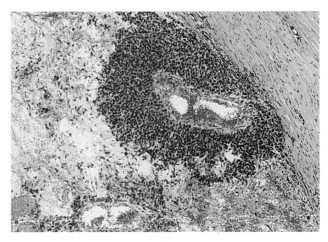

   A. RPE
   B. epithelioid cell malignant melanoma
   C. pseudorosette in retinoblastoma
   D. spindle cell melanoma
   E. necrotic malignant melanoma

CHAPTER 8

1. Goldmann-Favre disease is characterized by all of the following *except*:
   A. It is a vitreoretinal dystrophy.
   B. It causes night blindness.
   C. It causes ablation of the electroretinogram (ERG).
   D. It primarily affects the elderly.
   E. It leads to slow visual loss.

2. This photomicrograph shows the macular region. Which of the following observations cannot be used histologically to identify the macular region?

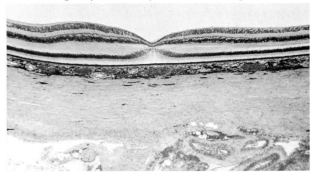

   A. Retinal thinning occurs at the fovea.
   B. The perifoveal area contains multilayered ganglion cells (six to eight layers).
   C. Cones are the predominant photoreceptor.
   D. The trypsin digest technique reveals a richly vascular central fovea that is clinically detectable by fluorescein angiography.
   E. The inferior oblique muscle inserts onto the posterior sclera near the macular region.

3. Hemorrhagic lesions of the macular region are frequently caused by or directly associated with all of the following *except:*
   A. histoplasmosis
   B. myopic choroidal degeneration
   C. Best's vitelliform dystrophy
   D. angioid streaks
   E. Kuhnt-Junius disease

4. The following illustration is a fluorescein angiogram of the fundus of a patient with preproliferative diabetic retinopathy. Which of the following ophthalmoscopic signs is *not* characteristic of background and/or preproliferative diabetic retinopathy?

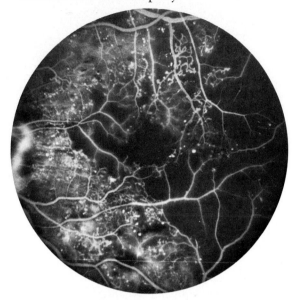

A. vitreous hemorrhage
B. yellow waxy exudates
C. venous dilatation and tortuosity
D. intraretinal microvascular abnormality (IRMA)
E. microaneurysms

5. A clinical finding common to both sickle cell disease of the eye and Eales' disease is:
A. a high incidence of both in the United States
B. bilateral eye involvement
C. midperipheral or peripheral distribution of retinal neovascularization
D. hemoglobinopathy
E. perivasculitis

6. All of the following are true about the pathogenesis of retinal detachments *except*:
A. It represents a reopening of embryonic lumen of optic vesicle.
B. It is inhibited by intraocular pressure holding the retina against the RPE.
C. It is inhibited near the fovea by the stronger attachments of cone outer segments to the RPE.
D. It is inhibited by microvilli of RPE cells attached to photoreceptor outer segments.
E. It is limited by the strong attachment of the retina at the ora serrata and optic nerve head.

7. In total central retinal artery occlusion:
A. The onset is typically insidious.
B. The cherry-red spot is histologically indistinguishable from that seen in Tay-Sachs disease.
C. Multiple flame-shaped hemorrhages often occur.
D. Retinal neuronal destruction may occur in as early as 90 minutes.
E. Extensive gliosis and retinal thickening occur late in the disease.

8. Angioid streaks sometimes are associated with:
A. pseudoxanthoma elasticum

B. bullous retinoschisis
C. age-related insufficiency of the choriocapillaris and retinal detachment
D. a benign degeneration that clinically looks like cobblestones
E. a correctable hyperopic shift

9. Following is a turn-of-the-century artist's drawing of a human fundus drawn with an inverted image as viewed by indirect ophthalmoscopy. Which of the following is true of the disease illustrated here?

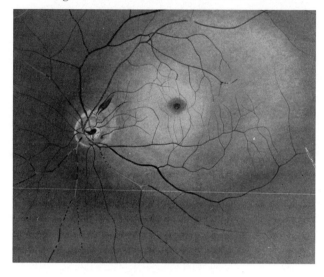

A. normal vision
B. mildly decreased visual fields
C. normal peripheral visual fields
D. slow loss of vision
E. rapid loss of vision

10. Histopathologic evidence of outer retinal degeneration would be expected in all of the following except:
A. RPE degeneration
B. glaucoma
C. choroidal vascular insufficiency
D. retinal detachment
E. retinis pigmentosa

11. Which is *not* characteristically associated with tractional retinal detachment?
A. congenital toxoplasmosis
B. Coats' syndrome
C. Eales' disease
D. vitreous loss during cataract surgery
E. retinopathy of prematurity (ROP, retrolental fibroplasia)

12. Which of the following is *not* a hallmark of presumed histoplasmic chorioretinitis?
A. focal peripheral retinal punched-out areas of scarring
B. peripapillary inflammation, pigmentary changes
C. disciform macular degeneration
D. bilateral eye involvement, although often asymmetric
E. ocular involvement usually occurring concomitantly with systemic disease

13. An important ocular finding that may occur in both toxoplasmosis and histoplasmosis is:

A. arcuate scotoma
B. a high incidence of peripapillary location of the inflammation
C. vitritis
D. keratic precipitates
E. intranuclear inclusion bodies

14. This is a PAS stain of the ciliary body (pars plicata) of a diabetic patient. Anterior segment changes in diabetes include all of the following *except*:

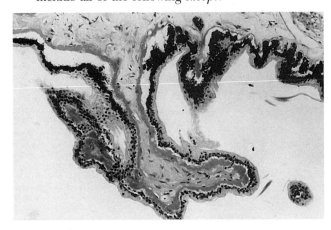

A. lacy vacuolation of iris pigment epithelium
B. thinning of ciliary pigment epithelial basement membrane
C. increased incidence of glaucoma
D. transient myopia with hyperglycemia
E. snowflake cataract

15. Proliferative retinopathy can be a result of all *except*:
A. central retinal artery occlusion
B. diabetes
C. Eales' disease
D. sarcoidosis
E. central retinal vein occlusion (venous stasis and hemorrhagic retinopathy)

16. This photomicrograph shows the typical micrographic appearance of an acute retinal vascular occlusion. Which of the following statements is true?

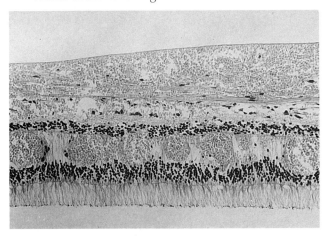

A. In the early stages photoreceptors undergo ischemic necrosis.
B. It usually is caused by atherosclerosis, not arteriolosclerosis.

C. It may spare the macula in 15% of cases because of the presence of the cilioretinal artery.
D. The condition illustrated in the photograph may progress toward neovascularization as a late sequela.
E. Occlusion often occurs just before emergence of the vessel from the optic nerve head.

17. Isolated retinitis (retinopathia) pigmentosa is characterized by which of the following?
A. It is an inflammatory reaction occurring in the retinal pigment epithelium.
B. It is an X-linked disease.
C. It usually is unilateral.
D. Formation of a bone spicular pattern yields findings similar to those of rubella pigmentary retinopathy.
E. Early changes are found in the outer half of the retina.

18. Which of the following causes of fundus pigmentation or pseudoretinitis pigmentosa does *not* histopathologically resemble true retinitis pigmentosa?
A. intrauterine rubella infection
B. trauma
C. syphilis
D. chloroquine toxicity
E. postretinal vascular occlusion

19. Which of the following statements is *not* true of the condition illustrated in this photomicrograph?

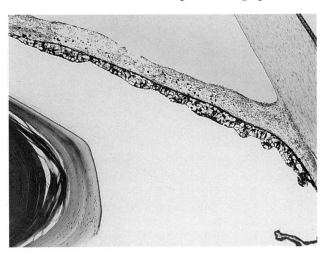

A. highly characteristic of diabetes
B. intraepithelial vacuoles contain glycogen
C. associated with "Schwarzwasser" (black water)
D. commonly seen in Coats' disease
E. worsened by very high blood glucose levels

20. Toxoplasmosis can be distinguished from histoplasmosis by all *except* the following:
A. It is characterized correctly as retinochoroiditis.
B. It is characterized correctly as a chorioretinitis.
C. Vitritis is more common in toxoplasmosis.
D. Arcuate scotomas are more likely with toxoplasmosis.
E. Congenital macular "colobomas" are thought to sometimes occur as a sequela to toxoplasmosis.

21. This electron micrograph shows a small retinal vessel. The cell labeled *P* is important:

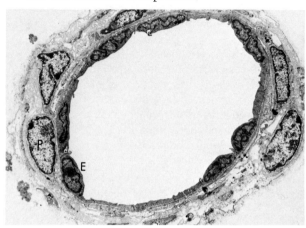

    A. in normal aging
    B. in Eales' disease
    C. in diabetic retinopathy
    D. in arteriolar occlusions
    E. in temporal arteritis

22. All of the following statements are true about cotton-wool spots *except*:
    A. They also are known as cytoid bodies.
    B. They are histopathologically clusters of ischemic bipolar cells.
    C. They are associated with hypertensive retinopathy.
    D. They are associated with lupus retinopathy.
    E. They are associated with proliferative diabetic retinopathy.

23. Which of the following does *not* predispose to retinal detachment?
    A. lattice or snail track degeneration
    B. granular tags
    C. cobblestone degeneration
    D. diabetic proliferative retinopathy
    E. trauma

24. Retinitis (retinopathia) pigmentosa may sometimes be associated with each of the following *except*:
    A. optic disc drusen
    B. astrocytic hamartomas of the optic nerve head
    C. keratoconus
    D. marginal corneal dystrophy
    E. situs inversus arteriosus

25. The subretinal space:
    A. is a true space, not a potential one
    B. is the vestige of the cavity of the embryonic optic vesicle
    C. is located external to the RPE
    D. is more likely to reopen or become detached anterior to the ora serrata because of the presence of cell junctions
    E. contains the nerve fiber layer

26. Following is an early fundus drawing. Which of the following is *not* a clinical feature of the disease illustrated?

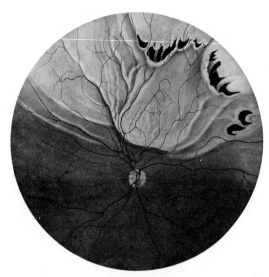

    A. The treatment is surgical.
    B. The subretinal fluid is composed of transudate from the choroid.
    C. It involves a retinal break.
    D. It rarely spontaneously resolves.
    E. The breaks often are shaped like horseshoes.

27. Retinal telangiectasia arterial macroaneurysms occur in all of the following *except*:
    A. Coats' disease
    B. Leber's disease
    C. Eales' disease
    D. hypertension
    E. von Hippel angiomatosis

28. Hereditary retinoschisis affecting the macula is associated with all *except*:
    A. nerve fiber layer disruption
    B. Goldman-Favre syndrome
    C. vitreous abnormalities
    D. schisis cavity at the level of the outer plexiform layer
    E. ERG abnormalities

29. Artifactitious retinal detachment that occurs during fixation is characterized histopathologically by which of the following?
    A. presence of subretinal fluid
    B. photoreceptor degeneration
    C. fragments of the apices of pigment cells clinging to photoreceptors
    D. cystoid degeneration
    E. glial membrane formation

30. Which of the following statements regarding sex-linked juvenile retinoschisis is *not* correct?
    A. Retinal detachment is rare.
    B. It is a potential source of significant visual loss.
    C. It is a bilateral process.
    D. The fovea almost always is involved.
    E. The congenital veils are caused by a split in the outer plexiform layer.

31. Proliferative diabetic retinopathy includes all of the following *except*:
    A. iris neovascularization
    B. retinal neovascularization
    C. choroidal neovascularization
    D. neovascularization of the disc
    E. neovascularization of the posterior pole

32. The changes noted in this fluorescein angiogram are compatible with which choice?

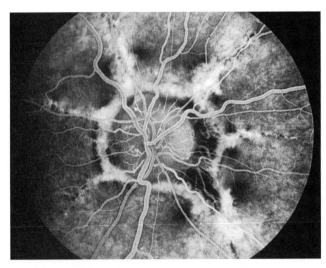

A. X-linked inheritance, afferently males
B. defective scotopic vision
C. pigment flecks confined to choroid
D. a tapetoretinal degeneration
E. associated with pseudoxanthoma elasticum

33. The pathogenesis of the foveal cherry-red spot seen in Tay-Sachs disease is caused by:
   A. lipid accumulation in perifoveal ganglion cells
   B. cloudy swelling of the inner retinal layers
   C. lipid accumulation in perifoveal photoreceptors
   D. mucopolysaccharide accumulation in perifoveal photoreceptors
   E. mucopolysaccharide accumulation in perifoveal ganglion cells

34. Following is a fluorescein angiogram of several lesions. The lesions are derived from:

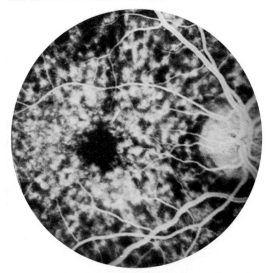

A. the nerve fiber layer, as a product of ganglion cells
B. the middle limiting membrane, caused by organization of degenerate Müller cells
C. the internal limiting membrane, as a product of Müller cells
D. Bruch's membrane, as a product of the RPE
E. Bruch's membrane, as a result of transudation of fluid from the choroid

35. Regardless of the instrument used, all forms of photocoagulation:

A. effectively occlude choriocapillaris channels
B. easily close intraretinal vessels
C. use hemoglobin as the prime source of light absorption and heat emission
D. primarily affect the inner layers of retina
E. prevent gliosis

36. The photograph shows original drawings of rhegmatogenous retinal detachment by Professor Jules Gonin. Note the areas of retinal degeneration and hole formation. Most detachments are of this type, but nonrhegmatogenous, exudative detachments may occur. Causes of exudative retinal detachment include all of the following *except*:

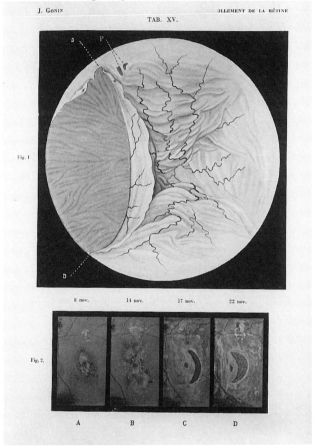

A. Harada's disease
B. sympathetic ophthalmia
C. toxemia of pregnancy
D. Goldmann-Favre disease
E. Coats' disease

37. Retinitis pigmentosa is characterized by all of the following *except*:
   A. Some types are caused by rhodopsin gene point mutations.
   B. It usually is bilateral and symmetric.
   C. Night blindness often is the first symptom.
   D. It is associated with posterior polar cataract.
   E. It usually is an autosomal dominant inheritance.

38. Central retinal artery occlusion is an example of all *except*:
   A. a hemorrhagic infarct
   B. a liquifactive infarct
   C. an anemic infarct

D. an inner retinal infarct

E. an ischemic infarct

39. Following is a fluorescein angiogram. Which of the following statements regarding the condition seen is correct?

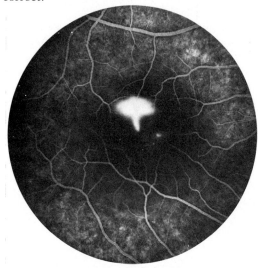

A. It represents a simple serous separation of the retina from the underlying pigment epithelium.

B. Neovascularization is common.

C. It usually affects older retired persons.

D. It results in severe visual loss.

E. It usually is located in the peripheral retina.

40. The vascular tissue highlighted in this photomicrograph is characterized by poorly formed junctional interconnection. This will cause extensive leakage. In normal cornea and retina free flow of fluid and solutes is limited by tight junctions (zonula occludens) or by gap junctions (zonula adherens) at all of the following *except*:

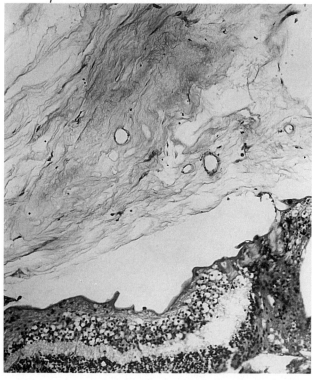

A. pigment epithelial cells

B. Bruch's membrane

C. endothelial cells of retinal capillaries

D. photoreceptor/Müller cell junctions

E. corneal endothelial cells

41. The following photomicrograph shows a condition that may be clinically mistaken for a malignant melanoma of the choroid. The lesion *least* likely to be mistaken for a posterior pole malignant melanoma is:

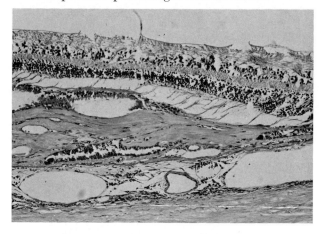

A. nevus

B. melanocytoma

C. central serous choroidopathy

D. disciform macular degeneration

E. pigment epithelial tumor

42. This fluorescein angiogram shows several lesions indicated by arrows just above the macula of a right eye. In later stages of the angiogram they remained unchanged in size. These lesions probably represent:

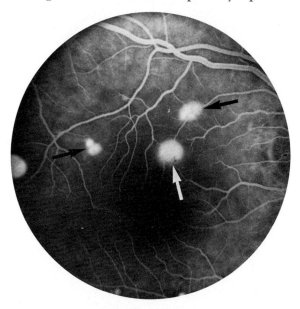

A. multiple discrete retinal hemangiomas

B. multifocal retinoblastoma

C. sensory retinal detachments

D. pigment epithelial detachments

E. hemorrhages

43. Which of the following retinitis (retinopathia) pig-

mentosa like syndromes is inherited in an autosomal dominant pattern?
- A. Lawrence-Moon-Bardet-Biedl syndrome
- B. Batten-Mayou syndrome
- C. Usher's syndrome
- D. Refsum's syndrome
- E. Hallgren's syndrome

44. Which of the following characterizes nerve fibers coursing through the nerve fiber layer?
- A. Myelination occurs.
- B. Macular fibers have the most superficial location as they enter the optic nerve.
- C. Cell bodies are located in the inner nuclear layer.
- D. Their axonal terminations form synapses with bipolar cell dendrites.
- E. There is a "spoke-wheel" pattern of convergence at the disc in the temporal quadrants.

45. The following cell is sometimes considered the third neuron of the sensory visual pathway:
- A. RPE
- B. ganglion cell
- C. bipolar cell
- D. lateral geniculate body cell
- E. photoreceptor cell

46. Following is a turn-of-the-century artist's drawing of the fundus of a patient with hypertensive retinopathy. Which of the following statements concerning the white lesions is *not* correct?

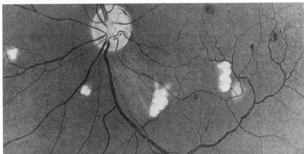

- A. They represent collections of leukocytes.
- B. They are also called lupus erythematosis cytoid bodies.
- C. They are common in hypertensive retinopathy.
- D. They may be present in diabetic retinopathy.
- E. They represent a collection of swollen nerve fibers caused by ischemia.

47. All of the following are true concerning sickle cell retinopathy *except:*

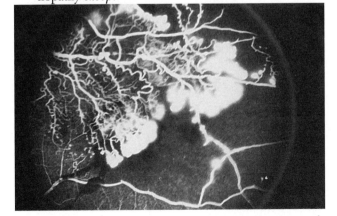

- A. more severe in sickle cell-C (SC)
- B. associated with arteriolar occlusion
- C. may create a fluorescein angiographic pattern similar to that seen in the photograph
- D. S-thalassemia disease is protective from retinopathy
- E. can lead to retinal detachment

48. The following illustrates a lesion of the pars plana. This lesion:

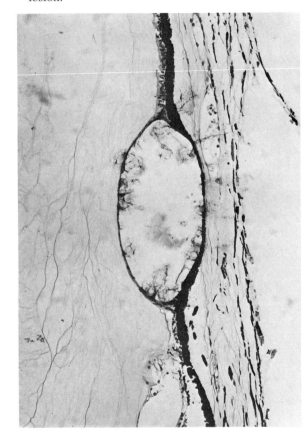

- A. typically contains mucopolysaccharides
- B. is a true cyst
- C. usually is congenital
- D. always is milky white in appearance after fixation
- E. typically predisposes to retinal detachment

49. Which of the following statements regarding degenerative (age-related) retinoschisis is *not* correct?
- A. It represents a splitting of the outer plexiform layer of the retina into two layers.
- B. It is a consequence of a coalescence of cavities of microcystoid degeneration.
- C. It most commonly involves the lower temporal quadrants bilaterally.
- D. It is located preequatorially.
- E. It does not cause a significant field defect.

50. Disciform macular degeneration is associated with all of the following *except:*
- A. toxoplasmosis
- B. histoplasmosis
- C. choroidal rupture
- D. rubella
- E. angioid streaks

CHAPTER 9

1. Which of the following statements concerning retinoblastoma genetics is *not* correct?
   A. The retinoblastoma gene is on the long arm of chromosome 13 (13q).
   B. The presence of one normal gene and one abnormal gene allows retinoblastoma to develop.
   C. The normal retinoblastoma gene stimulates the development of retinoblastoma.
   D. Retinoblastoma develops when both homologous loci of the suppressor gene become nonfunctional.
   E. Bilateral retinoblastoma can be sporadic or familial.

2. Which of the following statements about retinoblastoma is *not* correct?
   A. It is the most common intraocular malignancy of childhood.
   B. Most cases occur before the age of 3 years.
   C. In 40% to 50% of cases, it is inherited as an autosomal-dominant trait.
   D. There is no significant race or sex predilection.
   E. The incidence of retinoblastoma has been steadily decreasing in recent years.

3. Retinoblastoma often is bilateral in:
   A. familial cases
   B. sporadic cases
   C. X-linked recessive cases
   D. patients with Down syndrome
   E. patients with neuroblastoma

4. Which of the following statements concerning retinoblastoma is correct?
   A. It is derived from cells of the pars optica retinae, namely the outer neuroepithelial layer of the embryonic optic cup.
   B. The presence of multiple primary tumors in a single eye does not necessarily worsen prognosis.
   C. The cells primarily are of glial origin.
   D. Endophytic growth of tumor is derived from cells of the inner nuclear layer whereas exophytic growth is derived by proliferation of cells of the outer cellular layer(s).
   E. Undifferentiated retinoblastomas commonly form rosettes.

5. You are consulted by a local family physician for advice concerning the possible diagnosis of retinoblastoma in a child with leukokoria. Which of the following is *not* associated with retinoblastoma?
   A. increased levels of aqueous lactic dehydrogenase (LDH)
   B. the appearance seen in the following illustration

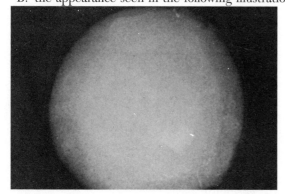

   C. rapid onset of secondary cataract
   D. an eye usually normal in size
   E. autosomal-dominant trait transmission

6. Which of the following is not a systemic manifestation of a phacomatosis?
   A. recurrent pulmonary infarction in Wyburn-Mason syndrome
   B. angiomyolipoma of kidney-Tuberous sclerosis
   C. hypernephroma-von Hippel Lindau
   D. pheochromocytoma-von Hippel Lindau
   E. acoustic neuroma-neurofibromatosis type II

7. Major factors influencing the prognosis for life in patients with retinoblastoma include all of the following *except*:
   A. rapidity of diagnosis
   B. size or mass of the tumor
   C. degree of vitreous and/or anterior chamber seeding
   D. degree of invasion of the optic nerve
   E. bilateral involvement

8. Retinoblastomas have many features in common with neuroblastomas *except*:
   A. Both are highly malignant neoplasms.
   B. Both tumors are of (medullary) neural tube origin.
   C. Both tumors may form rosettes.
   D. Both tumors produce 9 + 0 cilia when forming rosettes.
   E. Both tumors commonly arise in infants.

9. Common histopathologic features of retinoblastoma include all of the following *except*:
   A. dystrophic calcification in areas of necrosis
   B. potential for tumor cell hypopyon
   C. the structures seen in the following photomicrograph:

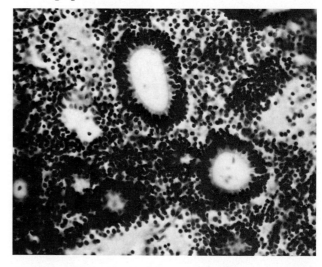

   D. basophilic staining nuclei with scant cytoplasm
   E. basophilic staining of tumor stromal vessel walls caused by permeation of calcium into the wall

10. Retinal folds may be seen in all the following *except*:
   A. *Toxocara canis*
   B. congenital falciform fold
   C. von Hippel-Lindau disease
   D. retinopathy of prematurity (retrolental fibroplasia)
   E. retinoblastoma

11. Of the following, the most common cause of leukokoria (pseudoretinoblastoma) is:
    A. Norrie's disease
    B. incontinentia pigmenti
    C. the disease illustrated in this fluorescein angiogram:

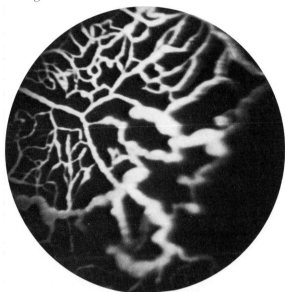

    D. coloboma of the choroid
    E. trisomy 13

12. A 7-year-old boy is referred to your office. Fundus examination and photography show a yellow retrolental mass with telangiectatic retinal vessels. Which of the following statements regarding this lesion is *not* correct?
    A. It is most often unilateral.
    B. It commonly is associated with intraretinal PAS-positive deposits.
    C. One mechanism of lesion formation is believed to be the loss of vascular endothelial cell tight junctions.
    D. It is nonfamilial.
    E. It is associated with basophilic staining of blood vessels walls.

13. Features of retinopathy of prematurity (retrolental fibroplasia) include all of the following *except*:
    A. The temporal portion of the peripheral retina is affected most often.
    B. The disease occasionally is seen in full-term infants.
    C. The vasoconstrictive phase of the disease commonly is followed by a vaso-obliterative phase.
    D. There is work suggesting a beneficial effect of vitamin E on the disease process.
    E. Later stages of the disease may include glaucoma.

14. Which of the following is matched incorrectly?
    A. choroidal cavernous hemangioma—Sturge Weber syndrome
    B. retinal capillary hemangioblastoma—von-Hippel Lindau syndrome
    C. angiofibroma—tuberous sclerosis
    D. astrocytic hamartoma—Wyburn-Mason syndrome
    E. all answers are correct

15. This photomicrograph of a retinoblastoma shows several features that should be analyzed when attempting to assign a prognosis to a given case. The *least* important histologic determinant of likelihood of recurrence after enucleation is:

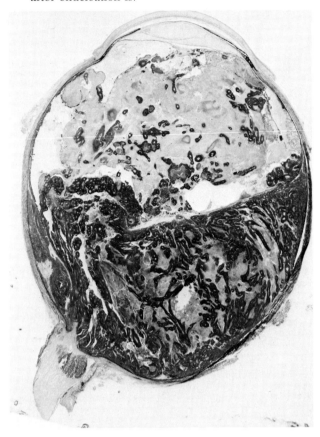

    A. calcification of the tumor
    B. anterior seeding of the tumor mass
    C. massive choroidal invasion of the tumor
    D. undifferentiated cell type
    E. tumor invasion of the optic nerve at the margin of surgical resection

16. In evaluating a child with leukocoria, one of the following is not characteristic of PHPV

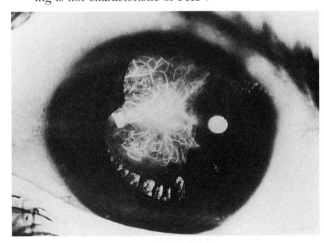

    A. microphthalmia
    B. no calcification on radiograph

C. elongated ciliary process
D. the lesions seen in this angiogram (p. 653)
E. early cataract

17. Which of the following is *not* a recognized cause of leukokoria?
A. PHPV
B. incontinentia pigmenti
C. retrolental fibroplasia
D. neurofibromatosis
E. Coats' disease

18. Features associated with retinopathy of prematurity (retrolental fibroplasia) include all of the following *except*:
A. relationship to premature birth
B. previous oxygen therapy
C. relative microphthalmia
D. calcification within the mass
E. centrally displaced ciliary processes

19. In a child with leukocoria, which of the following is true of toxocara canis?
A. Worms present in the leukocoria are pathogenomonic of toxocara canis.
B. The history reveals exposure to an adult dog.
C. The ocular disease is known as visceral larva migrans.
D. The presence of eosinophils and plasma cells in a retinal or vitreous abscess is sufficient for a diagnosis of nematode endophthalmitis.
E. The inflammation is related to the presence of the living organism.

20. All the following are characteristic of toxocariasis *except*:
A. The inflammatory mass in the macular region sometimes creates a "dragged disc."
B. The disease often is almost unilateral.
C. The diagnosis of nematode endophthalmitis often is confirmed with the finding of worms in the stool.
D. There is an eosinophilic granulomatous response associated with the infection.
E. After ingestion, the worms hatch in the small intestine.

21. This fluorescein angiogram was obtained on a patient with a history of bilateral ocular problems noted shortly after birth. The most likely diagnosis is:

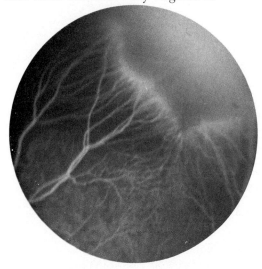

A. retinoblastoma
B. Coats' disease
C. retinopathy of prematurity (retrolental fibroplasia)
D. coloboma of the choroid
E. nematode endophthalmitis

22. Which of the following has autosomal-recessive inheritance?
A. Coats' syndrome
B. von Hippel-Lindau disease
C. ataxia telangiectasia
D. neurofibromatosis
E. tuberous sclerosis

23. A 9-year-old boy has a large retrolental mass in the right eye. The eye eventually is enucleated, and the histologic appearance is as illustrated. The boy has:

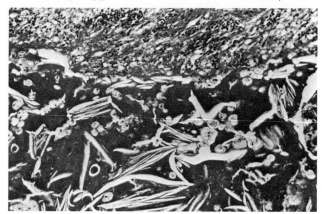

A. retinoblastoma
B. Coats' disease
C. PHPV
D. retrolental fibroplasia
E. toxocariasis

24. All of the following are inherited as autosomal dominant *except*:
A. tuberous sclerosis
B. Sturge-Weber syndrome
C. neurofibromatosis
D. von Hippel-Lindau angiomatosis
E. retinoblastoma

25. The second most common cause of spontaneous hyphema in children is
A. PHPV
B. tuberous sclerosis
C. retinoblastoma
D. Sturge-Weber syndrome
E. ataxia telangiactoria

26. Which of the following statements about Coats' disease is *not* correct?
A. Males are most commonly affected.
B. The peak incidence is at the end of the first decade of life.
C. It usually is bilateral.
D. Histologic examination shows subretinal and intraretinal deposits of cholesterol.
E. Intraretinal PAS-positive deposits are common.

27. The following illustration demonstrates histologic examination of an enucleated globe obtained from a young boy with a unilateral leukokoria and suspected

retinoblastoma. Findings confirmed the following diagnosis:

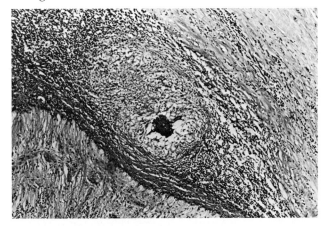

- A. Coats' disease
- B. toxocariasis (nematode endophthalmitis)
- C. incontinentia pigmenti
- D. PHPV
- E. retrolental fibroplasia

28. Incontinentia pigmenti is associated with all *except*:
    - A. intraepidermal vessicles on extremities
    - B. linear verrucous lesions
    - C. retrolental changes like exudative retinitis
    - D. disseminated pigmented skin lesions on the trunk
    - E. increased melanin in the basal layer of the epithelium

29. Which of the following conditions does *not* exhibit abnormal retinal embryogenesis and/or dysplasia that contributes to the pathogenesis of leukokoria?
    - A. Norrie's disease
    - B. trisomy 13
    - C. incontinentia pigmenti
    - D. X-linked retinoschisis
    - E. PHPV

30. Norrie's disease is characterized by all of the following *except*:
    - A. a defect in the development of the embryonic retina
    - B. retinal dysplasia with rosette formation
    - C. mental retardation
    - D. cerebral calcification
    - E. hearing impairment

31. Incontinentia pigmenti is characterized by:
    - A. exclusive male involvement
    - B. autosomal-dominant transmission
    - C. disseminated pigmentary disturbances of the skin
    - D. astrocytic hamartomas
    - E. choroidal hemangiomas

32. The findings of tuberous sclerosis include all of the following *except*:
    - A. adenoma sebaceum (angiofibroma)
    - B. epilepsy
    - C. mental deficiency
    - D. angiomyolipomas of the kidneys
    - E. choroidal hemangiomas

33. All are characteristics of Sturge-Weber syndrome *except*:
    - A. railroad track sign

    - B. choroidal capillary hemangioma
    - C. skin lesion of telangiectata vessels in dermis
    - D. intracranial (cerebellar) tumor
    - E. mental retardation less prevalent than in tuberous sclerosis

34. The most common intraocular lesion of tuberous sclerosis is:
    - A. astrocytic hamartoma
    - B. coloboma of the iris
    - C. optic nerve glioma
    - D. racemose hemangioma
    - E. heterochromia iridis

35. Following is an early artist's drawing of a human ocular fundus. Which of the following is *not* true of this condition?

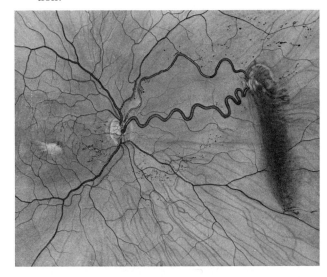

    - A. It occasionally may be fatal.
    - B. The primary lesion is a cavernous hemangioma.
    - C. It affects both sexes.
    - D. It is transmitted as an autosomal-dominant trait.
    - E. It is associated with cysts of the pancreas and kidney and with pheochromocytomas.

36. Common findings in neurofibromatosis include all of the following *except*:
    - A. café au lait spots
    - B. plexiform neuromas of the eyelids
    - C. bony enlargement of the orbit and pulsating encephalocele
    - D. glial hamartomas of the iris and retina
    - E. retinal angioneuroma

37. Norrie's disease is associated with the following *except*:
    - A. X-linked recessive
    - B. bilateral leukocoria
    - C. hearing impairment
    - D. unilateral preretinal white mass with hemorrhage
    - E. mental retardation

38. Regarding the brain findings of tuberous sclerosis, which of the following statements is *not* correct?
    - A. The brain lesions are analagous to those seen in the retinal lesions.
    - B. The lesions are characterized as choristomas.
    - C. The lesions rarely undergo malignant change.
    - D. The signs and symptoms of the disease usually become apparent by middle adulthood.

E. Intraocular lesions are caused by a proliferation of astrocytes.

39. A child with neurofibromatosis would have an increased incidence of all the following *except*:
    A. optic nerve glioma
    B. congenital glaucoma
    C. meningioma
    D. pheochromocytoma
    E. retinoblastoma

40. Which of the following is not consistent with a lesion of toxocara canis?
    A. bilateral white lesion
    B. may present as a retrolental intravitreal lesion forming a vitreous abscess
    C. a dragged disc
    D. may present as a localized peripheral retinal inflammatory mass
    E. may present as an isolated optic nerve lesion

41. The most common ocular finding in Sturge-Weber syndrome is:
    A. choroidal hemangioma
    B. astrocytic hamartoma
    C. plexiform neuroma
    D. retinal hemangioma
    E. pulsating exophthalmos

42. A mother brings her 17-year-old son to your office because of a swollen eye and ptosis. This boy has the disease shown in the following histologic section. The disease is:

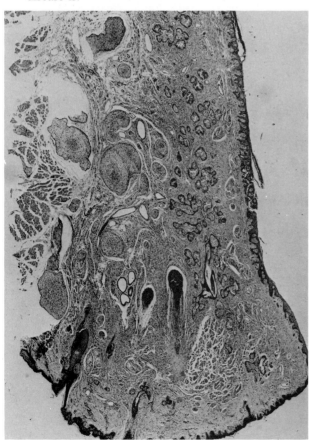

A. Sturge-Weber syndrome
B. tuberous sclerosis

C. neurofibromatosis
D. von Hippel-Lindau disease
E. Wyburn-Mason syndrome

43. Tuberous sclerosis has the following characteristics *except*:
    A. angiofibromas
    B. mental deficiency and epilepsy
    C. optic nerve lesions that may resemble the profile seen in this photomicrograph

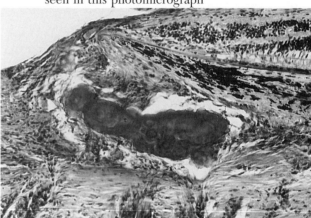

D. intracranial calcifications more common in patients with mental retardation than those with average intelligence
E. autosomal recessive

44. A mother brings her child to your office because of concern about his vision. The child has had a port-wine stain on the right side of his face since birth. Careful examination may reveal all of the following *except*:
    A. choroidal hemangioma in the right eye
    B. a chance of ipsilateral glaucoma
    C. intracranial hemangiomas
    D. angiofibroma (adenoma sebaceum)
    E. right-sided facial nevus flammeus

45. von Recklinghausen's disease or neurofibromatosis is associated with all of the following *except*:
    A. café au lait spots
    B. Lisch nodules
    C. thickened and myelinated corneal nerves
    D. central nervous system choristomas
    E. exophthalmos

46. Following is a high-power photomicrograph of a specimen obtained by enucleation from a child with leukokoria. The lesion is:

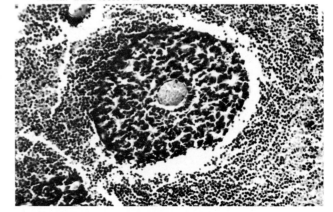

A. a Flexner-Wintersteiner rosette
B. a dystrophic calcification
C. a so-called pseudorosette
D. a Homer-Wright rosette
E. retrolental fibroplasia

47. All of the following involve the retina *except*:
   A. Wyburn Mason syndrome
   B. tuberous sclerosis
   C. von-Hippel Lindau angiomatosis
   D. Sturge-Weber syndrome
   E. the lesion seen in this photomicrograph

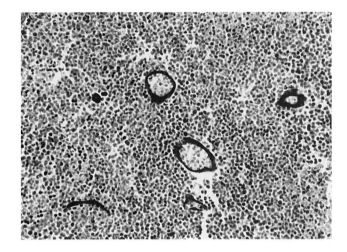

48. The differential diagnosis of this illustration includes all of the following *except*:

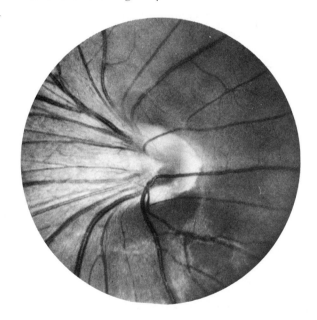

A. congenital falciform fold
B. a lesion that may be induced by a form of persistent hyaloid vasculature
C. astrocytic hamartoma in tuberous sclerosis
D. retrolental fibroplasia
E. dragged disc caused by *Toxocara canis*

49. Sturge-Weber syndrome is commonly associated with which of the following?

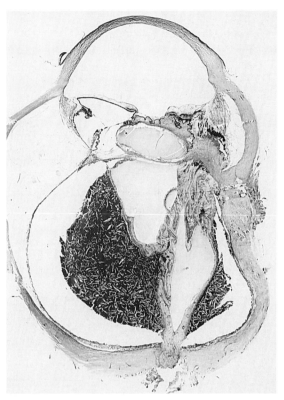

A. facial hemangioma generally limited to the distribution of all three divisions of the trigeminal nerve
B. a cavernous hemangioma of the retina
C. the lesion illustrated in this photomicrograph
D. mental retardation
E. glaucoma involving both eyes

50. All of the following statements regarding the lesion seen in the photomicrograph are true *except*:

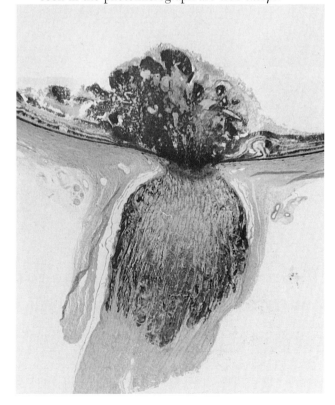

A. It can cause leukocoria.

B. Tumor hypopyon can occur.

C. Strabismus is the second most common sign of presentation.

D. The prognosis in this case probably is poor.

E. Microphthalmia is a common finding.

CHAPTER 10

1. The *major* blood supply to the disc in most of the prelaminar region, the lamina cribrosa, and the retrolaminar region is derived from the:

A. hyaloid artery

B. central retinal artery

C. posterior ciliary arteries

D. anterior ciliary arteries

E. external carotid artery

2. A disease that might cause late disappearance of the fundus lesion seen in this photograph is:

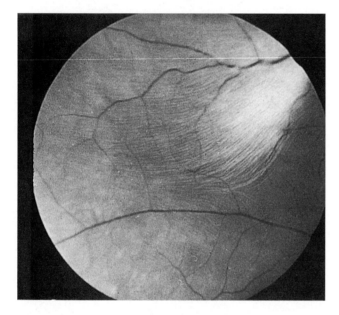

A. central retinal artery occlusion

B. toxoplasmosis

C. multiple sclerosis

D. glaucoma

E. congenital hereditary optic atrophy

3. Under normal circumstances:

A. Intraocular pressure is less than cerebrospinal fluid pressure.

B. Retrolaminar tissue pressure is greater than prelaminar tissue pressure.

C. Tissue pressure posterior to the lamina cribrosa is less than intraocular pressure.

D. Prelaminar tissue pressure is the same as cerebrospinal fluid pressure.

E. Intraocular pressure is less than prelaminar pressure.

4. Which of the following statements does *not* describe a function of atrocytes?

A. These cells function as the primary phagocyte or macrophage of the central nervous system, including the optic nerve.

B. These cells provide structural support to the optic nerve and retina.

C. These cells contribute to the nourishment of neuronal elements as an intermediary of metabolism.

D. The foot processes of these cells ensheathe the blood vessels within the nerve, contributing at least in part to the blood-brain barrier.

E. These cells contribute to the sheath of Bergmeister's papilla.

5. This photomicrograph shows a characteristic form of optic atrophy first described by Schnabel. In most types of optic atrophy, however, gliosis occurs. In gliosis of the optic nerve the glial cells:

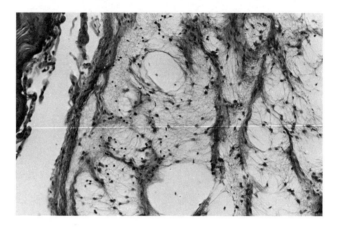

A. degenerate and are replaced by nerve parenchyma

B. appear in sagittal sections to be arranged within vertically oriented columns or rows of cells

C. degenerate and leave large cavernous spaces that often become filled with hyaluronic acid, as noted in the photomicrograph:

D. assume a random distribution throughout the nerve parenchyma

E. none of the above

6. The following sequence of cells represents the cell of origin of meningioma and optic glioma, respectively:

A. arachnoidal cell and astrocyte

B. astrocyte and arachnoidal cell

C. arachnoidal cell and oligodendroglial cell

D. oligodendroglial cell and astrocyte

E. meningiothial cell and oligodendroglial cell

7. Oligodendroglia are found anterior to the lamina cribrosa in which of the following conditions?

A. medullated retinal nerve fibers

B. multiple sclerosis

C. drusen

D. papilledema

E. meningioma

8. Which of the following statements concerning corpora amylacea is *correct*?

A. They stain positively with PAS stain.

B. They are more common in young children.

C. They are present in meningiomas of the optic nerve.

D. They are located within the meninges.

E. They also are called psammoma bodies.

9. This photomicrograph shows an atrophic optic nerve. Which of the following histopathologic findings is *not* seen in a typical case of optic atrophy?

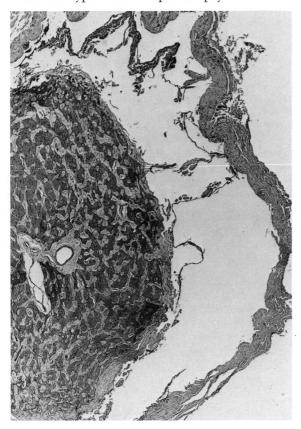

   A. loss of myelin
   B. loss of parallel architecture of the glial columns that are seen normally in sagittal sections
   C. loss of astrocytes
   D. widening of the space separating the optic nerve and the meninges
   E. thickening of the pial septa of the nerve

10. Optic atrophy that may create loss of central visual field of the ipsilateral eye and papilledema in the contralateral eye is called:
   A. pulseless disease (Takayasu's disease)
   B. Foster Kennedy syndrome
   C. Edinger-Westphal syndrome
   D. neuromyelitis optica (Devic's disease)
   E. pseudotumor cerebri

11. The cell of origin of a melanocytoma is:
   A. RPE
   B. epithelioid cells of an occult malignant melanoma within the optic nerve substance
   C. uveal dendritic melanocytes or their precursors
   D. migrated pigmented arachnoidal cells
   E. cells derived from the inner layer of the embryonic optic cup
   F. cells derived directly from the outer layer of the embryonic optic cup

12. A 29-year-old woman comes to your office for a routine eye examination. She has normal visual fields, except for a slightly enlarged blind spot, with a normal visual acuity of 20/20. However, while examining her fundus, you notice a mass, seen in the photograph below. The most likely diagnosis is:

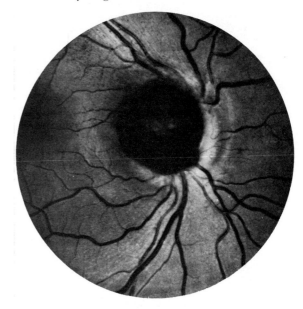

   A. malignant melanoma
   B. melanocytoma
   C. meningioma
   D. optic glioma
   E. retinoblastoma

13. Which of the following statements concerning papilledema is correct?
   A. It most commonly is unilateral.
   B. It is caused by an acute decrease in intracranial pressure.
   C. It sometimes is associated with hyperopia, especially in eyes of very short axial length.
   D. It may occur without disturbance of function, at least in early stages.
   E. It is not seen in any of the glaucomas.

14. A 25-year-old man is observed to have bilateral papilledema. His intraocular pressure is normal, and he has no history of vascular disease. His neurologic examination is negative. A spinal tap shows an increased intracranial pressure. Computed tomography (CT) scanning reveals no evidence of a space-occupying intracranial lesion. You decide that the papilledema is caused by either hypersecretion or by obstruction of resorption. This disease is called:
   A. Paget's disease
   B. meningitis
   C. Foster Kennedy syndrome
   D. malignant hypertension
   E. pseudotumor cerebri

15. The most common cause of Foster Kennedy syndrome is believed to be:
   A. tumor
   B. anterior ischemic optic neuropathy
   C. pseudotumor cerebri
   D. meningitis
   E. malignant hypertension

16. The fundus picture illustrated here:

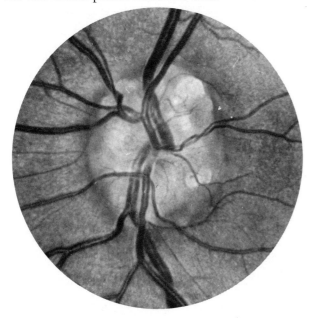

    A. often is visible ophthalmoscopically in young children
    B. represents an eosinophilic, PAS-positive deposit in Bruch's membrane
    C. usually is benign but may cause varying degrees of visual field defects and exudates or hemorrhages
    D. usually is unilateral
    E. involves mucopolysaccharide-rich excrescences of the pigment epithelium

17. Which of the following statements concerning the myelination of the optic nerve is *not* correct?
    A. Myelination begins during fetal life.
    B. Myelin in the central nervous system is the product of oligodendroglial cells.
    C. Myelinated nerve fibers normally are present and extend up to the posterior aspect of the lamina cribrosa.
    D. Myelination progresses anteriorly from the lateral geniculate body toward the globe.
    E. Myelination progresses posteriorly from the globe toward the lateral geniculate body.

18. A common reason for a misdiagnosis of a histologic biopsy of a temporal artery is:
    A. the presence of "skipped areas"
    B. the finding of giant cells within the biopsy vessel
    C. the finding of lymphocytes within the biopsy vessel
    D. narrowing of the lumina of the biopsy vessel
    E. thickening and pigmentation of the inner elastic lumina

19. A noticeable unilateral exophthalmos has developed in a 3-year-old otherwise healthy child. This has progressed slowly and has not been associated with pain. Vision in the involved eye is somewhat reduced. The eye is deviated downward and inward. Ophthalmoscopy reveals optic atrophy. The most likely diagnosis is:
    A. glioma of the optic nerve
    B. rhabdomyosarcoma

    C. malignant melanoma
    D. melanocytoma
    E. metatastic tumor

20. Following is a photomicrograph showing a particular pathologic state. Which of the following conditions would *not* cause this state?

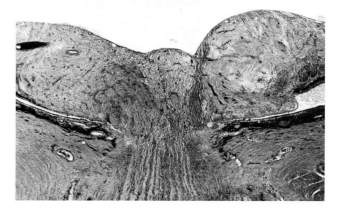

    A. acute glaucoma
    B. optic atrophy caused by methyl alcohol injection
    C. occlusion of the central retinal vein
    D. brain tumor
    E. malignant hypertension

21. Histologically a melanocytoma cell can be differentiated from an epithelioid cell of a malignant melanoma by which of the following?
    A. large and usually round cell
    B. polyhedral cell
    C. amount of pigment within the cell
    D. analysis of the nuclear cytoplasmic ratio
    E. presence of a distinct cell border

22. This is a photomicrograph of:

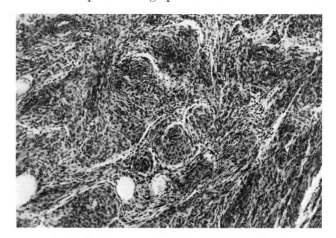

    A. malignant melanoma
    B. melanocytoma
    C. meningioma
    D. optic glioma
    E. retinoblastoma

23. The pathogenesis of papilledema may be:
    A. impairment of return of venous blood flow from the optic nerve

B. interruption of axoplasmic flow

C. increased viscosity of the cerebrospinal fluid

D. decreased tissue pressure in the prelaminar area

E. all of the above

24. All of the following are demyelinating diseases *except*:
    A. multiple sclerosis
    B. acute disseminated encephalomyelitis
    C. neuromyelitis optica (Devic's disease)
    D. myopic optic atrophy
    E. Schilder's disease

25. Papillitis (optic neuritis) differs from papilledema because:
    A. Papillitis usually is bilateral.
    B. The functional symptoms of papillitis usually are disproportionally greater than the disc changes would suggest.
    C. The visual impairment in papilledema usually is more extensive than in papillitis.
    D. Papillitis is associated less often with ocular pain than papilledema.
    E. None of the above.

26. Optic nerve gliomas show:
    A. slowly progressing proptosis
    B. optic nerve atrophy
    C. an enlarged optic foramen
    D. a tendency to cause a reactive meningothelial hyperplasia that may mimic a meningioma on CT scan or biopsy
    E. all of the above

27. Which of the following conditions would produce the most severe papilledema?
    A. pituitary tumor
    B. tumor of the frontal lobe
    C. tumor of the posterior fossa
    D. malignant melanoma
    E. melanocytoma

28. This fluorescein angiogram of the left eye of a middle-aged woman shows three separate discrete areas of hypofluorescence. One is at the inferior aspect of the disc, one is at the macula, and one is in the superior temporal quadrant. Note also the window defects (drusen) overlying this *latter* lesion. All three lesions were pigmented and flat. Possible cell types include:

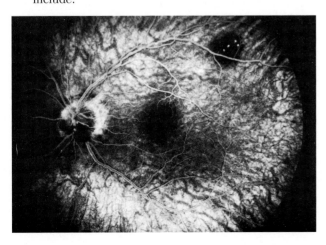

A. small spindle cells without nucleoli

B. balloon cells

C. plump, polyhedral cells

D. melanocytoma cells

E. all of the above

29. The cell of origin of myelin in the optic nerve is:
    A. oligodendroglia
    B. astroglia
    C. microglia
    D. pericytes of optic nerve capillaries
    E. retinal ganglion cells

30. Which of the following would *least* likely be seen in the early stages of multiple sclerosis?
    A. a deeply excavated optic nerve head
    B. a central scotoma
    C. impairment of color perception
    D. abnormal pupillary responses
    E. nystagmus

31. Which of the following may affect the prelaminar portion of the optic nerve?
    A. anterior ischemic optic neuropathy
    B. the disease shown in the following photomicrograph:

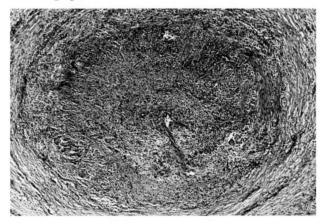

C. pulseless disease (Takayasu's disease)

D. arteriosclerosis

E. all of the above

32. Unilateral loss of vision developed suddenly in a 30-year-old woman; visual acuity decreased from 20/20 to 20/400. She reported a slight headache and some pain in the orbit when looking upward. She had no previous illness and no history of chronic disease. The most probable diagnosis is:
    A. optic glioma
    B. optic neuritis
    C. tumor of the frontal lobe
    D. pseudotumor cerebri
    E. papilledema

33. The tumor least likely to be considered in the differential diagnosis of epi- and peripapillary tumors and retrobulbar tumors of the optic nerve include:
    A. meningioma
    B. optic glioma
    C. medulloepithelioma
    D. melanocytoma
    E. malignant melanoma

34. This photomicrograph is most compatible with:

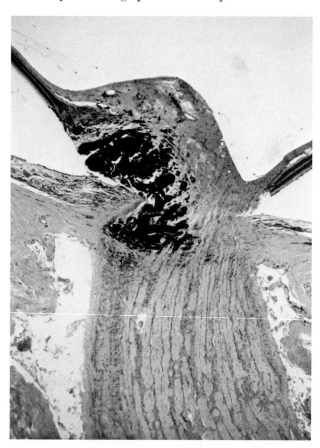

   A. an invasive peripapillary malignant melanoma invading the optic nerve head and deeper parenchyma
   B. a hyperplasia of the RPE
   C. calcified and partially buried drusen of the optic disc
   D. a benign, pigmented optic nerve tumor composed of spindle-shaped cells
   E. a lesion composed of plump, round polyhedral cells

35. All of the following cells generally are considered to be of neural crest origin *except*:
   A. arachnoidal cells
   B. dendritic melanocytes in the region of the lamina cribrosa
   C. astrocytes
   D. endothelial cells of optic nerve capillaries
   E. pigmented cells within the papillary choroid

36. Which of the following statements is incorrect in distinguishing arteritic (AION) and nonarteritic (NAION) anterior ischemic optic neuropathy?
   A. The development of cupping of the optic disc is associated more often with AION than NAION.
   B. NAION has a better long-term visual prognosis than AION.
   C. Amaurosis fugax occurs in a higher percentage of arteritic cases than nonarteritic cases.
   D. The scotomas associated with AION respect the horizontal midline whereas scotomas from NAION commonly respect the vertical midline.

   E. NAION generally occurs in younger individuals than AION.

37. Which of the following statements is true regarding the condition seen in this photomicrograph?

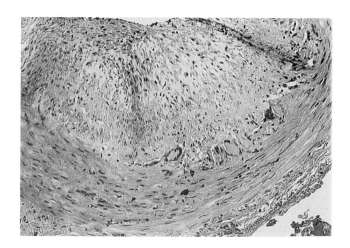

   A. The optic neuropathy in this condition usually is secondary to inflammatory occlusion of the ophthalmic artery on the involved side.
   B. Schnabel's atrophy is not seen in this condition.
   C. A Westergren sedimentation rate of 40 mm/hour is diagnostic of this condition.
   D. This condition may involve the cranial arteries, ophthalmic artery, the aorta, and the coronary arteries.
   E. The presence of giant cells is required for histopathologic diagnosis.

38. Which of the following statements is true?
   A. Optic nerve pallor in optic atrophy is caused by the replacement of transparent nerve fibers with white glial tissue and capillary dropout.
   B. The central retinal artery most commonly lies temporal because of the central retinal vein at the optic disc.
   C. Temporal crescents seen in myopia are the result of splitting of the retina caused by axial elongation.
   D. The border tissue of Jacoby separates the nerve fiber layer from the vitreous.
   E. The optic disc generally measures longer in the horizontal than vertical meridian.

39. Regarding psammoma bodies, which is not true?
   A. They are identified with heavy metal staining.
   B. They are "onion-like" structures of concentrically proliferating meningothelial cells.
   C. They can be seen in meningiomas.
   D. They may become calcified.
   E. They can become confused with nests of retinoblastoma tumor cells within the optic nerve.

40. Physiologic cupping
   A. is closely related to baseline intraocular pressure
   B. depends in part on the amount of resorption of glial tissue associated with Bergmeister' papilla

C. is typically seen more in hyperopia than myopia
D. results in paracentral scotomas
E. can be the result of cilioretinal artery occlusion

41. Regarding the lesions illustrated in this historic schematic illustration, which statement is *false*?

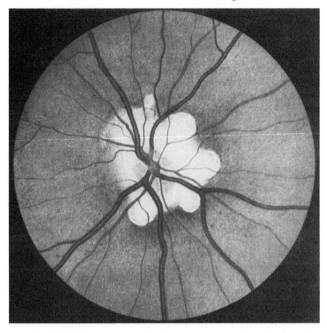

A. Drusen are more often associated with hyperopia.
B. Seventy-five percent of ophthalmolscopically visible drusen are bilateral.
C. Optic disc drusen may result in visual field loss.
D. They can be associated with chronic eye diseases.
E. They are seen most often in whites.

42. Choose the incorrectly matched item with its epidemiologic group.
A. temporal arteritis—women older than 55 years of age
B. multiple sclerosis—women 20 to 50 years of age
C. Schilder's disease—boys 2 to 12 years of age
D. orbital meningiomas—men 15 to 45 years of age
E. optic nerve glioma—children 2 to 12 years of age (slightly more in women)

43. Which of the following is not useful in differentiating melanocytoma from malignant melanoma?
A. embryologic origin
B. elevation of lesion
C. frequency in blacks
D. visual field loss
E. visual acuity loss

44. Regarding childhood optic gliomas, which is not true?
A. may cause progressive visual loss
B. represent a form of juvenile (grade I) pilocytic astrocytoma.
C. often undergo malignant degeneration
D. have features of congenital hamartomas
E. have hyperplasia of adjacent tissues such as the arachnoid

45. Which does not suggest orbital meningioma?
A. proptosis
B. optociliary shunt vessels
C. hyperostosis of the orbital walls
D. visual loss
E. chronic blepharitis

46. Which statement is not true regarding perineuritis?
A. There may be considerable loss of central vision with sparing of the peripheral fields.
B. It can be caused by extension of viral encephalitis.
C. It often is associated with orbital cellulitis.
D. The organisms of inflammatory infiltrates may enter the nerve via the pia septae and vessels.
E. Pyogenic bacteria, tuberculosis, and mycormycosis are significant infective agents.

47. Which of the following is not a demyelinating disease which can affect the optic nerve?
A. multiple sclerosis
B. Schilder's disease
C. Devic's disease
D. methyl alcohol toxicity
E. acute disseminated encephalomyelitis

48. Which of the following is not a possible cause of the condition seen in the photomicrograph?

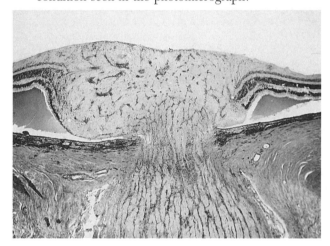

A. acute lowering of intraocular pressure
B. acute elevation of intraocular pressure
C. drusen
D. emphysema
E. brain tumor

49. Which of the following is correctly matched?
A. disc drusen—mostly unilateral
B. papilledma—more evident with high myopia
C. Paton's lines—concentric stripes from disc with papilledema
D. pseudotomor cerebri—collagen vascular disease
E. Foster Kennedy syndrome—bilateral papilledema

50. Which of the following statements is *incorrect*?
A. Optic nerve hypoplasia may be associated with coloboma.
B. Myelination of the optic nerve usually begins at limina cribrosa and progresses back to the lateral geniculate body.
C. Myelination normally is completed shortly after birth.
D. Peripapillary myelination results in an enlarged blind spot.
E. Oligodendrocytes are found anterior to the lamina cribrosa in medullated nerve fiber layer of the retina.

CHAPTER 11

1. Normally, which layer of the eyelid epidermis is the last to contain nuclei within the cells of that layer?
   A. granular layer (stratum granulosum)
   B. keratin layer (stratum corneum)
   C. prickle or squamous layer (stratum spinosum)
   D. malpighian layer
   E. basal cell layer (stratum germinativum)

2. Hyperkeratosis is defined as:
   A. thickening of the squamous cell layer
   B. retention of nuclei in the stratum corneum
   C. thickening of the stratum corneum
   D. occurrence of keratin in the basal cell layer
   E. loss of cohesion between epidermal cells

3. Choose the *incorrect* statement regarding the histology of the conjunctiva.
   A. Conjunctival epithelium, Tenon's capsule, corneal epithelium, and the crystalline lens all are derived embryologically from the surface ectoderm.
   B. The epithelium of the palpebral conjunctiva generally is nonkeratinized.
   C. The accessory lacrimal gland of Krause is located in the fornix of the upper lid.
   D. Goblet cells elaborate mucopolysaccharides that contribute to the mucin layer of the tear film—the innermost layer.
   E. The plica semilunaris is a rudimentary structure, analogous to the nictitating membrane found in certain animals.

4. The muscle that lies immediately posterior to the gray line at the posteroinferior aspects of the upper eyelid is:
   A. Müller's muscle
   B. the levator muscle
   C. the main bulk of the orbicularis muscle
   D. muscle of Riolan
   E. muscle of Steinmetz

5. Which gland is located within the tarsus?
   A. Zeis
   B. Moll
   C. Krause
   D. Wolfring
   E. meibomian

6. Which of the following statements regarding conjunctival follicles is *not* correct?
   A. They represent hyperplasia of lymphoid tissue.
   B. They contain small central arteries.
   C. They may represent a reaction to viral infection.
   D. They appear as lobular gray or white elevations.
   E. They will undergo hypertrophy in trachoma.

7. Which of the following criteria do *not* suggest or are *not* compatible with the diagnosis of conjunctival sarcoid?
   A. A biopsy of the lesion shows a noncaseating granuloma composed of epithelioid cells and/or giant cells.
   B. Empty spaces representing lipid droplets by H & E staining must be present.
   C. No specific organism can be demonstrated from the lesion after applying special stains.

D. The presence of Touton giant cells would not indicate sarcoidosis.
   E. Eosinophils usually are not prominent.

8. Choose the *correct* pairing regarding eyelid glands:
   A. Zeis—apocrine sweat—lid margin
   B. Krause—holocrine sebaceous—fornix
   C. Moll—apocrine sweat—lid margin
   D. Wolfring—accessory lacrimal gland—fornix
   E. meibomian—holocrine sebaceous—fornix

9. A disease characterized by the presence of recurrent, fleshy papillary conjunctival growths that show encapsulated sporangia by light microscopy is:
   A. rhinosporidiosis
   B. vernal conjunctivitis
   C. sardoidosis
   D. bulbous pemphigoid
   E. trachoma

10. Which of the following statements is *not* characteristic of ocular pemphigoid?
    A. It typically is a nonfatal entity.
    B. It may occur in an isolated fashion, as a complex of orogenital lesions, or associated with erythema multiforme; it also may be drug induced (Stevens-Johnson syndrome).
    C. The characteristic histopathologic feature is formation of intraepithelial bullae.
    D. It can form scar tissue leading to epiblepharon formation.
    E. It must be differentiated from pemphigus vulgaris.

11. The tarsus:
    A. provides structural support and is made of cartilage
    B. in the upper lid contains approximately 40 glands of Zeis
    C. allows on its posterior aspect an attachment for the levator aponeurosis
    D. lies posterior to a plane through the gray line
    E. is approximately 0.5 mm thick

12. Which of the following does *not* represent a solar-induced lesion?
    A. pingueculum
    B. actinic keratosis
    C. pterygium
    D. seborrheic keratosis
    E. basal cell carcinoma

13. Papillomas of the conjunctiva:
    A. are sun induced
    B. have no vascular stalk
    C. never recur and are eradicated easily by excision
    D. have a smooth surface
    E. are often induced virally

14. Which of the following histopathologic criteria clearly differentiates carcinoma in situ from squamous cell carcinoma of the conjunctiva?
    A. loss of squamous cell polarity
    B. an intact subepithelial basement membrane
    C. nuclear hyperchromatism
    D. hyperkeratosis
    E. atypical mitoses

15. Following is a photomicrograph of an invasive eyelid tumor. This tumor:

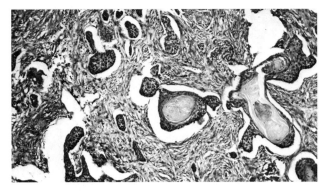

A. metastasizes early and distantly

B. behaves in a manner similar to squamous cell carcinoma of the internal organs, such as the esophagus

C. metastasizes by hematogenous spread

D. metastasizes by local lymphatic spread

E. is seen more commonly than carcinoma in situ

16. Trachoma is a major ocular disease characterized by:

A. primarily a papillary conjunctival reaction

B. inclusion bodies (Halberstaedter-Prowazek type) found mainly in polymorphonuclear neutrophils

C. the formation of Horner-Trantas spots at the superior limbus

D. formation of an Arlt's line, a scarring process, in late stages

E. little, if any, corneal involvement

17. Following is a photograph of a tumor. Which of the following pigmented epibulbar lesions is most likely to transform into this tumor?

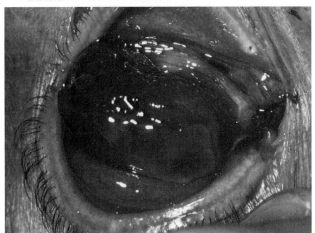

A. acquired melanosis oculi

B. nevus of Ota

C. subepithelial nevus

D. junctional nevus

E. congenital melanosis oculi

18. Pick the *incorrect* statement about mucocutaneous eruptions:

A. Pemphigus is potentially fatal.

B. The hallmark of ocular pemphigoid is acantholysis.

C. Intraepithelial bullae of pemphigus distinguish it from pemphigoid or Stevens-Johnson syndrome.

D. Ocular pemphigoid usually occurs in the absence of any systemic findings.

E. Most cases of Stevens-Johnson syndrome are found to be idiopathic.

19. This photomicrograph shows an eyelid lesion that clinically was raised and had central umbilication. The diagnosis is:

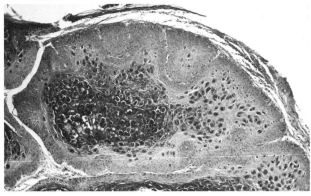

A. molluscum contagiosum

B. xanthelasma

C. keratoacanthoma

D. chalazion

E. cutaneous horn

20. Malignant melanoma of the conjunctiva:

A. metastasizes less commonly than skin melanoma

B. may arise de novo and is found most commonly on palpebral conjunctiva

C. may arise from acquired melanosis and even more commonly from melanosis oculi

D. is considered to be more malignant than skin melanoma

E. is a common end result of the nevus of Ota

21. Following is a photomicrograph of an eyelid lesion. Which of the following statements about this type of lesion is *not* correct?

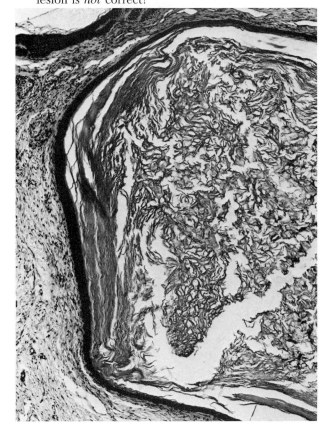

A. They are named according to the type of epithelium lining them.

B. When skin appendages are present in the outer lining, they are termed *dermoid cysts.*

C. Lesions that may show a similar consistency on palpation occasionally can result from a cavitated basal cell carcinoma.

D. The most common type is derived from the gland of Moll.

E. Epidermoid cyst cavities are filled with keratin.

22. Which of the following statements regarding microinvasive squamous cell carcinoma of the eyelid is correct?

A. Patients with this entity suffer less morbidity and mortality than those with the frankly invasive form.

B. The basement membrane is intact.

C. It also is called *Bowen's disease.*

D. It shows more cellular typism than frankly invasive carcinoma.

E. Patients have the same morbidity and mortality as those with the frankly invasive form.

23. This photomicrograph shows a common lesion of the eyelids and periocular skin. This type of lesion often is raised, "greasy," and pigmented. All of these possibilities must be considered in the differential diagnosis of this condition, but the pathologic picture shown in the photomicrograph confirms that this lesion is:

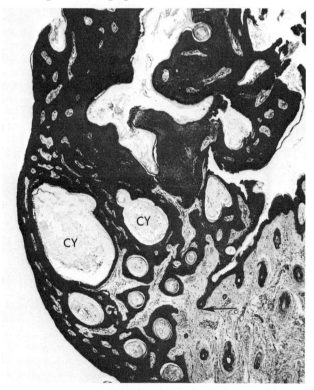

A. seborrheic keratosis

B. malignant melanoma

C. junctional nevus

D. compound nevus

E. intradermal nevus

24. Pick the *incorrect* statement regarding benign eyelid lesions:

A. Epidermoid and dermoid cysts often are filled with keratin.

B. Squamous papillomas often show acanthosis, hyperkeratosis, and parakeratosis.

C. Foam cells are lipid-laden histiocytes seen in xanthelasma.

D. Basal cell carcinoma can become cystlike and therefore can be confused with eyelid cysts.

E. Chalazia often contain Langerhans-type giant cells and also can show acute inflammation.

25. Following is a high-power photomicrograph of the edge of a lesion. Which of the following statements about this lesion is correct?

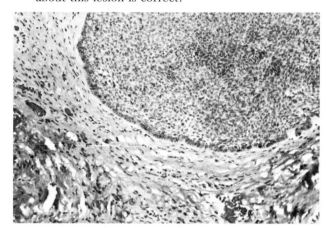

A. It usually involves the upper eyelid.

B. It is the most common malignant tumor of the eyelids.

C. It is common among blacks.

D. It commonly occurs on the conjunctiva.

E. Its morbidity and mortality are caused by high metastatic potential.

26. Which of the following lesions may show an ominous clinical appearance and may show significant epithelial cellular atypism microscopically but is not considered premalignant?

A. keratoacanthoma

B. actinic keratosis

C. Bowen's disease

D. microinvasive squamous cell carcinoma

E. the lesion(s) shown in the following illustration:

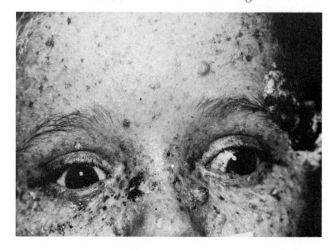

27. Horner-Trantas spots on the conjunctiva are composed of:
    A. lipid
    B. inclusion bodies
    C. polyorphonuclear neutrophils
    D. eosinophils
    E. sporangia

28. Pick the *incorrect* statement regarding basal cell carcinoma:
    A. The medial centhus is involved more frequently than the upper lid.
    B. It probably arises from basal cells in the epidermis.
    C. The palisade of peripheral nuclei provides a valuable clue to histologic recognition.
    D. It is rare in blacks.
    E. It can differentiate along many cellular lines, including sebaceous elements.

29. Clinically which of the following is *not* compatible with conjunctival carcinoma?
    A. an opaque appearance
    B. presence of dilated conjunctival vessels adjacent to the lesion
    C. the presence of a Bitot spot
    D. an irregular surface
    E. a sessile lesion

30. Clinically, stage I trachoma differs from stage II disease by:
    A. pannus formation
    B. demonstrable Halberstaedter-Prowazek inclusion bodies
    C. follicular hypertrophy
    D. duration of symptoms
    E. epithelial keratitis

31. A keratoacanthoma is a lesion that:
    A. is caused by a DNA virus
    B. has been called a "self-healing squamous cell carcinoma"
    C. exhibits solar elastosis
    D. has penetrated the epithelial basement membrane
    E. has malignant potential

32. Following is a photomicrograph of an eyelid lesion. Which of the following statements regarding this lesion is *not* correct?

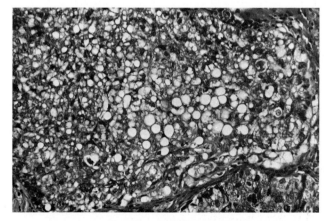

    A. It can be readily verified histopathologically by special staining techniques.
    B. It often is overlooked clinically because it may closely resemble other more common and less dangerous eyelid lesions.
    C. It seldom metastasizes.
    D. It occurs most frequently on the upper eyelids.
    E. It usually shows greater cellular anaplasia than a seborrheic keratosis.

33. This is a photomicrograph of a conjunctival lesion that some of the patient's clinicians diagnosed as a ligneous conjunctivitis. Which of the following histologic techniques would *not* help in arriving at the diagnosis?

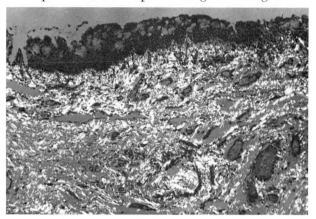

    A. thioflavine T
    B. Congo red
    C. polarizing filters
    D. Alcian blue
    E. crestyl violet

34. Following is a photograph of sebaceous cell carcinoma showing numerous oil-filled clear tumor cells. This tumor is characterized by all of the following, *except*:

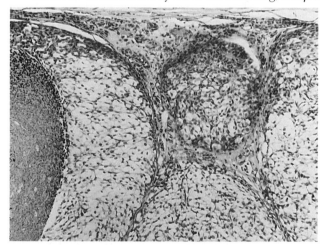

    A. The eyelid is the most common location in the body in which sebaceous cell carcinoma develops.
    B. It occurs most frequently on the upper lids.
    C. The caruncle is a potential source for this carcinoma.
    D. It has the potential for metastasis, therefore carrying a poor prognosis with up to approximately 25% mortality rate.
    E. Frozen sections of excised tumor stained with Congo red are helpful in identification.

35. Following is a photograph of a lesion that appeared

during childhood. Which of the following statements concerning this lesion is *not* correct?

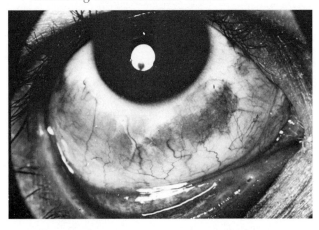

A. Eye lesions may coexist with periocular skin lesions.
B. This patient may have a nevus of Ota.
C. Subsequent transformation into a malignant melanoma of the conjunctiva is rare.
D. The lesion is composed of elements derived from the embryonic neural crest.
E. The lesion is composed of elements derived from embryonic mesoderm.

36. Concerning the anatomy of the eyelid:
  A. The glands of Wolfring are located at the superior border of the tarsus.
  B. The glands of Moll are part of the pilosebaceous unit.
  C. The gray line and the mucocutaneous junction are the same.
  D. The muscle of Riolan is part of the orbicularis oculi muscle and is situated near the lid margin.
  E. The upper lid contains approximately 20 meibomian glands and the lower lid contains approximately 40.

37. True statements about sebaceous carcinoma of the lid include all of the following *except*:
  A. Sebaceous tumors are more common on the upper lid.
  B. It occurs more frequently than in any other part of the skin.
  C. Most sebaceous tumors arise from the meibomian glands.
  D. Potential sources of abnormal sebaceous growths include the meibomian glands, glands of Zeis, and sebaceous glands associated with cilia and caruncle.
  E. Sebaceous growths are easily distinguished from recurrent chalazia.

38. The most common site of conjunctival squamous epithelial hyperplastic and neoplastic growths is the:
  A. limbal region
  B. caruncle
  C. plila semilunaris
  D. fornix
  E. palpebral conjunctiva

39. All of the following statements about the eyelid glands are true *except*:

A. The meibomian glands are holocrine, sebaceous glands located in the tarsus.
B. The glands of Zeis are apocrine sweat glands associated with cilia at the lid margin.
C. The glands of Krause are located at the fornix, and the glands of Wolfring are accessory lacrimal glands.
D. The glands of Krause are located at the fornix, and the glands of Wolfring are located at the upper margin of the tarsus.
E. The glands of Moll are apocrine glands.

40. True statements concerning microscopic pathologic terms include all of the following *except*:
  A. hyperkeratosis: thickening of the keratin layer or stratum corneum
  B. parakeratosis: retention of the nuclei in the keratin layer
  C. acanthosis: thickening of the granular layer
  D. acantholysis: loss of cohesion between cells of the epidermis as a result of breakdown of the intercellular bridges (desmosomes), which can cause vesicles and bullae
  E. dyskeratosis: abnormal maturation of the epidermis, often resulting in abnormal keratinization within individual cells anywhere in the squamous layer

41. False statements about dermoids, epibulbar hamartomas, and choristomas include all of the following *except*:
  A. They are congenital growths that most commonly occur at the nasal limbus.
  B. Most dermoids are cystic, but some may be solid.
  C. Dermoids commonly exhibit a rough irregular surface with abrupt margins.
  D. Dermoids are hamartomatous or choristomatous growths that are composed of derivative of epithelial or connective tissue elements believed to have become entrapped within facial clefts during embryogenesis.
  E. Dermoids always should be removed surgically because they are malignant lesions.

42. Which of the following statements is not true of follicles?
  A. They are a common reaction to virus infections.
  B. They clinically appear as gray or white lobular elevations.
  C. They are composed of lymphocytes with a vascular core in the germinal center.
  D. The central core is avascular.
  E. The central core contains germinal cells and macrophages.

43. Characteristic features of trachoma include all of the following *except*:
  A. Follicular hypertrophy is the hallmark of stage IIA.
  B. Arlt's line occurs in stage III.
  C. The causative organisms belong to the class Chlamydia.
  D. Halberstaedter-Prowazek inclusion bodies are best visualized with the Giemsa stain.
  E. Halberstaedter-Prowazek inclusion bodies are intranuclear inclusions that are sometimes seen in trachoma and inclusion conjunctivitis.

44. The following statements concerning mucocutaneous eruptions are false *except*:
    A. Pemphigus vulgaris is never fatal.
    B. Pemphigus vulgaris is characterized by subepithelial bullae within the skin and mucous membranes.
    C. Pemphigoid and Stevens-Johnson syndrome are characterized by bullae derived from a cleavage between the basal layer of the epithelium and the underlying stroma or dermis.
    D. The primary destructive process in ocular pemphigoid involves the epithelium.
    E. Stevens-Johnson syndrome usually occurs in the elderly, particularly women and usually is accompanied by general malaise, headache, fever, and upper respiratory infection.

45. Concerning the environmental degenerations of the cornea and conjunctiva, all of the following statements are correct *except*:
    A. Solar radiation is the most important environmental influence.
    B. Most show evidence of cellular atypism and are premalignant.
    C. Pingueculae and pterygia are characterized by degeneration of the subepithelial bulbar conjunctival stroma.
    D. Keratinoid degeneration consists of yellow-brown, drop-like, hyaline deposits, in the superficial corneal conjunctival stroma.
    E. Keratinoid degeneration usually occurs bilaterally and affects elderly persons with a history of outdoor exposure.

46. All of the following statements about xeroderma pigmentosum are incorrect *except*:
    A. Multiple malignant tumors often develop in the sun-exposed skin and conjunctiva, which ultimately may lead to metastasis and death.
    B. Xeroderma pigmentosum is inherited in an autosomal-dominant manner.
    C. Prevention of skin lesions rests primarily with alkylating chemotherapeutic agents.
    D. Most skin lesions become manifest in the early adult years.
    E. Skin tumors are almost exclusively basal cell carcinomas.

47. All of the following are correct statements regarding ocular and adnexal tumors *except*:
    A. Seborrheic keratosis is not a premalignant lesion.
    B. Squamous cell carcinoma is the most common tumor affecting the eyelids.
    C. Basal cell carcinomas are characterized histopathologically by formation of a "picket-fence" pattern of cells around lobules of tumor.
    D. The presence of an intrasclera nerve loop of Axenfeld must be considered in the differential diagnosis of an epibulbar pigmented lesion.
    E. Squamous cell carcinomas of the limbal conjunctiva may vary in clinical appearance from a clear-translucent mass to a dense white leukophakic lesion.

48. Basal cell carcinomas are derived from:
    A. melanocytic cells
    B. spindle cells
    C. basal cells
    D. primary epithelial germ cells
    E. Langerhan's cells

49. Which of the following statements is correct regarding concerning squamous cell carcinoma of the conjunctiva and eyelids?
    A. Highly invasive squamous cell carcinoma is common.
    B. It commonly metastasizes to distant foci.
    C. Carcinomas of sun-exposed surfaces tend to behave in a much less malignant manner than some internal squamous cell carcinomas, for example esophagus or lung.
    D. A squamous cell carcinoma in the temporal aspect of the upper lid would most likely drain in the submandibular lymph nodes.
    E. A squamous cell carcinoma in the nasal aspect of the lower lid would most likely drain into the preauricular lymph nodes.

50. True statements concerning nevi and malignant melanoma of the conjunctiva and eyelids include all of the following *except*:
    A. Most malignant melanomas of the conjunctiva occur at the eyelid margin.
    B. Conjunctival malignant melanomas are considered less malignant than melanomas of the eyelid.
    C. Dermal nevi of the eyelids are totally benign and possess no malignant potential.
    D. A compound nevus is one that exhibits junctional activity and also extends into the stroma or dermis.
    E. Two major criteria that differentiate a malignant melanoma from a compound nevus are cellular anaplasia and permeation of lymphoid channels.

ANSWERS

CHAPTER 1

1. (**C**) The sclera is white and opaque because of the random, irregular layering of its collagen fibers. In contrast the corneal collagen lamellae are arranged in a parallel manner, exhibiting a geometrically regular appearance, thus rendering the cornea transparent to incoming light. The corneal endothelium functions as a metabolic pump, thereby keeping the cornea in a state of relative dehydration, thus preventing edema. Regarding answer B, Descemet's membrane thickening and/or guttata formation actually may be associated with endothelial cell atrophy or loss. This can lead to corneal edema. With regard to answer D, a smooth corneal surface is more important in preventing irregular astigmatism rather than in maintaining transparency (pp. 1 and 59).

2. (**D**) All of the stains listed may be positive with transudates or exudates. Subretinal fluid almost always stains positive with eosin. Lipids such as cholesterol or lipid derived from serum or fluid breakdown products may stain positively with Oil red O. The PAS stain often is positive when substances such as glycogen or mucosubstances are present (Table 1-1, p. 4).

3. (**A**) All of the answers except A represent true PAS-positive basement membranes (p. 3). The external limiting "membrane" of the retina actually is composed of cell junctions of the zonula adherens type that interconnect retinal photoreceptors and Müller cells. Although Bruch's membrane, answer C, is actually a complex structure composed of five layers, two of these layers are composed of basement membrane material, and the membrane is therefore PAS positive by light microscopy (pp. 288 and 361).

4. (**E**) Stromal melanocytes in the iris are responsible for final iris color (p. 10), so answer E is false. The intensity of pigment cell pigmentation is relatively constant. Most increase in stromal pigmentation occurs after birth (p. 10). Stromal melanocytes are derived from the neural crest (p. 9) and reprint the cell or origin of uveal melanocytic neoplasm (see Chapter 7, p. 307). Albinism is discussed in Chapter 2 (p. 42). Answer D relates to the fact that the newborn iris is usually gray-blue.

5. (**C**) Glutaraldehyde provides the necessary preservation of subcellular structures and organelles that is desired for electron microscopy. Ten percent buffered neutral formalin and Bouin's fixative generally are used to prepare tissue for light microscopy (p. 6). Periodic acid-Schiff is not a fixative but a stain that is specific for glycoproteins and is useful in identifying basement membranes (p. 3).

6. (**B**) The inferior oblique muscle, which has a fleshy muscular insertion just temporal to the exit of the optic nerve, overlies the macula (Figs. 1-2 and 1-3 p. 2). This is a very important landmark in orienting the eye and identifying the right eye from the left during gross pathologic examination.

7. (**B**) The pigment epithelium is derived from the *outer* layer of the optic cup, and the multilayered sensory retina is derived from the *inner* layer. The cells at the anterior margin of the optic cup form the posterior pigment epithelium of the iris and the cells in the intermediate zone between the future iris and the future sensory retina from the ciliary body, which is the source of aqueous secretion. The optic cup is derived from the optic vesicle, which emanates from the diencephalic portion of the embryonic neural tube.

8. (**E**) The inferior oblique muscle has a direct muscular insertion into the sclera. It is identifiable at a point just temporal to the optic disc, near the site of the macular region. The superior oblique muscle is in the superotemporal quadrant and has a tendinous insertion (p. 2).

9. (**D**) The definitive adult vitreous is the *secondary vitreous* (Chapter 2, p. 29 and Chapter 8, p. 366), so answer D is false. The zonules are tertiary vitreous. A very important advance in anterior segment surgery, especially cataract surgery and intraocular lens implantation

occurred in the late 1970s when Pharmacia Corporation introduced Healon™, a hyaluronic acid obtained from rooster combs. This and other viscoelastics from various sources have proved to be very useful surgical adjuncts (p. 155).

10. (**D**) Rhabdomyosarcoma. Electron microscopy (p. 6) may be especially helpful in differentiating a rhabdomyosarcoma from other tumors by the detection of myofilaments and cross striations. Tissue should be submitted for both light and electron microscopy when a rhabdomyosarcoma is suspected.

11. (**C**) The PAS stain probably is the most important special stain used in ophthalmic pathology and stains basement membranes such as the lens capsule (and also, to some extent, the zonules as seen in the photomicrograph) pink to red. The Alcian blue stain also is used for mucopolysaccharides but is less useful in clearly differentiating basement membranes. The Prussian blue stain is used to identify iron. The trichrome stain is useful in identifying collagen, among other structures. The Sudan stain is used for fat (p. 3).

12. (**B**) The first retinal cells affected by retinal detachment are the rods and cones (p. 417), so A is true. E also is true because of pigment epithelium also lines the subepithelial space. Answer D also is true because the cells that line the embryonic vesicles (p. 7) are those that form the photoreceptors and retinal pigment epithelium. Damage to the inner retinal layers (toward the vitreous) such as the nerve fiber layer and inner plexiform layer is much more common after retinal vascular diseases (p. 370). Answer B is therefore false and therefore the correct answer to this question. Answers A, C, and D, connote common sequelae of retinal detachment.

13. (**E**) Congo red. This is a case of lattice corneal dystrophy; the "lattice lines" are compound of amyloid (p. 91). The various stains for the differentiation of amyloid are listed on pages 4 and 90.

14. (**D**) The dilator and sphincter muscles of the iris, like the erector pili muscle associated with hair follicles of the skin, have the rather unique distinction of being of ectodermal rather than mesodermal derivation.

15. (**D**) Answer D is the correct answer because the most common organisms found in acute vitreous abscesses are gram-positive bacteria. Answer A is incorrect because anaerobic cultures typically are used in the diagnosis of low-grade, *localized* endophthalmitis. This condition often is caused by Propionibacterium acnes, usually after cataract surgery (p. 164). Localized endophthalmitis probably is the most common cause of low-grade postoperative uveitis. It does not cause generalized destruction of the eye and vitreous abscess as occurs in a classic acute purulent endophthalmitis, as seen here. The acid fast stain (B) is used to identify mycobacterial infections such as tuberculosis. The GMS stain (C) is specific for fungi, which usually do not cause the acute pattern illustrated here. (p. 4). The von Kossa stain is positive for calcium (p. 4, Table 1-1).

16. (**B**) The retinal vascular endothelium is of mesodermal origin.

17. (**B**) All components of the anterior chamber angle outflow filtration apparatus are composed primarily of mesoderm (or mesectoderm). They do, however, contain neuroreceptors (from neuroectoderm) that respond to various pharmacologic agents used in the treatment of glaucoma (p. 10).

18. (**E**) The region under and just behind the insertion of the extraocular muscles is the weakest part of the outer layer of the eye. Knowledge of this fact is very important when performing strabismus surgery. These areas represent possible sites of rupture, either at surgery or after nonsurgical trauma (p. 59).

19. (**A**) The major iris circle is near the filtration apparatus but not within its boundaries. In most people it actually is situated within the anterior stroma of the ciliary body, near the ciliary sulcus rather than the iris itself (pp. 261 and 263).

20. (**D**) Answers A through C all connote conditions in which the eye shrinks to less than 24 to 25 mm in each diameter (p. 305), and therefore are incorrect answers. Answer E also is false because phthisis bulbi by definition connotes shrinkage (p. 305). Answer D is correct, because the typical change in glaucoma is one of insidious atrophy of the ocular tissues without shrinkage. In fact there often is

some enlargement of the globe, especially in congenital glaucoma (p. 273).

21. (**D**) All ocular pigment granules (including those within the retinal pigment epithelium, which are formed in situ within the optic cup, and the dendritic melanocytes of the uveal stroma, which are derived from the neural crest) are of neuroectodermal rather than mesodermal (mesectodermal) origin (pp. 9, 287, and 307).

22. (**E**) All of the above. Immunofluorescent methods, including the use of immunoperoxidase, may be used for the identification and localization of specific cells, tissues, or causative agents such as microbials (p. 6).

23. (**C**) The ciliary body is formed from three components of the embryo, namely 1) neuroectoderm of the embryonic optic cup that forms the two epithelium layers, 2) mesectoderm (neural-crest mesenchyme), which forms the bulk of the ciliary body stroma, and 3) mesoderm, which forms the anlage of the vasculature (p. 10). The adjacent zonules, derived partially from surface ectoderm, insert on the ciliary body but do not primarily take part in its formation (p. 29). Answers A and E are therefore false. Answer B is false because only neuroectoderm is not mentioned; Answer D is false because neuroectoderm is not mentioned (pp. 9 and 10).

24. (**B**) The pigment epithelium forms from the outer layer of the optic cup, and its granules develop in situ very early during gestation. They are therefore relatively mature by the time of birth (p. 9). Answers A and D are based on the fact that uveal stromal pigment within dendritic melanocytes is derived from the neural crest. This pigment migrates into the uvea and matures at a much later date, often several weeks or months after birth (pp. 10 and 287). Answer E relates to an important point useful to the ocular pathologist because an approximation of a person's age may be made by analysis of the cellularity of the uveal tract, particularly the stroma of the ciliary body (p. 10). The blue appearance of the sclera at birth is caused by the thinness and immaturity of the sclera, which permit visibility of the intraocular pigments.

25. (**B**) The Prussian (Berlin) blue stain for iron is invaluable for differentiation of intraocular pigments. Intraocular iron granules, such as occur in siderosis, in the various corneal iron lines (p. 82), after hemorrhage, or in foreign bodies, stain blue. Both iron and melanin may reveal varying hues of blue-brown-black in routine sections and thus may be difficult to differentiate in routine H & E sections. Melanin has no affinity for this stain and retains its yellow-brown appearance (p. 4). The Fontana stain (answer D) is a special stain for melanin pigment.

26. (**E**) Remnants of the trunk of the hyaloid artery and its sheath, Bergmeister's papilla, often are present on the optic nerve head for weeks, months, or even years after birth (p. 34). They usually do not create clinically significant sequelae. Answer A is discussed on p. 10 and answer B relates to continuing formation of lens sutures (p. 119, see also pp. 33 and 527).

27. (**A**) Masson's trichrome is positive for collagen and other substances, such as the deposits of granular stromal dystrophy (p. 89). Luxol fast blue is used to determine the presence of lipid material including myelin. Oil red O also is a stain for lipids. Alizarin red is used to determine the presence of calcium. The Congo red stain is positive for amyloid and therefore is useful to identify a *lattice* dystrophy of the corneal stroma (p. 91).

28. (**C**) All of the items except answer C usually are benign aging processes (p. 10). Circumferential deposits of lipid in the peripheral cornea, leaving a border of clear cornea around the lesion adjacent to the limbus, are benign and of no clinical consequence in elderly persons (arcus senilis, p. 62). However, a premature arcus, termed *arcus juvenilis,* in a child or adolescent may, in a small percentage of cases, signal a possibility of hyperlipidemia; therefore appropriate laboratory studies should be undertaken to evaluate this problem (p. 62).

29. (**C**) Answers A, B, D, and E clearly are false because they represent relatively benign conditions that rarely affect vision. They primarily involve peripheral structures only away from visual axis. Answer C

is the best answer, although most drusen are unassociated with visual loss. When drusen become associated with age-related macular generation, significant visual impairment occurs (p. 11).

30. (**E**) All of these are helpful in identifying amyloid (pp. 4 and 100).

31. (**C**) Hassall-Henle warts represent a physiologic aging process and do not affect vision. These are excrescences and thickenings of Descemet's membrane at the corneal periphery and do not involve the visual axis (pp. 11 and 61).

32. (**B**) The outer plexiform layer (pp. 11 and 363). These cysts are lined by Müller cells and contain mucopolysaccharides (see also p. 411).

33. (**E**) Phthisis bulbi is discussed in detail in Chapter 7 (p. 284). Answer B is correct because the intraocular bone most likely contains calcium, which cold be documented with the von Kossa or alizarin red stain (Table 1-1). All other answers are false. Alpha-1-antitrypsin (Table 1-2) is used to disprove hepatic carcinoma. The gridley stain is used to identify fungi; the calcofluor white stain is used to identify acanthamoeba organism (p. 4), and the Ziehl-Neelsen is used to identify acid-fast bacteria (see Tables 1-1 and 1-2).

34. (**A**) Because the macular region, and hence the tumor, is in the horizontal plane, obtaining a proper pupil-optic nerve section (so-called p-o section) of the lesion would require a horizontal section. A vertical section might cause the lesion to be missed completely. This demonstrates why clinical history and transillumination of the globe to identify the location of the lesion are so important (pp. 2 and 3).

35. (**A**) The vascular endothelium is derived from non-neural crest mesoderm (p. 10). Neural crest elements are important in the pathogenesis of tumors such as nevi and melanoma (p. 288) as well as the phacomatoses (p. 505).

36. (**C**) The important functions of the embryonic ocular fissure are to provide pathways for ingrowth of embryonic vessels into the eye and outgrowth of nervous elements from the eye into the brain via the optic nerve. Answer C correctly identifies that the fissure provides a pathway for growth of axons. Answer B would be correct because it identifies the grove necessary for growth of the hyaloid vessel, but the embryonic fissure is *ventral* rather than *dorsal* (p. 8). Answer A is false because the fissure does not primarily affect the the choroid, but rather is a primary defect of the neuroectodermal ectodermal optic cup (p. 8). Answer D is false because the closure of the fissure occurs at 6 weeks of gestation and is initiated in its midportion as opposed to the anterior and posterior portions (p. 8). Answer E is false because failure of closure of fissure results in formation of congenital colobomas (p. 9). Congenital falciform fold is discussed in Chapter 2 (p. 34).

37. (**C**) The most important reason to examine the vortex veins in eyes with suspected malignant melanoma is to rule out tumor extension. The most common route of extension of intraocular uveal melanoma is through the vortex veins or scleral emissaria (pp. 3 and 325).

38. (**B**) The embryonic fissure usually closes at approximately 6 weeks of gestation. This time corresponds to a crown-rump fetal length of approximately 15 mm. By 6 weeks the anlage of most body tissues are formed (p. 8 and p. 17).

39. (**E**) Polarizing filters are invaluable in evaluating structures or deposits that have a regular molecular structure (e.g., amyloid or answers A and B) and various types of foreign matter (answers C and D). Iron does not reveal a positive finding with this technique (pp. 4, 93, 95, 100, and 102).

40. (**C**) All cataract surgeons quickly realize that the posterior lens capsule is much thinner than the anterior or equatorial capsule, so the correct answer is C (pp. 119–120). The thickest portions of the capsule are at the anterior pole of the lens and at the equator (Fig. 4-7, p. 120). There is slight paracentral thinning of the anterior capsule forming a circular area of thinning approximately 5 to 6 millimeters in diameter (see Chapter 4, Fig. 4-7). This thinning actually may be useful because it coincides with the area where a continuous curvilinear capsulorhexis (CCC) commonly is performed during cataract surgery.

41. (**C**) This tumor belongs in the differential diagnosis of basal cell carcinoma (p. 589) versus squamous cell carcinoma (p. 592) versus sebaceous or meibomian carcinoma (p. 595). The latter is a tumor that often secretes a lipid material. When the lipid is found, it can be differentiated from other eyelid tumors. To demonstrate lipid within the tumor, one has to do a frozen section (to prevent leaching out of the lipid during paraffin processing) and a fat stain such as the oil red O stain. When the stain is positive, this is indicative of a sebaceous carcinoma diagnosis (pp. 4 and 595–597).

42. (**A**) Lange's fold is a common artifact appearance in newborn or fetal eyes. It is seen as the junction of the retina and pars plana of the ciliary body, probably caused by unequal shrinkage of retinociliary tissues during fixation. It is of no clinical or pathologic significance (p. 10).

43. (**C**) Optimally, the globe should be placed in fixative for 24 hours before it is distributed in any way (p. 3). It is not necessary to freeze the globe or cut a window to enhance entrance of fixative. The vitreous does not impede retinal fixation and should not be disrupted.

44. (**C**) All of the structures listed in answers A, B, D, and E continue anteriorly into the pars plana. The photoreceptors of the sensory retina actually begin to taper off in the peripheral retina and then disappear in the pars plana (p. 363).

45. (**E**) The two layers of the optic cup basically are formed by the ependyma of the neural tube having evaginated anteriorly from the brain proper. Thus a typical retinal detachment seen clinically simply represents an opening of this embryonic space, and therefore, all of the answers are correct (pp. 7 and 415).

46. (**A**) It is generally difficult to obtain an orientation by observation of the rectus muscles, so one counts on location of the two oblique muscles to determine the superior aspect of the globe and to determine whether it is a right eye or a left eye. The insertion of the superior oblique muscle is tendinous, whereas the inferior oblique muscle has a muscular insertion (p. 2).

47. (**C**) Answer A is true because the S-100 protein technique may be useful in identifying neural-crest derived cells (Color Plate 1-2). Answer B also is true because stains for mucopolysaccharide, such as Alcian blue, are helpful in diagnosing mucin-secreting adenocarcinomas. In answer C, the statement that Alcian blue is helpful is false. Most lung cancers are squamous cell or small-cell tumors that do not secrete mucin. Answer D is correct because metastatic intraocular tumors must be differentiated from primary uveal malignant melanomas (p. 328). Answer E also is correct because immunohistochemistry can help differentiate various cells of origin and cell types (Table 1-1, p. 4).

48. (**C**) This photomicrograph shows fungi within a vitreous abscess in a case of endophthalmitis. Silver stains such as GMS or other stains such as Gridley or PAS, all of which accentuate the cell wall of the organism, are useful in identifying such organisms (pp. 0, 0, and 00).

49. (**B**) Multiple sclerosis is a demyelinating disease, and the special stain for myelin is the Luxol fast blue stain. Normal myelin retains a blue color, whereas demyelinated plaques lose the affinity for the stain (pp. 4 and 546).

50. (**B**) Nucleic acids within nuclei. Hematoxylin imparts a basophilic or bluish hue to nuclear elements and structures containing nucleic acids (p. 4). Eosin is specific for most cytoplasmic organelles, such as mitochondria, which are stained light pink.

CHAPTER 2

1. (**E**) Keratoconus is not seen in Patau's syndrome (p. 45). Patau's syndrome is characterized by colobomatous microphthalmia (p. 45). Answers A, B, C, and D are true and describe keratoconus, either if associated with Down syndrome (p. 50) or as an isolated condition (Chapter 3, p. 85).

2. (**D**) The lesion pictured exhibits morning glory syndrome, which consists of an extensive excavation of the optic nerve head and peripapillary region, with peripapillary gliosis and pigmentary abnormalities. Some authorities consider this a form of optic nerve coloboma (p. 22). The congenital tilted disc syndrome is described on page 22,

and optic glioma is described on page 553. Answers B and C are considered on pages 533-534.

3. **(C)** Optic nerve glioma (p. 553) usually occurs sporadically or in association with phacomatosis such as neurofibromatosis (p. 509). All of the other lesions are associated with anomalous development of the apical forebrain (p. 16).

4. **(D)** The anterolateral outpouching or evagination of the primitive brainstem to form the optic vesicle is an early event of differentiation of the embryo, and any significant abnormality in this process may produce a severe ocular malformation, including anophthalmia, cyclopia, congenital cystic eye, and congenital nonattachment of the retina (pp. 14-17). Anterior chamber cleavage syndromes are described on page 35.

5. **(E)** The iris in this illustration is shortened, blunted, and rudimentary, representing a congenital defect. If this defect were confined to the inferonasal quadrant, it would fit the pattern of a typical coloboma (p. 18). A similar focal defect in any other quadrant of the eye would be considered an atypical coloboma (p. 24). Aniridia, either with or without Wilms' tumor (Miller syndrome), actually represents hypoplasia of the iris rather than true aplasia. Therefore aniridia also could assume this appearance (p. 27). Thus all of the answers could correlate with this photomicrograph.

6. **(A)** Macular colobomas, probably a misnomer, are very rare, but most cases are bilateral (p. 28). Answer A is therefore false. For lack of a better term they are classified as atypical colobomas (p. 24). Answers B through E are true. Some authors believe that most cases are postinflammatory-secondary to maternal infectious disease, for example by congenital toxoplasmosis (Chapter 8 p. 395).

7. **(B)** Defective closure of the embryonic ocular fissure, a process that usually is completed by the fourth to sixth weeks of gestation, produces the typical coloboma (p. 17).

8. **(D)** Medulloepithelioma is a tumor of the ciliary epithelium (p. 330). The ciliary body in trisomy 13 often has a coloboma and cartilage (p. 45).

9. **(D)** Embryonic fissure closure during normal embryogenesis begins in the midzone (approximate midequatorial region of the globe) and later extends posteriorly and anteriorly. Thus the fissure remains open for the longest time at the site of the future optic nerve head and iris, respectively. These sites are therefore susceptible for a longer period to noxious insults that might lead to malclosure of the fissure. This is the reason that colobomas involving the posterior aspect of the optic cup (disc and peripapillary retina) or the most anterior aspect (iris) are more common than those of the ciliary body and midfundus (pp. 8 and 17).

10. **(E)** Optic pits, a typical colobomas defects of the optic nerve are described on page 24. Answers A through D correctly describe optic pits.

11. **(E)** Optic pits (p. 24) are congenital defects of the optic nerve head that are considered atypical colobomas. Temporally located pits often are associated with serous detachment of the macula, macular edema, and, less commonly, macular hole. Visual field defects are relatively common if careful testing is done. The pathogenesis of the origin of the subretinal fluid still is unclear, although many authors believe that the fluid is derived from the vitreous that arrives in the subretinal space by passing through the colobomatous defect. Conclusive evidence is lacking of a communication with the meninges that would permit influx of cerebrospinal fluid.

12. **(A)** There is a statistically significant coexistence of aniridia and Wilms' tumor (nephroblastoma) (p. 26). Such a coexistence is not characteristic of familial aniridia.

13. **(A)** Although vision often is poor in eyes with a morning glory lesion, a sporadic and unilateral detachment of the thinned retina around the papillary lesion is the most common major complication.

14. **(A)** Congenital tilted disc is described and illustrated on page 22. Answer A is correct because area (1) shows elevation of the disc (nasal supertraction), area (2) shows colobomatous flattening or excavation of the disc, and area (3) shows a typical inferior-nasal conus (Fuchs' coloboma) (p. 24). This profile is very similar to the histopath-

ologic pictures seen with acquired myopic tilted disc, which is caused by mechanical stretching. (p. 41) The main difference is that the congenital tilted disc lesions generally face inferiorly—nasally (region of the embryonic ocular fissure, p. 17), whereas the acquired myopic tilted disc almost always faces temporally. Answers B through D are false because they do not connote the correct configuration of the disc and epipapillary structures.

15. **(D)** The *tertiary* vitreous is the precursor of the zonules of Zinn (suspensory ligament of the lens). It is unrelated to the primary vitreous. The tertiary vitreous probably is ectodermal, formed by a combination of neuroectodermal elements from the ciliary processes and surface ectodermal processes from the lens capsule (p. 29).

16. **(B)** Histopathologically one does not observe a decrease in pigment cells within the albinotic eye, but rather a partial (or rarely an absolute) lack of pigment granules within the cells of uveal and pigment of epithelial cells (p. 42). Therefore answer B is false. The most common reason that pigment formation is lacking is a disturbance of tyrosinase metabolism. Answers A and C through E are correct (p. 42).

17. **(B)** The glial sheath of Bergmeister (p. 30) envelopes the posterior one third of the hyaloid artery and begins to atrophy at approximately the seventh month of gestation. Remnants of portions of Bergmeister's papilla, such as seen in this photograph, are common but usually are clinically innocuous (p. 34). The circle of Zinn-Haller (answer D) is described on page 289.

18. **(B)** Simple myopia and myopic astigmatism are in part secondary to the posterior staphyloma that frequently occur in this condition, in effect increasing the axial length of the eye (p. 40).

19. **(E)** All of the answers A through D are correct (p. 34).

20. **(D)** Most cases of PHPV are isolated and sporadic with no apparent hereditary influence (p. 30).

21. **(A)** Serous macular detachment is a common finding in optic pits (p. 25).

22. **(A)** Congenital falciform fold is a rare cause of leukocoria, often bilateral, believed in some instances to be a variant PHPV. This condition is illustrated in Color Plate 2-14. Answers B through E are therefore true. Answer A is false because retinopathy of prematurity (ROP, retrolental fibroplasia), has a totally different pathogenesis. Retinopathy of prematurity is a disease primarily affecting the peripheral retina that occurs in low-birthweight multipremature babies—as opposed to congenital falciform fold that generally occurs in patients who do not have this history. Nematode endophthalmitis caused by *Toxocara canis* also may produce a picture of a "dragged disk" retinal fold.

23. **(B)** Leukokoria in PHPV (p. 32) is caused most commonly by a fibrovascular mass of tissue in the retrolental space. This fibrovascular membrane is derived from persistent and hyperplastic remnants of the embryonic vascular tunic of the lens (tunica vasculosa lentis).

24. **(E)** Persisent hydroplastic primary vitreous (PHPV) may be associated with adipose tissue metaplasia (pseudophakia lipomatosa, p. 33), peripheral retinal folds caused by traction on the retina by persistent fibrovascular remnants (p. 33), cataracts (usually caused by rupture of the posterior capsule) (p. 33), and elongated ciliary processes caused by shrinkage of the interciliary membrane.

25. **(D)** Answer D is not true because most cases usually occur spontaneously and sporadically (p. 43). Answers A,B,C, and E are true (p. 43).

26. **(A)** Untreated cases of PHPV commonly progress to phthisis bulbi and can have rapid progression of secondary complications such as glaucoma, repeated massive hemorrhages, and retinal detachment and atrophy (p. 33). Sympathetic ophthalmia (p. 298) is not a consequence of PHPV.

27. **(C)** "Classic" PHPV is a cause of unilateral leukocoria and, with the noteworthy exception of trisomy 13 (p. 45), is not associated with systemic abnormalities (p. 30). Modern vitrectomy techniques have improved the prognosis for vision, but the surgical technique may be difficult, and visual rehabilitation and avoidance of amblyopia are difficult.

28. (**D**) Answer D is false because although glaucoma sometimes occurs, there is not an *invariable* association with congenital glaucoma and aniridia (p. 27). Aniridia is an atypical iris coloboma, has two modes of occurrence (sporadic and autosomal dominant), and represents an iris hypoplasia rather than aplasia. Answers A through C are therefore true. Also answer E is true because its sporadic form can be associated with Wilms' tumor (Miller syndrome, (p. 26).

29. (**E**) This question emphasizes that the posterior aspect of the hyaloid system, including Bergmeister's papilla, not infrequently persists to varying degrees, leading to anomalies that usually are benign but that must be considered in the differential diagnosis of epipapillary and peripapillary lesions (pp. 33 and 34).

30. (**E**) The photomicrograph shows the classic appearance of Axenfeld's anomaly. In this group of answers the only eponym that does not fall into the category of anterior chamber cleavage syndromes is Schnabel's atrophy, which is described on page 278.

31. (**C**) Rieger's syndrome (p. 35) is associated more closely with corectopia and colobomas. All of the other listed choices are consistent with Axenfeld's anomaly (p. 35).

32. (**B**) In contrast to simple myopia, high pathologic myopia is characterized by all of the choices except a restrained myopic tendency after puberty. In high myopia the opposite often occurs. The nearsightedness may increase even more rapidly during adolescence, and the axial enlargement may slowly increase during adulthood into the 40s and 50s (p. 37).

33. (**B**) Persistent hydroplastic primary vitreous (PHPV) is an important cause of white pupil (leukocoria) (Chapters 2 and 9, p. 492). Answers A, C, D, and E are correct. Answer B is false. An important differential diagnostic difference is that eyes with PHPV commonly are microphthalmic, whereas eyes with retinoblastoma rarely are microphthalmic.

34. (**D**) Common peripapillary changes in pathologic myopia include tilted disc, myopic crescent, nasal supertraction, the loop of Weiss, and temporal flattening of the disc. The optic cup often is characterized by a relatively shallow physiologic excavation (p. 41).

35. (**E**) Neovascularization of the optic nerve head usually is not a complication of high myopia (p. 41).

36. (**E**) Another term for nevus of Ota is *oculo-dermal-melanocytosis* (p. 43). This form of *congenital* melanosis should be differentiated from the acquired form (p. 579), particularly with respect to the potential of forming conjunctival melanocytic neoplasms.

37. (**E**) The ocular changes in pathological myopia (p. 37) are generally based on axial elongation and stretching of the globe. Therefore answers A through D, all of which define conditions secondary to this, are correct. Answer E is false because the Förster-Fuchs' spot occurs at the macula rather than peripheral, again secondary to the elongation (p. 40).

38. (**C**) This section is a cut through a typical, inferonasal coloboma affecting the fundus where the embryonic fissure has not undergone proper closure (p. 17). The retina is reduced to a thin glial membrane, and there is total absence of retinal pigment epithelium and choroid. The sclera is seen below. The absence of pigment is responsible for the white color or "baring of the sclera" seen in a typical fundus coloboma (p. 19, Fig. 2-11). Myopic retinal degeneration is characterized by degenerative changes associated with pigmentary changes affecting the retina and choroid, findings that are not seen in this illustration (p. 41). The retina in trisomy 13 is characterized by a dysplasia, often with the formation of rosettes (p. 47). A congenital falciform fold (p. 34) shows a tentlike elevation of retinal tissue associated with a dragged disc rather than a thinned hypoplastic retina, as seen in this illustration.

39. (**A**) Ocular albinism usually is characterized by a normal number of pigment cells within the eye. However, a partial (or rarely, an absolute) lack of melanin granules within the uveal and pigment epithelial cells is the basic cause of the depigmentation. Common symptoms are photophobia, poor vision, and nystagmus, the latter two often being caused by maldevelopment of the fovea (p. 42).

40. (**A**) The morning glory is a well-known congenital syndrome (p. 22). Answers B and E are correct. Answer A is not true. Nonrhegmatogenous retinal detachment is a significant complication that can occur as a result of tugging by abnormal glial tissue on the thinned retina.

41. (**B**) All of the answers except answer B are characteristic of congenital melanosis oculi. An increased incidence of conjunctival malignant melanoma is not seen in the *congenital* form of melanosis oculi but rather is a feature of so-called *acquired* melanosis or precancerous melanosis (pp. 42 and 578). Answer D refers to oculodermal melanocytosis, or nevus of Ota.

42. (**E**) The iris "spots" in question can occur in normal and pathologic states (p. 50). These represent delicate fibrin proliferation on the anterior iris surface.

43. (**D**) Microphthalmia is associated with all of the conditions listed in answers A through C and E (p. 36). Answer D is false because nanophthalmia (p. 37) is a congenital retardation in growth of the eye in which the eye is smaller than normal but otherwise well developed without severe intraocular changes—as is the case in microphthalmia. In nanophthalmos all parts of the globe are reduced in size equally, but usually reveal an otherwise normal appearance.

44. (**B**) Intraocular cartilage within a coloboma of the ciliary body is highly characteristic of many eyes with trisomy 13 (p. 45). Although the eye may be extremely small and appear to represent an anophthalmia, a true *primary* anophthalmia, implying lack of formation of the original optic vesicle (p. 14), has not been reported in trisomy 13.

45. (**E**) All of the listed findings except melanosis oculi are classic features of trisomy 13 (p. 45).

46. (**D**) Trisomy 21 (Down syndrome) is characterized by intraocular lesions, including cataracts (60%), Brushfield's spot (85%), iris hypoplasia, and a higher incidence of keratoconus than occurs in the general population.

47. (**B**) Peters' anomaly is one of the conditions lumped in the group of anterior chamber cleavage syndromes (p. 35). Answer B is false because this condition usually is transmitted as autosomal recessive trait, with no relation to sex-linked transmission. Answers A and C through E are correct (p. 36).

48. (**A**) Although bona fide congenital, noninflammatory colobomas of the macula do exist and have been described in families (p. 28), most authors believe that the vast majority of so-called atypical colobomas of the macula are most likely postinflammatory, resulting from conditions such as toxoplasmosis or syphilis (p. 28).

49. (**A**) The Chédiak-Steinbrinck-Higashi syndrome is a special form of oculocutaneous tyrosinase-positive albinism, inherited as an autosomal-recessive trait that may be associated with leukocyte disturbances that may predispose to infections (p. 42). Heterochromic irides (p. 43) and congenital melanosis oculi (p. 42) are not forms of albinism.

50. (**E**) Anterior uveitis is not a typical complication of Down syndrome (p. 49). Answers A through D are common components of this syndrome (p. 50).

CHAPTER 3

1. (**D**) Axenfeld's nerve loop (p. 60) is a lesion that must be included in the differential diagnosis of primary or metastatic malignant melanoma of the uvea or ocular surface. In and of itself it is not pathologic, represents a loop that courses from the conjunctiva outward toward the sclera, and rarely is painful. Answers A, B, C, and E are therefore false.

2. (**A**) The sclera is approximately 0.45 mm thick at the limbus and 1.1 mm thick at the posterior pole (p. 61). Visible in the photomicrograph is a large fibrous wound track, the site of a perforation of the sclera after a bimedial recession procedure. This is located just posterior to the insertion of the medial rectus muscle. Therefore the danger of perforation is greatest at this site, where the sclera is thinnest.

3. (**E**) Goblet cells within the conjunctiva are responsible for much of the production of the inner mucopolysaccharide layer of the tear film (p. 60).

4. **(C)** Bowman's layer does not regenerate when broken (p. 61). Answers A, D, and E are incorrect because Bowman's layer is not a true basement membrane (p. 60) and is not produced by corneal epithelial cells. It is a modified portion of the anterior corneal stroma. Answer B is incorrect because Hassall-Henle warts are thickenings of Descemet's membrane (p. 61).

5. **(A)** Bowman's layer is an acellular layer of collagen and ground substance (p. 60). Often termed *Bowman's membrane,* it is not a true PAS-positive basement membrane but is considered a modification of the corneal stroma. It must be distinguished from the adjacent true basement membrane of the basal layer of corneal epithelium. A facet is described on page 99.

6. **(E)** Most cases of bans keratopathy are caused by dystrophic calcification of diseased tissue, but all of the conditions listed may cause metastatic calcific deposition into Bowman's layer (p. 61). Therefore answer E, all of the above, is correct.

7. **(D)** Unlike Bowman's layer, Descemet's membrane can regenerate after it has been damaged or destroyed as long as the endothelium is intact (p. 61).

8. **(B)** Acute fungal keratitis is a suppurative inflammation; the primary cell involved is the polymorphonuclear neutrophil. Chronic fungal keratitis may be granulomatous. Sympathetic ophthalmia (p. 298), chalazion (p. 583), and toxoplasmosis (p. 395) are diseases with granulomatous inflammation.

9. **(E)** Hassall-Henle warts are hyaline excrescences on Descemet's membrane located in the peripheral cornea that often occur with aging. In contrast to the centrally located guttata of Fuchs' dystrophy, which are similar in appearance histologically, they are clinically benign (pp. 61 and 92).

10. **(C)** Answers A, B, D, and E are correct (p. 84) Answer C is false. The technical definition of ectasia is a protrusion that does not include uvea, whereas a staphyloma connotes protrusion of tissue that contains uveal tissue (p. 84). It is true that most ectasis occur on the cornea, but answer C does not adhere to the strict technical definition (p. 84).

11. **(C)** The cells seen in the photomicrograph include giant cells and epithelioid cells that are characteristic of a granulomatous inflammation (p. 63). All of the answers except C, vitreous abscess, may contain either type of cell. The predominant cell in a vitreous abscess, which is a purulent, acute, nongranulomatous inflammatory process, is the polymorphonuclear neutrophil.

12. **(C)** Arcus juvenilis (composed of lipid infiltrates, p. 62). Anterior embryotoxon must be differentiated from posterior embryotoxon, a thickening and anterior displacement of Schwalbe's line (p. 35). An epithelial facet is described on page 99.

13. **(E)** This photomicrograph illustrates the anterior portion of the cornea showing total absence of the corneal epithelium, basement membrane, and Bowman's layer. This connotes an ulcer, in which the base of the ulcer is composed of necrotic, inflammatory debris. There is a diffuse infiltration of acute inflammatory cells throughout the entire portion of the corneal stroma. The densely staining areas represent huge bacterial colonies (p. 65). The presence of the bacterial colonies differentiates this from a viral keratitis (p. 68). Syphilitic interstitial keratitis is nonulcerative (p. 71), and Salzmann's nodular degeneration is a nonspecific lesion composed of collagenous tissue representing a sequela of other types of underlying disease (p. 78).

14. **(C)** This photomicrograph, a PAS stain, clearly shows two lesions: bullus keratopathy with separation of the epithelium from the stroma (above) and formation of a retrocorneal fibrous membrane (below), posterior to the PAS-positive Descemet's membrane (pp. 72 and 78). Bullous keratopathy is described on page 72. Answer A is false because there is no band keratopathy (p. 75). Answers B, C, and E are false because macular dystrophy represents a corneal stromal disorder (p. 89).

15. **(D)** The onset of a fungal keratitis often is delayed for 1 to 2 weeks or more after the initial injury (p. 66). The other answers all correctly apply to fungal keratitis.

16. **(A)** Answers B through E are true statements regarding Fuchs' dystrophy (p. 92). Answer A is false because most cases are not inherited (a rare autosomal-dominant case has been reported) and women are affected more frequently than men (p. 92).

17. **(D)** Two prominent plasmacytoid cells are visible in this illustration. The evolution of the plasma cell is described on page 63. The relative chronicity of a lesion may be judged histopathologically by the relative numbers of plasma cells versus plasmacytoid cells versus Russell bodies. To definitely classify these cells as eosinophils, one would have to identify a bilobed nucleus in at least one of the cells (p. 63).

18. **(D)** The inflammation is located primarily in the stroma, although the endothelium can decompensate late in the disease. Interstitial keratitis may be both unilateral or bilateral in acquired cases. It is caused by many diseases other than syphilis, including the nematode *Onchocerca volvulus* (p. 71).

19. **(E)** Answer E is incorrect because the giant cells are specific indicators of *granulomatous* chronic inflammation. (p. 71) Answers A through D all are correct, describing the basic morphology of four important types of inflammatory cells (pp. 63-65).

20. **(E)** The cause of Mooren's ulcer is unclear, but it is believed to be an autoimmune disease (p. 70). No causative organism has been demonstrated.

21. **(D)** Answer D is false because a pannus is defined as a limbal ingrowth and does not arise in situ. All of the other answers describe features of a pannus.

22. **(D)** Answers A, B, C, and D are true comments regarding the microcystic epithelial dystrophy (p. 86, and Table 3-2). Answer D is false because corneal hydration clearly is associated with microcyst formation (p. 86) Any condition that gives rise to increased corneal hydration may produce epithelial cysts. Excessive entry of fluid into the corneal epithelium may occur from either of two sources, the tear film or the aqueous. The latter follows decompensation of affected endothelial cells, allowing aqueous to penetrate into the cornea.

23. **(D)** This is an example of blood staining of the cornea following hyphema (p. 80). Clusters of erythrocytes and their breakdown products are visible in the anterior chamber immediately posterior to Descemet's membrane and a markedly degenerate corneal endothelium. The granular appearance seen within the corneal stroma itself is pathognomonic; these granules represent particles of hemoglobin derived from the erythrocytes in the anterior chamber. Keratic precipitate (p. 65) usually consists of larger mononuclear or epithelioid cells and is unrelated to the granularity of the stroma seen in this case. Similarly, retinoblastoma cells (p. 354) and acute inflammatory cells usually seen in a hypopyon (p. 65) would show a different morphology (i.e., small, hyperchromatic tumor cells in the former and polymorphonuclear neutrophils in the latter). The melanin deposits in Krukenberg's spindle (p. 80) are acellular and would appear histologically as delicate melanin granules deposited on the endothelial surface.

24. **(B)** Corneal edema (pp. 72 and 73) often is difficult to confirm microscopically by observing the stroma because routine processing typically creates artifactitious interlamellar clefts. Epithelial edema, however, is easily recognized microscopically as hydropic swelling of the cells, with both intracellular and extracellular edema, often leading to formation of intraepithelial microcysts.

25. **(C)** Answers A, B, and D are correct and describe various aspects of viral keratitis (p. 69). Answer C is false because viral uveitis associated with viral keratitis is not rare (p. 68).

26. **(A)** Epidemic keratoconjunctivitis (p. 71).

27. **(E)** Krukenberg's spindle (p. 80) is a deposit of uveal melanin pigment on the posterior surface of the cornea. Any lesion causing dispersion of pigment granules from the anterior uvea can predispose to Krukenberg's spindle. The pigment is carried by convection currents in the anterior chamber. The pigment dispersion syndrome consists of depigmentation and atrophy of iris epithelium, with consequent increased iris transillumination, trabecular meshwork pigmentation (Sampaolesi's line), and occasional pigmentary glaucoma. It is

found mainly in young male myopes and is caused by iris chafing by zonules.

28. (**C**) Answers A, B, D, and E, are true comments regarding granular corneal dystrophy (p. 89). Answer C is false because the opacities rarely extend to the limbus (p. 89).

29. (**A**) Krukenberg's spindles usually do not affect vision (p. 80). All of the other answers are correct.

30. (**A**) The Kayser-Fleischer ring (p. 83), although classically associated with Wilson's disease, also may be caused by an intraocular copper foreign body (chalcosis). It is a deposit of copper in Descemet's membrane. Answer C refers to Fleischer's line, which is an iron line seen at the base of the cone in keratoconus (p. 85).

31. (**E**) Although familial transmission of keratoconus has been reported, most cases of keratoconus are sporadic (p. 85).

32. (**C**) Answer C is incorrect. Lattice dystrophy (p. 91) has an intermediate prognosis. Granular dystrophy has the best prognosis because intervening areas of stroma are spared (p. 89). The diffuse stomal involvement characteristic of macular dystrophy causes earlier and more rapid deterioration of vision than the other two forms (p. 89).

33. (**B**) Answers A, C, D, and E are true, they describe various aspect of corneal dystrophy. The incorrect statement is answer B. By definition, dystrophies generally are isolated corneal lesions that are accompanied by systemic disease (p. 86). For example, the macular deposits in the cornea that occur with various mucopolysaccharides are therefore technically not primary dystrophies (p. 89).

34. (**C**) The mucopolysaccharide deposits in macular dystrophy (p. 89) are best visualized histologically with stains such as the Alcian blue technique. Masson trichrome stain is more useful in granular dystrophy (p. 89) of the cornea, where the lesions stain bright red. Note that in the photograph there is a slight separation of a thinned corneal epithelium from underlining Bowman's layer, indicating that this patient may be susceptible to corneal erosions. Lattice dystrophy is, however, the stromal dystrophy with which such erosions are most commonly associated (p. 91). The only stromal corneal dystrophy in which polarizing filters are useful is lattice dystrophy, where the amyloid deposits that form the lattice lines show distinct birefringence (p. 89). Because the deposits of mucopolysaccharides are diffuse within the superficial corneal stroma, as can be noted in the photomicrograph, diffuse clouding of the cornea occurs rapidly when compared with granular and lattice dystrophy, and these patients tend to have earlier loss of vision.

35. (**C**) Although a temporary conical deformation of the cornea resembling keratoconus may occur after long-term wearing of ill-fitting contact lenses, this does not represent a true keratoconus. Therefore it can be said that no iatrogenic causes have been demonstrated to date (p. 85).

36. (**C**) The corneal wound is through and through (perforating), whereas from the reference point of the entire globe, there is an entrance wound (penetration) but no exiting wound (p. 97).

37. (**E**) All of the statements regarding amyloidosis are true, therefore the answer is E (pp. 93 and 94).

38. (**B**) This globe shows the typical appearance of a vitreous abscess, in which the densely staining accumulation of purulent material is localized centrally in the retrolental space and is demarcated laterally by a total funnel-shaped retinal detachment. The densely staining material consists primarily of polymorphonuclear neutrophils, thus representing an example of acute, suppurative inflammation, from which organisms often can be cultured (p. 62). The abscess is preretinal rather than subretinal, there is no granulomatous component to this inflammation (no epithelioid cells and/or giant cells), and this disease is not chronic.

39. (**A**) Although rare exceptions occur, Hunter's and Sanfilippo's syndromes are the only two systemic mucopolysaccharidoses in which the cornea usually is spared (p. 99).

40. (**B**) A contusion injury does not connote penetration or perforation of the cornea or sclera. Therefore answer B is false (p. 102). Answers A, C, D, and E are true, each connoting sequelae of such an injury (p. 97).

41. (**D**) Trauma accounts for more than 75% of all globes processed in most ocular pathology laboratories (p. 97).

42. (**D**) Answers A, B, C, and E are true (p. 66). Answer D is false because the *definitive* treatment of this condition has not yet been determined. Multiple antibiotic combinations are being tested (p. 68).

43. (**C**) Cornea clouding may occur in congenital glaucoma (p. 272, answer B, anterior chamber cleavage syndrome (p. 35, answer D), congenital hereditary corneal dystrophy (p. 87), and hereditary Bowman' layer dysplasia (p. 94, answer E). Answer C is incorrect because, although some forms of systemic mucopolysaccharidoses do cause cornea clouding, Hurler's and Scheie's syndromes (p. 94 and Table 3-5) in particular cause cornea clouding. Sanfillipo's syndrome does not (p. 94, Table 3-5).

44. (**C**) A penetrating injury by definition extends only partially through the tissue of reference; a perforation is complete passage of a foreign object through the tissue of reference (p. 97). In this slide there is a total perforation of the cornea, but, because the question stated that there were no other defects in the cornea or sclera, that is, no exit wound, one must assume that there was no perforation of the eye. Because this is a through-and-through wound of the cornea, it cannot be considered a corneal penetration.

45. (**D**) Answer D is incorrect because there are numerous complications that may occur in the chronic phase, including recurrent corneal ulcerations, secondary cataract, secondary glaucoma, and loss of the tear film. Answers A, B, C, and E are correct (p. 104).

46. (**E**) This cornea shows numerous small droplets within the superficial stroma, which, in addition to the many synonyms listed in the question, also often are termed *droplet keratopathy* and *elastoid degeneration* (pp. 11 and 575). This lesion usually is caused by environmental influences.

47. (**D**) The iron lines are described on page 82, and answers B through E correctly describe four different lines. Answer A is false because corneal iron deposits usually occur anterial at the level of the epithelium, (p. 82) not at Descemet's membrane.

48. (**B**) Most normal tissues of the eye are nonbirefringent when viewed through polarizing lenses (p. 4). Several foreign bodies such as wood and many types of sutures are birefringent because of their particular molecular structure. Calcium oxalate crystals and amyloid also show birefringence, but deposits seen in granular dystrophy of the cornea do not (p. 89).

49. (**D**) Prussian blue imparts a blue color to iron (p. 4). Alcian blue and colloidal iron stains are used to identify mucopolysaccharides. The Luxol fast blue stain is a stain for myelin. The Mallory blue stain is applied to plastic-embedded tissues that are prepared for electron microscopic analysis. Therefore it is not in itself often used as a "special" stain (pp. 3 and 100).

50. (**D**) Answer D is false. Descemet's membrane can be damaged and wrinkled after all types of injury, contusion, and penetrating or perforating injury. The difference between penetration and perforation is described on page 97. Answers A through C and E are true. Sympathetic ophthalmia is described on page 298, phthisis bulbi is described on page 304, and epithelial ingrowth is described on page 98.

Chapter 4

1. (**B**) Lens fibers contain relatively few intracellular organelles. The lens receives most of its nourishment from the aqueous and vitreous (p. 120).

2. (**D**) Initially the sutures are Y shaped, but later in gestation they form more complicated dendritic patterns. The anterior Y is upright, and the posterior Y is inverted (p. 119).

3. (**C**) Growth of the lens throughout life is accomplished by the mitotic activity of the cells of the equatorial lens bow (pp. 117 and 119). Answer A is false because the cells of the anterior epithelium remain relatively stationary with minimal mitotic activity. Answer B is false because there are no cells situated on the posterior capsule, except in cases of posterior subcapsular cataract where epithelial cells and

bladder cells may migrate centrally from the equator. The only cells with significant mitotic activity are the newly formed cells of the equator. Older anterior and equatorial epithelial cells do not have germinal activity (answer E).

4. **(B)** The lens capsule is a true PAS-staining basement membrane secreted by the lens epithelium. It is thinnest posteriorly, a fact that is of clinical significance during both intracapsular (ICCE) or extracapsular (ECCE) lens extraction (p. 119).

5. **(E)** Soemmering's ring cataract has been described in detail on pages 121-125. It consists primarily of remnants of lens capsule and lens cortex, the latter forming the basic substance of the residual "doughnut" as viewed on gross examination or the peripheral thickenings on the "barbell" as seen histologically in the photomicrograph. In general all or most of the lens nucleus is resorbed in such cases.

6. **(A)** The lens capsule develops early as a derivative of the basement membrane of the original monolayer of cells that forms the lens vesicle after separation from the overlying surface ectoderm (p. 117). The lens sutures have nothing to do with the capsule but rather represent sites of juncture of lens fibers within the lens substance (p. 119).

7. **(D)** Mittendorf dots are light-gray opacities near the posterior pole. They are remnants of the tunica vasculosa lentis and usually do not significantly impair vision (pp. 30, 125, and 131).

8. **(C)** All answers except reduplication cataract are types of age-related cataracts. *Reduplication cataract* usually is used to designate a form of congenital lens opacity (pp. 125 and 126).

9. **(E)** All of the answers are correct. Phacoanaphylaxis (p. 136) and localized endophthalmitis (p. 163) represent crystalline lens-induced and infectious processes, respectively. It may be that these conditions actually are one and the same and that the infectious organisms actually create a tissue adjuvant to combine with the lens protein to cause the hypersensitivity reaction (p. 136). Problems with IOL manufacture and design—including such problems as sharp edges caused by inadequate polishing of the intraocular lens, residues of polishing compounds on the lens surface, problems with lens sterilizing, etc.—are rare today because of vast improvements in manufacturing over the past decade (pp. 139 and 140). Therefore the term "toxic lens syndrome," although entrenched in the literature and descriptive, does not correlate directly with etiology or pathogenesis.

10. **(A)** Snowflake cataracts are associated with diabetes (pp. 122 and 381). The sunflower cataract is associated with Wilson's disease or chalcosis (p. 84). A morgagnian cataract occurs in mature (ripe) cataracts when the cortex liquefies and the nucleus sinks inferiorly (p. 125).

11. **(C)** All except Hurler's syndrome are associated with cataracts. Visual loss in the mucopolysaccharidoses is caused more commonly by corneal clouding (p. 94).

12. **(E)** Marfan's syndrome is described on page 135. Retinal degenerations, such as those that occur in the retinitis pigmentosa syndrome (p. 402) or as a "salt-and-pepper" fundus, is not characteristic of this disease. The "salt-and-pepper" fundus may be a prominent feature in the rubella syndrome (p. 132).

13. **(D)** Hirschberg-Elsching pearls (p. 123) are clusters of swollen, proliferating epithelial cells situated in the anterior chamber and on adjacent structures. They characteristically occur after disruption of the lens capsule. This may be secondary to accidental trauma or may occur as a sequala to surgical procedures, e.g., planned or unplanned extracapsular lens extraction (ECCE). They morphologically resemble clusters of bladder cells, which also represent abnormal alterations of lens epithelium (p. 126).

14. **(E)** There are no nuclei in the center of the normal crystalline lens (p. 119). The germinal nuclei that cause constant laying down of lens fibers are situated at the equatorial lens bow. Only in pathologic states such as the rubella syndrome (p. 132) do nuclei persist, migrate, and become situated in the center of the lens (p. 126).

15. **(C)** The zonules course from the ciliary processes and the valleys between them to the surface of the equatorial lens capsule. As the ciliary muscle contracts during accommodation, the zonules relax,

that is, they become less taut (p. 120). Therefore answer C is a false statement.

16. **(D)** A Vossius ring is a circular pigmented ring on the anterior lens surface just behind the pupil. It consists of melanin deposits, usually caused by trauma or intraocular inflammation (p. 125).

17. **(D)** Steroids classically produce posterior subcapsular cataracts or diffuse cataracts (pp. 122 and 125).

18. **(B)** The thinnest portion of the lens capsule is clearly at the posterior capsule (p. 00). This is of major clinical significance for many reasons. In cataract surgery, both ICCE and ECCE, rupture of the posterior capsule increases the incidence of operative morbidity, for example, there is increased incidence of vitreous loss, possible subsequent retinal detachment, and other difficulties (p. 169). Rupture also can cause other problems such as difficulties in IOL fixation and subsequent decentration (pp. 151-161).

19. **(E)** Although all of the complications listed in answers A to D may occur after implantation of closed-loop anterior chamber IOLs, pseudophakic corneal decompensation, answer E, was by far the most common long-term complication after implantation of these lenses (pp. 146-151).

20. **(B)** The retrolental mass represents an endothelial proliferation derived from a persistence and hyperplasia of small vascular channels of the tunica vasculosa lentis (*small arrows*) (p. 29). Prenatal proliferative diabetic retinopathy has not been documented in children. This slide shows a very early embryo (first trimester of pregnancy). Retinopathy of prematurity occurs in premature infants but not at this very early stage. (p. 496). Lange's fold is an artifact described on page 11. A persistent Bergmeister papilla occurs at the level of the optic nerve head (p. 34), not near the lens.

21. **(D)** All of the diseases except Lowe's syndrome are well-documented causes of lens dislocation. The major findings in Lowe's syndrome are microphakia, spherophakia, wartlike excrescences on the capsule, cataracts, and congenital glaucoma (pp. 125 and 264).

22. **(E)** The maternal rubella syndrome is described on page 132. All of the listed conditions have been described in this syndrome except E, an abnormal electroretinogram. The "salt-and-pepper" fundus of the maternal rubella syndrome clearly differs from pigmentary retinopathy, such as is seen in retinopathia pigmentosa (p. 402) in that retinal degeneration does not occur and the electroretinogram is not disturbed.

23. **(B)** An anterior subcapsular fibrous plaque is caused by fibrous metaplasia of the anterior lens epithelium, which often is a reaction to irritation such as trauma or inflammation (p. 125). Some authors prefer the term *pseudometaplasia* because the cells that form the fibrous plaque have subtle morphologic features that differ slightly from those of the fibrocytes. Intralenticular hemorrhage is rare, and bladder cells represent sequelae of posterior migration of lens epithelium, which may lead to a posterior subcapsular cataract (p. 125).

24. **(E)** This slide shows the classic appearance of a so-called cocoon membrane in which debris is deposited around the surface of the optic of the intraocular lens, leading to obvious opacification (pp. 125 and 126). These membranes may be caused by inflammation, proliferation of iris tissue, proliferation of metaplastic residual lens epithelium after extracapsular extraction, organization of hemorrhage, or formation of a retrocorneal fibrous membrane (rare). Intraocular lens-induced posterior capsular membranes usually may be removed with reopening of the visual axis by the Nd:YAG laser, without necessitating removal of the IOL.

25. **(D)** All of the answers except D connote common features of maternal rubella syndrome. The important characteristic feature of maternal rubella syndrome emphasized in this question is the fact that there is a conspicuous absence of other *severe* congenital anomalies of the eye, such as anophthalmia, severe microphthalmia, and colobomas (pp. 131-133).

26. **(E)** Sampaolesi's line represents a pigmentation of the trabecular meshwork that is seen frequently in pseudoexfoliation syndrome (p. 136) and in pigmentary dispersion syndrome (p. 80). Answer A

describes Krukenberg's spindle (p. 80). Answer D describes a Vossius ring (p. 125).

27. (**E**) Answers A to D describe phacoanaphylactic endophthalmitis. Answer E refers to the cell more closely associated with phacolytic glaucoma (p. 136).

28. All of the conditions except C listed are significant causes of posterior chamber intraocular lens decentration (pp. 153-155). Ciliary sulcus fixation represents a symmetric fixation of loops at generally is not associated with decentration.

29. (**C**) All of the answers except C describe the classic findings of so-called true exfoliation of the lens capsule (glassblower's disease; p. 139). The photomicrograph actually shows dandruff-like particles characteristic of the pseudoexfoliation syndrome (glaucoma capsulare of Vogt; p. 136). The particles are derived from basement membrane, including 136e lens capsule and the ciliary epithelium. Similar particles also have been observed on basement membranes of vessels of the bulbar conjunctiva in affected patients.

30. (**C**) Epithelial cells are not normally seen on the posterior surface of the lens. Posterior migration and bladder cell formation are histopathologic signs in "senile" cataracts (p. 125). Cataracts secondary to fibrous plaques typically occur in the *anterior* subcapsular region (p. 125). Morgagnian globules may occur in many types of cataracts, anywhere within the lens substance, and represent a breakdown and liquefaction of lens protein (p. 125). Hirschberg-Elschnig pearls connote a proliferation of lens epithelial cells outside of the lens, caused by migration through the ruptured lens capsule (p. 123).

31. (**A**) The most common operation performed in the *industrialized* world today is implantation of rigid or foldable posterior chamber IOLs after ECCE or phacoemulsification. Therefore answers C and E are not true in terms of the truly rural developing world, where ICCE with spectacle rehabilitation still is the only therapy available. Therefore answer A is the correct one (p. 141). Answers B and E are false.

32. (**A**) The introduction of viscoelastics in the early 1980s (the first agent available was Healon,™ produced by Pharmacia Corporation) has provided major advances in allowing safe and effective surgery. Many surgeons prefer to use viscoelastics on a routine basis to protect tissue such as corneal endothelium and to manipulate tissue spaces for better cataract removal and intraocular lens implantation (p. 154). Answer B is, of course, false because closed-loop anterior chamber lenses have been shown to be inappropriate and have been removed from the market (pp. 146-151). Several complications, including posterior capsular opacification (PCO) and IOL decentration, are caused by proliferation of retained epithelial cells, so answer C also is clearly false. To date there is no medical therapy that has had a significant clinical effect on either cataract prevention or therapy of cataracts, so answer D is also false.

33. (**E**) Implantation in the capsular bag may be advantageous for all of the reasons listed (p. 155). Note in the scanning electron micrograph how clean the loop appears at the site where it had been surrounded by the lens capsule. There is no evidence of any type of polymer alteration (p. 153). Capsular bag fixation is mandatory for modern foldable IOLs.

34. (**A**) This type of lens is described on page 147. The pigmented tissue on the lens loops shows the sites where the lens made contact with the angle recess and the anterior iris surface. Modern flexible anterior chamber IOLs with footplates provide much better results than these older models (p. 148).

35. (**E**) The findings described in this question all occur in the uveitis-glaucoma-hyphema syndrome, or so-called UGH syndrome of Ellingson, a well-known complication of lens implantation (p. 162). Sharp edges of poorly manufactured lenses was a common culprit. The surface of the optic shown in this photograph is covered by numerous inflammatory cells, erythrocytes, and fibrous and proteinaceous debris.

36. (**E**) The development of CCC and hydrodissection in the mid 1980s and the introduction of viscoelastics were important factors in the evolution of modern capsular surgery, including small-incision procedures. The answers are discussed on pages 153, 155, and 156.

37. (**C**) It is not well known by most surgeons that an excellent means of enhancing removal of lens epithelial cells and cortex is by hydrodissection, which in effect represents a "hydro" polishing of the region of the fornix of the capsular bag (p. 156). Answer A is false because removal of anterior lens epithelial cells is not necessary. These cells participate more in the formation of anterior subcapsular fibrous cataract (p. 175) as opposed to classic posterior capsular opacifications. Answers B and D represent experimental approaches to combating this complication, but are not clinically available.

38. (**A**) Answers B to D are correct features of modern capsular all-PMMA IOLs (p. 157). Answer A is the correct choice in this case because most modern capsular lenses are 12.0 to 12.5 mm in total length, allowing a perfect "fit" into the capsular bag which averages 10.5 mm and 11.0 mm in diameter. The early 14-mm one-piece PMMA IOLs that appeared in the mid 1980s generally were rejected because they were too large, too rigid, and too difficult to insert.

39. (**C**) The best answer is C (p. 158), although surgeons now also are experimenting with modern foldable IOLs, such as an acrylic design for pediatric implantation. Ninety percent of the growth of the pediatric lens occurs within the first years of life (p. 158). Answer A is incorrect because IOL stabilization is achieved by good in-the-bag implantation. Answer B is incorrect because the major goal now is to attempt IOL implantation into every possible case. Answer D is incorrect because posterior capsular opacification and membrane formation still are relatively common in pediatric cataract surgery, and primary posterior capsulectomy is advisable until better techniques of preventing this complications are developed. Answer E is incorrect because the loop memory of polypropylene haptics is less than with a one-piece all-PMMA IOL, and haptic distortion and lens stability are not as assured.

40. (**C**) An often overlooked advantage of small incision surgery is the fact that the general safety of surgery is better (p. 158), e.g., lower incidence of endophthalmitis. Answers A, B, D, and E are definite advantages and speak for small incision-foldable lens surgery, but generally they are features that enhance the quality and efficacy of the procedures rather than the general safety of the procedure (pp. 158-161).

41. (**D**) In general a hydrophilic surface is most resistant to adherence of silicone oil and in many ways can be considered tissue friendly (p. 161). Adherence of silicone oil occurred to the greatest extent with silicone, so answer C is incorrect (p. 161). Adherence occurs to a lesser extent with standard PMMA and soft acrylic material, so these lenses are not totally immune to this complication; therefore answers A and B are incorrect. Answer E is incorrect because polypropylene is a haptic material and not an optic material.

42. (**B**) In this scenario, after a large can opener capsulectomy, "pea-podding" or exit from the capsular bag through a radial tear of the anterior capsular is a significant risk. This therefore creates a subsequent asymmetric fixation of the haptic (p. 156). Answers A and D are incorrect because although ciliary sulcus fixation is not the desired type with modern surgery, when both haptics are indeed in the ciliary sulcus decentration is not as severe as with asymmetric fixation. Answer C is incorrect because this actually represents the ideal type of implantation that helps to avoid decentration) and other complications and forms the basis of modern "capsular surgery."

43. (**E**) All of the answers are correct statements regarding modern concepts of cataract surgery in the developing world (p. 156).

44. (**C**) Answers A, B, and E are desirable features regarding small incision surgery, but are not critical to overall safety and avoidance of complications. Therefore they are incorrect (p. 161). Answer D also is incorrect because a CCC that is too small actually has several disadvantages, including difficulty of IOL insertion, and postoperative capsulorhexis contraction (p. 156). Answer C is the best answer because well-performed hydrodissection provides several positive functions including enhancing removal of lens material. This helps reduce such complication as posterior capsular opacification. The

latter complication used to occur in more than 50% of cases; the incidence of this probably is less than 20% with modern capsular "surgery."

45. **(E)** The photograph shows posterior capsular opacification. Note that the IOL was a three-piece design with polypropylene haptics, one of which has compressed over the optic. Answer E is correct because all of the answers are correct statements regarding means of avoiding or preventing this complication (p. 175). Copious hydrodissection allows thorough removal of cortex and cells (p. 156); all-PMMA lenses provide haptics with excellent memory and have good stability within the capsular bag (p. 155). A primary posterior capsulectomy does not prevent the complication but it will circumvent it by avoiding opacification over the visual axis (p. 156). The use of a biconvex IOL allows the posterior convex surface to provide a "barrier effect," which blocks ingrowth of epithelial cells into the visual axis by close opposition to the posterior capsule (p. 176). It recently has been postulated that IOLs made from acrylic materials may enhance the barrier effect.

46. **(E)** This photograph shows the almost perfect result after implantation of a foldable IOL into the capsular bag; thus all of the answers are correct (answer E). The outline of the CCC can be seen in the photograph, and it is clear that both lenses are placed symmetrically within the lens capsular bag. Because the capsular bag is almost free of retained lens material, it is likely that copious hydrodissection was performed prior to phacoemulsification. Modern soft material such as silicone, acrylic, and hydrogels show excellent biocompatibility. (p. 158)

47. **(E)** The choices listed A through D are viable alternatives for exchange or secondary implantation, therefore, answer E is correct. In general an anterior chamber lens is preferable for a surgeon who does not have extensive experience with the various sutured posterior chamber IOL implantation techniques. Sutured posterior chamber lenses are well suited for surgeons who frequently use this technique. They are especially amendable to implantation via an open sky-technique (p. 151).

48. **(C)** The high molecular weight PMMA used for one-piece (monoblock) all-PMMA IOLs has the best memory characteristics.[187] Both polypropylene and extruded PMMA have less memory retention, although extruded PMMA is less compressible than polypropylene. Answers A and B are therefore incorrect. Answers D and E are incorrect because hydrogel and silicone primarily are optic materials, although silicone is used in plate haptic IOLs where haptic memory is not a factor (p. 158).

49. **(A)** The correct answer is A because can opener capsulectomy rarely is used with modern capsular surgery (p. 156). Answer B through E are important procedures that have defined modern capsular surgery (pp. 156-157).

50. **(A)** The best answer is A because the Nd:YAG laser can cause direct damage to the posterior IOL surface. Answer B is false because the Nd:YAG laser is treatment rather than a cause of posterior capsular opacification. Answers C, D, and E are incorrect because these are rare complications of the Nd:YAG laser (pp. 178 and 179).

CHAPTER 5

1. **(C)** This is the one statement listed that is not true. Postoperative pain after PRK indeed peaks around 4 to 6 hours, but the pain frequently persists for a much longer period, up to 36 or 48 hours. All of the other statements are true (pp. 219)

2. **(D)** This photomicrograph shows a wound healing response after disruption of corneal epithelium basement membrane and Bowman's layer. This phenomenon can occur in all three of the listed surgical procedures. Therefore answer D is the correct one.

3. "Mini RK" does offer more structural integrity because there is much less tissue destruction (p. 210). After classic RK, the structural integrity of the cornea generally is not restored to normal and healing can take several years (pp. 210 and 211). The American technique is safer, but the Russian technique has a greater effect (p. 209).

4. **(E)** Answers A, B, C, and D are all well-known complications and side effects of radial keratotomy (pp. 210 and 212). Regression always occurs in the hyperopic direction and not toward myopia. Therefore, answer E is the correct choice.

5. **(E)** With the expansion of the ring the cornea will flatten; with constriction of the ring, the cornea will steepen. Small diameter rings cause deepening, larger diameter rings cause flattening (p. 225). The ring does not alter the structure of the central cornea, and the process is reversible.

6. **(E)** Production of all of these substances highlights the fact that there is a significant wound healing response after PRK (p. 220). Ongoing wound healing is one of the factors that can lead to complications such as unpredictability and haze.

7. **(A)** All of the answers except A are true, therefore, answer A is the correct choice. Bowman's layer normally does not regenerate when destroyed.

8. **(B)** A large epithelial plug often connotes a poorly performed radial keratotomy, forming after a wound gape (p. 210). The other items listed are not specific.

9. **(D)** Such hardware has been introduced in an attempt to create smoother ablation profiles (p. 218). The other choices are not true.

10. **(D)** Haze often is caused by deposition of scar tissue in the subepithelial scar zone (p. 220).

11. **(E)** Evidence of complete healing often requires 5 or more years (pp. 210 and 211).

12. **(E)** All of the substances, especially corticosteroids, have been used to moderate the human response (p. 220).

13. **(C)** The Dutch ophthalmologist Leendert Jan Lans was the first to describe an extensive experimental study in 1898 (p. 207). The classic work on RK by Sato in Japan occurred later during the 1930s (p. 207). Fyodorov and Durnev did their primary laboratory and clinical work in Russia in the 1960s and 1970s. Therefore, answers A, B, D, and E are incorrect.

14. **(E)** Intrastromal corneal implants are discussed on page 216.

15. **(A)** Undercorrection is the most common complication of PRK and generally can be managed by retreatment (p. 219). Answer B is incorrect because overcorrection is less common than undercorrection. Overcorrections commonly are managed by tapering or discontinuing postoperative steroids. Answers C and E are incorrect. Answer E is false because the subepithelial ingrowth and deposition of material from a Weck sponge are complications of LASIK (p. 225).

16. **(D)** All answers listed as A through C are correct regarding epikeratophakia (p. 216).

17. **(B)** Early IOLs were poorly designed and manufactured (p. 228). All of the other answers are false regarding phakic IOLs (p. 226).

18. **(C)** Although PTK may remove a scar, a new scar can be produced by the wound healing of the procedure itself and thus may cause visual effects (pp. 221-222). Answers A and B are incorrect because PTK is effective in treating these conditions. Answer D is incorrect because PTK has been shown to activate herpes simplex (p. 222). Answer E is incorrect because the posterior corneal endothelium is not directly affected by PTK.

19. **(E)** All of the stated reasons are responsible for relatively slow development of laser refractive surgery in the United States (p. 205).

20. **(D)** This is photomicrograph showing the formation of a large epithelial plug into the site of a gaping RK wound. Therefore, the correct answer is D. Answer A is incorrect because this can be of clinical significance. B is incorrect because the slide does not show evidence of bacteria. Answer C is incorrect because the lesion is at the epithelial level. Answer E is incorrect because no inflammation is present in the slide (p. 210).

21. **(D)** "Haze" is more common with higher attempted corrections (p. 00). Answers A, B, and C are false (p. 220).

22. **(C)** Sato, in Japan, used posterior corneal incisions, which at first glance appeared efficacious, but later showed complications (p. 207). Therefore answer C is the correct answer. Answers A, B, D, and E were important principles described by Lans in 1898 (p. 207).

23. (**E**) All items are potential or actual complications or side effects of RK (pp. 210 and 211).

24. (**A**) Transverse keratotomy is an incisional procedure designed to correct astigmatism (p. 212), so A is the correct answer. It often is used with cataract surgery, so answer B is incorrect. Answers C through E also are incorrect (p. 212).

25. (**C**) The wound healing response is a major factor in the refractive outcome of RK (p. 210). All the other answers are true.

26. (**D**) Closed-loop anterior chamber lenses were not successful (p. 228). Answer A is correct because the Baikoff and Kelman-Clemente designs represent modern, well-made anterior chamber lenses (p. 228). Answer B also is true because clear lens extraction is a viable option, although with this technique one loses accommodation (p. 226). One also can implant posterior chamber lenses in aphakic eyes (p. 230), so answer C is true. Answer E also is true because foldable IOLs can be used as phakic IOLs or with clear lens extraction (p. 226).

27. (**C**) Laser thermal keratoplasty has been introduced as a treatment for hyperopia (p. 221). Burns are placed in the paracentral cornea, so answer A is false. Answer B is false because the technique is not used for myopia (p. 221). Answer D is false because it creates its effect by steepening in the central cornea. Answer E is false because there is significant regression with this technique.

28. (**E**) Mathematical models are needed to predict the outcome (p. 225). Answers A to D do represent possible advantages, and therefore are not correct answers.

29. (**A**) Most of the patients who receive this procedure are myopes who have an increased propensity toward retinal detachment (p. 227). Answer B is false because posterior capsular opacification has been reduced in the incidence and is not a major safety hazard (p. 174). Answers C, D, and E are false because these are rare complication of modern capsular surgery (pp. 156 and 161).

30. (**B**) In LASIK, the refractive incisions are made with the accuracy and flexibility of the excimer laser. All the other answers are incorrect (p. 222)

31. (**E**) Phakic IOLs provide the most favorable long-term refractive stability and also are independent of corneal wound healing, so a) phakic IOL, b) phakic IOL would be the best choice; however, it is not listed as a choice. Of the listed choices, the best answer is E because LASIK is totally independent of the corneal epithelium-Bowman's layer wound healing process (p. 222). Answers A and B are false because radial keratotomy does not meet either criteria, and answer C is false because epikeratophakia does not meet the requirements (p. 216). Answer D is false because PRK is heavily dependent on the corneal epithelium-Bowman's layer wound healing process (p. 220).

32. (**E**) This is an electron micrograph of an activated keratocyte containing abundant endoplasmic reticulum that synthesizes collagen. It is situated in the anterior corneal stroma and is responsible for formation of delicate fibrous tissue at the interface (pp. 222 and 223).

33. (**E**) All of the answers are true facts regarding phakic IOL implantation (pp. 226 and 228).

34. (**C**) PRK does not require expert use of a microkeratome. All the other options actually are considered to be advantages of LASIK (p. 222).

35. (**C**) Excimer laser emits photons that are strongly absorbed by corneal tissue and penetrate less than the depth of a cell (p. 217). This allows various sizes of ablation. Answer A is false because thermal energy does not play a role. Answer B is incorrect because the laser does not function as well as a diamond blade acting as a "laser knife." Answer D is incorrect because the excimer laser is not a solid state laser. Answer E is incorrect because the laser is only successful in treating myopia up to approximately 6 D. LASIK is necessary for higher ranges (pp. 219 and 223).

36. (**E**) All the answers describe the wound healing response after PRK (p. 220).

37. (**C**) In the 1980s, Dr. Louis Ruiz added an automated gear system to Dr. Barraquer's microkeratome to control the speed of the pass across the cornea (p. 214). All other answers are incorrect.

38. (**E**) Epikeratophakia is reversible (p. 216). All the other items listed are true.

39. (**E**) All the listed answers are true regarding the Worst-Fechner lobster claw IOL (p. 229).

40. (**C**) Both RK and PRK can exhibit long-term fluctuation and volatility of vision (pp. 210 and 224). All other statements regarding possible advantages of RK are true (p. 208).

41. (**B**) Answer A is incorrect because the incisions are parallel to anterior surface of the cornea (p. 213). Answer C is incorrect because most cases to date have been performed for myopia. Answer D is incorrect because the lamellar procedure can be useful in treating high degrees of refractive error. Answer E is incorrect because Sato's pioneering work was done on radial keratotomy (p. 207).

42. (**A**) The healing at the junction is minimal, which is advantageous because this allows free passage of incoming light (p. 223; Color Plate 5-11). The wound healing process is not affected by epithelial mediators, so answer B is incorrect (p. 224). The fact that the reactive process is minimal makes answers C and E incorrect. The fibrosis occurs over a period more than 1 month, so answer D is incorrect.

43. (**A**) The use of an ablatable gel associated with PRK is very promising in the treatment of irregular corneal astigmatism or topography (p. 221). When the gel is placed on the regular cornea surface, the gel is then rendered smooth with an overlying contact lens. The laser is fooled into thinking it has treated a smooth surface so the hills and valleys are evened out. The other items mentioned are incorrect because they do not carry out a surface treatment that will smooth out the surface.

44. (**A**) There is less risk of continuing the incision into the central clear zone (p. 209). All other answers are false.

45. (**E**) Answers A through D correctly describe features of homoplastic keratomileusis (p. 215).

46. (**E**) Treatment is not indicated because the axial length of the eye still may be increasing during growth. The adult refraction is therefore usually not yet established at 12 years of age.

47. (**B**) LASIK is the best treatment listed here to treat higher ranges of myopia, as in this case (p. 223).

48. (**B**) This micrograph shows the typical scanning electron microscopic appearance after passage of the microkeratome (p. 214 and Fig. 5-7). Answers A, C, D, and E are false because these show different profiles.

49. (**B**) (See p. 224 and Fig. 5-10). Because the wound healing after LASIK occurs only at the incision site of the flap in the periphery, as soon as this reaction is complete there is no further wound healing. There is no subepithelial wound healing process centrally as occurs with PRK (p. 220). The graph shown in Fig. 5-10 indicates why answer A, C, and E are correct.

50. (**D**) This is a false statement because the numbers are reversed. During the past 15 years, more than one million RKs have been performed and more than 400,000 PRKs have been performed (p. 207). Answers A to C and E are correct statements.

CHAPTER 6

1. (**D**) Primary open-angle glaucoma, which affects approximately 1-2% of the population, is one of the most common causes of blindness (p. 268). It typically is bilateral. The photomicrograph shows a contusion angle deformity with severe angle recession, a cause of glaucoma that typically is unilateral (assuming that the blunt trauma that commonly causes such a lesion usually is unilateral) (p. 272). The glaucoma of Sturge-Weber syndrome usually is unilateral, ipsilateral, occurring on the same side as the facial portwine stain, which is characteristic of this syndrome (p. 513). Persistent hyperplastic primary vitreous almost is always unilateral (p. 30), as is uveal malignant melanoma.

2. (**C**) The large macrophages in phacolytic glaucoma that cause a particulate blockage of the trabecular meshwork contain protein derived from liquefaction of lens fibers caused by a mature cataract (p. 136). It has even been shown that glaucoma associated with such mature cataracts can occur *without* an influx of macrophages. A highly proteinaceous, viscous fluid derived from denatured lens fibers can enter the anterior chamber and apparently can cause decreased outflow in the absence of macrophages. Answers A and D are inflammatory cells; phacolytic glaucoma in the true sense of the word is not an "inflammatory" process. Answers B and E, implying that the macrophages contain either lipid or mucopolysaccharide, respectively, are not true because the main constituent of lens fibers is protein.

3. (**A**) Answer A is false because the volume of the adult anterior chamber is approximately 0.2 to 0.3 ml. The iris stroma differentiates from mesectoderm (p. 284), whereas the iris pigment epithelium differentiates from the primary neuroectoderm of the embryonic optic cuff (p. 284). The iris pigment epithelium forms one of the surface components of the blood-aqueous barrier (p. 261). The definitive filtration apparatus first appears just before birth (p. 261). A failure of recession of fetal iris processes is one of the factors responsible for the pathogenesis of the various anterior cleavage syndromes (p. 261).

4. (**C**) Atrophy of the inner retinal layers (including ganglion cells and nerve fiber layer) and glaucomatous atrophy of the optic nerve with deep cupping are by far the most common causes of blindness because of the various types of glaucoma (p. 278). Schnabel's cavernous atrophy (p. 278) also may be a sequela of glaucoma, but it is not nearly as common as answer C. Opacification of the cornea with degenerative pannus formation or band keratopathy often occurs in glaucoma and is a serious complication (p. 274) but not to the degree described in answer C. Answer B is incorrect because in glaucoma the inner retinal layers primarily are destroyed rather than the elements of the outer retina, such as the photoreceptors. Hemorrhage in the retina can occur in various types of glaucoma (e.g., splinter hemorrhages around the disc, associated with neovascular glaucoma in such diseases as central vein occlusion), but again this does not represent the most common cause of blindness that is represented in answer C.

5. (**E**) The retinal and optic nerve changes in glaucoma are described on page 276.

6. (**E**) The maintenance of corneal water content is regulated primarily by an active metabolic pump in the corneal endothelium. To prove that all the other answers are true, one only has to consider the effects of long-standing hypotony (p. 263). All the homeostatic mechanisms listed are compromised, leading to a typical, shrunken, distorted, soft eye with ciliary-choroidal detachment and the numerous well-known secondary sequelae of this syndrome.

7. (**E**) The aqueous in many ways can be considered analogous to cerebrospinal fluid; thus E is correct (p. 263). There are multiple outflow channels for the aqueous into the systemic circulation, including the episcleral collecting channels (p. 263). The aqueous itself is secreted by active metabolic activity within the ciliary epithelium, and this formation is therefore not passive (p. 262), Normal aqueous contains low levels of proteins. After breakdown of the blood aqueous barrier, for example, in climatory conditions, protein and cells may reach this barrier and enter the aqueous humor (pp. 162 and 262). Answer D is incorrect because the inner layer of the ciliary processes is nonpigmented (pp. 7 and 262).

8. (**B**) In low-tension glaucoma there probably is an imbalance between the normal relationship of intraocular pressure to the pressure in the posterior ciliary circulation (p. 264).

9. (**E**) All the causes listed may cause pupillary block and angle-closure glaucoma (p. 264).

10. (**D**) The lesions seen in this photograph are so-called glaukomflecken, which are associated most characteristically with attacks of acute glaucoma (p. 275).

11. (**A**) Answers B to E connote entities in which a morphologic shallowing or actual obliteration of the anterior chamber angle can occur (pp. 265-268). Ocular hypertension simply defines a stage in which morphologic changes are not evident but in which varying degrees of elevation of intraocular pressure are measured in the absence of obvious measurable functional, visual field, or ophthalmoscopic change (p. 263).

12. (**D**) See pages 276 and 537.

13. (**C**) All answers except C generally are associated with glaucoma of the narrow or closed-angle type. Most cases of congenital glaucoma are of the open-angle type (p. 272). Indeed, in some cases, the angles may appear to be even more "open" than usual because of stretching of the cornea, which leads to the characteristic dome-shaped appearance of the cornea. This type of change increases the volume of the anterior chamber.

14. (**B**) Glaucoma is not synonymous with ocular hypertension. Glaucoma is not a specific disease, but a collective term describing a condition in which anatomic and functional damage to the eye are caused by an abnormal relative or absolute increase in intraocular pressure (p. 263). The specific diagnosis of glaucoma should be differentiated from ocular hypertension, which is discussed on page 263. Most cases result from impaired aqueous outflow through the trabecular meshwork, although hypersecretion of aqueous may represent an uncommon cause (p. 263). The posterior sequelae of glaucoma are described on page 276.

15. (**A**) See pages 261-263 for a discussion of the anatomy and histology of the anterior chamber angel filtration structures and outflow channels.

16. (**E**) All of the statements are correct. The smallest sized pores of the trabecular meshwork, the juxtacanalicular apparatus, are situated immediately adjacent to Schlemm's canal (p. 263). Schwalbe's line, which may be prominent in normal situations and in pathologic situations such as the various anterior chamber cleavage syndromes, is the anterior termination of the trabecular meshwork (pp. 35 and 263). The trabecular meshwork is lined by a cellular layer, which commonly is termed an *endothelium* (others term this a *mesothelium* because these cells line a fluid-filled cavity analogous to pericardial or peritoneal mesothelium; p. 263).

17. (**D**) The marked degeneration of the ciliary processes with fibrosis, hyalinization, loss of epithelium, and dispersion and necrosis of pigment epithelium is secondary to cryocoagulation. This technique is used, often as a last resort, in the treatment of intractable neovascular glaucoma. The histopathologic appearances of sympathetic ophthalmia and Fuchs' adenoma are discussed on pages 298 and 329, respectively. Although an eye with end-stage glaucoma actually can become phthisic because of shutdown of the aqueous secretion product from the ciliary epithelium, this process would not create the markedly destructive changes seen in this photomicrograph. The dense pigment clumps in this illustration are derived from the pigmented layer of ciliary epithelium and have nothing do with pigment granules in pigmentary dispersion syndrome (p. 268).

18. (**E**) Answer E, all of the above, is correct. The various features of the ICE syndrome are described on page 266.

19. (**C**) The aqueous humor obviously passes initially through the trabecular meshwork and juxtacanalicular pores before entering Schlemm's canal (p. 263). All other answers are true, and maintenance of the homeostatic factors described in these answers is critical in preventing both glaucoma and hypotony.

20. (**C**) This is an angle totally closed by broad, peripheral anterior synechiae (p. 265).

21. (**A**) Corticosteroid-induced glaucoma is of the open-angle type. A tumor, ciliary body swelling, and phacomorphic glaucoma caused by swelling of the lens may induce an anterior displacement of the lens-iris diaphragm leading to angle closure. Organization of anterior chamber hemorrhage may create fibrous membranes that may lead to seclusion or occlusion of the pupil and secondary angle closure.

22. (**D**) The photomicrograph reveals Schnabel's cavernous optic atrophy. Schnabel's optic atrophy (p. 278) is most characteristically seen after acute and intense increases in intraocular pressure and may be seen in patients with anterior ischemic optic neuropathy (p. 544; e.g., associated with temporal arteritis). The basic cause is an imbalance between perfusion pressure in the posterior ciliary arteries and intraocular pressure. The cavernous spaces of Schnabel's atrophy cannot be observed clinically. The spaces contain hyaluronic acid derived from the vitreous rather than a serous fluid or lipid. Familial transmission is not a direct factor in the pathogenesis of this lesion.

23. (E) Answer E, all of the above, is correct. Primary open-angle glaucoma is described on page 268. Regarding answer B, primary open-angle glaucoma is certainly a relative if not an absolute contraindication for implantation of an anterior chamber IOL, in which the lens is placed within the narrow confines of the anterior chamber. Damage to outflow channels may be caused by the presence of loops or haptics in the angle recess (p. 162).

24. (E) Schwalbe's line forms the *anterior* margin of the filtration apparatus. The internal and external scleral sulci are indentations in the sclera at the limbus. The term "spaces of Fontana" is outdated, connoting the pores within the trabecular meshwork. There is no such thing as a pectinate ligament or ligament of Fontana in humans (p. 263).

25. (C) The characteristics of angle recession are described on page 271. All the other answers are common features of congenital glaucoma. Atrophia bulbi should be differentiated from phthisis bulbi (p. 304). It is a common misconception that an atrophic globe has to be small. On the contrary, many "atrophic" globes are large and are secondary to absolute glaucoma. This is especially true in congenital glaucoma and even to some extent in adult glaucoma. In the latter, the enlargement of the globe is not as great, but in many cases the measurements of the globe may be greater than normal because of stretching of the sclera.

26. (D) All the answers are correct except D (p. 272). There is no evidence that endothelial cells undergo an enlargement in congenital glaucoma.

27. (A) Iridodialysis is caused by trauma. All the other answers are well-known sequelae of increased intraocular pressure (pp. 273–278).

28. (E) The trabecular meshwork and most other structures of the aqueous outflow channels are derived from mesectoderm, not surface ectoderm (pp. 9 and 261). The other answers are correct features of congenital glaucoma (p. 272).

29. (E) The small pores at the juxtacanalicular region are the most susceptible to particulate blockage or occlusion (pp. 263).

30. (E) The lesion seen in the drawing is a so-called contusion rosette (p. 270), formed because of separation of lens fibers around the lens sutures. This is a frequent sequel to blunt trauma. Note the dendritic branching pattern of the sutures in this drawing. In a patient with this type of injury, a contusion angle deformity can develop, and angle-recession glaucoma has the potential to develop; angle-recession glaucoma typically is an open-angle glaucoma, but it also may evolve into closed-angle glaucoma. Therefore all of the answers must be considered true.

31. (E) Buphthalmos is a significant feature of congenital glaucoma (p. 272). Corneal edema may occur after long-standing pressure elevations or in acute glaucoma (p. 274). Glaukomflecken are multiple, white punctate opacities appearing in the subcapsular cortex, usually occurring after sudden acute rises in pressure (p. 274).

32. (B) These two cells, measuring approximately 40 μm in diameter, are much larger than most chronic inflammatory cells. They contain small benign-appearing nuclei and show a foamy cytoplasm. These are the macrophages that pick up liquefied lens protein from mature cataracts and lead to particulate blockage of the trabecular meshwork (p. 136). Bona fide inflammatory cells would be observed if this were a case of phacoanaphylactic endophthalmitis (p. 136). Cells in the anterior chamber typically would not be seen in answer C to E.

33. (B) Phacolytic glaucoma is a form of open-angle glaucoma in which there is particulate blockage of the trabecular meshwork by macrophages. Angle closure and pupillary block are not primary factors in this condition. Simple iridectomy would therefore be inappropriate (p. 136).

34. (B) All of the answers except B are correct and represent retinal and optic nerve changes occurring as sequelae to intraocular pressure increase (p. 276). Answer B is false because vessels normally are only present in the inner half of the retina; the outer half is basically vessel free (p. 364).

35. (C) All of the answers except C are causes of possible lens-induced glaucoma (pp. 135 and 136). True exfoliation, or glassblower's disease (p. 139), does not cause glaucoma.

36. (A) This statement is false because the future anterior chamber is not a space lined by two endothelial layers (p. 261). Answers B, C, and D are true statements regarding embryogenesis and growth of the angle (p. 261). Answer E also is true because congenital glaucoma (p. 272) and the anterior chamber cleavage syndrome (p. 35) are two important malformations.

37. (B) Answer B is not correct because the scleral spur consists of collagenous tissue situated posterior to the canal of Schlemm (p. 263). Answers A, and C through E are correct statements regarding the anatomy of the anterior chamber angle (p. 261).

38. (D) Answers A, B, C, and E all are causes of secondary open-angle glaucoma and therefore are not correct (pp. 268 and 272). Answer D is the correct one because diabetes mellitus is not a cause of secondary open-angle glaucoma. Diabetes with rubeosis may cause closed-angle neovascular glaucoma (p. 381).

39. (E) Seclusion of the pupil is created by posterior synechia between the iris and crystalline lens or anterior vitreous face (p. 265). Answers A through D are correct statements regarding angle-closure glaucoma and pupillary block (p. 265).

40. (E) All of the statements are correct regarding ICE syndrome (p. 266).

41. (C) Haab's striae are breaks in Descemet's membrane, not Bowman's layer, therefore, making answer C false (pp. 73 and 273). Answer A is true because the photomicrograp shows a globe with buphthalmos. Answers B, D, and E also are true (p. 273).

42. (E) All the lesions mentioned may create a disc appearance that may mimic, glaucomatous optic atrophy (pp. 19, 22, and 24).

43. (D) Answer D is false because thickening of the ciliary body basement membrane is more characteristic of changes of diabetes mellitus (p. 381). Answers A, B, C, and E are correct and describe sequelae of various types of glaucoma, including pigmentary glaucoma (p. 268) and acute glaucoma with glaukomfled (p. 274).

44. (E) All the statements are true about the ICE syndrome (p. 266).

45. (A) The most common inherited pattern of primary open-angle glaucoma is autosomal dominant (p. 268).

46. (D) The ciliary processes are situated in the posterior chamber (p. 263). All other statements define structures that line portions of the anterior chamber (p. 263).

47. (E) All the statements are true (p. 261).

48. (E) All answers are true statements regarding the ciliary body (p. 262).

49. (A) Answer A is the correct one because the statement is false. Glaucoma actually occurs in the minority of cases after trauma. Answers B through E are true statements regarding posttraumatic glaucoma (p. 271).

50. (E) All these statements are true regarding congenital glaucoma (p. 272).

CHAPTER 7

1. (C) The posterior pigment epithelium of the iris is derived from the anterior portion of the embryonic optic cup (p. 284). The pigment granules arise in situ within the optic cup epithelium very early in gestation (p. 287), as contrasted to stromal melanocytes, which arise from the neural crest and complete their migration into the uvea shortly after birth (p. 287).

2. (A) Sympathetic ophthalmia is described on page 298. All of the answers are true except A. Phacoanaphylaxis sometimes is associated with a sympathizing response, but in general the distinct entities of sympathetic ophthalmia and phacoanaphylaxis (p. 136) differ in pathogenesis and clinical and pathologic characteristics.

3. (D) Epithelioid cells and giant cells are by definition seen in granulomatous inflammation (p. 294). The polymorphonuclear neutrophil is seen in acute suppurative inflammation. Eosinophils may be seen to varying degrees in uveitis but are most prominent in allergic conditions (e.g., vernal conjunctivitis) (p. 572) or in association with intraocular parasites such as *Toxocara canis* (p. 499).

4. (A) Although varying cell types may be seen in chronic nongranulomatous uveitis, the best answer in this selection is A. Lymphocytes and plasma cells and their derivatives are most prominent in such cases (p. 291).

5. **(E)** By definition, the main criterion differentiating endophthalmitis from panophthalmitis is the presence or absence of significant involvement of the sclera. In panophthalmitis the sclera and even the surrounding orbital tissues may be involved in the acute inflammatory process (p. 291).

6. **(D)** Granulomatous uveitis is associated with both Vogt-Koyanagi-Harada syndrome and sympathetic ophthalmia. Vogt-Koyanagi-Harada syndrome sometimes is associated with central nervous system involvement and alopecia, and shows an increased incidence in Asians and blacks. Both conditions typically are bilateral (pp. 298, 299, and 300).

7. **(B)** The photomicrograph shows several Touton giant cells (p. 295). These often are similar in appearance to a classic Langhans' giant cell but are characterized by deposits of lipid circumferentially around the rim of the cell between the row of nuclei and the cell membrane. The lipid is recognizable in routine sections as a foamy material because of the fact that lipid is leached out during routine paraffin processing. The granulomatous mass usually affects the skin and the iris. This condition is thought to be the most common cause of spontaneous hyphema in childhood (p. 395). The microcysts of toxoplasmosis are described on (pages 395-396). Giant cells also may be seen in sympathetic ophthalmia, tuberculosis, and sarcoidosis, but they are not of the Touton variety.

8. **(C)** Sympathetic ophthalmia (p. 298) classically occurs after a perforating injury to the globe with prolapse of uveal tissue. It has long been believed that an allergic reaction to this uveal pigment was the basic cause of the sympathetic response. Recent studies have challenged this theory. The final answer is not known, but some authors believe that the responsible antigen may be derived from a portion of retinal photorceptors.

9. **(B)** All of the findings described, including the problem of "dry eyes" are compatible with sarcoidosis. "Dry eyes" may be caused by lacrimal infiltration by sarcoid granulomas (pp. 293 and 571).

10. **(A)** Dendritic melanocytes are derived from the embryonic neural crest (p. 287) and not from the optic cup epithelium. Medulloepitheliomas of the ciliary body are described on page 332. Dendritic melanocytes (or their precursors) are the cell of origin of uveal malignant melanoma (p. 287).

11. **(E)** Optic glioma generally is a retrobulbar lesion and does not involve the choroid (p. 553). Metastatic carcinoma, sympathetic ophthalmia, and diffuse flat malignant melanoma are obvious important causes of a diffusely thickened choroid. Also, this finding must be considered in patients with phacoanaphylactic uveitis even though the primary inflammatory reaction actually surrounds the lens. This is because a certain percentage of these patients, who likewise typically have suffered from penetrating ocular trauma, may develop a concurrent sympathetic ophthalmia (pp. 298-299).

12. **(A)** Dalén-Fuchs nodules (p. 299) are highly characteristic, if not pathognomonic, of sympathetic ophthalmia. They represent "cannonball pilelike" clusters of cells at the level of the pigment epithelium.

13. **(D)** Although involvement of the lens may occur in advanced cases with severe involvement of the lens, all other types of lens changes involving the cortex are seen more commonly in uveitis. The peripheral cortex is more exposed to inflammatory changes in the surrounding aqueous and adjacent tissues.

14. **(D)** The condition described in answer D is more typical of a melanocytoma of the optic nerve head (pp. 308 and 550) as opposed to a malignant melanoma. The "double" circulation, the mushroom or collar-button shape of the lesion, and a significant elevation of the lesion should suggest the possibility of a malignancy. A history of breast carcinoma should suggest a metastatic lesion to the choroid (p. 328).

15. **(D)** The nests of cells within the tumor are most compatible with metastatic adenocarcinoma. The lumina of the neoplastic glandular elements contain mucin. Adenocarcinoma from the breast is the most

common tumor metastatic to the choroid in females. Squamous cell carcinoma of the lung is the most common malignant tumor metastatic to the choroid in males (p. 328). A diffuse flat malignant melanoma usually has a more homogeneous cellular pattern than is seen in this photomicrograph (p. 317).

16. **(C)** Although residual lens epithelial cells, seen, for example, after extracapsular lens extraction, may proliferate and undergo a fibrous metaplasia that may contribute to a cyclitic membrane, the lens capsule itself is acellular and not capable of proliferation. Therefore answer C is the least likely to be correct. All of the other answers connote processes in which cellular proliferation and formation of a true cyclitic membrane may occur (p. 304). The residual lens capsule may be caught up within a cyclitic membrane, but it does not have the capacity to elaborate the cellular elements necessary to form the membrane.

17. **(B)** The best answer in this group is B, bronchogenic carcinoma, certainly the most common metastatic lesion to the choroid in males. This probably will increase in incidence as more females smoke. Metastatic malignant melanoma of the skin, prostate carcinoma, and carcinoma of the ovary are less common sources of metastases. Answer D is false because most breast tumors are adenocarcinomas rather than sarcomas. Adenocarcinoma of the breast is the most common cause of ocular metastases in females (p. 328).

18. **(C)** Although intraocular bone formation is one of the hallmarks of phthisis bulbi (p. 305), it is believed that the bone is derived as an osseous metaplasia of the retinal pigment epithelium (p. 305).

19. **(D)** The differentiation of uveal melanocytes derived from the neural crest (answer D) and the formation of the pigmented epithelia (answers A, C, and E) of the eye derived from the optic cup are described on pages 284, 285-288, and 306-308. Answer B is incorrect because none of the pigmented cells or tumors of the eye arise from mesectoderm.

20. **(A)** Most iris malignant melanomas may be cured by simple excision, have a good prognosis, and generally are composed of cells with a relatively "benign" cell type, that is, spindle cells. They generally do not require extensive surgery and rarely metastasize (pp. 325-328).

21. **(E)** The electroretinogram measures retinal function and is not helpful in evaluation of underlying choroidal masses. All the other ancillary tests and features listed help in assessing a choroidal lesion and in diagnosing malignant melanoma (pp. 311-312).

22. **(E)** The condition described in this series of answers is sarcoidosis (p. 293). All the answers are true except E. The lack of a hilar mass on chest radiograph does *not* rule out this disease.

23. **(B)** The most common site of extension of uveal melanoma is the liver. Hematogenous extension often occurs by way of the vortex veins. Retinoblastoma, however, usually spreads by local extension into the optic nerve and cranial cavity or by blood-borne metastasis to bones and other body tissues (p. 226).

24. **(A)** This is a photomicrograph of a "mushroom" or "collar-button" melanoma. This configuration is almost diagnostic of malignant melanoma, connoting a growth of the tumor through a ruptured Bruch's membrane. The other lesions mentioned seldom form this typical "mushroom" configuration (p. 312).

25. **(E)** All of these possibilities are important criteria and must be assessed together in estimating a prognosis for a patient with uveal malignant melanoma (pp. 310-327).

26. **(E)** All of these conditions are associated with granulomatous uveitis, which is characterized by epithelioid cells and giant cells (pp. 291-302).

27. **(A)** Although many features are important in establishing prognosis, including size of the lesion and epibulbar extension, the cell type of a melanoma, when taken alone, also is an important indicator. All of the answers are correct except A. A melanoma with a pure epithelioid cell type theoretically has a worse prognosis than a melanoma that consists of a combination of spindle B and epithelial cells. Although exceptions occur, answer A is the most appropriate for this question (pp. 320-325).

28. (**E**) Adenocarcinoma of the breast is the most common tumor in females that may metastasize to the eye. This may change, however, because the incidence of lung cancer in women has increased markedly in recent years as a result of more widespread cigarette smoking by women. The most common tumor metastatic to the eye in males is bronchogenic carcinoma. Genitourinary tract carcinomas frequently metastasize to the choroid, and sometimes is hard to differentiate primary from metastatic melanoma within the choroid by histologic examination (pp. 328-329).

29. (**E**) All of the answers except E refer to various microscopic features that may be seen in medulloepitheliomas (p. 330). This tumor represents a neuroepithelial tumor, usually arising from the ciliary body. The epithelium is derived embryologically from the embryonic neural tube (p. 7), and the epithelial elements listed in answers A, B, and D reflect this derivation. The epithelium secretes a stroma, which represents an abortive attempt to form embryonic vitreous (pp. 28 and 366). Medulloepitheliomas do not form organized lens substance.

30. (**E**) The condition in question is juvenile xanthogranuloma (pp. 294-295). All of the answers are correct except E. *Toxocara canis* has not been implicated in the pathogenesis.

31. (**A**) All of the answers are correct except A. The overwhelming majority of medulloepitheliomas arise at the ciliary body, being classified as neuroepithelial tumors of the ciliary body. Rarely they may arise at the posterior pole or at the optic nerve head (p. 333).

32. (**C**) Although exceptions occur, most authors differentiate between childhood forms of neuroepithelial tumors of the ciliary body (medulloepithelioma) and those tumors occurring in adults (adenoma or adenocarcinoma). All the answers relate to the latter type except C, which refers to medulloepithelioma (pp. 330-333).

33. (**A**) Phthisis bulbi is associated with bone formation, secondary to an osseous metaplasia of ocular tissues such as pigmented epithelium (p. 304). Answers A, D, and E represent variations of neuroepithelial tumors of the ciliary body that on occasion may form cartilage, not bone (p. 333). Trisomy 13 is characterized by formation of cartilage in a coloboma of the ciliary body (p. 45).

34. (**D**) This slide shows a diffuse flat lesion, which could be compatible with a metastatic lesion, a leukemic infiltrate, or a diffuse flat melanoma (p. 318). The overall picture is most compatible with the latter. Medulloepitheliomas arise or usually are localized at the ciliary body (p. 330). Melanocytomas rarely are so extensive and most commonly arise at or near the optic nerve head (p. 308).

35. (**D**) Numerous tumor giant cells, which clearly are recognizable as epithelioid cells, are present in this microscopic section. Therefore answer D is the only tenable answer in this case. The Callendar classification of uveal melanomas is discussed on page 320.

36. (**C**) Prompt nucleation of the injured eye is the best way to prevent sympathetic ophthalmia, so answer C is correct (pp. 298-299). Improved techniques of wound closure, choroid-steroid therapy, and immunosuppresive therapy may be useful adjuncts, but the optimal treatment in severe cases is to remove the exciting eye. Therefore answers A, B, and E are incorrect. Experimental models of sympathetic ophthalmia has suggested that the Retinal S indigent maybe causative to this condition, but therapy based on this finding has not been developed. Therefore answer D also is incorrect.

37. (**D**) Answer D is incorrect because caseating granulomas are characteristic of tuberculosis; the granuloma of sarcoidosis is typically noncaseous (p. 293). Answers A, B, C, and E are correct because they may be associated with sarcoid chorioretinitis (p. 293).

38. (**D**) The retinal vessels are mesodermal in origin and therefore are not associated with neural crest cells, so answer D is incorrect (Chapter 2, p. 28). Answers A and C are correct, that is, neural crest cells give rise to dendritic melanocytes. Answer B is correct because neural crest cells give rise to neural glial elements such as Schwann cells. The array of tumorous conditions seen in the phacomatoses can be explained best by noting that most of these are of neural crest origin (pp. 9 and 288).

39. (**C**) The spectrum of diseases characterized as Langerhans' cell histiocytosis (histiocytosis X) may include the findings listed in answers A, B, D, and E (p. 295). Answer C is false because a nevoxanthoendothelioma is not seen in the classic histiocytosis X syndromes, but rather in juvenile xanthogranuloma (p. 294).

40. (**E**) The answer is E because all of the listed conditions represent relatively *serious* or advanced conditions that generally are not amenable to local resections (pp. 312 and 327).

41. (**E**) All these answers are true. The anatomy of the cellular vasculature is described on page 289, and the anatomy of the retinal vessel is described on page 363. Anterior ischemic optic neuropathy, an occlusive or inflammatory disease affecting the posterior ciliary vessels, is described in Chapter 10 (p. 543).

42. (**B**) The classification of Apple and Blodi is based on the concept that tumors often evolve from a relatively benign into a more malignant form, especially noted as tumor doubling time increases. The only correct answer in this group is B (p. 310). Answer A is incorrect because Phase A melanoma are on the more benign end of the spectrum. Answer C is incorrect because the metastatic potential between Phase A and Phase B is not equal, but much greater for Phase B to emerse. Answer D is incorrect because collar-button morphology (p. 315) indicates a more advanced tumor.

43. (**B**) The VKH syndrome most commonly presents as bilateral uveitis, so answer B is correct. (p. 299). It is most common in Asians, blacks, and Native Americans. It often causes exudative retinal attachment and usually is sporadic and not inherited. Therefore answers A, C, and D are false. Answer E also is incorrect because sympathetic ophthalmia and VKH syndrome may have a very similar form of granulomatis inflammation, and Dalén-Fuchs' nodules may be present in both conditions (p. 299).

44. (**C**) One of the criteria helpful in the diagnosis of malignant melanoma is a so-called double circulation. This represents an overlying retinal vasculature plus vessel within the tumor stroma, usually best observed with fluorescein angiography (p. 313). A double circulation usually rules out choroidal nervus, so answer E is incorrect. Answers A, B, and D are incorrect. Phthisis bulbi is described on page 304, acute endophthalmitis is described on page 290, and retinal hemangioma is described on page 310.

45. (**E**) This photomicrograph illustrates postperforation acute, purulent endophthalmitis with a vitreous abscess (p. 290). Therefore answer E is correct. Answer A is incorrect because sympathetic ophthalmia consists of a granulomatous inflammation in which the response is confined to the uvea (p. 298). Hemophthalmos (answer B) implies intraocular hemorrhage. Answer C is incorrect because it *P. acnes* organism causes a localized, often reversible endophthalmitis within the lens capsular bag after cataract surgery (p. 163). Answer D also is incorrect in that phacoanaphylactic endophthalmitis represents a reaction to lens protein after rupture of the lens capsule, so the general reaction is focused around the region of the crystalline lens (p. 136).

46. (**D**) Intraocular cartilage formation is not seen in phthisis bulbi, but rather there is osseous metaplasia and bone formation (p. 305). Intraocular cartilage formation can be observed in trisomy 13 (Patau's syndrome) (p. 45) and in medulloepithelioma (p. 330) Answers A, B, C, and E all are correct (p. 304).

47. (**A**) Answer A is correct because the dilator and sphincter muscle of the iris are unique, that is, they arrive from ectoderm (like the erector pili) of the skin, as opposed to mesoderm or mesectoderm (p. 285). Answer B is incorrect because the final iris color is determined by the melanin contact of intrastromal dendritic melanocyte (p. 287) Answer C is incorrect because the iris epithelium develops from the optic cups, not the iris stroma.

48. (**C**) The answer is C because chronic anterior segment ischemia syndrome can be associated with segmental iris atrophy and necrosis (p. 302) See also page 266 for description of essential iris atrophy. Answer A, B, D, and E all are incorrect. Phthisis bulbi medullo epithelioma (diktyoma) are unrelated conditions (pp. 304 and 330).

The denervation of the iris and heterochromia iridium (p. 43) generally do not cause these changes.

49. (**E**) The three conditions lumped together under the term Langerhans' cell histiocytosis (histiocytosis X) are the Hand-Schuller Christian syndrome, eosinophilic granuloma, and Letterer-Siwe disease. All the answers are true (p. 295).

50. (**E**) Answer E is correct because the photograph shows a necrotic malignant melanoma (p. 324). Note how relatively viable tumors are situated around intratumor stromal vessels. The tumor mass away from the vessels is necrotic and has lost staining characteristics. Answer A is incorrect because the photograph does not resemble RPE; also anaplasia of this cell type is very rare. Answer B also is incorrect because although part of necrotic cell mass may contain epithelioid cells, they are not recognizable in the section (p. 324). Answer C is incorrect because this tumor is not a retinoblastoma. However, the pathogenesis of a necrotic melanoma is similar to that of the pseudorosette and retinoblastoma (p. 487) in which viable tumor cells cluster around the tumors stromal vessels. Answer D is incorrect because a spindle cell melanoma shows a different pattern of elongated, often palisading cells (p. 320)

CHAPTER 8

1. (**D**) Answers A, B, C, and E correctly describe Goldmann-Favre disease (p. 422). Answer D is incorrect because the disease usually affects young people.

2. (**D**) The trypsin digest technique will reveal a rich intraretinal capillary network in the perifoveal zones. The central fovea is devoid of vessels (so-called foveal avascular zone; p. 365).

3. (**C**) Best's vitelliform dystrophy (p. 428) is a form of exudative central detachment of the macula in which pigmentation can occur in the end stages, but which is unrelated to hemorrhage except for rare cases. It is thought that the deposits are secondary to a product of abnormally proliferating pigment epithelial cells. Histoplasmosis (p. 394), myopic choroidal degeneration (p. 41), angioid streaks (p. 429), and Kuhnt-Junius disease (p. 442) often are associated with hemorrhagic lesions of the macula.

4. (**A**) The changes in background and preproliferative diabetic retinopathy are mostly intraretinal. Vitreous hemorrhage usually occurs in proliferative retinopathy after vitreal traction on neovascular fronds (p. 376).

5. (**C**) As opposed to diabetic retinopathy, in which much of the proliferative process occurs nearer to the posterior pole, the retinopathy of both sickle cell disease (p. 384) and Eales' disease (p. 386) most commonly affects the midperipheral and peripheral retina. Eales' disease is uncommon in the United States but is endemic in India. Its pathogenesis is unknown, but it is not caused by a hemoglobinopathy. It usually is unilateral. Perivasculitis is not a primary feature of sickle cell retinopathy.

6. (**C**) Answers A, B, D, and E are true statements regarding retinal detachment (p. 415). Answer C is incorrect because the attachment of cone outer segments to the RPE actually are less secure than photoreceptor attachments elsewhere. Therefore the fovea region is vulnerable not only to general retinal detachment, but also to local, central detachment of the neuroepithelium, for example, central serous chorioretinopathy (p. 434).

7. (**D**) Studies in monkeys have shown that extensive neuronal destruction may occur as early as 90 minutes after central arterial occlusion (p. 386). The onset of signs in central artery occlusion usually is acute. The cherry-red spot seen in central retinal artery occlusion is caused by ischemia of the retina in the macular region (p. 387), whereas the cherry-red spot of Tay-Sachs disease is caused by deposits of sphingolipids within ganglion cells in the macular region (p. 423). Answers C and E are characteristic findings of central retinal vein occlusion (p. 390).

8. (**A**) Angioid streaks (p. 429) represent defects in Bruch's membrane. Because elastic tissue primarily is affected, systemic diseases producing elastic tissue degeneration, such as pseudoxanthoma elasticum, sometimes are associated with these lesions.

9. (**E**) This is an illustration of central retinal arterial occlusion showing extensive pallor and cloudy swelling of the fundus, particularly temporally, with formation of a cherry-red spot. This condition often causes rapid and not infrequently irreversible loss of vision (p. 386). Note a small, flame-shaped hemorrhage near the disc. There is a "box car effect" of blood within retinal arterioles signifying stagnation of flow. There is generalized arteriolar attenuation.

10. (**B**) Answer B is the answer of choice because certain diseases such as glaucoma and retinal vascular diseases primarily and initially affect the inner retinal layers (pp. 276, 360, 363, and 366). Answers A, C, D, and E all are conditions that primarily affect the outer (photoreceptor) layers.

11. (**B**) In Coats' syndrome the detachment usually is exudative, caused by accumulation of fluid or exudate in or below the sensory retina in the absence of the retinal break (p. 415). All the other conditions may be direct causes of tractional retinal detachment (p. 416), in which traction is exerted from the vitreous in front of the retina, thus causing detachment in the absence of the retinal break.

12. (**E**) Answers A to D are correct, and this disease is described on page 394. The condition is termed *presumed* because it rarely occurs in association with systemic histoplasmosis affecting other organ systems. In most cases the ocular findings occur in patients without historical, clinical, or histopathologic evidence of exposure to the organism, and the organism itself has only been demonstrated histologically in very few human eyes.

13. (**B**) Both toxoplasmosis (p. 395) and the presumed ocular histoplasmosis syndrome (p. 394) are characterized, among other features, by a high incidence of peripapillary involvement. Toxoplasmosis causes more retinal destruction with vitreous involvement, hence the formation of arcuate scotomas and the presence of vitritis, both of which are not typical of histoplasmosis. Toxoplasmosis also may cause anterior uveitis with keratic precipitates. These organisms are not viruses, and intranuclear inclusion bodies are not seen in either condition.

14. (**B**) This photograph illustrates a common and typical *thickening* of the basement membrane of ciliary body, occurring in diabetes. Therefore B is the answer because thinning of the membrane does not occur. Answers A and C through E are associated with diabetes mellitus (p. 374).

15. (**A**) The central retinal artery rarely is associated with proliferative retinopathy (p. 386), although it has been described because this condition causes ischemia or hypoxia to the retina. All the other conditions listed are classic causes of proliferative retinopathy. Diabetic retinopathy (pp. 372 and 374) must be added to this list.

16. (**D**) This photograph shows marked hemorrhage distributed throughout the inner retinal layers, which extends outward, It represents a hemorrhagic retinopathy (central venous occlusion, (p. 390). Answer D is therefore the correct answer. Neovascularization is not a typical sequela of central retinal artery occlusion. Answers A, B, C, and E all are true regarding central retinal arterial occlusion (p. 386).

17. (**E**) The primary site of involvement in any form of retinitis (retinopathia) pigmentosa is at the level of photoreceptor-pigment epithelium (p. 411). Rubella pigmentary retinopathy (p. 132) does not show a bone spicular pattern but rather a diffuse "salt-and-pepper" fundus, which does not cause a change in the electroretinogram. Although the term *retinitis* is used, the condition is not inflammatory in origin. All three major patterns of familial transmission may be seen, and retinitis pigmentosa usually is bilateral.

18. (**A**) The "salt-and-pepper" pigmentary retinopathy of maternal rubella syndrome is caused by alternating hyperplasia and hypoplasia of the RPE. There is no migration of the retinal pigment epithelial melanin into the sensory retina, a process that would lead to formation of the bone spicule pattern (p. 132). In contrast, all other answers are diseases that may exhibit a migration of retinal pigment epithelial melanin into the sensory retina (pp. 402-407).

19. (**D**) The photograph illustrates lacy vacuolization of the iris pigment epithelium, an occasional complication of severe diabetes mellitus (p. 380). Note also advanced peripheral anterior synechiae, indicative of secondary glaucoma. Answers A, B, C, and E are true because

they all relate to diabetes. Coats' disease is not a cause of lacy vacuolization (p. 493).

20. **(B)** Presumed histoplasmic chorioretinitis (p. 394) is characterized by a triad of peripapillary inflammation and atrophy, pigment proliferation, peripheral scars, and (less often) disciform detachment of the macula. The primary target tissue is the choroid, as opposed to cases of toxoplasmosis in which the lesion typically is a retinochoroiditis. Toxoplasmosis (p. 395) retinochoroiditis often is associated with cells in the vitreous and formation of arcuate scotomas. It is believed that some cases of congenital "macular colobomas" are caused by intrauterine inflammation, such as may be caused by toxoplasmosis.

21. **(C)** The lumina of retinal capillaries and small vessels are lined by endothelial cells (*E* in this photograph). The cell labeled *P* represents a pericyte or "mural cell," which is situated outside the endothelial basement membrane and forms a basement membrane of its own. The normal ratio of endothelial cells to pericytes and retinal capillaries is 1:1. In diabetic retinopathy there is a characteristic dropout of pericytes (p. 375). Conversely, a gradual loss of endothelial cells occurs as a normal aging process.

22. **(B)** Cotton-wool spots are clusters of fusiform, swollen axons in the retinal nerve fiber layer. They often are designated as cytoid bodies (answer A) and they frequently occur in the diseases listed in C, D, and E. Answer B is the correct answer because these spots do not originate from bipolar cells (pp. 371 and 372).

23. **(C)** Cobblestone degeneration is described on page 412. It is the only listed answer that has not been implicated as causative in the pathogenesis of retinal detachment (p. 415).

24. **(E)** Retinitis (retinopathia) pigmentosa syndromes are retinal dystrophies that may occur as isolated conditions, may be heredofamilial, and may be associated with all of the conditions listed in answers A through D (p. 402). Situs inversus arteriosus is not infrequently associated with a tilted disc syndrome (p. 22). In situs inversus the vessels emerge from the temporal rather than the nasal side of the disc and course nasally before sweeping out in the usual temporal distribution.

25. **(B)** The subretinal space is a potential cavity situated between the RPE and the neurosensory retina and is the vestige of the cavity of the embryonic vesicle (answer B) (pp. 7 and 354-357). Detachment anterior to the ora serrata usually is localized (e.g., typical cysts of the pars plana [p. 410] because of the presence of cell junctions that attach the two layers of the ciliary epithelium).

26. **(B)** This is a turn-of-the-19th-century artist's drawing of a rhegmatogenous retinal detachment with numerous horseshoe tears (p. 413). The subretinal fluid is derived from the vitreous. The fluid passes through the retinal defects into the subretinal space, thus separating the retina from the underlying pigment epithelium. The condition is caused by breaks that often are horseshoe-shaped, as illustrated here. Spontaneous resolution is rare, and the treatment is surgical.

27. **(E)** Macroaneurysms occur in all the conditions listed in answers A through D (pp. 382 and 493). They do not occur in von Hippel-Lindau angiomatosis (p. 506).

28. **(D)** The vitreoretinal dystrophies that have in common the formation of a schisis cavity at the level of the neurofiber layer and ganglion cell layer, accompanied by vitreous anomalies, are described on page 422. Only juvenile sex-linked retinoschisis and Goldman-Favre recessive vitreal retinal dystrophy affect the macular region. The Wagner-Stickler dystrophy does not affect the macular region, Answer D is correct because the schisis cavity is not situated at the level of the outer plexiform layer but rather in the neurofiber layer.

29. **(C)** When artifactitious detachment of the retina occurs during fixation and processing, the photoreceptors are "wrenched away" from the apices of the RPE, and one sees fragments of pigment attached to the photoreceptors (p. 418). A true detachment is a "clean break" with no pigment attached to the photoreceptors. All the other findings (answers A, B, C, and E) are characteristic sequelae of more or less long-standing in vivo retinal detachment (p. 418).

30. **(E)** As opposed to so-called senile schisis, which arises in areas of peripheral microcystoid degeneration (p. 410), the split in the retina in juvenile retinal schisis occurs at the level of the nerve fiber layer (p. 422).

31. **(C)** Diabetic proliferative retinopathy typically consists of neovascularization and fibrous tissue proliferation intraretinally, on the retinal surface, and on the surface of the optic disc. This often is with extension of disc or retinal vessels into the vitreous. Subpigment epithelial and choroidal neovascularization is not a characteristic finding (p. 376).

32. **(E)** Answer E is correct. This fluorescein angiogram illustrates angioid streaks, which may be associated with pseudoxanthoma elasticum (p. 429). Answers A through D are more compatible with choroideremia I (p. 407).

33. **(A)** The whitish discoloration of the fundus in the perifoveal region around the central cherry-red spot in Tay-Sachs disease is caused by deposits of sphingolipids within ganglion cells (p. 424). The ganglion cell layer is stratified in the perifoveal region (p. 358). The central fovea itself is spared because it contains no ganglion cells and readily transmits the red color of the underlying choroid. Cloudy swelling applies to the changes seen in retinal arterial occlusion. Mucopolysaccharides have no role in the pathogenesis of Tay-Sachs disease.

34. **(D)** This fluorescein angiogram shows multiple drusen, which are visible as multiple areas of hyperfluorescence. The hyperfluorescence is caused by both a "window defect" resulting from degeneration of the overlying pigment epithelium and probably by an uptake of fluorescein dye within the drusen themselves. Drusen are mildly eosinophilic, PAS-positive, hyaline excrescence on Bruch's membrane. They are derived secondary to a secretory and degenerative process involving the RPE (p. 426).

35. **(A)** The melanin within the RPE is the primary site of light absorption and heat emission with all forms of photocoagulation (p. 447). All modalities in clinical usage can readily occlude choriocapillaris channels. When relatively mild xenon arc, argon laser, or krypton laser burns are applied, they only affect the areas immediately surrounding the pigment epithelium, that is, the choriocapillaris and the outer layers of the retina. Mild burns thus usually spare the nerve fiber layer.

36. **(D)** The diseases listed in answers A, B, C, and E are causes of exudative retinal detachment (p. 415). Goldmann-Favre disease is a vitreoretinal dystrophy and is not a cause of exudative retinal detachment (p. 422).

37. **(E)** Answer E is correct because the statement is not true. Retinitis pigmentosa usually is inherited as an autosomal recessive trait (p. 402). Answers A to D are all true of this disease.

38. **(A)** A central venous occlusion (venous stasis and hemorrhagic retinopathy) causes of a hemorrhagic infarct (p. 390). All the other answers apply to central retinal arterial occlusion (p. 386).

39. **(A)** This fluorescein angiogram is characteristic of central serous chorioretinopathy (p. 434). The illustration shows leakage of dye from the choriocapillaris through a defect in Bruch's membrane, creating the "smokestack" effect, with lateral spreading of the dye superiorly. This condition most commonly affects the macula region of younger or middle-aged persons, and severe visual loss is extremely rare.

40. **(B)** This slide shows a typical histopathologic appearance of preretinal neovascularization, in which new-formed vessels have incomplete junctional inner connections. The RPE (answer A), endothelial cells of normal retinal capillaries (answer C), junctions between photoreceptor and Müller's cells (or external limiting membrane) (answer D), and the corneal endothelial cells (answer E) all have various intercellular junctions (pp. 357-361). Bruch's membrane (answer B) does not limit flow of fluid and solids because no junctions are present. Bruch's membrane therefore allows passive fluid movements.

41. **(C)** The photomicrograph shows the histopathologic appearance of a classic disciform macular degeneration (p. 442). Because these lesions often contain foci of dispersed RPE and/or blood breakdown products with formation of hemosiderin, they may be pigmented and elevated and mimic malignant melanoma. In cases of eccentric (nonmacular) disciform lesions, the frequency of erroneous diagnosis is higher because the ophthalmologist is more accustomed to seeing

this process in the macular region. Choroidal nevi, melanocytoma, and pigment epithelial tumors all may mimic a malignant melanoma (Chapter 7). A central serous choroidopathy usually is easily recognizable by ophthalmoscopy or slitlamp examination with the contact lens because the subretinal space contains fluid rather than solid tumor tissue. Also, a defect in the underlying Bruch's membrane can be demonstrated by fluorescein angiography.

42. **(D)** This angiogram shows the classic appearance of well-circumscribed pigment epithelial detachments. They do not increase in size, even in later stages of the angiogram (p. 435). The configuration seen here is not compatible with retinal hemangiomas (von Hippel-Lindau disease) or with choroidal hemangioma. Foci of hemorrhage would cause a hypofluorescenee because of blockage of the choroid by the overlying hemorrhage.

43. **(C)** The most common inheritance pattern of the various retinitis (retinopathia) pigmentosa syndromes is autosomal recessive, including all of the conditions listed in A, B, D, and E (p. 404). Answer C is correct because Usher's syndrome is inherited in an autosomal dominant fashion (p. 406).

44. **(B)** Nerve fibers within the nerve fiber layer are the axons of ganglion cells (p. 358). Peripherally located ganglion cells have their axons running deep in the layer, whereas the central ganglion cells (particularly in the posterior pole) send out axons that course more superficially. They are unmyelinated until they reach the lamina cribrosa, except in cases of medullated or myelinated nerve fibers in which oligodendroglia are present (pp. 532 and 534). They synapse with nuclei of cells in the lateral geniculate body. The fibers course in an "arcuate" direction temporally because they must pass around the fovea. The "spoke-wheel" pattern is seen nasally.

45. **(B)** B is correct (p. 357 and Fig. 8-2). The photoreceptor cell is the first neuron in the series of synapses within the visual pathway, the bipolar cell is the second neuron, the ganglion cell is the third neuron, and the final synapse occurs in the fourth neuron in the lateral geniculate body.

46. **(A)** Several "cotton-wool" exudates or cytoid bodies are seen in this drawing. These are not true exudates; rather they are collections of swollen, dilated nerve fiber layer axons that have undergone an ischemic necrosis secondary to the underlying disease (p. 372). They may be especially prominent in conditions such as hypertensive retinopathy and lupus erythematosus. They also may be seen in association with yellow, waxy exudates (p. 376) in diabetic retinopathy. Note also the attenuation of arterioles, advanced arteriovenous crossing changes, and flame-shaped hemorrhages in this illustration.

47. **(D)** The photograph illustrates extensive retinal neovascularization that can occur with a wide variety of diseases including diabetic retinopathy and sickle cell retinopathy (pp. 376 and 384). Answers A, B, C, and E are true concerning sickle cell retinopathy. Answer D is incorrect because S-thalassemia may be associated with proliferative retinopathy.

48. **(A)** This illustration shows a typical cyst of the pars plana (p. 409). This is not a true cyst but represents a splitting of the inner nonpigmented layer of ciliary epithelium from the outer pigmented layer. It is thus analogous to a detachment of the sensory retina from the underlying pigment epithelium. Just as mucopolysaccharides are present within the space between photoreceptors and pigment epithelium, the space within a typical cyst of the pars plana contains a mucopolysaccharide, specifically hyaluronic acid. This photomicrograph shows an Alcian blue stain in which the smudgy material within the cyst demonstrates the mucopolysaccharide (answer A). This Alcian blue stain also clearly demonstrates vitreous fibrils and ground substance (seen to the left in this illustration). They are benign and do not predispose to retinal detachment. They are not considered to be true cysts because they are not lined by a single continuous epithelium. They are not congenital but begin to appear and increase in numbers after adolescence. Milky-white pars plana cysts (as viewed by gross examination after fixation) may be similar in appearance histologically but are seen only in conditions characterized by formation of abnormal proteins, such as multiple myeloma or in states

of increased immunoglobulin formation (p. 409). The milky-white appearance is caused by denaturation of the protein after formalin fixation.

49. **(E)** Answers A to D are highly characteristic of degenerative age-related retinoschisis (p. 410). Answer E is incorrect because the splitting of the retina causes an absolute scotoma subtending the involved area. This clinical finding may help differentiate this entity from a retinal detachment, in which the scotoma typically is relative rather than absolute.

50. **(D)** There are multiple causes of disciform (age-related) macular degeneration, which generally occurs in the absence of obvious preexisting disease, (p. 442) but also occurs secondary to many conditions (p. 444). Rubella (answer D) is the only condition listed that is not typically associated with macular degeneration (p. 132).

CHAPTER 9

1. **(C)** Answer C is not correct (p. 480). Answers A, B, D, and E correctly describe the various aspects of genetics of retinoblastoma (p. 482).

2. **(E)** All of the answers are correct about retinoblastoma except E. Because of improved cure rates, with more survivors, the incidence of retinoblastoma is increasing. This leads to an ever-increasing number of births of infants with genetically transmitted retinoblastoma (p. 480).

3. **(A)** Retinoblastoma is bilateral in 25% to 30% of cases, and bilaterality almost always indicates the heritable form (p. 480). Retinoblastoma is not inherited as an X-linked recessive trait but is inherited as an autosomal-dominant trait with incomplete penetrance. Association with Down syndrome and neuroblastoma is rare and generally coincidental.

4. **(B)** Multiple primary tumors in a single eye differ significantly from multiple deposits of tumor along the retinal surface that occur during seeding of the tumor. The latter connotes a poorer prognosis. The presence of multiple primary tumors is not necessarily an ominous finding (p. 484). A retinoblastoma is derived from the cells of the *inner* layer of the optic cup (pp. 7 and 482). The cells primarily are of neural origin. The rule that endophytic growths are derived from cells of the inner nuclear layer and exophytic growths are derived by proliferation of cells of the outer cellular layers is not a hard and fast one. Formation of rosettes by convention usually connotes tumor cell differentiation, as opposed to an undifferentiated tumor.

5. **(C)** "Retrolental" causes of leukokoria such as PHPV, retinopathy of prematurity (retrolental fibroplasia), or an anterior vitreous abscess caused by *Toxocara canis* may induce a secondary cataract caused by close proximity to the lens. In contrast, retinoblastomas characteristically arise posterior to the ora serrata and thus usually spare the lens in early stages. Opacification of the lens therefore usually only ensues when the tumor enlarges and/or there is anterior seeding or anterior growth of the tumor toward the lens region. Answers A, D, and E are well-established criteria of retinoblastoma (p. 481). Answer B refers to a dental radiograph of an enucleated retinoblastoma. The diffuse, white opacification indicates intense calcification of the tumor, a finding that is characteristic of retinoblastoma (p. 488).

6. **(A)** Tuberous sclerosis sometimes is associated with angiomyelolipoma of the kidney (B) (p. 505). Von Hippel-Lindau disease may be associated with hypernephroma and pheochromocytoma (answers C and D) (p. 506). Neurofibromatosis may have an associated acoustic narooma (answer E). In this case, answer A is the answer of choice because Wyburn-Mason syndrome has nothing to do with recurrent pulmonary infarction (p. 514).

7. **(E)** Bilateral involvement typically signifies a familial form of hereditary transmission but not necessarily a poor prognosis. The prognosis is determined by the status of the tumor in the worst eye. In many cases the eye with the largest tumor can be treated by enucleation, whereas the opposite eye may be saved by local therapy such as radiation (p. 491). All the other answers are important in determining the prognosis of retinoblastoma.

8. **(D)** The retinoblastoma is by definition a tumor of photoreceptor elements. As noted on page 485, photoreceptors contain cilia with

a typical 9 + 0 pattern. This is not present in neuroblastomas, which are not tumors derived from photoreceptor elements. All the other answers are true for both neoplasms.

9. **(E)** The peculiar basophilic staining of tumor stromal vessels walls (illustrated on p. 488) is not caused by calcium but rather by permeation of DNA into the wall. This nucleic acid is derived from necrosis and release of this substance from degenerating tumor cells. This phenomenon occurs in only a few forms of cancer. All the other answers are characteristic features of retinoblastoma. The photomicrograph shows classic Flexner-Wintersteiner rosettes (pp. 484-490).

10. **(C)** *Toxocara canis* (p. 499), congenital falciform fold (p. 34), retinopathy of prematurity (retrolental fibroplasia) (p. 496), and retinoblastoma (p. 480), *are all conditions in which traction folds created by the intraocular lesion may occur.* Answers A, B, D, and E are thus true statements. Answer C, von Hippel-Lindau disease is the correct answer to this question because this condition is not typically associated with retinal folds (p. 506).

11. **(C)** This fluorescein angiogram shows the presence of dilated, telangiectatic blood vessels. This profile, when present in association with leukokoria, should conjure a suspicion of Coats' disease. Of the answers mentioned in this question, Coats' disease is the most common cause of leukokoria. Answers A, B, and E all are extremely rare. Colobomas of the choroid are not as rare, but only massive defects are sufficient to cause a clinical leukokoria (p. 493).

12. **(E)** The condition described here is Coats' syndrome, which usually is unilateral, commonly is associated with intraretinal PAS-positive deposits caused by loss of structural integrity of the vascular wall, and frequently is nonfamilial. It usually occurs in infants or juveniles in the absence of other systemic findings. In retinoblastoma, a deposition of DNA occurs. These breakdown products of retinoblastoma cells cause a basophilic staining of the walls of blood vessels. This is a frequent finding retinoblastoma (p. 488) and is quite unique to the tumor. It rarely, if ever, is observed in Coats' syndrome (p. 493).

13. **(C)** The vasoconstrictive phase of retinopathy of prematurity usually is not followed by a vaso-obliterative phase, and the neovascularization occurs because of lack of formation of adequate gap junctions between the vasoformative spindle cells of the peripheral human retina (p. 498). All the other answers regarding retinopathy of prematurity are true (p. 496).

14. **(D)** Wyburn-Mason syndrome is a vascular malformation of the retina (p. 514) and has nothing to do with astrocytic hamartomas. Astrocytic hamartomas are more characteristic of tuberous sclerosis, as are angiofibromas (C) (p. 505). Answers A and B list correct lesions associated with Sturge-Weber syndrome (p. 513) and von Hippel-Lindau syndrome (p. 506), respectively.

15. **(A)** Many retinoblastomas undergo greater or lesser degrees of calcification within the tumor. Thus these changes generally are not of foremost importance in the determination of prognosis. All the other answers are definite factors that must be evaluated in assessing a prognosis (p. 489). Some tumors show seeding and/or hypopyon formation. These tumors often are necrotic. *Mild* choroidal invasion probably is not significant, but when the choroidal invasion is massive, it must be taken into consideration. The accompanying photomicrograph shows several features pointing toward a poor prognosis, including the very large size of the tumor that fills the entire globe, anterior seeding and necrosis, and, although the surgical margin is free, invasion into the optic nerve parenchyma (p. 490).

16. **(E)** This angiogram shows the vessels of the tunica vasculosa lentis, an indication of PHPV, described on page 493. Answers A to D are characteristic findings of this condition. Answer E is incorrect because the lens generally is clear in early stages and only becomes cataractous in the late stages, usually after invasion through the posterior capsule by the fibrovascular mass (p. 30).

17. **(D)** Although neurofibromatosis may cause myriad intraocular lesions, including hamartomas, it rarely causes a leukokoria (p. 509). All the other answers are well-known causes of a white pupil.

18. **(D)** All answers except D are highly characteristic of retrolental fibroplasia (p. 497). As opposed to retinoblastoma (p. 488), calcification

within the eye is not a classic radiographic, echographic, or histopathologic sign of retrolental fibroplasia. This can be an important differentiating feature when the history is vague or when an advanced lesion with opaque media is present.

19. **(D)** Answer D is a true statement regarding nematode endophthalmitis (p. 499). Answers A, B, C, and E are incorrect statements about this disease (p. 499).

20. **(C)** The finding of worms in the stool in association with the ocular disease is rare in nematode endophthalmitis (p. 499). All the other answers are true regarding this condition.

21. **(C)** This fluorescein angiogram shows myriad tufts of delicate new vessels in the retinal periphery, a phenomenon that represents the basic pathogenesis of formation of the retrolental membrane seen in retinopathy of prematurity (retrolental fibroplasia) (p. 496). Abnormal vessels may be seen overlying and within retinoblastomas and are important in Coats' disease, but the pattern seen here is not typical of these diseases.

22. **(C)** Ataxia telangiectasia (p. 515) has autosomal recessive inheritance (p. 00), so answer C is correct. Answers B, D, and E are diseases with an autosomal dominant inheritance pattern (pp. 505, 506, and 509). Coats' syndrome does not have a well-described pattern of hereditary transmission in Coats' disease (p. 493).

23. **(B)** The photomicrograph illustrated here clearly is from a case of Coats' disease. The degenerate gliotic retina is at the top of the figure, and the subretinal fluid contains multiple cholesterol clefts that are highly characteristic of this disease (p. 494). Numerous lipid- and hemosiderin-laden macrophages also are present. The remaining diseases listed are discussed in Chapter 9.

24. **(B)** All the phacomatoses except Sturge-Weber syndrome are inherited as autosomal dominant (pp. 509 and 513). Retinoblastoma also may be heritable, often transmitted as an autosomal-dominant trait with incomplete penetrance (p. 480).

25. **(C)** The most common cause of spontaneous hyphema in children is juvenile xanthogranuloma (nevoxanthoendothelioma) (p. 294). Retinoblastoma also causes this lesion (p. 480). Answers A, B, D, and E are not causes of spontaneous hyphema (pp. 505, 513, and 515).

26. **(C)** Coats' disease (p. 493) typically is unilateral, most commonly occurring in boys within the first decade of life. The three histopathologic hallmarks of this disease include retinal vascular anomalies such as telangiectasia, subretinal and intraretinal deposition of cholesterol, and formation of intraretinal PAS-positive deposits (pp. 495 and 496). The primary lesion probably is a defect in retinal vascular endothelial cells.

27. **(B)** The photomicrograph shows an inflammatory mass that, in this case, is present in the vitreous in front of an anteriorly displaced retina (lower left of the figure). It is in the retrolental area and is undergoing organization and fibrosis. There is a calcified, densely staining remnant of an organism in the center. Although not clear on this photomicrograph, many of the surrounding cells are eosinophils. The only answer that fits this pattern is B, nematode endophthalmitis (p. 499). The remaining answers are diseases that do not show this type of inflammatory process.

28. **(E)** Incontinentia pigmenti is a rare cause of leukocoria that is characterized by a depletion of melanin in basal layer of the epithelium, with subsequent deposition into the underlying dermis (p. 502). Answers A to D are correct statements regarding this condition (pp. 502 and 503).

29. **(E)** Persistent hyperplastic primary vitreous (PHPV) clearly is a disease caused by abnormal development of the mesodermally derived embryonic intraocular vasculature (p. 29). Although the pathogenesis of the intraocular lesions of the other four conditions is unclear, they usually show signs of either primary or secondary maldevelopment of the sensory retina (pp. 500-504).

30. **(D)** All the answers regarding Norrie's disease (p. 501) are true except that this condition typically does not cause cerebral calcification. The latter lesion is more characteristically seen in the Sturge-Weber syndrome (pp. 513-514).

31. **(C)** Determination of the pathogenesis of leukokoria in a child with puzzling fundus changes can be aided by careful examination of the skin if the lesion is caused by incontinentia pigmenti. The various skin lesions and ocular findings are briefly outlined on page 502. Incontinentia pigmenti occurs in females only, and tumors or hamartomas are not present in this disease.

32. **(E)** Answers A to C represent the classic triad of tuberous sclerosis. Angiomyolipomas of the kidneys also are seen frequently in this syndrome. Choroidal hemangiomas are associated with the Sturge-Weber syndrome (p. 513).

33. **(D)** The Sturge-Weber syndrome is described on page 513 and answers A, B, C, and E are correct findings of this condition. Answer D is the correct answer because it does not describe the Sturge-Weber syndrome, but is more compatible with the cerebellar hemangioblastoma (Lindau tumor) in von Hippel-Lindau disease (p. 506).

34. **(A)** Tuberous sclerosis was named for the rootlike (tuber) appearance of the cerebral lesions. These lesions are astrocytic hamartomas, similar in composition to the ophthalmoscopically visible masses that are situated on or near the optic nerve or in the nerve fiber layer of the retina. A classic *retrobulbar* optic nerve glioma (as opposed to the ophthalmoscopically visible fundus glial hamartomas) occasionally may occur, but it certainly is not the most common intraocular lesion. Answers B, D, and E are incorrect (p. 505).

35. **(B)** The artist's drawing is a clear example of a von Hippel tumor of the retina with a feeder and a draining vessel. In this case hemorrhage has occurred from the lesion. The tumor mass itself is not a cavernous hemangioma, but is a hemangioblastoma. The histopathologic appearance of this entity is demonstrated clearly on page 509. All the other answers are true in the von Hippel-Lindau syndrome. Fatality may occur because of complications of the Lindau tumor within the cerebellum (p. 506; Fig. 9-41).

36. **(E)** All of the answers except E are important findings of von Recklinghausen's neurofibromatosis (p. 509).

37. **(D)** Norrie's disease is an X-linked recessive condition that is associated with hearing impairment, mental retardation, and bilateral leukocoria. Therefore answers A, B, C, and E correctly describe this condition (p. 501). Answer D is the best correct answer because this condition generally is bilateral (p. 501).

38. **(B)** Tuberous sclerosis (p. 505) is a condition in which the brain and fundus lesions represent astrocytic hamartomas. Therefore B is the correct answer because the lesions are not choristomas. The brain lesions are analogous to the retinal astrocytic hamartomas and rarely undergo a malignant change.

39. **(E)** Patients with neurofibromatosis have a higher incidence of all of the conditions mentioned in answers A to D. An increased incidence of retinoblastoma in association with neurofibromatosis is not established. Such a correlation would *not* be expected because retinoblastoma arises from neuroblasts of the sensory retina derived in situ from the optic cup, whereas the lesions of neurofibromatosis arise from a separate embryologic origin, namely the neural crest (p. 288).

40. **(A)** Answer B through E are correct, representing varying forms for which *Toxocara canis* may present (p. 499). Answer A is the correct answer to this question because most lesions of nematode endophthalmitis are unilateral.

41. **(A)** A choroidal hemangioma is an important finding in the Sturge-Weber syndrome (p. 514). The hemangioma is usually of the cavernous type and may be associated with an ipsilateral portwine stain of the skin and glaucoma. Answer D (retinal hemangioma) is incorrect; a retinal hemangioma is seen in von Hippel-Lindau disease. Astrocytic hamartomas of the ocular fundus are more characteristic of tuberous sclerosis (p. 505). Plexiform neuroma and pulsating exophthalmos are more characteristic of neurofibromatosis (p. 509).

42. **(C)** This photomicrograph shows a sagittal section through the eyelid. The epithelial surface is on the right, and the sebaceous glands forming the meibomian or tarsal plate are readily recognizable. Between the tarsal plate and the bundles of orbicularis muscle (*left*) are several round tumefactions, which show the histopathologic appearance of a plexiform neurofibroma (p. 511). Grossly this tumor would appear

as a "bag of worms," but in cross section, as seen here, it is manifest as multiple circular nests of tissue showing small spindle-shaped nuclei. The other phakomatoses listed here are described on pages 505 to 516.

43. **(E)** Tuberous sclerosis characteristically is associated with facial angiofibromas, mental deficiency, epilepsy, and intracranial calcification that is more common in patients with mental retardation than those patients with average intelligence. Therefore answers A, B, and D are correct. Answer C also is correct because intraretinal or intraoptic nerve lesions such as the hamartomatous drusen associated with calcification, as seen in this photograph, often occur in this disease (p. 505). Answer E is the correct answer to this question because the inheritance pattern tuberous sclerosis is autosomal dominant (p. 505).

44. **(D)** Adenoma sebaceum is part of the triad of characteristic findings of tuberous sclerosis (p. 505). The triad consists of adenoma sebaceum, epilepsy, and mental deficiency. The remaining answers all are classic features of Sturge-Weber syndrome (p. 513).

45. **(D)** All the items mentioned here might be associated with von Recklinghausen's disease except that most of the central nervous system lesions are *hamartomas* rather than *choristomas*. The latter two terms are defined on page 505.

46. **(C)** True Flexner-Wintersteiner rosettes of retinoblastoma have been illustrated and diagrammed on pages 482 to 489. This photomicrograph shows a cluster of viable, deeply staining tumor cells surrounding a central vessel, whereas the tissues peripheral to this area (remote from the vessel) show degeneration and loss of chromatin (pyknosis and necrosis). This has classically been termed a *pseudorosette*, although the term is a poor one because it should be distinguished clearly from the Flexner-Wintersteiner rosette. The latter connotes a degree of differentiation of the tumor, whereas the presence of so-called psuedorosettes does not have any relationship to tumor differentiation (p. 487). Homer-Wright rosettes frequently are seen in adrenal neuroblastomas and not in retinoblastomas.

47. **(D)** The illustration is a high-power microphotograph of an undifferentiated necrotic retinoblastoma with deposition of basophilic material in the walls of tumor vessel (p. 486). Therefore answer E is true because retinoblastoma obviously involves the retina. Answer D, Sturge-Weber syndrome, is the only condition listed that does not involve the retina (p. 513), so this is the correct answer (p. 513). Answer A, Wyburn-Mason syndrome, represents a primary vascular anomaly in the retina (p. 514). Answer C, von Hippel-Lindau angiomatosis, consists of a hemangioblastoma (von Hippel tumor) within the retina (p. 506). Glial hamartomas may occur in retina and optic nerve in tuberous sclerosis, answer B (p. 505). The fundus lesion of Sturge-Weber syndrome is a *choroidal* hemangioma (p. 514).

48. **(C)** This fundus photograph shows a so-called dragged disc with formation of a retinal fold extending temporally in this right eye, leading to deformity of the disc. All of the conditions except C can cause such a profile. Some cases of so-called congenital falciform fold (p. 34) may be explained by a form of so-called posterior persistent hyperplastic primary vitreous. Retrolental fibroplasia and dragged disc caused by *Toxocara canis* are considered on pages 499 and 500, respectively.

49. **(D)** Mental retardation does occur, although with respect to the amount of cerebral calcification, it is not as severe as might be expected (p. 513). The facial hemangioma generally is limited to the first two divisions of the trigeminal nerve. The cavernous hemangioma typically affects the choroid rather than the retina. The globe illustrated shows a large subretinal mass with numerous cholesterol clefts, indicative of Coats' disease, not Sturge-Weber syndrome. Glaucoma typically involves the same side as the skin lesion.

50. **(E)** This photomicrograph demonstrates an epiperipapillary retinoblastoma with extensive invasion into the parenchyma of the optic nerve. Therefore answer D is true because optic nerve invasion connotes poor prognosis. Retinoblastoma of course, causes leukocoria (answer A), can cause a tumor hypopyon (answer B) due to seeding of tumor cells into the anterior chamber (p. 481), and, because of

visual loss, may cause strabismus (answer C). Answer E is incorrect because microphthalmia is a rare finding in retinoblastoma (p. 36). This helps differentiate it from several other causes of leukocoria that often are associated microphthalmia (pp. 492-505).

CHAPTER 10

1. (**C**) The major blood supply to the optic disc, with the exception of the superficial nerve fiber layer, is derived from the posterior ciliary arteries (p. 532). This is important in the pathogenesis of the optic nerve lesion in various conditions, including glaucoma and anterior ischemic optic neuropathy (p. 544).

2. (**C**) This is a fundus photograph showing medullated (myelinated) retinal nerve fibers. On rare occasions, it has been noted that a demyelinating disease such as multiple sclerosis has caused disappearance of this lesion. (p. 546).

3. (**C**) Normally the retrolaminar pressure is less than the intraocular pressure. When the retrolaminar pressure (or cerebrospinal fluid pressure) exceeds the intraocular pressure (answer A), papilledema develops.

4. (**A**) Microglia, not astrocytes, function as the primary phagocytes of the central nervous system (p. 532). All the other answers are true. The sheath of Bergmeister's papilla is glial in nature and probably also contains astrocytes (p. 527).

5. (**D**) Gliosis, which in sagittal histologic sections is characterized by a random "salt-and-pepper" distribution of glial cells throughout the optic nerve parenchyma, is an important feature of optic atrophy (p. 548). Answer A is wrong because glial cells actually replace optic nerve parenchyma. Answer B describes the *normal* appearance of vertically oriented columns or rows of cells within the optic nerve in nonpathologic states (p. 531). The photomicrograph shows a degeneration of optic nerve substance leading to a special form of optic atrophy. Schnabel's cavernous optic atrophy (p. 548).

6. (**A**) Arachnoidal (meningiothial) cells and astrocytes are the cells of origin of meningioma and optic glioma, respectively. Answer B has a reverse order. The oligodendroglial cell is the cell that is responsible for the formation of myelin and is the cell of origin for oligodendrogliomas (p. 552).

7. (**A**) Oligodendroglia, the cells that elaborate the myelin sheaths of axons in the central nervous system (as opposed to Schwann cells in the peripheral nervous system), normally are found only posterior to the lamina cribrosa in the optic nerve. They are found anterior to the lamina cribrosa when myelinated (medullated) retinal nerve fibers are present (p. 534; Fig. 10-11). In patients with multiple sclerosis associated with medullated nerve fibers, the fundus lesion may diminish during the demyelination process.

8. (**A**) Corpora amylacea are PAS-positive bodies within the parenchyma of the optic nerve that probably occur as an aging process (p. 531). The difference between corpora amylacea and corpora arenacea (psammoma bodies) (pp. 531 and 552) must be understood.

9. (**C**) In most types of optic atrophy there actually is an *increase* in the number of astrocytes (gliosis). All the other answers are characteristic features of advanced optic atrophy. The widening of the meningeal space seen here occurs because of loss of substance of the optic nerve parenchyma (p. 548).

10. (**B**) There are at least two causes of the Foster Kennedy syndrome (p. 539). First the classic explanation is a process caused by an intracranial tumor leading to direct pressure of the tumor on the intracranial part of one optic nerve, thus creating a unilateral atrophy on the same side as the tumor. In addition, the same tumor may lead to increased intracranial pressure and cause papilledema in the opposite eye. The Foster Kennedy syndrome also may be seen as a sequela to AION. This occurs when a previously involved eye has reached a chronic stage and the optic nerve becomes atrophic. If involvement of the other eye then occurs at a later date, it may assume the appearance of a swollen disc (acute AION) in the other eye (p. 544).

11. (**C**) The uveal dendritic melanocytes or their neural crest precursors are the cells of origin melanocytoma. Answers A, B, and E represent cells derived from an epithelial layer, which do not contribute to melanocytoma. Answer B is totally false because a true melanocytoma is totally benign and not related to malignant melanoma. Answer D also is false because melanocytomas are not related to meningiothelial (arachnoidal) cells.

12. (**B**) Melanocytomas are benign pigmented tumors that usually arise at the optic nerve head or in the adjacent region (p. 550). Although varying in degree of pigmentation, most melanocytomas are jet black. Malignant melanoma is the most important tumor in the differential diagnosis. Meningiomas and optic gliomas usually occur in the retrolaminar optic nerve. Retinoblastomas are not pigmented.

13. (**D**) Papilledema, in its early stages, often occurs without loss of visual acuity or field loss, or with only minimal loss of function, such as enlargement of the blind spot (p. 537). It usually is bilateral and more commonly associated with an increased intracranial pressure. A pseudopapilledema picture may be seen in eyes with hyperopia (p. 540). A picture of papilledema sometimes is seen in association with acute glaucoma (p. 276).

14. (**E**) Pseudotumor cerebri is characterized by a fundus picture resembling that of bilateral papilledema without other findings except for increased cerebrospinal fluid pressure of obscure origin. The pathogenesis of this syndrome is unclear, but it may be caused by either hypersecretion or by obstruction of cerebrospinal fluid resorption. All the other answers have been ruled out by the clinical and laboratory examinations mentioned in the question (p. 540).

15. (**A**) The classic Foster-Kennedy syndrome connotes unilateral optic atrophy associated with an ipsilateral tumor (caused by direct pressure on the intracranial part of the optic nerve) and a papilledema on the opposite side (p. 539). Myopia may cause a similar pattern, as may an anterior ischemic optic neuropathy. In the latter condition, one eye may progress to optic atrophy because of a previous attack of the condition, whereas the opposite eye reveals a papilledema-like appearance due to active inflammatory disease (p. 544).

16. (**C**) This fundus picture shows classic drusen of the optic nerve head (p. 534). These usually are relatively benign but may cause varying degrees of visual field defects and hemorrhages. They are observed rarely in children and usually are bilateral. Answers B and E refer to a different type of drusen, that is, fundus drusen of the RPE and Bruch's membrane (p. 426).

17. (**E**) Myelination progresses from the lateral geniculate body to the optic nerve and reaches the lamina cribrosa approximately at the time of birth. This process is described on page 534. However, the intrauterine growth of the axon (which is ensheathed by the myelin) moves in the opposite direction, beginning with the ganglion cell of the retina, which forms their cell body, passing posterior through the optic chiasm and optic tracts, and ending in a dendritic synapse with the fourth neuron within the lateral geniculate body (p. 527).

18. (**A**) Because the inflammatory involvement of the biopsied artery may be sporadic, leaving intervening areas of normal tissue, multiple sections of the vessel must be studied to compensate for the presence of "skipped areas" (p. 545).

19. (**A**) Optic gliomas (p. 553) usually occur during the first decade of life. The most common signs are unilateral exophthalmos, loss of vision, and strabismus. Papilledema and later optic atrophy are common findings. Many authors consider these lesions to be hamartomas, which, after a period of growth, may stabilize and not cause further symptoms. Therefore we recommend conservative treatment in such cases (p. 555). Malignant melanoma and melanocytoma are intraocular lesions that would have been identified by ophthalmoscopy; furthermore, they usually are not seen at this age. Rhabdomyosarcoma and metastatic tumor to the orbit probably would show a history of more rapid progression.

20. (**B**) This photomicrograph shows the classic histopathologic appearance of papilledema (p. 537). All of the answers except B represent conditions that may cause such a swelling of the optic disc. A papilledema may progress to optic atrophy, but the optic atrophy caused by methyl alcohol ingestion is not associated with such elevation of the nerve head (p. 542).

21. (**D**) All the other answers also may apply to a malignant melanoma, but the most important factor is the study of the nucleus, including evidence of mitotic activity, and the nuclear cytoplasmic ratio (p. 310).

22. (**C**) This photomicrograph shows the classic "whorled" cellular pattern characteristic of meningoma (p. 552). Note the nests of meningothelial cells derived from the arachnoid layer of the meninges that produces this tumor. Optic nerve meningiomas may be primary within the sheaths of the nerve itself or may be secondary to invasion of the optic nerve from surrounding structures. Although none are present in this section, many meningiomas contain numerous psammoma bodies or corpora arenacea (p. 552). The histopathologic appearance of the other tumors in this question are described on pages 320, 484, 550, and 553.

23. (**E**) Papilledema (p. 537) may be caused by an impairment of venous return at the disc or by an interruption of axoplasmic flow, caused by increased retrolaminar pressure. Increased viscosity of cerebrospinal fluid (e.g., in meningitis, where a cellular infiltrate may be present in the fluid) may cause an elevation of intracranial pressure, leading to papilledema. A decreased tissue pressure in the prelaminar area (e.g., in hypotony) also may produce a picture of papilledema (p. 538).

24. (**D**) Myopic optic atrophy is not an example of a primary demyelinating disease, whereas all of the other answers are (p. 41).

25. (**B**) The functional symptoms of papillitis or optic neuritis (a sudden loss of vision) usually are disproportionately greater than the disc changes would suggest (p. 542). The reverse often is true regarding papilledema. With papilledema there may be no, or only moderate, visual impairment (p. 537).

26. (**E**) All these answers may apply to optic gliomas (p. 553). It is particularly important to be aware that a significant reactive meningothelial hyperplasia may be observed in this condition. When a biopsy is obtained, this could lead to an erroneous diagnosis of meningioma if the tissue sampling is not adequate.

27. (**C**) The most severe papilledema would result from a tumor of the posterior fossa. This occurs because such tumors encroach on the cerebral aqueduct and the fourth ventricle and could lead to a relatively rapid increase in intraocular pressure and papilledema (p. 538).

28. (**E**) This eye contains three flat, pigmented, benign "nevi." All the cell types listed could be seen in any of these lesions histopathologically. The optic nerve lesion alone shows the classic features of a melanocytoma (p. 550). The other two lesions could be spindle cell nevi (p. 309), but melanocytomas (which also are essentially benign nevi) can occur in the choroid and on the optic nerve; thus a melanocytoma cell type (compatible with C) also would be possible in these two lesions.

29. (**A**) The oligodendroglial cell is the cell of origin of myelin (p. 532). Astrocytes generally are supporting elements, microglia generally appear in inflammatory states, and pericytes provide structural integrity to capillary walls (p. 532). There normally is no myelin in the retina, and retinal ganglion cells have nothing to do with formation of myelin.

30. (**A**) Multiple sclerosis in its early stages usually causes retrobulbar neuritis, so changes on the optic nerve head, especially excavation, would be unlikely (p. 546). The other answers are common clinical features of this disease.

31. (**E**) This photomicrograph of a temporal artery shows classic features of temporal arteritis, including massive infiltration of inflammatory cells and obliteration of the lumen. A few giant cells also are present, but these are difficult to see in this section. Therefore all the answers are correct. All these conditions may cause an AION (p. 545). Partial or complete occlusion with compromise of the blood supply from the posterior ciliary circulation is the common denominator in the pathogenesis of AION.

32. (**B**) The clinical features in this patient are highly suggestive of optic neuritis (p. 541).

33. (**C**) Although medulloepithelioma of the optic nerve head region may rarely occur, it would belong very low in a list of the differential diagnoses of epi- and peripapillary and retrobulbar tumors of the optic nerve. All the other tumors are relatively more common and must be considered more likely.

34. (**E**) This photomicrograph shows the classic histologic appearance of a melanocytoma (p. 550). Although bleached preparations are necessary to establish a final diagnosis, the appearance seen here is almost pathognomonic. A melanocytoma is a benign lesion composed of plump, round polyhedral cells that may, at first glance, appear to invade the retina and optic nerve, as seen in this section. Answer D would be correct except for the fact that the typical melanocytoma cell is not spindle shaped. Drusen of the optic nerve head are illustrated on page 534 and in Fig. 10-12. Melanocytomas may cause some elevation of the optic disc, as seen in this illustration, and may show gradual growth, thus confusing the diagnosis. In such cases, epipapillary or peripapillary malignant melanoma has to be considered.

35. (**D**) In general, vessels are considered mesodermal in origin, whereas all the other mentioned cell types (arachnoidal cells, melanocytes, astrocytes, and choroidal pigmented cells) generally are considered to be of neural crest origin.

36. (**D**) The scotomas associated with each type of AION are variable, and they include altitudinal defects, central scotomas, segmental defects, arcuate scotomas, vertical defects, and peripheral contractions. (p. 544) These various lesions occur with both types. Answers A, B, C, and E are incorrect because they are indeed true facts (p. 544).

37. (**A**) This is a photomicrograph showing temporal arteritis. Because the optic neuropathy often is secondary to inflammatory involvement of the ophthalmic artery on the involved side, answer A is correct. Answer B is incorrect because Schnabel's optic atrophy is not seen infrequently in this condition. Regarding answer C, a sedimentation rate of 40 mm/hour the first hour suggests this etiology, and a temporal artery biopsy is indicated. Regarding answer D, this is a disease of small to medium size arteries as opposed to larger arteries such as the aorta. Answer E is incorrect because the diagnosis can be made in the presence of nonspecific inflammatory cells or epithelioid cells even in the absence of giant cells.

38. (**A**) Answer A describes an important component of optic atrophy (p. 547). Answer B is false because the artery most commonly lies nasal to the vein (p. 529). Answer C is false because temporal crescents in myopia are secondary to tractional stretching as the globe enlarges (p. 44). Answer D is false because the tissue of Jacoby separate the prelaminar region from the adjacent choroid and not the vitreous (p. 529). Answer E is false because the optic nerve head generally is longer in the vertical meridian (p. 527).

39. (**A**) Psammoma bodies are best identified with the PAS stain, not with heavy metal stains (p. 531). Answers B to E are all true statements regarding psammoma bodies (p. 531).

40. (**B**) The degree of reabsorption of glial tissue associate with Bergmeister's papilla is in part responsible for the depth of the physiologic cup (p. 533).

41. (**A**) Drusen rarely are associated with a specific refractive error such as hyperopia (p. 536). Answers B to E are true regarding optic nerve drusen, and therefore do not represent the correct answer to this question (p. 534).

42. (**D**) Orbital meningiomas occur much more commonly in females (p. 554). The other answers are correct matches.

43. (**A**) Although these lesions have a specific embryologic origin from uveal melanocytes in the neural crest (p. 550), this information is not useful in clinical differentiation. Answers B to E are therefore incorrect answers because these are indeed useful clinical features in differentiating these two tumors (p. 552).

44. (**C**) Statement C is false because childhood optic gliomas rarely undergo malignant degeneration (p. 555). Answers A, B, D, and E are all true facts regarding this tumor (p. 553).

45. (**E**) Chronic blepharitis is not a typical finding of orbital meningiomas (p. 552). Answers A through D are all typical findings of this disease (p. 552).

46. (**A**) Because the loss of central vision is not a primary event after perineuritis, answer A is the correct choice. Answers B to E are correct features regarding this condition, which essentially represents an involvement of leptomeninges around the nerve, usually caused by extension from adjacent orbital or ocular structures (p. 542).

47. (**D**) Methyl alcohol toxicity represents a toxic degeneration (p. 542). Answers A, C, and E all represent demyelinating diseases (p. 542).

48. (**C**) All the answers except C (drusen) may cause optic nerve swelling, as seen in this photograph). Therefore, the correct answer (p. 537) is C.

49. (**C**) Paton's lines represent concentric stripes around the disc associated with papilledema (p. 537). A is false because drusen usually are bilateral (p. 536), answer B is false because papilledema is not more evident with myopia (p. 537). Answer D is false because pseudotumor cerebri is a form of benign intracranial hypertension and not related to collagen disease (p. 539). Answer E is false because the Foster Kennedy syndrome applies an optic atrophy on one side and a contralateral disc swelling (p. 539).

50. (**B**) Statement B is false. Myelination begins at the lateral geniculate body and proceeds toward the lamina cribosa during embryogenesis (p. 534). Answer A, C, D, and E are correct features regarding myelination and medullated nerve fibers (p. 534).

CHAPTER 11

1. (**A**) As squamous cells migrate to the surface from the basal layer, they lose their nuclei in the granular layer where keratinization begins to occur. The "granular substance" is composed of products of broken-down squamous cell nuclei (p. 566). The keratin layer is, on the whole, devoid of nuclei except in pathologic states (parakeratosis).

2. (**C**) Hyperkeratosis is a thickening of the stratum corneum, usually caused by too rapid a growth and maturation of the epidermis, either because of a benign process such as a hyperkeratotic subcutaneous horn or because of a premalignant or malignant process such as squamous cell carcinoma (p. 566). Thickening of the squamous cell layer is termed *acanthosis*. Retention of nuclei in the stratum corneum, or keratin layer, is termed *parakeratosis*. Occurrence of abnormal keratin in the basal cell layer or deeper layers of the prickle cell layer is termed *dyskeratosis*. A loss of cohesion between epidermal cells with breakdown of intercellular junctions, creating spaces within the epidermis, is termed *acantholysis* (p. 566).

3. (**A**) Conjunctival epithelium, corneal epithelium, and the crystalline lens all are derived embryologically from the surface ectoderm (p. 563). However, the underlying Tenon's capsule is not. All of the other answers are true with regard to the anatomy and physiology of the eyelids (pp. 563-565).

4. (**D**) The striated muscle of Riolan is one of four parts of the orbicularis oculi muscle. Some authors believe that the force of this muscle tends to direct the posterior-inferior aspect of the upper lid toward the globe, thus maintaining normal contact with the epibulbar surface (p. 567).

5. (**E**) The meibomian glands are located within the tarsus and differ from other sebaceous glands in the body because they are not associated with a hair follicle and each individual gland connects with the external surface via a long duct (p. 567). The glands of Zeis (sebaceous) and Moll (apocrine) are located near the lid margin. The sebaceous glands of Zeis are associated with cilia. The accessory lacrimal gland of Krause is located in the fornix, and the accessory lacrimal gland of Wolfring is situated just above the tarsal plate (p. 568).

6. (**B**) The central portions of follicles contain germinal centers and are avascular; therefore they are lymphocytic follicles (p. 568). Papillae, however, contain vessels that show extensive arborization and typically fill the core of the papillary projections.

7. (**B**) A description of a granulomatous inflammation containing prominent lipid droplets should arouse awareness of a chalazion (p. 583). This inflammatory reaction is, by definition, a foreign-body granulomatous reaction against liberated fat from the meibomian glands of the tarsal plate. Answers A and C are true concerning conjunctival sarcoid (p. 571). The presence of Touton giant cells (p. 295) does

not indicate sarcoidosis. These typically are present in xanthomatous diseases. Eosinophils are also *not* prominent in sarcoid. They characteristically are seen in allergic or parasitic conditions (p. 63).

8. (**C**) The gland of Moll is an apocrine sweat gland that is situated at the lid margin. The other important glands of the eyelid, namely the meibomian gland and the glands of Zeis, Krause, and Wolfring, are described on page 567.

9. (**A**) Rhinosporidiosis is a rare cause of conjunctival papillomatosis in this country, but it is common in many third world nations. This condition is considered on page 572.

10. (**C**) The bullae, or vesicles, that may be seen in ocular pemphigoid occur in the subepithelial region, that is, between the basal layer of epithelium and the underlying stroma. The vesicles of pemphigus vulgaris are intraepithelial, forming as a result of acantholysis. This group of conditions defined as "mucocutaneous eruptions" are considered on page 572.

11. (**D**) The tarsus lies just posterior to a plane through the gray line. All the other answers relating to the anatomy of the tarsus are incorrect (p. 567).

12. (**D**) Seborrheic keratosis is a benign, often hyperpigmented and greasy-appearing elevated hyperkeratotic lesion. It is not sun induced or environmentally induced and, in contrast to all of the other answers, often occurs on nonexposed areas of the body (p. 588).

13. (**E**) Many papillomas of the conjunctiva probably are virally induced. They typically have an irregular surface and often contain a central vascular stalk. Viral papillomas are recurrent and difficult to eradicate with excision or cryotherapy. A papilloma with its cellular atypia sometimes can histopathologically resemble a true neoplasm (p. 585).

14. (**B**) Carcinoma in situ of the conjunctiva (sometimes termed *Bowen's disease*) and invasive squamous cell carcinoma may share all of the listed characteristics, with the exception of answer B. A carcinoma in situ remains intraepithelial, with no invasion through the basement membrane, whereas a microinvasive or an invasive carcinoma shows penetration through this structure into the underlying stroma (p. 593).

15. (**D**) This photomicrograph shows a well-differentiated squamous cell carcinoma. Notice the nest of hyperchromatic cells, abundant stroma, and, in particular, the presence's of multiple keratin pearls that identify this as a squamous cell tumor (pp. 592 and 594). In general, squamous cell carcinomas of the conjunctiva and eyelids, particularly well-differentiated lesions such as these, behave less aggressively than those of other structures, for example, internal organs such as the esophagus. When lymphatic metastases occur, they often are local, with extension most commonly toward preauricular or submandibular lymph nodes (p. 592).

16. (**D**) An Arlt's line is a manifestation of a late scarring process in trachoma (p. 571). The primary reaction in trachoma is a follicular conjunctivitis. The inclusion bodies of the Halberstaedter-Prowazek type generally are found in conjunctiva epithelial cells as opposed to polymorphonuclear neutrophils. Corneal involvement, of course, does occur in trachoma. Horner-Trantas spots are associated with vernal conjunctivitis (p. 572).

17. (**A**) This photograph shows an aggressive, recurrent, large malignant melanoma of the conjunctiva. The various forms of congenital melanosis oculi (answers B and E) rarely show malignant transformation. Although nevi of the conjunctiva in some instances may become malignant, one must keep a special watch on patients with acquired (previously termed *precancerous*) melanosis oculi (p. 578). With constant vigil and appropriate excision of recurrences, disastrous complications, as seen here, can be avoided. However, when the lesion is massive, widespread, and progresses toward more malignant cell types, an outcome as seen here occasionally ensues.

18. (**B**) The hallmark of ocular pemphigoid is a subepithelial bullous change, as opposed to intraepithelial acantholysis, which occurs in pemphigus. All other answers are true (p. 572).

19. (**A**) This is the classic histopathologic picture of molluscum contagiosum, showing marked acanthosis of the epithelium with formation of myriad inclusion bodies that have completely replaced individual

cells. These inclusions are composed of nucleic acid derived from the DNA virus (p. 583). Keratoacanthoma is a lesion that also is characterized by a central umbilication in many cases but shows an entirely different cellular pattern, namely cellular aptyalism, which may mimic a squamous cell carcinoma (p. 592). Xanthelasma (p. 584), chalazion (p. 583), and cutaneous horn (p. 585) show no resemblance to this lesion.

20. **(A)** Conjunctival malignant melanomas are locally infiltrative but metastasis locally or to distant foci is not as common as in primary skin melanomas (p. 579). All the other answers are incorrect.

21. **(D)** Although many authorities consider the gland of Moll the most common source of eyelid cysts, we have found that eyelid cysts are either derived from simple eccrine sweat glands (sudoriferous cyst) or represent epidermoid cysts (misnamed sebaceous cysts), as seen in this photomicrograph (p. 586). Because the gland of Moll (p. 587) is of the apocrine type, showing secretions that are elaborated from the apex of the cell, such a histopathologic profile must be seen within a cyst to consider its origin from this gland. All the other answers are true with regard to various types of cysts. Basal cell carcinoma can cavitate and clinically mimic a simple cyst (p. 589).

22. **(A)** *Micro-invasive squamous cell carcinoma of the eyelid* is a term used by some surgeons and pathologists to define lesions that cannot be considered carcinoma in situ (equivalent to answers B and C) but which also have been shown to be much less invasive and malignant than the frankly invasive type (answers D and E). Patients with early tiny foci of microinvasion clearly suffer less morbidity and mortality than those with the frankly invasive form (p. 593).

23. **(A)** The problem of this question is the differential diagnosis of pigmented lesions of the skin. A seborrheic keratosis (p. 588) usually has a characteristic pattern in that it is elevated above the skin as if it were "tacked on" to the skin and also has a "greasy," often keratinized appearance, which usually makes it easy to differentiate from the other pigmented lesions. The photomicrograph shows how the seborrheic keratosis is elevated above the skin, which is at the lower right. The arrow demarcates the margin of skin (*right*) and the lesion itself. The mass contains hyperchromatic cells and extends upward as a papillomatous growth. These lesions classically contain so-called pseudohorn cysts (*CY*), which represent intraepithelial foci of hyperkeratosis. These are pathognomonic for the histopathologic diagnosis. This lesion is one of the most common, albeit benign, lesions seen on the eyelid and periocular skin.

24. **(D)** The best answer here is D. All these statements actually are true, but basal cell carcinoma is not a benign eyelid lesion, the primary focus of this question (pp. 583 and 589).

25. **(B)** Although identification of this tissue may be difficult in this photomicrograph, there is one clue to the diagnosis. The main mass to be observed is in the upper right portion of the photograph and is composed of a monotonous array of numerous small cells with moderately hyperchromatic nuclei. The most distinguishing feature is the formation of a so-called picket fence or palisading arrangement of cells around the edge of the mass, thus indicating a diagnosis of basal cell carcinoma. The tumor has caused a degree of reactive fibrosis of the surrounding tissue within the dermis. Basal cell carcinoma accounted for 79% of the malignant tumors of the eyelids seen in our study quoted in the text (Apple DJ and Stewart L, unpublished data, p. 589). It typically affects fair-skinned people, is located more commonly on the lower eyelid or medial canthus, and rarely, if ever, occurs on the conjunctiva. Its morbidity results from local invasion; it rarely metastasizes.

26. **(A)** A keratoacanthoma usually is a clinically characteristic lesion with a central umbilication on its surface that, both clinically and pathologically, may show an appearance of squamous cell carcinoma. However, most of these lesions regress within a matter of months and therefore actually should not be considered premalignant. Another term for this condition is *self-healing squamous cell carcinoma.* All the other lesions mentioned definitely may be considered premalignant and may lead to squamous cell carcinoma. This photograph of the child (answer E) shows an illustration of xeroderma pigmento-

sum. The latter is an inherited condition in which multiple forms of tumors, both benign and malignant, may simultaneously occur or randomly crop up over a period of time, especially after exposure to the sun (p. 594).

27. **(D)** Horner-Trantas spots seen in vernal conjunctivitis (p. 572) are composed primarily of eosinophils.

28. **(B)** The cell of origin of a basal cell carcinoma is an embryonic stem cell that is situated in the basal cell layer of the epidermis but does not come from the basal cells themselves. All the other answers are true (p. 591).

29. **(C)** All the answers except C may be compatible with conjunctival carcinoma. A Bitot spot has nothing to do with carcinoma but rather represents a localized plaque of hyperkeratotic conjunctiva seen in vitamin A deficiency. The spot often contains *Corynebacterium xerosis* (diphtheroids) within the lesion (p. 577).

30. **(C)** Follicular hypertrophy is the hallmark of stage IIA of the MacCallan classification of trachoma (p. 569).

31. **(B)** Another term for a keratoacanthoma is "self-healing squamous cell carcinoma" (p. 592).

32. **(C)** This is a photomicrograph of a sebaceous, or meibomian, carcinoma of the upper eyelid. In addition to the numerous hyperchromatic tumor cells, the most characteristic feature is the presence of large, empty, or vacuolated spaces that contain lipid. With routine paraffin sections such as this, these spaces are empty, but after frozen section technique and staining with special stains for lipids such as oil red O or Sudan stain, the lipid is readily identified (p. 595). These tumors are indeed carcinomas and, if not adequately treated, may metastasize in a significant percentage of cases. Because of their location in the tarsus and because of their lipid content, which may occasionally cause a yellow appearance, these lesions occasionally are confused with chalazion and therefore are treated inadequately. Tissue obtained from any recurrent "chalazion" should be submitted for pathologic analysis to rule out the possibility of this tumor. Because the number of meibomian glands is approximately twice as great on the upper eyelids as on the lower lids, the upper lid is the most frequent site of the tumor; indeed, this site is the most common site of sebaceous carcinoma in the body (p. 595).

33. **(D)** This photomicrograph shows bulbar conjunctiva as viewed through crossed polarizing lenses. The epithelium is seen at the top, and deposits of birefringent material are seen throughout the subepithelial stroma. This pattern is consistent with amyloid (p. 93). All of the stains or techniques listed are used to identify amyloid except D, Alcian blue. This stain is used to identify mucopolysaccharides (p. 4).

34. **(E)** Congo red stain is for amyloid and not for lipid secretions, such as those that occur in sebaceous cell carcinoma. All the other answers are true regarding this tumor (pp. 4 and 595).

35. **(E)** This illustration shows congenital melanosis oculi, which may involve the uvea, sclera, or episclera. When the surrounding skin is involved, it is termed *nevus of Ota.* Transformation into a malignant melanoma of the conjunctiva is not a worry. Because pigment elements are derived from the neural crest rather than the mesoderm, E is the only incorrect answer (p. 578).

36. **(D)** The muscle of Riolan is part of the orbicularis oculi muscle and is situated near the lid margin (p. 567). Answer A is false because the gland of Krause is located at the superior border of the tarsus (p. 568). Answer B is false because the glands of Moll are apocrine glands (p. 568). Answer C is false because the gray line is situated anterior the mucocutaneous junction (p. 567). Answer E is false because the upper lid contains 40 meibomian glands and the lower lid contains approximately 20. This fact is of clinical importance; meibomian carcinomas are much more common in the upper lids (p. 595).

37. **(E)** It sometimes is difficult to distinguish recurrent chalazion from sebaceous growths (p. 583). Answers A through D all are true statements regarding this tumor (p. 595).

38. **(A)** Most conjunctival lesions originate at the limbus (p. 577). Answers B through E are incorrect because these are less common sites of origin.

39. (**B**) The glands of Zeis actually are sebaceous glands (p. 567). Answers A and C through E are true and therefore are not correct answers to the question (pp. 567-568).

40. (**C**) Acanthosis represents a thickening of the entire squamous epithelium rather than the granular layer only (p. 566). Answers A, B, D, and E are true statements and therefore represent incorrect answers (p. 566).

41. (**D**) This is a correct statement regarding dermoids (p. 568). Answers A through C and E are incorrect statements regarding dermoids.

42. (**C**) The central portion of a follicle is not vascular (p. 568). Answers A, B, D, and E are true statements.

43. (**E**) Answers A through D all are true statements regarding trachoma (p. 569). Answer E is the correct one in this case because it is false. These inclusion bodies are cytoplasmic rather than the nuclear (p. 571).

44. (**C**) This statement represents true information regarding the mucocutaneous eruptions (p. 572). Answers A, B, D, and E all are false statements.

45. (**B**) Most of the lesions classified as environmental degenerations do not show premalignant or malignant change (p. 574). Answers A, C, D, and E are all true statements regarding environmental degeneration.

46. (**A**) This is a true statement regarding this disease (p. 594). Answers B through E all are false.

47. (**B**) Basal cell carcinoma actually is the most common malignant tumor involved in the ocular adnexa (p. 589). All the other answers are true (pp. 588 and 593). The nerve loop of Axenfeld (pp. 56, 60, and 326), especially if ensheathed by pigment, should be distinguished from an infiltrative pigmented tumor.

48. (**D**) Basal cell carcinomas are derived from epithelial germ layers that reside primarily within the basal cell layer of epithelium (p. 589). Thus answer D is more precise than answer C. Answers A, B, and D are incorrect.

49. (**C**) Carcinomas of sun-exposed surfaces tend to behave in a much less malignant manner than similar carcinomas arising from such internal as the esophagus or lung (p. 592). Answers A, B, D, and E are incorrect. The lymphatic draining of the lids is illustrated in Fig. 11-24 (p. 578).

50. (**A**). Answers B through E are true statements (p. 578). Therefore answer A, a false statement, is the correct choice.

INDEX

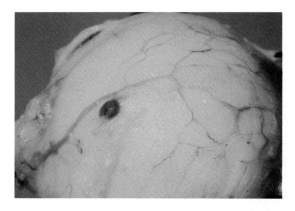

Color Plate 1-1. Gross photograph of an eye with small extension of choroidal malignant melanoma.

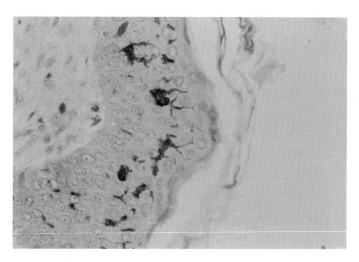

Color Plate 1-2. Photomicrograph of a biopsy of normal skin. Note brown-staining cells within the skin epithelium. These are normal Langerhan's cells derived from the neural crest (S-100 stain × 80.) (Courtesy Amy Scott, MD and H.L. Hennis, MD.)

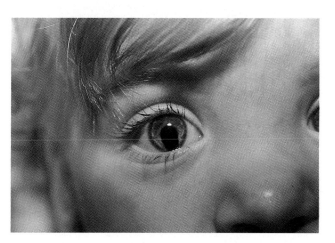

Color Plate 2-1. Typical (inferior nasal) coloboma of the iris. (Courtesy M. Edward Wilson, MD, Charleston, SC).

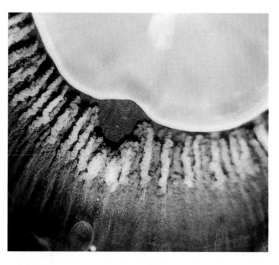

Color Plate 2-2. Lens coloboma, posteroinferior view. Note the four maldeveloped ciliary processes and adjacent defective zonules inferiorly. (From Daicker B: Anatomie und Pathologie der menschlichen retino-ziliaren Fundusperipherie, Basel, 1972, S. Karger, AG.)

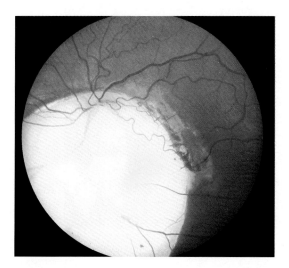

Color Plate 2-3. Typical coloboma of the fundus, involving not only the inferonasal retinochoroid but also the entire optic disc.

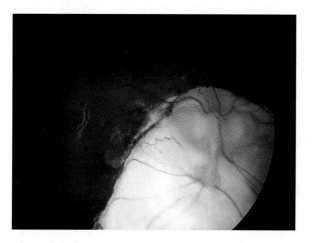

Color Plate 2-4. Fundus photograph of an eye with a massive typical coloboma, not only involving the inferior nasal fundus, but also involving and encompassing the optic nerve head.

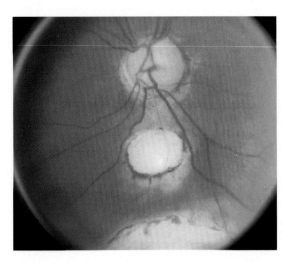

Color Plate 2-5. Typical fundus coloboma. Partial closure of the fissure has occurred, with patches of relatively normal retina sandwiched between the white defects (bridge coloboma).

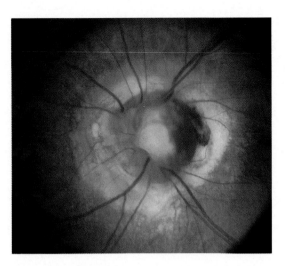

Color Plate 2-6. Optic nerve coloboma (morning glory syndrome) with posterior protrusion of tissue through the defect forming an ectatic cyst.

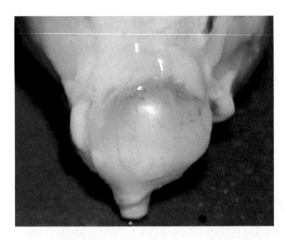

Color Plate 2-7. Morning glory syndrome: gross photograph from the posterior aspect showing an ectatic cystlike protrusion and the optic nerve (*below*).

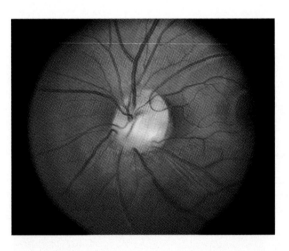

Color Plate 2-8. Congenital tilted disc syndrome with inferior crescent (Fuchs' coloboma).

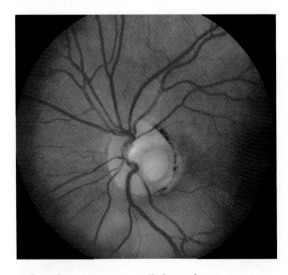

Color Plate 2-9. Temporally located optic pit.

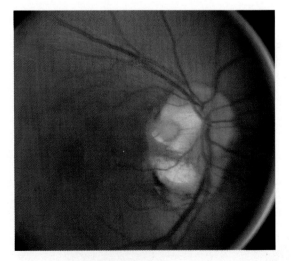

Color Plate 2-10. Optic pit, temporal aspect, associated with a typical inferior coloboma of the disc. Note the serous detachment of the sensory retina and the macular hole. (Compare with Fig. 2-18.)

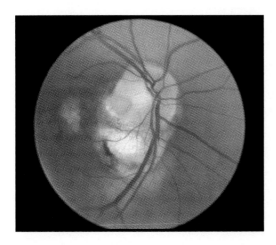

Color Plate 2-11. Fundus photograph of an eye with two types of optic nerve coloboma—a typical inferior coloboma and crescent (Fuchs' coloboma) and a temporal optic pit.

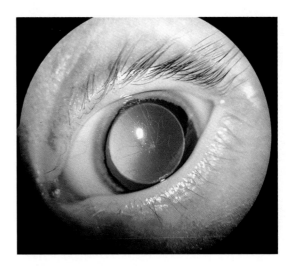

Color Plate 2-12. Congenital aniridia.

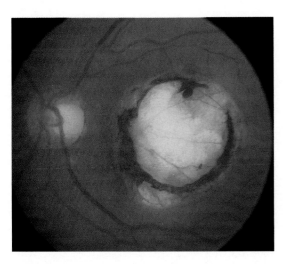

Color Plate 2-13. Atypical coloboma of the macula. Many such lesions with peripheral pigment clumping probably are inflammatory in origin.

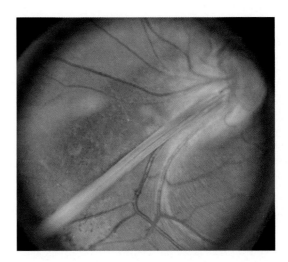

Color Plate 2-14. Congenital falciform fold, which occasionally may be induced by persistence and traction from the posterior hyaloid vasculature.

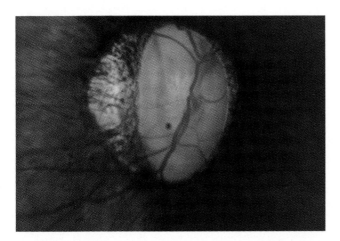

Color Plate 2-15. Acquired tilted disc in high myopia. Note the temporal crescent caused by mechanical stretching of the ocular tunics as the globe elongates.

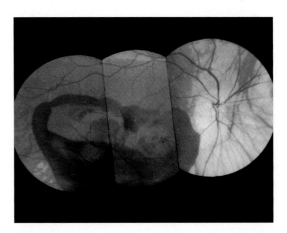

Color Plate 2-16. Severe myopia with retinochoroidal atrophy and hemorrhage.

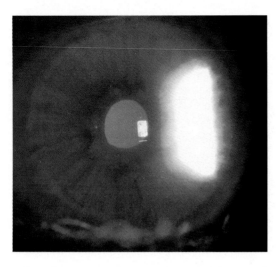

Color Plate 2-17. Albinism: iris viewed by transillumination. (Courtesy Kirk Packo, MD, Chicago, IL.)

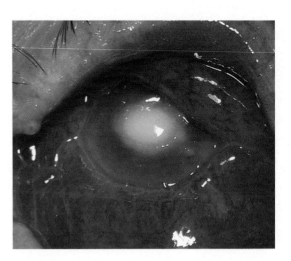

Color Plate 3-1. Bacterial corneal ulcer with an acute, purulent inflammatory reaction.

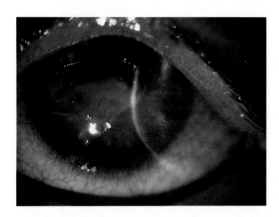

Color Plate 3-2. *Acanthamoeba* keratitis. (Courtesy Joel Sugar, MD.)

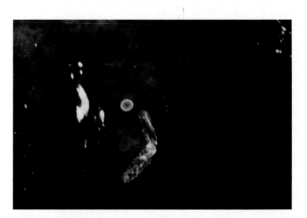

Color Plate 3-3. *Acanthamoeba* keratitis (Calcoflour White stain). (Courtesy Mark O. M. Tso, MD, and Joel Sugar, MD.)

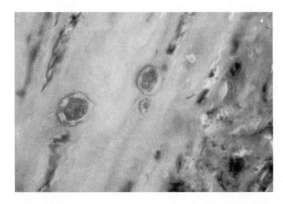

Color Plate 3-4. Photomicrograph of the *Acanthamoeba* organism (PAS stain; original magnification × 200). (Courtesy Mark O. M. Tso, MD.)

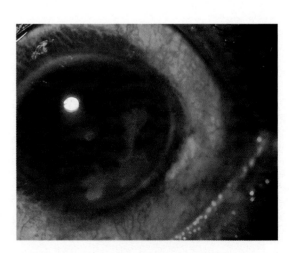

Color Plate 3-5. Herpes simplex, dendritic ulcer.

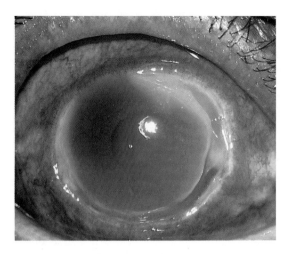

Color Plate 3-6. Mooren's ulcer.

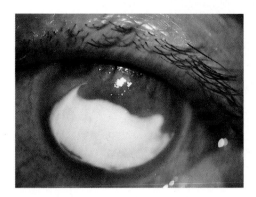

Color Plate 3-7. Clinical photograph of an eye of a patient with neurotrophic keratopathy in whom a severe band-shaped keratopathy developed after extracapsular cataract extraction (ECCE) and intraocular lens (IOL) implantation.

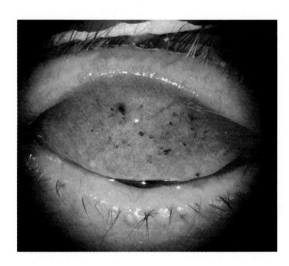

Color Plate 3-8. Adrenochrome pigmentation of the conjunctiva.

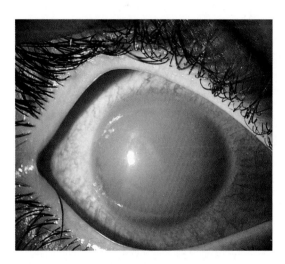

Color Plate 3-9. Bloodstaining of the cornea.

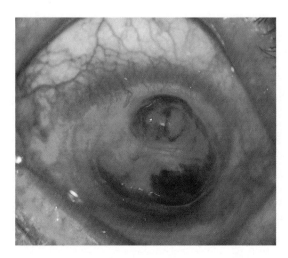

Color Plate 3-10. Corneal staphyloma (grapelike appearance), with uveal prolapse into the anteriorly protruding cornea.

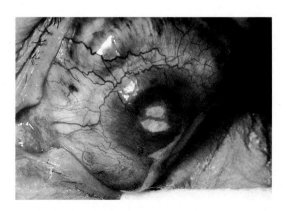

Color Plate 3-11. Scleral staphyloma associated with corneal melting caused by collagen disease.

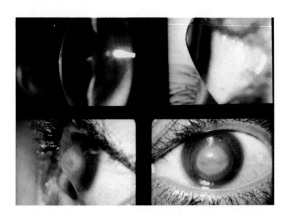

Color Plate 3-12. Keratoconus showing corneal hydrops and scarring.

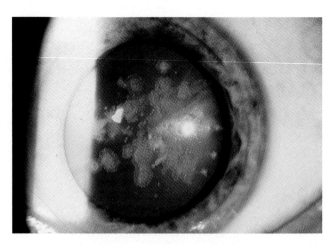

Color Plate 3-13. Autosomal-dominant granular corneal dystrophy. Note ``bread crumb'' corneal stromal lesions.

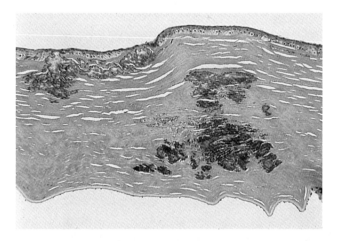

Color Plate 3-14. Photomicrograph of the cornea (same case as Color Plate 3-13). The individual granular lesions stain intensely positive (red) with the trichrome stain. Corneal stromal collagen stains blue (Masson trichrome stain, × 150). (Courtesy Timothy Powers, MD.)

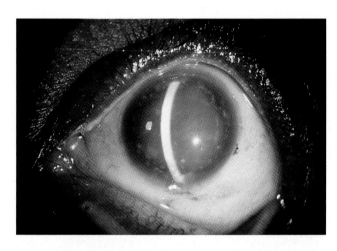

Color Plate 3-15. Autosomal recessive macular corneal dystrophy. Note diffuse haze throughout the corneal stroma.

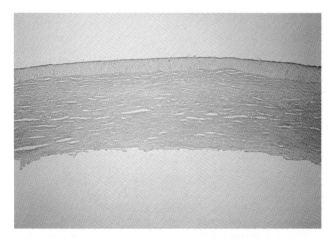

Color Plate 3-16. Photomicrograph of cornea (same case as Color Plate 3-15). Note diffuse infiltration of blue-staining mucopolysaccharide material (Alcian blue stain, × 125). (Courtesy Timothy Powers, MD.)

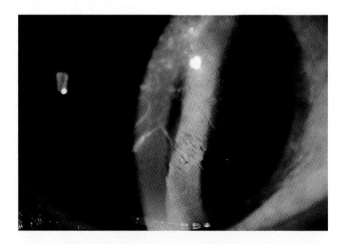

Color Plate 3-17. Autosomal-dominant lattice corneal dystrophy. The discrete lattice lines are deposits of amyloid within the stroma.

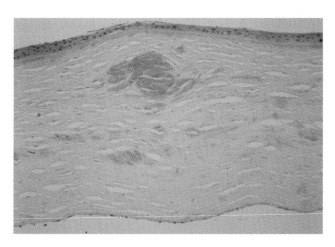

Color Plate 3-18. Photomicrograph of the cornea (same case as Color Plate 3-17). The lattice (amyloid) lesions reveal positive staining with the Congo red technique (Congo red, × 160). (Courtesy Timothy Powers, MD.)

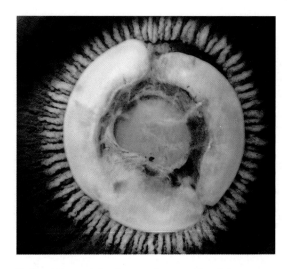

Color Plate 4-1. Gross photograph of Soemmering's ring cataract and encircling ciliary processes viewed from behind. A thin, weblike residual lens capsule is present centrally. (From Daicker B: Anatomie und Pathologie der menschlichen retinoziliaren Fundusperipherie, Basel, 1972, S. Karger, AG.)

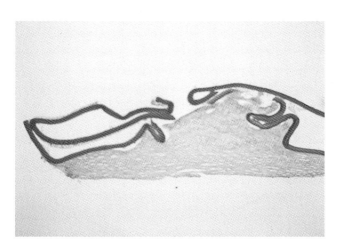

Color Plate 4-2. Photomicrograph of an anterior subcapsular cataract secondary to uveitis, removed during capsulorhexis and phacoemulsification. Note the dense fibrous plaque underneath the overlying anterior capsule (PAS stain × 150).

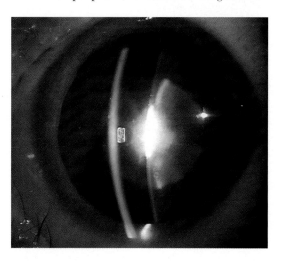

Color Plate 4-3. Slitlamp view of a combined anterior polar and nuclear cataract.

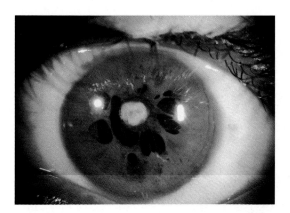

Color Plate 4-4. Congenital anterior polar cataract associated with remnants of the pupillary membrane.

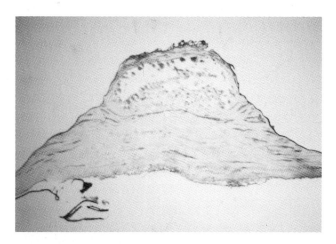

Color Plate 4-5. Photomicrograph of the histologic appearance of a congenital anterior polar cataract. Note that the main bulk of the mass is composed of dense fibrouslike tissue, secondary to pseudofibrous metaplasia of the anterior lens epithelium. The apex of the specimen contains calcium, an unusual material formed by long-term dystrophic calcification (PAS stain × 150).

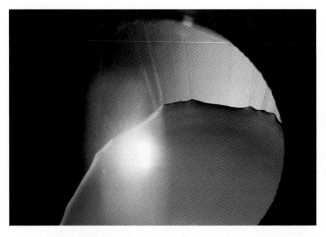

Color Plate 4-6. Congenital lens displacement secondary to homocystinura, with inferior displacement (Courtesy M. Edward Wilson, MD).

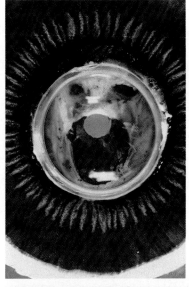

Color Plate 4-7. Gross photograph viewed from behind of an eye obtained postmortem showing the implantation site of a Ridley intraocular lens. To the time of this patient's death, almost 30 years after implantation, the patient's visual acuity remained 20/20 in both eyes. Note the good centration and clarity of the all-polymethylmethacrylate (PMMA) optic in the central visual axis. The lens in this eye was implanted by Dr. W. Reese and Dr. T. Hamdi of Philadelphia.

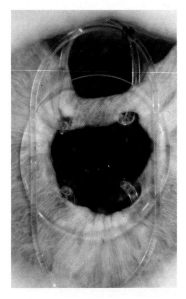

Color Plate 4-8. Clinical photograph of a correctly positioned Binkhorst four-loop iris clip lens, well centered in an eye with good visual acuity. There is moderate pupillary distortion and sphincter erosion. Note the iris-fixation suture superior to the site of the large iridectomy.

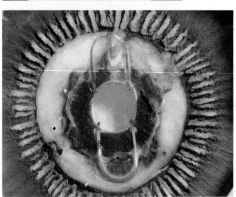

Color Plate 4-9. Gross photograph viewed from behind of an autopsy globe containing a two-loop iridocapsular IOL. Note the rod that helps to secure the lens to the iris through the iridectomy. An outer Soemmering's ring is present, but the visual axis remains clear. The optic is well centered.

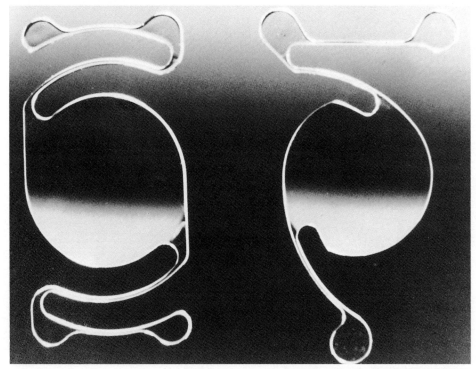

Color Plate 4-10. Modern one-piece, all-PMMA Kelman style anterior chamber lenses, four-point and three-point fixation designs. Note excellent polishing and tissue-friendly Choyce-Kelman–style footplates. These represent modern state-of-the-art lenses that should be distinguished clearly from the earlier, unsatisfactory closed loop anterior chamber lenses. (Courtesy Peter Clemente, MD, Munich, Germany.)

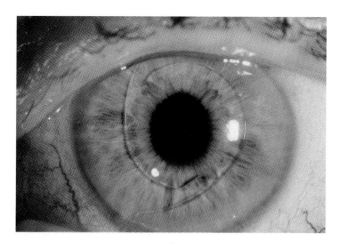

Color Plate 4-11. Clinical photograph of a three-point fixation style anterior chamber lens showing an excellent result (Courtesy Peter Clemente, MD, Munich, Germany).

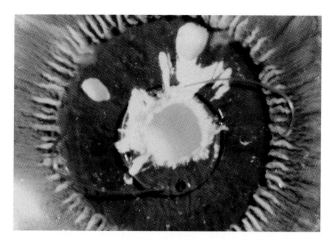

Color Plate 4-12. Gross photograph viewed from behind of an eye obtained postmortem showing the implantation of an iris-fixated sutured posterior chamber intraocular lens. Sutured lenses are excellent when implanted by experienced surgeons, especially as an exchange or during penetrating keratoplasty with an open sky. Anterior chamber lenses probably are equally efficacious for secondary implantation.

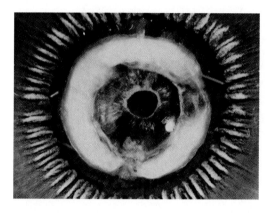

Color Plate 4-13. Gross photograph viewed from behind of an autopsy eye containing a modified J-loop posterior chamber IOL fixated in the ciliary sulcus. The lens optic is well centered, and the ocular media are clear. Note the almost complete Soemmering's ring in the equatorial region around the lens optic.

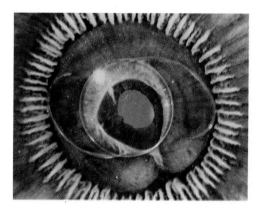

Color Plate 4-14. Gross photograph viewed from behind of an autopsy eye showing a Sinskey-style modified J-loop posterior chamber IOL implanted within the lens capsular bag. The optic is well centered, the visual axis is clear, and there is only minimal regeneration of cortex in scattered areas. There is moderate haziness or opacity at the margins of the anterior capsulotomy, which does not encroach on the visual axis.

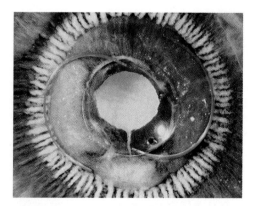

Color Plate 4-15. Gross photograph viewed from behind of an autopsy eye showing an "in-the-bag" placement of a Simcoe C-loop-style posterior chamber IOL. The optic is well centered and the loops conform to the circumference of the lens capsular bag. There is moderate retention of cortical material throughout several clock hours in the periphery, but the central visual axis remains clear.

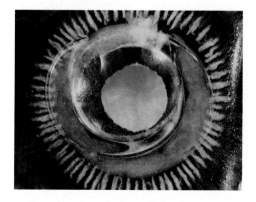

Color Plate 4-16. Gross photograph viewed from behind of an autopsy eye showing a one-piece, all-PMMA–style posterior chamber IOL of the Arnott-Jaffe style. Both loops are implanted in the capsular bag, and the modified C-style loops show moderate compression to conform to the diameter and shape of the capsular bag. The central visual axis is clear. The optic is well centered, and a mild amount of regenerative cortical material is in the periphery, outside the optic.

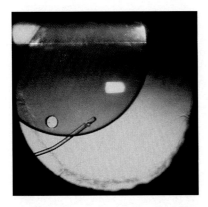

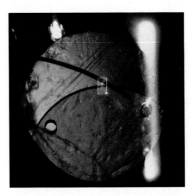

Color Plate 4-17. Clinical retroillumination photograph of a malpositioned posterior chamber lens. During implantation, a wide 8-mm anterior capsulotomy was performed, seen below and to the left through the dilated pupil. The surgeon may have been unable to see the edges of the capsular flaps during lens insertion to achieve symmetrical loop fixation. Alternately, because the large capsulotomy left only an extremely small anterior flap, one of the loops could have slipped from the capsular bag during dialing of the IOL or the immediate postoperative period (pea podding).

Color Plate 4-18. Clinical photograph of a sunset syndrome, with the upper edge of the optic, two positioning holes, and a large portion of the superior loop within the pupil. This lens was implanted in the ciliary region but was decentered because of a zonular rupture.

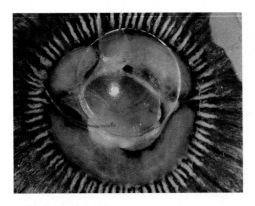

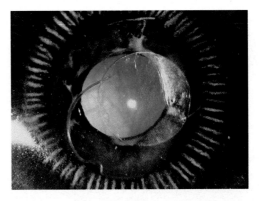

Color Plate 4-19. Gross photograph viewed from behind of an autopsy eye showing a posterior chamber IOL in which both loops were implanted within the ciliary sulcus. Note the marked decentration of the optical component in a direction perpendicular to the long axis of the lens loops.

Color Plate 4-20. Gross photograph viewed from behind of a posterior chamber IOL implanted with one loop in the capsular bag and the opposite loop in the ciliary sulcus. Note the marked optic decentration with the edge of the optic, a portion of the loop, and a positioning hole within the pupillary aperture.

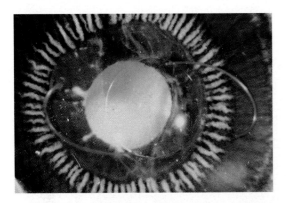

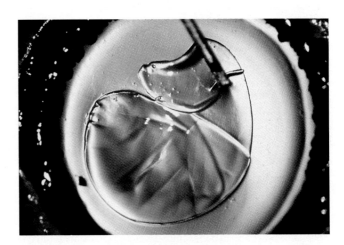

Color Plate 4-21. Gross photograph viewed from behind of an autopsy eye in which the loop on the left was implanted in the capsular bag and the opposite modified J loop was implanted neither in the ciliary sulcus nor the capsular bag but rather extended through the zonules on to the pars plana. Note that this asymmetric fixation leads to extensive decentration so that the edge of the optic is within the pupillary aperture.

Color Plate 4-22. Gross photograph (surgeon's view, cornea and iris removed) of a porcine eye showing the capsulorhexis procedure. Notice the smooth edges of the anterior capsular tear, which is the key feature of this procedure.

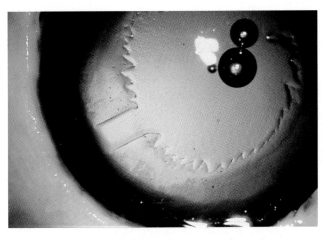

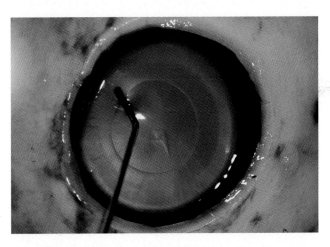

Color Plate 4-23. Gross photograph (surgeon's view, cornea and iris removed) of a human eye obtained postmortem, showing experimentally performed can-opener capsulectomy, with typical radial tears to the equator of the anterior capsule. After clinical can-opener anterior capsulectomy, one to five radial tears invariably occur. (Courtesy of Ehud Assia, MD.)

Color Plate 4-24. Gross photograph (surgeon's view, cornea and iris removed) of a human eye obtained postmortem showing experimental hydrodissection. In this case the cannula is placed immediately under the anterior capsule (cortical cleaving hydrodissection). Hydrodissection is one of the most important maneuvers that helps reduce the incidence of posterior capsular opacification.

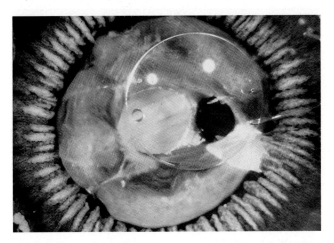

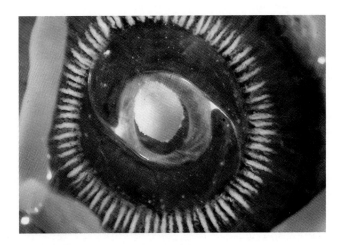

Color Plate 4-25. Gross photograph viewed from behind (Miyake view) of an eye obtained postmortem showing an IOL that had been implanted in the early 1980s. Note marked decentration because of asymmetric fixation as well as advanced posterior capsular opacification. Contrast this to Color Plate 4-26.

Color Plate 4-26. Gross photograph viewed from behind (Miyake view) of a human eye obtained postmortem with an IOL implanted in the 1990s using modern capsular surgery with hydro dissection, continuous curvilinear capsulorhexis (CCC), and a modern one-piece, all-PMMA capsular lens. Note excellent centration and excellent cortical cleanup, with absence of residual cortical material.

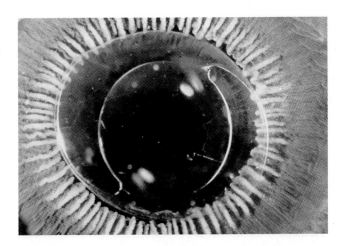

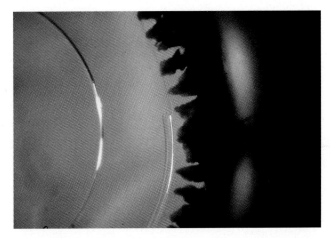

Color Plate 4-27. Gross photograph from behind (Miyake view) of a human eye obtained postmortem with a modern one-piece, all-PMMA capsular IOL implanted experimentally. Note excellent centration and a perfect fit within the capsular bag.

Color Plate 4-28. Another eye showing an IOL of the design illustrated in Color Plate 4-27 (Miyake view). Note excellent fit of the lens haptic in the equatorial fornix of the capsular bag adjacent to the ciliary body.

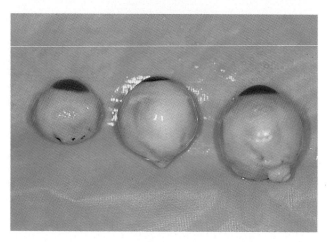

Color Plate 4-29. Gross photograph of three human eyes obtained postmortem at different ages. Left = newborn, middle = age 2 years, right = adult. Most eye growth occurs within the first 18 months to 2 years. (From Wilson ME et al.[999])

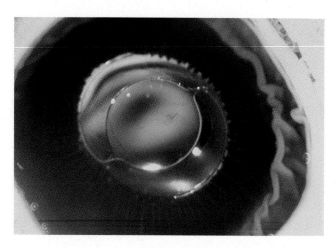

Color Plate 4-30. Gross photograph from behind of an eye obtained postmortem from a 2-year-old child, experimentally implanted using the technique of Miyake with a 12-mm, one-piece, all-PMMA IOL in the capsular bag. Note excellent fit in the capsular bag. (From Bluestein EC et al.[535])

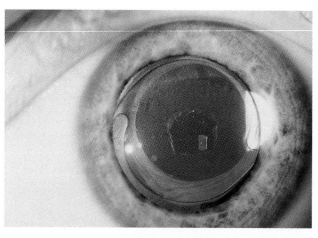

Color Plate 4-31. Clinical photograph of the eye of a 12-year-old boy who had lens implantation at 8 years of age and required Nd:YAG capsulotomy 4 years later. (Courtesy M. Edward Wilson, MD, Charleston, SC.)

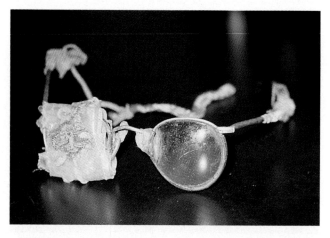

Color Plate 4-32. Photograph of a badly damaged aphakic spectacle demonstrating graphically the immense problem with surgical aphakia in developing world countries. Aphakic spectacles cause unacceptable visual aberrations and may be damaged (as in this case) or lost. The patient is deprived of visual rehabilitation. There is a need to move toward IOL implantation in the developing world as rapidly as possible. (Courtesy Marilyn Skudder, MD, Tanzania, Africa.)

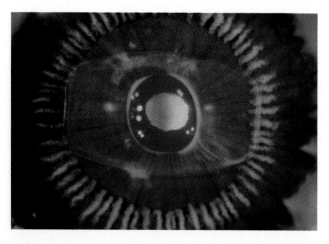

Color Plate 4-33. Gross photograph viewed from behind (Miyake view) of an eye obtained postmortem containing a well-implanted STAAR-Chiron style silicone plate IOL, with excellent cortical removal and centration.

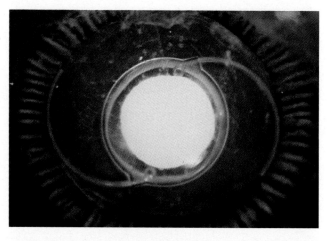

Color Plate 4-34. Gross photograph viewed from behind (Miyake view) of an eye obtained postmortem containing a well-implanted Allergan Medical Optics three-piece silicone IOL. The lens is well centered, and cortical cleanup has been excellent.

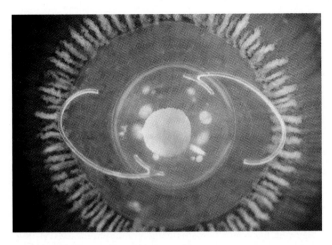

Color Plate 4-35. Gross photograph viewed from behind (Miyake view) of an eye obtained postmortem containing a STAAR Surgical Corporation three-piece IOL with polyimide haptics. The lens is well centered and positioned in a clean capsular bag.

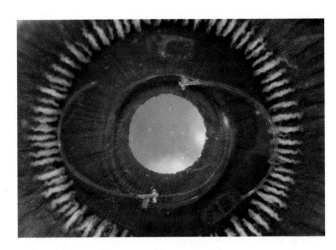

Color Plate 4-36. Gross photograph viewed from behind (Miyake view) of a well-implanted Alcon AcrySof™ acrylic IOL. The lens is well-centered in the capsular bag after thorough cortical removal.

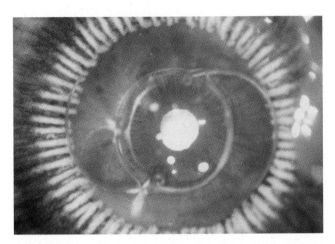

Color Plate 4-37. Gross photograph viewed from behind (Miyake view) of a human eye obtained postmortem containing a well-implanted Allergan Medical Optics three-piece silicone IOL after excellent cortical cleanup (compare with Color Plate 4-38).

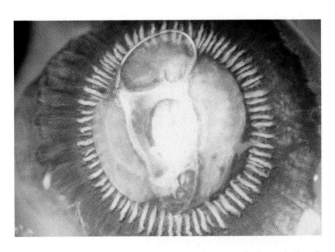

Color Plate 4-38. Gross photograph viewed from behind (Miyake view) of an Allergan Medical Optics three-piece silicone IOL implanted after poor surgery with poor cortical cleanup (compare with Color Plate 4-37).

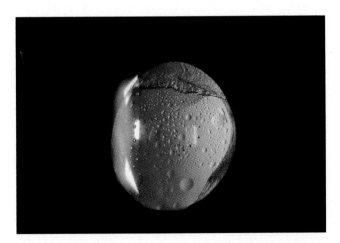

Color Plate 4-39. Clinical photograph of a patient with a silicone IOL who later required vitreoretinal surgery with silicone oil. Note the dense bubbles covering the optic surface, which impaired vision and also the surgeon's view into the eye. (From Apple DJ et al.[462])

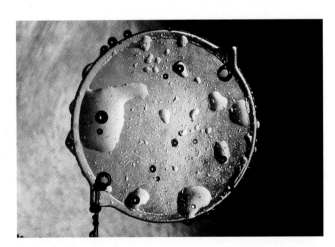

Color Plate 4-40. Gross photograph of an explanted silicone IOL with adherent silicone oil. Adherence of silicone oil represents a problem that hopefully can be solved by new research on optical surface biomaterials. (From Apple DJ et al.[462])

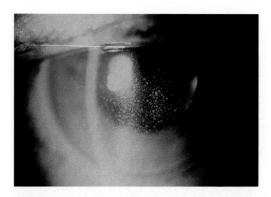

Color Plate 4-41. Postoperative slitlamp photograph of an eye implanted with a modified J-loop posterior chamber lens. The patient experienced an inflammatory reaction during the first postoperative week, which progressed to a persistent hypopyon and "toxic lens syndrome." Numerous keratic precipitates are seen. The eye was enucleated, and a diagnosis of phakoanaphylactic endophthalmitis was made. In this case, no bacteria suggesting infectious endophthalmitis were cultured or observed in sections.

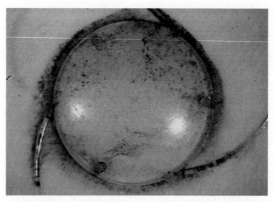

Color Plate 4-42. Gross photograph of a Dubroff Model IOL removed because of uveitis-glaucoma-hyphema (UGH) syndrome. Note the copious amounts of blood on the surface of the lens optic and loops. Contact of the components of the pseudophakos with the iris was responsible for the breakdown of the blood-aqueous barrier and hemorrhage that occurred.

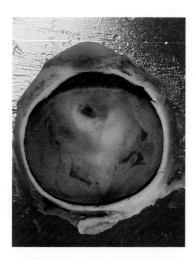

Color Plate 4-43. Gross photograph of an eye from a 19-year-old, 9 months postimplantation of a PC-IOL for traumatic cataract. The classic features of endophthalmitis with vitreous abscess are visible. Note the funnel-shaped retinal detachment. The preretinal space contains a yellow, purulent exudate, and the subretinal space contains a serosanguinous exudate. The cornea is opaque, and a dense membrane is in the retrocorneal region. *Staphylococcus epidermidis* was cultured.

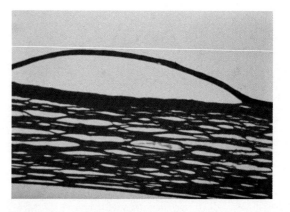

Color Plate 4-44. Photomicrograph of a cornea showing a large, bullous separation of the epithelium from the underlying stroma. An unlicensed Choyce copy anterior chamber lens was implanted in 1983, but head trauma led to rotation and movement of the lens within the eye, causing subsequent uveitis and a secondary glaucoma. The patient underwent removal of the IOL and a penetrating keratoplasty 1 year after surgery. (PAS stain; original magnification × 50.)

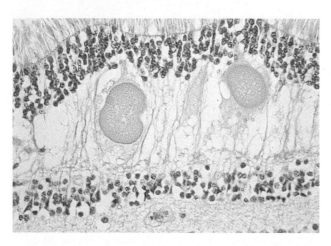

Color Plate 4-45. High-power photomicrograph of a retina with pseudophakic cystoid macular edema. Note eosinophilic deposits in the outer plexiform layer (H&E × 150).

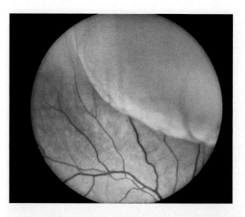

Color Plate 4-46. Fundus photograph of an eye into which an anterior chamber IOL has been implanted after intracapsular cataract extraction (ICCE). Note that a superior nasal retinal detachment has occurred. The detachment is seen as a bullous separation and elevation of the sensory retina (*upper left*). Currently pseudophakic retinal detachment is a very uncommon complication of cataract surgery and IOL implantation.

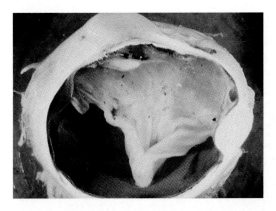

Color Plate 4-47. Gross photograph of an eye implanted with a posterior chamber IOL. There is postoperative retinal detachment. This complication is now rare after modern capsular surgery.

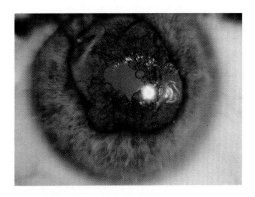

Color Plate 4-48. Retroillumination photograph of an enucleated eye with a ciliary sulcus-fixated posterior chamber lens. A low-grade anterior segment inflammation developed in the patient, which caused formation of posterior synechiae, leading to marked pupil distortion. Numerous epithelial pearls are seen. An Nd:YAG posterior capsulotomy was performed, but the pupillary zone is almost completely reopacified by a membrane formed from residual equatorial lens epithelial cells. (Courtesy John M. Maggiano, MD, Santa Ana, CA.)

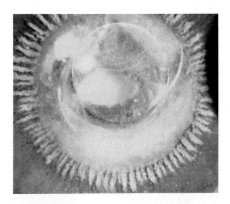

Color Plate 4-49. Gross photograph viewed from behind of a postmortem eye with a posterior chamber IOL fixated in the ciliary sulcus. Cortical cleanup was incomplete, and a diffuse Soemmering's ring is present. There are milky-white cortical remnants and epithelial pearls in the periphery and across the pupillary axis. The IOL is decentered slightly, and the pupil is horizontally oval. An iridectomy is seen (*upper left*).

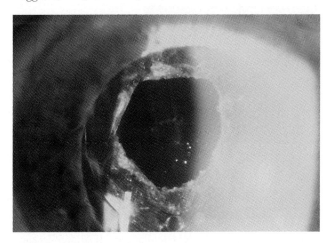

Color Plate 4-50. Eye of a patient who required Nd:YAG laser secondary posterior capsulotomy, a procedure that can cause secondary complications such as damage to the IOL, disruption of vitreoretinal structures, and inflammation.

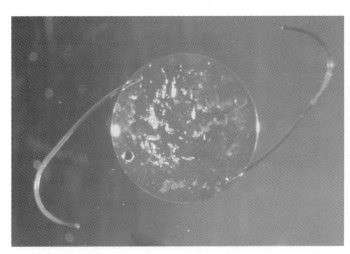

Color Plate 4-51. Gross photograph of an IOL from a patient who had excessive Nd:YAG laser treatment and required explantation. This illustrates the damage that the laser can cause to the IOL optic.

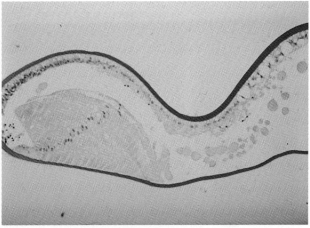

Color Plate 4-52. Photomicrograph of an evacuated capsular bag from an experimental rabbit model showing how both anterior epithelial cells and cells from the equatorial lens bow can remain in the eye after routine ECCE. Removal of cells and cortical material can be enhanced markedly with hydrodissection (PAS stain × 100).

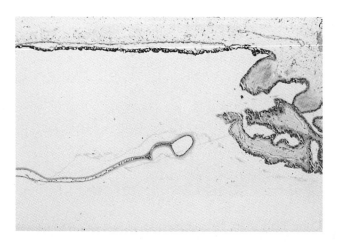

Color Plate 4-53. Photomicrograph of the anterior segment of an eye containing a well-fixated lens in the capsular bag (the haptic rests in the circular empty space at the right equatorial fornix). Note that the anterior and posterior capsules are directly opposed to each other, with almost no remaining cortical material–an example of excellent cleanup after hydrodissection (H&E × 50).

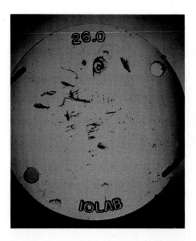

Color Plate 4-55. Nd:YAG laser-damaged IOL after explantation. Opacities up to 100 μm in diameter are scattered throughout the visual axis, which account for glare and reduced visual acuity experienced by the patient. (From Bath PE et al: J Cataract Refract Surg 13:309, 1987.)

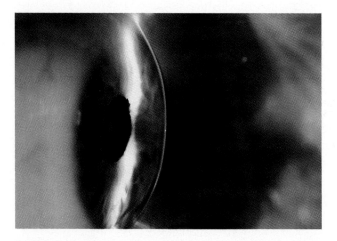

Color Plate 5-2. Post-RK, cornea, too flat. Refraction shifted from −6 diopters (D) preoperative to +5 D postoperative. (Courtesy Kerry D. Solomon, MD, Charleston, SC.)

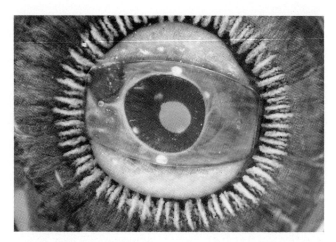

Color Plate 4-54. Gross photograph viewed from behind (Miyake view) of a human eye obtained postmortem containing a silicone plate IOL. This case represents vividly the concept of barrier effect or "no space–no cells." Extensive cortical remnants remain in the equator above and below the region of the lens. The bulk of the IOL optic is in contact with the posterior capsule prohibiting growth into the visual axis. The minimal haze over the haptic of the lens and around the continuous curvilinear capsulorhexis (CCC) represents retained anterior epithelial cells and is not part of the posterior capsular opacification (PCO) process.

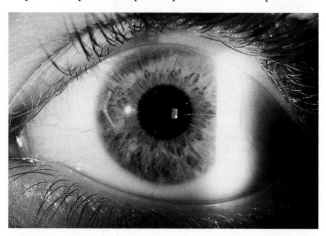

Color Plate 5-1. Sixteen cut radial keratomy (RK). Most modern RK is done with fewer incisions, for example, mini RK with four small incisions. (Courtesy Kerry D. Solomon, MD, Charleson, SC.)

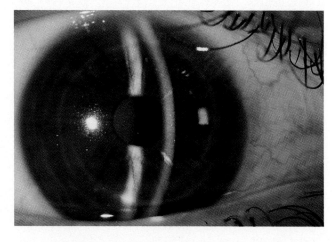

Color Plate 5-3. Post-RK with epithelial plugs and scarring (inferior cut in slitlamp beam). This lesion correlates with the histopathologic patterns seen in Figs. 5-4 and 5-5. (Courtesy Kerry D. Solomon, MD, Charleson, SC.)

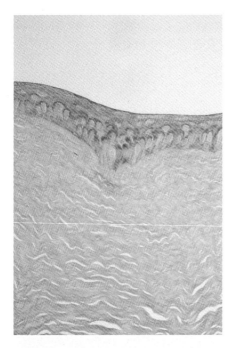

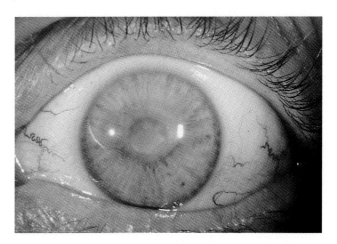

Color Plate 5-5. Opacity of cornea, pretherapeutic (homoplastic) automated lamellar keratotomy (ALK). (Courtesy Kerry D. Solomon, MD, Charleson, SC.)

Color Plate 5-4 Photomicrograph of rabbit cornea after well-performed RK showing a small epithelial plug (facet) representing excellent wound healing (H&E ×100).

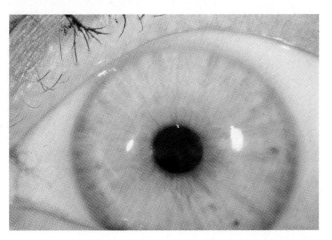

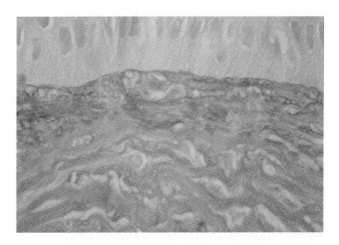

Color Plate 5-7. Photomicrograph of rabbit cornea after experimental photorefractive keratectomy (PRK). Note the laying down of mucoid substances (blue) that occurs during the healing process.

Color Plate 5-6. Same cornea as Color Plate 5-5, post-therapeutic ALK with total removal of the opacity. (Courtesy Kerry D. Solomon, MD, Charleson, SC.)

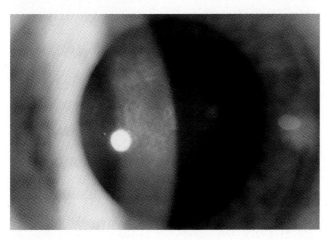

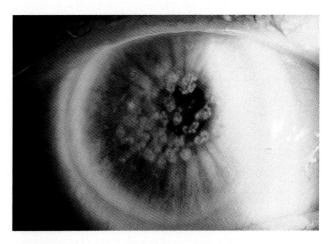

Color Plate 5-8. Corneal haze after PRK, a complication related to excessive and poorly controlled wound healing response. (Courtesy Kerry D. Solomon, MD, Charleson, SC.)

Color Plate 5-9. Cornea with granular stromal dystrophy (see Color Plates 3-13 and 3-14), prephototherapeutic keratectomy (PTK). (Courtesy Kerry D. Solomon, MD, Charleson, SC.)

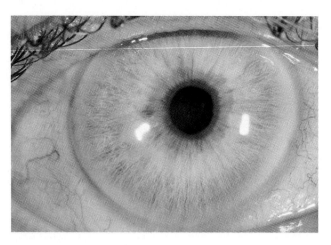

Color Plate 5-10. Same cornea as in Color Plate 5-9, showing removal of opacities after PTK. (Courtesy Kerry D. Solomon, MD, Charleson, SC.)

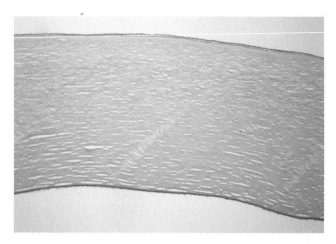

Color Plate 5-11. Photomicrograph of a human cornea grown in organ culture post-laser in situ keratomileusis (LASIK) demonstrating excellent healing with almost no evidence of scarring or disruption at the interface of the anterior and posterior corneal stromal lamellae.

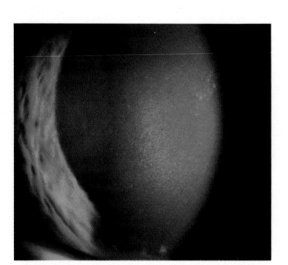

Color Plate 6-1. Krukenberg spindle. (Courtesy Kirk Packo, MD, Chicago, IL.)

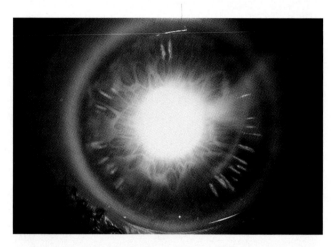

Color Plate 6-2. Clinical photograph of a human eye from a patient with pigmentary dispersion syndrome and glaucoma. Note transillumination defects at the site of contact of the zonules with the iris pigment epithelium. (Courtesy David Campbell, MD, Hanover, NH.)

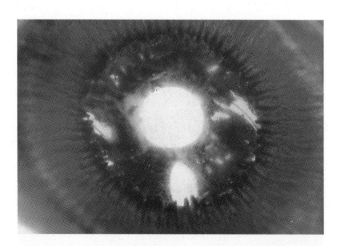

Color Plate 6-3. Gross photograph of an eye obtained postmortem demonstrating secondary iatrogenic pigmentary dispersion and pigmentary glaucoma. The IOL haptics are adjacent to and chafe the iris pigment epithelium. This is more common after ciliary sulcus fixation and is rare after capsular (in-the-bag) haptic placement.

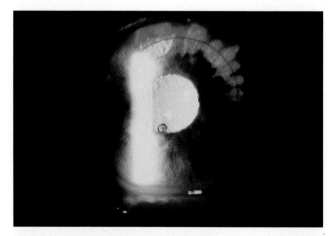

Color Plate 6-4. Clinical photograph of an eye obtained from a patient with IOL-induced pigmentary glaucoma. In this case, the dispersion of pigment was caused by chafing against the edge of a poorly finished IOL optic. This edge is visible in the region of the transillumination defect. This complication is now very rare with capsular bag fixation.

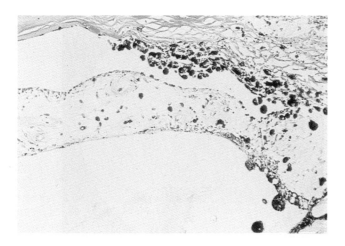

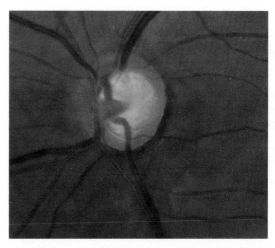

Color Plate 6-5. Photomicrograph of the anterior segment of an eye from a patient with IOL-induced pigmentary dispersion syndrome and pigmentary glaucoma. Notice the absence of posterior iris pigment epithelium that was caused by chafing against the ciliary sulcus-fixated IOL optic. The dispersed pigment accumulates in the anterior chamber outflow structures, which may create a clinical appearance of a Sampolesi's line (trichrome stain × 200).

Color Plate 6-6. Chronic open-angle glaucoma with optic atrophy. Discontinuity of the superior temporal vein is apparent; a segment of the vessel disappears under the edge. Note inferior notch at 6 o'clock position.

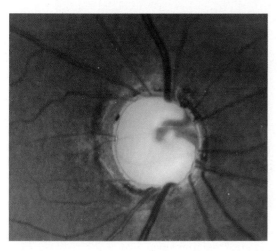

Color Plate 6-7. Glaucomatous optic atrophy with significant pathologic excavation of the optic cup.

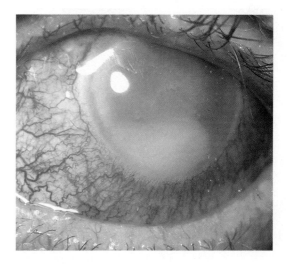

Color Plate 7-1. Acute, nongranulomatous anterior keratouveitis, showing subconjunctival injection and white exudate within the anterior chamber.

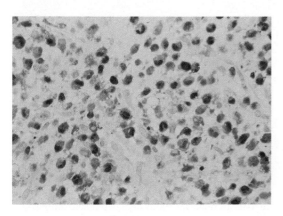

Color Plate 7-2. Photomicrograph of eosinophilic granuloma showing positive S-100 protein. (S-100 stain × 300.) (Courtesy Amy Scott, MD, and H. L. Hennis, MD.)

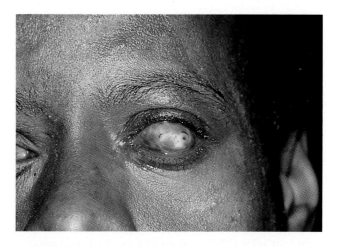

Color Plate 7-3. Clinical photograph of a patient with a severe perforating injury to the left eye (inciting eye) globe that resulted in uveal prolapse. Sympathetic response occurred in the opposite (right) eye. (Courtesy Timothy Powers, MD.)

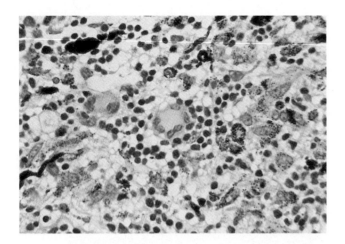

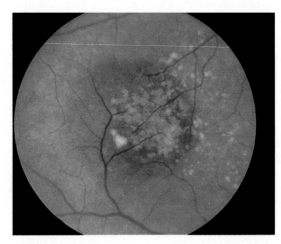

Color Plate 7-4. Sympathetic ophthalmia. Photomicrograph through the choroid of the sympathizing eye of the patient illustrated in Color Plate 7-3. There is a diffuse infiltration of lymphocytes, plasma cells, epithelioid cells, and giant cells, characteristic of granulomatous inflammation. (Courtesy Timothy Powers, MD.)

Color Plate 7-5. Benign choroidal nevus, associated with degenerative changes of the overlying pigment epithelium.

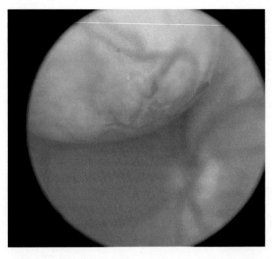

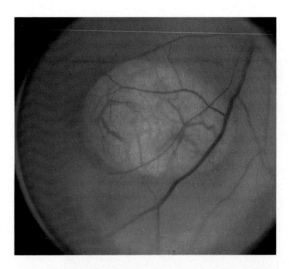

Color Plate 7-6. Highly elevated, pigmented choroidal malignant melanoma. The fundus and optic nerve are posterior to the plane of focus.

Color Plate 7-7. Amelanotic melanoma of the choroid. The tumor contains a rich vascular plexus.

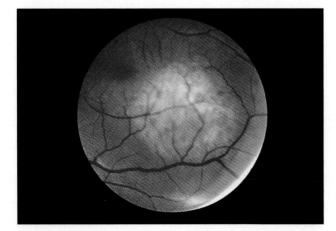

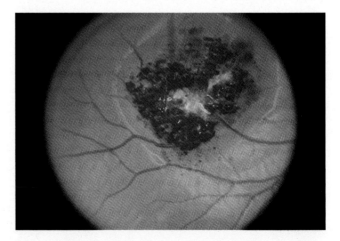

Color Plate 7-8. Choroidal hemangioma, slightly inferior-temporal to the left macula. This amelanotic lesion reveals a pale, pink color that is emitted from the vessels within the choroid.

Color Plate 7-9. Retinal cavernous hemangioma, manifested as a brilliant purple lesion. See Fig. 7-31 for a fluorescein angiogram of this lesion.

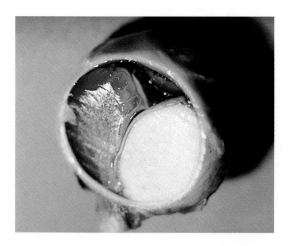

Color Plate 7-10. Gross photograph of an amelanotic malignant melanoma of the choroid. A massive serous detachment of the adjacent retina has occurred.

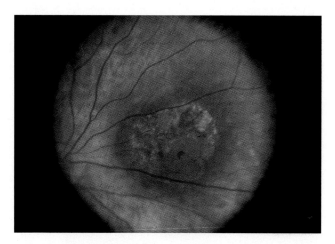

Color Plate 7-11. Hypertrophy of the retinal pigment epithelium. This large, deeply pigmented lesion is situated superiornasal to the disc. This lesion is relatively flat, benign, and nonprogressive.

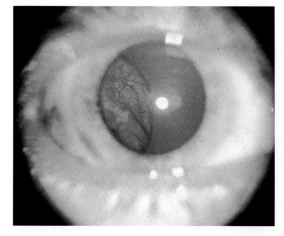

Color Plate 7-12. Malignant melanoma of the ciliary body and anterior choroid.

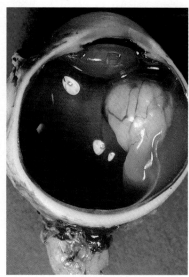

Color Plate 7-13. Gross photograph of the malignant melanoma in Color Plate 7-12. The adjacent sensory retina has undergone serous detachment.

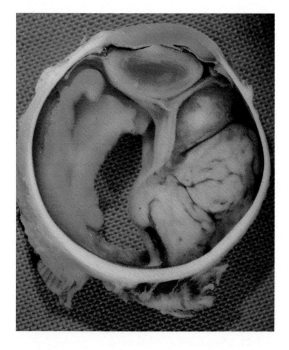

Color Plate 7-14. Gross photograph of a moderately pigmented malignant melanoma of the choroid, with a total funnel-shaped detachment of the retina.

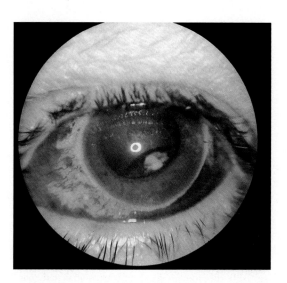

Color Plate 7-15. Malignant melanoma of the ciliary body. An extracapsular cataract extraction (ECCE) (note white residual retained lens cortex) was performed with the intention of implanting an IOL.

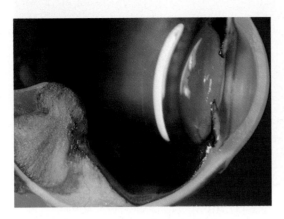

Color Plate 7-16. Gross photograph of a "mushroom" or "collarbutton" choroidal melanoma. The degree of pigmentation varies within the tumor mass.

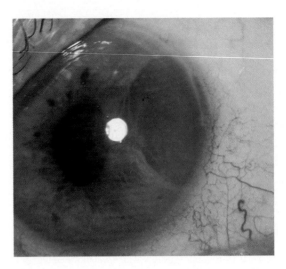

Color Plate 7-17. Malignant melanoma of the iris and ciliary body. When the iris root is involved, one must rule out involvement posterior to the angle recess.

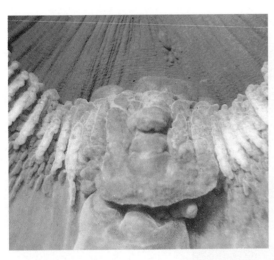

Color Plate 7-18. Gross photograph of a small ciliary body malignant melanoma. (From Daicker B: Anatomie und Pathologie der menschlichen retino-ziliaren Fundusperipherie, Basel, 1972, S. Karger, AG.)

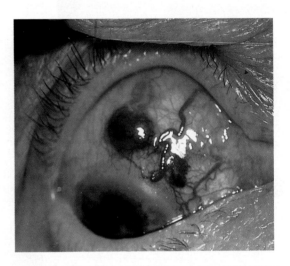

Color Plate 7-19. Malignant melanoma of the ciliary body with epibulbar extension. The episcleral vessels are dilated.

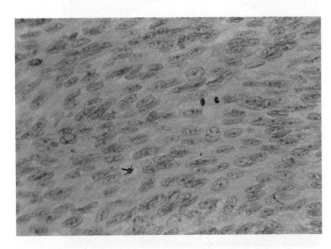

Color Plate 7-20. Photomicrograph of a choroidal malignant melanoma. Note parallel arrangement of spindle B cells arranged in a syncytium, with prominent nuclei and occasional mitoses.

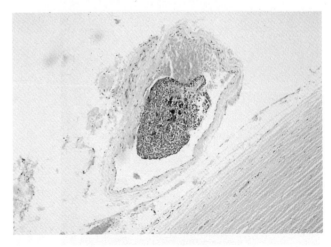

Color Plate 7-21. Photomicrograph through an episcleral vessel containing choroidal malignant melanoma cells. This demonstrates the pattern of dissemination through ocular emissaria.

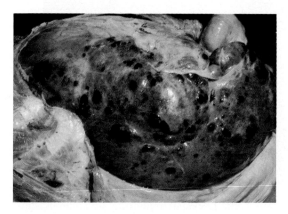

Color Plate 7-22. Greatly enlarged (7000 g vs. the normal 1200 g) liver at autopsy, containing myriad nodules of pigmented, metastatic, choroidal malignant melanoma.

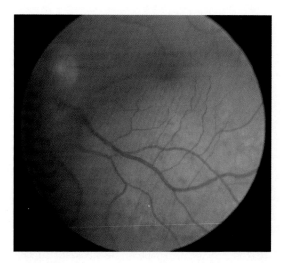

Color Plate 7-23. Bronchogenic carcinoma metastatic to the choroid in a woman who is a heavy smoker. Most such tumors are relatively flat and diffuse, and multiple deposits may occur.

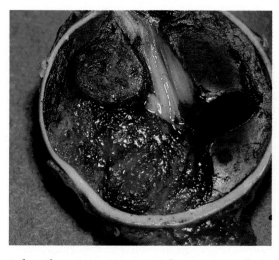

Color Plate 7-24. Metastatic adenocarcinoma from the lung. The retina is totally detached. The "shiny" gelatinous appearance of the tumor is caused by secretion of mucin.

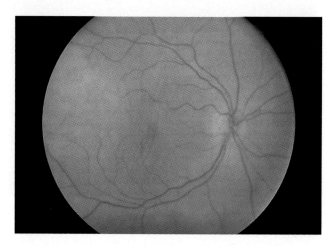

Color Plate 7-25. Fundus photograph of an amelanotic elevated choroidal mass. The eye was enucleated for suspected malignant melanoma. Pathologic analysis revealed a follicular adenocarcinoma, metastatic from the thyroid. (Courtesy Timothy Powers, MD.)

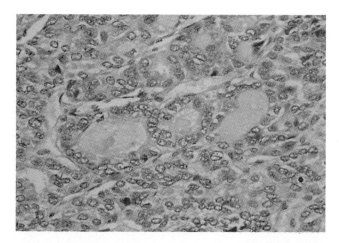

Color Plate 7-26. Photomicrograph of the metastatic thyroid carcinoma illustrated in Color Plate 7-25. The origin from thyroid tissue is evidenced by the presence of multiple colloid-filled follicles. (Courtesy Timothy Powers, MD.)

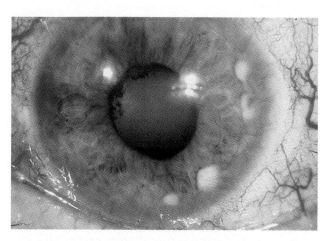

Color Plate 7-27. Multiple "seedlets" within the anterior segment and vitreous that were found at autopsy to be secondary to metastatic adenoid cystic carcinoma originating in the sinuses. (Courtesy Timothy Powers, MD.)

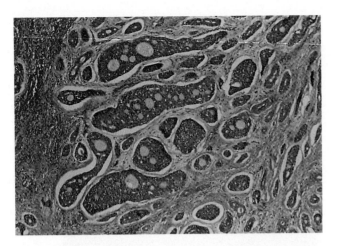

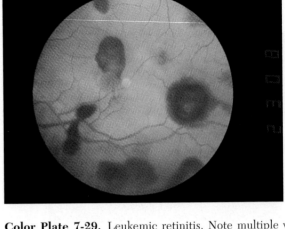

Color Plate 7-28. Photomicrograph of the metastatic adenoid cystic carcinoma (same case as illustrated in Color Plate 7-27). (Courtesy Timothy Powers, MD.)

Color Plate 7-29. Leukemic retinitis. Note multiple white-centered hemorrhages.

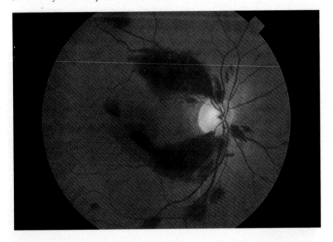

Color Plate 7-30. Leukemic retinitis. Note multiple white-centered hemorrhages.

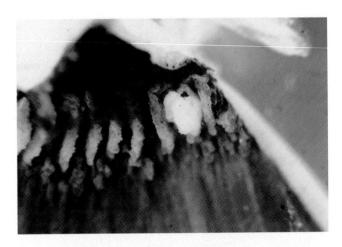

Color Plate 7-31. Gross photograph of an adult human eye obtained postmortem showing the microscopic appearance of a solitary Fuchs' adenoma involving the pars plicata. (Courtesy Louis Karp, MD.)

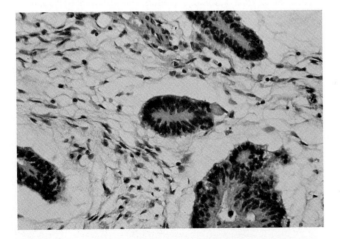

Color Plate 7-32. Photomicrograph illustrating the two major components of a medulloepithelioma, namely 1) an epithelial component composed of rows or chords cuboidal cells resembling those found in the neural tube of the embryonic eye and 2) an interstitial fibrillar matrix composed of elongated spindle-shaped cells with delicate fibrils. This stroma contains a hyaluronic acid-rich ground substance that represents an attempt by the tumor to form embryonic vitreous.

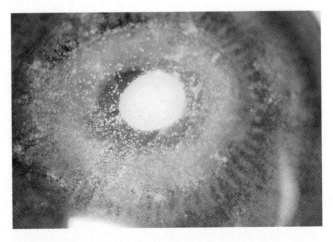

Color Plate 8-1. Gross photograph viewed from behind of a human eye obtained postmortem showing asteroid hyalosis.

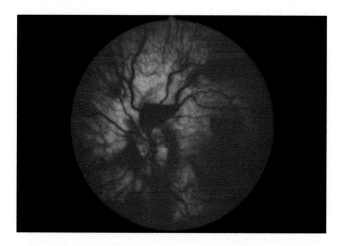

Color Plate 8-2. Fundus photograph of an infant eye with "shaken baby syndrome." Note the florid intraretinal and preretinal hemorrhages involving all quadrants of the fundus. (Courtesy M. Edwards Wilson, MD, Charleston, SC.)

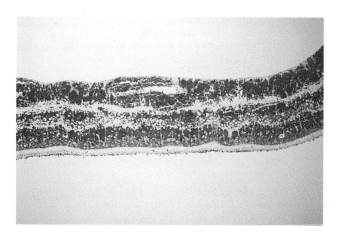

Color Plate 8-3. Photomicrograph, same patient with "shaken baby syndrome" as in Color Plate 8-2, showing diffuse acute hemorrhage throughout all retinal layers.

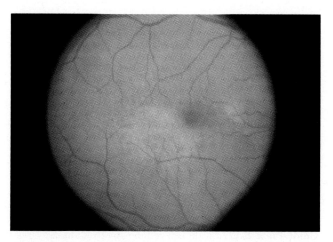

Color Plate 8-4. Retinal phototoxicity caused by light from a surgical operating microscope. This is a fundus photograph of the right eye of a patient who has had two operations. The first was cataract removal and the second was a vitrectomy. Note two discrete yellow lesions appearing at the level of the pigment epithelium. See Fig 8-16 for a fluorescein angiogram.

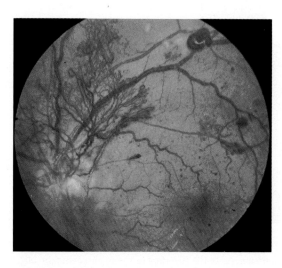

Color Plate 8-5. Proliferative diabetic retinopathy with venous "beading" and florid neovascularization.

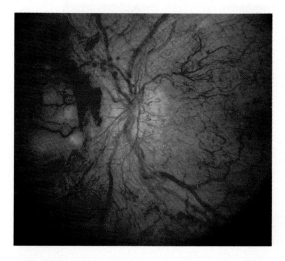

Color Plate 8-6. Proliferative diabetic retinopathy with extensive neovascularization and hemorrhage.

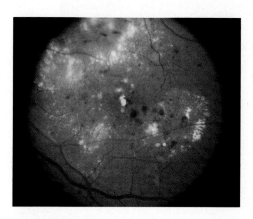

Color Plate 8-7. Fundus photograph showing severe diabetic retinopathy.

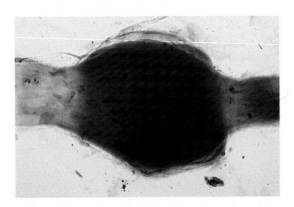

Color Plate 8-8. Trypsin digest preparation showing a "cuff" macroaneurysm. Note the fusiform swelling of the vessel. (Trypsin digest preparation, PAS and hematoxylin stain, × 250.) (Reprinted with permission from Fichte C, Streeten BW, and Friedman AH: Am J Ophthalmol 85(4):509, 1978, with the permission of the authors and the *American Journal of Ophthalmology*. Copyright The Ophthalmic Publishing Company.)

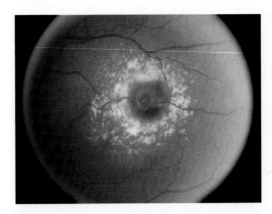

Color Plate 8-9. Fundus photograph of a macroaneurysm showng moderately extensive circinate exudation.

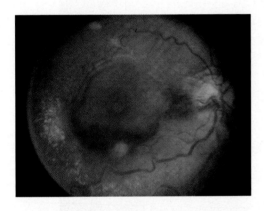

Color Plate 8-10. Fundus photograph showing a temporal macroaneurysm. Note the bleeding of the macroaneurysm at the level of the inferior temporal artery.

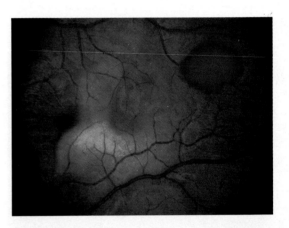

Color Plate 8-11. Sickle cell retinopathy (S-C disease), right eye, showing a "salmon" patch and an old infarction of the macular region.

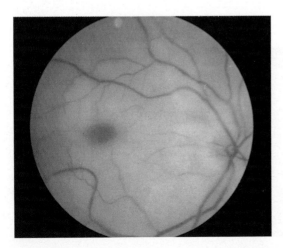

Color Plate 8-12. Occlusion of the central retinal artery with "cloudy swelling" of the retina and a macular cherry-red spot.

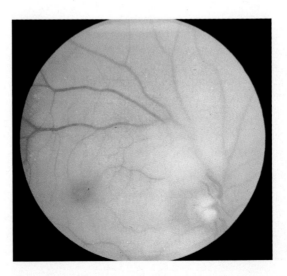

Color Plate 8-13. Classic clinical appearance of central retinal artery occlusion with formation of a cherry-red spot.

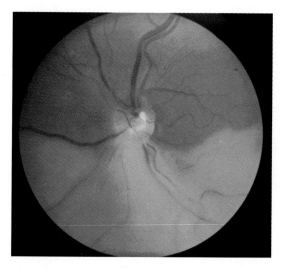

Color Plate 8-14. Occlusion of the arterial supply to the lower hemisphere of the fundus, with typical ``cloudy swelling'' inferiorly.

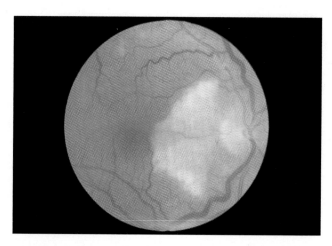

Color Plate 8-15. Cilioretinal artery occlusion, right eye. Note the area of white discoloration between the optic disc and the macula, representing acute ischemic necrosis of the inner retinal layers (see Fig. 8-41).

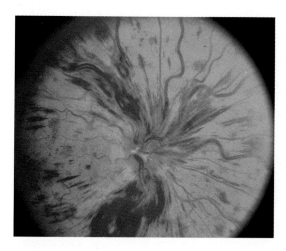

Color Plate 8-16. Occlusion of the central retinal vein (hemorrhagic retinopathy), with formation of flame-shaped hemorrhages in all quadrants.

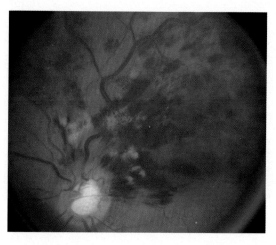

Color Plate 8-17. Acute occlusion of the superior temporal branch vein, with formation of flame-shaped hemorrhages.

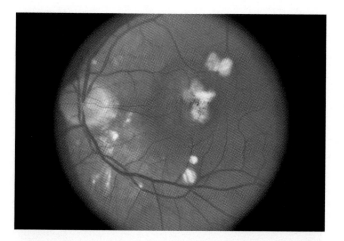

Color Plate 8-18. Ocular histoplasmosis with submacular neovascularization in the left eye. The triad of peripapillary atrophy, macular involvement, and peripheral lesions was present in both eyes of this patient.

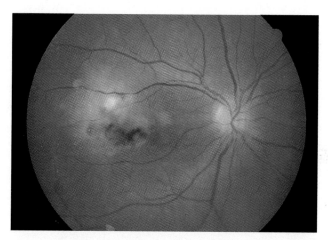

Color Plate 8-19. Acute and healed toxoplasmosis. Note both an acute white lesion and an adjacent healed, pigmented scar.

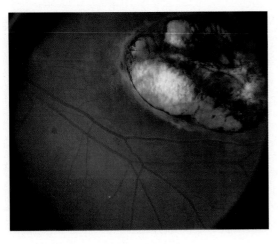

Color Plate 8-20. Healed toxoplasmosis.

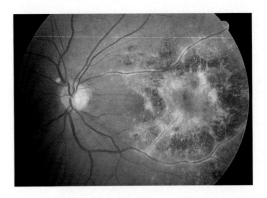

Color Plate 8-21. Fundus photograph of a patient with acquired immune deficiency syndrome (AIDS) and cytomegalic inclusion retinitis.

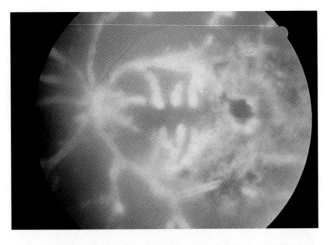

Color Plate 8-22. Acquired immune deficiency syndrome, retinopathy. Patient had cytomegalic conclusion retinitis and sheathing of retinal venules (periphlebitis).

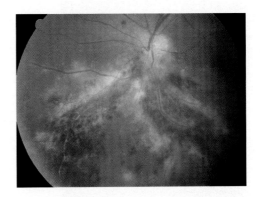

Color Plate 8-23. Fundus photograph from a patient with AIDS and cytomegalic inclusion retinitis showing a hemorrhagic, exudative, and necrotic retinitis.

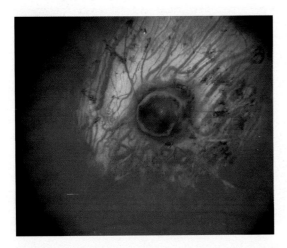

Color Plate 8-24. Pseudoretinitis pigmentosa (posttraumatic migration of the retinal pigment epithelium), with intraocular gravel foreign body.

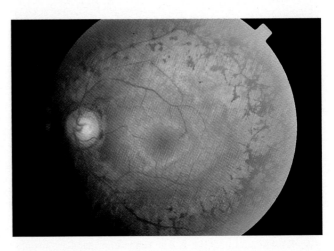

Color Plate 8-25. Clinical photograph of moderately advanced retinitis pigmentosa.

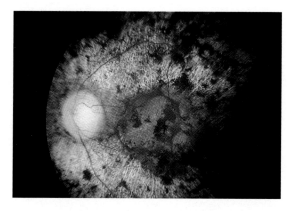

Color Plate 8-26. Clinical photograph of advanced retinitis pigmentosa. (Courtesy Lowrey P. King, MD, Charleston, SC.)

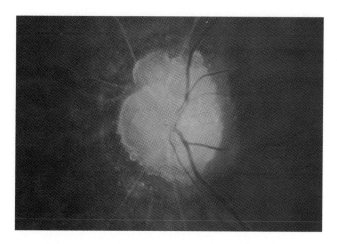

Color Plate 8-27. Drusen of the optic nerve head in retinitis pigmentosa. Note attenuated obliterated peripapillary retinal vessels.

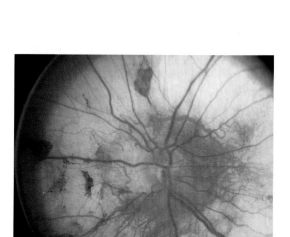

Color Plate 8-28. Choroideremia. The white sclera is visible as a result of atrophy of the retinal pigment epithelium and choroid.

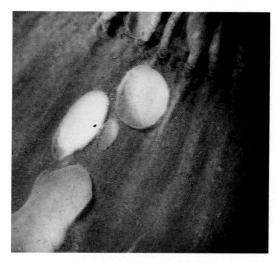

Color Plate 8-29. Multiple myeloma: gross photograph. Milky-white pleural cysts of the pars plana are viewed from behind. The ciliary processes are seen at the upper right. (From Daicker B: Anatomie und Pathologie der menschlichen retinoziliaren Fundusperipherie, Basel, 1972, S. Karger, AG.)

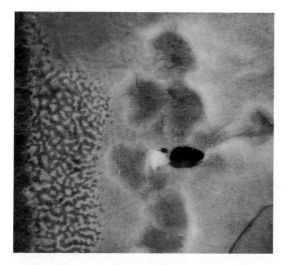

Color Plate 8-30. Peripheral retina at the ora serrata (*left*). Note the honeycomb region of microcystoid degeneration near the ora and an operculated flap tear in an area of atrophic retina. (From Daicker B: Anatomie und Pathologie der menschlichen retinoziliaren Fundusperipherie, Basel, 1972, S. Karger, AG.)

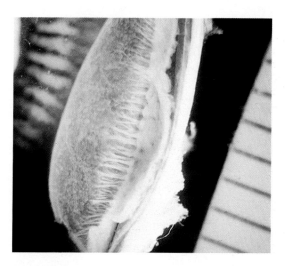

Color Plate 8-31. Gross photograph of a peripheral retina showing senile retinoschisis arising from microcystoid degeneration. Residual Müller cell columns are visible. (From Daicker B: Anatomie und Pathologie der menschlichen retino-ziliaren Fundusperipherie, Basel, 1972, S. Karger, AG.)

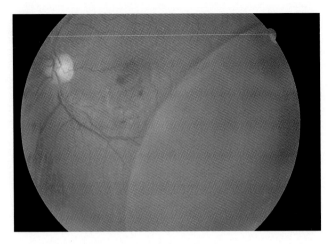

Color Plate 8-32. Peripheral reticular microcystic retinoschisis, adult form. This patient presented with age-related macular degeneration. She also was found to have this lesion. It consists of a bullous separation of layers in the nerve fiber layer.

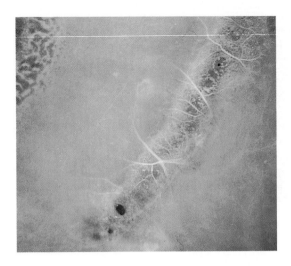

Color Plate 8-33. Gross photograph of lattice degeneration showing crisscrossing white lattice lines, background hyperpigmentation, and a developing retinal hole. (From Daicker B: Anatomie und Pathologie der menschlichen retino-ziliaren Fundusperipherie, Basel, 1972, S. Karger, AG.)

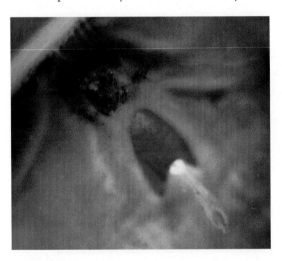

Color Plate 8-34. Gross photograph of a peripheral retinal horseshoe tear with a tuft of retina protruding into the vitreous (*below*). (From Daicker B: Anatomie und Pathologie der menschlichen retino-ziliaren Fundusperipherie, Basel, 1972, S. Karger, AG.)

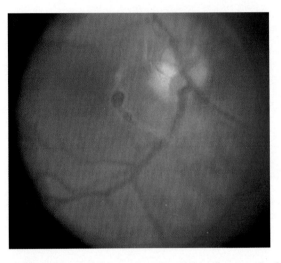

Color Plate 8-35. Posterior vitreous detachment. The filmy vitreous face obscures the retina except at the hole (Vogt's ring) inferotemporal to the disc.

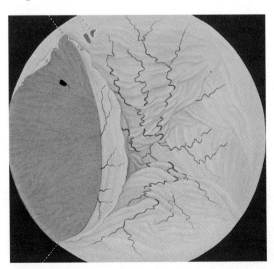

Color Plate 8-36. Fundus drawing from the classic monograph of Professor Jules Gonin, showing a giant retinal tear with associated retinal detachment. (From Gonin J: Le décollement de la rétine: pathogenie, traitement, Lausanne, 1934, Librairie Payot & Cie.)

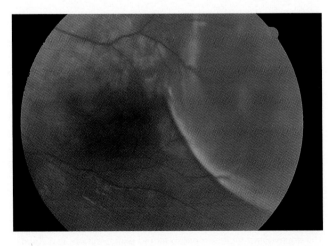

Color Plate 8-37. Nonrhegmatogenous detachment associated with pre-eclampsia. Such a detachment usually follows termination of the pregnancy.

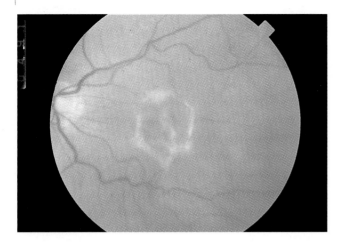

Color Plate 8-38. Epiretinal membrane, visible as a white "fibroglial" membrane.

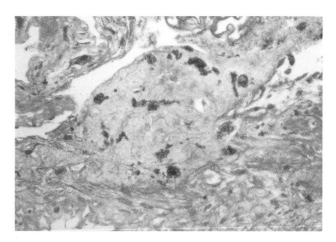

Color Plate 8-39. Epiretinal membrane, composed primarily of a fibrous component (blue stain), admixed with pigment epithelial pigment and scattered glial tissue (burgandy color) (Masson trichrome stain × 400).

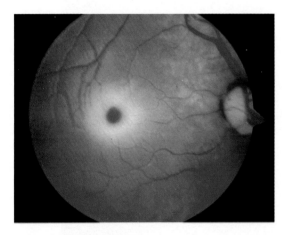

Color Plate 8-40. Tay-Sachs' disease with a classic cherry-red spot.

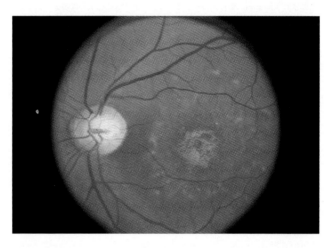

Color Plate 8-41. Stargardt's macular dystrophy (fundus flavi-maculatus). Note the "beaten metal" appearance of the macular region and the typical associated yellow lesions surrounding the left macula. These are believed to be composed of mucopolysaccharide material.

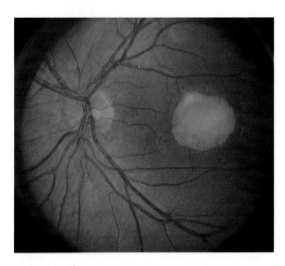

Color Plate 8-42. Best's vitelliform macular dystrophy with egg-yolk appearance.

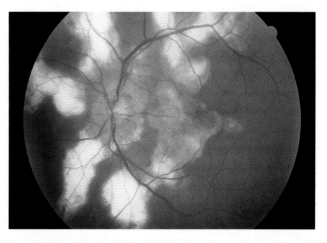

Color Plate 8-43. Serpiginous (geographic) choroiditis with multiple "geographic" areas of atrophy.

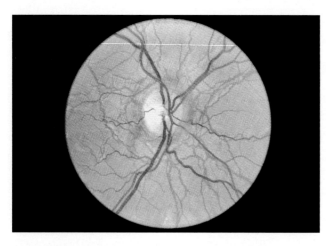

Color Plate 8-44. Angioid streaks.

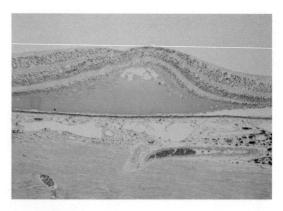

Color Plate 8-45. Photomicrograph of a serous detachment of the retina at the macula.

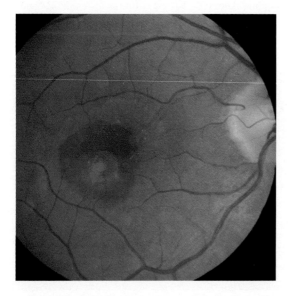

Color Plate 8-46. Subpigment epithelial neovascularization of the macular region. At the center is a greenish discoloration surrounded by a rim of hemorrhage.

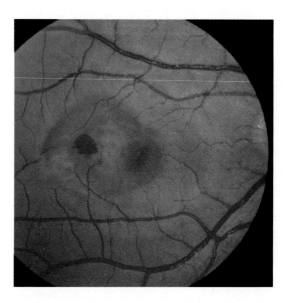

Color Plate 8-47. Subretinal neovascularization at the macula.

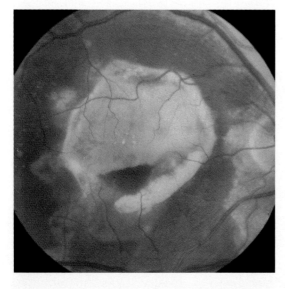

Color Plate 8-48. Hemorrhagic macular degeneration (Junius-Kuhnt type), showing superficial and deep hemorrhage. The boat-shaped hemorrhage connotes a fresh preretinal bleed.

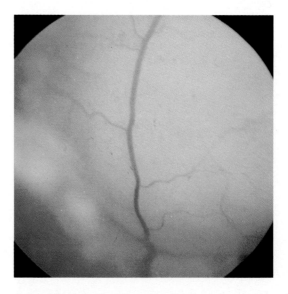

Color Plate 8-49. Eccentric disciform lesion, mimicking an amelanotic choroidal malignant melanoma.

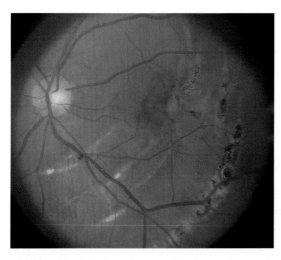

Color Plate 8-50. Multiple traumatic choroidal ruptures with macular hemorrhage. Typical crescent-shaped choroidal defects that bare the underlying sclera are present.

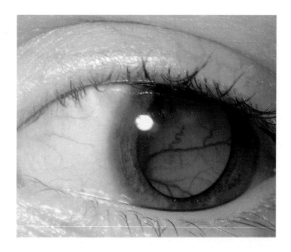

Color Plate 9-1. Retinoblastoma, exophytic growth. The retrolental white mass (leukokoria, or white pupil) is a common initial sign. The anteriorly displaced retinal vessels are clearly visible.

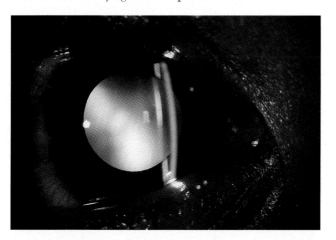

Color Plate 9-2. Fundus photograph of the eye of a child with advanced retinoblastoma that fills the vitreous cavity. (Courtesy M. Edward Wilson, MD, Charleston, SC.)

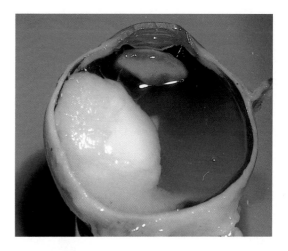

Color Plate 9-3. Retinoblastoma. The tumor is typically light gray to white. The cut surface may be smooth but more commonly reveals a granular or cobblestone appearance.

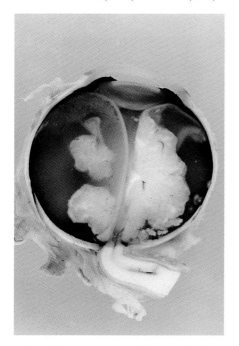

Color Plate 9-4. Gross photograph of an eye with retinoblastoma, exophytic type. There is total retinal detachment, and the tumor is situated in the subretinal space.

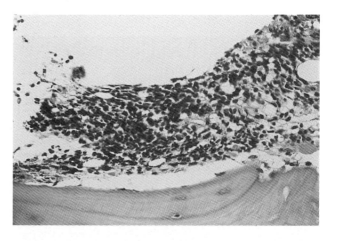

Color Plate 9-5. Photomicrograph of a retinoblastoma, metastatic to the femur. The primary ocular tumor was misdiagnosed as Coats' disease, and the globe was eviscerated, leaving residual tumor. The child died less than 1 year later with widespread metastasis, including the one illustrated here. Exenteration is not recommended for leukocoria (H & E, ×250). (Courtesy Timothy Powers, MD.)

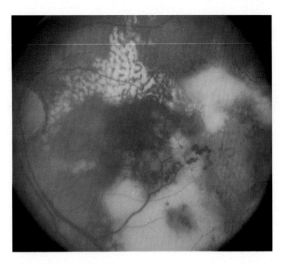

Color Plate 9-6. Coats' syndrome. The multiple yellow-white retinal and subretinal lipid deposits must be differentiated from multifocal retinoblastoma.

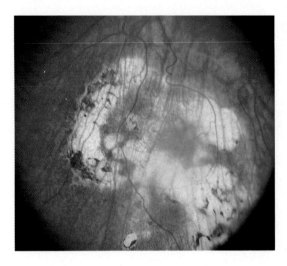

Color Plate 9-7. Probable spontaneous regression of a retinoblastoma. The necrotic tumor has a white, chalky appearance with peripheral pigmentation.

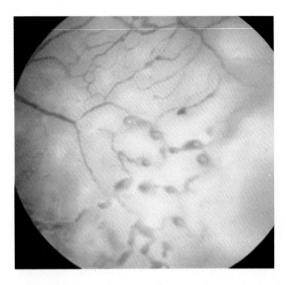

Color Plate 9-8. Coats' syndrome with retinal vascular telangiectasia and massive outpouring of lipid.

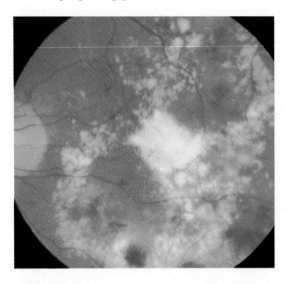

Color Plate 9-9. Coats' syndrome with deposition of lipid.

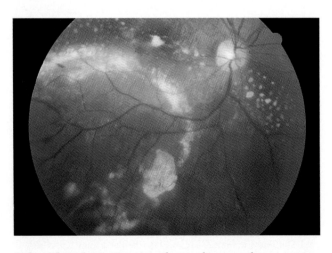

Color Plate 9-10. Coats' syndrome showing a large circinate ring of yellow exudate inferiotemporally.

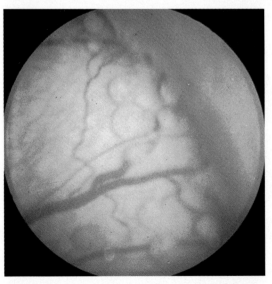

Color Plate 9-11. Retrolental fibroplasia (retinopathy of prematurity), with multiple vascular tufts posterior to a peripheral avascular zone. (From Garoon O et al. [357])

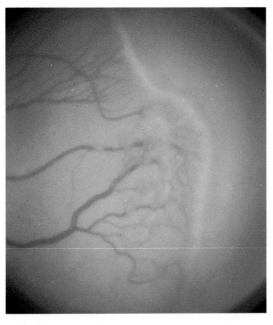

Color Plate 9-12. Retrolental fibroplasia (retinopathy of prematurity). The superotemporal periphery shows vascular tufts just posterior to an arteriovenous shunt. (From Garoon O et al.[357])

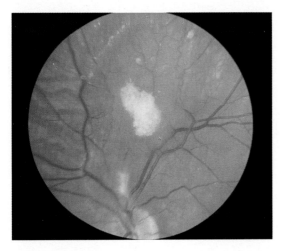

Color Plate 9-14. "Mulberry" or "tapioca" lesion of tuberous sclerosis. This astrocytic hamartoma is a benign proliferation of retinal astrocytes, similar to a glial nodules of the brain. (Courtesy John Hattenhauer, MD, Wausau, WI.)

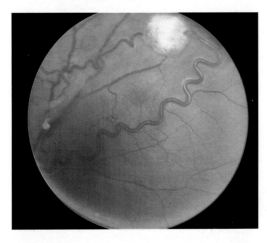

Color Plate 9-16. Von Hippel-Lindau disease. The round, sharply circumscribed hemangioblastoma is at the upper right. Afferent and efferent vessels are visible. (Courtesy Charles Vygantas, MD.)

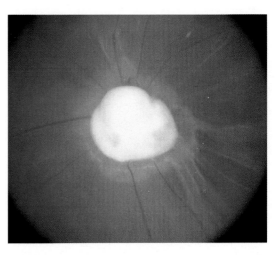

Color Plate 9-13. Epipapillary inflammatory mass caused by *Toxocara canis* (nematode endopthalmitis).

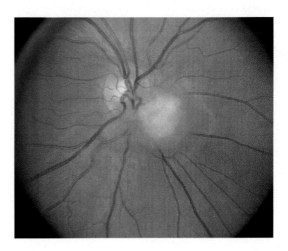

Color Plate 9-15. Tuberous sclerosis (peripapillary astrocytic hamartoma.)

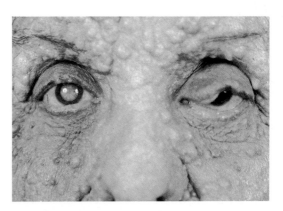

Color Plate 9-17. Von Recklinghausen's neurofibromatosis multiple subcutaneous nodules and S-shaped ptosis. (Courtesy Nick Mamalis, MD, University of Utah.)

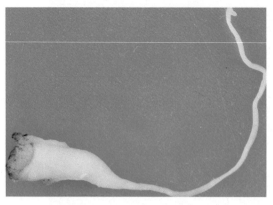

Color Plate 9-18. Solitary neurofibroma arising from the fourth cranial nerve: gross photograph of excised specimen. (Courtesy Nick Mamalis, MD, University of Utah.)

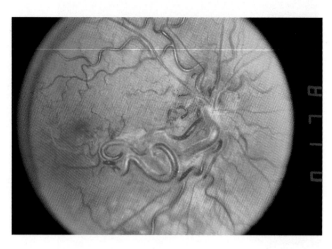

Color Plate 9-19. Wyburn-Mason syndrome (racemose hemangiomas of the retina). (See Figs. 9-60 and 9-61.)

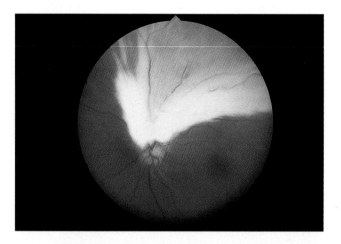

Color Plate 10-1. Extensive myelinated (medullated) nerve fiber layer. (Courtesy M. Edward Wilson, MD, Charleston, SC.)

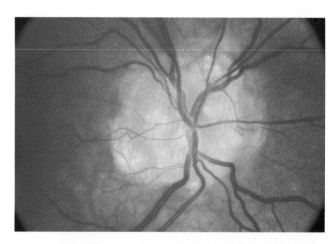

Color Plate 10-2. Drusen of the optic disc. Note the multiple yellow hyaline bodies involving all quadrants of the nerve head. (Courtesy Bernard Reznick, Pentield, NY.)

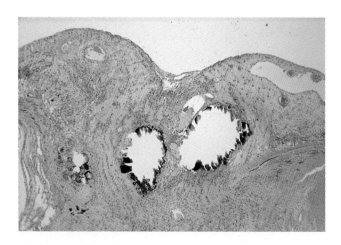

Color Plate 10-3. Drusen of optic nerve head, photomicrograph. Areas of calcification are present as clear empty spaces that have formed during processing (H & E, × 175).

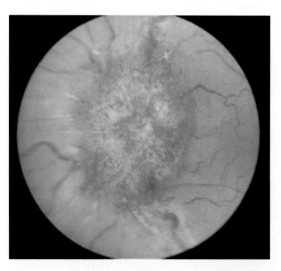

Color Plate 10-4. Papilledema, with dilated, tortuous, congested vessels; blurry disc margins, and nerve fiber layer hemorrhages.

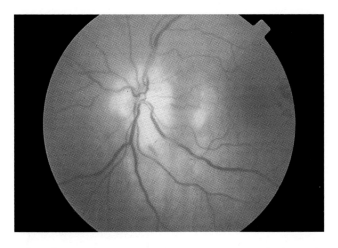

Color Plate 10-5. Anterior ischemic optic neuropathy (AION) associated with temporal arteritis.

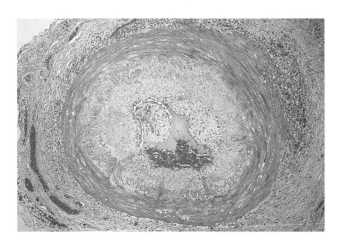

Color Plate 10-6. Photomicrograph of temporal artery (same case as Color Plate 10-5) showing extensive inflammatory cell infiltrate of all layers, with partial occlusion of the vessel lumen (H & E, × 250).

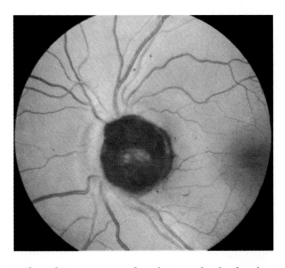

Color Plate 10-7. Fundus photograph of a deeply pigmented, slightly elevated melanocytoma of the optic nerve head.

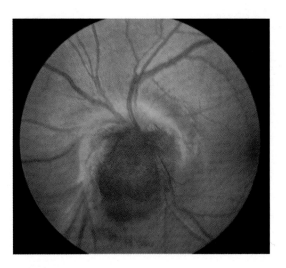

Color Plate 10-8. Melanocytoma of the optic nerve head showing significant elevation. This benign growth must be differentiated from peripapillary choroidal malignant melanoma. (Courtesy Terry Ernest, MD.)

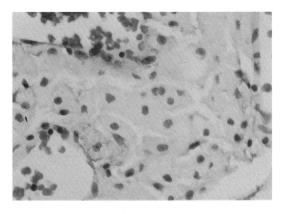

Color Plate 10-9. Bleached histologic preparation showing round to polyhedral melanocytoma cells with small, normochromic nuclei and abundant cytoplasm.

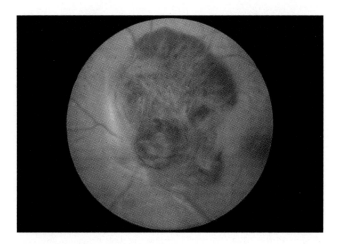

Color Plate 10-10. Epiperipapillary pigmented mass consistent with choroidal malignant melanoma.

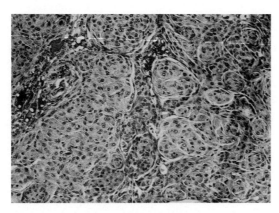

Color Plate 10-11. Photomicrograph of a meningioma arising from the arachnoid around the optic nerve. The numerous nests of tumor cells have a "whorled" appearance.

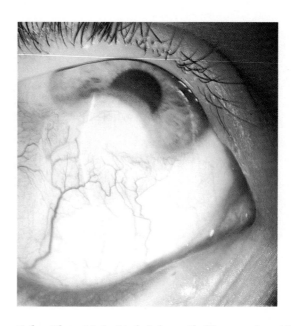

Color Plate 11-1. Limbal dermoid. (Courtesy Lee Allen and Ogden Frazier, University of Iowa.)

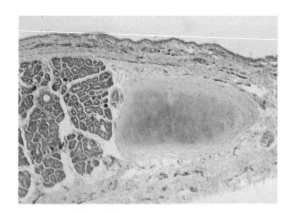

Color Plate 11-2. Photomicrograph of a limbal dermoid. This choristomatous growth contains the lacrimal gland (*left*) and hyaline cartilage (*right*).

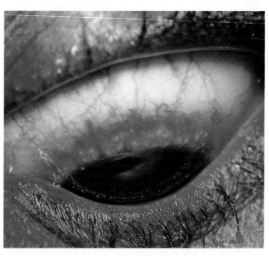

Color Plate 11-3. Vernal conjunctivitis. The white flecks along the superior limbus are clusters of inflammatory cells, primarily eosinophils termed Horner-Trantas spots.

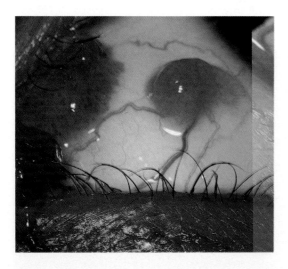

Color Plate 11-4. Multiple squamous papillomas of the conjunctiva in a child. These lesions probably are caused by a virus and may be recurrent.

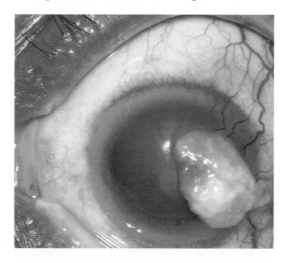

Color Plate 11-5. Carcinoma in situ of the cornea and conjunctiva. The white, glistening appearance of the surface (leukoplakia) is a result of hyperkeratosis of the neoplastic epithelium.

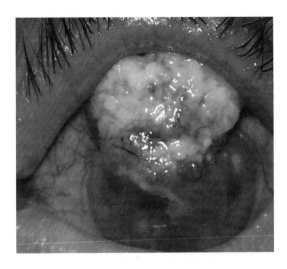

Color Plate 11-6. Advanced squamous cell carcinoma of the bulbar conjunctiva. Note the lobulated or fungating appearance of the tumor.

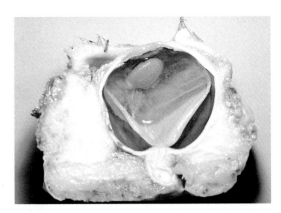

Color Plate 11-7. Exenteration specimen showing squamous cell carcinoma of the medial canthus, apparent as a white infiltrating growth (*left*) into the orbit.

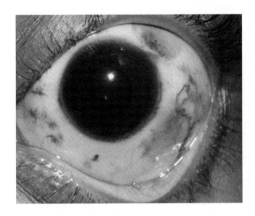

Color Plate 11-8. Congenital melanosis oculi. There is patchy hyperpigmentation of the sclera and episclera.

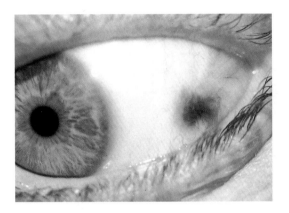

Color Plate 11-9. Benign hyperpigmentation of the bulbar conjunctiva in a woman. The onset occurred during pregnancy. (Courtesy K. Abrams, MD, New Orleans, LA.)

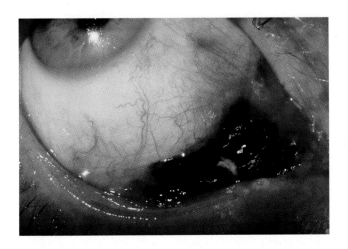

Color Plate 11-10. Primary, malignant melanoma of the conjunctiva emanating from the inferior fornix.

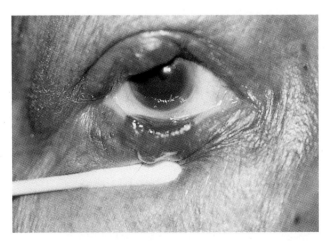

Color Plate 11-11. Kaposi's sarcoma involving both upper and lower conjunctiva. This case was unusual because it involved an elderly black woman who did not have AIDS. (Courtesy Gene R. Howard, MD, Qun Peng, MD, and Erik Skoog, MD, Charleston, SC.)

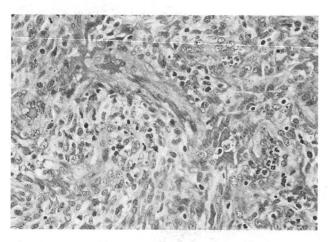

Color Plate 11-12. Photomicrograph of Kaposi's sarcoma (same case as Color Plate 11-11) showing typical proliferation of vascular elements, spindle-shaped cells, and fibrocytes, with a background infiltrate of chronic inflammatory cells. (Courtesy Qun Peng, MD, and Erik Skoog, MD, Charleston, SC.)

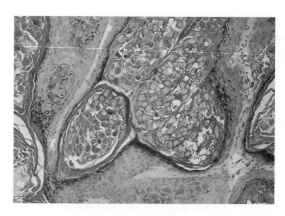

Color Plate 11-13. Photomicrograph of acanthotic eyelid epithelium from a case of molluscum contagiosum. Large DNA-containing inclusions are visible.

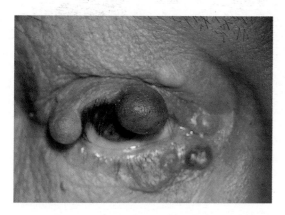

Color Plate 11-14. Multiple eyelid cysts. The walls may rupture, leading to hemorrhage or creating a granulomatous inflammatory reaction. Xanthoma palpebrarum also is apparent.

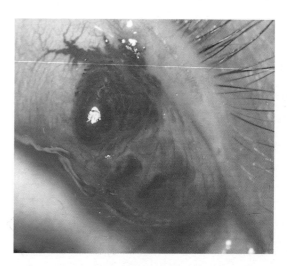

Color Plate 11-15. Hemangioma of the palpebral conjunctiva of the upper eyelid.

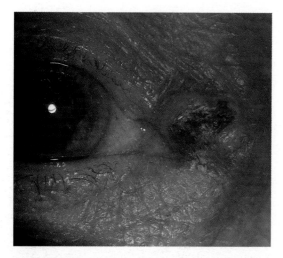

Color Plate 11-16. Basal cell carcinoma of the medial canthus. The medial aspect of the eye is the second-most common site of origin of this tumor. The central portion of the lesion is ulcerated and surrounded by a slightly raised pearly border.

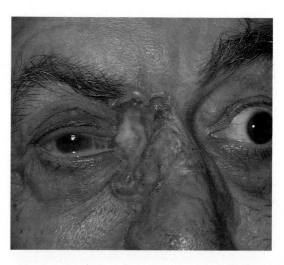

Color Plate 11-17. Recurrent necrotic, ulcerated basal cell carcinoma of the medial canthus. The lesion was in an advanced state when the patient was first examined.

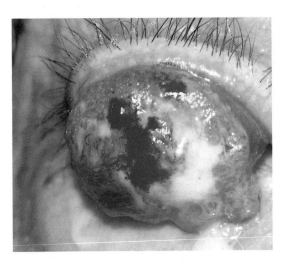

Color Plate 11-18. Squamous cell carcinoma of the upper eyelid with ulceration and purulent necrosis. A 2-year follow-up examination revealed no recurrence.

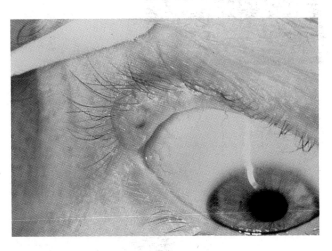

Color Plate 11-19. Superior temporal mass subsequently diagnosed as sebaceous carcinoma. (Courtesy Timothy Powers, MD.)

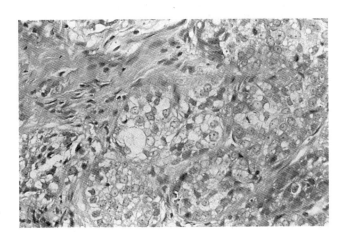

Color Plate 11-20. Photomicrograph of the lesion illustrated in Color Plate 11-19. There are numerous hyperchromatic tumor cells and numerous empty clear spaces. These unstained vacuoles are foci where lipid material was extracted from the cell during processing through paraffin (H & E, ×200). (Courtesy Timothy Powers, MD.)

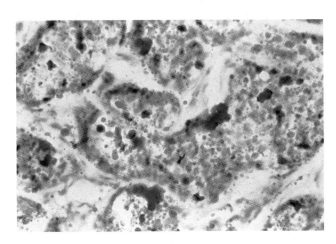

Color Plate 11-21. Photomicrograph (same case as Color Plates 11-19 and 11-20). The lipid material that is elaborated by the tumor is seen as bright red droplets (frozen section, oil red O stain, × 200). (Courtesy Timothy Powers, MD.)